Medical Radiology

Radiation Oncology

Series Editors

Nancy Y. Lee
Jiade J. Lu

Medical Radiology - Radiation Oncology is a unique series that aims to document the most innovative technologies in all fields within radiology, thereby informing the physician in practice of the latest advances in diagnostic and treatment techniques.

The contents range from contemporary statements relating to management for various disease sites to explanations of the newest techniques for tumor identification and of mechanisms for the enhancement of radiation effects, with the emphasis on maximizing cure and minimizing complications.

Each volume is a comprehensive reference book on a topical theme, and the editors are always experts of high international standing. Contributions are included from both clinicians and researchers, ensuring wide appeal.

Branislav Jeremić
Editor

Advances in Radiation Oncology in Lung Cancer

Third Edition

Volume I

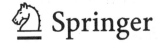

Editor
Branislav Jeremić
School of Medicine
University of Kragujevac
Kragujevac, Serbia

ISSN 0942-5373　　　　　ISSN 2197-4187　(electronic)
Medical Radiology
ISSN 2731-4715　　　　　ISSN 2731-4723　(electronic)
Radiation Oncology

ISBN 978-3-031-34846-4　　　ISBN 978-3-031-34847-1　(eBook)
https://doi.org/10.1007/978-3-031-34847-1

© The Editor(s) (if applicable) and The Author(s), under exclusive license to Springer Nature Switzerland AG 2005, 2011, 2023

This work is subject to copyright. All rights are solely and exclusively licensed by the Publisher, whether the whole or part of the material is concerned, specifically the rights of translation, reprinting, reuse of illustrations, recitation, broadcasting, reproduction on microfilms or in any other physical way, and transmission or information storage and retrieval, electronic adaptation, computer software, or by similar or dissimilar methodology now known or hereafter developed.
The use of general descriptive names, registered names, trademarks, service marks, etc. in this publication does not imply, even in the absence of a specific statement, that such names are exempt from the relevant protective laws and regulations and therefore free for general use.
The publisher, the authors, and the editors are safe to assume that the advice and information in this book are believed to be true and accurate at the date of publication. Neither the publisher nor the authors or the editors give a warranty, expressed or implied, with respect to the material contained herein or for any errors or omissions that may have been made. The publisher remains neutral with regard to jurisdictional claims in published maps and institutional affiliations.

This Springer imprint is published by the registered company Springer Nature Switzerland AG
The registered company address is: Gewerbestrasse 11, 6330 Cham, Switzerland

For
Aleksandra and Marta.

Preface

Worldwide, there is an estimated 19.3 million new cancer cases with almost 10.0 million cancer deaths occurred in 2020. Lung cancer is now the second most commonly diagnosed cancer, with an estimated 2,206,771 new cases annually occurring. It, however, remains the leading cause of cancer death, with an estimated 1.8 million deaths (18%). Due to continuing efforts of the tobacco industry shifting its focus from developed to a developing world, more than 50% of new cases continue to occur in the latter one in the past decade. It is, therefore, not unexpectedly a big burden to national health care systems worldwide with hundreds of thousands of patients succumbing to it every year.

Radiation therapy remains the cornerstone of modern treatment approaches, regardless of histology and stage of the disease. It is used in both curative and palliative setting, being the most cost-effective treatment option in lung cancer. Recent decades witnessed important technological and biological developments which enabled continuous and efficient adaptation to the growing demands to offer precision medicine in the twenty-first century. Together with other two treatment modalities, surgery and systemic therapy, it successfully evolves focusing on both patient and society needs. Indeed, there seems to be very few competitors among medical disciplines that have so broadly embraced scientific novelties such as computer-driven technological aspects as is the case with radiation therapy.

This, updated and third edition of the book initially published in 2004 and 2011, respectively, remains focused upon constant research and development in the field of radiation oncology as the indispensable part of our comprehensive and hopefully orchestrated approach in the diagnosis and treatment of lung cancer. While the intervening 10 years may deem too short for any major leaps in this field, I am sure this third edition will stand the test of time as the necessary checkpoint in the global development in this field.

To demonstrate this premise, while many chapters of the first and the second edition respectively remained, many are updated and, furthermore, many are completely new additions, bringing more substance to keep the pace with the most recent scientific achievements in the field, becoming new standards of care almost daily. Various, non-radiation oncology aspects are again included in the book with the same goal. Ultimately, the book is composed in such a way to enable both radiation oncologists and other lung cancer specialists benefit from reading it.

As with the previous two efforts, I have had great pleasure and very much privilege of having a distinguished faculty joining me. They dedicated their professional lives to the fight against lung cancer, having continuously provided substantial contribution in this field. They painstakingly focused on more comprehensive understanding of basic premises of biology and technology, its successful incorporation in the diagnosis and treatment of the disease and finally ending up in state-of-the-art approaches in the third decade of the new millennium.

I would also like to thank my former and current staff colleagues with whom I have collaborated around the world, especially those still living and working in developing countries. From such collaboration, I grew up not only as a better and more mature medical professional but also a better human being. I would also like to express my gratitude to Alexander von Humboldt Foundation, Bonn, Germany, for their continuous support since 1998. Without them all it would simply be impossible to imagine both the final shape of the book and its timely delivery.

Belgrade, Serbia   Branislav Jeremić

Contents

Volume I

Part I Basic Science of Lung Cancer

Genomic Alterations in Lung Cancer 3
Daniel Morgensztern

Epigenetic Events in Lung Cancer 17
Octavio A. Romero and Montse Sanchez-Cespedes

Part II Clinical Investigations

Interventional Pulmonology 35
Branislav Perin and Bojan Zarić

Pathology of Lung Cancer 45
Mari Mino-Kenudson

Role of Radiologic Imaging in Lung Cancer 67
Salome Kukava and George Tsivtsivadze

Place and Role of PET/CT in the Diagnosis and Staging
of Lung Cancer 85
Salome Kukava and Michael Baramia

Surgical Staging of Lung Cancer 113
Jarrod Predina, Douglas J. Mathisen, and Michael Lanuti

Part III Basic Treatment Considerations

Surgical Workup and Management of Early-Stage
Lung Cancer 131
Stephanie H. Chang, Joshua Scheinerman, Jeffrey Jiang,
Darian Paone, and Harvey Pass

Radiation Biology of Lung Cancer 151
Jose G. Bazan

Radiation Time, Dose, and Fractionation in the Treatment
of Lung Cancer 171
David L. Billing and Andreas Rimner

**Optimizing Lung Cancer Radiotherapy Treatments
Using Personalized Dose-Response Curves** 189
Joseph O. Deasy, Jeho Jeong, Maria Thor, Aditya Apte,
Andrew Jackson, Ishita Chen, Abraham Wu, and Andreas Rimner

Tumor Motion Control 213
Hiroki Shirato, Shinichi Shimizu, Hiroshi Taguchi,
Seishin Takao, Naoki Miyamoto, and Taeko Matsuura

PET and PET/CT in Treatment Planning 237
Michael MacManus, Sarah Everitt, and Rodney J. Hicks

Target Volume Delineation in Non-small Cell Lung Cancer....... 255
Jessica W. Lee, Haijun Song, Matthew J. Boyer,
and Joseph K. Salama

The Radiation Target in Small Cell Lung..................... 271
Gregory M. M. Videtic

Radiation Sensitizers 285
Mansi K. Aparnathi, Sami Ul Haq, Zishan Allibhai,
Benjamin H. Lok, and Anthony M. Brade

Radioprotectors in the Management of Lung Cancer............ 303
Zhongxing Liao, Ting Xu, and Ritsuko Komaki

Chemotherapy for Lung Cancer............................. 321
Mariam Alexander, Elaine Shum, Aditi Singh,
and Balazs Halmos

Targeted Therapies in Non-small Cell Lung Cancer............. 347
Jessica R. Bauman and Martin J. Edelman

Immunotherapy of Lung Cancer............................. 371
Igor Rybkin and Shirish M. Gadgeel

**Combined Radiotherapy and Chemotherapy:
Theoretical Considerations and Biological Premises**............. 385
Michael K. Farris, Cole Steber, Corbin Helis,
and William Blackstock

**Mechanisms of Action of Radiotherapy and Immunotherapy
in Lung Cancer: Implications for Clinical Practice**.............. 399
Kewen He, Ugur Selek, Hampartsoum B. Barsoumian,
Duygu Sezen, Matthew S. Ning, Nahum Puebla-Osorio,
Jonathan E. Schoenhals, Dawei Chen, Carola Leuschner,
Maria Angelica Cortez, and James W. Welsh

**Part IV   Current Treatment Strategies in Early-Stage
Non-small Cell Lung Cancer**

**Early Non-small Cell Lung Cancer: The Place of Radical
Non-SABR Radiation Therapy** 417
Tathagata Das and Matthew Hatton

**Never-Ending Story: Surgery Versus SBRT in
Early-Stage NSCLC** 433
James Taylor, Pamela Samson, William Stokes,
and Drew Moghanaki

**Stereotactic Ablative Radiotherapy for Early-Stage
Lung Cancer** 445
Dat T. Vo, John H. Heinzerling, and Robert D. Timmerman

**Role of Postoperative Radiation Therapy in Non-Small
Cell Lung Cancer** 471
Alexander K. Diaz and Chris R. Kelsey

**The Role of Thermal Ablation in the Treatment of Stage
I Non-small Cell Lung Cancer** 483
Roberto B. Kutcher-Diaz, Aaron Harman, and John Varlotto

**Part V Current Treatment Strategies in Locally Advanced
and Metastatic Non-small Cell Lung Cancer**

Lung Dose Escalation 507
Kenneth E. Rosenzweig

**Multimodality Treatment of Stage IIIA/N2 NSCLC:
Why Always NO to Surgery?** 517
Branislav Jeremić, Ivane Kiladze, and Slobodan Milisavljevic

**Multimodality Treatment of Stage IIIA/N2 Non-Small
Cell Lung Cancer: When YES to Surgery** 533
Sean All and David J. Sher

**Combined Radiation Therapy and Chemotherapy as an
Exclusive Treatment Option in Locally Advanced Inoperable
Non-small Cell Lung Cancer** 547
Branislav Jeremić, Pavol Dubinsky, Slobodan Milisavljević,
and Ivane Kiladze

**Optimizing Drug Therapies in the Maintenance Setting After
Radiochemotherapy in Non-small Cell Lung Cancer** 571
Steven H. Lin and David Raben

**Prophylactic Cranial Irradiation in Non-small Cell
Lung Cancer** 581
Hina Saeed, Monica E. Shukla, and Elizabeth M. Gore

**Palliative External Beam Thoracic Radiation Therapy
of Non-small Cell Lung Cancer** 597
Stein Sundstrøm

**Intraoperative Radiotherapy in Lung Cancer: Methodology
(Electrons or Brachytherapy), Clinical Experiences, and
Long-Term Institutional Results** 605
Felipe A. Calvo, Javier Aristu, Javier Serrano, Mauricio Cambeiro,
Rafael Martinez-Monge, and Rosa Cañón

Brachytherapy for Lung Cancer 623
Raul Hernanz de Lucas, Teresa Muñoz Miguelañez,
Alfredo Polo, Paola Lucia Arrieta Narvaez,
and Deisy Barrios Barreto

**Oligometastatic Disease: Basic Aspects and Clinical
Results in NSCLC** 637
Gukan Sakthivel, Deepinder P. Singh, Haoming Qiu,
and Michael T. Milano

Part VI Current Treatment Strategies in Small Cell Lung Cancer

**Radiation Therapy in Limited Disease Small Cell
Lung Cancer** 651
Branislav Jeremić, Ivane Kiladze, Pavol Dubinsky,
and Slobodan Milisavljević

**Role of Thoracic Radiation Therapy in Extensive Disease
Small Cell Lung Cancer** 667
Branislav Jeremić, Mohamed El-Bassiouny, Ramy Ghali,
Ivane Kiladze, and Sherif Abdel-Wahab

Prophylactic Cranial Irradiation in Small Cell Lung Cancer 677
William G. Breen and Yolanda I. Garces

Volume II

Part VII Treatment in Specific Patient Groups and Other Settings

Radiation Therapy for Lung Cancer in Elderly................. 691
Erkan Topkan, Ugur Selek, Berrin Pehlivan, Ahmet Kucuk,
and Yasemin Bolukbasi

Radiation Therapy for Intrathoracic Recurrence of Lung Cancer . 717
Yukinori Matsuo, Hideki Hanazawa, Noriko Kishi,
Kazuhito Ueki, and Takashi Mizowaki

Treatment of Second Lung Cancers 739
Reshad Rzazade and Hale Basak Caglar

Radiation Therapy for Brain Metastases 755
Dirk Rades, Sabine Bohnet, and Steven E. Schild

**Radiation Therapy for Metastatic Lung Cancer: Bone
Metastasis and Metastatic Spinal Cord Compression**............ 779
Begoña Taboada-Valladares, Patricia Calvo-Crespo, and Antonio
Gómez-Caamaño

Radiation Therapy for Metastatic Lung Cancer: Liver Metastasis . 795
Fiori Alite and Anand Mahadevan

**Advances in Supportive and Palliative Care for
Lung Cancer Patients**..................................... 809
Michael J. Simoff, Javier Diaz-Mendoza, A. Rolando Peralta,
Labib G. Debiane, and Avi Cohen

Part VIII Other Intrathoracic Malignancies

Thymic Cancer 833
Gokhan Ozyigit and Pervin Hurmuz

Advances in Radiation Therapy for Malignant Pleural Mesothelioma 849
Gwendolyn M. Cramer, Charles B. Simone II, Theresa M. Busch, and Keith A. Cengel

Primary Tracheal Tumors 863
Shrinivas Rathod

Pulmonary Carcinoid 879
Roshal R. Patel, Brian De, and Vivek Verma

Part IX Treatment-Related Toxicity

Hematological Toxicity in Lung Cancer 907
Francesc Casas, Diego Muñoz-Guglielmetti, Gabriela Oses, Carla Cases, and Meritxell Mollà

Radiation Therapy-Induced Lung and Heart Toxicity 925
Soheila F. Azghadi and Megan E. Daly

Spinal Cord 941
Timothy E. Schultheiss

Radiation Therapy-Related Toxicity: Esophagus 955
Srinivas Raman and Meredith Giuliani

Brain Toxicity 969
C. Nieder

Part X Quality of Life Studies and Prognostic Factors

Patient-Reported Outcomes in Lung Cancer 987
Newton J. Hurst Jr, Farzan Siddiqui, and Benjamin Movsas

Importance of Prognostic Factors in Lung Cancer 1001
Lukas Käsmann

Part XI Technological Advances in Lung Cancer

Intensity-Modulated Radiation Therapy and Volumetric Modulated Arc Therapy for Lung Cancer 1021
Jacob S. Parzen and Inga S. Grills

Image-Guided Radiotherapy in Lung Cancer 1049
Julius Weng, Patrick Kupelian, and Percy Lee

Heavy Particles in Non-small Cell Lung Cancer: Protons 1059
Charles B. Simone II

Heavy Particles in Non-small Cell Lung Cancer: Carbon Ions 1075
S. Tubin, P. Fossati, S. Mori, E. Hug, and T. Kamada

The Role of Nanotechnology for Diagnostic and Therapy Strategies in Lung Cancer 1093
Jessica E. Holder, Minnatallah Al-Yozbaki,
and Cornelia M. Wilson

Part XII Clinical Research in Lung Cancer

Translational Research in Lung Cancer 1113
Haoming Qiu, Michael A. Cummings, and Yuhchyau Chen

Radiation Oncology of Lung Cancer: Why We Fail(ed) in Clinical Research? 1135
Branislav Jeremić, Nenad Filipović, Slobodan Milisavljević,
and Ivane Kiladze

Randomized Clinical Trials: Pitfalls in Design, Analysis, Presentation, and Interpretation 1147
Lawrence Kasherman, S. C. M. Lau, K. Karakasis, N. B. Leighl,
and A. M. Oza

Part I
Basic Science of Lung Cancer

Genomic Alterations in Lung Cancer

Daniel Morgensztern

Contents

1 Introduction.. 3
2 NSCLC.. 5
3 EGFR.. 7
4 ALK.. 8
5 ROS1... 8
6 BRAF... 9
7 MET... 9
8 RET.. 10
9 NTRK... 11
10 HER2... 11
11 KRAS... 11
12 FGFR... 12
13 **Small Cell Lung Cancer**................................. 12
14 **Conclusion**.. 12
References... 12

Abstract

Lung cancer is a heterogeneous disease characterized by genomic alterations in oncogenes and tumor suppressor genes. The increased use of genomic profile has allowed a better understanding of the lung cancer biology and the development of targeted therapies with improved efficacy and toxicity profile compared to standard cytotoxic chemotherapy. Nevertheless, most of the targetable alterations occur in patients with adenocarcinoma histology and virtually all patients develop tumor progression after the initial benefit from targeted therapy indicating that novel approaches are still needed to continue to improve the outcomes for patients with advanced-stage lung cancer.

1 Introduction

Cancer is a term used to denote a set of diseases characterized by autonomous expansion and spread of a somatic clone. Unlike normal cells that carefully control the production and release of signals for cell growth and division, cancer cells deregulate these signals, usually through the binding of growth factors to surface receptors containing intracellular tyrosine kinase domain (TKD), which transmit the signals through multiple-branched signaling pathways that regulate the cell cycle and growth (Hanahan and Weinberg 2011). The sustained proliferative signaling may occur by increased production of growth factor ligands leading to autocrine proliferative stimulation, increased levels of receptor proteins in the cell surface making the cells more responsive to the limited amounts of growth factor ligands, or structural alterations in the

D. Morgensztern (✉)
Division of Medical Oncology, Department of Medicine, Washington University School of Medicine, St. Louis, MO, USA
e-mail: danielmorgensztern@wustl.edu

receptor molecules leading to ligand-independent activation. In addition to increasing growth-stimulating signals, cancer cells are also capable of inactivating tumor suppressor genes that inhibit cell proliferation such as *TP53* and *RB*.

The multistage process of lung tumorigenesis occurs through progressive accumulation of mutations with dominant gain of function in oncogenes and loss of function in tumor suppression genes (Salehi-Rad et al. 2020). The DNA sequence of most normal cell genomes, including cancer cells, acquires a set of alterations compared to its progenitor fertilized egg. These alterations are collectively termed somatic mutations, which, unlike the germline mutations which are inherited from the parents, are not transmitted to offspring (Stratton et al. 2009). The mutations found in the cancer cell genome are accumulated over the lifetime of the patient, some of them acquired when the ancestors of the cancer cell were biologically normal. The somatic mutations in the cancer cells are classified as driver mutations when conferring growth advantage. Passenger mutations in contrast have not been selected, do not confer clonal growth advantage, and do not contribute to cancer development. They are found in cancer genomes because somatic mutations without functional consequences often occur during cell division. Cells that acquire a driver mutation often already have biologic inert somatic mutations in their genome, which are carried along in the clonal expansion at some point during the lineage of cancer development. It should be noted however that there are differences between drive gene and driver gene mutation. A driver gene is one that contains driver gene mutations. However, driver genes may also contain passenger mutations (Vogelstein et al. 2013).

Somatic mutations in cancer genomes occur due to a slight infidelity of DNA replication, defective DNA repair, exogenous or endogenous mutagen exposures, or enzymatic DNA modification (Alexandrov et al. 2013). The major classes of genomic alterations involved in the development of cancer, including lung cancer, include point mutations, copy number alterations, and translocations (Macconaill and Garraway 2010). Point mutations involve a single base and may be subdivided into transitions, when a pyrimidine is replaced by another pyrimidine (T to C or vice versa) or a purine is replaced by another purine (A to G or vice versa), whereas transversions are defined by base replacement from purine to pyrimidine or vice versa (Clark et al. 2019). Nonsynonymous mutations alter the encoded amino acid sequence of a protein and may be classified as missense, nonsense, indels, and splice site. In missense mutations, a single-nucleotide change results in amino acid substitution whereas in nonsense mutations, a single-nucleotide substitution results in the production of a stop codon (UAA, UAG, and UGA). Indels represent the insertion or deletion of one or more bases from the DNA sequence. The consequences of indels depend on the location and length of the alteration. With insertions or deletions close to the 3′ end of the gene, most of the DNA sequence remains intact and a functional protein can still be made. Deletions and insertions may be particularly harmful when the number of missing or extra base pairs is not a multiple of three. This occurs because the codons consist of groups of three base pairs and the insertion or deletion of one or two bases, which constitute the frameshift mutations, will completely alter the subsequent DNA sequence with profound alterations in the protein function. In contrast, with the addition or deletion of three bases or one of the multiples of three, the reading frame will be retained with the protein unchanged with the exception of the amino acids gained or deleted. Splice-site mutations occur at the intron-exon boundary and fall on either the consensus intronic dinucleotide splice donor GT at the 5′ splice site or the splice acceptor AG at the 3′ splice site (Jayasinghe et al. 2018). Transcriptional changes may also occur with mutations beyond the intron-exon boundary. In synonymous or silent mutations, the alteration in the DNA sequence has no predicted effect on the phenotype and may occur in the noncoding DNA, introns (except for splice-site recognition sequences), or third base of the codons. Genomic amplification is the selective increase in the copies of a gene from the two copies present in the normal diploid genome in a restricted region of a chromosome arm, which may involve one or multiple genes (Stratton et al. 2009). This definition does not include multiple copies of entire chromosomes or entire genomes which would also increase the number of copies for each gene (Santarius et al. 2010). Genomic rearrangements arise from breaks in chromosomes that are aberrantly joined and include duplications, deletions, inversions, and translocations (Clark et al. 2019; Anderson et al. 2018). Translocations are rearrangements where a section of DNA is removed from its original position and inserted in another location, either in the same or in a different chromosome. Gene rearrangements, including translocations and deletions, may lead to the creation of fusion genes, which are hybrid genes formed when two independent genes become juxtaposed (Latysheva and Babu 2016).

2 NSCLC

Both adenocarcinoma and squamous cell carcinoma of the lung are among the cancer types with the highest frequency of mutations, with increased cytosine-to-adenosine (C>A) nucleotide transversions which are a signature of exposure to cigarette smoke (Alexandrov et al. 2013; Kandoth et al. 2013). Data from the Cancer Genome Atlas showed mean rates of somatic mutations in adenocarcinomas and squamous cell carcinomas of 8.9 and 8.1 mutations per megabase, respectively (The Cancer Genome Atlas Research Network 2012, 2014). Targetable alterations in NSCLC include epidermal growth factor receptor (*EGFR*) mutations, anaplastic lymphoma kinase (*ALK*) fusions, *ROS-1* fusions, *BRAF* V600E mutation, *RET* fusions, *MET* exon 14 skipping mutations, and *NTRK* fusions (Hanna et al. 2021). Emerging targets include *KRAS* G12C, *HER2* exon 20 insertions, and high-level *MET* amplification.

Methods for genomic profile in lung cancer include Sanger sequencing, polymerase chain reaction (PCR), fluorescent in situ hybridization (FISH), immunohistochemistry (IHC), and next-generation sequencing (NGS) (Garrido et al. 2020). NGS, also called massive parallel sequencing, allows the evaluation of large amounts of genomic information. Before the development of NGS, tumor genotyping was performed only on hotspots, defined as genomic loci known to be frequently mutated in cancer (Gagan and Van Allen 2015). The clinical sample for NGS may be from tissue, including formalin-fixed paraffin-embedded or fresh frozen tissue, or peripheral blood, also known as liquid biopsy, with the use of circulating tumor DNA (ctDNA). ctDNA is the fraction of cell-free DNA (cfDNA) that originates from tumor cells. cfDNA also contains germline DNA released into the peripheral blood from normal cells throughout the body (Corcoran and Chabner 2018). Commercially available NGS sequencing platforms such as FoundationOne, Caris, Tempus, and OncomineDx are based on next-generation sequencers, mostly Illumina and Ion Torrent (Gong et al. 2018). These platforms typically cover hundreds of genes and detect mutations, copy number variation, and fusions, and some offer additional IHC analyses and have a turnaround time of 7–14 days. Guardant360 is an FDA-approved liquid biopsy method that uses Illumina platform with high concordance with tissue-based genotype (Odegaard et al. 2018). Actionable alterations tested in the Guardant360 73-gene panel include *EGFR* mutation, *ALK* fusion, *ROS1* fusion, *BRAF* V600E mutation, *RET* fusion, *MET* amplification, *MET* exon 14 skip mutation, and *HER2* mutation among others (Leighl et al. 2019). NGS may be used for the detection of all actionable driver alterations in NSCLC, whereas the Sanger method and PCR may be used for mutations including those occurring on *EGFR*, *BRAF*, *HER2*, and *MET*. FISH may be used to detect gene rearrangements in *ALK*, *ROS1*, *RET*, and *NTRK* as well as *HER2* and *MET* amplifications whereas IHC may be used to infer the presence of some of the gene rearrangements (Garrido et al. 2020).

Many of the driver alterations in NSCLC occur in genes encoding tyrosine kinases, including *EGFR*, *HER2*, *ALK*, *ROS1*, and *MET*. Kinases are proteins that catalyze the addition of phosphate groups to other molecules such as proteins or lipids and are essential to nearly all signal transduction pathways. The signaling cascades are propagated by the addition of the γ-phosphate from ATP transferred to the hydroxyl groups of serine, threonine, or tyrosine residues (Tong and Seeliger 2015). Protein kinases may be subdivided into transmembrane receptor tyrosine kinases (RTKs) and nonreceptor tyrosine kinases. RTKs enable communication between cells and the extracellular environment (Trenker and Jura 2020). They are composed of an N-terminal extracellular domain, a single transmembrane domain, an intracellular region that contains the juxtamembrane regulatory region, a TKD, and a carboxy-terminal tail (Du and Lovly 2018). RTKs are activated by specific ligands which lead to receptor dimerization or oligomerization, leading to a conformational change that allows transphosphorylation of each TKD and release of cis-inhibition. The transphosphorylation sites allow the binding of SH2 and PTB domain containing signaling proteins which lead to recruitment of additional signaling molecules and regulation of downstream signaling pathways including MAPK, PI3K, and JAK-STAT. Since protein kinases regulate key processes such as cellular proliferation, survival, and migration, they are frequent targets of oncogenic alterations (Fleuren et al. 2016). The disturbance of the tightly controlled RTK activity by mutations may lead to constitutional activation of the receptors independent of the presence of the ligands with abnormal downstream signaling. The identification of driver alterations through tumor genotyping allows the individualization of therapy for patients, particularly in those tyrosine kinase alterations treated with matched tyrosine kinase inhibitors (TKIs), which are associated with increased efficacy and better toxicity profile compared to standard cytotoxic chemotherapy (Table 1) (Hanna et al. 2021; Herbst et al. 2018).

In the Lung Cancer Mutation Consortium study evaluating multiplex assays in adenocarcinoma, 1007 and 733 patients were tested for at least 1 and 10 oncogene drivers, respectively (Kris et al. 2014). Among the 733 patients tested for all 10 oncogene drivers, the most common alterations included *KRAS* mutation (25%), EGFR exon 19 deletion (10%), *ALK* rearrangements, and EGFR L858R (6%). In the CRISP study conducted in Germany, 3717 patients were prospectively evaluated for 9 genes (Griesinger et al. 2021). Among the 2921 patients with non-squamous histology, 7.8% were not tested and 37.8% had no alterations. Of the patients tested, the most common alterations were *TP53* mutations (51.4%), *KRAS* mutations (39.2%), and *EGFR* mutations (15.1%). Alterations in *MET*, *ALK*, *ROS1*, *RET*, and *HER2* were observed in 9.3%, 5.5%, 3.1%, 2.1%, and 3.9% of patients, respectively. In a study evaluating 4064 patients with NSCLC from the Foundation Medicine database, the median age was 66 years, 51.9% were female, 79.9% were white, 79.3% had a

Table 1 Targetable alterations in NSCLC

Alteration	Selected treatment options
Established biomarkers	
Sensitizing *EGFR* mutations	Gefitinib (Mok et al. 2009), erlotinib (Rosell et al. 2012), afatinib (Yang et al. 2015), dacomitinib (Wu et al. 2017), osimertinib (Soria et al. 2018)
ALK rearrangements	Alectinib (Peters et al. 2017), brigatinib (Camidge et al. 2018), lorlatinib (Shaw et al. 2020)
ROS1 rearrangements	Crizotinib (Shaw et al. 2014), entrectinib (Drilon et al. 2020a)
BRAF V600E mutations	Dabrafenib plus trametinib (Planchard et al. 2017)
MET exon 14 skipping mutations	Capmatinib (Wolf et al. 2020), tepotinib (Paik et al. 2020)
RET rearrangements	Selpercatinib (Drilon et al. 2020b), pralsetinib (Gainor et al. 2020)
NTRK fusions	Larotrectinib (Drilon et al. 2018b), entrectinib (Doebele et al. 2020)
Emerging biomarkers	
High-level *MET* amplification	Crizotinib (Landi et al. 2019), capmatinib (Wolf et al. 2020)
HER2 mutations	Ado-trasutumab (Li et al. 2018)
KRAS G12C	Sotorasib (Hong et al. 2020)

history of smoking, 59.9% had stage IV disease, 77.6% had nonsquamous histology, 21.4% had squamous histology, and 4.6% had NSCLC not otherwise specified (NOS) (Singal et al. 2019). The most common driver alterations were in *KRAS* (29.6%), followed by *EGFR* (17.2%), *BRAF* (4.9%), *MET* (4.6%), *HER2* (4.5%), *ALK* (3.1%), *RET* (1.7%), and *ROS1* (1%). The median age was lower in patients with *ALK* translocations (58 years) and higher in those with *MET* alterations (71 years). *EGFR, ALK, ROS1, RET,* and *HER2* were more common in patients without a history of smoking. All alterations were more common in patients with nonsquamous histology. In the French Cooperative Thoracic Intergroup, 17,664 patients with NSCLC underwent molecular profiling (Barlesi et al. 2016). Most patients were smokers or former smokers (81%) and adenocarcinoma was the most common histology (76%), followed by NSCLC NOS or other (16%), squamous (5%), and large-cell carcinoma (3%). The most common alterations were *KRAS* mutations (29%), *EGFR* mutations (11%), and *ALK* rearrangements (5%). Among patients with adenocarcinoma, *KRAS* mutations, *EGFR* mutations, and *ALK* rearrangements were detected in 32%, 12%, and 5%, respectively.

3 EGFR

The epidermal growth factor receptor (EGFR) is a member of the EGFR RTK family that also includes HER2, HER3, and HER4 (Lemmon et al. 2014; Sharma et al. 2007). The receptor contains an extracellular region which spans from amino acid residues 1 to 620, four domains named I to IV, a short extracellular juxtamembrane region, a transmembrane region, a short intracellular juxtamembrane region, a TKD, a carboxy-terminal tail spanning from amino acid residues 953 to 1186, and tyrosine autophosphorylation sites. The TKD includes amino acid residues 688–728 (coded by exon 18), 729–761 (coded by exon 19), 762–823 (coded by exon 20), and 824–875 (coded by exon 21). EGFR is activated by the binding of one of the ligands including epidermal growth factor (EGF), transforming growth factor-α (TGF-α), amphiregulin (ARG), epigen (EGN), heparin-binding EGF (HB-EGF), epiregulin (EPR), and betacellulin (BTC). Heterozygous mutations clustering in the ATP-binding pocket of the TKD may lead to constitutive EGFR activation and ligand independence (Lynch et al. 2004; Paez et al. 2004). The most common *EGFR* mutations, representing approximately 90% of the cases, include deletions in exon 19 affecting the LREA sequence from residues 746 to 750 and a leucine-to-arginine substitution at position 858 on exon 21 (L858R) (Rosell et al. 2009). Less common mutations include G719X (G719A, G719S, or G719C) in exon 18, other mutations in exon 18 or 21, and mutations or insertions in exon 20 (Sharma et al. 2007). Exon 20 insertions are the most prevalent of the uncommon mutations, accounting for approximately 10% of *EGFR* mutations (Kosaka et al. 2017). Patients with tumors harboring EGFR mutations, with the exception of most exon 20 insertions, are usually responsive to EGFR tyrosine kinase inhibitors (TKIs), including the first-generation gefitinib and erlotinib, second-generation afatinib and dacomitinib, and third-generation drug osimertinib (Mok et al. 2009; Rosell et al. 2012; Yang et al. 2015; Wu et al. 2017; Soria et al. 2018). With the exception of the A763ins FQEA, *EGFR* exon 20 insertions are usually resistant to first- and second-generation EGFR TKIs (Robichaux et al. 2018). Possible treatment options for patients with *EGFR* exon 20 insertions include poziotinib, mobocertinib, and amivantamab (JNJ-61186372) (Remon et al. 2020).

Among patients treated with first-generation or second-generation EGFR TKIs, the most common mechanism of acquired resistance is the C-to-T base-pair mutation leading to a change from methionine to threonine at position 790 (T790M), which occurs in approximately 50–60% of cases (Westover et al. 2018). Other less common mechanisms include *MET* gene amplification, *HER2* amplification, small cell lung cancer transformation, and other mutations. In contrast, there is no dominant mechanism of acquired resistance to osimertinib, which may be subdivided according to the EGFR dependence

(Leonetti et al. 2019; Schmid et al. 2020). EGFR-dependent mechanisms are represented by additional *EGFR* mutations whereas EGFR-independent mechanisms involve lineage plasticity, activation of an additional pathway, and acquired cell cycle gene alterations. Although there are some differences depending on whether osimertinib is given as the first-line treatment for previously treated patients, the most common mechanisms for acquired resistance include mutations in *EGFR*, *BRAF* V600E, *PIK3CA*, and *KRAS*; *MET* amplifications; transformation to small cell lung cancer (SCLC); and amplifications of the cell cycle genes *CCND1*, *CCND2*, *CCNE1*, *CDK4*, or *CDK6*. Point mutations in the *EGFR* cysteine residue at position 797 (C797), which is the covalent binding site for osimertinib, represent the most common mechanism of EGFR-dependent acquired resistance. The C979S mutation may develop in the same allele as T790M (*cis*) or separate alleles (*trans*), with the former associated with resistance to EGFR TKIs, whereas the latter may still be sensitive for early-generation drugs and be targeted with a combination of first- and third-generation EGFR TKIs (Vokes and Janne 2017). A promising therapy for patients with C797S mutation is the bispecific EGFR/MET antibody amivantamab and patients with triple-*EGFR* mutations including the original sensitizing mutation, T790M and C797S, could benefit from the combination of brigatinib plus cetuximab (Wang et al. 2020). Several other resistant secondary genomic alterations may potentially be targeted including *MET* exon 14 mutations, *MET* amplification, *BRAF* mutation, and *ALK* and *RET* fusions (Piper-Vallillo et al. 2020).

4 ALK

The anaplastic lymphoma kinase (*ALK*) gene is located on chromosome 2p and encodes for a transmembrane receptor tyrosine kinase that is involved in early neurodevelopment (Le and Gerber 2017; Katayama et al. 2015). In adult humans ALK is normally restricted to low levels in the small intestine, nervous system, and testes where the function remains unclear. *ALK* rearrangements, which lead to constitutive activation of the kinase, are most common in younger patients with adenocarcinoma. Among the multiple fusion partners for ALK, the most common is *EML4*. Current treatment options for patients with *ALK* rearrangements include the first-generation TKI crizotinib; second-generation alectinib, ceritinib, and brigatinib; and third-generation lorlatinib (Solomon et al. 2014; Peters et al. 2017; Soria et al. 2017; Camidge et al. 2018; Shaw et al. 2020). Secondary *ALK* mutations may hinder the TKI binding to the kinase and alter the kinase conformation or its ATP-binding affinity. Resistant *ALK* mutations occur in approximately 20% of patients treated with crizotinib with the percentage increasing to approximately 50% in those treated with one of the second-generation drugs (Gainor et al. 2016; Lin et al. 2017). Due to structural differences among the ALK TKIs, there are some differences in efficacy for the second-generation drugs according to the secondary mutation. The most common *ALK* resistance mutation in patients treated with alectinib or ceritinib is the G1002R which is associated with resistance to all ALK inhibitors except for lorlatinib. The sequential treatment with successive generations of TKIs is associated with the acquisition of secondary mutations after each line of therapy and development of treatment-refractory compound *ALK* mutations (Dagogo-Jack et al. 2019a).

5 ROS1

The *ROS1* gene is located on 6q22.1 and its tyrosine kinase domain has considerable homology with other members of the insulin receptor RTKs, particularly ALK (Facchinetti et al. 2017; Drilon et al. 2021). The 3′ regions of ROS1 may be fused with multiple 5′ gene partners, with the most common being *CD74*, with the in-frame fusion of the N-terminal portion of the partner gene with the intracellular kinase domain region of *ROS1*. ROS1 activation results in the stimulation of several signaling pathways including PI3K, MAPK, and JAK-STAT3. In NSCLC, *ROS1* fusions are detected in approximately 1% of NSCLCs, mostly in younger, never-smokers with adenocarcinoma. There are several active TKIs for patients with *ROS1* fusions including crizotinib, entrectinib, ceritinib, lorlatinib, and repotrectinib (Hanna et al. 2021; Shaw et al. 2014; Drilon et al. 2020a).

6 BRAF

The *BRAF* gene codes for a nonreceptor serine/threonine kinase, activated downstream of the Ras protein (Marchetti et al. 2011). When activated, RAF kinases, including BRAF, phosphorylate and activate MEK1 and MEK2 kinases with subsequent activation of ERK1 and ERK2 kinases (Yaeger and Corcoran 2019). Somatic mutations have been described in multiple solid tumors and may be subdivided into three general classes (Yaeger and Corcoran 2019). Class I is the most common and occurs in *BRAF* V600, representing over 90% of *BRAF* mutations. Among the *BRAF* V600, the most common mutation is V600E in exon 15 where a T1799 point mutation leads to a valine-to-glutamate substitution at codon 600 (V600E) (Yaeger and Corcoran 2019; Nguyen-Ngoc et al. 2015). These mutations are characterized by constitutively activated BRAF kinase capable of signaling as a monomer and capable of activating the MAPK pathway independent of RAS activity. Non-V600E mutations include class II mutations which signal through dimers and are independent of RAS activation and class III mutations which signal through dimers and require RAS activity. In a study evaluating 236 patients with NSCLC harboring *BRAF* mutations, 107 (45%) had class I, 75 (32%) had class II, and 54 (23%) had class III mutations (Dagogo-Jack et al. 2019b). Among the patients evaluated, 213 (90.2%) had adenocarcinoma histology and 9 (3.8%) had squamous cell carcinoma. The current approved drugs for the treatment of *BRAF* mutations selectively inhibit BRAF monomers, being active only against class I mutations (Yaeger and Corcoran 2019). Treatment options for *BRAF* V600E mutations in NSCLC include the BRAF inhibitors vemurafenib and dabrafenib, with the latter being used as a single agent or in combination with the MEK inhibitor trametinib (Hyman et al. 2015; Planchard et al. 2016, 2017).

7 MET

The MET gene is located on chromosome 7q21-q31 and encodes for c-MET, a tyrosine kinase receptor (Friedlaender et al. 2020). Binding of the ligand hepatocyte growth factor (HGF) leads to MET dimerization and autophosphorylation with the activation of several downstream pathways including PI3K, MAPK, STAT and JNK, and FAK, with the regulation of cell survival, proliferation, and epithelial-to-mesenchymal transformation. MET activation may occur through mutations, amplifications, overexpression, fusions, and HGF overstimulation.

Activating *MET* mutations may occur at the kinase domain, extracellular domain, and intronic spice sites flanking exon 14, with the latter representing the most common alteration. The *MET* exon 14 (*MET*ex14) encodes part of the juxtamembrane domain containing Y1003, which is the c-Cbl E3 ubiquitin ligase-binding site (Drilon et al. 2017; Guo et al. 2020). Upon MET activation, the phosphorylation of Y1003 residue of the exon 14 mediates the binding of c-Cbl E3 ligase, leading to ubiquitination and degradation of MET in an autoregulatory negative feedback loop. Mutations in gene positions for splicing out introns flanking *MET*ex14, either at the donor or acceptor sites flanking exon 14, result in *MET*ex14 skipping and production of a truncated MET receptor lacking the Y1003 c-CbL binding site causing decreased degradation and accumulation as an active ligand-receptor complex on the cell surface. The resulting shortened MET receptor retains affinity for HGF and catalytic activity with sustained activation of downstream signaling pathways and oncogenesis. A similar effect on c-Cbl E3 ligase can occur with Y1003 point mutations. In a large comprehensive genome profiling study involving 11,205 patients, *MET*ex14 was identified in 298 cases (2.7%) (Schrock et al. 2016). The median age of the patients with *MET*ex14 alterations was 73 years and the tumors were more common in adenosquamous histology (8.2%) followed by sarcomatoid (7.7%), NSCLC not otherwise specified (3%), adenocarcinoma (2.9%), and squamous cell carcinoma (2.1%). The *MET*ex14 alterations included base substitutions in 51.6%, most commonly in the splice donor, and indels in 47.7%, most commonly in the splice acceptor. Treatment options for patients with *MET*ex14 mutations include crizotinib, capmatinib, and tepotinib (Landi et al. 2019; Wolf et al. 2020; Paik et al. 2020).

An increase in the *MET* copy number may occur through polysomy or focal amplification (Friedlaender et al. 2020; Guo et al. 2020). *MET* polysomy occurs in the presence of more than two copies of chromosome 7 resulting in an increase in the copies of its genes including *MET*, *EGFR*, and *BRAF*. In contrast, *MET* amplifications are caused by focal copy number gains without chromosome 7 duplication. The distinction between polysomy and focal amplification is important since the latter is more likely to be associated with oncogenic *MET* addiction. Since the simple determination of the gene copy number per cell does not differentiate between *MET* polysomy and amplification, a more commonly used FISH method involves the calculation of *MET* to the centromeric portion of chromosome 7 (CEP7). *MET* amplifications occur in 1–6% of patients with NSCLC and the degree of amplification may be subdivided according to the *MET*-to-CEP7 ratios into low (1.8 to 2.2), intermediate (>2.2 to <5), and high (≥5), with the higher ratios and gene copy numbers associated with increased response rates to targeted therapy. *MET* amplifications may be targeted with crizotinib or capmatinib (Landi et al. 2019; Wolf et al. 2020).

MET overexpression detected by immunohistochemistry (IHC) may be quantified by intensity from negative (0) to strong (3+) or with the *H*-score which is calculated by multiplying the percentages of positive cells by their score with the range of result from 0 to 300. MET overexpression may potentially be targeted with antibody drug conjugates including telisotuzumab vedotin (Strickler et al. 2018). *MET* fusions are rare in NSCLC but may be responsive to crizotinib (Plenker et al. 2018).

8 RET

The *RET* gene is located on 10q11.2 and encodes an RTK that plays important roles in the development of the kidney and nervous system, regulation of hematopoietic cells, and spermatogenesis (Subbiah et al. 2020). The RET ligands belong to the GFL family which includes GDNF, nurturing, artemin, and persephin, which bind to GDNF family receptor-α (GFRα), with the GFL-GFRα complex mediating RET homodimerization and trans-autophosphorylation of tyrosine residues with the activation of several pathways including MAPK, PI3K, JAK-STAT, PKA, and PKC (Drilon et al. 2018a). Aberrant *RET* activation in cancer may occur through chromosomal rearrangements that generate fusion genes containing the RET kinase domain, gain-of-function missense mutations, and increased expression of the wild-type gene (Subbiah et al. 2020). *RET* rearrangements leading to ligand-independent constitutional activation of the RET kinase occur in approximately 2% of patients with lung cancer, with the most common partners being KIF5B and CCDC6. For patients with NSCLC harboring *RET* rearrangements, the selective RET inhibitors selpercatinib (LOXO-292) (Drilon et al. 2020b) and pralsetinib (BLU-667) (Gainor et al. 2020) are more effective than multitarget tyrosine kinase inhibitors such as cabozantinib and vandetanib (Hanna et al. 2021; Subbiah and Cote 2020). Resistance to selpercatinib or pralsetinib occurs mostly from RET-independent mechanism with *MET* gene amplification being a potentially targetable alteration with the use of cabozantinib or with combinations involving MET inhibitors (Lin et al. 2020). Acquired RET mutations such as in the solvent residue G810 (R, S, V, or V) or the gatekeeper residue V804 have also been reported and could potentially be targeted with novel RET inhibitors (Solomon et al. 2020).

The multikinase inhibitor TPX-0046 inhibits the RET solvent but not the gatekeeper mutations.

9 NTRK

The *NTRK* genes 1, 2, and 3 encode the tropomyosin-receptor kinase (TRK) A, B, and C, respectively (Vaishnavi et al. 2015). The TRK pathway plays important roles in the nervous system development. *NTRK* fusions are uncommon, can be found in multiple adult pediatric tumor types including lung cancer, and may be targeted with TKIs including larotrectinib and entrectinib (Drilon et al. 2018b; Doebele et al. 2020).

10 HER2

HER2 is a member of the EGFR family of RTKs and may be altered in multiple solid tumors through amplification, overexpression, and mutation. In NSCLC, amplifications, overexpression, and mutations are observed in approximately 2–3%, 2.5%, and 1–3% of patients, respectively (Oh and Bang 2020). Approximately 90% of the *HER2* mutations in patients with NSCLC are located on exon 20, with a predominance of insertions. The most common alteration is a 12-base-pair in-frame insertion YVMA (p.A775_G776insYVMA) (Eng et al. 2016). *HER2* exon 20 insertions are usually resistant to EGFR TKIs including erlotinib, gefitinib, afatinib, dacomitinib, neratinib, and osimertinib. Possible treatment options for patients with *HER2*-mutated NSCLC include ado-trastuzumab emtansine, trastuzumab deruxtecan, poziotinib, and pyrotinib (Li et al. 2018; Rolfo and Russo 2020; Koga et al. 2018).

11 KRAS

RAS genes, which include *KRAS*, *NRAS*, and *HRAS*, encode small membrane-bound guanine nucleotide proteins that have high affinity for guanosine diphosphate (GDP) and guanosine triphosphate (GTP) switching between GTP-bound active and GDP-bound inactive stages (Burns et al. 2020; Moore et al. 2020; Elez and Tabernero 2020). In normal cells, RAS is activated by growth factor receptors, including EGFR, which promote the exchange of GDP for GTP in an effect mediated by guanine nucleotide exchange factors (GEFs), including son-of-sevenless (SOS). GTP-bound RAS activates several downstream pathways including MAPK and PI3K. SHP2 binds to SOS1 and GRB2 increasing the RAS nucleotide exchange. GTPase-activating proteins (GAPs) including neurofibromin (NF-1) increase the hydrolysis of GTP leading to the conversion to the inactive GDP-bound state. Missense single-base *RAS* mutations in codons 12, 13, or 61 disrupt the GAP-mediated GTP hydrolysis and allow the accumulation of RAS in the GTP-bound state with constitutive signaling activation. *KRAS* accounts for approximately 85% of all *RAS* mutations and the most common oncogenic *KRAS* mutations occur at codon 12, with less frequent mutations in codons 13 and 61. In Western populations with NSCLC, *KRAS* G12C accounts for 40–55% of the *KRAS* mutations and occurs in approximately 12–14% of patients. In contrast to the other *KRAS* mutations, the substitution of glycine to cysteine on codon 12 (*KRAS* G12C) is associated with preserved GTPase activity. This highest level of GTPase activity for *KRAS* G12C compared to other oncogenic *RAS* mutations may be explored with the use of covalent inhibitors that bind to KRAS-G12C in the GDP-bound state and prevent the conversion of the mutant protein to the GTP-bound state. Treatment options for patients with *KRAS* G12C mutations may include the direct inhibitors sotorasib (AMG-510) (Hong et al. 2020), MRTX849, JNJ-74699157, or LY3499446. Inhibition of SOS or SHP2 decreases the rate of GDP-to-GTP exchange and has been tested both as single agents and in combinations with direct KRAS inhibitors. Since RAS activates both PI3K and MAPK pathways, combinations of direct KRAS G12C with PI3K, AKT, MEK, or ERK inhibitors are currently being tested.

12 FGFR

Fibroblast growth factor receptors (FGFRs) constitute a family of four RTKs (FGFR1–4) that mediate cellular signaling when bound to one of the fibroblast growth factors (FGFs), regulating many cellular functions including cell cycle progression, metabolism, survival, proliferation, and differentiation (Desai and Adjei 2016). Targetable FGFR alterations include gene amplifications, somatic mutations, and chromosomal fusions. *FGFR1* is located on 8q12 and amplifications have been described in 17% of patients with squamous cell carcinoma, 6% of those with small cell lung cancer, and 1% of those with adenocarcinoma (Babina and Turner 2017; Katoh 2019). Both *FGFR2* and *FGFR3* mutations may be found in 3% of squamous cell lung cancer and several of these mutations drive cellular transformation (Liao et al. 2013). In a large study evaluating 26,054 NSCLC specimens, *FGFR* fusions retaining the kinase domain were detected in 0.2% of the cases (Qin et al. 2019). Fusions were more common in squamous cell carcinoma (0.59%) than adenocarcinoma (0.12%). The most common fusion was *FGFR3-TACC3*, which accounted for all 21 positive squamous cell carcinoma cases. *FGFR*-altered tumors may be treated with TKIs including FGFR inhibitors and multikinase inhibitors.

13 Small Cell Lung Cancer

Small cell lung cancer (SCLC) accounts for approximately 15% of the lung cancer cases and is characterized by the simultaneous inactivation of tumor suppressor genes *TP53* and *RB1* (George et al. 2015). Other findings detected in tissue or ctDNA include alterations in *FGFR1*, PI3K pathway, *MYC*, and NOTCH pathway (George et al. 2015; Rudin et al. 2012; Devarakonda et al. 2019). Several classifications have been proposed in an attempt to differentiate subgroups of SCLC. In the most recent classification, SCLC is subdivided into four groups including SCLC-A, SCLC-N, SCLC-Y, and SCLC-P based on the increased expression of achaete-scute homolog 1 (ASCL1), NeuroD1, YAP1, and POU2F3, respectively (Rudin et al. 2019). Delta-like ligand 3 (DLL3) is a downstream target of ASCL1 and may be targeted with antibody drug conjugates, bispecific T-cell engagers, or chimeric antigen receptor T-cell therapy (Morgensztern et al. 2019; Poirier et al. 2020). *MYC* amplification in SCLC may be associated with sensitivity to aurora kinase inhibitors (Owonikoko et al. 2020).

14 Conclusion

The increasing use of molecular profiling, particularly with the advent of NGS, has allowed a better understanding of the molecular biology of lung cancer and the development of novel therapies matching the genomic alteration. Although virtually all patients eventually developed tumor progression while receiving targeted therapy, new mechanisms of acquired resistance have been unveiled for most of the genomic alterations and novel treatments are being developed. For patients with small cell lung cancer, recent data increased the knowledge of the molecular heterogeneity and subgroups based on the RNA expression of transcription regulators may allow a better understanding of the tumor biology with the development of effective targeted therapies.

References

Alexandrov LB, Nik-Zainal S, Wedge DC et al (2013) Signatures of mutational processes in human cancer. Nature 500:415–421

Anderson ND, de Borja R, Young MD et al (2018) Rearrangement bursts generate canonical gene fusions in bone and soft tissue tumors. Science 361:eaam8419

Babina IS, Turner NC (2017) Advances and challenges in targeting FGFR signalling in cancer. Nat Rev Cancer 17:318–332

Barlesi F, Mazieres J, Merlio JP et al (2016) Routine molecular profiling of patients with advanced non-small-cell lung cancer: results of a 1-year nationwide programme of the French Cooperative Thoracic Intergroup (IFCT). Lancet 387:1415–1426

Burns TF, Borghaei H, Ramalingam SS et al (2020) Targeting KRAS-mutant non-small-cell lung cancer: one mutation at a time, with a focus on KRAS G12C mutations. J Clin Oncol 38:4208–4218

Camidge DR, Kim HR, Ahn MJ et al (2018) Brigatinib versus crizotinib in ALK-positive non-small-cell lung cancer. N Engl J Med 379:2027–2039

Clark D, Pazdernik N, McGehee M (2019) Mutations and repair. In: Molecular biology. Academic, San Diego, CA, pp 832–879

Corcoran RB, Chabner BA (2018) Application of cell-free DNA analysis to cancer treatment. N Engl J Med 379:1754–1765

Dagogo-Jack I, Rooney M, Lin JJ et al (2019a) Treatment with next-generation ALK inhibitors fuels plasma ALK mutation diversity. Clin Cancer Res 25:6662–6670

Dagogo-Jack I, Martinez P, Yeap BY et al (2019b) Impact of BRAF mutation class on disease characteristics and clinical outcomes in BRAF-mutant lung cancer. Clin Cancer Res 25:158–165

Desai A, Adjei AA (2016) FGFR signaling as a target for lung cancer therapy. J Thorac Oncol 11:9–20

Devarakonda S, Sankararaman S, Herzog BH et al (2019) Circulating tumor DNA profiling in small-cell lung cancer identifies potentially targetable alterations. Clin Cancer Res 25:6119–6126

Doebele RC, Drilon A, Paz-Ares L et al (2020) Entrectinib in patients with advanced or metastatic NTRK fusion-positive solid tumours: integrated analysis of three phase 1–2 trials. Lancet Oncol 21:271–282

Drilon A, Cappuzzo F, Ou SI et al (2017) Targeting MET in lung cancer: will expectations finally be MET? J Thorac Oncol 12:15–26

Drilon A, Hu ZI, Lai GGY et al (2018a) Targeting RET-driven cancers: lessons from evolving preclinical and clinical landscapes. Nat Rev Clin Oncol 15:151–167

Drilon A, Laetsch TW, Kummar S et al (2018b) Efficacy of larotrectinib in TRK fusion-positive cancers in adults and children. N Engl J Med 378:731–739

Drilon A, Siena S, Dziadziuszko R et al (2020a) Entrectinib in ROS1 fusion-positive non-small-cell lung cancer: integrated analysis of three phase 1–2 trials. Lancet Oncol 21:261–270

Drilon A, Oxnard GR, Tan DSW et al (2020b) Efficacy of selpercatinib in RET fusion-positive non-small-cell lung cancer. N Engl J Med 383:813–824

Drilon A, Jenkins C, Iyer S et al (2021) ROS1-dependent cancers - biology, diagnostics and therapeutics. Nat Rev Clin Oncol 18:35–55

Du Z, Lovly CM (2018) Mechanisms of receptor tyrosine kinase activation in cancer. Mol Cancer 17:58

Elez E, Tabernero J (2020) The effective targeting of KRAS(G12C) elusiveness. Cancer Cell 38:785–787

Eng J, Hsu M, Chaft JE et al (2016) Outcomes of chemotherapies and HER2 directed therapies in advanced HER2-mutant lung cancers. Lung Cancer 99:53–56

Facchinetti F, Rossi G, Bria E et al (2017) Oncogene addiction in non-small cell lung cancer: focus on ROS1 inhibition. Cancer Treat Rev 55:83–95

Fleuren ED, Zhang L, Wu J et al (2016) The kinome 'at large' in cancer. Nat Rev Cancer 16:83–98

Friedlaender A, Drilon A, Banna GL et al (2020) The METeoric rise of MET in lung cancer. Cancer 126:4826–4837

Gagan J, Van Allen EM (2015) Next-generation sequencing to guide cancer therapy. Genome Med 7:80

Gainor JF, Dardaei L, Yoda S et al (2016) Molecular mechanisms of resistance to first- and second-generation ALK inhibitors in ALK-rearranged lung cancer. Cancer Discov 6:1118–1133

Gainor JF, Curigliano G, Kim D-W et al (2020) Registrational dataset from the phase I/II ARROW trial of pralsetinib (BLU-667) in patients (pts) with advanced RET fusion+ non-small cell lung cancer (NSCLC). J Clin Oncol 38:9515–9515

Garrido P, Conde E, de Castro J et al (2020) Updated guidelines for predictive biomarker testing in advanced non-small-cell lung cancer: a National Consensus of the Spanish Society of Pathology and the Spanish Society of Medical Oncology. Clin Transl Oncol 22:989–1003

George J, Lim JS, Jang SJ et al (2015) Comprehensive genomic profiles of small cell lung cancer. Nature 524:47–53

Gong J, Pan K, Fakih M et al (2018) Value-based genomics. Oncotarget 9:15792–15815

Griesinger F, Eberhardt W, Nusch A et al (2021) Biomarker testing in non-small cell lung cancer in routine care: analysis of the first 3,717 patients in the German prospective, observational, nation-wide CRISP Registry (AIO-TRK-0315). Lung Cancer 152:174–184

Guo R, Luo J, Chang J et al (2020) MET-dependent solid tumours - molecular diagnosis and targeted therapy. Nat Rev Clin Oncol 17:569–587

Hanahan D, Weinberg RA (2011) Hallmarks of cancer: the next generation. Cell 144:646–674

Hanna NH, Robinson AG, Temin S et al (2021) Therapy for stage IV non-small-cell lung cancer with driver alterations: ASCO and OH (CCO) Joint Guideline Update. J Clin Oncol 39(9):1040–1091

Herbst RS, Morgensztern D, Boshoff C (2018) The biology and management of non-small cell lung cancer. Nature 553:446–454

Hong DS, Fakih MG, Strickler JH et al (2020) KRAS(G12C) inhibition with sotorasib in advanced solid tumors. N Engl J Med 383:1207–1217

Hyman DM, Puzanov I, Subbiah V et al (2015) Vemurafenib in multiple nonmelanoma cancers with BRAF V600 mutations. N Engl J Med 373:726–736

Jayasinghe RG, Cao S, Gao Q et al (2018) Systematic analysis of splice-site-creating mutations in cancer. Cell Rep 23:270–281.e3

Kandoth C, McLellan MD, Vandin F et al (2013) Mutational landscape and significance across 12 major cancer types. Nature 502:333–339

Katayama R, Lovly CM, Shaw AT (2015) Therapeutic targeting of anaplastic lymphoma kinase in lung cancer: a paradigm for precision cancer medicine. Clin Cancer Res 21:2227–2235

Katoh M (2019) Fibroblast growth factor receptors as treatment targets in clinical oncology. Nat Rev Clin Oncol 16:105–122

Koga T, Kobayashi Y, Tomizawa K et al (2018) Activity of a novel HER2 inhibitor, poziotinib, for HER2 exon 20 mutations in lung cancer and mechanism of acquired resistance: an in vitro study. Lung Cancer 126: 72–79

Kosaka T, Tanizaki J, Paranal RM et al (2017) Response heterogeneity of EGFR and HER2 exon 20 insertions to covalent EGFR and HER2 inhibitors. Cancer Res 77:2712–2721

Kris MG, Johnson BE, Berry LD et al (2014) Using multiplexed assays of oncogenic drivers in lung cancers to select targeted drugs. JAMA 311:1998–2006

Landi L, Chiari R, Tiseo M et al (2019) Crizotinib in MET-deregulated or ROS1-rearranged pretreated non-small cell lung cancer (METROS): a phase II, prospective, multicenter, two-arms trial. Clin Cancer Res 25:7312–7319

Latysheva NS, Babu MM (2016) Discovering and understanding oncogenic gene fusions through data intensive computational approaches. Nucleic Acids Res 44:4487–4503

Le T, Gerber DE (2017) ALK alterations and inhibition in lung cancer. Semin Cancer Biol 42:81–88

Leighl NB, Page RD, Raymond VM et al (2019) Clinical utility of comprehensive cell-free DNA analysis to identify genomic biomarkers in patients with newly diagnosed metastatic non-small cell lung cancer. Clin Cancer Res 25:4691–4700

Lemmon MA, Schlessinger J, Ferguson KM (2014) The EGFR family: not so prototypical receptor tyrosine kinases. Cold Spring Harb Perspect Biol 6:a020768

Leonetti A, Sharma S, Minari R et al (2019) Resistance mechanisms to osimertinib in EGFR-mutated non-small cell lung cancer. Br J Cancer 121:725–737

Li BT, Shen R, Buonocore D et al (2018) Ado-trastuzumab emtansine for patients with HER2-mutant lung cancers: results from a phase II basket trial. J Clin Oncol 36:2532–2537

Liao RG, Jung J, Tchaicha J et al (2013) Inhibitor-sensitive FGFR2 and FGFR3 mutations in lung squamous cell carcinoma. Cancer Res 73:5195–5205

Lin JJ, Riely GJ, Shaw AT (2017) Targeting ALK: precision medicine takes on drug resistance. Cancer Discov 7:137–155

Lin JJ, Liu SV, McCoach CE et al (2020) Mechanisms of resistance to selective RET tyrosine kinase inhibitors in RET fusion-positive non-small-cell lung cancer. Ann Oncol 31:1725–1733

Lynch TJ, Bell DW, Sordella R et al (2004) Activating mutations in the epidermal growth factor receptor underlying responsiveness of non-small-cell lung cancer to gefitinib. N Engl J Med 350:2129–2139

Macconaill LE, Garraway LA (2010) Clinical implications of the cancer genome. J Clin Oncol 28:5219–5228

Marchetti A, Felicioni L, Malatesta S et al (2011) Clinical features and outcome of patients with non-small-cell lung cancer harboring BRAF mutations. J Clin Oncol 29:3574–3579

Mok TS, Wu YL, Thongprasert S et al (2009) Gefitinib or carboplatin-paclitaxel in pulmonary adenocarcinoma. N Engl J Med 361:947–957

Moore AR, Rosenberg SC, McCormick F et al (2020) RAS-targeted therapies: is the undruggable drugged? Nat Rev Drug Discov 19:533–552

Morgensztern D, Besse B, Greillier L et al (2019) Efficacy and safety of rovalpituzumab tesirine in third-line and beyond patients with DLL3-expressing, relapsed/refractory small-cell lung cancer: results from the phase II TRINITY study. Clin Cancer Res 25:6958–6966

Nguyen-Ngoc T, Bouchaab H, Adjei AA et al (2015) BRAF alterations as therapeutic targets in non-small-cell lung cancer. J Thorac Oncol 10:1396–1403

Odegaard JI, Vincent JJ, Mortimer S et al (2018) Validation of a plasma-based comprehensive cancer genotyping assay utilizing orthogonal tissue- and plasma-based methodologies. Clin Cancer Res 24:3539–3549

Oh DY, Bang YJ (2020) HER2-targeted therapies - a role beyond breast cancer. Nat Rev Clin Oncol 17:33–48

Owonikoko TK, Niu H, Nackaerts K et al (2020) Randomized phase II study of paclitaxel plus alisertib versus paclitaxel plus placebo as second-line therapy for SCLC: primary and correlative biomarker analyses. J Thorac Oncol 15:274–287

Paez JG, Janne PA, Lee JC et al (2004) EGFR mutations in lung cancer: correlation with clinical response to gefitinib therapy. Science 304:1497–1500

Paik PK, Felip E, Veillon R et al (2020) Tepotinib in non-small-cell lung cancer with MET exon 14 skipping mutations. N Engl J Med 383:931–943

Peters S, Camidge DR, Shaw AT et al (2017) Alectinib versus crizotinib in untreated ALK-positive non-small-cell lung cancer. N Engl J Med 377:829–838

Piper-Vallillo AJ, Sequist LV, Piotrowska Z (2020) Emerging treatment paradigms for EGFR-mutant lung cancers progressing on osimertinib: a review. J Clin Oncol. https://doi.org/10.1200/JCO.19.03123

Planchard D, Kim TM, Mazieres J et al (2016) Dabrafenib in patients with BRAF(V600E)-positive advanced non-small-cell lung cancer: a single-arm, multicentre, open-label, phase 2 trial. Lancet Oncol 17:642–650

Planchard D, Smit EF, Groen HJM et al (2017) Dabrafenib plus trametinib in patients with previously untreated BRAF(V600E)-mutant metastatic non-small-cell lung cancer: an open-label, phase 2 trial. Lancet Oncol 18:1307–1316

Plenker D, Bertrand M, de Langen AJ et al (2018) Structural alterations of MET trigger response to MET kinase inhibition in lung adenocarcinoma patients. Clin Cancer Res 24:1337–1343

Poirier JT, George J, Owonikoko TK et al (2020) New approaches to SCLC therapy: from the laboratory to the clinic. J Thorac Oncol 15:520–540

Qin A, Johnson A, Ross JS et al (2019) Detection of known and novel FGFR fusions in non-small cell lung cancer by comprehensive genomic profiling. J Thorac Oncol 14:54–62

Remon J, Hendriks LEL, Cardona AF et al (2020) EGFR exon 20 insertions in advanced non-small cell lung cancer: a new history begins. Cancer Treat Rev 90:102105

Robichaux JP, Elamin YY, Tan Z et al (2018) Mechanisms and clinical activity of an EGFR and HER2 exon 20-selective kinase inhibitor in non-small cell lung cancer. Nat Med 24:638–646

Rolfo C, Russo A (2020) HER2 mutations in non-small cell lung cancer: a Herculean effort to hit the target. Cancer Discov 10:643–645

Rosell R, Moran T, Queralt C et al (2009) Screening for epidermal growth factor receptor mutations in lung cancer. N Engl J Med 361:958–967

Rosell R, Carcereny E, Gervais R et al (2012) Erlotinib versus standard chemotherapy as first-line treatment for European patients with advanced EGFR mutation-positive non-small-cell lung cancer (EURTAC): a multicentre, open-label, randomised phase 3 trial. Lancet Oncol 13:239–246

Rudin CM, Durinck S, Stawiski EW et al (2012) Comprehensive genomic analysis identifies SOX2 as a frequently amplified gene in small-cell lung cancer. Nat Genet 44:1111–1116

Rudin CM, Poirier JT, Byers LA et al (2019) Molecular subtypes of small cell lung cancer: a synthesis of human and mouse model data. Nat Rev Cancer 19:289–297

Salehi-Rad R, Li R, Paul MK et al (2020) The biology of lung cancer: development of more effective methods for prevention, diagnosis, and treatment. Clin Chest Med 41:25–38

Santarius T, Shipley J, Brewer D et al (2010) A census of amplified and overexpressed human cancer genes. Nat Rev Cancer 10:59–64

Schmid S, Li JJN, Leighl NB (2020) Mechanisms of osimertinib resistance and emerging treatment options. Lung Cancer 147:123–129

Schrock AB, Frampton GM, Suh J et al (2016) Characterization of 298 patients with lung cancer harboring MET exon 14 skipping alterations. J Thorac Oncol 11:1493–1502

Sharma SV, Bell DW, Settleman J et al (2007) Epidermal growth factor receptor mutations in lung cancer. Nat Rev Cancer 7:169–181

Shaw AT, Ou SH, Bang YJ et al (2014) Crizotinib in ROS1-rearranged non-small-cell lung cancer. N Engl J Med 371:1963–1971

Shaw AT, Bauer TM, de Marinis F et al (2020) First-line lorlatinib or crizotinib in advanced ALK-positive lung cancer. N Engl J Med 383:2018–2029

Singal G, Miller PG, Agarwala V et al (2019) Association of patient characteristics and tumor genomics with clinical outcomes among patients with non-small cell lung cancer using a clinicogenomic database. JAMA 321:1391–1399

Solomon BJ, Mok T, Kim DW et al (2014) First-line crizotinib versus chemotherapy in ALK-positive lung cancer. N Engl J Med 371:2167–2177

Solomon BJ, Tan L, Lin JJ et al (2020) RET solvent front mutations mediate acquired resistance to selective RET inhibition in RET-driven malignancies. J Thorac Oncol 15:541–549

Soria JC, Tan DS, Chiari R et al (2017) First-line ceritinib versus platinum-based chemotherapy in advanced ALK-rearranged non-small-cell lung cancer (ASCEND-4): a randomised, open-label, phase 3 study. Lancet 389:917–929

Soria JC, Ohe Y, Vansteenkiste J et al (2018) Osimertinib in untreated EGFR-mutated advanced non-small-cell lung cancer. N Engl J Med 378:113–125

Stratton MR, Campbell PJ, Futreal PA (2009) The cancer genome. Nature 458:719–724

Strickler JH, Weekes CD, Nemunaitis J et al (2018) First-in-human phase I, dose-escalation and -expansion study of telisotuzumab vedotin, an antibody-drug conjugate targeting c-Met, in patients with advanced solid tumors. J Clin Oncol 36:3298–3306

Subbiah V, Cote GJ (2020) Advances in targeting RET-dependent cancers. Cancer Discov 10:498–505

Subbiah V, Yang D, Velcheti V et al (2020) State-of-the-art strategies for targeting RET-dependent cancers. J Clin Oncol 38:1209–1221

The Cancer Genome Atlas Research Network (2012) Comprehensive genomic characterization of squamous cell lung cancers. Nature 489:519–525

The Cancer Genome Atlas Research Network (2014) Comprehensive molecular profiling of lung adenocarcinoma. Nature 511:543–550

Tong M, Seeliger MA (2015) Targeting conformational plasticity of protein kinases. ACS Chem Biol 10:190–200

Trenker R, Jura N (2020) Receptor tyrosine kinase activation: from the ligand perspective. Curr Opin Cell Biol 63:174–185

Vaishnavi A, Le AT, Doebele RC (2015) TRKing down an old oncogene in a new era of targeted therapy. Cancer Discov 5:25–34

Vogelstein B, Papadopoulos N, Velculescu VE et al (2013) Cancer genome landscapes. Science 339:1546–1558

Vokes NI, Janne PA (2017) Resistance in trans-ition. J Thorac Oncol 12:1608–1610

Wang Y, Yang N, Zhang Y et al (2020) Effective treatment of lung adenocarcinoma harboring EGFR-activating mutation, T790M, and cis-C797S triple mutations by brigatinib and cetuximab combination therapy. J Thorac Oncol 15:1369–1375

Westover D, Zugazagoitia J, Cho BC et al (2018) Mechanisms of acquired resistance to first- and second-generation EGFR tyrosine kinase inhibitors. Ann Oncol 29:i10–i19

Wolf J, Seto T, Han JY et al (2020) Capmatinib in MET exon 14-mutated or MET-amplified non-small-cell lung cancer. N Engl J Med 383:944–957

Wu YL, Cheng Y, Zhou X et al (2017) Dacomitinib versus gefitinib as first-line treatment for patients with EGFR-mutation-positive non-small-cell lung cancer (ARCHER 1050): a randomised, open-label, phase 3 trial. Lancet Oncol 18:1454–1466

Yaeger R, Corcoran RB (2019) Targeting alterations in the RAF-MEK pathway. Cancer Discov 9:329–341

Yang JC, Wu YL, Schuler M et al (2015) Afatinib versus cisplatin-based chemotherapy for EGFR mutation-positive lung adenocarcinoma (LUX-Lung 3 and LUX-Lung 6): analysis of overall survival data from two randomised, phase 3 trials. Lancet Oncol 16:141–151

Epigenetic Events in Lung Cancer

Octavio A. Romero
and Montse Sanchez-Cespedes

Contents

1 Introduction 18
2 **Classification of the Epigenetic Modifications** 18
2.1 DNA Methylation 18
2.2 Regulators of the Chromatin Structure: Histone Modifiers 18
2.3 Regulators of the Chromatin Structure: Chromatin Remodeling Complexes 21
3 **Landscape of the Epigenetic Abnormalities in Lung Cancer** 21
3.1 Aberrant DNA Methylation 22
3.2 Gene Abnormalities Affecting Chromatin Remodelers: The SWI/SNF Complex 23
3.3 Abnormalities in Histone Modifiers 24
4 **Epigenetic-Based Therapeutic Strategies in Lung Cancer** 25
4.1 DNA Methyltransferase Inhibitors 25
4.2 Histone Deacetylase Inhibitors 26
4.3 Other Epigenetic Inhibitors 27
5 **Conclusions and Future Directions** 28
References 28

Abstract

The term epigenetics refers to the study of heritable and reversible changes in the genome that modulate gene expression without altering the DNA sequence. These mechanisms comprise the addition of methyl groups to a cytosine within a CpG dinucleotide, referred to as DNA methylation, posttranslational and covalent modifications of the histone proteins, and chromatin remodeling. The different epigenetic events elicit structural and functional changes within chromatin that determine many different cellular processes and response to environmental modifications through the control of gene expression. Abnormal epigenetic states can predispose to or cause human diseases, including cancer. In cancer cells, alterations in DNA methylation or genetic alterations in histone protein modifiers or in chromatin remodelers promote changes in the expression levels of important genes and genome instability, thus contributing to cancer development. In this chapter, the different epigenetic processes that are disrupted in cancer cells are described with special focus on the genetic abnormalities that disturb chromatin stability to promote lung cancer development.

O. A. Romero · M. Sanchez-Cespedes (✉)
Cancer Genetics Group, Josep Carreras Leukemia
Research Institute (IJC), Barcelona, Spain
e-mail: oromero@carrerasresearch.org;
mscespedes@carrerasresearch.org

1 Introduction

Although all the different types of cells that make up our body have exactly the same genome, with the exception of the cells of the immune and reproductive system, they have different gene expression profiles and specific functions, depending on the tissue or organ to which the cell belongs. These differences among cells that have identical genetic background are made possible through the epigenetic modifications of the DNA. To fit within the nucleus, the DNA is tightly packaged to form a compact structure called chromatin and eventually into very large, high-order structures, called chromosomes. Within the chromatin, the DNA is wrapped into structural units called nucleosomes, composed by about 150 base pairs of DNA and histone proteins (Khorasanizadeh 2004). There are five different histones: H1, H2A, H2B, H3, and H4, all of them positively charged proteins that interact with the negatively charged phosphate backbone of the DNA. The nucleosome is constituted by two H3 and two H4 proteins, which form a tetramer that combines with two H2A/H2B dimers to form the histone core. There is an additional histone, a linker histone (e.g., histone H1 or H5), that has a structural function in the stabilization of the nucleosome. In order to respond to a variety of endogenous and exogenous stimuli, the chromatin needs to be highly dynamic and allow accessibility to the DNA when needed. The accessibility to the DNA is controlled by changes in DNA methylation, by posttranslational modifications in the histone proteins and by ATP-dependent chromatin remodelers (Kouzarides 2007).

2 Classification of the Epigenetic Modifications

2.1 DNA Methylation

DNA methylation is the chemical modification of a methyl group to the 5-carbon position of a cytosine that occurs almost exclusively in cytosines located 5′ to a guanine. These pairs of nucleotides are referred to as CpG dinucleotide. In normal cells, the CpG dinucleotides are found across the genome both sparsely distributed and sprinkled throughout the genome, with these CpGs usually being methylated. Alternatively, CpGs can be found well grouped in clusters, known as CpG islands, which are normally found at promoters (Jones and Taylor 1980). CpG islands are defined as stretches of DNA 500–1500 base pairs long with a CG:GC ratio of more than 0.6. Around half of the gene promoters in humans contain CpG islands. The methylation of CpG islands is associated with the suppression of gene expression.

DNA methylation was the first epigenetic modification to be discovered, after studying the molecular processes that are involved in mammalian chromosome X-inactivation (Riggs 1975). Nowadays it is well established that DNA methylation plays a role in a number of processes including embryonic development, genetic imprinting, cell differentiation, and tumorigenesis (Jones and Taylor 1980). In mammals, CpG methylation is driven by three enzymes with DNA methyltransferase activity: DNMT1, which methylates daughter DNA strands after DNA replication, and DNMT3A and DNMT3B (Jones and Baylin 2007).

2.2 Regulators of the Chromatin Structure: Histone Modifiers

Chromatin accessibility is regulated by opposite epigenetic modifications that promote or repress chromatin packaging levels. Owing to these modifications, chromatin can be found in two varieties: heterochromatin, typically highly condensed, gene poor, and transcriptionally silent, and euchromatin, less condensed, gene rich, and transcriptionally active. The balance between these two states of the chromatin structure plays a key role in embryonic development, cell differentiation, and cell fate, among others. An abnormal regulation of the transition between the two states of the chromatin causes disruptions in these processes, contributing to the incidence of diverse diseases, including cancer (Khorasanizadeh 2004).

The control of chromatin accessibility is a dynamic process consisting of covalent modifications of the histone proteins which includes methylation, phosphorylation, acetylation, ubiquitylation, and sumoylation. There are different sets of proteins that catalyze (so-called writers), remove (so-called erasers), and recognize (so-called readers) each of the different chemical modifications in the histones. Writers include histone acetyltransferases and histone methyltransferases whereas erasers include histone deacetylases and histone demethylases. Figure 1 shows a schematic representation of the different histone modifications and the enzymes that catalyze each of them. Finally, the readers are those proteins or complexes of proteins, such as the chromatin remodeling complexes, that recognize the different histone modifications, through specialized domains (Kouzarides 2007).

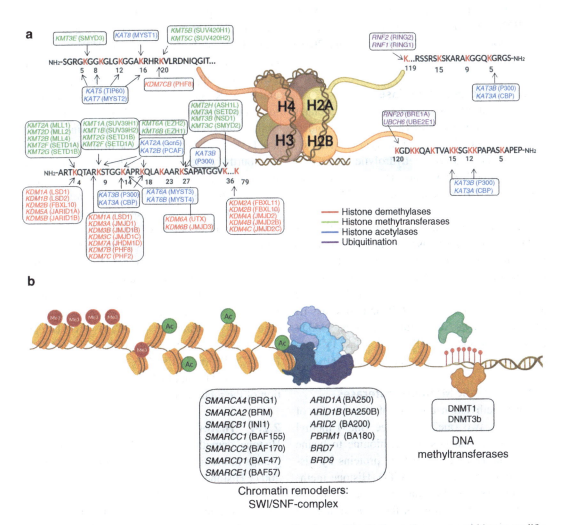

Fig. 1 (**a**) Schematic representation of a nucleosome, with the different histones (H2A, H2B, H3, and H4), histone tails, and DNA (double helix in brown). A selection of different histone-modifying enzymes and some of their lysine (K) substrates is also included. For simplification, the chemical modification at the arginine (R) residues has not been included here. (**b**) Schematic representation of the chromatin with the nucleosomes and histone modifications (*Me3* trimethylation, *Ac* acetylation). The picture highlights the SWI/SNF-chromatin remodeling complex, with a list of different components and of DNA methylation and corresponding methyltransferases. (Created with BioRender.com)

2.2.1 Histone Acetyltransferases

Histone acetylation occurs by the enzymatic addition of an acetyl group (COCH3), in highly conserved lysine residues, from acetyl coenzyme A. This modification is almost invariably associated with the activation of transcription. The modifying enzymes involved in histone acetylation are called histone acetyltransferases (HATs) and they play a critical role in controlling histone H3 and H4 acetylation. There are more than 20 different HATs which have been classified into five different families: GNAT1, MYST, TAFII250, P300/CBP, and nuclear receptor coactivators such as ACTR (Gong et al. 2016) (Fig. 1a).

2.2.2 Histone Deacetylases

The reversal of histone acetylation correlates with transcriptional repression and it is undertaken by the histone deacetylase (HDAC) enzymes that catalyze the hydrolytic removal of acetyl groups from H3 and H4 lysine residues (Fig. 1a). HDACs lack intrinsic DNA-binding activity and are recruited to target genes via their direct association with transcriptional activators and repressors, as well as their incorporation into large multiprotein transcriptional complexes. At least four classes of HDACs have been identified so far. Class I include HDAC1–3 and 8. Class II are comprised of HDAC4–7, 9, and 10. Class III enzymes, known as sirtuins, require NAD+ cofactors and include SIRTs 1–7. Class IV contains only HDAC11 (Haberland et al. 2009).

2.2.3 Histone Methyltransferases

Histone methylation consists of the transfer of one (me1), two (me2), or three (me3) methyl groups from S-adenosyl-L-methionine to lysine or arginine residues of histone proteins by histone methyltransferases (HMTs). Histone methylation is associated to transcriptional activation or repression depending on the residue and the degree of methylation. Thus, the substrate and product specificities of HMTs define the biological roles of these enzymes in the transcriptional regulation (Fig. 1a). Most HMTs present an evolutionarily conserved catalytic domain named SET (Su(var) 3–9, enhancer of zeste, trithorax), which transfers the methyl groups from S-adenosyl-L-methionine onto the N group of a lysine in substrate proteins. In the last decades, next-generation sequencing technologies have allowed the determination of the histone methylation patterns throughout the mammalian genomes.

The enhancer of zeste homolog 2 (EZH2) is a histone lysine methyltransferase that together with zeste 12 (SUZ12) and with embryonic ectoderm development (EED) proteins constitutes the polycomb repressive complex 2. EZH2 mediates trimethylation of H3K27me3 (referring to the trimethylation at the 427th lysine of H3) at promoters to silence the expression of a wide variety of genes, including many involved in lineage differentiation (Ringrose and Paro 2004). Other histone modifications such as H3K4me3 (referring to the trimethylation at the fourth lysine of H4) and H3K4me2 (referring to the di-methylation at the fourth lysine of H3) are highly enriched in transcriptionally active regions or in active promoters whereas H3K4me1 (referring to the mono-methylation at the fourth lysine of H3) is mostly found in enhancer regions. On the other hand, histone methylation can also take place in the arginine residues, in histones H3 and H4, promoting transcriptional activation (Del Rizzo and Trievel 2014). This modification is mediated by a family of seven different types of histone arginine methyltransferases (PRMTs). PRMTs can also be classified into type I (CARM1, PRMT1, PRMT2, PRMT3, PRMT6, and PRMT8) and type II (PRMT5 and PRMT7), based on the position of the methyl group addition.

2.2.4 Histone Demethylases

Histone demethylases (HDMs) remove methyl groups in modified histone proteins (Kouzarides 2007). Histone demethylation is catalyzed by two distinct families of HDMs that both employ oxidative mechanisms. One of them is the lysine-specific demethylase LSD1 (*KDM1A*) family that demethylates lysine residues through a flavin adenine dinucleotide (FAD)-dependent amine oxidase reaction. The other one is the Jumonji domain-containing (JmjC domain) histone demethylases (JMJD2, JMJD3/UTX, and

JARIDs) which demethylate histones in a Fe^{2+}/2-oxoglutarate (2OG)-dependent manner (Klose et al. 2006). The specific amino acid residue and the degree of methylation determine the demethylation enzyme in charge. For example, KDM1 is specific for methylated H3K4, removing methyl groups from H3K4me1 and H3K4me2 but not from H3K4me3, which is catalyzed by KDM5A/B (Zhang et al. 2015). All members of KDM4 family are H3K9 (referring to the ninth lysine of H3) demethylases. The epigenetic mark H3K4me3 recruits and stimulates KDM4C to remove the repressive H3K9me3 mark. KDM6A and KDM6B are histone H3K27 demethylases (Zhang et al. 2015) (Fig. 1a).

2.3 Regulators of the Chromatin Structure: Chromatin Remodeling Complexes

Chromatin remodeling complexes act in healthy adult tissues, during embryonic development and in cell differentiation processes in order to enable dynamic access to packaged DNA and to tailor nucleosome composition in chromosomal regions. For example, chromatin remodeling is needed to fully package the genome after DNA replication or to provide DNA accessibility in packaged regions to allow gene expression. The wide variety of chromatin remodeling complexes that exist allows for a number of different mechanisms to remodel chromatin (Clapier and Cairns 2009). To break the histone-DNA contacts, remodelers can slide nucleosomes, eject histone octamers, remove H2A-H2B dimers, and replace dimers, using the energy from the ATP hydrolysis. Based on the identity of its catalytic subunit, four families of chromatin remodeling complexes have been described: SWI/SNF, ISWI (imitation SWI), Mi-2/NuRD (nucleosome remodeling deacetylase), and INO80/SWR1 (inositol/choline-responsive element-dependent gene activation mutant 80) (Hargreaves and Crabtree 2011).

The SWI/SNF complex is currently the best characterized, and has traditionally been described to have a tumor suppressor role. This complex was originally described in yeast as the complex critical for cellular responses to mating-type switching (SWI) or sucrose fermentation (SNF) (Biegel et al. 2014). In mammals, the SWI/SNF (switch/sucrose nonfermentable) chromatin remodeling complex is combinatorially assembled into 10–15-subunit multimers from the products of 29 genes, including 1 ATPase, either the *SMARCA4* (BRG1) or the *SMARCA2* (BRM), and additional subunits with specialized protein domains that enable to interact with chromatin and/or DNA substrates (Fig. 1b). The SWI/SNF complex contributes to the control of lineage-specific gene expression, being involved in cell differentiation and tissue specification either in adult or in embryonic tissues. Moreover, the complex has been reported to participate in the reprogramming of somatic cells (Kim et al. 2015). The effect of SWI/SNF on some of these processes is related to its involvement in the regulation of the function of hormone and nuclear receptors, some of them important for normal lung development, such as retinoids, corticoids, thyroid, and estrogen receptors, among others (Cardoso and Lü 2006).

3 Landscape of the Epigenetic Abnormalities in Lung Cancer

Over the last decades, in parallel with the advent of next-generation sequencing technologies, our understanding of the catalogue of mutations in oncogenes and tumor suppressor genes in lung cancer has greatly increased (Sondka et al. 2018). Recurrent mutations in oncogenes, leading to a constitutive activation of the coded proteins, are now known to affect many proteins, specially enzymes with tyrosine kinase activity in non-small cell lung cancer (NSCLC) from nonsmokers, such as ALK, EGFR, HER2, MET, RET, and ROS (Saito et al. 2016). These constitute targets for therapeutic intervention with specific tyrosine kinase inhibitors. Other oncogenes, such as KRAS or tumor suppressor genes such as TP53 or STK11, affect mostly NSCLC from smokers. On the other side, the small cell lung cancer (SCLC) type commonly harbors loss-of-function mutations at tumor suppressor genes such as *TP53* and *RB1* and genetic activation, due to gene amplification, of the well-known oncogenes *MYC*, *MYCL*, and *MYCN* (Blanco et al. 2009). Neither of these is therapeutically approachable.

In the last few years, alterations affecting genes that regulate the structure of the chromatin have been described in many types of cancer, including lung cancer. These include genetic inactivation of different components of the SWI/SNF complex, especially of the gene coding for the ATPase of the complex, *SMARCA4* (Medina et al. 2008; Romero and Sanchez-Cespedes 2014). Furthermore, genetic alterations and abnormal expression of genes coding for different histone modifier enzymes have also been found in lung cancer. Importantly, small molecule inhibitors targeting some of these molecules are currently available or being developed for specific molecularly defined subsets of lung cancer patients. In the next paragraphs the epigenetic alterations and genetic alterations in epigenetic controllers that have been found in lung cancer are described.

3.1 Aberrant DNA Methylation

Like main types of cancer, lung cancer also arises as the result of accumulation of genetic alterations along with epigenetic abnormalities. Somatic gene mutations or copy number alterations play a well-known role in oncogenesis but the epigenetic alterations are, in fact, more frequent than somatic mutations (Jones and Baylin 2007). The main abnormalities in DNA methylation that take place in cancer cells are changes in global hypomethylation and hypermethylation at CpG islands in specific gene promoters.

DNA hypomethylation was the initial epigenetic abnormality recognized in human tumors (Feinberg and Vogelstein 1983). DNA hypomethylation refers to the loss of DNA methylation in CpGs within a particular region of the genome. In cancer, when the loss of methylation encompasses gene regions, including transcription control sequences, it can promote the transcriptional activation of genes with an oncogenic role. For example, this has recently been described as the mechanism by which genes that show oncogenic properties, such as cancer testis antigens (CEA), that exhibit a methylated promoter region in normal cells, can become reactivated in cancer cells (De Smet et al. 1999). On the other hand, hypomethylation of highly repeated DNA sequences, which comprise approximately half of the genome, is largely responsible for the global DNA hypomethylation that is observed so frequently in cancers (Feinberg and Vogelstein 1983). This alteration has been shown to affect chromosomal stability and to promote DNA rearrangements and chromosomal alterations in several tumor types (Feinberg and Vogelstein 1983; Ehrlich 2010).

As opposed to DNA hypomethylation, abnormal CpG hypermethylation in cancer cells mostly occurs in CpG islands within promoter regions and it is associated with the repression of the expression of a wide variety of tumor suppressor genes, such as genes involved in growth, adhesion, apoptosis, cell cycle, differentiation, signaling, and transcription (Jones and Baylin 2007). Promoter hypermethylation has been proposed to affect the elongation efficiency and the prevention of spurious initiations of transcription (Zilberman et al. 2007). Tumor suppressor gene inactivation through promoter methylation, often referred to as hypermethylation, is a hallmark of lung cancer and is an early event in the carcinogenic process (Esteller 2007). Some of the best studied genes in the context of promoter methylation in lung cancer include *CDKN2A*, *RASSF1A*, *APC*, *RARβ*, *CDH1*, *CDH13*, *DAPK*, and *MGMT* (Esteller 2007). CDKN2A is perhaps the tumor suppressor which shows inactivation by either promoter hypermethylation, point mutations, or homozygous intragenic deletions in lung cancer, mostly NSCLC, with estimates for the prevalence of all these alterations of around 60% (Sanchez-Cespedes et al. 1999).

3.2 Gene Abnormalities Affecting Chromatin Remodelers: The SWI/SNF Complex

Inactivating mutations at *SMARCB1* (also SNF5) were the first reported in human cancer in a chromatin remodeler, linking chromatin remodeling and cancer development. In human tumors *SMARCB1* mutations affect a large proportion of malignant rhabdoid tumors (MRTs), a pediatric and highly lethal form of cancer that arises primarily in kidney and brain, choroid plexus carcinomas, and rare cases of pediatric brain tumors (Versteege et al. 1998). *SMARCB1* is, therefore, a bona fide tumor suppressor gene, biallelically inactivated, mostly with mutations that predict truncated proteins. The mutations arise either somatically or in the germ line conferring, in the latter case, a cancer predisposition syndrome. Mutations at *SMARCB1* can also affect lung cancer, although at a relative low frequency (Romero and Sanchez-Cespedes 2014). Alongside *SMARCB1*, mutations in SMARCA4 were identified a few years later in different types of cancers (Medina et al. 2008; Romero and Sanchez-Cespedes 2014). *SMARCA4* inactivating mutations affect about one-fourth of the NSCLCs and from 2% to 5% of the SCLCs. These mutations are especially predominant in pulmonary sarcomatoid carcinomas (Rekhtman et al. 2020; Frühwald et al. 2021). Moreover, over the past 5 years, sequencing studies of solid tumors revealed that two tumor types, small cell carcinoma of the ovary, hypercalcemic type (SCCOHT), and *SMARCA4*-deficient thoracic sarcomas, feature genetic loss of *SMARCA4* in nearly 100% of the cases (Tischkowitz et al. 2020). Genetic alterations at other members of the SWI/SNF complex have also been reported in human lung cancer. The *SMARCE1* (encoding the BAF57 protein), *PBRM1* (encoding the BAF180), *SMARCF1* (also called ARID1A, encoding the BAF250 protein), and *ARID2* (encoding BAF200) are among the most representative (Romero and Sanchez-Cespedes 2014) (Table 1). All the alterations affecting these genes are inactivating, thus impairing the function of the SWI/SNF complex.

The tumor suppressor nature of these genes is also strongly supported by animal models and functional observations. For example, homozygous knockout mice for Smarcb1 experience embryonic lethality and, similarly to what happens in humans, heterozygous Smarcb1-mutant mice develop tumors that look similar to human MRTs (Roberts et al. 2000). Likewise, Smarca4 heterozygous mutant mice have an increased risk of developing cancer, although these are prone to developing epithelial tumors at different locations. Complementary to these data, mice that carry heterozygous inactivation of Smarca4 in the lung also develop tumors in response to carcinogens (Bultman et al. 2008). As abovementioned, the SWI/SNF complex is involved in cell differentiation and tissue specification (Romero and Sanchez-Cespedes 2014). Given these functions, it is very likely that these observations indicate that abrogation of the SWI/SNF complex activity during cancer development enables the cancer cell to maintain undifferentiated gene expression programs.

Maintenance of stem-associated programs of gene expression and loss of cell differentiation, acquired by the cancer cell through the inactivation of the SWI/SNF complex, could also be related to the impaired ability of the cell to respond to nuclear receptor signaling. For example, the response to retinoic acid and corticoids, essential compounds controlling embryonic development and tissue specification, is impaired in *SMARCA4*-mutant lung cancer cells (Romero et al. 2012, 2017). Although the involvement of the SWI/SNF complex in controlling cell differentiation is well known, it may not be the only mechanism by which its inactivation contributes to carcinogenesis. In this regard, the SWI/SNF complex is involved in other cell processes such as in early embryonic development, in DNA repair, in cell migration, and in cell cycle (Romero and Sanchez-Cespedes 2014). Supporting this, the SWI/SNF interacts physically with known tumor suppressors and oncoproteins (RB1, BRCA1, MYC), which might be impaired in can-

Table 1 Examples of genetic alterations at epigenetic modifying enzymes in lung cancer

Enzyme	Lung cancer type	References
Histone demethylases		
KDM6A (UTX)	NSCLC	Liu et al. (2012)
Histone methyltransferases		
ESET (SETDB1)	NSCLC	Rodriguez-Paredes et al. (2014)
KMT2A (MLL1)	NSCLC and SCLC	Liu et al. (2012), Peifer et al. (2012)
KMT2B (MLL4)	NSCLC	Govindan et al. (2012)
KMT2C (MLL3)	NSCLC	Govindan et al. (2012)
KMT2D (MLL2)	NSCLC and SCLC	Liu et al. (2012), Pleasance et al. (2010), Augert et al. (2017), Pereira et al. (2017)
KMT2G (SETD1B)	NSCLC	Pereira et al. (2017), Pros et al. (2020)
KMT2H (ASH1L)	NSCLC	Liu et al. (2012)
KMT3A (SETD2)	NSCLC	Cancer Genome Atlas Research Network (2014), Pros et al. (2020)
KMT3F (WHSC1L1)	NSCLC	Govindan et al. (2012)
SETD9	NSCLC	Pereira et al. (2017)
Histone acetyltransferases		
CREBBP	SCLC	Peifer et al. (2012), George et al. (2015)
EP300	SCLC	Peifer et al. (2012)
SWI/SNF-chromatin remodeling complex		
ARID1A (BAF250A)	NSCLC	Cancer Genome Atlas Research Network (2014)
ARID2 (BAF200)	NSCLC	Manceau et al. (2013)
PBRM1 (BAF180)	NSCLC	Pereira et al. (2017)
SMARCA4 (BRG1)	NSCLC and SCLC	Medina et al. (2008)
SMARCB1 (INI1, SNF5)	Squamous cell carcinoma of the pleura	Yoshida et al. (2018)

cer carrying inactivation of the complex. Regarding *MYC*, several observations point toward a functional relationship between this oncogene and the SWI/SNF complex. By one hand, in lung cancer, mutations at *SMARCA4* and at other members of the SWI/SNF do not tend to coexist with oncogenic activation of MYC (Medina et al. 2008). Moreover, the SWI/SNF complex is known to be required for the *MYC* function in activating gene transcription (Romero et al. 2012). All these experimental evidences support that both *MYC* and SWI/SNF exert a similar biological function during tumorigenesis.

3.3 Abnormalities in Histone Modifiers

Epigenetic gene silencing through histone modification is an important mechanism that causes loss of gene expression and mediates, along with genetic mutations, the initiation and progression of human cancer. The polycomb group (PcG) of proteins are involved in the maintenance of embryonic and adult stem cells and repression of key tumor suppressor pathways, which might contribute to their oncogenic function (Ringrose and Paro 2004). In lung cancers, the polycomb component EZH2, a methyltransferase that catalyzes the trimethylation of H3K27, has been found to be upregulated both at the mRNA and protein levels. Activating mutations at this gene have also been reported in some types of cancer, further supporting its oncogenic role (Kim and Roberts 2016). The use of drugs that inhibit the activity of this enzyme has been proposed to be therapeutically beneficial (Sparmann and van Lohuizen 2006). Similarly, gene mutations, either inactivating mutations, activating mutations, or mutations with still unknown effect, have been reported in other lysine methyltransferases such as *KMT2A* (also *MLL1*), *KMT2B* (also *MLL4*), *KMT2C* (also *MLL3*), *KMT2D* (also *MLL2*), and *KMT2G* (also *SETD1B*) in different types of cancer, such as those of the large intestine, endometrium, and lung (Rao and Dou 2015; Wang et al. 2017) (Table 1). Moreover, mutations in *KMT2D* (also MLL2) are found in about 17% of SCLC (Augert et al. 2017). In general, in lung cancer, mutations at these epigenetic modifiers are more common in SCLC as compared to NSCLC. Some of these proteins are extremely large in size. For this reason, caution must be exercised when stating that a certain gene is genetically inactivated/activated in cancer since, in some cases, the presence of mutations can be generated as a consequence of genetic instability associated with tumor development. Conversely, genetic inactivation of some lysine demethylases (KDMs) has also been reported in cancer. *KDM6A* (UTX) was first reported as a highly mutated histone H3K27 demethylase in a survey of different human cancers and cancer cell lines including lung cancer (Wang and Shilatifard 2019).

4 Epigenetic-Based Therapeutic Strategies in Lung Cancer

During the last decades, the therapeutic landscape for lung cancer has evolved significantly and now includes a wide range of molecularly targeted therapies and immune checkpoint inhibitors. However, there remains a subset of patients who do not benefit from these therapies. Moreover, after the initial response to these therapies, many of the patients eventually experience disease progression. Thus, there is a pressing need for new strategies for the treatment of lung cancer. At the same time, the accumulated knowledge about the anomalies that affect DNA methylation, histone modification, and chromatin remodeling in cancer cells opens up new avenues for the development of new therapeutic strategies. Next, we provide an overview of the therapeutic approaches based on epigenetic alterations that have been proposed to date and their current status in the management of patients with lung cancer (see also Table 2).

4.1 DNA Methyltransferase Inhibitors

Broadly speaking, most epigenetic therapies consist of chemical compounds that inhibit the activity of the enzymes that catalyze or remove the posttranslational modifications of histone proteins or the DNA methylation. Alternatively, the epigenetic-based therapeutics can also be designed to prevent the recognition of these enzymes by specific adaptor proteins. As mentioned above, among the first and most prominent type of epigenetic alterations in lung cancer is the promoter hypermethylation of CpG islands that leads to transcriptional silencing of tumor suppressor genes. In this regard, it has been known for a long time that DNA methyltransferase (DNMT) inhibitors can effectively induce DNA demethylation and promote the reactivation of gene expression of the epigenetically silenced genes (Egger et al. 2004). The 5-azacytidine and 5-aza-2′-deoxycytidine, first synthesized by Sorm et al. (1964), were the first drugs that showed to suppress the activity of DNMTs. Both are incorporated into DNA and inhibit DNA methylation because the DNMT, as it prepares to methylate cytosines, will form a covalent intermediate and become irreversibly bound to the 5-azacytidine and 5-aza-2′-deoxycytidine residues. There are several FDA-approved DNMT inhibitor drugs in cancer treatment. Clinical trials using the first-generation inhibitors 5-azacytidine (Vidaza) and 2′-deoxy-5-azacytidine (Decitabine) have shown clinical response in myelodysplastic syndrome and acute myeloid leukemias; however, their activity has been limited in solid tumors. Second-generation DNMT inhibitors, which are largely prodrugs of azacitidine with improved pharmacokinetic and pharmacodynamic properties, have been pursued and some are undergoing investigation in a number of solid tumors (Mohammad et al. 2019).

Table 2 Summary of clinical trials involving epigenetic-related drugs, as a single agent or in combination, in lung cancer

Agent/s	Patient characteristics	Phase	Effects	References
Single agents				
Decitabine (DNA demethylating)	Stages III–IV NSCLC. Refractory to standard therapies	Phase I	Establishment of maximum tolerated doses. No objective responses	Schrump et al. (2006)
Vorinostat (HDAC inhibitor)	Stages IIIB–IV NSCLC. Progression after chemotherapy	Phase II	No objective responses. 57% of the patients experienced SD	Traynor et al. (2009)
Romidepsin (HDAC inhibitor)	SCLC. Progression after chemotherapy	Phase II	No objective responses. 19% of the patients experienced SD	Schrump et al. (2008)
Combinations				
Vorinostat/carboplatin/paclitaxel (HDAC inhibitor/chemotherapy)	Stages IIIB–IV. NSCLC	Phase II	A trend to vorinostat enhancing the efficacy of chemotherapy	Ramalingam et al. (2010)
5-Aza/entinostat (DNA demethylating/HDAC inhibitor)	Progression after chemotherapy. Metastatic NSCLC	Phase I/II	Objective responses in 4% of the patients. Strong antitumor activity in two patients	Juergens et al. (2011)
Vorinostat/radiation (HDAC inhibitor/radiation)	NSCLC with up to 4 brain metastases	Phase I	Trial to determine the maximum tolerated dose. Not conclusive	Choi et al. (2017)
Vorinostat/pembrolizumab (HDAC inhibitor/immunotherapy)	Pretreated advanced NSCLC patients	Phase I/Ib	Well-tolerated and preliminary antitumor activity	Gray et al. (2019)
Entinostat/erlotinib (HDAC inhibitor/tyrosine kinase inhibitor)	Stages IIIB–IV. NSCLC	Phase II	Does not improve the outcome of patients when compared with erlotinib monotherapy	Witta et al. (2012)
Vorinostat/gefitinib (HDAC inhibitor/tyrosine kinase inhibitor)	BIM deletion/EGFR-mutant NSCLC	Phase I	Determination of the safety of vorinostat-gefitinib combination and pharmacodynamic biomarkers of vorinostat activity	Takeuchi et al. (2020)

4.2 Histone Deacetylase Inhibitors

Complementary, and in addition to DNMT inhibitors, inhibitors of histone deacetylases (HDAC) have also contributed to the shaping of epigenetic cancer therapy. Because aberrant HDAC activity is implicated in a variety of cancers, HDAC inhibitors (HDACi) have been developed as potential anticancer therapies. There is a high number of developmental drugs to target the HDAC family of enzymes, which exhibit antiproliferative activities in human lung cancer cells, increasing cell cycle arrest or apoptosis (Mamdani and Jalal 2020). Suberoylanilide hydroxamic acid-SAHA or vorinostat (Zolinza®) was among the first HDACi to be approved by the FDA. Other HDACi include belinostat (Beleodaq®), romidepsin (Istodax®), panobinostat (Farydak®), and entinostat, among others. Despite the plethora of preclinical evidence, the clinical trials with HDACi as single agents in NSCLC have demonstrated only modest efficacy (Reid et al. 2004; Schrump et al. 2008; Traynor et al. 2009). Consequently, and also based on preclinical evidences showing synergistic activity of drug combinations, clinical trials have been performed to harness the full therapeutic potential of HDACi in lung cancer treatment. The combination of an HDACi such as belinostat, vorinostat, or panobinostat with the cytotoxic chemotherapeutics carboplatin, paclitaxel, or etoposide has shown therapeutic advantages; however, the toxicities of these agents, especially myelosuppression and gastrointestinal toxicity, prevent a wider application in clinical practice (Mamdani and Jalal 2020). On the other hand, several studies in lung cancer cell lines support that HDACi may increase the efficacy of ionizing radiation. To build on these observations, several clinical trials are underway (Mamdani and Jalal 2020). HDACi demonstrate synergy with not only conventional treatment modalities such as chemotherapy and radiation, but also molecularly targeted therapies such as immune checkpoint inhibitors (ICIs). The efficacy and wide use of these new therapeutics in lung cancer treatment have prompted a growing interest in the combination of HDACi with ICIs. There are several ongoing trials evaluating the combination of different HDACi (e.g., vorinostat, entinostat, panobinostat) with ICIs. In some cases, the preliminary data is encouraging. The results of these trials, including the long-term outcomes of the patients and the degree of the putative associated toxicities, are awaited (Mamdani and Jalal 2020). Further, the use of specific tyrosine kinase inhibitors (TKIs) against growth factor receptors, such as EGFR, ALK, RET, ROS, and MET, among others, in lung cancer patients with tumors carrying genetic activation at each specific receptor is, nowadays, the standard of care. There have been some clinical trials reporting benefits in the overall survival of the patients after combining TKIs against EGFR with HDACi, in patients that had relapse to TKIs (Mamdani and Jalal 2020; Takeuchi et al. 2020).

4.3 Other Epigenetic Inhibitors

As abovementioned, the acetylation of lysine residues at the N-terminal of histones is associated with the activation of transcription through opening of chromatin architecture. This allows for assembly of transcriptional complexes by recruiting proteins with bromodomain and extra-terminal (BET) domains such as BRD2, BRD3, and BRD4. These proteins are linked to human cancers, such as NUT midline carcinoma which frequently carries genetic activation due to BRD–NUT fusions (Delmore et al. 2011). The finding that BET family proteins play a critical role in the transcriptional activation and have oncogenic potential suggested that BET proteins may be potential therapeutic targets in cancer. One of these is the JQ1 (Filippakopoulos et al. 2010), a BET inhibitor that suppresses cell growth in a variety of cancer cell lines in the context of an activated MYC, through either chromosomal translocation or gene amplification (Mertz et al. 2011). These inhibitors have also shown antiproliferative capabilities when tested in lung cancer cell lines. In NUT midline carcinoma and in hematological malignancies BET inhibitors have showed therapeutic benefits; however, the data from various solid tumor trials do not look as promising (Mohammad et al. 2019). Additional small molecule BET protein inhibitors have been developed and are being tested preclinically and in clinical trials (Mohammad et al. 2019).

Among histone methyltransferases as therapeutic targets, inhibitors of EZH2 have shown the most promising results, both preclinically and in clinical trials. As previously mentioned, EZH2 is a histone methyltransferase responsible for the trimethylation of H3K27me3. It is the catalytic subunit of the polycomb repressive complex 2 (PRC2), responsible for repressing transcription. Activating mutations in EZH2 are found in some types of lymphomas (Kim and Roberts 2016) whereas, in lung cancer, high levels of EZH2 have been reported, especially in SCLC. Preclinical studies have shown that high levels of EZH2 are associated with acquired chemotherapeutic resistance in SCLC (Gardner et al. 2017). These observations prompted the development of EZH2 inhibitors for cancer treatment and the initiation of clinical trials. In clinical trials, the use of the most advanced agent targeting EZH2, tazemetostat, suggests impressive response rates in follicular lymphoma but not in other lymphomas that have EZH2 genetic activation (Mohammad et al. 2019). Tazemetostat has also been tested in solid tumors such as in mesotheliomas, which lack the deubiquitinase complex component BAP1, and in malignant rhabdoid tumors, which lack the SWI/SNF complex component SMARCB1, but limited clinical activity has been observed to date.

5　Conclusions and Future Directions

Genetic abnormalities in multiple components of complexes involved in epigenetic regulation are common in lung cancer and have been shown to be essential for its development. A large proportion of these alterations are inactivating mutations, which makes their use as therapeutic targets difficult. Given the widespread presence of these alterations in all types of lung cancer and in other common solid tumors, there is an urgent need to develop selective strategies aimed at identifying and addressing the vulnerabilities of cancer cells that contain inactivation of these epigenetic regulators. In today's era, with the availability of a wide variety of high-performance technologies, this is an achievable goal.

References

Augert A, Zhang Q, Bates B, Cui M, Wang X, Wildey G, Dowlati A, MacPherson D (2017) Small cell lung cancer exhibits frequent inactivating mutations in the histone methyltransferase KMT2D/MLL2: CALGB 151111 (Alliance). J Thorac Oncol 12(4):704–713

Biegel JA, Busse TM, Weissman BE (2014) SWI/SNF chromatin remodeling complexes and cancer. Am J Med Genet 166:350–366

Blanco R, Iwakawa R, Tang M, Kohno T, Angulo B, Pio R, Montuenga LM, Minna JD, Yokota J, Sanchez-Cespedes M (2009) A gene-alteration profile of human lung cancer cell lines. Hum Mutat 30(8):1199–1206

Bultman SJ, Herschkowitz JI, Godfrey V, Gebuhr TC, Yaniv M, Perou CM et al (2008) Characterization of mammary tumors from Brg1 heterozygous mice. Oncogene 27:460–468

Cancer Genome Atlas Research Network (2014) Comprehensive molecular profiling of lung adenocarcinoma. Nature 511(7511):543–550

Cardoso WV, Lü J (2006) Regulation of early lung morphogenesis: questions, facts and controversies. Development 133(9):1611–1624

Choi CYH, Wakelee HA, Neal JW, Pinder-Schenck MC, Yu HM, Chang SD, Adler JR, Modlin LA, Harsh GR, Soltys SG (2017) Vorinostat and concurrent stereotactic radiosurgery for non-small cell lung cancer brain metastases: a phase 1 dose escalation trial. Int J Radiat Oncol Biol Phys 99(1):16–21

Clapier CR, Cairns BR (2009) The biology of chromatin remodeling complexes. Annu Rev Biochem 78:273–304

De Smet C, Lurquin C, Lethé B, Martelange V, Boon T (1999) DNA methylation is the primary silencing mechanism for a set of germ line- and tumor-specific genes with a CpG-rich promoter. Mol Cell Biol 19(11):7327–7335

Del Rizzo PA, Trievel RC (2014) Molecular basis for substrate recognition by lysine methyltransferases and demethylases. Biochim Biophys Acta 1839:1404–1415

Delmore JE et al (2011) BET bromodomain inhibition as a therapeutic strategy to target c-Myc. Cell 146:904–917

Egger G, Liang G, Aparicio A, Jones PA (2004) Epigenetics in human disease and prospects for epigenetic therapy. Nature 429:457–463

Ehrlich M (2010) DNA hypomethylation in cancer cells. Epigenomics 1:239–259

Esteller M (2007) Epigenetic gene silencing in cancer: the DNA hypermethylome. Hum Mol Genet 16 Spec No 1:R50–R59

Feinberg AP, Vogelstein B (1983) Hypomethylation of ras oncogenes in primary human cancers. Biochem Biophys Res Commun 111(1):47–54

Filippakopoulos P, Qi J, Picaud S, Shen Y, Smith WB, Fedorov O, Morse EM, Keates T, Hickman TT, Felletar I, Philpott M, Munro S, McKeown MR, Wang Y, Christie AL, West N, Cameron MJ, Schwartz B, Heightman TD, La Thangue N, French CA, Wiest O, Kung AL, Knapp S, Bradner JE (2010) Selective inhibition of BET bromodomains. Nature 468(7327):1067–1073

Frühwald MC, Nemes K, Boztug H, Cornips MCA, Evans DG, Farah R, Glentis S, Jorgensen M, Katsibardi K, Hirsch S, Jahnukainen K, Kventsel I, Kerl K, Kratz CP, Pajtler KW, Kordes U, Ridola V, Stutz E, Bourdeaut F (2021) Current recommendations for clinical surveillance and genetic testing in rhabdoid tumor predisposition: a report from the SIOPE Host Genome Working Group. Fam Cancer 20(4):305–316

Gardner EE, Lok BH, Schneeberger VE, Desmeules P, Miles LA, Arnold PK, Ni A, Khodos I, de Stanchina E, Nguyen T, Sage J, Campbell JE, Ribich S, Rekhtman N, Dowlati A, Massion PP, Rudin CM, Poirier JT (2017) Chemosensitive relapse in small cell lung cancer proceeds through an EZH2-SLFN11 axis. Cancer Cell 31(2):286–299

George J, Lim JS, Jang SJ, Cun Y, Ozretić L, Kong G, Leenders F, Lu X, Fernández-Cuesta L, Bosco G, Müller C, Dahmen I, Jahchan NS, Park KS, Yang D, Karnezis AN, Vaka D, Torres A, Wang MS, Korbel JO, Menon R, Chun SM, Kim D, Wilkerson M, Hayes N, Engelmann D, Pützer B, Bos M, Michels S, Vlasic I, Seidel D, Pinther B, Schaub P, Becker C, Altmüller J, Yokota J, Kohno T, Iwakawa R, Tsuta K, Noguchi M, Muley T, Hoffmann H, Schnabel PA, Petersen I,

Chen Y, Soltermann A, Tischler V, Choi CM, Kim YH, Massion PP, Zou Y, Jovanovic D, Kontic M, Wright GM, Russell PA, Solomon B, Koch I, Lindner M, Muscarella LA, la Torre A, Field JK, Jakopovic M, Knezevic J, Castaños-Vélez E, Roz L, Pastorino U, Brustugun OT, Lund-Iversen M, Thunnissen E, Köhler J, Schuler M, Botling J, Sandelin M, Sanchez-Cespedes M, Salvesen HB, Achter V, Lang U, Bogus M, Schneider PM, Zander T, Ansén S, Hallek M, Wolf J, Vingron M, Yatabe Y, Travis WD, Nürnberg P, Reinhardt C, Perner S, Heukamp L, Büttner R, Haas SA, Brambilla E, Peifer M, Sage J, Thomas RK (2015) Comprehensive genomic profiles of small cell lung cancer. Nature 524(7563):47–53

Gong F, Chiu LY, Miller KM (2016) Acetylation reader proteins: linking acetylation signaling to genome maintenance and cancer. PLoS Genet 12(9):e1006272

Govindan R, Ding L, Griffith M, Subramanian J, Dees ND, Kanchi KL, Maher CA, Fulton B, Fulton L, Wallis J, Chen K, Walker J, McDonald S, Bose R, Ornitz D, Xiong D, You M, Dooling DJ, Watson M, Mardis ER, Wilson RK (2012) Genomic landscape of non-small cell lung cancer in smokers and never-smokers. Cell 150(6):1121–1134

Gray JE, Saltos A, Tanvetyanon T, Haura EB, Creelan B, Antonia SJ, Shafique M, Zheng H, Dai W, Saller JJ, Chen Z, Tchekmedyian N, Goas K, Thapa R, Boyle TA, Chen DT, Beg AA (2019) Phase I/Ib study of pembrolizumab plus vorinostat in advanced/metastatic non-small cell lung cancer. Clin Cancer Res 25(22):6623–6632

Haberland M, Montgomery RL, Olson EN (2009) The many roles of histone deacetylases in development and physiology: implications for disease and therapy. Nat Rev Genet 10(1):32–42

Hargreaves DC, Crabtree GR (2011) ATP-dependent chromatin remodeling: genetics, genomics and mechanisms. Cell Res 21(3):396–420

Jones PA, Baylin SB (2007) The epigenomics of cancer. Cell 128(4):683–692

Jones PA, Taylor SM (1980) Cellular differentiation, cytidine analogs and DNA methylation. Cell 20:85–93

Juergens RA, Wrangle J, Vendetti FP, Murphy SC, Zhao M, Coleman B, Sebree R, Rodgers K, Hooker CM, Franco N, Lee B, Tsai S, Delgado IE, Rudek MA, Belinsky SA, Herman JG, Baylin SB, Brock MV, Rudin CM (2011) Combination epigenetic therapy has efficacy in patients with refractory advanced non-small cell lung cancer. Cancer Discov 1(7):598–607

Khorasanizadeh S (2004) The nucleosome: from genomic organization to genomic regulation. Cell 116:259–272

Kim KH, Roberts CW (2016) Targeting EZH2 in cancer. Nat Med 22(2):128–134

Kim KH et al (2015) SWI/SNF-mutant cancers depend on catalytic and non-catalytic activity of EZH2. Nat Med 21:1491–1496

Klose RJ, Kallin EM, Zhang Y (2006) JmjC-domain containing proteins and histone demethylation. Nat Rev Genet 7(9):715–727

Kouzarides T (2007) Chromatin modifications and their function. Cell 128(4):693–705

Liu J, Lee W, Jiang Z, Chen Z, Jhunjhunwala S, Haverty PM, Gnad F, Guan Y, Gilbert HN, Stinson J, Klijn C, Guillory J, Bhatt D, Vartanian S, Walter K, Chan J, Holcomb T, Dijkgraaf P, Johnson S, Koeman J, Minna JD, Gazdar AF, Stern HM, Hoeflich KP, Wu TD, Settleman J, de Sauvage FJ, Gentleman RC, Neve RM, Stokoe D, Modrusan Z, Seshagiri S, Shames DS, Zhang Z (2012) Genome and transcriptome sequencing of lung cancers reveal diverse mutational and splicing events. Genome Res 22(12):2315–2327

Mamdani H, Jalal SI (2020) Histone deacetylase inhibition in non-small cell lung cancer: hype or hope? Front Cell Dev Biol 8:582370

Manceau G, Letouzé E, Guichard C, Didelot A, Cazes A, Corté H, Fabre E, Pallier K, Imbeaud S, Le Pimpec-Barthes F, Zucman-Rossi J, Laurent-Puig P, Blons H (2013) Recurrent inactivating mutations of ARID2 in non-small cell lung carcinoma. Int J Cancer 132(9):2217–2221

Medina PP, Romero OA, Kohno T, Montuenga LM, Pio R, Yokota J, Sanchez-Cespedes M (2008) Frequent SMARCA4/SMARCA4-inactivating mutations in human lung cancer cell lines. Hum Mutat 29(5):617–622

Mertz JA, Conery AR, Bryant BM, Sandy P, Balasubramanian S, Mele DA, Bergeron L, Sims RJ III (2011) Targeting MYC dependence in cancer by inhibiting BET bromodomains. Proc Natl Acad Sci U S A 108(40):16669–16674

Mohammad HP, Barbash O, Creasy CL (2019) Targeting epigenetic modifications in cancer therapy: erasing the roadmap to cancer. Nat Med 25(3):403–418

Peifer M, Fernandez-Cuesta L, Sos ML et al (2012) Integrative genome analyses identify key somatic driver mutations of small-cell lung cancer. Nat Genet 44(10):1104–1110

Pereira C, Gimenez-Xavier P, Pros E, Pajares MJ, Moro M, Gomez A, Navarro A, Condom E, Moran S, Gomez-Lopez G, Graña O, Rubio-Camarillo M, Martinez-Martí A, Yokota J, Carretero J, Galbis JM, Nadal E, Pisano D, Sozzi G, Felip E, Montuenga LM, Roz L, Villanueva A, Sanchez-Cespedes M (2017) Genomic profiling of patient-derived xenografts for lung cancer identifies B2M inactivation impairing immunorecognition. Clin Cancer Res 23(12):3203–3213

Pleasance ED, Stephens PJ, O'Meara S, McBride DJ, Meynert A, Jones D, Lin ML, Beare D, Lau KW, Greenman C, Varela I, Nik-Zainal S, Davies HR, Ordoñez GR, Mudie LJ, Latimer C, Edkins S, Stebbings L, Chen L, Jia M, Leroy C, Marshall J, Menzies A, Butler A, Teague JW, Mangion J, Sun YA, McLaughlin SF, Peckham HE, Tsung EF, Costa GL, Lee CC, Minna JD, Gazdar A, Birney E, Rhodes MD, McKernan KJ, Stratton MR, Futreal PA, Campbell PJ (2010) A small-cell lung cancer genome with complex signatures of tobacco exposure. Nature 463(7278):184–190

Pros E, Saigi M, Alameda D, Gomez-Mariano G, Martinez-Delgado B, Alburquerque-Bejar JJ, Carretero J, Tonda R, Esteve-Codina A, Catala I, Palmero R, Jove M, Lazaro C, Patiño-Garcia A, Gil-Bazo I, Verdura S, Teulé A, Torres-Lanzas J, Sidransky D, Reguart N, Pio R, Juan-Vidal O, Nadal E, Felip E, Montuenga LM, Sanchez-Cespedes M (2020) Genome-wide profiling of non-smoking-related lung cancer cells reveals common RB1 rearrangements associated with histopathologic transformation in EGFR-mutant tumors. Ann Oncol 31(2):274–282

Ramalingam SS, Maitland ML, Frankel P, Argiris AE, Koczywas M, Gitlitz B, Thomas S, Espinoza-Delgado I, Vokes EE, Gandara DR, Belani CP (2010) Carboplatin and paclitaxel in combination with either vorinostat or placebo for first-line therapy of advanced non-small-cell lung cancer. J Clin Oncol 28(1):56–62

Rao RC, Dou Y (2015) Hijacked in cancer: the KMT2 (MLL) family of methyltransferases. Nat Rev Cancer 15:334–346

Reid T, Valone F, Lipera W, Irwin D, Paroly W, Natale R et al (2004) Phase II trial of the histone deacetylase inhibitor pivaloyloxymethyl butyrate (Pivanex, AN-9) in advanced non-small cell lung cancer. Lung Cancer 45:381–386

Rekhtman N, Montecalvo J, Chang JC, Alex D, Ptashkin RN, Ai N, Sauter JL, Kezlarian B, Jungbluth A, Desmeules P, Beras A, Bishop JA, Plodkowski AJ, Gounder MM, Schoenfeld AJ, Namakydoust A, Li BT, Rudin CM, Riely GJ, Jones DR, Ladanyi M, Travis WD (2020) SMARCA4-deficient thoracic sarcomatoid tumors represent primarily smoking-related undifferentiated carcinomas rather than primary thoracic sarcomas. J Thorac Oncol 15(2):231–247

Riggs AD (1975) X inactivation, differentiation, and DNA methylation. Cytogenet Cell Genet 14:9–25

Ringrose L, Paro R (2004) Epigenetic regulation of cellular memory by the Polycomb and Trithorax group proteins. Annu Rev Genet 38:413–443

Roberts CW, Galusha SA, McMenamin ME, Fletcher CD, Orkin SH (2000) Haploinsufficiency of Snf5 (integrase interactor 1) predisposes to malignant rhabdoid tumors in mice. Proc Natl Acad Sci U S A 97:13796–13800

Rodriguez-Paredes M, Martinez de Paz A, Simó-Riudalbas L, Sayols S, Moutinho C, Moran S, Villanueva A, Vázquez-Cedeira M, Lazo PA, Carneiro F, Moura CS, Vieira J, Teixeira MR, Esteller M (2014) Gene amplification of the histone methyltransferase SETDB1 contributes to human lung tumorigenesis. Oncogene 33(21):2807–2813

Romero OA, Sanchez-Cespedes M (2014) The SWI/SNF genetic blockade: effects in cell differentiation, cancer and developmental diseases. Oncogene 33(21):2681–2689

Romero OA et al (2012) The tumour suppressor and chromatin-remodelling factor SMARCA4 antagonizes Myc activity and promotes cell differentiation in human cancer. EMBO Mol Med 4:603–616

Romero OA, Verdura S, Torres-Diz M, Gomez A, Moran S, Condom E, Esteller M, Villanueva A, Sanchez-Cespedes M (2017) Sensitization of retinoids and corticoids to epigenetic drugs in MYC-activated lung cancers by antitumor reprogramming. Oncogene 36(9):1287–1296

Saito M, Shiraishi K, Kunitoh H, Takenoshita S, Yokota J, Kohno T (2016) Gene aberrations for precision medicine against lung adenocarcinoma. Cancer Sci 107(6):713–720

Sanchez-Cespedes M, Reed AL, Buta M, Wu L, Westra WH, Herman JG, Yang SC, Jen J, Sidransky D (1999) Inactivation of the INK4A/ARF locus frequently coexists with TP53 mutations in non-small cell lung cancer. Oncogene 18(43):5843–5849

Schrump DS, Fischette MR, Nguyen DM, Zhao M, Li X, Kunst TF, Hancox A, Hong JA, Chen GA, Pishchik V, Figg WD, Murgo AJ, Steinberg SM (2006) Phase I study of decitabine-mediated gene expression in patients with cancers involving the lungs, esophagus, or pleura. Clin Cancer Res 12(19):5777–5785

Schrump DS, Fischette MR, Nguyen DM, Zhao M, Li X, Kunst TF et al (2008) Clinical and molecular responses in lung cancer patients receiving Romidepsin. Clin Cancer Res 14:188–198

Sondka Z, Bamford S, Cole CG, Ward SA, Dunham I, Forbes SA (2018) The COSMIC Cancer Gene Census: describing genetic dysfunction across all human cancers. Nat Rev Cancer 18(11):696–705

Sorm F, Pískala A, Cihák A, Veselý J (1964) 5-Azacytidine, a new, highly effective cancerostatic. Experientia 20(4):202–203

Sparmann A, van Lohuizen M (2006) Polycomb silencers control cell fate, development and cancer. Nat Rev Cancer 6:846–856

Takeuchi S, Hase T, Shimizu S, Ando M, Hata A, Murakami H et al (2020) Phase I study of vorinostat with gefitinib in BIM deletion polymorphism/epidermal growth factor receptor mutation double-positive lung cancer. Cancer Sci 111:561–570

Tischkowitz M, Huang S, Banerjee S, Hague J, Hendricks WPD, Huntsman DG, Lang JD, Orlando KA, Oza AM, Pautier P, Ray-Coquard I, Trent JM, Witcher M, Witkowski L, McCluggage WG, Levine DA, Foulkes WD, Weissman BE (2020) Small-cell carcinoma of the ovary, hypercalcemic type-genetics, new treatment targets, and current management guidelines. Clin Cancer Res 26(15):3908–3917

Traynor AM, Dubey S, Eickhoff JC, Kolesar JM, Schell K, Huie MS et al (2009) Vorinostat (NSC# 701852) in patients with relapsed non-small cell lung cancer: a Wisconsin Oncology Network phase II study. J Thorac Oncol 4:522–526

Versteege I, Sévenet N, Lange J, Rousseau-Merck MF, Ambros P, Handgretinger R et al (1998) Truncating mutations of hSNF5/INI1 in aggressive paediatric cancer. Nature 394:203–206

Wang L, Shilatifard A (2019) UTX mutations in human cancer. Cancer Cell 35(2):168–176

Wang SP et al (2017) A UTX-MLL4-p300 transcriptional regulatory network coordinately shapes active enhancer landscapes for eliciting transcription. Mol Cell 67:308–321.e6

Witta SE, Jotte RM, Konduri K, Neubauer MA, Spira AI, Ruxer RL, Varella-Garcia M, Bunn PA Jr, Hirsch FR (2012) Randomized phase II trial of erlotinib with and without entinostat in patients with advanced non-small-cell lung cancer who progressed on prior chemotherapy. J Clin Oncol 30(18):2248–2255

Yoshida K, Fujiwara Y, Goto Y, Kohno T, Yoshida A, Tsuta K, Ohe Y (2018) The first case of SMARCB1 (INI1) - deficient squamous cell carcinoma of the pleura: a case report. BMC Cancer 18(1):398

Zhang T, Cooper S, Brockdorff N (2015) The interplay of histone modifications - writers that read. EMBO Rep 16(11):1467–1481

Zilberman D, Gehring M, Tran RK, Ballinger T, Henikoff S (2007) Genome-wide analysis of Arabidopsis thaliana DNA methylation uncovers an interdependence between methylation and transcription. Nat Genet 39(1):61–69

Part II

Clinical Investigations

Interventional Pulmonology

Branislav Perin and Bojan Zarić

Contents

1 Introduction 35
2 **Diagnostic Techniques** 36
2.1 Autofluorescence Videobronchoscopy 36
2.2 Narrow-Band Imaging 37
2.3 Endobronchial Ultrasound 37
2.4 Recent Diagnostic Techniques in Interventional Pulmonology 38
3 **Therapeutic Techniques** 40
3.1 Techniques with Immediate Effect 40
3.2 Techniques with Delayed Effect 42
References 42

Abstract

Interventional pulmonology is an important aspect of thoracic oncology with established place and role in both diagnostic and treatment domain of lung cancer invading central airways (trachea and principal bronchi). While success ratio of interventional techniques is reported to vary in different studies, they remain a vital part of armamentarium with excellent potential and perspective. Increase in number and variety of these techniques led to the development of internationally accepted guidelines for their use. Of diagnostic techniques, white light bronchoscopy, autofluorescence videobronchoscopy, narrow-band imaging, and endobronchial ultrasound have mostly been used in the past. Newer diagnostic techniques, such as electromagnetic navigation, bronchoscopic navigation using cone bean computed tomography, confocal fluorescence microscopy (endoscopy), optical coherence tomography, and ultrathin bronchoscopy, had also shown promise in this field. Of therapeutic techniques with immediate effect, laser photoresection, electrocautery, and argon plasma coagulation remain standard approaches in this domain, while therapeutic techniques with delayed effect, such as balloon dilatation (bronchoplasty), endobronchial brachytherapy cryotherapy, and photodynamic therapy, have also been used with success and, if properly managed, very low toxicity. They are being presented in detail in other chapters.

B. Perin (✉) · B. Zarić
Institute for Pulmonary Diseases of Vojvodina, Clinic for Pulmonary Oncology, Faculty of Medicine, University of Novi Sad, Novi Sad, Serbia
e-mail: branislavperin@gmail.com

1 Introduction

Several past decades witnessed interventional pulmonology techniques firmly establishing its place in both diagnostic and treatment domain of lung cancer invading central airways (trachea and principal bronchi). While success ratio of interventional techniques is reported to vary in different studies, they remain a vital part of armamentarium with excellent potential and perspective. Increase in number and variety of these techniques led to the development of internationally accepted guidelines for their use. Accumulated knowledge showed that the choice of specific interventional technique in the treatment of lung cancer patients with central airway obstruction (CAO) depended on several factors, including patient's general condition and comorbidities, type and characteristics of airway stenosis, as well as availability of techniques and trained personnel. To extend this, recent technological advances, namely robotic bronchoscopy, were seen as the final evolutionary step in the development of interventional pulmonology. With a mounting evidence of its efficacy and safety, it might happen that in the near future state-of-the-art bronchoscopy suites will be majorly equipped with robotic-guided instruments (Kent et al. 2020; Ho et al. 2021).

Interventional techniques can broadly be divided into diagnostic and therapeutic. The former includes, among others, white light bronchoscopy (WLB), autofluorescence bronchoscopy (AFB), narrow-band imaging (NBI) bronchoscopy, endobronchial ultrasound (EBUS), and electromagnetic navigation bronchoscopy, while the latter are divided into those with imminent effect on CAO and those with delayed effect. Therapeutic techniques can be either curative or palliative. In cases of carcinoma in situ or early invasive lung cancer, a variety of techniques, such as photodynamic therapy (PDT), cryotherapy, electrocautery (EC), argon plasma coagulation (APC), and brachytherapy, can have curative potential. In cases of early-stage lung cancer, bronchoscopic treatment requires precise and accurate staging of the disease, using all available state-of-the-art techniques such as positron emission tomography, endobronchial ultrasound, and autofluorescence or narrow-band imaging. Their joint goal is to make a distinction between noninvasive and invasive bronchial carcinoma and to determine nodal status with reliable accuracy.

Palliative techniques are primarily aimed at relief of symptoms of malignant CAO. Those with imminent effect are laser resection, electrocautery, argon plasma coagulation, and placement of tracheobronchial stents. After such an initial treatment and reopening of the airway, subsequent therapeutic interventions can also take place. Techniques with delayed effect can improve the control of symptoms and quality of life (QoL), and, when combined with chemoradiation, can have significant impact on disease-free and overall survival.

Since every symptomatic malignant CAO is considered potentially fatal, prompt and thorough bronchoscopic evaluation should lead to establishing firm indication for a technique that offers the fastest airway desobstruction. A multidisciplinary team consisting of interventional pulmonologist, anesthesiologist, thoracic surgeon, radiologist, and oncologist should timely act to indicate and execute the appropriate technique. As a prerequisite, any institution deemed to be at the level capable to offer such approach need to have not only modern facility but also a variety of interventional techniques and, most importantly, well-trained personnel available at any time (Colt and Murgu 2010; Sutedja 2003; Wahidi et al. 2007).

2 Diagnostic Techniques

2.1 Autofluorescence Videobronchoscopy

One of many systems of autofluorescence bronchoscopy designed for thorough examination of bronchial mucosa is called autofluorescence imaging videobronchoscopy (AFI). By integrating autofluorescence and videobronchoscopy clear images of normal and pathologically altered bronchial mucosa are provided. Major indications for AFI include detection of precancerous lesions and evaluation of early-stage lung cancer. In addition to it, evaluation of tumor extension or follow-up after surgical resection are slowly but definitely finding its place in daily clinical practice in busy and modern departments worldwide. However, clear distinction between healthy and pathologically altered mucosa and rapidly gaining knowledge and skill of the user-friendly technique make this technology also favored among young and inexperienced bronchoscopists. On the other side, one must clearly identify low specificity in detection of premalignant lesions and early-stage lung cancer as the major disadvantage of AFI. However, backscattered light analysis, ultraviolet spectra, fluorescence-reflectance, or dual digital systems is increasingly and successfully used to improve the detection rate. Additionally, quantitative image analysis improves objectivity and minimizes observer errors. Majority of clinicians and researchers, however, agree that one of the most appropriate solutions is integration of AFI and narrow-band imaging (NBI) into one videobronchoscope. Recent years saw successful incorporation of autofluorescence and white light videobronchoscopy into one scope, making it, therefore, easy to switch between the two modes of examination: normal mucosa appears green AFI, while pathologically altered one appears as magenta or red-brownish (Yarmus and Feller-Kopman 2010; Yasufuku 2010).

Two meta-analyses summarized previous experiences. Sun et al. (2011) evaluated the use of AFI in both bronchial preneoplasia and lung cancer. There was a lower pool-relative specificity of AFI plus WLB which was 0.65. However, the pool-relative sensitivity of combined AFI and WLB was 2.04 for preneoplasia and 1.15 for invasive lung cancer, confirming significantly better sensitivity of AFI over WLB. Chen et al. (2011) revealed pooled sensitivity and specificity of AFI to be 90% and 56%, respectively, while corresponding values for WLB were 66% and 69%. However, the difference in specificity was not significant (66% vs. 69%). While both meta-analyses showed superiority of AFI over WLB, its low specificity remains a major disadvantage toward its widespread use in daily clinical practice.

2.2 Narrow-Band Imaging

Narrow-band imaging (NBI) is an endoscopic technique designed for the detection of pathologically altered submucosal and mucosal microvascular patterns (Chauhan et al. 2021). The combination of magnification videobronchoscopy and NBI proved to be of a great potential in the detection of both precancerous and cancerous lesions. Recent meta-analyses (Iftikhar and Musani 2015; Zhu et al. 2017) confirmed supremacy of NBI over white light videobronchoscopy in the detection of premalignant and malignant lesions, although in some of them (Zhu et al. 2017) the specificities of the two modalities did not differ significantly, while others showed that combining AFI and NBI does not significantly improve test performance characteristics (Iftikhar and Musani 2015). Pathological patterns of capillaries in bronchial mucosa are known as Shibuya's descriptors (dotted, tortuous, and abrupt ending blood vessels). More randomized trials are necessary to firmly confirm the place of NBI in the diagnostic algorithm, and more trials are needed to evaluate the relation of NBI to AFI, and WLB. Considering the fact that NBI examination of the tracheobronchial tree is easy, reproducible, and clear to interpret, NBI videobronchoscopy increasingly plays an important role in the lung cancer detection and staging as it provides a better contrast on the mucosal surface, reduces examination time, and eliminates futile biopsies.

NBI enables better visualization of the bronchial mucosa and differentiation between malignant and nonmalignant tissue and proves to be more efficient in the detection of precancerous lesions, especially angiogenic squamous dysplasia (ASD) than the WLB alone. Additionally, knowledge and skill generation is fast and that fact makes the NBI useful even when used by an inexperienced bronchoscopist. It is believed that the combination of NBI with AFI will give even better results in lung cancer detection.

2.3 Endobronchial Ultrasound

Two major types of endobronchial ultrasound (EBUS) are linear and radial (Liam et al. 2021). The former one is commonly used for mediastinal staging of lung cancer, during real-time TBNA (transbronchial needle aspiration). It enables the bronchoscopist to visualize lymph nodes even <1 cm in maximal diameter, allowing, therefore, accurate nodal staging. While this technique is known to be completely complementary with mediastinoscopy, however, real-time EBUS-guided TBNA is helpful in mediastinal restaging deemed necessary after neoadjuvant chemoradiation. Insertion of the probe through the working channel of the diagnostic bronchoscope is enabled by radial endobronchial probe. It has demonstrated additional advantage due to enabling excellent insight into the pulmonary parenchyma and is being increasingly used for the diagnosis of peripheral lung cancers, as well as in cases when assessment of tumor penetration into the bronchial wall is needed. Owing to the fact that up to nine layers of bronchial wall can be visualized by radial EBUS, this technique is irreplaceable for the assessment of bronchial wall in early-stage lung cancer.

Comparative images of WLB, AFI, NBI, and radial EBUS on the same lesion are presented in Figs. 1, 2, 3, and 4.

2.4 Recent Diagnostic Techniques in Interventional Pulmonology

Several newly developed techniques entered the arena of diagnostic interventional pulmonology in the last years. Bronchial navigation method

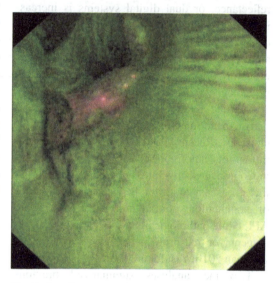

Fig. 2 Autofluorescence imaging (AFI) videobronchoscopy image of the tumor in the distal part of intermediary bronchus

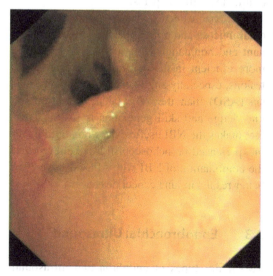

Fig. 1 White light videobronchoscopy image of the tumor in the distal part of intermediary bronchus

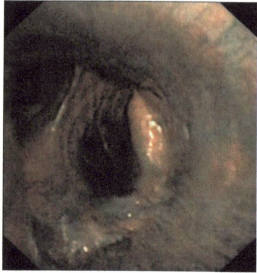

Fig. 3 Narrow-band imaging videobronchoscopy image of the tumor in the distal part of intermediary bronchus

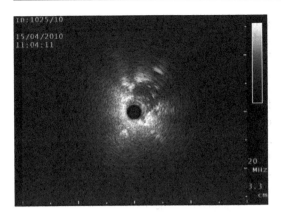

Fig. 4 Linear endobronchial ultrasound (EBUS) image of the tumor in the distal part of intermediary bronchus

using a magnetic field (electromagnetic navigation: EMN) to link the navigation system and the actual bronchoscope in real time has appeared. This new technique, electromagnetic navigational bronchoscopy (ENB) promises accurate navigation to peripheral pulmonary target lesion (Usuda 2018). However, Ost et al. (2016) used the AQuIRE (ACCP Quality Improvement Registry, Evaluation, and Education) registry to conduct a multicenter study of consecutive patients who underwent transbronchial biopsy (TBBx) for the evaluation of peripheral lesions. Unadjusted for other factors, the diagnostic yield was 63.7% when no radial endobronchial ultrasound (r-EBUS) and no EMN were used, 57.0% with r-EBUS alone, 38.5% with EMN alone, and 47.1% with EMN combined with r-EBUS. In multivariate analysis, peripheral transbronchial needle aspiration (TBNA), larger lesion size, nonupper lobe location, and tobacco use were associated with increased diagnostic yield, whereas EMN was associated with lower diagnostic yield. In order to improve this approach, a novel EMN system utilizing novel tip-tracked instruments for endobronchial [electromagnetic navigation bronchoscopy (ENB)] as well as transthoracic lung biopsy [electromagnetic-guided transthoracic needle aspiration (EMTTNA)] was developed. The system provides real-time feedback as well as the ability to biopsy lesions outside of the airway. These advances have the potential to improve diagnostic yield over previous EMN systems. Belanger et al. (2019) used a novel EMN platform for biopsy and/or fiducial marker (FM) placement. The combined diagnostic yield was 78%. EMTTNA provided a diagnosis for five patients in whom the ENB biopsy results were negative. Diagnostic yield by nodules <20, 20 to 30, and >30 mm in size was 30/45 (67%), 27/30 (90%), and 16/18 (89%), respectively. Sixty-five patients underwent FM placement with a total of 133 FM placed. The authors concluded that this novel tip-tracked EMN system incorporating both ENB and EMTTNA can guide biopsy and FM placement with a high degree of success and with a low complication rate. They have, however, warned that multicentered prospective trials were required to develop algorithmic approaches to combine ENB and EMTTNA into a single procedure. Another form of bronchoscopic navigation utilized cone beam computed tomography (CBCT), as this approach was basically three-dimensional (3D) and offered additional advantage. Verhoeven et al. (2021) assessed whether CBCT imaging can improve navigation and diagnosis of peripheral lesions by two clinical workflows with a cross-over design: (1) a primary CBCT and radial endobronchial ultrasound mini probe imaging-based approach and (2) a primary electromagnetic navigation (EMN) and radial endobronchial ultrasound mini probe imaging-based approach. The primary CBCT approach and primary EMN approach had 76.3% and 52.2% navigation success, respectively. Addition of EMN to the CBCT approach increased navigation success to 89.9%. Addition of CBCT imaging to the EMN approach significantly increased navigation success to 87.5% per lesion. The overall diagnostic accuracy per patient was significantly lower than the navigation success, being 72.4%. The authors concluded that CBCT imaging is a valuable addition to navigation bronchoscopy. However, although overall navigation success was high, the diagnostic accuracy remains to be improved, indicating that future research should focus on improving the tissue acquisition methodology. Confocal fluorescence microscopy (endoscopy) (Rakotomamonjy et al. 2014; Chowdhury et al. 2015), optical coherence tomography (Michel et al. 2010; Shostak et al.

2018; Goorsenberg et al. 2020), and ultrathin bronchoscopy (Matsuno et al. 2011; Liu et al. 2019; Kinoshita et al. 2019) had also shown promise in this field.

3 Therapeutic Techniques

3.1 Techniques with Immediate Effect

3.1.1 Nd:YAG and Ho:YAG Laser Photoresection

One of the most explored principles in interventional pulmonology is known as LASER (light amplification of stimulated emission of radiation) (Unger 1985; Duhamel and Harrell II 2001; Colt et al. 2013). It delivers energy in the form of heat to the target tissues, leading to its vaporization, coagulation, and necrosis. Several types of lasers are used in practice (Nd:YAG, CO_2, argon, dye, diode, YAP:Nd), but only Nd:YAG (neodymium:yttrium aluminum garnet) is widely used in pulmonology. The effects of laser beam on target tissue depend on several factors, including power density, absorption, and scattering ratio of soft tissues as well as delivery system. It must clearly be stressed that one of the most important factors determining its biological effect is the wavelength of the laser light, because it determines the absorption though the effect of delivered heat energy on the tissue. The wavelength of Nd:YAG laser is 1064 nm; it is in invisible range of infrared region and needs a pilot light (usually red) for its guidance.

Due to intraluminal growth of malignant or benign tissue, malignant or nonmalignant CAO represents the major indication for laser photoresection. Ideal for laser resections are the lesions situated centrally (trachea and main bronchi), being short in length (≤ 4 cm), having visible distal bronchial lumen and functional lung distal to the obstruction.

Nd:YAG laser resection is usually performed using either flexible bronchoscopy alone or in the combination of rigid and flexible bronchoscopy under general anesthesia. As a precaution, oxygen concentration should be kept under 40% in order to prevent airway fire. The initial power setting is usually about 40 W, with pulse duration of 0.5–1 s. The tip of the probe is aimed 1 cm proximally and parallel to the lesion. One can manipulate tissue effect of Nd:YAG laser by adjusting either the power setting or by moving the tip of the probe further or closer to the target lesion. However, cautious approach is always suggested as the depth of penetration of laser beam is not immediately visible, requesting, therefore, frequent reanalysis of the lesion.

Holmium:YAG (Ho:YAG) laser resection accomplishes the same effects with more precision than Nd:YAG (Squiers et al. 2014; Mudambi et al. 2017; Shepherd and Radchenko 2019). Ho:YAG provides better accuracy than Nd:YAG in spite of the fact that physical characteristics of holmium laser enable the bronchoscopist to perform more aggressive intervention but with the confidence that tissue damage is visible in real time. Ho:YAG can be also preformed via flexible or rigid bronchoscopy. Accumulated evidence shows that the Ho:YAG, having all the advantages of Nd:YAG including excellent coagulative properties, however, is being superior due to better accuracy and precision.

Absolute contraindication for any laser resection includes existence of extraluminal disease, while relative contraindications include severe heart (recent myocardial infarction, ventricular arrhythmias, conduction abnormalities, hypotension, or decompensated heart failure) and severe obstructive lung disease, but extensive tumor involvement, unresolved coagulopathies, and sepsis as well.

The complications of laser resection are generally rare and include intraoperative and postoperative hypoxemia, hemorrhage, airway perforation, airway fire (burns), pneumothorax, and fistulae formation. Treatment is almost always successful and the patient should be observed in the recovery room for a reasonable period of time to timely observe possible bronchospasm or laryngospasm. With adequate precaution measures taken, complication rate is usually less than 5%.

3.1.2 Electrocautery

Electrocautery (EC) represents a contact form of electrosurgery (Lee et al. 2002; Chaddha et al. 2019; Mahajan et al. 2020). As a result of voltage difference between the tip of the probe and the tissue electrons flow between these two surfaces. Electrons are then transmitted through a tiny gap of air between these two surfaces. Created electrical current affects the target tissue in the form of heat, causing its coagulation, carbonization, or vaporization. The current leaves the body through a grounding plate, usually applied on patient's arm. The power setting, tissue resistance, time of application, and the applied mode of EC govern the effects of EC. While low voltage, low power, and high amperage cause coagulation, high voltage, high power, and low amperage cause carbonization. EC has two operating modes, "cut" mode and "blended" mode; the latter one is preferred due to its ability to combine cutting and coagulation. Some authors propose distinguishing EC coagulation in three types: soft—to avoid carbonization, hard—for deeper tissue penetration, and spray—for surface hemostasis. EC is indicated in the same cases as laser resection is, and EC is more often used as a cheaper alternative. CAO due to benign or malignant disease is the most common indication for its use. Absolute contraindications are extraluminal disease and a pacemaker due to their susceptibility to electrical interference.

EC can be carried out either via rigid or flexible bronchoscopy, and with the combination of these two techniques as well. While rigid bronchoscopy EC requires general anesthesia, analgosedation modality can be used in flexible bronchoscopy EC. A specially isolated ceramic-tip flexible bronchoscope is used for EC, and the patient is electrically grounded with a pad or a plate. Necessary precaution measures mandate limiting inhaled oxygen fraction and avoiding flammable materials (plastic endotracheal tube or tracheobronchial stents). Several types of EC probes designed to achieve wanted effects on target tissue exist. While blunt probe is usually used for coagulation and carbonization, the knife causes coagulation and blend, and snare is designed for blend. The amount of histologic tissue damage in the targeted tissue significantly correlates with the extent of coagulation of EC.

Among possible complications of EC airway perforation, electrical shocks and hemorrhage are of potential concern, although only mild hemorrhage has been reported in published studies. To avoid or minimize these, established precaution measures include limited power setting (40 W), low inspired oxygen concentration ($\leq$40%), short burst time ($\leq$2 s), and the use of isolated bronchoscope. Being a cheap and safe technique for urgent airway debulking, EC represents a good alternative to laser resection.

3.1.3 Argon Plasma Coagulation

Argon plasma coagulation (APC) represents a form of noncontact electrosurgery that uses high voltage spark (5000–6000 V) to ionize Argon gas, which is then transformed into plasma in order to create electrical current (Bolliger et al. 2006; Miller et al. 2013; Mahajan et al. 2020). Monopolar current of ionized plasma affects target tissue in the form of heat, leading to coagulation and necrosis in target tissue. Since plasma seeks the way of least resistance, it targets wide surface of tissue directly. Closed current circuit is necessary for Argon plasma to flow; therefore, the tip of the probe must be situated less than 1 cm from the tissue. If the distance between the tip of the probe and the tissue is >1 cm, the circuit will be open with the consequential effect being lost. The current leaves the body through a grounding plate usually situated under patient's lower back.

The effect of APC depends on power setting, application time, and conductivity of the tissue. Coagulated tissues have higher resistance, and higher resistance lowers conductivity and limits penetration. At power setting of 40–120 W and burst time less than 2 s, the penetration depth is limited to <5 mm. One of the major benefits of APC, in contrast to laser or electrocautery, is successful treatment of the lesions situated laterally to the probe or the lesions "around the corner." Disadvantages of APC include low penetration ability; therefore, the treatment of bulky tumor masses APC is not recommended as likely to be inefficient. If such case, however, occurs, then other interventional techniques must follow APC. In order to remove all the necrotic debris from the airways, repeated bronchoscopic check-ups are frequently required.

Indications for APC are similar to EC or laser resections. They include intrinsic airway obstruction due proliferation of malignant or benign tissue. Most suitable lesions are those with large endobronchial component with visible distal bronchial lumen and functional pulmonary tissue. The major indication for APC is hemostasis in hemoptysis, since APC affects wide surface. APC is also successfully used in resection of granulation tissue proliferating through the pores of metallic stent, including the treatment of respiratory papillomatosis and posttransplantation benign tracheobronchial stenosis. There are no absolute contraindications for APC use, except for extraluminal disease. Relative contraindications are the same as for laser resections and EC.

Although APC can be performed via flexible bronchoscopy alone, the combination of flexible and rigid bronchoscopy, however, enables better control of bursts and adequate removal of debris during the intervention. The technique is usually performed under general anesthesia, requiring necessary precautions for its safe performance. Oxygen concentration should be under 40% and all flammable materials, e.g., silicone stents or endotracheal tube, should be avoided. Initial settings for application of APC include power at 30–80 W, burst time of 2–3 s, and argon gas flow 0.3–2 L/min. The flexible probes for APC are 1.5 or 2.3 mm in diameter and usually 200 cm long, and they easily pass through working channel of flexible bronchoscope. The tip of the probe must protrude at least 1 cm off the tip of the bronchoscope. It makes the visualization field clear and prevents possible burning of the bronchoscope. The probe must be kept 1 cm from the target tissue in order to keep the flow of plasma. During the procedure, attempt should be always made to remove the debris with forceps or with suction.

Possible and serious complications include airway perforation (pneumomediastinum or pneumothorax), airway fire, and damage to the bronchoscope. However, the incidence of these complications is less than 1%. By limiting the oxygen concentration on <40%, keeping power settings <80 W, and securing that application time is <5 s, one can effectively minimize the probability of these complications. APC is a recommendable technique for the management of hemoptysis and for removing CAO.

3.2 Techniques with Delayed Effect

There are several techniques that have delayed effect. Balloon dilatation (bronchoplasty), endobronchial brachytherapy, cryotherapy, and photodynamic therapy have all been used with success and, if properly managed, very low toxicity. They are all presented in detail in other chapters.

References

Belanger AR, Burks AC, Chambers DM et al (2019) Peripheral lung nodule diagnosis and fiducial marker placement using a novel tip-tracked electromagnetic navigation bronchoscopy system. J Bronchology Interv Pulmonol 26:41–48

Bolliger CT, Sutedja TG, Strausz J, Freitag L (2006) Therapeutic bronchoscopy with immediate effect: laser, electrocautery, argon plasma coagulation and stents. Eur Respir J 27:1258–1271

Chaddha U, Hogarth DK, Murgu S (2019) Bronchoscopic ablative therapies for malignant central airway obstruction and peripheral lung tumors. Ann Am Thorac Soc 16:1220–1229

Chauhan NK, Elhence P, Deokar K et al (2021) Vascular patterns on narrow band imaging (NBI) video bronchoscopy of lung cancer patients and its relationship with histology: an analytical cross-sectional study. Adv Respir Med 89:30–36

Chen W, Gao X, Tian Q et al (2011) A comparison of autofluorescence bronchoscopy and white light bronchoscopy in detection of lung cancer and preneoplastic lesions: a meta-analysis. Lung Cancer 73:183–188

Chowdhury R, Amin A, Bhattacharyya K (2015) Intermittent fluorescence oscillations in lipid droplets in a live normal and lung cancer cell: time-resolved confocal microscopy. J Phys Chem B 119:10868–10875

Colt HG, Murgu SD (2010) Interventional bronchoscopy from bench to bedside: new techniques for early lung cancer detection. Clin Chest Med 31:29–37

Colt HG, Murgu SD, Korst RJ, Slatore CG, Unger M, Quadrelli S (2013) Follow-up and surveillance of the patient with lung cancer after curative-intent therapy: diagnosis and management of lung cancer, 3rd ed: American College of Chest Physicians evidence-based clinical practice guidelines. Chest 143(5 Suppl):e437S–e454S

Duhamel DR, Harrell JH II (2001) Laser bronchoscopy. Chest Surg Clin N Am 11:769–789

Goorsenberg A, Kalverda KA, Annema J, Bonta P (2020) Advances in optical coherence tomography and confocal laser endomicroscopy in pulmonary diseases. Respiration 99:190–205

Ho E, Agrawal A, Hogarth DK, Murgu S (2021) What should we realistically expect from robotic bronchoscopy in the near future? J Thorac Dis 13: 405–408

Iftikhar IH, Musani AI (2015) Narrow-band imaging bronchoscopy in the detection of premalignant airway lesions: a meta-analysis of diagnostic test accuracy. Ther Adv Respir Dis 9:207–216

Kent AJ, Byrnes KA, Chang SH (2020) State of the art: robotic bronchoscopy. Semin Thorac Cardiovasc Surg 32:1030–1035

Kinoshita T, Effat A, Gregor A et al (2019) A novel laser fiberscope for simultaneous imaging and phototherapy of peripheral lung cancer. Chest 156:571–578

Lee P, Kupeli E, Mehta AC (2002) Therapeutic bronchoscopy in lung cancer. Laser therapy, electrocautery, brachytherapy, stents, and photodynamic therapy. Clin Chest Med 23:241–256

Liam CK, Lee P, Yu CJ, Bai C, Yasufuku K (2021) The diagnosis of lung cancer in the era of interventional pulmonology. Int J Tuberc Lung Dis 25:6–15

Liu N, Kan J, Cao W et al (2019) Metagenomic next-generation sequencing diagnosis of peripheral pulmonary infectious lesions through virtual navigation, radial EBUS, ultrathin bronchoscopy, and ROSE. J Int Med Res 47:4878–4885

Mahajan AK, Ibrahim O, Perez R, Oberg CL, Majid A, Folch E (2020) Electrosurgical and laser therapy tools for the treatment of malignant central airway obstructions. Chest 157:446–453

Matsuno Y, Asano F, Shindoh J et al (2011) CT-guided ultrathin bronchoscopy: bioptic approach and factors in predicting diagnosis. Intern Med 50:2143–2148

Michel RG, Kinasewitz GT, Fung K-M, Keddissi JI (2010) Optical coherence tomography as an adjunct to flexible bronchoscopy in the diagnosis of lung cancer: a pilot study. Chest 138:984–988

Miller SM, Bellinger CR, Chatterjee A (2013) Argon plasma coagulation and electrosurgery for benign endobronchial tumors. J Bronchology Interv Pulmonol 20:38–40

Mudambi L, Miller R, Eapen GA (2017) Malignant central airway obstruction. J Thorac Dis 9(Suppl 10):S1087–S1110

Ost DE, Ernst A, Lei X et al, AQuIRE Bronchoscopy Registry (2016) Diagnostic yield and complications of bronchoscopy for peripheral lung lesions. Results of the AQuIRE Registry. Am J Respir Crit Care Med 193(1):68–77.

Rakotomamonjy A, Petitjean C, Salaün M, Thiberville L (2014) Scattering features for lung cancer detection in fibered confocal fluorescence microscopy images. Artif Intell Med 61:105–118

Shepherd RW, Radchenko C (2019) Bronchoscopic ablation techniques in the management of lung cancer. Ann Transl Med 7:362

Shostak E, Hariri LP, Cheng GZ, Adams DC, Suter MJ (2018) Needle based optical coherence tomography to guide transbronchial lymph node biopsy. J Bronchology Interv Pulmonol 25:189–197

Squiers JJ, Teeter WA, Hoopman JE et al (2014) Holmium:YAG laser bronchoscopy ablation of benign and malignant airway obstructions: an 8-year experience. Lasers Med Sci 29:1437–1443

Sun J, Garfield DH, Lam B et al (2011) The value of autofluorescence bronchoscopy combined with white light bronchoscopy compared with white light alone in the diagnosis of intraepithelial neoplasia and invasive lung cancer: a meta-analysis. J Thorac Oncol 6:1336–1344

Sutedja G (2003) New techniques for early detection of lung cancer. Eur Respir J 21:57–66

Unger M (1985) Neodymium:YAG laser therapy for malignant and benign endobronchial obstructions. Clin Chest Med 6:277–290

Usuda J (2018) Virtual bronchoscopic navigation (VBN) and electromagnetic navigation system. Kyobu Geka 71:843–849

Verhoeven RLJ, Fütterer JJ, Hoefsloot W, van der Heijden EHFM (2021) Cone-beam CT image guidance with and without electromagnetic navigation bronchoscopy for biopsy of peripheral pulmonary lesions. J Bronchology Interv Pulmonol 28:60–69

Wahidi MM, Herth FJF, Ernst A (2007) State of the art: interventional pulmonology. Chest 131:261–274

Yarmus L, Feller-Kopman D (2010) Bronchoscopes of the twenty-first century. Clin Chest Med 31(1):19–27

Yasufuku K (2010) Early diagnosis of lung cancer. Clin Chest Med 31:39–47

Zhu J, Li W, Zhou J et al (2017) The diagnostic value of narrow-band imaging for early and invasive lung cancer: a meta-analysis. Clinics (Sao Paulo) 72:438–448

Pathology of Lung Cancer

Mari Mino-Kenudson

Contents

1 Introduction 46
2 **Adenocarcinoma** 47
2.1 Background 47
2.2 Major Adenocarcinoma Patterns 47
2.3 Adenocarcinoma Variants 49
2.4 Nonmucinous Adenocarcinoma Classification 50
2.5 Grading of Lung Adenocarcinoma 51
2.6 Staging Issues Associated with Adenocarcinoma 51
3 **Squamous Cell Carcinoma** 52
3.1 Background 52
3.2 Histology of Squamous Cell Carcinoma ... 52
3.3 Differentiation of Primary Squamous Cell Carcinoma of the Lung from Metastatic Squamous Cell Carcinoma 54
4 **Adenosquamous Carcinoma** 54
5 **Pleomorphic Carcinoma** 54
6 **Neuroendocrine Neoplasms of the Lung** ... 55
6.1 Background 55
6.2 Histology of Neuroendocrine Neoplasms ... 55
6.3 Immunohistochemistry for Neuroendocrine Neoplasms 58
6.4 Ki-67 Proliferative Index for Pulmonary Neuroendocrine Neoplasms 58
7 **Molecular Diagnostics in NSCLC and Triage of Limited Tissue Samples for Comprehensive Diagnosis** 59
8 **Pathology Assessment of Post-Neoadjuvant Resections for NSCLC** 60
References 61

M. Mino-Kenudson (✉)
Pulmonary Pathology Service, Department of Pathology, Massachusetts General Hospital, Harvard Medical School, Boston, MA, USA
e-mail: mminokenudson@partners.org

Abstract

Treatment for patients with advanced non-small cell lung cancer (NSCLC) has expanded to include histology-based chemotherapy, targeted therapy, and immunotherapy in the past two decades along with the rapidly advanced molecular diagnostic testing. As such, accurate subtyping of lung carcinomas has become of paramount importance for appropriate patient management. In addition, a systematic approach to histologic classification of lung adenocarcinoma has been implemented in the past decade and is proven to stratify patient outcomes after resection. Thus, in this chapter, histologic classification of adenocarcinoma will be discussed in detail, along with a brief discussion of squamous cell carcinoma histology including the differentiation from adenocarcinoma and other histologic types in morphologically undifferentiated tumors in particular. A few other histologic types that are pertinent to therapeutic decision-making will also be described, and a multimodality approach for a comprehensive diagnosis of advanced NSCLC including predictive biomarker testing will be discussed. Finally, given that the scope of this publication is radiation oncology, the chapter will end with a discussion on pathology assessment of post-neoadjuvant resections for NSCLC.

1 Introduction

The current World Health Organization (WHO) classification recognizes multiple subtypes of lung carcinoma (Table 1) (WHO Classification of Tumours Editorial Board 2021). Of those, adenocarcinoma, squamous cell carcinoma, small cell carcinoma, and large cell carcinoma comprise the vast majority of lung carcinomas and have traditionally been classified into non-small cell and small cell carcinomas based on differences in some clinical characteristics and response to treatment regimens between the two entities (Travis et al. 2004). Further subtyping non-small cell lung carcinoma (NSCLC) was of little clinical relevance in the past, but given the advancement of treatment for lung cancer including histology-based chemotherapy, targeted therapy, and immunotherapy, classification of non-small cell lung carcinoma (NSCLC) into squamous and nonsquamous subtypes has become of clinical importance (NCCN 2021a). In addition, the incidence of large cell carcinoma that is defined as undifferentiated, non-small cell carcinoma has significantly declined in the last 30 years, likely reflecting changes in the use of immunohistochemistry in pathology practice (Cardarella et al. 2012). Therefore, the scope of this chapter will focus on the pathology and evolving issues of adenocarcinoma and squamous cell carcinoma. The evolving issues include changes in pathology tumor (pT) stage descriptors as well as histologic diagnosis, subtyping, and molecular testing on small tissue samples obtained by interventional radiologists and pulmonologists. In particular, morphologically undifferentiated non-small cell carcinoma in small biopsies or cytology specimens (non-small cell carcinoma, NOS, equivalent to large cell carcinoma in resections) require immuno-

Table 1 2021 World Health Organization classification of malignant epithelial tumors and neuroendocrine neoplasms of the lung including preinvasive lesions

Epithelial tumors
Preinvasive glandular lesions
Atypical adenomatous hyperplasia
Adenocarcinoma in situ
Adenocarcinomas
Minimally invasive adenocarcinoma
Adenocarcinoma of lung, invasive nonmucinous
Invasive mucinous adenocarcinoma
Colloid adenocarcinoma
Fetal adenocarcinoma
Enteric-type adenocarcinoma
Squamous precursor lesions
Squamous dysplasia and carcinoma in situ
Squamous cell carcinomas
Squamous cell carcinoma
Lymphoepithelial carcinoma
Large cell carcinoma
Sarcomatoid carcinomas
Pleomorphic carcinoma
Pulmonary blastoma
Carcinosarcoma
Others
Adenosquamous carcinoma
NUT carcinoma
Thoracic SMARCA4-deficient tumor
Salivary gland-type tumors
Pleomorphic adenoma
Adenoid cystic carcinoma
Epithelial-myoepithelial carcinoma
Hyalinizing clear cell carcinoma
Myoepithelioma and myoepithelial carcinoma
Neuroendocrine neoplasms
Preinvasive lesion
Diffuse idiopathic pulmonary neuroendocrine cell hyperplasia
Neuroendocrine tumor
Carcinoid/neuroendocrine tumor
Neuroendocrine carcinoma
Small cell (lung) carcinoma
Large cell neuroendocrine carcinoma

histochemistry workup to further subtype and differentiate squamous vs. nonsquamous cell carcinoma, if possible, while tumor tissue needs to be conserved for molecular testing in patients with advanced tumors. In addition, adenosquamous carcinoma, pleomorphic carcinoma, and neuroendocrine neoplasm classification will be briefly discussed since they are pertinent to therapeutic decision-making. The chapter will end with a brief discussion on the histologic assessment of post-neoadjuvant resections for NSCLC.

2 Adenocarcinoma

2.1 Background

Histologically, invasive adenocarcinoma is highly heterogenous and more than one histologic pattern can be seen in up to 90% of all lung adenocarcinomas (Travis et al. 2004). In the 2004 WHO classification, "mixed subtype" reflected the intratumoral heterogeneity (Travis et al. 2004), but this nonspecific approach with the majority of tumors classified into the subtype failed to convey prognostic information associated with the histologic patterns. The 2011 International Association for the Study of Lung Cancer (IASLC)/American Thoracic Society (ATS)/European Respiratory Society (ERS) international multidisciplinary classification of lung adenocarcinoma recognizes five major patterns (nonmucinous lepidic [former bronchioloalveolar; BAC], acinar, papillary, micropapillary, and solid) along with four variants (mucinous lepidic [former mucinous BAC], colloid, fetal, and enteric type) (Travis et al. 2011). This classification was adopted by the 2015 WHO classification that recommends recording each pattern identified in the tumor in 5–10% increments and rendering a diagnosis based on the predominant pattern (Table 2) (Travis et al. 2015). The most updated WHO classification recognizes complex glandular pattern, which has typically been classified into acinar pattern, as one associated with worse patient survival after resection (WHO Classification of Tumours Editorial Board 2021; Moreira et al. 2014, 2020). This semiquantitative pattern classification allows reproducible prognostic stratification (Eguchi et al. 2014) and aids in differentiating between intrapulmonary metastasis and multiple synchronous and/or metachronous primaries in the setting of multiple tumor nodules (Nicholson et al. 2018).

Table 2 Classification of adenocarcinoma

Preinvasive lesions
Atypical adenomatous hyperplasia (usually ≤0.5 cm)
Adenocarcinoma in situ (≤3 cm, formally bronchioloalveolar carcinoma [BAC])[a]
• Nonmucinous
• Mucinous
• Mixed mucinous/nonmucinous
Minimally invasive adenocarcinoma (≤3 cm lepidic-predominant tumor with ≤0.5 cm invasion)[a]
• Nonmucinous
• Mucinous
• Mixed mucinous/nonmucinous
Invasive adenocarcinoma[a]
• Lepidic adenocarcinoma (lepidic-predominant tumor with entire size >3 cm and/or >0.5 cm invasion)
• Acinar adenocarcinoma
• Papillary adenocarcinoma
• Micropapillary adenocarcinoma
• Solid adenocarcinoma
Variant of invasive adenocarcinoma
• Invasive mucinous adenocarcinoma (formally mucinous BAC)
• Colloid adenocarcinoma
• Fetal adenocarcinoma
• Enteric-type adenocarcinoma

The tumor is classified in accordance with the predominant pattern and invasive size. Of note, non-lepidic-predominant tumors and those with pleural and/or vascular invasion and presence of necrosis and/or tumor spreading in airspaces are classified as invasive adenocarcinoma irrespective of the invasive size

[a] A proportion of each pattern identified in the tumor is measured with 5–10% increments. Non-lepidic patterns are considered invasive patterns, and an invasive size is determined based on the largest dimension of the invasive component, if the invasion is confined to a single focus, or the largest dimension of the entire tumor size x% of non-lepidic patterns (collectively)/100, if the invasion is present in multiple foci

2.2 Major Adenocarcinoma Patterns

Nonmucinous lepidic pattern (Fig. 1a) is characterized by pneumocytic cells (type II pneumocytes or club cells) growing along the alveolar structures. It is often associated with septal thickening by inflammatory cell infiltrates, but tumor cells should not be seen in the stroma of alveolar walls (in situ pattern). Lepidic predominant tumors typically exhibit minimal to mild cytologic atypia with

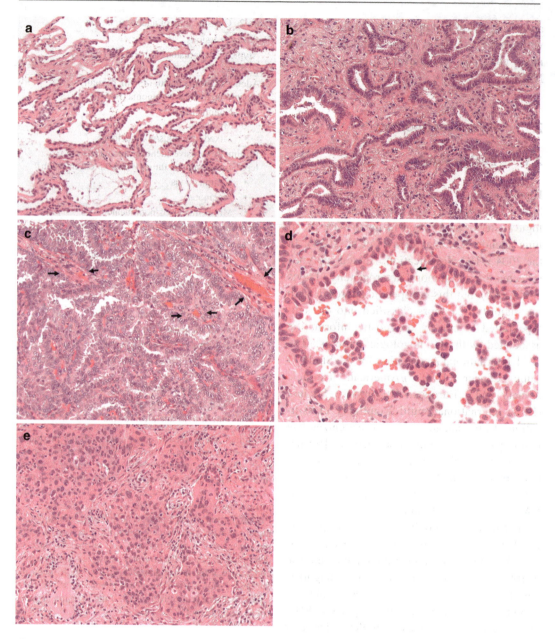

Fig. 1 (**a**) Lepidic pattern characterized by pneumocytes with mild cytologic atypia growing along the preexisting alveolar walls without stomal invasion (Hematoxylin & Eosin stain, ×200). (**b**) Acinar pattern consisting of oval or slightly jagged glands in the background of fibroelastotic stroma replacing the alveolar parenchyma (Hematoxylin & Eosin stain, ×200). (**c**) Papillary pattern demonstrating growth of glandular cells along fibrovascular cores (arrows) (Hematoxylin & Eosin stain, ×200). (**d**) Micropapillary pattern characterized by floret-like small clusters of tumor cells without fibrovascular cores floating within an air space (Hematoxylin & Eosin stain, ×400). (**e**) An example of solid pattern demonstrating nests of polygonal tumor cells in the background of fibroinflammatory stroma (Hematoxylin & Eosin stain, ×200). In this case, a TTF-1-positive and p40-negative immunoprofile supports the diagnosis of lung adenocarcinoma

mildly enlarged hyperchromatic nuclei (WHO Classification of Tumours Editorial Board 2021).

Acinar pattern (Fig. 1b) exhibits round to oval glands or more jagged structures with central luminal spaces surrounded by tumor cells. Mucin can be seen within tumor cells and/or in glandular spaces. The neoplastic glands invade into myofibroblastic stroma and/or replace the background alveolar parenchyma opposed to preserved alveolar architecture seen in lepidic pattern (WHO Classification of Tumours Editorial Board 2021). Notably, complex glandular patterns, including cribriform and fused acinar patterns, that have been classified into acinar pattern appear to harbor more aggressive tumor biology associated with worse patient outcomes (Moreira et al. 2014). Of those, cribriform pattern is characterized by nests of tumor cells with sieve-like perforation, while fused glands with irregular borders, back-to-back glands without intervening stroma, or ribbon-like formations are classified as fused gland pattern (Moreira et al. 2014).

Papillary pattern (Fig. 1c) is characterized by growth of glandular cells along fibrovascular cores (WHO Classification of Tumours Editorial Board 2021). Papillary pattern may be difficult to differentiate from lepidic, acinar, or micropapillary pattern and may be in continuity with those patterns (Shih et al. 2019; Thunnissen et al. 2012). Further, there is a morphologic spectrum of papillary pattern based on size of papillae and nuclear grade that is reflected to patient survival (Warth et al. 2016).

Micropapillary pattern (Fig. 1d) is composed of tumor cells forming papillary tuffs without fibrovascular cores resembling florets. Ring-like structures floating within alveolar spaces are also classified into this pattern, and micropapillary pattern may be seen within the stroma (stromal invasion) (WHO Classification of Tumours Editorial Board 2021; Ohe et al. 2012). The recently recognized filigree pattern consists of tumor cells growing in delicate, lace-like, narrow stacks of three or more cells without fibrovascular cores and has expanded the morphologic spectrum of micropapillary pattern (Emoto et al. 2019).

Solid pattern (Fig. 1e) consists of polygonal tumor cells in nests or sheets without recognizable lepidic, acinar, papillary, or micropapillary architecture. It mimics nonkeratinizing squamous cell carcinoma as described later in the chapter; thus, it is important to confirm glandular differentiation by pneumocyte marker expression (thyroid transcription factor-1 [TTF-1] and/or Napsin A) along with negative or focal p40 expression by immunohistochemistry (Thunnissen et al. 2014; Yatabe et al. 2019) or demonstration of intracytoplasmic mucin in ≥5 tumor cells per two high-power fields with PAS/d or mucicarmine stain (Travis et al. 2011). Notably, mucin-producing lung adenocarcinoma tends to be negative for TTF-1 (Yatabe et al. 2019).

2.3 Adenocarcinoma Variants

Variant patterns consist of mucinous lepidic, colloid, fetal, and enteric type. These patterns can be predominant or focal in the background of the major patterns. When predominant, the tumors are classified as invasive mucinous/mixed mucinous and nonmucinous adenocarcinoma, colloid adenocarcinoma, fetal adenocarcinoma (low- or high-grade) or enteric-type adenocarcinoma, respectively. These variants are very rare except invasive mucinous/mixed mucinous and nonmucinous adenocarcinoma, and morphologically mimic nonpulmonary adenocarcinomas. For instance, enteric-type adenocarcinoma resembles colorectal adenocarcinoma and low-grade fetal adenocarcinoma, endometrioid adenocarcinoma. Therefore, the possibility of metastasis from an extrapulmonary site needs to be excluded before rendering the diagnosis (WHO Classification of Tumours Editorial Board 2021; Yatabe et al. 2020).

Of adenocarcinoma variants, invasive mucinous adenocarcinoma is relatively common (3–10% of resected adenocarcinomas) (WHO Classification of Tumours Editorial Board 2021) and is characterized by a columnar and/or goblet cell morphology with abundant intracytoplasmic mucin and basally located nuclei growing in a lepidic pattern. Tumor cells typically lack significant pleomorphism. The surrounding airspaces are often filled with mucin. Invasive mucinous adenocarcinoma often shows lepidic predominant growth but usually contains invasive foci including acinar, papillary, micropapillary, solid, and complex glandular patterns that often exhibit less intracytoplasmic mucin than a lepidic component. Tumors with a mixture of mucinous and nonmucinous components should be classified as invasive mixed mucinous and nonmucinous adenocarcinoma, if each component comprises ≥10% of the tumor (WHO Classification of Tumours Editorial Board 2021; Geles et al. 2015). Notably, metastasis from mucin-producing tumors, including pancreatobiliary, upper and lower GI, and GYN primaries, may show a morphology similar to invasive mucinous adenocarcinoma (Yatabe et al. 2019).

2.4 Nonmucinous Adenocarcinoma Classification

Nonmucinous adenocarcinomas are classified into adenocarcinoma in situ (AIS) that is a preinvasive lesion, minimally invasive adenocarcinoma (MIA), and invasive adenocarcinoma based on the size of entire tumor, invasive size, and predominant pattern (WHO Classification of Tumours Editorial Board 2021; Travis et al. 2011).

If the tumor measuring 3 cm or smaller is composed only of nonmucinous lepidic pattern, it is classified as AIS, nonmucinous, while the presence of invasion, defined as tumor cells infiltrating myofibroblast stroma, and/or the presence of any of the non-lepidic patterns, leads to the diagnosis of invasive adenocarcinoma. Of those, a small (≤3 cm) lepidic predominant tumor with invasive size of ≤5 mm is classified as MIA (Table 2) (Travis et al. 2015) that follows excellent prognosis similar to AIS (100% 5-year disease-free survival [DFS]) (Eguchi et al. 2014). AIS and MIA could also exhibit a mucinous or mixed mucinous and nonmucinous morphology, but such tumors are extremely rare (Travis et al. 2015). Notably, lymphovascular and pleural invasion, tumor spreading through airspaces surrounding adjacent normal lung parenchyma (STAS), and tumor necrosis are all considered exclusion criteria for AIS and MIA. Of those, STAS is a recently recognized pathologic feature defined as tumor cells within air spaces in the lung parenchyma beyond the edge of the main tumor and has been associated with shorter DFS and overall survival (OS) not only in adenocarcinoma but also in other major types of lung carcinomas (airspace invasion) (Mino-Kenudson 2020; Shih and Mino-Kenudson 2020).

The rest of nonmucinous adenocarcinomas are classified into lepidic, acinar, papillary, micropapillary, and solid adenocarcinomas based on the predominant pattern, and they reportedly comprise 2.4–27%, 14–45%, 8.9–41%, 0–16%, and 6.7–28% of resected early-stage lung adenocarcinomas, respectively (Eguchi et al. 2014). The wide range of reported prevalence seen in each subtype is likely attributed to significant interobserver variability in the diagnosis of these patterns (Shih et al. 2019; Thunnissen et al. 2012).

It is important to note that the diagnosis of AIS and MIA cannot be made in biopsy or cytology specimens that represent only a small fraction of the entire tumor. In general, all patterns present in the biopsy specimen should be listed along with the diagnosis of adenocarcinoma. For instance, a biopsy from a small tumor proven to be AIS on resection would show adenocarcinoma with lepidic pattern (WHO Classification of Tumours Editorial Board 2021).

2.5 Grading of Lung Adenocarcinoma

Lung carcinomas have traditionally been classified into well, moderately, and poorly differentiated based on cytomorphologic features with no clear definitions for adenocarcinoma in particular. After introduction of the IASLC/ATS/ERS international multidisciplinary classification of lung adenocarcinoma, multiple studies have shown the association of predominant patterns with survival in lung adenocarcinomas (Eguchi et al. 2014). Lepidic predominant adenocarcinomas have excellent prognosis (>90% 5-year DFS following curative resection), followed by acinar or papillary predominant adenocarcinomas (70–80% 5-year DFS). Micropapillary or solid predominant adenocarcinomas are biologically aggressive with 25–70% 5-year DFS after curative resection (Eguchi et al. 2014). Accordingly, lepidic adenocarcinoma is considered well differentiated, acinar and papillary adenocarcinomas, moderately differentiated, and micropapillary and solid adenocarcinomas, poorly differentiated. More recently, it has been shown that tumors with predominant complex glandular patterns have poor prognosis similar to micropapillary and solid adenocarcinomas (Moreira et al. 2014). Further, the presence of micropapillary and/or solid patterns, even as a small component, indicates worse prognosis (Hwang et al. 2014; Lee et al. 2015). Thus, a new grading system (the IASLC grading system) for invasive lung adenocarcinoma that concerns both predominant pattern and a proportion of high-grade patterns has been proposed (Table 3) (WHO Classification of Tumours Editorial Board 2021; Moreira et al. 2020).

Table 3 The IASLC grading system for invasive lung adenocarcinoma

Grade	Differentiation	Patterns
1	Well differentiated	Lepidic predominant with <20% high-grade pattern[a]
2	Moderately differentiated	Acinar or papillary predominant with <20% high-grade pattern[a]
3	Poorly differentiated	Any tumor with ≥20% high-grade pattern[a]

[a] High-grade patterns include micropapillary, solid, and complex glandular patterns

2.6 Staging Issues Associated with Adenocarcinoma

In accordance with the updated cancer staging systems (Amin et al. 2017; Sobin et al. 2017), invasive size is used to determine tumor stage (pT) in nonmucinous lung adenocarcinomas with lepidic pattern, irrespective of its predominance, while nonmucinous adenocarcinomas without lepidic pattern, mucinous adenocarcinomas, and other types of lung carcinoma are staged based on entire tumor size (Amin et al. 2017). It is a reflection of accumulating data in the literature to suggest that invasive size is a better predictor of survival than total tumor size in lung adenocarcinoma (Travis et al. 2016; Tsutani et al. 2013). If the invasive area is in a single focus, the invasive size can be easily measured in the largest dimension of the focus. Unfortunately, however, lung adenocarcinomas with a lepidic component often have multiple invasive foci scattered over multiple histology sections. In such tumors, the invasive size can be estimated as follows: the entire size of the tumor × the total percentage of non-lepidic/invasive components/100 (WHO Classification of Tumours Editorial Board 2021). Notably, a significant difference between the tumor size depicted by radiology imaging and the (invasive) tumor size measured in a resection specimen and used to determine pT stage may be seen in some nonmucinous adenocarcinomas (Travis et al. 2016).

Another issue that warrants a discussion is staging of multiple nodules that are not uncommon in patients with lung adenocarcinomas in particular (Nicholson et al. 2018). The multiple nodules are essentially classified as intrapulmonary metastasis and multiple primary lung cancers, and single pT stage is determined based on the locations of nodules in the intrapulmonary metastasis setting, while multiple primary cancers are individually staged (Amin et al. 2017). Histologic differentiation of intrapulmonary metastasis from multiple primary tumors is relatively straightforward in resection specimens and is based on major histologic pattern, other pattern percentages, and cytologic (cell size, nuclear pleomorphism, nuclear size, mitotic rates, etc.) and stromal features (Nicholson et al. 2018). However, 20–25% of cases with multiple nodules show discordant interpretations as to whether they are clonally related between molecular testing (NGS) and histologic assessment in small biopsy specimens in particular (Chang et al. 2019); thus, it is important to lower a threshold for molecular testing in this context.

3 Squamous Cell Carcinoma

3.1 Background

Lung squamous cell carcinomas typically originate in central airways; however, recent series have shown increasing prevalence of peripheral squamous cell carcinomas, which are becoming as common as central squamous cell carcinomas (Funai et al. 2003).

Invasive squamous cell carcinomas consist of conventional squamous cell carcinomas, both keratinizing and nonkeratinizing, and basaloid squamous cell carcinoma. Conventional squamous cell carcinomas are defined as malignant epithelial tumors showing keratinization and/or intercellular bridges that arise from bronchial epithelium (WHO Classification of Tumours Editorial Board 2021). Basaloid squamous cell carcinoma is composed of cytologically undifferentiated, small cells that exhibit a squamous marker expression and appears to have worse prognosis than that of other NSCLC (Moro et al. 1994; Moro-Sibilot et al. 2008).

One of important issues involving squamous cell carcinomas is to differentiate nonkeratinizing and basaloid tumors from their mimickers. Another issue is to differentiate primary from metastatic tumors since patients with prior history of squamous cell carcinoma of other sites, such as head and neck, esophagus, or cervix, may develop squamous cell carcinoma in the lung.

3.2 Histology of Squamous Cell Carcinoma

Keratinizing squamous cell carcinoma (Fig. 2a) is characterized by the presence of keratinization and/or intercellular bridges. The keratinization includes layered keratin and cytoplasmic keratin of individual tumor cells. Keratin pearl formation may also be seen. These features vary with the degree of differentiation; well-differentiated tumors exhibit prominent keratinization and intercellular bridges, while those features are found only focally in poorly differentiated tumors (Cardesa et al. 2005).

Nonkeratinizing squamous cell carcinoma (Fig. 2b, c) typically lacks maturation in the epithelial nests and does not generally show evidence of keratinization, although some degree may be seen (Chan et al. 2005). It may exhibit an "undifferentiated non-small cell carcinoma" morphology with a squamous linage revealed by immunohistochemistry. Thus, nonkeratinizing squamous cell carcinoma can be confused with large cell carcinoma or solid adenocarcinoma, in particular, that with pseudosquamous features (Kadota et al. 2014). Given the differences in molecular alterations and response to some therapeutic regimens between squamous and nonsquamous carcinomas, it is important to achieve accurate subtyping with immunohistochemistry for adenocarcinoma (TTF-1 ± Napsin A) and

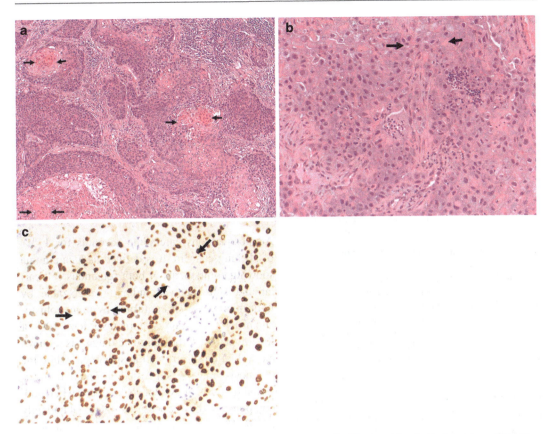

Fig. 2 (a) Keratinizing squamous cell carcinoma characterized by tumor cells growing in irregular nests in the background of fibroinflammatory stroma. Scattered areas with keratinization (arrows) are evident (Hematoxylin & Eosin stain, ×100). (b, c) Nonkeratinizing squamous cell carcinoma demonstrating polygonal cells forming irregular nests (b: Hematoxylin & Eosin stain, ×200). The "undifferentiated non-small cell carcinoma" morphology requires immunohistochemistry workup to confirm a squamous lineage. In this case, diffusely positive p40 and negative TTF-1 expressions have confirmed the diagnosis (c: p40 immunostain, ×200)

squamous (p40) markers (Table 4) ± mucin histochemistry (WHO Classification of Tumours Editorial Board 2021).

Basaloid squamous cell carcinoma is characterized by a proliferation of small cells with lobular architecture or anastomotic trabecular growth and prominent peripheral palisading of tumor nuclei. The tumor may or may not have a small component (<50%) of unequivocal keratinizing and/or nonkeratinizing squamous cell carcinoma (Brambilla et al. 2015a). The basaloid features consist of scant cytoplasm, a high nuclear/cytoplasmic (N/C) ratio, and hyperchromatic nuclei that lack prominent nucleoli. The tumor exhibits abundant mitotic activity (15–50 per 2 mm^2) and high Ki-67 proliferative index (50–80%). Comedo-type necrosis is common, and rosette may be seen in one-third of cases, but nuclear molding is essentially absent. Most basaloid squamous cell carcinomas have hyalinized or mucoid stroma (Brambilla et al. 1992). Given the small size of tumor cells with a high N/C ratio, and possible peripheral palisading and/or rosette-like structures, basaloid squamous cell carcinoma may be confused with small cell carcinoma, NUT carcinoma, or large cell neuroendocrine carcinoma (WHO Classification of Tumours Editorial Board 2021). Appropriate immunohistochemistry and/or molecular workup is important to exclude the possibility of those mimickers before

Table 4 Initial diagnostic immunohistochemical panel for morphologically undifferentiated NSCC in small biopsies or cytology specimens

TTF-1	p40	Positive cell population	Diagnosis
+[a] to +++	− or +	Same cell population	NSCC, favor adenocarcinoma
−	+ in ≥50%	N/A	NSCC, favor squamous cell carcinoma
−[b]	− or <50%	N/A	NSCC, NOS[c]
+ to ++	+ at any extent	Separate cell populations	NSCC, NOS, possible adenosquamous carcinoma

NSCC non-small cell carcinoma, *N/A* not applicable, *NOS* not otherwise specified

[a] A small fraction of tumor cells staining
[b] Since 15–20% of lung adenocarcinomas are TTF-1 negative, additional immunohistochemistry for Napsin A and/or mucin stain are helpful to rule out adenocarcinoma
[c] The possibility of metastasis from extrapulmonary sites needs to be excluded in TTF-1 (and Napsin A/mucin stain)-negative and p40-negative tumors

rendering the diagnosis of basaloid squamous cell carcinoma (WHO Classification of Tumours Editorial Board 2021; French 2012).

3.3 Differentiation of Primary Squamous Cell Carcinoma of the Lung from Metastatic Squamous Cell Carcinoma

The differentiation between primary pulmonary squamous cell carcinoma and a metastasis from extrapulmonary organs can be challenging since squamous cell carcinomas from different sites lack distinct morphologic features. In addition, the degree of keratinization and growth pattern may change after chemotherapy and/or radiation therapy in particular. To date, there is no immunostain that is useful for the distinction of primary from metastatic squamous cell carcinomas of the lung and it often requires genetic testing including HPV genotyping (Yatabe et al. 2020; Bishop et al. 2012; Chang et al. 2015; Weichert et al. 2009; Yanagawa et al. 2013). As a surrogate marker for high-risk HPV infection, strong p16 staining in squamous cell carcinomas is typically seen in uterine cervix or a subset of oropharyngeal squamous cell carcinomas, but approximately 20% of NSCLC exhibit diffuse and strong p16 expression despite the lack of HPV infection; thus, its role in excluding pulmonary origin is limited (Bishop et al. 2012; Chang et al. 2015).

4 Adenosquamous Carcinoma

Adenosquamous carcinoma accounts for 1–3% of all lung cancers. It is defined as a carcinoma showing components of both squamous cell carcinoma and adenocarcinoma, recognizable by light microscopy or confirmed by immunohistochemistry, with each comprising at least 10% of the tumor. Thus, the definitive diagnosis requires an evaluation of a resection specimen, while the diagnosis may be suggested in small or excisional biopsies or cytology specimens when both components have been sampled abundantly (WHO Classification of Tumours Editorial Board 2021). Although adenosquamous carcinoma has morphologically distinct components, both share driver mutations, indicating their clonal relationship (Wang et al. 2014; Vassella et al. 2015; Amer et al. 2017). It is important to report a minor (<10%) component of adenocarcinoma, if present, since the tumor may harbor targetable genetic alterations irrespective of the adenocarcinoma proportion (Wang et al. 2014; Rekhtman et al. 2012; Pan et al. 2014).

5 Pleomorphic Carcinoma

Pleomorphic carcinoma along with carcinosarcoma and pulmonary blastoma belong to sarcomatoid carcinoma of the lung. Given that the latter two are extremely rare, only pleomorphic carcinoma, which accounts for 2–3% of resected non-small cell lung cancers, is briefly discussed here (WHO Classification of Tumours Editorial Board 2021).

Pleomorphic carcinoma is a poorly differentiated NSCLC (adenocarcinoma, squamous cell carcinoma and/or large cell carcinoma) with at least a 10% component of spindle and/or neoplastic giant cells, or a carcinoma consisting entirely of spindle and/or neoplastic giant cells. Thus, the definitive diagnosis requires an evaluation of a surgical specimen, while the possibility can be suggested in small or excisional biopsies or cytology specimens, if the specific morphology is identified. When present, adenocarcinoma, squamous cell carcinoma, and/or large cell carcinoma components should be mentioned in the pathology report (WHO Classification of Tumours Editorial Board 2021) since it may determine adjuvant treatment regimens.

Genetic alterations are driven by the NSCLC component, particularly adenocarcinoma (Fallet et al. 2015; Terra et al. 2016; Schrock et al. 2017). Interestingly, a significant subset of pleomorphic carcinomas harbor *MET* exon 14 skipping mutations (Liu et al. 2016; Kwon et al. 2017), and the majority (60–90%) exhibits PD-L1 expression that is often more intense in the sarcomatoid areas (Schrock et al. 2017; Lococo et al. 2017; Nakanishi et al. 2019). An evaluation of these biomarkers is of paramount importance in advanced tumors in particular, since patients with pleomorphic carcinoma often suffer resistance to conventional chemotherapy and low responsiveness to radiotherapy (Martin et al. 2007; Yendamuri et al. 2012).

6 Neuroendocrine Neoplasms of the Lung

6.1 Background

Neuroendocrine neoplasms of the lung have traditionally been classified into low-grade (typical carcinoid), intermediate-grade (atypical carcinoid), and high-grade (small cell carcinoma [SCLC] and large cell neuroendocrine carcinoma [LCNEC]) malignancies. However, accumulating evidence has shown significant differences in association with diffuse idiopathic pulmonary neuroendocrine cell hyperplasia (DIPNECH), association with NSCLC, clinical behavior and molecular alterations between carcinoid tumors and high-grade neuroendocrine carcinomas (Table 5); thus, the two groups are now considered biologically distinct (Travis et al. 2015; Fernandez-Cuesta et al. 2014; George et al. 2015; Marchevsky and Walts 2015).

6.2 Histology of Neuroendocrine Neoplasms

Carcinoid tumors (Fig. 3a) are characterized by neuroendocrine morphology, and relatively uniform, polygonal cells with moderate to abundant eosinophilic cytoplasm, fine ("salt and pepper") chromatin, and inconspicuous nucleoli. The neuroendocrine morphology is characterized by organoid nesting and/or trabecular patterns, rosette-like structures and/or peripheral palisading. In addition, spindle cell growth is not uncommon in the peripheral tumors in particular. The tumor stroma is typically vascular-rich. Carcinoid tumors are classified into typical and atypical forms, and the latter is differentiated from the former based on the presence of 2–10 mitoses per 2 mm^2 and/or presence of necrosis. The necrosis is usually punctate opposed to large zonal one of high-grade neuroendocrine carcinomas. Prominent pleomorphism and/or conspicuous nucleoli may be seen in typical carcinoid and likely represent degenerative changes, thus should not be considered as supportive features for atypical carcinoid (Travis et al. 2015).

Small cell carcinoma (Fig. 3b) typically exhibits a sheet-like diffuse growth of small cells with a high N/C ratio. The aforementioned classic neuroendocrine architectural patterns are less common. The tumor cells have been designated as small cells using the arbitrarily criterion of nuclear size <3 times the diameter of the nuclei in resting lymphocytes (Colby et al. 1995); however, considerable variation in the nuclear size (den Bakker et al. 2010; Marchevsky et al. 2001) as well as scattered pleomorphic giant tumor

Table 5 Pathologic and molecular features of neuroendocrine neoplasms of the lung

	Typical carcinoid	Atypical carcinoid	LCNEC	Small cell carcinoma
Mitoses per 2 mm^2	0–1	2–10	>10	>10
Necrosis	–	+/– focal/punctate, if present	+	+
Neuroendocrine architecture	+	+	+	–/+
Pattern of pancytokeratin staining	Diffuse cytoplasmic		Dot-like, perinuclear or diffuse cytoplasmic	
NE marker expression				
Synaptophysin	Mostly +	Mostly +	+ in 60%	+ in 60%
Chromogranin A	Mostly +	Mostly +	+ in 60%	+ in 45%
CD56	Mostly +	Mostly +	+ in 90%	+ in 90%
Any of the above	100%	100%	Approximately 100%	+ in 90–95%
INSM1	+ in 100%	+ in 100%	+ in 85%	+ in 85%
TTF-1 expression	+ in up to 30%, often expressed in peripheral tumors	+ in up to 50%	+ in 40–60%	+ in 90%
Ki-67 proliferative index	<5%	<20%	45–70%	65–100%
Possible precursor	DIPNECH		Pluripotent cells, possibly shared with NSCLC	
Combined with a NSCLC component	–		–/+	
Molecular profile	Mutations in covalent histone modifiers or subunits of the SWI/SNF complex		Two major (SCLC-like and NSCLC-like) and one minor (carcinoid-like) types	Concurrent *TP53* mutation and RB loss

DIPNECH diffuse idiopathic pulmonary neuroendocrine cell hyperplasia, *LCNEC* large cell neuroendocrine carcinoma, *NE* neuroendocrine, *NSCLC* non-small cell lung cancer, *SCLC* small cell lung cancer, *SWI/SNF* SWItch/Sucrose Non-Fermentable

cells may be seen. The tumor cells usually exhibit round, ovoid, or spindled nuclei, and nuclear chromatin is finely granular ("salt and pepper") with absent or inconspicuous nucleoli. Nuclear molding is common in small biopsy samples in particular. By definition, the tumor harbors at least 10 mitoses/2 mm^2, and mitotic activity is usually brisk (median of 80 mitoses/2 mm^2) (Brambilla et al. 2015b). Apoptotic activity is also significant and, if examined, ki-67 labeling is >50% (Brambilla et al. 2015b; Pelosi et al. 2005). In larger specimens (excisional biopsies and resections), the tumor cells may be larger, and classic neuroendocrine architecture patterns, prominent nucleoli and/or extensive necrosis may be seen.

Rare tumors exhibit a predominant small cell carcinoma morphology with an element of non-small cell carcinoma (including squamous cell carcinoma, adenocarcinoma, large cell carcinoma, LCNEC, and less commonly sarcomatoid carcinoma) and are classified as combined small cell carcinoma (Travis et al. 2015).

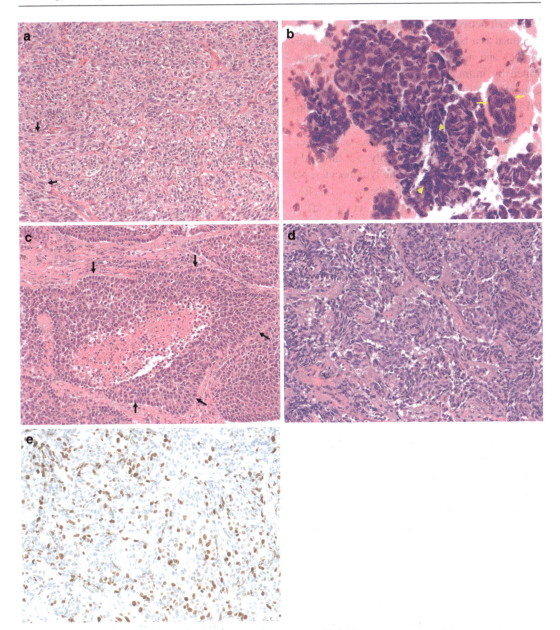

Fig. 3 (**a**) Typical carcinoid consisting of uniform polygonal cells with a moderate amount of eosinophilic cytoplasm in nests with intervening vascular-rich stroma. Scattered foci with a spindle cell morphology (arrows) are present, but no mitoses or necrosis are seen in this case (Hematoxylin & Eosin stain, ×200). (**b**) A biopsy demonstrating small cell carcinoma characterized by small cells with a high N/C ratio, fine chromatin, inconspicuous nucleoli, nuclear molding (arrows), and crush artifact (arrow heads) (Hematoxylin & Eosin stain, ×400). (**c**) Large cell neuroendocrine carcinoma with polygonal cells with ample eosinophilic cytoplasm demonstrating a neuroendocrine morphology characterized by a nesting pattern and peripheral palisading (arrows). Comedo necrosis is also evident (Hematoxylin & Eosin stain, ×200). (**d**, **e**) An example of atypical carcinoid with increased proliferation. The tumor maintains a carcinoid morphology (**d**: Hematoxylin & Eosin stain, ×200), but Ki67 proliferative index is 38% in this case, higher than expected to see in atypical carcinoid (<20%) (**e**: Ki-67 immunostain, ×200)

Large cell neuroendocrine carcinoma (Fig. 3c) is defined as a NSCLC with neuroendocrine morphology and neuroendocrine differentiation confirmed by immunohistochemistry (see the next section) and/or electron microscopy (Travis et al. 2015). The combination of solid nests with multiple rosette-like structures leading to a cribriform pattern is not uncommon and mimics adenocarcinoma. Tumor cells are typically >3 times the diameter of the nuclei in resting lymphocytes, but significant overlap in cell size between LCNEC and SCLC exits (den Bakker et al. 2010; Marchevsky et al. 2001). Thus, moderate to ample, often eosinophilic cytoplasm and prominent nucleoli are more important features to differentiate LCNEC from SCLC. By definition, the tumor harbors >10 mitoses/2 mm^2, and mitotic activity is usually brisk (median 70 mitoses/2 mm^2) (WHO Classification of Tumours Editorial Board 2021). The tumor often shows large areas of necrosis. Similar to combined SCLC, any amounts of non-small cell carcinomas in the background of LCNEC leads to the diagnosis of combined LCNEC.

It is important to note that 10–20% of NSCLCs, most commonly adenocarcinoma, exhibit neuroendocrine marker expression by immunohistochemistry despite the absence of neuroendocrine morphology. Such tumors are not classified as LCNEC given their biology similar to conventional NSCLC (Ionescu et al. 2007; Sterlacci et al. 2009).

6.3 Immunohistochemistry for Neuroendocrine Neoplasms

Expression of neuroendocrine marker(s) is required for the diagnosis of LCNEC. While immunohistochemistry workup is not a requisite for the diagnosis of SCLC or carcinoid tumor, it is often applied to differentiate from their mimickers including basaloid squamous cell carcinoma (vs. SCLC). The most commonly used panel of neuroendocrine markers include synaptophysin, chromogranin A, and CD56/NCAM1. Of those, chromogranin A is positive in ≥90% of typical carcinoid tumors, 60–70% of atypical carcinoid and LCNEC, but significantly less sensitive (approximately 45% positive) for SCLC, while 60–70% of pulmonary neuroendocrine neoplasms, regardless of grade, is immunoreactive to synaptophysin. CD56 is more sensitive in high-grade neuroendocrine carcinomas in particular, but less specific for neuroendocrine differentiation (Yatabe et al. 2019). Positive staining of any of these neuroendocrine markers combined with unequivocal neuroendocrine morphology is suggestive of the diagnosis of a neuroendocrine neoplasm, although caution should be made with interpreting tumors labeling for CD56 alone given its lower specificity. Importantly, SCLC may be negative for all of these markers in 5–10% of cases (WHO Classification of Tumours Editorial Board 2021). The recently introduced Insulinoma-associated protein 1 (INSM1) has been shown to be a more reliable marker in the setting of SCLC in particular (Mukhopadhyay et al. 2019; Kriegsmann et al. 2020). It is important to note that TTF-1 expression has been reported in 50% of LCNEC and 90–95% of SCLC as well as a fraction of carcinoid tumors; however, it is not specific for a pulmonary origin in the setting of SCLC and LCNEC (Kaufmann and Dietel 2000; Matoso et al. 2010). Finally, the vast majority of SCLC show concurrent loss of Rb protein and p53 overexpression or null expression (Onuki et al. 1999; Beasley et al. 2003). The alterations of those markers in LCNEC support small cell carcinoma-like biology (Rekhtman et al. 2016).

6.4 Ki-67 Proliferative Index for Pulmonary Neuroendocrine Neoplasms

Ki-67 proliferative index is usually <5% in typical carcinoid and <20% in atypical carcinoid tumors (Pelosi et al. 2014). While Ki-67 proliferation rates of up to 30% have been reported in atypical carcinoid, the rate is constantly >30% and typically >40% in LCNEC with some cases exhibiting high proliferation rate (≥80%), and the rate ranges from 65% to 100% in SCLC

(Pelosi et al. 2005). Different from the GI/pancreas neuroendocrine neoplasm classification, however, a Ki-67 proliferate index is not part of the current diagnostic criteria for lung neuroendocrine neoplasms, particularly in the distinction of atypical vs. typical carcinoid tumors (Pelosi et al. 2014; Swarts et al. 2017; Marchio et al. 2017), and the role of Ki-67 is rather limited to differentiating a carcinoid tumor from SCLC or LCNEC in crushed biopsy or cytology samples (Pelosi et al. 2005). Notably, tumors with carcinoid-like morphology and mitotic activity exceeding 10 mitoses/2 mm^2 are not uncommon in metastatic setting, and such tumors often exhibit Ki-67 proliferative index of >20% (Fig. 3d, e). While they likely correspond to G3 tumors in the GI/pancreas neuroendocrine neoplasm classification, they are classified as LCENC with the current WHO classification (WHO Classification of Tumours Editorial Board 2021). Thus, future work is warranted to determine how to fit these tumors into the classification and address the predictive and/or prognostic roles of Ki-67 proliferative index in pulmonary neuroendocrine neoplasms (Pelosi et al. 2014).

7 Molecular Diagnostics in NSCLC and Triage of Limited Tissue Samples for Comprehensive Diagnosis

Treatment for patients with advanced NSCLC has expanded to include histology-based chemotherapy, targeted therapy, and immunotherapy in the past two decades. Similarly, molecular diagnostic testing has rapidly advanced in the past decade with the advent of new massively parallel sequencing technologies such as next-generation sequencing (Suster and Mino-Kenudson 2020). In 2013, the College of American Pathologists (CAP), IASLC, and the Association for Molecular Pathology (AMP) created a set of guidelines for the molecular testing of lung cancer specimens (Lindeman et al. 2013), which were updated in 2018 and then endorsed by the American Society of Clinical Oncology (ASCO) (Lindeman et al. 2018; Kalemkerian et al. 2018). The guidelines recommend that molecular testing be available at centers where patients with lung cancer are treated, and *EGFR*, *ALK*, and *ROS1* be tested on nonsquamous NSCLC as well as squamous cell carcinoma with clinical features suggesting the presence of an oncogenic driver mutation (young age and/or never or light smoking history). Testing for *BRAF, MET, RET, ERBB2 (HER2)*, and *KRAS* mutations should also be offered, if possible. The National Comprehensive Cancer Network (NCCN) recommends the similar approach for advanced or metastatic disease and also includes PD-L1 testing to guide potential immunotherapy (NCCN 2021b). In general, testing can be accomplished either as part of broad molecular profiling or with sequential testing using smaller panels (including smaller targeted sequencing assays, fluorescent in situ hybridization [FISH], and/or polymerase chain reaction-based assays). The broad molecular profiling can also identify uncommon alterations with available therapies, such as *NTRK* rearrangements. In addition, large panels can provide information on tumor mutational burden which is an emerging biomarker for immunotherapy (Alexander et al. 2018) as well as genetic alterations that may indicate resistance to a variety of therapies including *SKT11* and *KEAP1* mutations (Skoulidis et al. 2018; Sitthideatphaiboon et al. 2021; Shang et al. 2021). The advantage of smaller directed panels is a shorter turnaround time that allows for faster clinical decision-making (Evrard et al. 2019).

For advanced NSCLC, multiple modalities are required to achieve a comprehensive diagnosis including histological assessment, immunohistochemistry for histologic subtyping of NSCLC, NOS on morphology and that for predictive biomarkers (PD-L1 and ALK & ROS1) in an appropriate setting, as well as molecular testing. Given that small biopsy and/or cytology specimens may be only tissue samples available for these patients, specimen handling is of paramount importance. In addition, hydrochloric acid used in standard decalcification procedures degrades nucleic acids and prevents many types of molecular testing; thus, care should be taken when triaging material obtained from bone (Choi et al. 2015). If tissue is limited, the minimum panel of immunostains (p40 and TTF-1 ± Napsin A) ± a mucin stain should be used for the initial diagnosis, if needed, and the remaining tissue should be preserved for predictive biomarker immunohistochemistry and molecular testing (WHO Classification of Tumours Editorial Board 2021).

8 Pathology Assessment of Post-Neoadjuvant Resections for NSCLC

Neoadjuvant therapy has increasingly been used in the management of patients with resectable stage IB to IIIA NSCLC or under evaluation in clinical trials. Major pathologic response (MPR, defined as viable tumor cells occupying ≤10% of the pretreatment tumor area [tumor bed] in resection specimens) has been adopted as a surrogate biomarker for survival in neoadjuvant trials (Hellmann et al. 2014; Blumenthal et al. 2018), since radiographic imaging methods based on Response Evaluation Criteria in Solid Tumor (RECIST) have proven unreliable in predicting residual tumor viability after neoadjuvant therapy (Lee et al. 2010; William Jr. et al. 2013). Thus, it is important to standardize pathology assessments of post-neoadjuvant resections to achieve accurate and reproducible quantification of residual viable tumor. Unfortunately, however, there are no uniform approaches to specimen preparation, gross examination and sampling of pretreated tumors as well as the histologic assessment and calculation of residual viable tumor. Further, quantification of residual viable disease may require consideration of the type of treatment—chemotherapy ± radiation vs. immunotherapy vs. targeted therapy (Cottrell et al. 2018). In addition, cutoffs for MPR may be different between adenocarcinoma and squamous cell carcinoma (Qu et al. 2019; Zens et al. 2021). While these issues warrant further investigations, there are two commonly used recommendations for pathology assessment of NSCLC specimens resected after neoadjuvant chemotherapy ± radiation (Table 6) (Pataer et al. 2012; Travis et al. 2020). In accordance with both recommendations, necrosis (Fig. 4a, b), fibrosis (Fig. 4c), inflammation, and other stromal changes are considered response to neoadjuvant therapy and are excluded from residual tumor volume. Interestingly, therapy-related necrosis is strictly

Table 6 Summary of published recommendations for pathologic assessment of NSCLC resection specimens post-neoadjuvant chemotherapy ± radiation

Recommendation	Pataer et al. (2012)	Travis et al. (2020)
Composition of tumor bed (sum to 100%)	• RVT • Necrosis • Stromal tissue	• RVT • Necrosis • Stromal tissue
Mature fibrosis w/o evidence of "regression"	Part of stroma	Part of stroma
Specimen processing	At least 1 section per 1 cm; otherwise, not specified	A slab with the largest dimension of tumor bed entirely submitted + 1 section per 1 cm from the remaining tumor bed[a]
Sections to include for %RVT calculation	All sections from tumor bed of the primary tumor	All sections from tumor bed of the primary tumor
Calculation of final %RVT score for the primary tumor	Determined in each slide individually; then, averaged across slides w/ tumor	By summing RVT and tumor bed area across all slides w/ tumor
MPR	≤10% residual viable tumor	≤10% residual viable tumor
CR	0% residual viable tumor based on the assessment of the primary tumor	0% residual viable tumor including LNs
LN assessment	Not specified	The above method could be applied for LNs

NSCLC non-small cell carcinoma, IASLC International Association for the Study of Lung Cancer, RVT residual viable tumor, MPR major pathologic response, CR complete response, LN lymph node

[a] If the tumor is ≤3 cm, the tumor bed + adjacent nonneoplastic lung parenchyma is entirely submitted

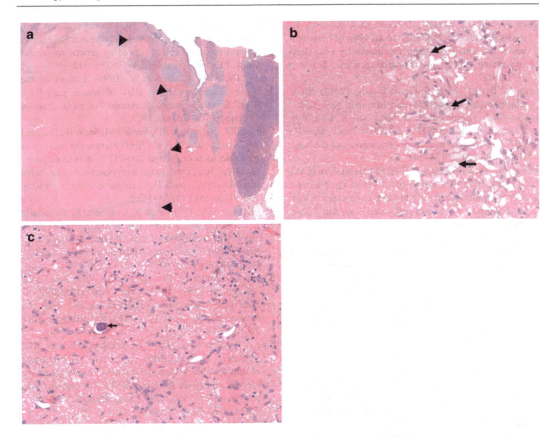

Fig. 4 (**a, b**) A case with biopsy-proven lung adenocarcinoma with a metastasis to the adrenal gland treated with neoadjuvant chemotherapy (2 cycle of cisplatin and pemetrexed). Preoperative CT scan showed stable disease in both the lung and adrenal gland, but only a large necrotic tumor (arrow heads) was identified in a lobectomy specimen (**a**: Hematoxylin & Eosin stain ×20). A high-power view reveals macrophages with foamy cytoplasm surrounding the necrotic mass (arrows), but viable tumor cells are not identified (**b**: Hematoxylin & Eosin stain ×400). The adrenal gland also showed a lesion completely replaced by fibrosis (pCR). (**c**) An example of biopsy-proven lung squamous cell carcinoma treated with neoadjuvant chemotherapy + radiation. The tumor bed only shows fibroelastosis with scattered calcifications (arrow) and no viable tumor cells (pathologic complete response) (Hematoxylin & Eosin stain ×400)

defined in the recommendation by Pataer et al., but not in the IASLC recommendation (Travis et al. 2021; Weissferdt et al. 2020). Further, % residual tumor volume (%RTV) is calculated in each section from tumor bed and results of all sections are averaged together to determined mean value for %RTV in the former, while %RTV is measured collectively in all sections from tumor bed in the latter (Pataer et al. 2012; Travis et al. 2020). It is important to note that MPR has been correlated with longer OS and DFS in studies applying the Pataer's recommendation that has also been shown to have a high interobserver agreement between two observers, while correlation of MPR with patient outcomes and interobserver agreements need to be confirmed in the ongoing and/or future studies following the IASLC recommendation (Pataer et al. 2012; Travis et al. 2020; Weissferdt et al. 2020, 2021).

References

Alexander M, Galeas J, Cheng H (2018) Tumor mutation burden in lung cancer: a new predictive biomarker for immunotherapy or too soon to tell? J Thorac Dis 10(Suppl 33):S3994–S3998

Amer W, Toth C, Vassella E, Meinrath J, Koitzsch U, Arens A et al (2017) Evolution analysis of heterogeneous non-small cell lung carcinoma by ultra-deep sequencing of the mitochondrial genome. Sci Rep 7(1):11069

Amin M, Byrd D, Edge S, Green F (eds) (2017) AJCC cancer staging manual, 8th edn. Springer, New York

Beasley MB, Lantuejoul S, Abbondanzo S, Chu WS, Hasleton PS, Travis WD et al (2003) The P16/cyclin D1/Rb pathway in neuroendocrine tumors of the lung. Hum Pathol 34(2):136–142

Bishop JA, Ogawa T, Chang X, Illei PB, Gabrielson E, Pai SI et al (2012) HPV analysis in distinguishing second primary tumors from lung metastases in patients with head and neck squamous cell carcinoma. Am J Surg Pathol 36(1):142–148

Blumenthal GM, Bunn PA Jr, Chaft JE, McCoach CE, Perez EA, Scagliotti GV et al (2018) Current status and future perspectives on neoadjuvant therapy in lung cancer. J Thorac Oncol 13(12):1818–1831

Brambilla E, Moro D, Veale D, Brichon PY, Stoebner P, Paramelle B et al (1992) Basal cell (basaloid) carcinoma of the lung: a new morphologic and phenotypic entity with separate prognostic significance. Hum Pathol 23(9):993–1003

Brambilla E, Lantuejoul S, Butnor KJ, Caporaso NE, Chen G, Chou TY et al (2015a) Basaloid squamous cell carcinoma. In: Travis WD, Brambilla E, Burke AP, Marx A, Nicholson AG (eds) WHO classification of tumours of the lung, pleura, thymus and heart. IARC Press, Lyon, France, pp 56–58

Brambilla E, Beasley MB, Austin JHM, Capelozzi VL, Chirieac LR, Devesa SS et al (2015b) Small cell carcinoma. In: Travis WD, Brambilla E, Burke AP, Marx A, Nicholson AG (eds) WHO classification of tumours of the lung, pleura, thymus and heart. IARC Press, Lyon, France, pp 63–68

Cardarella S, Ortiz TM, Joshi VA, Butaney M, Jackman DM, Kwiatkowski DJ et al (2012) The introduction of systematic genomic testing for patients with non-small-cell lung cancer. J Thorac Oncol 7(12):1767–1774

Cardesa A, Gal A, Nadal A (2005) Squamous cell carcinoma. In: Barnes L, Eveson JW, Reichart P (eds) WHO classification of tumours: head and neck tumours. IARC Press, Lyon, France, pp 118–121

Chan JKC, Bray F, McCarron PF (2005) Nasopharyngeal carcinoma. In: Barnes L, Eveson JW, Reichart P (eds) WHO classification of tumours: head and neck tumours. Lyon, France, IARC Press, pp 85–97

Chang SY, Keeney M, Law M, Donovan J, Aubry MC, Garcia J (2015) Detection of human papillomavirus in non-small cell carcinoma of the lung. Hum Pathol 46(11):1592–1597

Chang JC, Alex D, Bott M, Tan KS, Seshan V, Golden A et al (2019) Comprehensive next-generation sequencing unambiguously distinguishes separate primary lung carcinomas from intrapulmonary metastases: comparison with standard histopathologic approach. Clin Cancer Res 25(23):7113–7125

Choi SE, Hong SW, Yoon SO (2015) Proposal of an appropriate decalcification method of bone marrow biopsy specimens in the era of expanding genetic molecular study. J Pathol Transl Med 49(3):236–242

Colby TV, Koss M, Travis W (1995) Tumors of the lower respiratory tract. atlas of tumor pathology, Third Series, Fascicle 13. Armed Forces Institute of Pathology, Washington, DC

Cottrell TR, Thompson ED, Forde PM, Stein JE, Duffield AS, Anagnostou V et al (2018) Pathologic features of response to neoadjuvant anti-PD-1 in resected non-small-cell lung carcinoma: a proposal for quantitative immune-related pathologic response criteria (irPRC). Ann Oncol 29(8):1853–1860

den Bakker MA, Willemsen S, Grunberg K, Noorduijn LA, van Oosterhout MF, van Suylen RJ et al (2010) Small cell carcinoma of the lung and large cell neuroendocrine carcinoma interobserver variability. Histopathology 56(3):356–363

Eguchi T, Kadota K, Park BJ, Travis WD, Jones DR, Adusumilli PS (2014) The new IASLC-ATS-ERS lung adenocarcinoma classification: what the surgeon should know. Semin Thorac Cardiovasc Surg 26(3):210–222

Emoto K, Eguchi T, Tan KS, Takahashi Y, Aly RG, Rekhtman N et al (2019) Expansion of the concept of micropapillary adenocarcinoma to include a newly recognized filigree pattern as well as the classical pattern based on 1468 stage I lung adenocarcinomas. J Thorac Oncol 14(11):1948–1961

Evrard SM, Taranchon-Clermont E, Rouquette I, Murray S, Dintner S, Nam-Apostolopoulos YC et al (2019) Multicenter evaluation of the fully automated PCR-based Idylla EGFR mutation assay on formalin-fixed, paraffin-embedded tissue of human lung cancer. J Mol Diagn 21(6):1010–1024

Fallet V, Saffroy R, Girard N, Mazieres J, Lantuejoul S, Vieira T et al (2015) High-throughput somatic mutation profiling in pulmonary sarcomatoid carcinomas using the LungCarta Panel: exploring therapeutic targets. Ann Oncol 26(8):1748–1753

Fernandez-Cuesta L, Peifer M, Lu X, Sun R, Ozretic L, Seidel D et al (2014) Frequent mutations in chromatin-remodelling genes in pulmonary carcinoids. Nat Commun 5:3518

French CA (2012) Pathogenesis of NUT midline carcinoma. Annu Rev Pathol 7:247–265

Funai K, Yokose T, Ishii G, Araki K, Yoshida J, Nishimura M et al (2003) Clinicopathologic characteristics of peripheral squamous cell carcinoma of the lung. Am J Surg Pathol 27(7):978–984

Geles A, Gruber-Moesenbacher U, Quehenberger F, Manzl C, Al Effah M, Grygar E et al (2015) Pulmonary mucinous adenocarcinomas: architectural patterns in correlation with genetic changes, prognosis and survival. Virchows Arch 467(6):675–686

George J, Lim JS, Jang SJ, Cun Y, Ozretic L, Kong G et al (2015) Comprehensive genomic profiles of small cell lung cancer. Nature 524(7563):47–53

Hellmann MD, Chaft JE, William WN Jr, Rusch V, Pisters KM, Kalhor N et al (2014) Pathological response after neoadjuvant chemotherapy in resectable non-small-cell lung cancers: proposal for the use of major pathological response as a surrogate endpoint. Lancet Oncol 15(1):e42–e50

Hwang I, Park KU, Kwon KY (2014) Modified histologic classification as a prognostic factor in pulmonary adenocarcinoma. Int J Surg Pathol 22(3): 212–220

Ionescu DN, Treaba D, Gilks CB, Leung S, Renouf D, Laskin J et al (2007) Nonsmall cell lung carcinoma with neuroendocrine differentiation—an entity of no clinical or prognostic significance. Am J Surg Pathol 31(1):26–32

Kadota K, Nitadori J, Woo KM, Sima CS, Finley DJ, Rusch VW et al (2014) Comprehensive pathological analyses in lung squamous cell carcinoma: single cell invasion, nuclear diameter, and tumor budding are independent prognostic factors for worse outcomes. J Thorac Oncol 9(8):1126–1139

Kalemkerian GP, Narula N, Kennedy EB, Biermann WA, Donington J, Leighl NB et al (2018) Molecular testing guideline for the selection of patients with lung cancer for treatment with targeted tyrosine kinase inhibitors: American Society of Clinical Oncology endorsement of the College of American Pathologists/International Association for the Study of Lung Cancer/Association for Molecular Pathology Clinical Practice Guideline Update. J Clin Oncol 36(9):911–919

Kaufmann O, Dietel M (2000) Expression of thyroid transcription factor-1 in pulmonary and extrapulmonary small cell carcinomas and other neuroendocrine carcinomas of various primary sites. Histopathology 36(5):415–420

Kriegsmann K, Zgorzelski C, Kazdal D, Cremer M, Muley T, Winter H et al (2020) Insulinoma-associated protein 1 (INSM1) in thoracic tumors is less sensitive but more specific compared with synaptophysin, chromogranin A, and CD56. Appl Immunohistochem Mol Morphol 28(3):237–242

Kwon D, Koh J, Kim S, Go H, Kim YA, Keam B et al (2017) MET exon 14 skipping mutation in triple-negative pulmonary adenocarcinomas and pleomorphic carcinomas: an analysis of intratumoral MET status heterogeneity and clinicopathological characteristics. Lung Cancer 106:131–137

Lee HY, Lee KS, Hwang HS, Lee JW, Ahn MJ, Park K et al (2010) Molecularly targeted therapy using bevacizumab for non-small cell lung cancer: a pilot study for the new CT response criteria. Korean J Radiol 11(6):618–626

Lee G, Lee HY, Jeong JY, Han J, Cha MJ, Lee KS et al (2015) Clinical impact of minimal micropapillary pattern in invasive lung adenocarcinoma: prognostic significance and survival outcomes. Am J Surg Pathol 39(5):660–666

Lindeman NI, Cagle PT, Beasley MB, Chitale DA, Dacic S, Giaccone G et al (2013) Molecular testing guideline for selection of lung cancer patients for EGFR and ALK tyrosine kinase inhibitors: guideline from the College of American Pathologists, International Association for the Study of Lung Cancer, and Association for Molecular Pathology. J Thorac Oncol 8(7):823–859

Lindeman NI, Cagle PT, Aisner DL, Arcila ME, Beasley MB, Bernicker EH et al (2018) Updated molecular testing guideline for the selection of lung cancer patients for treatment with targeted tyrosine kinase inhibitors: guideline from the College of American Pathologists, the International Association for the Study of Lung Cancer, and the Association for Molecular Pathology. J Thorac Oncol 13(3):323–358

Liu X, Jia Y, Stoopler MB, Shen Y, Cheng H, Chen J et al (2016) Next-generation sequencing of pulmonary sarcomatoid carcinoma reveals high frequency of actionable MET gene mutations. J Clin Oncol 34(8): 794–802

Lococo F, Torricelli F, Rossi G, Alifano M, Damotte D, Rapicetta C et al (2017) Inter-relationship between PD-L1 expression and clinic-pathological features and driver gene mutations in pulmonary sarcomatoid carcinomas. Lung Cancer 113:93–101

Marchevsky AM, Walts AE (2015) Diffuse idiopathic pulmonary neuroendocrine cell hyperplasia (DIPNECH). Semin Diagn Pathol 32(6):438–444

Marchevsky AM, Gal AA, Shah S, Koss MN (2001) Morphometry confirms the presence of considerable nuclear size overlap between "small cells" and "large cells" in high-grade pulmonary neuroendocrine neoplasms. Am J Clin Pathol 116(4):466–472

Marchio C, Gatti G, Massa F, Bertero L, Filosso P, Pelosi G et al (2017) Distinctive pathological and clinical features of lung carcinoids with high proliferation index. Virchows Arch 471(6):713–720

Martin LW, Correa AM, Ordonez NG, Roth JA, Swisher SG, Vaporciyan AA et al (2007) Sarcomatoid carcinoma of the lung: a predictor of poor prognosis. Ann Thorac Surg 84(3):973–980

Matoso A, Singh K, Jacob R, Greaves WO, Tavares R, Noble L et al (2010) Comparison of thyroid transcription factor-1 expression by 2 monoclonal antibodies in pulmonary and nonpulmonary primary tumors. Appl Immunohistochem Mol Morphol 18(2):142–149

Mino-Kenudson M (2020) Significance of tumor spread through air spaces (STAS) in lung cancer from the pathologist perspective. Transl Lung Cancer Res 9(3):847–859

Moreira AL, Joubert P, Downey RJ, Rekhtman N (2014) Cribriform and fused glands are patterns of high-grade pulmonary adenocarcinoma. Hum Pathol 45(2):213–220

Moreira AL, Ocampo PSS, Xia Y, Zhong H, Russell PA, Minami Y et al (2020) A grading system for invasive pulmonary adenocarcinoma: a proposal from the International Association for the Study of Lung Cancer Pathology Committee. J Thorac Oncol 15(10):1599–1610

Moro D, Brichon PY, Brambilla E, Veale D, Labat F, Brambilla C (1994) Basaloid bronchial carcinoma. A histologic group with a poor prognosis. Cancer 73(11):2734–2739

Moro-Sibilot D, Lantuejoul S, Diab S, Moulai N, Aubert A, Timsit JF et al (2008) Lung carcinomas with a basaloid pattern: a study of 90 cases focusing on their poor prognosis. Eur Respir J 31(4):854–859

Mukhopadhyay S, Dermawan JK, Lanigan CP, Farver CF (2019) Insulinoma-associated protein 1 (INSM1) is a sensitive and highly specific marker of neuroendocrine differentiation in primary lung neoplasms: an immunohistochemical study of 345 cases, including 292 whole-tissue sections. Mod Pathol 32(1): 100–109

Nakanishi K, Sakakura N, Matsui T, Ueno H, Nakada T, Oya Y et al (2019) Clinicopathological features, surgical outcomes, oncogenic status and PD-L1 expression of pulmonary pleomorphic carcinoma. Anticancer Res 39(10):5789–5795

NCCN (2021a) National Comprehensive Cancer Network guidelines. NCCN, Philadelphia

NCCN (2021b) National Comprehensive Cancer Network guidelines V. 2.2021

Nicholson AG, Torkko K, Viola P, Duhig E, Geisinger K, Borczuk AC et al (2018) Interobserver variation among pathologists and refinement of criteria in distinguishing separate primary tumors from intrapulmonary metastases in lung. J Thorac Oncol 13(2): 205–217

Ohe M, Yokose T, Sakuma Y, Miyagi Y, Okamoto N, Osanai S et al (2012) Stromal micropapillary component as a novel unfavorable prognostic factor of lung adenocarcinoma. Diagn Pathol 7:3

Onuki N, Wistuba II, Travis WD, Virmani AK, Yashima K, Brambilla E et al (1999) Genetic changes in the spectrum of neuroendocrine lung tumors. Cancer 85(3):600–607

Pan Y, Wang R, Ye T, Li C, Hu H, Yu Y et al (2014) Comprehensive analysis of oncogenic mutations in lung squamous cell carcinoma with minor glandular component. Chest 145(3):473–479

Pataer A, Kalhor N, Correa AM, Raso MG, Erasmus JJ, Kim ES et al (2012) Histopathologic response criteria predict survival of patients with resected lung cancer after neoadjuvant chemotherapy. J Thorac Oncol 7(5):825–832

Pelosi G, Rodriguez J, Viale G, Rosai J (2005) Typical and atypical pulmonary carcinoid tumor overdiagnosed as small-cell carcinoma on biopsy specimens: a major pitfall in the management of lung cancer patients. Am J Surg Pathol 29(2):179–187

Pelosi G, Rindi G, Travis WD, Papotti M (2014) Ki-67 antigen in lung neuroendocrine tumors: unraveling a role in clinical practice. J Thorac Oncol 9(3):273–284

Qu Y, Emoto K, Eguchi T, Aly RG, Zheng H, Chaft JE et al (2019) Pathologic assessment after neoadjuvant chemotherapy for NSCLC: importance and implications of distinguishing adenocarcinoma from squamous cell carcinoma. J Thorac Oncol 14(3):482–493

Rekhtman N, Paik PK, Arcila ME, Tafe LJ, Oxnard GR, Moreira AL et al (2012) Clarifying the spectrum of driver oncogene mutations in biomarker-verified squamous carcinoma of lung: lack of EGFR/KRAS and presence of PIK3CA/AKT1 mutations. Clin Cancer Res 18(4):1167–1176

Rekhtman N, Pietanza MC, Hellmann MD, Naidoo J, Arora A, Won H et al (2016) Next-generation sequencing of pulmonary large cell neuroendocrine carcinoma reveals small cell carcinoma-like and non-small cell carcinoma-like subsets. Clin Cancer Res 22(14):3618–3629

Schrock AB, Li SD, Frampton GM, Suh J, Braun E, Mehra R et al (2017) Pulmonary sarcomatoid carcinomas commonly harbor either potentially targetable genomic alterations or high tumor mutational burden as observed by comprehensive genomic profiling. J Thorac Oncol 12(6):932–942

Shang X, Li Z, Sun J, Zhao C, Lin J, Wang H (2021) Survival analysis for non-squamous NSCLC patients harbored STK11 or KEAP1 mutation receiving atezolizumab. Lung Cancer 154:105–112

Shih AR, Mino-Kenudson M (2020) Updates on spread through air spaces (STAS) in lung cancer. Histopathology 77(2):173–180

Shih AR, Uruga H, Bozkurtlar E, Chung JH, Hariri LP, Minami Y et al (2019) Problems in the reproducibility of classification of small lung adenocarcinoma: an international interobserver study. Histopathology 75(5):649–659

Sitthideatphaiboon P, Galan-Cobo A, Negrao MV, Qu X, Poteete A, Zhang F et al (2021) STK1/LKB1 mutations in NSCLC are associated with KEAP1/NRF2-dependent radiotherapy resistance targetable by glutaminase inhibition. Clin Cancer Res 27(6):1720–1733

Skoulidis F, Goldberg ME, Greenawalt DM, Hellmann MD, Awad MM, Gainor JF et al (2018) STK11/LKB1 mutations and PD-1 inhibitor resistance in KRAS-mutant lung adenocarcinoma. Cancer Discov 8(7):822–835

Sobin L, Gospodarowicz M, Wittekind C (eds) (2017) TNM classification malignant tumours, 8th edn. Wiley-Blackwell, Oxford

Sterlacci W, Fiegl M, Hilbe W, Auberger J, Mikuz G, Tzankov A (2009) Clinical relevance of neuroendocrine differentiation in non-small cell lung cancer assessed by immunohistochemistry: a retrospective study on 405 surgically resected cases. Virchows Arch 455(2):125–132

Suster DI, Mino-Kenudson M (2020) Molecular pathology of primary non-small cell lung cancer. Arch Med Res 51(8):784–798

Swarts DR, Rudelius M, Claessen SM, Cleutjens JP, Seidl S, Volante M et al (2017) Limited additive value of the Ki-67 proliferative index on patient survival in World Health Organization-classified pulmonary carcinoids. Histopathology 70(3):412–422

Terra SB, Jang JS, Bi L, Kipp BR, Jen J, Yi ES et al (2016) Molecular characterization of pulmonary sarcomatoid carcinoma: analysis of 33 cases. Mod Pathol 29(8):824–831

Thunnissen E, Beasley MB, Borczuk AC, Brambilla E, Chirieac LR, Dacic S et al (2012) Reproducibility of histopathological subtypes and invasion in pulmonary adenocarcinoma. An international interobserver study. Mod Pathol 25(12):1574–1583

Thunnissen E, Noguchi M, Aisner S, Beasley MB, Brambilla E, Chirieac LR et al (2014) Reproducibility of histopathological diagnosis in poorly differentiated NSCLC: an international multiobserver study. J Thorac Oncol 9(9):1354–1362

Travis WD, Muller-Hermelink HK, Harris CC, Hammar SP, Brambilla C, Pugatch B (2004) WHO tumours pathology and genetics of tumours of the lung, pleura, thymus and heart, 3rd edn. IARC Press, Lyon, France

Travis WD, Brambilla E, Noguchi M, Nicholson AG, Geisinger KR, Yatabe Y et al (2011) International Association for the Study of Lung Cancer/American Thoracic Society/European Respiratory Society International multidisciplinary classification of lung adenocarcinoma. J Thorac Oncol 6(2):244–285

Travis WD, Brambilla E, Burke AP, Marx A, Nicholson AG (2015) WHO classification of tumours of the lung, pleura, thymus and heart, 4th edn. IARC Press, Lyon, France

Travis WD, Asamura H, Bankier AA, Beasley MB, Detterbeck F, Flieder DB et al (2016) The IASLC Lung Cancer Staging Project: proposals for coding T categories for subsolid nodules and assessment of tumor size in part-solid tumors in the forthcoming eighth edition of the TNM classification of lung cancer. J Thorac Oncol 11(8):1204–1223

Travis WD, Dacic S, Wistuba I, Sholl L, Adusumilli P, Bubendorf L et al (2020) IASLC multidisciplinary recommendations for pathologic assessment of lung cancer resection specimens after neoadjuvant therapy. J Thorac Oncol 15(5):709–740

Travis WD, Dacic S, Sholl LM, Wistuba II (2021) Pathologic assessment of lung squamous cell carcinoma after neoadjuvant immunotherapy. J Thorac Oncol 16(1):e9–e10

Tsutani Y, Miyata Y, Mimae T, Kushitani K, Takeshima Y, Yoshimura M et al (2013) The prognostic role of pathologic invasive component size, excluding lepidic growth, in stage I lung adenocarcinoma. J Thorac Cardiovasc Surg 146(3):580–585

Vassella E, Langsch S, Dettmer MS, Schlup C, Neuenschwander M, Frattini M et al (2015) Molecular profiling of lung adenosquamous carcinoma: hybrid or genuine type? Oncotarget 6(27):23905–23916

Wang R, Pan Y, Li C, Zhang H, Garfield D, Li Y et al (2014) Analysis of major known driver mutations and prognosis in resected adenosquamous lung carcinomas. J Thorac Oncol 9(6):760–768

Warth A, Muley T, Harms A, Hoffmann H, Dienemann H, Schirmacher P et al (2016) Clinical relevance of different papillary growth patterns of pulmonary adenocarcinoma. Am J Surg Pathol 40(6):818–826

Weichert W, Schewe C, Denkert C, Morawietz L, Dietel M, Petersen I (2009) Molecular HPV typing as a diagnostic tool to discriminate primary from metastatic squamous cell carcinoma of the lung. Am J Surg Pathol 33(4):513–520

Weissferdt A, Pataer A, Vaporciyan AA, Correa AM, Sepesi B, Moran CA et al (2020) Agreement on major pathological response in NSCLC patients receiving neoadjuvant chemotherapy. Clin Lung Cancer 21(4):341–348

Weissferdt A, Pataer A, Swisher SG, Heymach JV, Gibbons DL, Cascone T et al (2021) Controversies and challenges in the pathologic examination of lung resection specimens after neoadjuvant treatment. Lung Cancer 154:76–83

WHO Classification of Tumours Editorial Board (2021) Thoracic tumours, WHO classification of tumours series, vol 5, 5th edn. IARC Press, Lyon, France

William WN Jr, Pataer A, Kalhor N, Correa AM, Rice DC, Wistuba II et al (2013) Computed tomography RECIST assessment of histopathologic response and prediction of survival in patients with resectable non-small-cell lung cancer after neoadjuvant chemotherapy. J Thorac Oncol 8(2):222–228

Yanagawa N, Wang A, Kohler D, Santos Gda C, Sykes J, Xu J et al (2013) Human papilloma virus genome is rare in North American non-small cell lung carcinoma patients. Lung Cancer 79(3):215–220

Yatabe Y, Dacic S, Borczuk AC, Warth A, Russell PA, Lantuejoul S et al (2019) Best practices recommendations for diagnostic immunohistochemistry in lung cancer. J Thorac Oncol 14(3):377–407

Yatabe Y, Borczuk A, Cooper W, Dacic S, Kerr K, Moreira A et al (eds) (2020) IASLC atlas of diagnostic immunohistochemistry. IASLC, Denver, CO

Yendamuri S, Caty L, Pine M, Adem S, Bogner P, Miller A et al (2012) Outcomes of sarcomatoid carcinoma of the lung: a Surveillance, Epidemiology, and End Results Database analysis. Surgery 152(3):397–402

Zens P, Bello C, Scherz A, Koenigsdorf J, Pollinger A, Schmid RA et al (2021) A prognostic score for non-small cell lung cancer resected after neoadjuvant therapy in comparison with the tumor-node-metastases classification and major pathological response. Mod Pathol 34:1333–1344

Role of Radiologic Imaging in Lung Cancer

Salome Kukava and George Tsivtsivadze

Contents

1 Introduction, Technical Advances... 67
2 Diagnosis of Lung Cancer/Solitary Pulmonary Nodule... 68
3 T Staging/NSCLC... 71
4 N Staging/NSCLC... 72
5 M Staging/NSCLC... 75
6 CT in Treatment Response Assessment and Follow-Up of NSCLC... 78

References... 83

Abstract

Computed tomography (CT) of the chest is the cornerstone of the diagnosis and staging of lung cancer. The advantages of CT in imaging the thorax are its cross-sectional format, superior density resolution, and wide dynamic range. Today's CT scanners combine fast acquisition, fast data reconstruction, and very high spatial resolution. The aim of the current chapter is to review the role of contrast-enhanced MDCT in the diagnosis and staging of lung cancer and characterization of solitary pulmonary nodules.

Abbreviations

LLL   Left lower lobe
LUL   Left upper lobe
NSCLC   Non-small cell lung cancer
RECIST Response evaluation criteria in solid tumors
RLL   Right lower lobe
RML   Right middle lobe
RUL   Right upper lobe

1 Introduction, Technical Advances

Computed tomography (CT) of the chest is the cornerstone of the diagnosis and staging of lung cancer. CT was introduced in the 1970s of the twentieth century and has developed rapidly since its introduction. Basic components of a CT system consist of a gantry that contains the moving X-ray tube and detectors, a table supporting the patient, a computer, and a viewing console. The following CT systems can be distinguished: incremental or conventional CT, spiral or helical CT, and multidetector or multislice CT. MDCT is characterized by faster acquisition and high

S. Kukava (✉) · G. Tsivtsivadze
Department of Computed Tomography, Acad. F. Todua Clinic, Tbilisi, Georgia
e-mail: salome_kukava@yahoo.com; giacivciv@yahoo.com

spatial resolution. The advantages of CT in imaging the thorax are its cross-sectional format, superior density resolution, and wide dynamic range. Thus, the lung, soft tissue, and bone can be imaged in detail simultaneously with a single exposure. There have been important technical improvements like the development of spiral CT and MDCT. Today's CT scanners combine fast acquisition, fast data reconstruction, and very high spatial resolution.

2 Diagnosis of Lung Cancer/Solitary Pulmonary Nodule

The primary tumor can have a wide range of appearances on CT. NSCLCs can be centrally located masses invading the mediastinal structures or peripheral lesions invading the chest wall. Tumors can have smooth, lobulated, or irregular and spiculated margins. They can be totally solid or with central necrosis and cavitation. Sometimes tumor can present as a ground glass opacity or the combination of solid and ground glass opacities. Bronchoscopy or image-guided (CT-guided) biopsy is necessary to obtain the tissue sample and confirm the morphologic diagnosis.

Lung cancer can be incidentally detected in an asymptomatic patient. It is referred to as a solitary pulmonary nodule (SPN).

The NCCN guidelines recommend low-dose chest CT for screening of individuals with high risk of lung cancer (NCCN.org n.d.). The recommendations are based on a large, randomized trial—The National Lung Screening Trial (NLST). Total of 53,454 persons at high risk for lung cancer at 33 U.S. medical centers were enrolled in the study from August 2002 through April 2004. Participants randomly underwent three annual screenings with either low-dose CT (26,722 participants) or single-view PA chest radiography (26,732). The mortality decreased with low-dose CT (247 in the low-dose CT group vs. 309 deaths in the radiography group), representing a relative reduction in mortality of 20.0% (95% CI, 6.8–26.7; $p = 0.004$). Authors concluded that screening with the use of low-dose CT reduces mortality from lung cancer (National Cancer Institute (NCI) 2011).

Solitary pulmonary nodule is defined as a round opacity less than or equal to 3 cm, surrounded by a lung parenchyma, not associated with atelectasis, lymph node enlargement, pneumonia, and pleural effusion. The term "pulmonary mass" is used for lesions more than 3 cm, malignant probability of which is considerably higher (Erasmus et al. 2000a, b). Differential diagnoses of SPN on CT include neoplastic lesions (benign and malignant), inflammatory lesions (infectious and noninfectious), and vascular and congenital lesions (Table 1) (Erasmus et al. 2000a). SPNs can be completely solid or may contain component of ground glass attenuation, which are referred to as subsolid nodules (Erasmus et al. 2000a, b) (Figs. 1, 2, and 3).

While evaluating SPN, patient's risk factors, such as age, smoking history, family history of malignancy, and history of exposure to asbestos or radioactive material, must be taken into consideration. MDCT plays a pivotal role in evaluating morphologic characteristics and growth pattern of nodules on serial images. In order to minimize the radiation exposure of the patient, low-dose techniques have been recommended for surveillance of lung nodules. Morphologic characteristics of SPN on conventional imaging include size, growth, margins, location, calcification, attenuation, fat, air bronchogram, and cavitation (Erasmus et al. 2000a, b).

Typically, benign nodules have well-defined, smooth margins (Fig. 4), whereas malignant nodules have irregular, spiculated margins and a lobular contour (Fig. 5). Increase in the size of the nodule positively correlates with the likelihood of malignancy; however, a small nodule diameter does not exclude malignancy. Benign patterns of calcification include diffuse, central (a bull's-eye appearance), laminated, and popcorn. Diffuse, central, and laminated patterns are usually seen in granulomatous infections, but lung metastases from chondrosarcomas or osteosarcomas can also be associated with the same patterns of calcification (Fig. 6). Cavitation may occur in both infectious and inflammatory conditions, as well as in malignancies (Fig. 7). Smooth, thin walls are typically seen in

Table 1 Differential diagnosis for solitary pulmonary nodule

Malignant neoplasms	Bronchogenic carcinoma
	Carcinoid tumor
	Pulmonary lymphoma
	Pulmonary sarcoma
	Solitary metastases
Benign neoplasms	Hamartoma
	Adenoma
	Lipoma
Infectious inflammatory	Granuloma (tuberculous/fungal)
	Nocardia infection
	Round pneumonia
	Abscess
Noninfectious inflammatory	Rheumatoid arthritis
	Wegener's granulomatosis
	Sarcoidosis
Vascular	Arteriovenous malformation
	Infarction
	Hematoma
Congenital	Bronchial atresia
Miscellaneous	External object
	Pseudotumor
	Pleural thickening

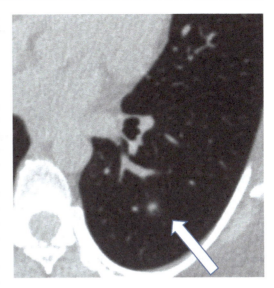

Fig. 2 Subsolid solitary pulmonary nodule in the LLL

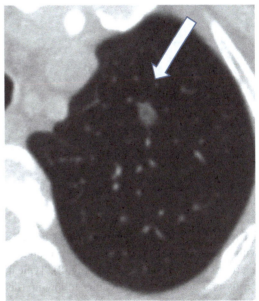

Fig. 3 8 mm Ground glass solitary pulmonary nodule in the LUL

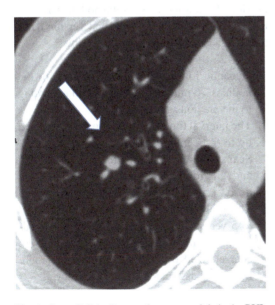

Fig. 1 8 mm Solid solitary pulmonary nodule in the RUL

benign lesions, whereas thick, irregular walls are seen in malignant lesions. Fat attenuation is seen in hamartomas. Enhancement pattern and increase of attenuation more than 20 HU after IV contrast administration is associated with malignancy. The radiological finding defined as air bronchogram is more frequently observed in malignant lung tumors than in benign nodules (Erasmus et al. 2000a, b).

Perifissural nodules are a separate entity and likely represent intrapulmonary lymph nodes. On

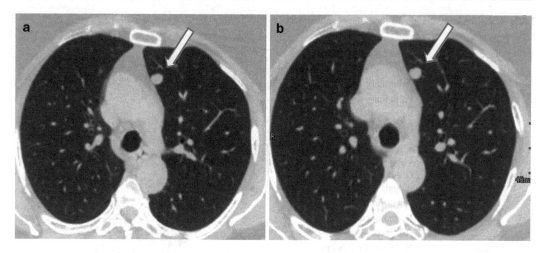

Fig. 4 10 mm Round nodule in the LUL, segment III, with smooth, sharp margins (**a**), remains stable over a year period (**b**)

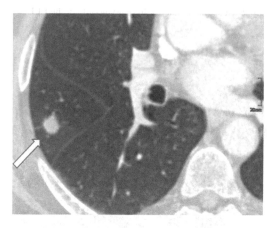

Fig. 5 15 mm Peripheral solid SPN with spiculated margins

CT images they are solid, homogeneous nodules with a smooth margin, can be oval or rounded, lentiform or triangular in shape (Fig. 8). Typical perifissural nodules do not require follow-up (de Hoop et al. 2012).

While addressing the measurement of the SPN, international guidelines recommend the measurements be obtained on the same transverse, coronal, or sagittal reconstructed image, whichever plane reveals the greatest dimensions. Manual 2D caliper measurements should be rounded to the nearest whole millimeter. In part-solid (subsolid) nodules both the total nodule and the solid component dimensions should be measured separately, both using the abovementioned averaging technique (Fig. 9).

Several international guidelines address the recommendations on the management of SPN. These include the Fleischner Society Guideline, Guideline from American College of Radiology (Lung RADS), and the British Thoracic Society Guideline (Callister et al. 2015), (Figs. 10, 11, and 12). Fleischner Society guidelines were first introduced in 2005. New version with introduction of a new term—subsolid nodule was published in 2013, and recent updated version dates to 2017. The basic changes are as follows:

1. Dynamic follow-up is recommended for the nodules >6 mm (instead of >4 mm according to the previous guidelines).
2. The interval time for follow-up was increased up to 6–12 months (instead of 3–6 months). Scans done within 3 months are not effective and are related to the excessive radiation dose.
3. The total time for follow-up was increased up to 5 years. This applies to the subsolid nodules, which according to various data are characterized by slow growth and are more frequently associated with malignancy.

In conclusion, 6 mm nodules in low-risk patients do not require follow-up; in high-risk patients the optimal time interval for follow-up is 12 months.

CT-guided needle biopsy is used to confirm the morphologic diagnosis, as CT provides a

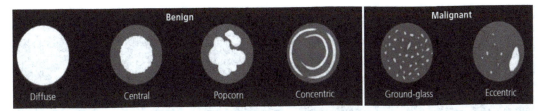

Fig. 6 Patterns of nodule calcification. (Am Fam Physician. Evaluation of the Solitary Pulmonary Nodule. 2015;92(12):1084–1091. 2015 American Academy of Family Physicians)

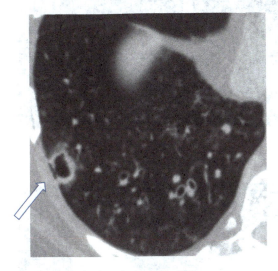

Fig. 7 20 mm Cavitary lesion in the RLL

good visualization of all thoracic structures. CT-guided biopsy is the procedure of choice for sampling peripheral nodules (<2 cm in diameter) as the yield for transbronchial needle biopsy, in the absence of an endobronchial lesion, is 50–80%. CT-guided biopsy has an accuracy for diagnosing malignancy of 80–95% (Klein et al. 1996; Salazar and Westcott 1993).

3 T Staging/NSCLC

CT with intravenous contrast is the imaging modality of choice for evaluating patients with lung cancer. Currently the lung cancer is staged according to eighth TNM developed by the International Association for the Study of Lung Cancer (IASLC), which used both retrospective and prospective clinical information for the creation of a large database of more than 100,000 patients. It describes the anatomic extent of the tumor by TNM system: T for characteristics of the primary tumor, N for nodal involvement, and M for (distant) metastasis (Detterbeck et al. 2017). The classification is used to discriminate patients that are appropriately treated in a certain way (Fig. 13).

MDCT has been the cornerstone of lung cancer staging, with MRI being superior for local staging of Pancoast tumor.

The T descriptor describes the local extent of tumor, involving the tumor size, invasion of adjacent structures, endobronchial location and distance from the carina, and presence of satellite nodules. CT scan is the most commonly used imaging modality for T staging. T1, T2, T3, and some T4 tumors are considered to be technically resectable. Invasion of the chest wall does not preclude surgical excision. An important role of CT is to help the surgeon to know preoperatively whether chest wall invasion is very likely. Obliteration of the extrapleural fat, great degree of pleural contact, and pleural thickening are signs that make pleural invasion very likely. It has also been reported that change in the relative location between the peripheral tumor and the chest wall with deep inspiration and expiration (respiratory shift at CT) indicates lack of parietal invasion. Mediastinal invasion is an important criterion in deciding resectability. Tumoral invasion of the mediastinal pleura and the fatty tissue is classified as stage T3 and it does not preclude resection; however, infiltration/gross invasion of the mediastinal great vessels with encasement, distortion of the vascular structures of the mediastinum, and invasion of esophagus, trachea, and vertebral body are staged as T4 and make the tumor unresectable (Purandare and Rangarajan 2015; Verschakelen et al. 2002) (Figs. 14, 15, 16, 17, and 18).

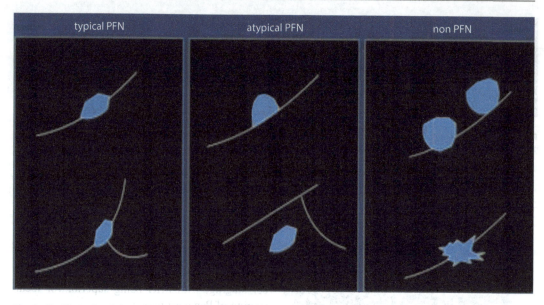

Fig. 8 Perifissural nodules. (Adapted from source de Hoop et al. 2012)

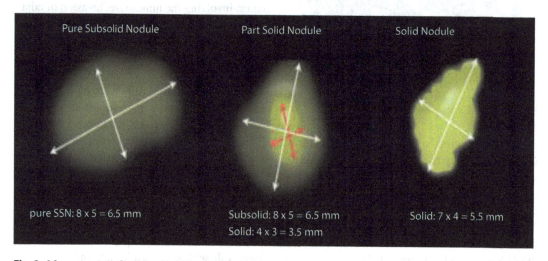

Fig. 9 Measurements of solid, subsolid, and ground glass nodules. (Adapted from source MacMahon et al. 2017)

4 N Staging/NSCLC

Accurate N staging is an important prognostic factor and is critical in deciding the treatment options. One system describing mediastinal lymph node map was proposed by the American Thoracic Society (ATS) surgeons using the Mountain–Dressler system (Fig. 19).

Hilar, interlobar, lobar, segmental, and subsegmental lymph nodes are referred as N1 disease. Ipsilateral mediastinal nodes are considered as N2 disease and it includes nodes in the upper paratracheal, prevascular, lower paratracheal, subcarinal, paraesophageal, and pulmonary ligament regions. Involvement of ipsilateral or contralateral supraclavicular lymph nodes or involvement of contralateral mediastinal, hilar/interlobar, or peripheral lymph nodes is classified as N3 disease. One of the important changes introduced in the new IASLC map is the shifting of boundary between the right and left sides of the mediastinum to the left lateral border of the trachea.

Fleischner Society 2017 Guidelines for Management of Incidentally Detected Pulmonary Nodules in Adults

A: Solid Nodules*

Nodule Type	<6 mm (<100 mm³)	6–8 mm (100–250 mm³)	>8 mm (>250 mm³)	Comments
Single				
Low risk†	No routine follow-up	CT at 6–12 months, then consider CT at 18–24 months	Consider CT at 3 months, PET/CT, or tissue sampling	Modules <6mm do not require follow-up in low-risk patients (recommendation 1A).
High risk†	Optional CT at 12 months	CT at 6–12 months, then CT at 18–24 months	Consider CT at 3 months, PET/CT, or tissue sampling	Certain patients at high risk with suspicious nodule morphology, upper lobe location, or both may warrant 12-month follow-up (recommendation 1A)
Multiple				
Low risk†	No routine follow-up	CT at 3–6 months, then consider CT at 18–24 months	CT at 3–6 months, then consider CT at 18–24 months	Use most suspicious nodule as guide to management. Follow-up intervals may vary according to size and risk (recommendation 2A).
High risk†	Optional CT at 12 months	CT at 3–6 months, then at 18–24 months	CT at 3–6 months, then at 18–24 months	Use most suspicious nodule as guide to management. Follow-up intervals may vary according to size and risk (recommendation 2A).

Fig. 10 Guidelines for management of incidental pulmonary nodules detected on CT images. (From the Fleischner Society 2017; Radiology: Volume 284: Number 1—July 2017 source MacMahon et al. 2017)

Fleischner Society 2017 Guidelines for Management of Incidentally Detected Pulmonary Nodules in Adults

B: Subsolid Nodules*

Nodule Type	<6 mm (<100 mm³)	≥6 mm (>100 mm³)	Comments
Single			
Ground glass	No routine follow-up	CT at 6–12 months to confirm persistance, then CT every 2 years until 5 years	In certain suspicious nodules <6 mm, consider follow-up at 2 and 4 years. If solid component(s) or growth develops, consider resection. (Recommendations 3A and 4A).
Part solid	No routine follow-up	CT at 3–6 months to confrim persistance. If unchanged and solid component remains <6mm, annual CT should be performed for 5 years.	In practice, part-solid nodules cannot be defined as such until ≥6mm, and nodules <6mm do not usually require follow-up. Persistent part-solid nodules with solid components ≥6 mm should be considered highly suspicious (recommendations 4A-4C)
Multiple	CT at 3–6 months, If stable, consider CT at 2 and 4 years.	CT at 3–6 months. Subsequent management based on the most suspicious nodule(s).	Multiple <6mm pure ground-glass nodules are usually benign, but consider follow-up in selected patients at high risk at 2 and 4 years (recommendation 5A).

Fig. 11 Guidelines for management of incidental pulmonary nodules detected on CT images. (From the Fleischner Society 2017; Radiology: Volume 284: Number 1—July 2017 source MacMahon et al. 2017)

Category Descriptor	Lung-RADS Score	Findings	Management	Risk of Malignancy	Est Population Prevalence
Incomplete	0	Prior chest CT examination(s) being located for comparison	Additional lung cancer screening CT images and/or comparison to prior chest CT examinations is needed	n/a	1%
		Part or all of lungs cannot be evaluated			
Negative — No nodules and definitely benign nodules	1	No lung nodules	Continue annual screening with LDCT in 12 months	< 1%	90%
		Nodule(s) with specific calcifications: completed, central, popcorn, concentric rings and fat containing nodules			
Benign Appearance or Behavior — Nodules with a very low likelihood of becoming a clinically active cancer due to size or lack of growth	2	Perifissural nodule(s): *(See Footnote 11)* < 10 mm (524 mm^3)			
		Solid nodule(s): < 6 mm (< 113 mm^3) new < 4 mm (< 34 mm^3)			
		Part solid nodule(s): < 6 mm total diametere (< 113 mm^3) on baseline screening			
		Non solid nodule(s) (GGN): <30mm (< 14137 mm^3) OR ≥ 30 mm (≥ 14137 mm^3) and unchanges or slowly growing			
		Category 3 or 4 nodules unchanged for ≥ 3 months			
Probably Benign — Probably benign finding(s) - short trrm follow up suggested; includes nodules with a low likelihood of becoming a clinically active cancer	3	Solid nodule(s): ≥ 6 to < 8 mm (≥ 113 to < 268 mm^3) at baseline OR new 4 mm to < 8 mm (34 to < 113 mm^3)	6 month LDCT	1-2%	5%
		Part solid nodule(s): ≥ 6 mm total diameter (≥ 113 mm^3) with solid component < 6 mm (< 113 mm^3) OR new < 6 mm total diameter (< 113 mm^3)			
		Non solid nodule(s): (GGN) ≥ 30 mm (≥ 14137 mm^3) on baseline CT or new			
Suspicious — Findings for which additional diagnostic testing is recommended	4A	Solid nodule(s): ≥ 8 to < 15 mm (≥ 268 to < 1767 mm^3) at baseline OR growing < 8 mm (< 268 mm^3) OR new 6 to < 8 mm (113 to < 268 mm^3)	3 month LDCT; PET/CT may be used when there is a ≥ 8 mm (≥ 268 mm^3) solid component	5-15%	2%
		Part solid nodule(s): ≥ 6 mm (≥ 113 mm^3) with solid component ≥ 6mm to < 8mm (≥ 113 to <268mm^3) OR with a new or growing < 4 mm (< 34 mm^3) solid component			
		Endobronchial nodule			
Very Suspicious — Findings for which additional diagnostic testing and/or tissue sampling is recommended	4B	Solid nodule(s) ≥ 15 mm (≥ 1767 mm^3) OR new or growing, and ≥8mm (≥ 268 mm^3)	Chest CT with or without contrast, PET/CT and/or tissue sampling depending on the *probability of malignancy and comorbidities. PET/CT may be used when there is a ≥ 8 mm (≥ 268 mm^3) solid component. For new large nodules that develop on an annual repeat screening CT, a 1 month LDCT may be recommended to address potentially infectious or inflammatory conditions	> 15%	2%
		Part solid nodule(s) with: a solid component ≥ 8mm (≥ 268 mm^3) OR a new or growing ≥4 mm (≥ 34 mm^3) solid component			
	4X	Category 3 or 4 nodules with additional features or imaging findings that increases the suspicion of malignancy			
Other — Clinically Significant or Potentially Clinically Significant Findings (non lung cancer)	S	Modifier - may add on to category 0-4 coding	As appropriate to the specific finding	n/a	10%

Fig. 12 Lung CT Screening Reporting and Data System (Lung-RADS); American college of radiology

The presence of mediastinal lymphadenopathy is crucial in evaluating the resectability of the disease. N1 and N2 disease may be resectable (usually after induction chemotherapy); however, N3 disease is considered to be inoperable. Size of the lymph node is the criterion used on CT scan to differentiate between benign and malignant nodes. A node with short axis diameter of more than 1 cm is generally considered to be malignant. The use of size cutoff, however, can be erroneous, as enlarged

TNM 7th EDITION	TNM 8th EDITION
T	
-	Tis
-	Tmi
-	Tss
T1a (≤2 cm)	T1a (≤1 cm)
T1b (>2-3 cm)	T1b (>1-2 cm)
	T1c (>2-3 cm)
T2a (>3-5 cm)	T2a (>3cm but ≤4cm)
T2b (>5-7 cm)	T2b (>4cm but ≤5cm)
T3 (>7 cm)	T4
T3 - atelectasis/pneumonitis involving whole lung)	T2 atelectasis/pneumonitis irrespective of involving lobe or whole lung
T3 tumor involving the main bronchus <2cm distance to carina	T2 -tumor involving the main bronchus irrespective of distance to carina
T3 -invasion of the diaphragm	T4 (invasion of the diaphragm)
N No changes	
M M1b - distant metastasis	M1b - single extrathoracic metastasis
	M1c - multiple extrathoracic metastasis

Fig. 13 Changes in the eighth edition of TNM classification of lung cancer. (Source: Radiologyassistant.nl)

inflammatory nodes will be called malignant and small cancerous nodes will be called benign. Results are worse in those populations where granulomatous diseases, such as histoplasmosis, tuberculosis, or fungal diseases, are endemic. Results are also worse in tumors such as adenocarcinomas or undifferentiated tumors, which are more aggressive and more likely to harbor microscopic metastasis. Generally, the false-negative rate of CT increases with higher T-status and is also higher in adenocarcinoma compared with squamous cell carcinoma (Purandare and Rangarajan 2015; Verschakelen et al. 2002). According to the two meta-analyses the CT has combined sensitivity of 60–83%, specificity of 77–82%, and accuracy of 75–80% for mediastinal staging (Dales et al. 1990; Dwamena et al. 1999) (Figs. 20, 21, 22, and 23).

5 M Staging/NSCLC

Most common sites for distant metastasis of lung cancer are the adrenal glands, liver, bones, and brain. According to the current TNM system, metastatic disease is classified as M1a or intrathoracic metastasis (malignant pleural effusion, pleural metastases, pericardial disease, and pulmonary nodules in the contralateral lung), M1b (single extrathoracic metastasis, including single nonregional lymph node), and M1c or extrathoracic metastasis (multiple metastasis in one or

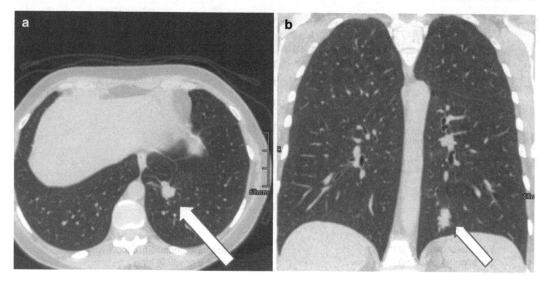

Fig.14 (a) 20 mm Solid tumor with irregular spiculated margins in the posterior basal segment of LLL. (b) Coronal reconstruction at the same level (T1 peripheral tumor)

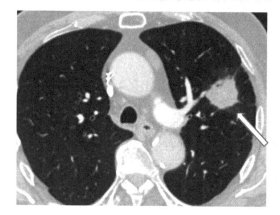

Fig. 15 36 mm LUL soft tissue mass with irregular, spiculated margins (T2 peripheral tumor)

more organs). CT is a valuable tool to assess thoracic as well as extrathoracic sites. Sider et al. demonstrated CT evidence of extrathoracic tumor spread in 24 of 95 (25%) patients with newly diagnosed non-small cell lung cancer and N0 disease at thoracic CT. These included metastases to the brain, bone, liver, adrenals, and soft tissue (Sider and Horejs 1988). Intrathoracic metastases can be detected on CT scan with a high degree of accuracy.

CT compared to ultrasound better demonstrates hepatic regions that are difficult to assess with US and can distinguish more accurately between metastatic disease and benign lesions. Contrast-enhanced CT allows contrasts dynamics in the liver to be optimized and spiral CT has increased ability to detect hepatic metastases (Yeh and Rabinowitz 1980).

CT examination used for staging of bronchogenic carcinoma should include the upper abdomen to evaluate the adrenal glands as they are a frequent site of metastasis and if solitary resection of isolated adrenal metastasis in an otherwise operable lung cancer improves survival (Sider and Horejs 1988). However, not infrequently, adrenal masses identified on CT in patients with lung carcinoma are adenomas (Porte et al. 2001). Most incidental nonfunctioning adenomas are <3 cm in diameter and of homogenous low attenuation (<10 HU on non-contrast-enhanced images), because of their fat content. Adrenal nodules with HU value of <10 on an unenhanced CT scan are suggestive of an adenoma with a high specificity (96–100%). When adrenal lesions do not meet these criteria, non-contrast-enhanced, contrast-enhanced, and delay CT images are necessary. Dynamic contrast-enhanced CT scan showing absolute contrast washout >60% and relative washout >40% on delayed imaging is indicative of an adenoma. For indeterminate adrenal lesions in

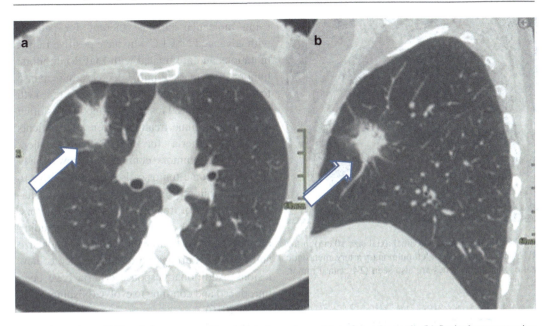

Fig. 16 (a) 40 mm RUL soft tissue mass with spiculated margins and transfissural growth. (b) Sagittal reconstruction at the same level demonstrates transfissural growth through the minor fissure

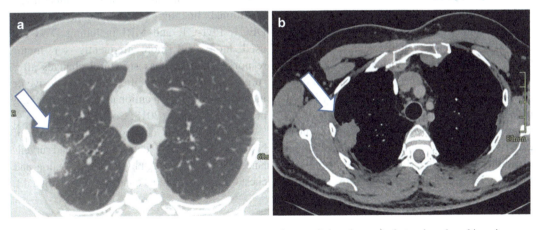

Fig. 17 (a) 40 mm RUL peripheral mass with broad base toward costal pleura. (b) Mediastinal window at the same level shows obliteration of the extrapleural fat, great degree of pleural contact that makes pleural invasion very likely (T3 peripheral tumor)

patients with known malignancy PET/CT, biopsy or resection is necessary (Oliver et al. 1984; Boland et al. 1998; Korobkin et al. 1996; Caoili et al. 2000; Mayo-Smith et al. 2017) (Figs. 24, 25, and 26).

HRCT (high-resolution computed tomography) is best at demonstrating lymphangitic carcinomatosis and malignant infiltration of the lymphatics and perilymphatic connective tissue. Typical finding is interlobular septal thickening, which is irregular and nodular (Fig. 27). Subpleural nodules, thickening of interlobar fissures, and pleural effusion may also be present.

MRI is considered to be superior to CT scan in the evaluation of brain metastases (Yokoi et al. 1999). It is the best imaging modality for identifying brain metastases, as well as liver and adrenal metastasis.

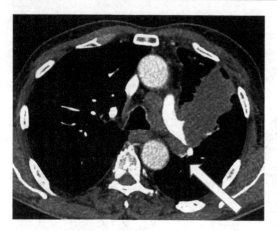

Fig. 18 A large tumor (maximal axial size 10 cm) in the RUL with encasement of left pulmonary artery, metastatic station 4L lymph nodes are also seen (T4 central tumor, N2 disease)

6 CT in Treatment Response Assessment and Follow-Up of NSCLC

After treatment of lung cancer, it is necessary to evaluate treatment response, detect residual tumor or recurrence, and further plan the correct strategy. In routine clinical practice and in clinical trials, lung cancer response to therapy is evaluated with unidimensional measurements by CT using RECIST 1.1. However, these morphological criteria have some limitations (measurement variability, tumor heterogeneity), especially in the era of targeted and immunotherapy. In case of using molecular targeted therapy for patients with advanced NSCLC who have positive EGFR mutations and are treated with EGFR inhibitors, tumors show marked initial decrease in response to therapy but subsequently demonstrate regrowth because of acquired resistance. Oncologists often decide to continue treatment even after patients meet the criteria for RECIST progression, because their tumors continue to grow slowly suggesting some tumor cells remain sensitive to EGFR inhibitors. Because of the unique mechanism of action of immune checkpoint inhibitors, atypical response patterns are noted, including response after an initial increase in tumor size and response during or after appearance of new lesions. Additional response criteria have been introduced and continue to evolve (Nishino 2018; Coche 2016).

Structural changes after surgery or radiotherapy often are inconclusive or indeterminate on conventional anatomic imaging modalities. Additional imaging biomarkers provided by DECT, PET-CT, and MRI including DWI are used more and more frequently for tumor response evaluation as structural changes after surgery or radiotherapy often are inconclusive or indeterminate on conventional anatomic imaging modalities (Nishino 2018; Coche 2016).

As recurrence is common after treatment of NSCLC, the NCCN guidelines recommend surveillance with history and physical examination and chest CT with or without contrast (NCCN.org n.d.).

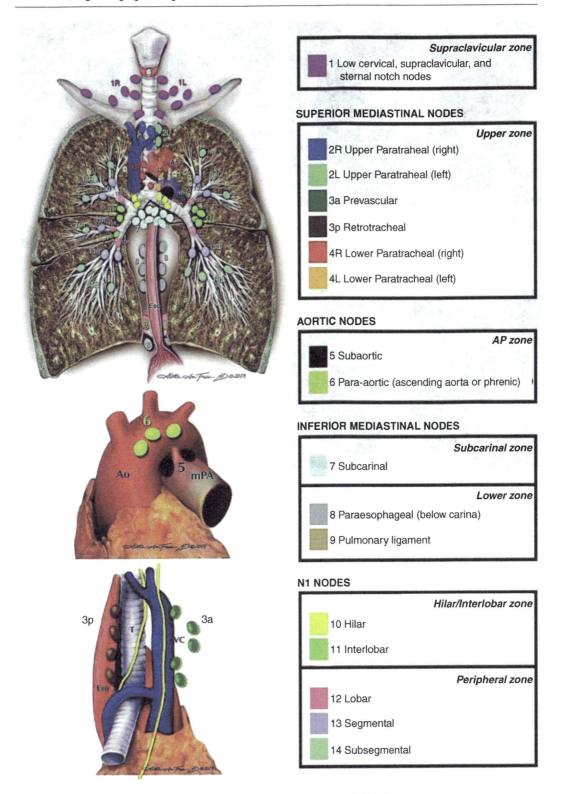

Fig. 19 Mediastinal lymph node stations. (Adapted from source Rusch et al. 2009)

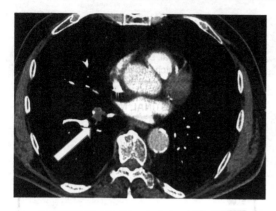

Fig. 20 15 mm Station 10R (right hilar) metastatic lymph node, suggesting N1 disease

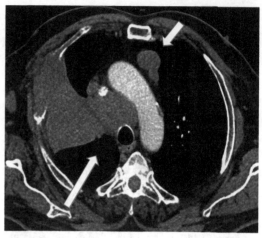

Fig. 22 Right upper lobe central tumor, with chest wall invasion and enlarged (metastatic) right lower paratracheal (station 4R) and para-aortic (station 6) lymph nodes, suggesting N3 disease

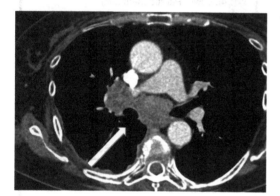

Fig. 21 30 mm Station 10R and station 7 enlarged metastatic lymph nodes, suggesting N2 disease

Role of Radiologic Imaging in Lung Cancer

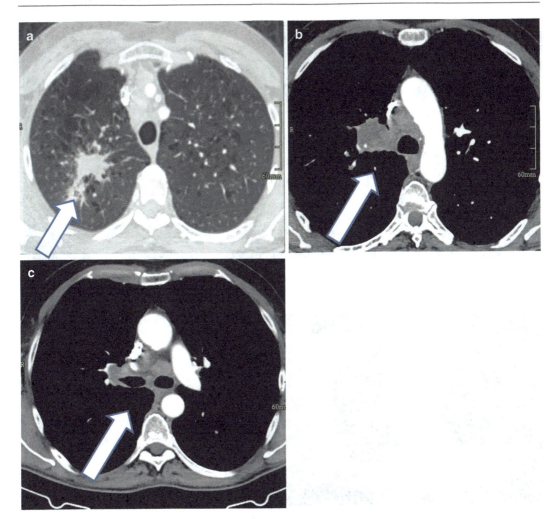

Fig. 23 RUL peripheral tumor (**a**), with enlarged metastatic ipsi- (**b**) and contralateral (**c**) mediastinal lymph nodes, suggesting N3 disease

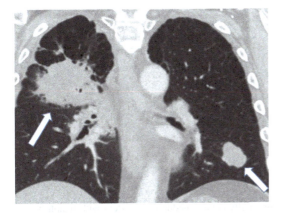

Fig. 24 RUL central tumor, with metastatic lesion in the contralateral lung, suggesting M1a disease

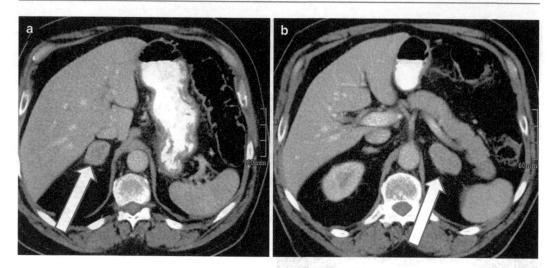

Fig. 25 Bilateral adrenal metastasis (**a**, **b**), suggesting M1c disease

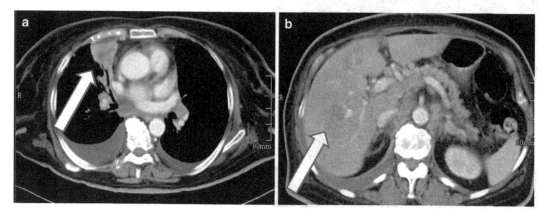

Fig. 26 RML central tumor (**a**) with multiple liver metastasis (**b**), suggesting M1c disease

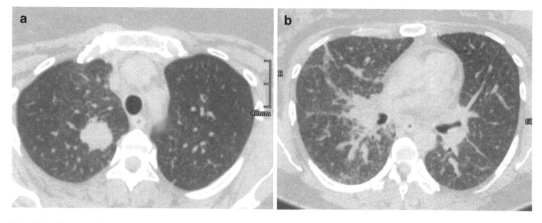

Fig. 27 65 year-old female with 30 mm RUL soft tissue mass, with irregular margins, morphologically proven BAC (**a**), bilateral interlobar septal thickening and multiple perilymphatic nodules, consistent with lymphangitic carcinomatosis (**b**)

References

Boland GW et al (1998) Characterization of adrenal masses using unenhanced CT: an analysis of the CT literature. AJR Am J Roentgenol 171:201–204

Callister MEJ, Baldwin DR, Akram AR, Barnard S, Cane P, Draffan J, Franks K, Gleeson F, Graham R, Malhotra P, Prokop M, Rodger K, Subesinghe M, Waller D, Woolhouse I, British Thoracic Society Pulmonary Nodule Guideline Development Group; British Thoracic Society Standards of Care Committee (2015) British Thoracic Society guidelines for the investigation and management of pulmonary nodules. Thorax. https://doi.org/10.1136/thoraxjnl-2015-207168

Caoili EM et al (2000) Delayed enhanced CT of lipid-poor adrenal adenomas. AJR Am J Roentgenol 175:1411–1415

Coche E (2016) Evaluation of lung tumor response to therapy: current and emerging techniques. Diagn Interv Imaging 97:1053–1065

Dales RE, Stark RM, Raman S (1990) Computed tomography to stage lung cancer. Approaching a controversy using meta-analysis. Am Rev Respir Dis 141:1096–1101

de Hoop B, van Ginneken B, Gietema H, Prokop M (2012) Pulmonary perifissural nodules on CT scans: rapid growth is not a predictor of malignancy. Radiology 265(2):611–616

Detterbeck FC, Boffa DJ, Kim AW, Tanoue LT (2017) The eighth edition lung cancer stage classification. Chest 151(1):193–203

Dwamena BA, Sonnad SS, Angobaldo JO, Wahl RL (1999) Metastases from non-small cell lung cancer: mediastinal staging in the 1990s—meta-analytic comparison of PET and CT. Radiology 213:530–536

Erasmus JJ, Connolly JE, McAdams HP et al (2000a) Solitary pulmonary nodules: Part I. Morphologic evaluation for differentiation of benign and malignant lesions. Radiographics 20:43–58

Erasmus JJ, McAdams HP, Connolly JE (2000b) Solitary pulmonary nodules: Part II. Evaluation of the indeterminate nodule. Radiographics 20:43–58

Klein JS, Salomon G, Stewart EA (1996) Transthoracic needle biopsy with a coaxially placed 20-gauge automated cutting needle: results in 122 patients. Radiology 198:715–720

Korobkin M et al (1996) Differentiation of adrenal adenomas from nonadenomas using CT attenuation values. AJR Am J Roentgenol 166:531–536

MacMahon H et al (2017) Guidelines for management of incidental pulmonary nodules detected on CT images: from the Fleischner Society 2017. Radiology. https://doi.org/10.1148/radiol.2017161659

Mayo-Smith WW et al (2017) Management of incidental adrenal masses: a white paper of the ACR Incidental Findings Committee. J Am Coll Radiol 14(8):1038–1044

National Cancer Institute (NCI) (2011) The National Lung Screening Trial Research Team reduced lung-cancer mortality with low-dose computed tomographic screening. N Engl J Med 365:395–409. https://doi.org/10.1056/NEJMoa1102873

NCCN guidelines for lung cancer screening: https://www.nccn.org/professionals/physician_gls/pdf/lung_screening.pdf

NCCN clincal practice guidelines in Oncology: Non-Small Cell Lung Cancer: https://www.nccn.org/professionals/physician_gls/pdf/nscl.pdf

Nishino M (2018) Tumor response assessment for precision cancer therapy: response evaluation criteria in solid tumors and beyond. asco.org/edbook. ASCO EDUCATIONAL BOOK

Oliver TW et al (1984) Isolated adrenal masses in non-small cell bronchogenic carcinoma. Radiology 153:217–218

Porte H et al (2001) Resection of adrenal metastases from non-small cell lung cancer: a multicenter study. Ann Thorac Surg 71:981–985

Purandare NC, Rangarajan V (2015) Imaging of lung cancer: implications on staging and management. Indian J Radiol Imaging 25(2):109–120. https://doi.org/10.4103/0971-3026.155831

Rusch VW, Asamura H, Watanabe H, Giroux DJ, Rami-Porta R, Goldstraw P, on Behalf of the Members of the IASLC Staging Committee (2009) The IASLC Lung Cancer Staging Project: a proposal for a new international lymph node map in the forthcoming seventh edition of the TNM classification for lung cancer. J Thorac Oncol 4:568–577

Salazar AM, Westcott JL (1993) The role of transthoracic needle biopsy for the diagnosis and staging of lung cancer. Clin Chest Med 14:99–110

Sider L, Horejs D (1988) Frequency of extrathoracic metastases from bronchogenic carcinoma in patients with normal-sized hilar and mediastinal lymph nodes on CT. AJR Am J Roentgenol 151:893–895

Verschakelen JA, Bogaert J, De Wever W (2002) Computed tomography in staging for lung cancer. Eur Respir J 19(Suppl. 35):40s–48s. https://doi.org/10.1183/09031936.02.00270802

Yeh HC, Rabinowitz JG (1980) Ultrasonography and computed tomography of the liver. Radiol Clin North Am 18:321–338

Yokoi K et al (1999) Detection of brain metastasis in potentially operable non-small cell lung cancer: a comparison of CT and MRI. Chest 115:714–719

Place and Role of PET/CT in the Diagnosis and Staging of Lung Cancer

Salome Kukava and Michael Baramia

Contents

1 Introduction, Technical Advances, Radiopharmaceuticals, and Clinical Applications of PET 85
2 Diagnosis of Lung Cancer/Solitary Pulmonary Nodule 87
3 T Staging/NSCLC 90
4 N Staging/NSCLC 93
5 M Staging/NSCLC 96
6 FDG PET and PET/CT in Treatment Response Assessment and Follow-Up of NSCLC 100
7 The Prognostic Value of FDG PET/CT 106
8 The Effect of FDG PET and PET/CT on the Management of Patients with NSCLC/Cost-Effectiveness of FDG PET and PET/CT 106
9 FDG PET and PET/CT in SCLC 106
10 Pitfalls, False-Negative and False-Positive Results 108
References 108

S. Kukava (✉)
Acad. F. Todua Clinic, Tbilisi, Georgia
e-mail: salome_kukava@yahoo.com

M. Baramia
Department of PET/CT, Department of Radition Oncology, Todua Clinic, Tbilisi, Georgia
e-mail: mbaramia@yahoo.com

Abstract

Positron emission tomography is a sensitive and specific method of molecular imaging. The application of PET in oncology developed gradually and nowadays the most widely used radiopharmaceutical in oncologic studies is the F18-labeled glucose (FDG). The introduction of integrated PET/CT scanners provides information about both anatomy (CT) and function (PET). The fused images from PET/CT greatly assist image interpretation and offer more accurate staging and diagnosis. However, there are a number of limitations. In this chapter we review the role of FDG PET and FDG PET/CT in the diagnosis, staging, and treatment response assessment of lung cancer.

1 Introduction, Technical Advances, Radiopharmaceuticals, and Clinical Applications of PET

Introduction of hybrid PET/CT scanner provides information about both anatomy (CT) and function (PET). The fused images from PET/CT greatly assist image interpretation and offer more accurate staging and diagnosis of oncologic diseases (Fig. 1). Modern hybrid PET/CT scanners are equipped with 16- or 64-slice MDCT, which makes it possible to acquire diagnostic, high-

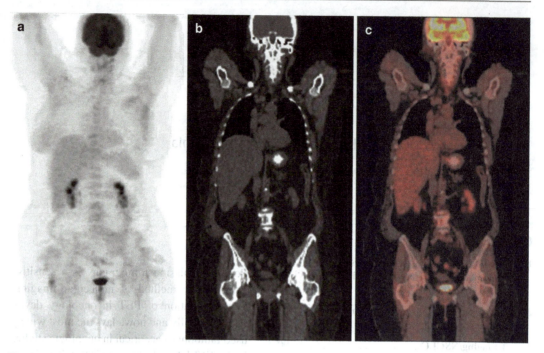

Fig. 1 PET, CT, and fused images (a–c)

quality CT images. Many institutions have protocols, which incorporate contrast-enhanced CT, and thus provide the full diagnostic whole-body images with "one-stop-shop" principle.

The benefits of PET/CT over PET and CT acquired separately are already documented in thousands of publications. A recent innovation introduced is the continuous bed motion acquisition instead of the conventional step-and-shoot approach, termed the mCT flow.

F18, a cyclotron-produced radiopharmaceutical, has the half-life of 110 min, which makes it possible to produce and then transport it from the supplier to the distant center, having enough radioactivity to perform a scan.

The application of PET in oncology developed gradually and nowadays the most widely used radiopharmaceutical in oncologic studies is the F18-labeled glucose (FDG). Evidence suggests that malignant tumor cells use anaerobic glycolysis and thus glucose as the major source of energy, the phenomenon known as Warburg effect. The uptake of FDG by the cell is facilitated by glucose transporters (GLUT1), located on the surface of the cell. Within the cell FDG is converted to FDG-6-phosphate by enzyme hexokinase, but it becomes trapped in a metabolic trap and undergoes no further reaction. The accumulation and distribution of FDG are then measured by PET scanner detector cameras. High glucose utilization by a majority of cancer types has led to a wide use of FDG and subsequently FDG PET has become the principal clinical PET procedure for detecting, staging, and assessing treatment response of cancer.

The intensity of FDG uptake can be measured visually, by comparing FDG uptake in a region of interest to the background activity (mediastinal blood pool, liver) or measuring a semiquantitative parameter—standardized uptake value (SUV). The SUV value can vary considerably and depends on injected activity, patient weight, blood glucose level, postinjection uptake time, respiratory motion, and different scanner parameters. Data suggest that both methods can be used with equal accuracy.

2 Diagnosis of Lung Cancer/Solitary Pulmonary Nodule

Solitary pulmonary nodule is a frequent, often incidental radiological finding and is defined as a round opacity less than or equal to 3 cm, surrounded by a lung parenchyma, not associated with atelectasis, lymph node enlargement, pneumonia, and pleural effusion. The term "pulmonary mass" is used for lesions more than 3 cm, the malignant probability of which is considerably higher. Differential diagnoses of SPN on CT include neoplastic lesions (benign and malignant), inflammatory lesions (infectious and noninfectious), and vascular and congenital lesions. SPNs can be completely solid or may contain a component of ground-glass attenuation, which are referred to as subsolid nodules. MDCT plays a pivotal role in evaluating morphologic characteristics and growth pattern of nodules on serial images.

Since the introduction of F-fluorodeoxyglucose positron emission tomography (18F-FDG PET), it has been extensively evaluated in patients with an indeterminate solitary pulmonary nodule. In 2001 in the meta-analysis of more than 40 studies Gould et al. showed that PET had sensitivity and specificity of approximately 90% for detecting malignant nodules with a diameter of 10 mm or larger (Gould et al. 2001). However, PET has a number of limitations. In a study by Nomori et al. the sensitivity (10%) and specificity (20%) of PET for evaluating ground-glass opacities were significantly lower than those for evaluating solid nodules (90% and 71%, respectively) (Nomori et al. 2004). In addition to the dimensions and morphologic characteristics (solid vs. subsolid) of the solitary pulmonary nodule, false-negative results can be obtained in case of tumors with low metabolic activity (e.g., carcinoid tumors and adenocarcinoma in situ, formerly known as bronchoalveolar carcinoma) (Erasmus et al. 1998).

The increased FDG uptake in the nodule can be assessed visually or by measuring standardized uptake value (SUV), being the most common semiquantitative method for evaluating pulmonary lesions. In a retrospective study of 140 patients, Grgic et al. evaluated the pulmonary nodules with the visual interpretation and with different cutoff points of standardized uptake value (SUVmax). The SUVmax values were higher in malignant nodules compared with benign nodules (SUVmax: 9.7 ± 5.5 vs. 2.6 ± 2.5; $p < 0.01$). More than 90% of pulmonary nodules with SUVmax <2.0 proved to be benign. The greatest diagnostic accuracy was obtained with a SUVmax cutoff point of 4 (Grgic et al. 2010).

One technique that has been evaluated in pulmonary nodules is dual-time-point FDG PET, obtaining images and measuring SUV at standard 60 min after injection and late-phase images at approximately 120 min after FDG injection. Matthies et al. evaluated 36 patients with that modality. There was a significant increase of SUV ($20.5 \pm 8.1\%$) in malignant nodules ($p < 0.01$) (Matthies et al. 2002). These results were not confirmed in studies conducted in endemic areas for tuberculosis (Sathekge et al. 2010; Kim et al. 2008). A meta-analysis including 8 studies showed that the accuracy of 18F-FDG PET/CT was similar between the standard protocol and the two-phase protocol, although the latter was found to have slightly higher specificity (Zhang et al. 2013).

The introduction of integrated PET/CT scanners has enabled the near-simultaneous acquisition of functional and anatomic data, which has increased the diagnostic accuracy. In a study comparing PET/CT and helical dynamic CT

(HDCT) for the evaluation of SPNs, PET/CT was more sensitive (96% vs. 81%) and more accurate (93% vs. 85%) than HDCT (Yi et al. 2006). Kim et al. published a study involving a population in the United States comparing the accuracy of CT vs. PET vs. PET/CT in the characterization of SPN, and the accuracy was 74%, 74%, and 93%, respectively (Kim et al. 2007).

In a retrospective analysis of 754 patients (705 pathologically proven lung cancer) Feng et al. reported the diagnostic accuracy of PET/CT to be 93.5%, and the false-positive rate to be 6.50%. Among the false-positive patients, inflammatory pseudotumor (42.86%) and tuberculoma (36.74%) were the most pathological types. In the positive detection group, adenocarcinoma (57.16%) and squamous carcinoma (33.19%) were the main histological types (Feng et al. 2017).

In conclusion, the combination of anatomical and metabolic data significantly improves the diagnostic accuracy of the characterization of pulmonary nodule. However, misregistration between CT and PET introduces artifacts and quantitative errors, which may lead to an underestimation of the SUV and false-negative results (Beyer et al. 2003). Most recent strategy to improve the respiratory mismatch between CT and PET images includes respiratory-gated CT for attenuation correction of PET (Pan et al. 2005) (Figs. 2, 3, and 4).

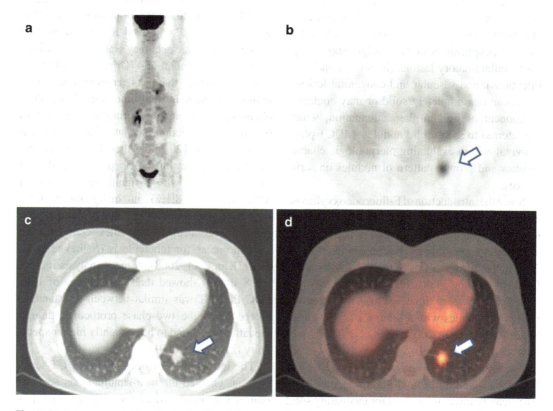

Fig. 2 Forty-one-year-old female with incidental finding on chest CT, hypermetabolic LLL SPN; MIP, PET, axial CT, axial fused images (**a–d**); postoperative morphology revealed adenocarcinoma

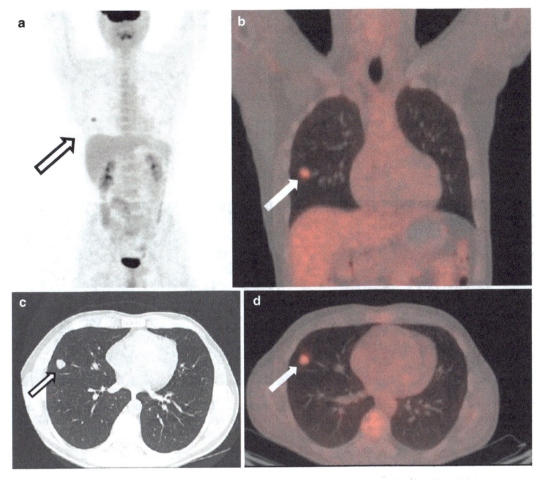

Fig. 3 Thirty-seven-year-old male, with incidental finding on chest CT, RML SPN, with moderately increased metabolic activity, suspicious for malignancy; MIP, fused coronal, axial CT, axial fused images (**a–d**); morphology revealed atypic carcinoid

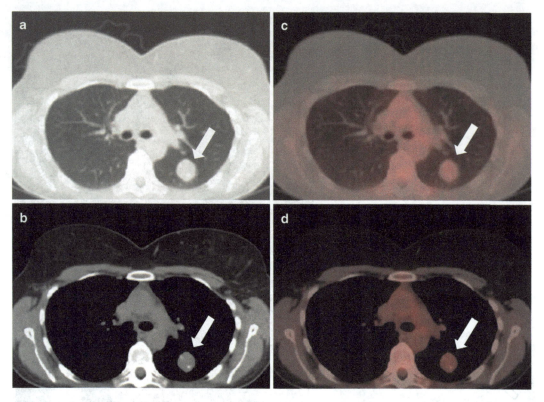

Fig. 4 Thirty-eight-year-old female with incidental finding on chest CT, LUL SPN, without increased metabolic activity suggesting benign process, follow-up recommended. CT (**a**, **b**) and fused PET/CT (**c**, **d**) images

3 T Staging/NSCLC

The lung cancer stage classification is developed by the International Association for the Study of Lung Cancer (IASLC). It describes the anatomic extent of the tumor by TNM system. The classification is used to select patients that are appropriately treated in a certain way.

MDCT has been the cornerstone of lung cancer staging, with MRI being superior for local staging of Pancoast tumor. PET, due to its low spatial resolution, does not add much value for the assessment of local spread and resectability, as it does not add more information about anatomical details. FDG PET/CT, however, provides that information by combining anatomical and functional data. Antoch et al. compared the accuracy of PET/CT in the staging of NSCLC with PET alone and CT alone and proved its superiority. Primary tumor stage was correctly identified in more patients with PET/CT than with either PET alone or CT alone. Similar results were obtained by De Wever et al. in 2007 in a retrospective study of 50 patients (Antoch et al. 2003; De Wever et al. 2007) (Figs. 5 and 6). PET/CT also allows to differentiate metabolically active tumor from peritumoral inflammation or atelectasis (Lardinois et al. 2003; De Wever et al. 2009), which is successfully used for planning radiotherapy treatment by distinguishing tumor from nondamaged tissues, thus preserving uninvolved lung. (Fig. 7).

FDG PET/CT can be used to guide biopsy and accurately localize "the hottest"—hypermetabolic regions of tumor that yield the useful diagnostic information. Studies have shown that using FDG PET/CT to guide transthoracic biopsy helps to find the most viable portion of the lesion and thus increases the rate of accurate diagnosis (Purandare et al. 2013; İntepe et al. 2016; Collins et al. 2000) (Fig. 8).

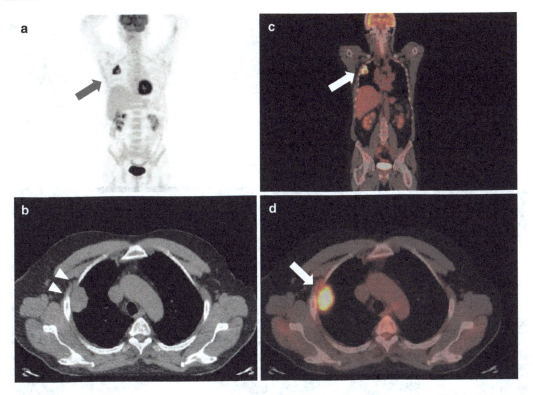

Fig. 5 Fifty-nine-year-old male, with morphologically proven NSCLC, hypermetabolic peripheral RUL lesion (arrow), with signs of visceral and parietal pleural invasion (arrowheads), metabolic stage T3 N0 M0

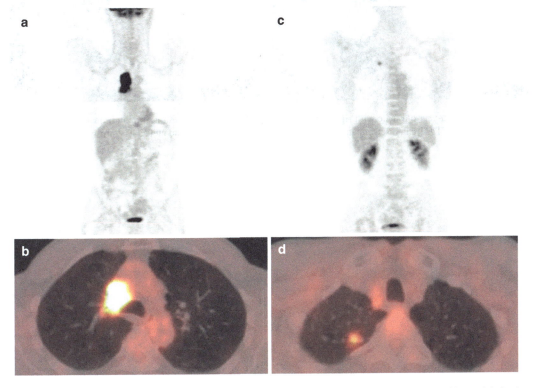

Fig. 6 Fifty-nine-year-old male, with morphologically proven NSCLC (**a**, **b**), hypermetabolic satellite nodule in the same lobe (**c**, **d**), suggesting T2 disease

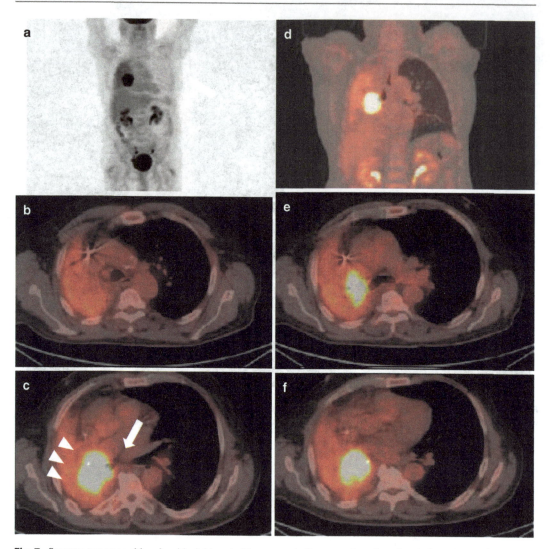

Fig. 7 Seventy-two-year-old male with right central hypermetabolic tumor, invasion of main bronchus and right lung atelectasis, FDG PET/CT can discriminate well between viable tumor (arrow) and atelectasis (arrowheads)

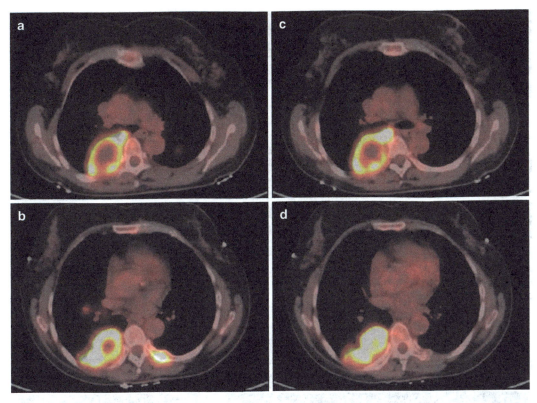

Fig. 8 Fifty-eight-year-old female, RLL peripheral hypermetabolic mass, with chest wall invasion, ultrasound-guided biopsy was inconclusive, due to central necrosis and low diagnostic yield, malignant hemangioendothelioma was confirmed after PET-based biopsy

4 N Staging/NSCLC

The anatomic imaging, like CT, uses the size criteria for mediastinal and hilar staging, with 1 cm being the threshold for metastatic involvement. The limitations of these criteria are the normal-size lymph nodes, infiltrated with tumor cells and enlarged lymph nodes due to benign causes. Numerous studies have reported comparisons of FDG PET and CT for lymph node staging in NSCLC, demonstrating its superiority. Gould et al. performed a meta-analysis comparing FDG PET and CT in mediastinal staging of NSCLC in both normal-size and enlarged lymph nodes. PET was more sensitive but less specific for enlarged lymph nodes (sensitivity 100%, specificity 78%), and less sensitive but more specific for normal-size lymph nodes (sensitivity 82%, specificity 93%) (Gould et al. 2003). These data demonstrate the superiority of PET for normal-size malignant and enlarged benign lymph nodes (Figs. 9 and 10).

Anatomic-metabolic correlation and fusion of FDG PET and CT allow better localization of involved lymph nodes, better delineation of primary tumor from adjacent lymph nodes, and differentiation of mediastinal and hilar lymph nodes (Vansteenkiste et al. 1998). Results from several studies comparing the accuracy of integrated FDG PET/CT with PET alone and CT alone for mediastinal staging of NSCLC show pooled average sensitivity, specificity, positive predictive value, negative predictive value, and accuracy of PET/CT of 73%, 80%, 78%, 91%, and 87%, respectively (De Wever et al. 2009). Lardinois et al. and Cerfolio et al. have documented in their studies better and correct evaluation of N status with integrated PET/CT than with PET alone

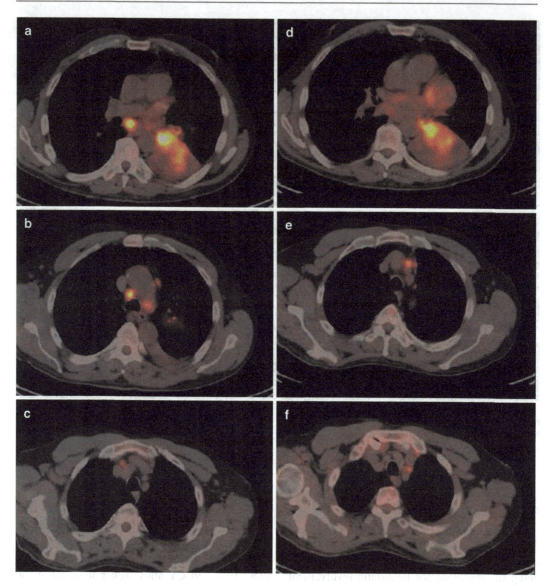

Fig. 9 Seventy-three-year-old male, with NSCLC, left central hypermetabolic tumor, with peripheral LLL atelectasis, subcentimetric hypermetabolic ipsi- (**a, e, f**) and contralateral (**b, c**) mediastinal lymphadenopathy, suggesting N3 disease

(Lardinois et al. 2003; De Wever et al. 2009; Cerfolio et al. 2004a). A meta-analysis of 17 eligible studies was performed by Birim et al., and all the 17 studies reported a better accuracy of FDG PET when compared with CT in detecting mediastinal lymph node metastases (Birim et al. 2005). A retrospective study of 159 patients with NSCLC and evaluation of 1001 nodal stations by Bille et al. reported that the accuracy of PET/CT for detecting metastatic lymph nodes was 80.5% on a per-patient basis, and 95.6% on per-nodal-station basis. With regard to N2/N3 disease, PET/CT accuracy was 84.9% and 95.3% on a per-patient basis and per-nodal-station basis, respectively (Billé et al. 2009). Wang et al. reported that the negative predictive value of FDG PET/CT for

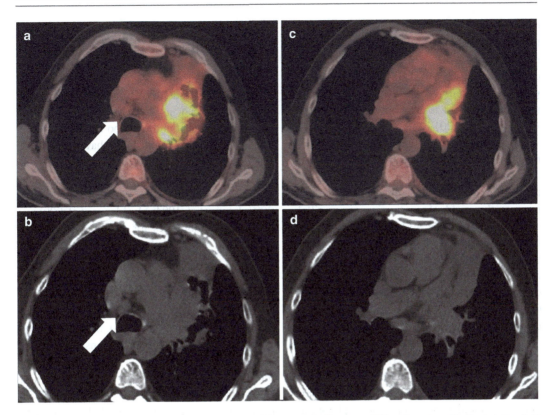

Fig. 10 Sixty-three-year-old male with the left central hypermetabolic tumor (T4), enlarged mediastinal station 4, 7 lymph nodes w/o increased metabolic activity (arrow), suggesting reactive changes

mediastinal metastases was 94% in T1 disease, suggesting a low yield from routine invasive staging procedures (Wang et al. 2012). The retrospective study by Zhou et al. included 54 patients with T1-2N0M0 NSCLC who had undergone 18F-FDG PET/CT before surgery. Occult nodal metastasis was detected in 25.9% (14/54) of the patients. The authors identified that combining tumor size with SUVmax offered some predictive ability—for tumors >2.5 cm with SUVmax >4.35, there was an 88.9% chance of detecting occult lymph node metastases (Zhou et al. 2017). In a multicenter study Li et al. reported an excellent negative predictive value of 18F-FDG PET/CT (91%) in the mediastinal evaluation of early-stage T1-2N0 tumors and thus in identifying patients for SBRT (Li et al. 2012). The comparison between PET and CT has also been done in a prospective setting. A Japanese multicenter study showed statistically significant improvement in the diagnostic accuracy of mediastinal lymph node metastasis with integrated FDG PET/CT (Kubota et al. 2011).

However, besides the recent advances in technology, FDG PET/CT remains by far not the perfect method with possible false-negative (low tumor load, micrometastasis, or small size) and false-positive results (inflammation). In a meta-analysis by Wang et al. the NPV of FDG PET for mediastinal lymph node involvement was 89% in T2 disease, and the authors recommended invasive staging procedures before the initiation of any active treatment in this subgroup of patients with adenocarcinoma histology, or high FDG uptake in primary lesions due to high risk of nodal metastasis (Wang et al. 2012). Gao et al. evaluated 284 patients with T1-2N0 disease staged with FDG PET/CT between 2011 and 2015. They concluded that invasive mediastinal staging should be strongly encouraged in central tumors and solid T2 tumors because of the 10% risk of occult nodal metastasis. However, for patients with peripheral T1 tumors or peripheral T2 tumors with a ground-glass component, invasive staging after a negative PET/CT is discouraged due to its low yield (Gao et al. 2017). In a meta-analysis of 14 studies by Langen et al. negative PET scan resulted in a post-PET probability for N2 disease of 5% for LN <15 mm, suggesting that these patients should be planned for thoracotomy because the yield of mediastinoscopy will be extremely low, while post-PET probability for N2 disease was 21% for LN ≥16 mm, suggesting that these patients should be planned for mediastinoscopy (Langen et al. 2006). In a retrospective review of Lee et al. the PPV of PET/CT was only 56%, with the increase in false-positive results being associated with inflammatory and infectious conditions (Lee et al. 2007). The PPV 64% of FDG PET/CT in mediastinal staging was reported by Darling et al. (2011). Such data prove the need for pathologic confirmation of mediastinal lymph node abnormalities (EBUS or EUS with FNA or invasive mediastinal staging) before planning thoracotomy and radical surgical treatment.

Attempts have been made to increase the accuracy of FDG PET/CT. A meta-analysis of eight studies (including 654 patients) showed the better performance of dual-time-point PET/CT in mediastinal staging; however, it has not been implemented in routine protocols so far (Shen et al. 2015) (Fig. 11).

5 M Staging/NSCLC

One of the most important roles of whole-body FDG PET and PET/CT is to detect distant metastasis and thus accurately stage the lung cancer, by segregation of patients who have distant spread and cannot be cured from those who can benefit from radical treatment. Several studies have proven that FDG PET detects unsuspected distant metastasis in 5% to 29% of cases (Marom et al. 1999; Pieterman et al. 2000; Saunders et al. 1999; Stroobants et al. 2003; Lewis et al. 1994; MacManus et al. 2001).

Most common sites for distant metastasis of lung cancer are adrenal glands, liver, bones, and brain. In a retrospective study of 94 patients, Kumar et al. reported the sensitivity, specificity, and accuracy of FDG PET for detecting adrenal metastatic disease to be 93%, 90%, and 92%, respectively (Kumar et al. 2004). Brady et al. proposed an algorithm combining density measurement on non-CE CT (HU >10) and a SUV threshold (SUV >3.1) to define malignancy. In a study of 147 patients this algorithm for PET/CT proved to be more specific than PET or CT alone without loss in sensitivity (Brady et al. 2009). A recent meta-analysis of nine studies to evaluate the diagnostic accuracy of FDG PET/CT for the detection of adrenal metastasis in patients with lung cancer showed the pooled sensitivity and specificity of 89% and 90%, respectively (Wu et al. 2017).

FDG PET is superior to bone scintigraphy in the detection of osseous metastasis, as the lesions are mostly osteolytic rather than osteoblastic. In a meta-analysis of 14 articles, Liu et al. reported

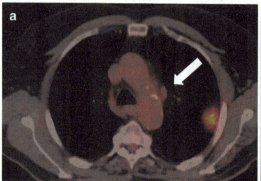 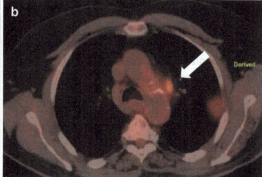

Fig. 11 Seventy-year-old male with peripheral hypermetabolic LUL tumor (T3), subcentimetric station 5 lymph node shows increased metabolic activity (arrow) on dual-time-point imaging 60 min (**a**) and 120 min (**b**) postinjection

FDG PET to be the best modality to detect bone metastasis in patients with lung cancer, both on a per-patient basis and a per-lesion basis; MRI had the highest specificity on a per-lesion basis. For the subgroup analysis of FDG PET, PET/CT was shown to be better than PET (Liu et al. 2011). PET/CT adds to the value of PET by demonstrating the skeletal changes associated with malignancy, trauma, or degenerative changes and improves sensitivity and specificity. In a meta-analysis of patients with lung cancer, the authors found that FDG PET/CT and FDG PET were more accurate for the diagnosis of bone metastases than MRI or bone scintigraphy (Qu et al. 2012).

FDG PET is also valuable in the detection of liver metastasis, indeterminate on conventional imaging modalities (Hustinx et al. 1998). FDG PET is limited in detecting brain metastasis due to its high glucose uptake in brain tissue and high background activity; thus FDG PET is not sensitive enough to exclude brain metastases. MRI (or CT) remains the method of choice to stage the brain, although there are patients with accidentally detected brain hypermetabolic lesions, confirmed to be metastases (Fig. 25).

With the introduction of hybrid PET/CT systems, the integrated information acquired simultaneously at the same time, on the same table, is more accurate than that of either PET or CT alone. In studies using integrated PET/CT, although limited in detection of brain metastases, the modality was significantly better than CT or PET alone for extrathoracic metastases (De Wever et al. 2009; Cerfolio et al. 2004a) (Figs. 12, 13, 14, and 15).

FDG PET is also effective in detecting pulmonary metastasis. CT has higher anatomical and spatial resolution and is less affected by respiratory motion. So integrated PET/CT is effective to identify lung lesions with minimal FDG uptake (Fig. 16). In the results of a 2013 meta-analysis of 56 studies to evaluate the diagnostic value of FDG PET/CT in patients with NSCLC, Wu et al. concluded that FDG PET/CT confers significantly higher sensitivity and specificity than contrast-enhanced CT and higher sensitivity than FDG PET in staging NSCLC (Wu et al. 2013).

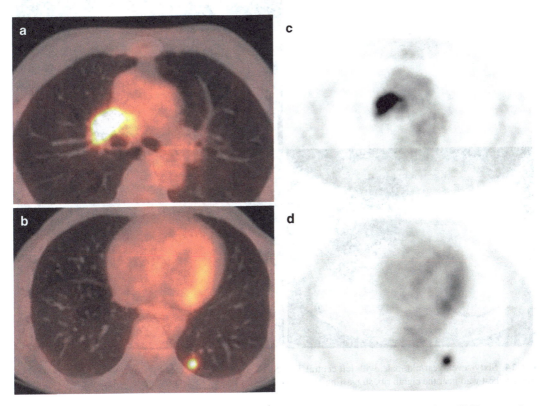

Fig. 12 Sixty-seven-year-old male, with right central NSCLC, hypermetabolic nodule in contralateral LLL, suggesting M1a disease

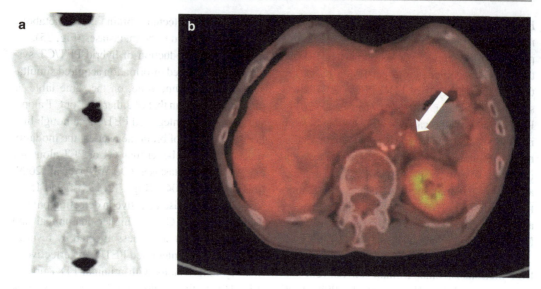

Fig. 13 Sixty-nine-year-old male, with left central NSCLC (**a**), unsuspected hypermetabolic lesion of the left adrenal gland (**b**), suggesting M1 disease

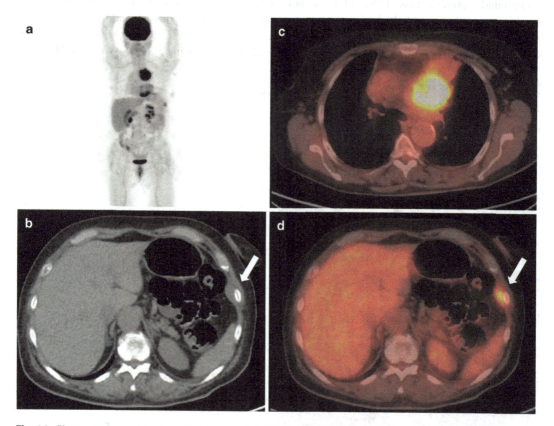

Fig. 14 Sixty-seven-year-old male, with left central T4 NSCLC (**a, c**), unsuspected hypermetabolic lesion (arrow) in the left chest wall near the eighth rib, suggesting M1 disease

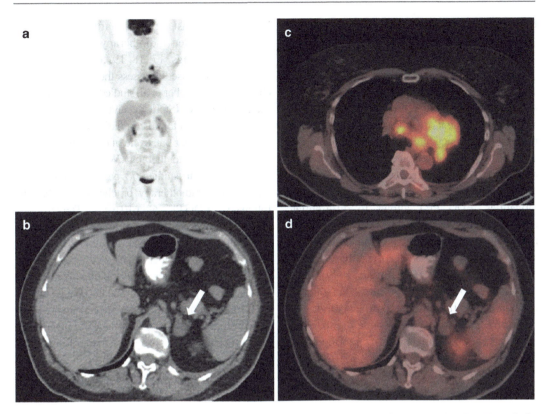

Fig. 15 Sixty-year-old female with LUL central hypermetabolic tumor (**a, c**), hypermetabolic ipsi- and contralateral mediastinal lymphadenopathy, left adrenal lesion considered to be metastatic shows no increased metabolic activity (**b, d** arrow), the patient was downstaged

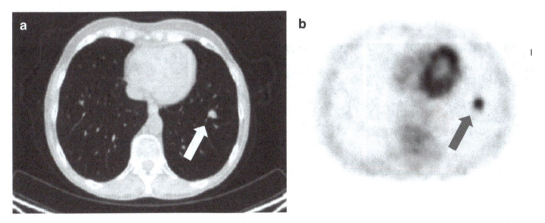

Fig. 16 Seventy-six-year-old female with a history of NSCLC, suspected LLL metastasis, 9 mm nodule (arrow) on CT (**a**) shows increased FDG uptake on PET (**b**), respiratory-gated PET/CT

6 FDG PET and PET/CT in Treatment Response Assessment and Follow-Up of NSCLC

After treatment of lung cancer it is necessary to evaluate treatment response, detect residual tumor or recurrence, and further plan the correct strategy. Structural changes after surgery or radiotherapy often are inconclusive or indeterminate on conventional anatomic imaging modalities. FDG PET allows to differentiate between fibrosis/necrosis and residual or recurrent tumor after both surgery and radiotherapy and its sensitivity is higher than that of other imaging modalities (Bury et al. 1999). It is important to perform PET scan in an optimal time interval after radiotherapy or surgery to minimize false-positive results due to inflammatory changes. Erasmus and Patz reported high accuracy (78–98%) for the detection of recurrence when there is delay between treatment and PET scan at least 2 months after surgery and 4–6 months after radiotherapy (Erasmus and Patz Jr 1999) (Figs. 17, 18, 19, and 20).

FDG PET is used to assess the effectiveness of chemotherapy. Weber et al. studied 57 patients with stage IIIB and IV NSCLC receiving platinum-based chemotherapy and found correlation between metabolic response after one cycle of chemotherapy and overall response to therapy (Weber et al. 2003). MacManus et al. studied 73 patients who underwent radical radiotherapy or chemo/radiotherapy followed by FDG PET after 10 weeks. The response assessment by FDG PET was found to be superior to CT in predicting survival duration (MacManus et al. 2003). In another study of 56 patients the decrease in SUV after adjuvant treatment was a more accurate predictor than was the change in size on CT (Cerfolio et al. 2004b). Several studies confirm the high diagnostic performance of FDG PET/CT in metabolic response assessment of lung cancer with high NPV (Sheikhbahaei et al. 2016; Kremer et al. 2016; Moon et al. 2013).

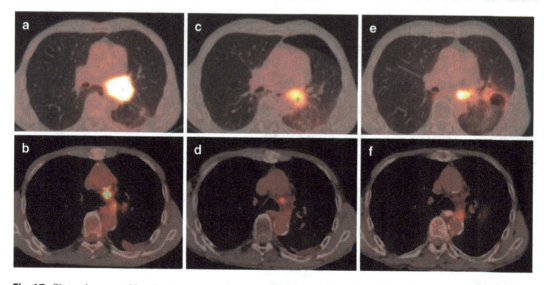

Fig. 17 Sixty-nine-year-old male, treated with chemoradiotherapy for the left central T4, N3 NSCLC (**a**, **b**), follow-up fused FDG PET/CT images show marked decrease in size and activity of primary tumor (**c**) and mediastinal lymph node (**d**), but subsequent imaging residual metabolic activity of primary tumor (**e**), whereas complete response of mediastinal lymph node is noted (**f**)

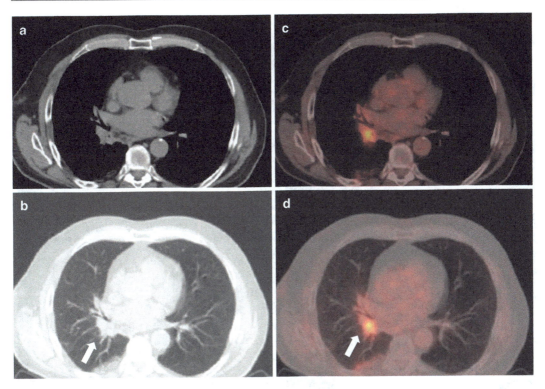

Fig. 18 Seventy-year-old male treated with radical radiotherapy for T2 N2 right NSCLC, follow-up axial CT images (**a, b**) are inconclusive, axial fused PET/CT images (**c, d**) show residual metabolic activity, consistent with residual malignancy, confirmed by bronchoscopy and morphology

PET Response Evaluation Criteria in Solid Tumors has been shown to be a better predictor of histopathologic response than anatomic response criteria, such as WHO criteria and RECIST 1.1 (Wahl et al. 2009). Recently, new PET-based structured qualitative treatment response criteria (Hopkins criteria) have been proposed with inter-reader agreement and high accuracy (Sheikhbahaei et al. 2016) (Fig. 21).

In a meta-analysis of 13 studies including 1035 patients with lung cancer He et al. reported that PET/CT and PET were superior modalities for the detection of lung cancer recurrence compared to conventional imaging modalities, and PET/CT was superior to PET (He et al. 2014).

In a study of 90 patients Dane et al. confirmed that PET/CT was more sensitive than CT alone in the detection of recurrence 1 year after lobectomy for all patients included in the study, and the higher sensitivity was related to the superiority of PET/CT in identifying extrathoracic masses and a new hypermetabolic pulmonary nodule (Dane et al. 2013). In a prospective study of 358 patients Choi et al. studied the effectiveness of postoperative follow-up FDG PET/CT compared with chest CT and found the added value of FDG PET/CT as in 37% of cases (19 patients) recurrence was confirmed only by FDG PET/CT (Choi et al. 2011) (Figs. 22, 23, 24, and 25).

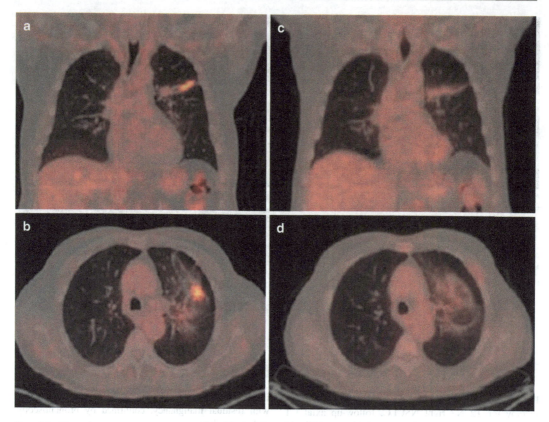

Fig. 19 Sixty-six-year-old male treated for the left NSCLC, follow-up FDG PET images show complete metabolic response and only fibrosis/necrosis in irradiated area; pretreatment (**a**, **b**) and posttreatment fused PET/CT images (**c**, **d**)

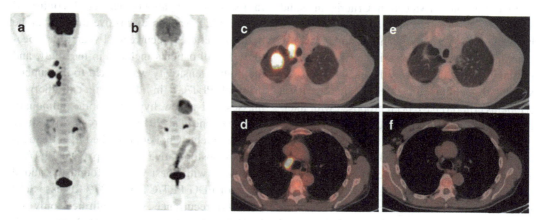

Fig. 20 Sixty-two-year-old male with NSCLC, treated with chemotherapy and immunotherapy, shows complete metabolic response and disappearance of metabolically active lesions; pretreatment (**a**, **c**, **d**) and posttreatment MIP and fused (**b**, **e**, **f**) images

Fig. 21 Hopkins criteria. (Source: Sheikhbahaei S, Mena E, Marcus C, Wray R, Taghipour M, Subramaniam R. 18F-fluorodeoxyglucose PET/CT: therapy response assessment interpretation (Hopkins criteria) and survival outcomes in lung cancer patients. *J Nucl Med* 2016; 57:855–860)

Score	Description	
1	^{18}F-FDG uptake less than mediastinal blood pool consistent with complete metabolic response	Negative
2	Focal ^{18}F-FDG uptake greater than mediastinal blood pool but less than liver, consistent with likely complete metabolic response	Negative
3	Diffuse ^{18}F-FDG uptake greater than mediastinal blood pool or liver consistent with probable inflammation	Negative
4	Focal ^{18}F-FDG uptake greater than liver consistent with likely residual disease	Positive
5	Focal and intense ^{18}F-FDG uptake consistent with residual disease	Positive

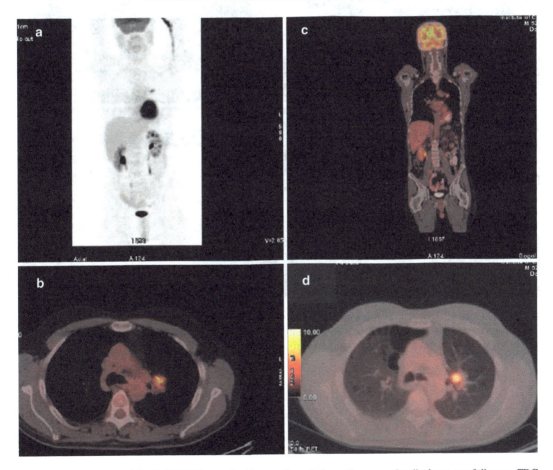

Fig. 22 Fifty-two-year-old with NSCLC treated with neoadjuvant chemotherapy and radical surgery, follow-up FDG PET/CT images show local recurrence with no distant spread, MIP (**a**), coronal (**c**), and axial fused (**b**, **d**) images

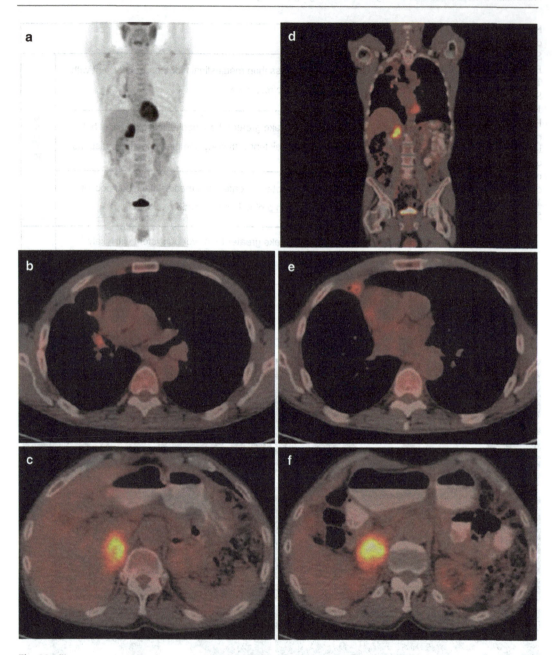

Fig. 23 Sixty-two-year-old male treated with radical surgery for the right T2N1 NSCLC; restaging of a patient with FDG PET/CT—no metabolically active tumor in primary location (**b**, **e**) and oligoprogression in the right adrenal, MIP (**a**), coronal fused (**d**), axial fused (**c**, **f**) images

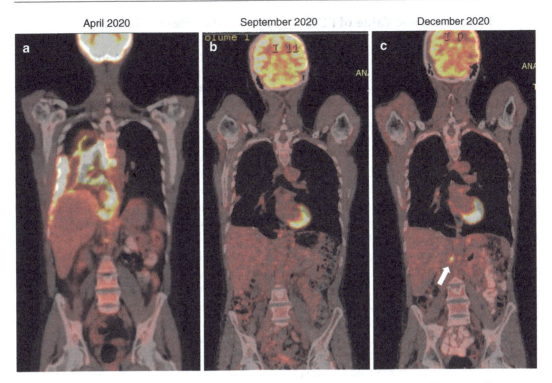

Fig. 24 Four-year-old male, with NSCLC, treated with chemo- and immunotherapy, pretreatment fused (**a**) image shows widespread disease, complete response on post-treatment fused PET/CT image (**b**); distant oligoprogression in paracaval lymph node (arrow) on subsequent fused PET/CT (**c**) scan

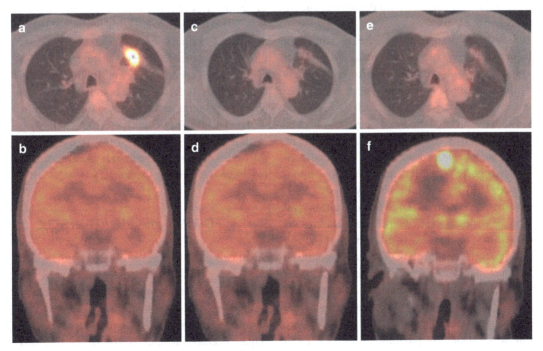

Fig. 25 Sixty-three-year-old male treated with immunotherapy for T4N2M1 left NSCLC, axial fused PET CT images (**a, c, e**) show complete metabolic response in lungs, coronal fused PET CT images (**b, d, f**) show incidental hypermetabolic brain lesion; oligoprogression was proved by brain MRI

7 The Prognostic Value of FDG PET/CT

The potential prognostic value of FDG PET and SUVmax for primary lung cancer has been widely reported in various studies including various staged and treated populations. In a meta-analysis of 24 studies Paesmans et al. concluded that patients with a tumor demonstrating a higher metabolic activity and higher SUV have shorter survival than patients with a tumor with a lower glucose metabolic rate (Paesmans et al. 2010). In a meta-analysis, Na et al. reported that the SUVmax in the primary tumor both before and after RT was able to predict patient outcome and overall survival (Na et al. 2014). FDG PET also provides prognostic value and correlates with survival rates of patients with treated lung cancer (Patz Jr et al. 2000; Eschmann et al. 2007). Induction chemotherapy can be used as a neoadjuvant therapy prior to consolidative radiotherapy. A study of 31 patients reported a complete response on FDG PET following induction chemotherapy for locally advanced, unresectable NSCLC to be a more powerful prognostic marker for survival compared to partial response on CT (Decoster et al. 2008).

SUVmax is the most widely used parameter for diagnosis and response assessment due to its higher reproducibility and availability. However, it only measures a single volumetric pixel within the tumor. Volumetric parameters, such as MTV and TLG, have been introduced and investigated recently. In a meta-analysis of 36 studies Liu et al. investigated the prognostic value of maximal standardized uptake value (SUVmax), metabolic tumor volume (MTV), and total lesion glycolysis (TLG) on disease-free survival (DFS) and overall survival (OS) in surgical NSCLC patients. The results showed that high values of SUVmax, MTV, and TLG predicted a higher risk of recurrence or death in patients with surgical NSCLC. Thus, FDG PET/CT can be used to select patients at high risk of disease recurrence or death who may benefit from more aggressive treatments (Liu et al. 2016). Lee et al. also evaluated the prognostic value of MTV in patients with NSCLC treated definitively and reported tumor burden as assessed by MTV yields prognostic information on survival beyond that of established prognostic factors (Lee et al. 2012).

8 The Effect of FDG PET and PET/CT on the Management of Patients with NSCLC/Cost-Effectiveness of FDG PET and PET/CT

According to numerous earlier studies FDG PET changes management of patients with NSCLC by upstaging and detecting unsuspected metastasis or downstaging and excluding benign lesions, especially important being the exclusion of futile surgery. A randomized study evaluated 188 patients and found the relative reduction of 51% in the futile surgery in patients staged with PET with no extra cost (Van Tinteren et al. 2002). A prospective multicenter trial by Kubota et al. reported strategy modification rate of 72% for the patients with lung cancer, before and after FDG PET/CT, higher than previously reported rates (Kubota et al. 2015). Both prospective and retrospective studies have demonstrated high management impact with the introduction of integrated FDG PET/CT in patients with NSCLC intended for primary surgery or definitive RT, including significant percentage of avoided futile surgeries due to disease upstaging (Gregory et al. 2012; Kung et al. 2017; Takeuchi et al. 2014).

Several authors have addressed the cost-effectiveness of FDG PET and integrated PET/CT for lung cancer staging and found that it was cost effective over CT alone both in terms of correct TNM staging and assessment of resectability (Scott et al. 1998; Dietlein et al. 2000; Schreyogg et al. 2010). They concluded that costs for PET/CT were within the commonly accepted range for diagnostic tests or therapies.

9 FDG PET and PET/CT in SCLC

Small-cell lung cancer is divided into limited-stage and advanced diseases. Limited-stage disease can be treated with curative chemoradiotherapy or in selected cases with surgery, advanced-stage disease requires systemic chemotherapy. Accurate staging is crucial for the selection of correct treatment options as well as the stage is an important prognostic factor. The role of FDG and FDG PET/CT in SCLC has not yet been fully established but several studies have addressed this question as

SCLC is an aggressive neuroendocrine tumor and is considered to be FDG avid. Brink et al. evaluated the role of FDG PET in the staging of SCLC and reported that the sensitivity was significantly superior to that of CT in the detection of extrathoracic lymph node involvement and distant metastases except to the brain. The change of the stage lead to significant changes in treatment (Brink et al. 2004). Bradley et al. prospectively evaluated 24 patients with limited-stage SCLC and reported that FDG PET upstaged disease in 8% of cases and detected unsuspected nodal metastasis in 25% of cases, and thus altered radiation therapy plan (Bradley et al. 2004). In a more recent study Azad et al. reported that FDG PET altered management in 12 of 46 (26%) patients (Azad et al. 2010).

Hybrid imaging using 18F-FDG PET/CT, providing both functional and morphological data, has been demonstrated to be superior to 18F-FDG PET alone (Fischer et al. 2007). The most recent meta-analysis of nine studies showed that integrated FDG PET/CT can lead to significant changes in SCLC staging and thus can alter management in 5–21.9% of cases. This is majorly related to the better diagnostic accuracy of 18F-FDG PET/CT compared to conventional imaging methods in detecting distant metastases (except for brain), as functional abnormalities detected by 18F-FDG PET usually precede anatomical abnormalities (Martucci et al. 2020).

Kamel et al. tried to evaluate the impact of FDG PET on the management of patients with SCLC. PET led to change in the management in 29% of patients, either by upstaging the disease or by downstaging by excluding mediastinal involvement or distant metastasis; it also led to the change in radiation treatment plan. In the setting of restaging after therapy PET correctly identified all patients with total remission and progressive disease, and 11 of 12 patients with residual disease (Ehab et al. 2003). Few studies have addressed the role of FDG in treatment response assessment in SCLC (Yamamoto et al. 2009; Ziai et al. 2013). As in NSCLC, FDG PET can have prognostic value in SCLC (Lee et al. 2009; Pandit et al. 2003) (Fig. 26).

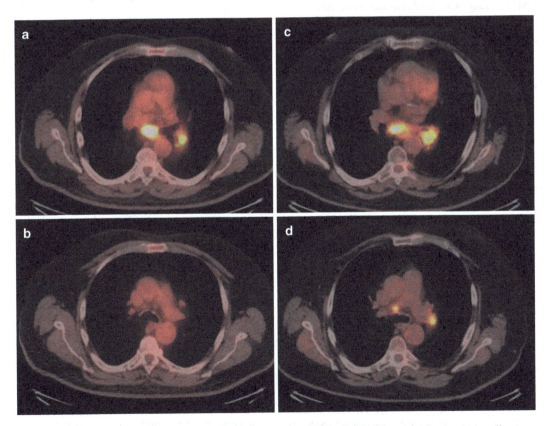

Fig. 26 Sixty-three-year-old male with metastatic SCLC, treated with chemo-immunotherapy, fused axial FDG PET/CT images show metabolic progression of initially involved mediastinal lymph nodes (**a, c**) as well as progression in subcentimetric mediastinal lymph nodes (**b, d**)

10 Pitfalls, False-Negative and False-Positive Results

There are a number of limitations of FDG PET/CT in lung cancer. False-positive results are not infrequent and inflammatory disease is one of the known confounders in FDG PET/CT studies. A retrospective study of patients with lung cancer revealed that false-positive results included inflammatory pseudotumor (43%), tuberculoma (37%), and organizing pneumonia (6%) (Feng et al. 2017). False-positive lymph nodes may also be related to the presence of interstitial pneumonitis, previous tuberculosis, silicosis, and emphysema (Konishi et al. 2003; Betancourt-Cuellar et al. 2015; Al-Sarraf et al. 2008). These studies demonstrate an important limitation of FDG PET/CT, and confirm that PET-positive lymph nodes still require pathological confirmation by mediastinoscopy (Shiraki et al. 2004). In the posttreatment setting false-positive results may be associated with post-radiotherapy inflammation, particularly after SBRT (Zhang et al. 2012; Hoopes et al. 2007).

False-negative findings at PET can be the result of a small size of the nodule, low cellular density in lesions such as carcinoma in situ, or low metabolic activity and low tumor avidity for FDG. Positron emission tomography has been shown to be less sensitive for the characterization of smaller lung lesions. This may be at least in part due to respiratory motion, which causes a significant underestimation of 18F-FDG uptake (Liu et al. 2009). Tumors of certain histologic phenotypes, such as bronchoalveolar carcinoma and well-differentiated tumors, have shown to be less 18F-FDG avid (Vesselle et al. 2008).

References

Al-Sarraf N et al (2008) Lymph node staging by means of positron emission tomography is less accurate in non-small cell lung cancer patients with enlarged lymph nodes: analysis of 1,145 lymph nodes. Lung Cancer 60:62–68

Antoch G et al (2003) Non-small cell lung cancer: dual-modality PET/CT in preoperative staging. Radiology 229:526–533

Azad A et al (2010) High impact of 18F-FDG PET on management and prognostic stratification of newly diagnosed small cell lung cancer. Mol Imaging Biol 12:433–451

Betancourt-Cuellar SL et al (2015) Pitfalls and limitations in non-small cell lung cancer staging. Semin Roentgenol 50(3):175–182

Beyer T, Antoch G et al (2003) Dual-modality PET/CT imaging: the effect of respiratory motion on combined image quality in clinical oncology. Eur J Nucl Med Mol Imaging 30(4):588–596

Billé A et al (2009) Preoperative intrathoracic lymph node staging in patients with non-small-cell lung cancer: accuracy of integrated positron emission tomography and computed tomography. Eur J Cardiothorac Surg 36(3):440–445

Birim O et al (2005) Meta-analysis of positron emission tomographic and computed tomographic imaging in detecting mediastinal lymph node metastases in non-small cell lung cancer. Ann Thorac Surg 79:375–382

Bradley JD et al (2004) Positron emission tomography in limited-stage small-cell lung cancer: a prospective study. J Clin Oncol 22(16):3248–3254

Brady MJ et al (2009) Adrenal nodules at FDG PET/CT in patients known to have or suspected of having lung cancer: a proposal for an efficient diagnostic algorithm. Radiology 250:523–530

Brink I et al (2004) Impact of [18F]FDG-PET on the primary staging of small-cell lung cancer. Eur J Nucl Med Mol Imaging 31(12):1614–1620

Bury T et al (1999) Value of FDG-PET in detecting residual or recurrent nonsmall cell lung cancer. Eur Respir J 14:1376–1380

Cerfolio RJ et al (2004a) The accuracy of integrated PET-CT compared with dedicated PET alone for the staging of patients with non-small cell lung cancer. Ann Thorac Surg 78:1017–1023

Cerfolio RJ et al (2004b) Repeat FDG-PET after neoadjuvant therapy is a predictor of pathologic response in patients with non-small cell lung cancer. Ann Thorac Surg 78(6):1903–1909

Choi SH et al (2011) Positron emission tomography-computed tomography for postoperative surveillance in non-small cell lung cancer. Ann Thorac Surg 92:1826–1832; discussion, 1832

Collins BT et al (2000) Initial evaluation of pulmonary abnormalities: CT-guided fine needle aspiration biopsy and fluoride-18 fluorodeoxyglucose positron emission tomography correlation. Diagn Cytopathol 22:92–96

Dane B et al (2013) PET/CT vs. non-contrast CT alone for surveillance 1-year post lobectomy for stage I non-small-cell lung cancer. Am J Nucl Med Mol Imaging 3:408–416

Darling GE et al (2011) Positron emission tomography-computed tomography compared with invasive mediastinal staging in non-small cell lung cancer: results of mediastinal staging in the early lung positron emission tomography trial. J Thorac Oncol 6(8):1367–1372

De Wever W et al (2007) Additional value of PET-CT in the staging of lung cancer: comparison with CT alone, PET alone and visual correlation of PET and CT. Eur Radiol 17:23–32

De Wever W, Stroobants S et al (2009) Integrated PET/CT in the staging of non-small cell lung cancer: technical aspects and clinical integration. Eur Respir J 33:201–212

Decoster L et al (2008) Complete metabolic tumor response, assessed by 18-fluorodeoxyglucose positron emission tomography (18FDG-PET), after induction chemotherapy predicts a favourable outcome in patients with locally advanced non-small cell lung cancer (NSCLC). Lung Cancer 62(1):55–61

Dietlein M, Weber K et al (2000) Cost-effectiveness of FDG-PET for the management of potentially operable non-small cell lung cancer: priority for a PET-based strategy after nodal-negative CT result. Eur J Nucl Med 27:1598–1609

Ehab M et al (2003) Whole-body 18F-FDG PET improves the management of patients with small cell lung cancer. J Nucl Med 44(12):1911–1917

Erasmus JJ, Patz EF Jr (1999) Positron emission tomography imaging in the thorax. Clin Chest Med 20(4):715–724

Erasmus JJ, McAdams HP et al (1998) Evaluation of primary pulmonary carcinoid tumors using FDG PET. AJR Am J Roentgenol 170(5):1369–1373

Eschmann SM et al (2007) 18F-FDG PET for assessment of therapy response and preoperative re-evaluation after neoadjuvant radio-chemotherapy in stage III non-small cell lung cancer. Eur J Nucl Med Mol Imaging 34(4):463–471

Feng M et al (2017) Retrospective analysis for the false positive diagnosis of PET-CT scan in lung cancer patients. Medicine (Baltimore) 96(42):e7415

Fischer BM et al (2007) A prospective study of PET/CT in initial staging of small-cell lung cancer: comparison with CT, bone scintigraphy and bone marrow analysis. Ann Oncol 18:338–345

Gao SJ et al (2017) Indications for invasive mediastinal staging in patients with early nonsmall cell lung cancer staged with PET-CT. Lung Cancer 109:36–41

Gould MK, Maclean CC et al (2001) Accuracy of positron emission tomography for diagnosis of pulmonary nodules and mass lesions: a meta-analysis. JAMA 285(7):914–924

Gould MK et al (2003) Test performance of positron emission tomography and computed tomography for mediastinal staging in patients with non-small-cell lung cancer: a meta-analysis. Ann Intern Med 139(11):879–892

Gregory DL et al (2012) Effect of PET/CT on management of patients with non–small cell lung cancer: results of a prospective study with 5-year survival data. J Nucl Med 53:1007–1015

Grgic A, Yiksel Y, Gruschel A et al (2010) Risk stratification of solitary pulmonary nodules by means of PET using (18)F-fluorodeoxyglucose and SUV quantification. Eur J Nucl Med Mol Imaging 37:1087–1094

He YQ et al (2014) Diagnostic efficacy of PET and PET/CT for recurrent lung cancer: a meta-analysis. Acta Radiol 55:309–317

Hoopes DJ et al (2007) FDG-PET and stereotactic body radiotherapy (SBRT) for stage I non-small-cell lung cancer. Lung Cancer 56:229–234

Hustinx R et al (1998) Clinical evaluation of whole-body 18F-fluorodeoxyglucose positron emission tomography in the detection of liver metastases. Ann Oncol 9(4):397–401

İntepe YS et al (2016) Our transthoracic biopsy practices accompanied by the imaging process: the contribution of positron emission tomography usage to accurate diagnosis. Acta Clin Belg 71:214–220

Kim SK et al (2007) Accuracy of PET/CT in characterization of solitary pulmonary lesions. J Nucl Med 48:214–220

Kim IJ, Lee JS et al (2008) Double-phase 18F-FDG PET-CT for determination of pulmonary tuberculoma activity. Eur J Nucl Med Mol Imaging 35:808–814

Konishi J et al (2003) Mediastinal lymph node staging by FDG-PET in patients with nonsmall cell lung cancer: analysis of false-positive FDG-PET findings. Respiration 70(5):500–506

Kremer R et al (2016) FDG PET/CT for assessing the resectability of NSCLC patients with N2 disease after neoadjuvant therapy. Ann Nucl Med 30:114–121

Kubota K et al (2011) Additional value of FDG-PET to contrast enhanced-computed tomography (CT) for the diagnosis of mediastinal lymph node metastasis in non-small cell lung cancer: a Japanese multicenter clinical study. Ann Nucl Med 25(10):777–786

Kubota K et al (2015) Impact of FDGPET findings on decisions regarding patient management strategies: a multicenter trial in patients with lung cancer and other types of cancer. Ann Nucl Med 29(5):431–441

Kumar R et al (2004) 18F-FDG PET in evaluation of adrenal lesions in patients with lung cancer. J Nucl Med 45:2058–2062

Kung BT et al (2017) The pearl of FDG PET/CT in preoperative assessment of patients with potentially operable non–small-cell lung cancer and its clinical impact. World J Nucl Med 16(1):21–25

Langen AJ et al (2006) The size of mediastinal lymph nodes and its relation with metastatic involvement: a meta-analysis. Eur J Cardiothorac Surg 29:26–29

Lardinois D, Weder W et al (2003) Staging of non-small-cell lung cancer with integrated positron-emission tomography and computed tomography. N Engl J Med 348:2500–2507

Lee BE et al (2007) Advances in positron emission tomography technology have increased the need for surgical staging in non-small cell lung cancer. J Thorac Cardiovasc Surg 133:746–752

Lee YJ et al (2009) High tumor metabolic activity as measured by fluorodeoxyglucose positron emission tomography is associated with poor prognosis in limited and extensive stage small-cell lung cancer. Clin Cancer Res 15:2426–2432

Lee P et al (2012) Metabolic tumor volume is an independent prognostic factor in patients treated definitively for non-small-cell lung cancer. Clin Lung Cancer 13(1):52–58

Lewis P et al (1994) Whole-body 18F-fluorodeoxyglucose positron emission tomography in preoperative evaluation of lung cancer. Lancet 344:1265–1266

Li X et al (2012) Mediastinal lymph nodes staging by 18F-FDG PET/CT for early stage non-small cell lung cancer: a multicenter study. Radiother Oncol 102(2):246–245

Liu C et al (2009) The impact of respiratory motion on tumor quantification and delineation in static PET/CT imaging. Phys Med Biol 54:7345–7362

Liu T et al (2011) Fluorine-18 deoxyglucose positron emission tomography, magnetic resonance imaging and bone scintigraphy for the diagnosis of bone metastases in patients with lung cancer: which one is the best? A meta-analysis. Clin Oncol (R Coll Radiol) 23(5):350–358

Liu J et al (2016) Prognostic value of 18F-FDG PET/CT in surgical non-small cell lung cancer: a meta-analysis. PLoS One 11(1):e0146195

MacManus MP et al (2001) High rate of detection of unsuspected distant metastases by PET in apparent stage III non-small cell lung cancer: implications for radical radiation therapy. Int J Radiat Oncol Biol Phys 50:287–293

MacManus MP, Hicks RJ et al (2003) Positron emission tomography is superior to computed tomography scanning for response-assessment after radical radiotherapy or chemoradiotherapy in patients with non-small-cell lung cancer. J Clin Oncol 21(7):1285–1292

Marom EM, McAdams HP, Erasmus JJ et al (1999) Staging non-small cell lung cancer with whole-body PET. Radiology 212:803–809

Martucci F, Traglia G et al (2020) Impact of 18F-FDG PET/CT in staging patients with small cell lung cancer: a systematic review and meta-analysis. Front Med 6:336

Matthies A, Hickeson M et al (2002) Dual time point 18FFDG PET for the evaluation of pulmonary nodules. J Nucl Med 43:871–875

Moon SH et al (2013) Metabolic response evaluated by 18F-FDG PET/CT as a potential screening tool in identifying a subgroup of patients with advanced non-small cell lung cancer for immediate maintenance therapy after first-line chemotherapy. Eur J Nucl Med Mol Imaging 40:1005–1013

Na F et al (2014) Primary tumor standardized uptake value measured on F18-Fluorodeoxyglucose positron emission tomography is of prediction value for survival and local control in non-small-cell lung cancer receiving radiotherapy: meta-analysis. J Thorac Oncol 9(6):834–842

Nomori H, Watanabe K et al (2004) Evaluation of F-18 fluorodeoxyglucose (FDG) PET scanning for pulmonary nodules less than 3 cm in diameter, with special reference to the CT images. Lung Cancer 45(1):19–27

Paesmans M et al (2010) Primary tumor standardized uptake value measured on fluorodeoxyglucose positron emission tomography is of prognostic value for survival in non-small cell lung cancer: update of a systematic review and meta-analysis by the European Lung Cancer Working Party for the International Association for the Study of Lung Cancer Staging Project. J Thorac Oncol 5(5):612–619

Pan T, Mawlawi O et al (2005) Attenuation correction of PET images with respiration-averaged CT images in PET/CT. J Nucl Med 46(9):1481–1487

Pandit N et al (2003) Prognostic value of [18F] FDG-PET imaging in small cell lung cancer. Eur J Nucl Med Mol Imaging 30:78–84

Patz EF Jr et al (2000) Prognostic value of thoracic FDG PET imaging after treatment for non-small cell lung cancer. AJR Am J Roentgenol 174(3):769–774

Pieterman RM, van Putten JW et al (2000) Preoperative staging of non-small-cell lung cancer with positron-emission tomography. N Engl J Med 343(4):254–261

Purandare NC et al (2013) 18F-FDG PET/CT-directed biopsy: does it offer incremental benefit? Nucl Med Commun 34:203–210

Qu X et al (2012) A meta-analysis of 18FDG-PET-CT, 18FDG-PET, MRI and bone scintigraphy for diagnosis of bone metastases in patients with lung cancer. Eur J Radiol 81(5):1007–1015

Sathekge MM, Maes A et al (2010) Dual time-point FDG PET/CT for differentiating benign from malignant solitary pulmonary nodules in a TB endemic area. S Afr Med J 100:598–601

Saunders CA, Dussek JE et al (1999) Evaluation of fluorine-18-fluorodeoxyglucose whole body positron emission tomography imaging in the staging of lung cancer. Ann Thorac Surg 67:790–797

Schreyogg J et al (2010) Cost-effectiveness of hybrid PET/CT for staging of non–small cell lung cancer. J Nucl Med 51(11):1668–1675

Scott WJ et al (1998) Cost-effectiveness of FDG-PET for staging non–small lung cancer: a decision analysis. Ann Thorac Surg 66(6):1876–1883

Sheikhbahaei S, Mena E, Marcus C, Wray R, Taghipour M, Subramaniam R (2016) 18F-fluorodeoxyglucose PET/CT: therapy response assessment interpretation (Hopkins criteria) and survival outcomes in lung cancer patients. J Nucl Med 57:855–860

Shen G et al (2015) Diagnostic value of dual time-point 18F-FDG PET/CT versus single time-point imaging for detection of mediastinal nodal metastasis in non-small cell lung cancer patients: a meta-analysis. Acta Radiol 56(6):681–687

Shiraki N et al (2004) False-positive and true negative hilar and mediastinal lymph nodes on FDG-PET–radiological-pathological correlation. Ann Nucl Med 18:23–28

Stroobants S et al (2003) Additional value of whole-body fluorodeoxyglucose positron emission tomography in the detection of distant metastases of non-small cell lung cancer. Clin Lung Cancer 4:242–247

Takeuchi S et al (2014) Impact of initial PET/CT staging in terms of clinical stage, management plan, and prognosis in 592 patients with non-small-cell lung cancer. Eur J Nucl Med Mol Imaging 41(5):906–914

Van Tinteren H et al (2002) Effectiveness of positron emission tomography in the preoperative assessment of patients with suspected non-small-cell lung cancer: the PLUS multicentre randomised trial. Lancet 359(9315):1388–1393

Vansteenkiste JF, Stroobants SG et al (1998) FDG-PET scan in potentially operable non-small cell lung cancer: do anatometabolic PET-CT fusion images improve the localisation of regional lymph node metastases? The Leuven Lung Cancer Group. Eur J Nucl Med 25(11):1495–1501

Vesselle H et al (2008) Relationship between non-small cell lung cancer FDG uptake at PET, tumor histology, and Ki-67 proliferation index. J Thorac Oncol 3:971–978

Wahl RL, Jacene H, Kasamon Y, Lodge MA (2009) From RECIST to PERCIST: evolving considerations for PET response criteria in solid tumors. Nucl Med 50:122S–150S

Wang J, Welch K et al (2012) Negative predictive value of positron emission tomography and computed tomography for stage T1-2N0 non-small-cell lung cancer: a meta-analysis. Clin Lung Cancer 13(2):81–89

Weber WA, Petersen V et al (2003) Positron emission tomography in non-small-cell lung cancer: prediction of response to chemotherapy by quantitative assessment of glucose use. J Clin Oncol 21(14):2651–2657

Wu Y et al (2013) Diagnostic value of fluorine 18 fluorodeoxyglucose positron emission tomography/computed tomography for the detection of metastases in non-small-cell lung cancer patients. Int J Cancer 132(2):E37–E47

Wu Q et al (2017) The utility of FDG PET/CT for the diagnosis of adrenal metastasis in lung cancer: a PRISMA-compliant meta-analysis. Nucl Med Commun 38(12):1117–1124

Yamamoto Y et al (2009) Early assessment of therapeutic response using FDG PET in small cell lung cancer. Mol Imaging Biol 11:467–472

Yi CA, Lee KS et al (2006) Tissue characterization of solitary pulmonary nodule: comparative study between helical dynamic CT and integrated PET/CT. J Nucl Med 47(3):443–450

Zhang X et al (2012) Positron emission tomography for assessing local failure after stereotactic body radiotherapy for non-small-cell lung cancer. Int J Radiat Oncol Biol Phys 83:1558–1565

Zhang L et al (2013) Dual time point 18FDG-PET/CT versus single time point 18FDG-PET/CT for the differential diagnosis of pulmonary nodules: a meta-analysis. Acta Radiol 54:770–777

Zhou X et al (2017) Potential clinical value of PET/CT in predicting occult nodal metastasis in T1-T2N0M0 lung cancer patients staged by PET/CT. Oncotarget 8:82437–82445

Ziai D et al (2013) Therapy response evaluation with FDG-PET/CT in small cell lung cancer: a prognostic and comparison study of the PERCIST and EORTC criteria. Cancer Imaging 13(1):73–80

Surgical Staging of Lung Cancer

Jarrod Predina, Douglas J. Mathisen, and Michael Lanuti

Contents

1 Introduction 114
2 TNM Staging System for Lung Cancer 114
3 T-Stage Evaluation 114
4 N-Stage Evaluation 116
4.1 Mediastinoscopy 117
4.2 Endobronchial Ultrasound (EBUS) 120
4.3 Esophageal Ultrasound (EUS) 122
4.4 Anterior Mediastinotomy (Chamberlain Procedure) 122
4.5 Thoracoscopy (VATS) 123
4.6 Supraclavicular (Scalene) Lymph Node Biopsy 124
4.7 Comparative Data for Surgical Staging 124
5 M-Stage Evaluation 125
6 General Recommendations 125
7 Conclusions 126
References 126

Abstract

The idiom "name it, stage it, treat it" is perhaps no more relevant (and confusing) than when applied to the management of lung cancer. In this chapter we focus on the second task of this dogma, which involves staging. We specifically provide an overview of the current TNM staging classifications for lung cancer, a description of various invasive mediastinal staging modalities, the evidence supporting invasive mediastinal staging procedures, and general recommendations for the thoracic oncology community at large.

Abbreviations

CT	Computed tomography
DWI	Diffusion-weighted imaging
EBUS	Endobronchial ultrasound
EUS	Endoscopic ultrasound
FDG	Fluorodeoxyglucose (^{18}F)
FNA	Fine needle aspirate
MRI	Magnetic resonance imaging
PET	Positron emission tomography
STIR	Short tau inversion-recovery
TBNA	Transbronchial needle aspiration
TNM	Tumor-node-metastasis
VATS	Video-assisted thoracic surgery

J. Predina
Cardiothoracic Surgery, Massachusetts General Hospital, Boston, MA, USA

D. J. Mathisen · M. Lanuti (✉)
Division of Thoracic Surgery, Massachusetts General Hospital, Harvard Medical School, Boston, MA, USA
e-mail: MLanuti@mgh.harvard.edu

1 Introduction

Lung cancer staging is continuously evolving as technological advances improve both imaging and surgical techniques. The goal of staging is to stratify patients into treatment and prognostic categories. The goal of staging is to identify patients who can benefit from surgery and to avoid surgery in those patients who are not likely to benefit. Lung cancer staging should include a diagnostic quality CT, a PET to evaluate the mediastinal lymph nodes and exclude extrathoracic or bone metastases, and liberal use of surgical staging [mediastinoscopy, endobronchial ultrasound (EBUS) and/or esophageal ultrasound-guided needle aspiration of lymph nodes (EUS-FNA), mediastinotomy, and video-assisted thoracoscopy (VATS)] in most patients. These modalities each have different sensitivity and specificity for lymph node staging (discussed further in this chapter). Techniques for the identification and subsequent staging of lung cancer have improved; however, no single modality has been able to noninvasively confirm the presence of lymph node metastases with perfect accuracy. In addition to patient triage, molecular analysis of tissue obtained during staging may support the use of systemic therapy regimens incorporating targeted therapies (e.g., therapies targeting mutant-EGFR or ALK) or immunotherapy (namely checkpoint inhibitors) (Yuan et al. 2019; Forde et al. 2018).

Surgical staging is only one component of a multimodal approach, and information should be integrated with imaging techniques such as FDG-PET, high-resolution CT, and less commonly thoracic MRI. "Surgical staging" often relies on a combination of information resulting from pathologic review of preoperatively sampled specimens and intraoperative findings during resection. For the purposes of this review, we will focus on surgical approaches that obtain tissue for pathologic assessment and not those findings found during definitive resection.

2 TNM Staging System for Lung Cancer

The tumor-node-metastasis (TNM) staging system is the primary system used for lung cancer and has undergone multiple revisions since first described in 1986 by Clifton Mountain and colleagues at the University of Texas, MD Anderson Cancer Center (Mountain 1986). The current eighth edition staging system for lung cancer (revised in 2018, and summarized in Tables 1 and 2) has been validated in a data set of 94,708 lung cancer patients who were treated in 16 countries between 1999 and 2010, with the majority of patients from Europe and Asia. The contribution of patients from North America, Australia, and South America was disappointingly low at ≤5% (Detterbeck et al. 2017). As compared to the seventh TNM edition, the eighth TNM edition improves upon prognostication and incorporates imaging studies, particularly CT scans (Detterbeck 2018). It is the basis by which treatment strategies are constructed and is highly reliant upon accurate staging information.

3 T-Stage Evaluation

Characteristics which impact the T-stage include tumor size, location, presence of airway obstruction, and/or invasion into surrounding intrathoracic and mediastinal structures (as noted in Table 1). Methods for ascertaining the T-stage include primarily preoperative axial imaging and intraoperative assessment. The most common preoperative imaging modalities include CT and MRI. In general, high-resolution CT provides a comprehensive evaluation of the tumor and its involvement of intrathoracic structures; however, MRI can provide enhanced soft tissue clarity and sometimes delineate invasion in situations in which the tumor approaches mediastinal and thoracic inlet structures. Although FDG-PET is useful in determining metastatic involvement, this modality provides little additional information specific to the T-stage of a given lesion.

Table 1 TNM eighth edition international lung cancer staging system

T: Primary tumor	
Tx	Primary tumor cannot be assessed, or tumor proven by presence of malignant cells in sputum or bronchial washings but not visualized by imaging or bronchoscopy
T0	No evidence of primary tumor
Tis	Carcinoma in situ
T1	Tumor ≤3 cm surrounded by lung or visceral pleura without bronchoscopic evidence of invasion more proximal than the lobar bronchus (i.e., not in the main bronchus)[a]
T1a(mi)	Minimally invasive adenocarcinoma[b]
T1a	Tumor ≤1 cm
T1b	Tumor >1 cm but ≤2 cm
T1c	Tumor >2 cm but ≤3 cm
T2	Tumor >3 cm but ≤5 cm or tumor with any of the following features[c]
T2a	**Tumor >3 cm but ≤4 cm**
T2b	**Tumor >4 cm but ≤5 cm**
T3	**Tumor >5 cm but ≤7 cm in greatest dimension** or associated with separate tumor nodule(s) in the same lobe as the primary tumor or directly invades any of the following structures: chest wall (including the parietal pleura and superior sulcus tumors), phrenic nerve, parietal pericardium
T4	**Tumor >7 cm in greatest dimension** or associated with separate tumor nodule(s) in a different ipsilateral lobe than that of the primary tumor or invades any of the following structures: **diaphragm**, mediastinum, heart, great vessels, trachea, recurrent laryngeal nerve, esophagus, vertebral body, and carina
N: Regional lymph node involvement	
Nx	Regional lymph nodes cannot be assessed
N0	No regional lymph node metastasis
N1	Metastasis in ipsilateral peribronchial and/or ipsilateral hilar lymph nodes and intrapulmonary nodes, including involvement by direct extension
N2	Metastasis in ipsilateral mediastinal and/or subcarinal lymph node(s)
N3	Metastasis in contralateral mediastinal, contralateral hilar, ipsilateral or contralateral scalene, or supraclavicular lymph node(s)
M: Distant metastasis	
M0	No distant metastasis
M1	Distant metastasis present
M1a	Separate tumor nodule(s) in a contralateral lobe; tumor with pleural or pericardial nodule(s) or malignant pleural or pericardial effusion[d]
M1b	Single extrathoracic metastasis[e]
M1c	Multiple extrathoracic metastases in one or more organs

Adapted from the American Joint Committee on Cancer, eighth edition Lung Cancer Staging manual, 2018, Chicago, IL (Detterbeck et al. 2017)
TNM tumor, node, metastasis; *Tis* carcinoma in situ; *T1a(mi)* minimally invasive adenocarcinoma
[a] The uncommon superficial spreading tumor of any size with its invasive component limited to the bronchial wall, which may extend proximal to the main bronchus, is also classified as T1a
[b] Solitary adenocarcinoma, ≤3 cm with a predominately lepidic pattern and ≤5 mm invasion in any one focus
[c] T2 tumors with these features are classified as T2a if ≤4 cm in greatest dimension or if size cannot be determined, and T2b if >4 cm but ≤5 cm in greatest dimension
[d] Most pleural (pericardial) effusions with lung cancer are due to tumor. In a few patients, however, multiple microscopic examinations of pleural (pericardial) fluid are negative for tumor and the fluid is non-bloody and not an exudate. When these elements and clinical judgment dictate that the effusion is not related to the tumor, the effusion should be excluded as a staging descriptor
[e] This includes involvement of a single distant (nonregional) lymph node

In a review by Cagemi and colleagues, CT provided a sensitivity of 38–97% for detection of T3 lesions and 31–78% for T4 lesions (Cangemi et al. 1996). With regard to MRI, sensitivity approaches 85% and accurately determining the highest T-stage (Manfredi et al. 1996). MRI has greatly contributed to the clinical staging of superior sulcus tumors which can involve subclavian vessels, the brachial plexus, recurrent nerve, or sympathetic chain.

Invasive procedures may be necessary in circumstances in which axial imaging does not provide a clear determination of the T-stage of a specific lesion, and that local invasion may preclude an upfront surgical resection. Endoscopic

Table 2 Eighth edition international lung cancer staging system

T/M	Subcategory	N0	N1	N2	N3
T1	T1a	IA1	IIB	IIIA	IIIB
	T1b	IA2	IIB	IIIA	IIIB
	T1c	I13	IIB	IIIA	IIIB
T2	T2a	IB	IIB	IIIA	IIIB
	T2b	IIA	IIB	IIIA	IIIB
T3	T3	IIB	IIIA	IIIB	IIIC
T4	T4	IIIA	IIIA	IIIB	IIIC
M1	M1a	IVA	IVA	IVA	IVA
	M1b	IVA	IVA	IVA	IVA
	M1c	IVB	IVB	IVB	IVB

Adapted from the American Joint Committee on Cancer, eighth edition Lung Cancer Staging manual, 2018, Chicago, IL (Detterbeck et al. 2017)

ultrasound (EUS) and endobronchial ultrasound (EBUS) have proven to be safe and minimally invasive options for locally invasive lesions with proximity to the esophagus and airways; however, sensitivity does not appear to be dramatically superior to axial imaging (sensitivity 85–90%) (Varadarajulu et al. 2004). Surgical exploration, most commonly video-assisted thoracic surgery (VATS), is the gold standard for such an evaluation as it allows both direct visual and tactile feedback and may demonstrate either upstaging or downstaging of the T-stage in 25–50% of the those patients with ambiguous imaging (Sebastian-Quetglas et al. 2003). Diagnostic thoracotomy should be avoided due to an unnecessary risk of morbidity.

4 N-Stage Evaluation

The N-stage of a given lesion is determined by the involvement of lymph nodes which span from the supraclavicular region to the diaphragm. Lymph nodes are divided into 14 stations or levels, with the most current IASLC map describing lymph node involvement described in Fig. 1 and Table 3.

Lymph node metastases portend a worse prognosis, and rates of curative surgical resection are significantly influenced by mediastinal lymph node involvement. In general, the presence of lymph node involvement requires adjuvant therapy when surgery is employed or definitive nonoperative therapy. As such, determination of nodal involvement is key for both prognostication and treatment planning purposes. There are a number of imaging modalities and surgical approaches useful for nodal assessment and are described below.

Imaging may suggest nodal metastases, but suspicious lesions typically require tissue sampling for confirmation. CT has historically yielded an overall sensitivity of 59% (range, 20–81%) and an overall specificity of 78% (range, 44–100%) (McCloud et al. 1992). PET evaluation of the mediastinum for stage I and II NSCLC has yielded a sensitivity as high as 85% and specificity of 88% (Reed et al. 2003). PET is associated with negative predictive value for the mediastinum of 87%, whereas the positive predictive value is 56%. Specificity of PET is limited as both neoplastic and inflammatory nodes can have increased FDG uptake, while sensitivity is limited by the inability to reproducibly characterize metabolic activity of lesions smaller than 10 mm (Predina et al. 2017; Silvestri et al. 2007a). Accurate detection of hilar nodal involvement in lung cancer has historically been difficult, but with CT-PET and more widespread use of EBUS transbronchial needle aspiration biopsy (see discussion regarding EBUS below), pathologic correlation has proven that PET has a role in identifying N1 disease.

The widespread use and availability of PET-CT fusion imaging has increased the proportion of patients found to have additional lesions that contraindicate surgical treatment; however, suspicious imaging typically requires tissue confirmation to exclude a false-positive examination. In a sentinel study from Switzerland in 2003, the authors studied PET-CT in 50 patients with NSCLC. Integrated PET-CT provided additional information in 41% of patients and was significantly more accurate in precise staging compared with CT alone, PET alone, or visual correlation of PET and CT (Lardinois et al. 2003). This technology has been evaluated in the literature with increasing frequency.

MRI of the lung has historically been challenged by poor spatial resolution and high

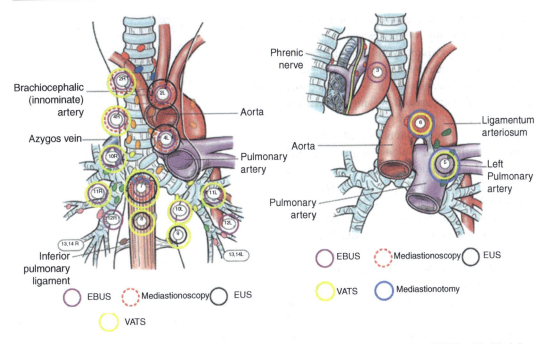

Fig. 1 Map depiction of thoracic lymph node stations according to accessibility by common staging modalities EBUS (endobronchial ultrasound), cervical mediastinoscopy, esophageal ultrasound (EUS), mediastinotomy, and video-assisted thoracic surgery (VATS). (*Modified from Mountain* CF, *Dresler CM. Regional lymph node classification for lung cancer staging. Chest* **1997**; *111:1718–1723c* (Mountain 1986))

Table 3 Thoracic Lymph node station nomenclature

Supraclavicular zone
Station 1—Low cervical, supraclavicular, and sternal notch nodes
Superior mediastinal nodes
Station 2—Upper Paratracheal
Station 3a—Prevascular; Station 3p—Retrotracheal
Station 4—Lower Paratracheal
Aortic nodes
Station 5—Subaortic
Station 6—Para-aortic (ascending or phrenic nodes)
Inferior mediastinal nodes
Station 7—Subcarinal
Station 8—Paraesophageal
Station 9—Pulmonary ligament
N1 nodes
Station 10—Hilar
Station 11—Interlobar
Station 12—Lobar
Station 13—Segmental
Station 14—Subsegmental

noise-to-contrast ratio and has traditionally been reserved for characterizing mediastinal masses or detecting tumor invasion into the chest wall, mediastinum, vasculature structures, diaphragm, pericardium, or bone. A recent report suggests that new MR techniques such as diffusion-weighted imaging (DWI) and short tau inversion-recovery turbo spin echo (STIR) sequences can improve upon the accuracy of PET/CT for distinguishing benign from malignant lymph nodes (Ohno et al. 2011). In these studies, STIR and DWI have sensitivities of 82.8% and 75.2%, respectively, and overall accuracy of 86.8% and 84.4%. Furthermore, PET-MRI is the newest modality that is being evaluated for lung cancer staging and may incrementally be more accurate compared to PET-CT (Klenk et al. 2014).

4.1 Mediastinoscopy

The gold standard for staging nodal disease within the mediastinum is cervical mediastinoscopy which was developed by Harken and associates in 1954 and then promulgated by Carlens in 1959 and later Pearson in 1965 (Carlens 1959).

Carlens and Pearson recognized that mediastinoscopy was not only for lung cancer staging but also for the diagnosis of lymphoma, metastatic disease from an extrathoracic origin, infectious etiologies, and sarcoidosis. It is the modality upon which all comparisons of lymph node accuracy are currently analyzed.

Mediastinoscopy should be considered in any patient harboring a suspicious lung nodule with enlarged (>1 cm in short axis measured on CT) or fluorine-18-labeled deoxyglucose (FDG)-avid mediastinal lymph nodes (N2 or N3), those with central tumors, and those with peripheral tumors ≥3 cm. T1 tumors with an aggressive histology (i.e., large cell neuroendocrine, carcinosarcoma, small cell, pleomorphic carcinomas, micropapillary adenocarcinomas) should also undergo mediastinoscopy. Peripheral T1a–c lesions (tumors <3 cm) with PET-negative mediastinal lymph nodes can be regarded as the one exception to the routine use of mediastinoscopy (Detterbeck et al. 2013). Mediastinoscopy is the procedure of choice for lung cancer staging (*endorsed by the American College of Chest Physicians, and European Society of Thoracic Surgeons*); however, endoscopic techniques such as EBUS or EUS-FNA are recognized as modalities where a cytologic diagnosis can be achieved to initiate a treatment strategy. If EBUS or EUS-directed biopsies are negative in a pathologically enlarged or FDG-avid mediastinal lymph node, mediastinoscopy is still mandatory.

With regard to the procedure itself, mediastinoscopy is a day procedure that allows for sampling of level 2, level 4, and level 7 lymph nodes (see Fig. 1) through a cervical incision. This procedure should be performed in a hospital setting that allows for the rare, but catastrophic, circumstance for hemorrhage. The patient is positioned supine on the operating room table where the head is placed at the top of the bed. After establishing general endotracheal anesthesia, the neck is extended, and a small incision is made superior to the sternal notch (Fig. 2). Dissection is carried down through the strap muscles and to the pretracheal alveolar plane. This pretracheal plane is then developed with a combination of blunt dissection with a finger and sharp dissection using surgical scissors. The mediastinoscope is then inserted into the pretracheal tunnel which allows the surgeon to explore the length of the trachea and both mainstem bronchi for nodal sampling (Fig. 3).

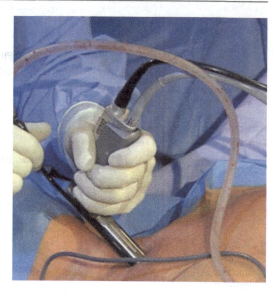

Fig. 2 Cervical mediastinoscopy with suction cautery. (Obtained from Video mediastinoscopy copyright 2011 Endo Press Tuttlingen, Germany, email endopress@t-online.de)

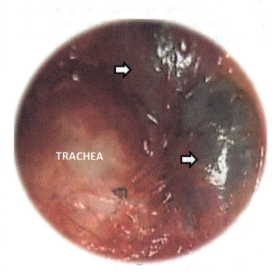

Fig. 3 Intraoperative photo of video mediastinoscopy dissection of level 4R lymph node (arrow) during cervical mediastinoscopy. (Courtesy of M. Lanuti)

The paratracheal adipose tissue is carefully surveyed to identify lymph node stations 2, 4, and 7 as depicted in Fig. 3. Nodes are identified by a color and consistency difference. For example, surrounding mediastinal fat is yellow, while nodes are typically anthracotic (black) or more pearly in color when involved with inflammatory or bulky malignant processes. Nodes are often more "full" and firm, while mediastinal fat is typically flimsy and quite soft. Particular care is taken when retrieving specimens near the tracheobronchial angles because of the proximity of the azygos vein and apical branch of the pulmonary artery on the right and the recurrent laryngeal nerve on the left. The right main pulmonary artery is observed superior to the carina and can be injured with cautery while achieving hemostasis from biopsies of subcarinal lymph nodes.

The efficacy of mediastinoscopy has been well established in the assessment of enlarged mediastinal lymph nodes with 100% specificity and ~90% sensitivity. In patients with known or suspected lung cancer, the routine use of mediastinoscopy can change the plan of care in up to 25% of patients. Large studies confirm false-negative rates from 5% to 8% as demonstrated in Table 3 (Hammoud et al. 1999; Park et al. 2003; Lemaire et al. 2006). The false-negative rate of mediastinoscopy may be attributed to the diligence of the surgeon dissecting and sampling the nodes. Ideally, five nodal stations (stations 2R, 4R, 7, 2L, and 4L) should be routinely examined (refer to Fig. 2), with a least one node sampled from each station unless none are present after dissection in the region of a particular nodal station. Video mediastinoscopy compared to conventional mediastinoscopy appears to yield some improvement in sensitivity (92%) and false-negative rates (7%) (Ergene et al. 2012; Adebibe et al. 2012) and appears to have a threefold increase in the ability to identify N2/N3 involvement when present (Turna et al. 2013).

Routine mediastinoscopy remains somewhat controversial in that many lung cancer treatment centers use the modality selectively. A national survey of 729 hospitals (31% teaching or university hospitals, 38% community cancer centers, 46% comprehensive community cancer centers) sponsored by the American College of Surgeons identified more than 11,668 patients whose initial management included surgical therapy for lung cancer (Little et al. 2005). The mediastinum was evaluated preoperatively with mediastinoscopy in only 27% of these surgical patients and only 26% underwent a staging PET. The underuse of aggressive mediastinal staging in both academic and community lung cancer care is sobering. Additionally, troublesome is that only 42% had lymph nodes sampled at any mediastinal level during surgery.

The incidence of complications for mediastinoscopy across large series is extremely low (summarized in Table 4). The most common injury occurring during mediastinoscopy is temporary left recurrent laryngeal nerve palsy/dysphonia, which occurs in approximately 3% of patients (~1% are permanent injuries) (Call et al. 2016). This can be observed with traction injury from the scope or as a result of thermal injury from cautery (Roberts and Wadsworth 2007). Because of these concerns, cautery is typically avoided along the left paratracheal space to avoid thermal injury to the recurrent laryngeal nerve. Catastrophic hemorrhage can be observed during mediastinoscopy (<1%); however, most bleeding is minor and can be controlled with

Table 4 Morbidity and mortality reported in large studies of patients undergoing mediastinoscopy for lung cancer

Study	N	No. with lung cancer	No. (%) with false-negative results	No. (%) of complications	No. (%) deaths
Turna, 2013	433	433	35 (8.1%)	23 (5.3)	0
Lemaire, 2006	2145	1019	56 (5.5)	23 (1.07)	1 (0.05)
Park, 2003	3391	NA	NA	14 (0.04)	0
Hammoud, 1999	2137	947	76 (8.0)	12 (0.06)	4 (0.2)

NA not applicable

transient packing or partial withdrawal of the scope to tamponade the mediastinum. If significant bleeding occurs, the mediastinoscope is packed and left in place for at least 10 min and gently removed. If bleeding is uncontrolled, sternotomy with cardiopulmonary bypass may be necessary for repair. Esophageal injury is extremely uncommon and can be encountered in association with aggressive biopsy at the low left paratracheal or subcarinal space. This injury may not be immediately recognized, and the patient may present postoperatively with mediastinal air, mediastinitis, or pleural effusion. Pneumothorax (0.1%) can be observed when violating the parietal pleura and is not often associated with a parenchymal injury. If there is a recognized lung parenchymal injury, tube thoracostomy must be implemented. Other uncommon complications include tracheobronchial injury, stroke, mediastinitis, thoracic duct injury, or death (Lemaire et al. 2006).

There are several modifications to the standard cervical mediastinoscopy to enhance surgical staging. Two such examples are mediastinopleuroscopy and extended cervical mediastinoscopy. Mediastinopleuroscopy begins using a standard neck incision and tracheal exposure and incorporates deliberate entry into the pleural spaces for additional sampling of pleural fluid, pleural lesions, or lung nodules (Deslauriers et al. 1976). Extended cervical mediastinoscopy also utilizes a standard cervical incision, but also includes creation of a tunnel over the aortic arch to approach the subaortic space. The sensitivity of this approaches ranges from 45% to 51% and a complication rate of 0.3% (Detterbeck et al. 2007). Despite relatively low rates of complication, there are dramatic implications of the rare injury to the innominate or carotid artery, left main pulmonary artery, left recurrent laryngeal nerve, and left phrenic nerve. Because of these complexities, the level 5 and 6 nodal stations are more commonly accessed via anterior mediastinotomy (Chamberlain procedure) or VATS with improved visualization (see below for further discussion).

4.2 Endobronchial Ultrasound (EBUS)

Since being developed in the early 1990s, EBUS has quickly gained popularity as an invasive diagnostic modality for assessing lymph node stations situated in the mediastinum (stations 2, 4, and 7) and hilum (stations 10, 11, and 12) (Hurter and Hanrath 1992). EBUS has been adapted and modified to better fit its current role in lung cancer staging by Yasufuku and colleagues at the University of Toronto over the previous decades (Yasufuku et al. 2004). In the current era, EBUS has replaced cervical mediastinoscopy and has become the most common initial staging procedure of the mediastinum (Krantz et al. 2018). EBUS is performed utilizing a specialized bronchoscope which is equipped with (1) a working channel which accommodates various biopsy needles and (2) either a radial (360° cross-sectional view) or more commonly linear (180° directional view) ultrasound probe with color Doppler capabilities (Fig. 4). The working channel is large enough to accommodate specialized needles (range 25, 22, 21, and 19 G) which allow for nodal or tumor sampling via transbronchial needle aspiration (TBNA) (Fig. 5). The maximum distance this needle can traverse is approximately ~4–5 cm but depends on the device being deployed.

Real-time EBUS transbronchial needle aspiration is utilized for sampling mediastinal and hilar

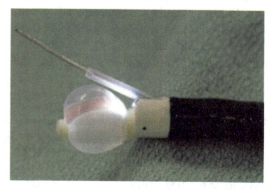

Fig. 4 Linear endobronchial ultrasound with balloon inflated and 22-G needle passed through the working channel. (Origin M. Lanuti)

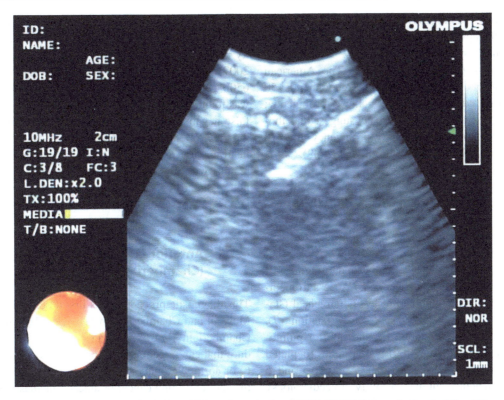

Fig. 5 Endobronchial ultrasound transbronchial needle aspiration (EBUS-TBNA) biopsy of subcarinal (level 7) mediastinal lymph node. (Origin M. Lanuti)

lymph nodes or concerning lesions in close proximity to the airway (Herth et al. 2008a). The utilization of Doppler ultrasound helps identify intervening vessels and is routinely used before needle puncture. EBUS is most commonly performed in an outpatient setting with either conscious sedation or general anesthesia. Fine needle aspiration is performed by passing a needle through the tracheal or bronchial wall into adjacent lymph nodes or central or perihilar parenchymal masses under real-time ultrasound control. Specimens can be smeared on glass and fixed with ethanol or sprayed with Cytofix for cytologic evaluation. Additional specimens can be placed in 10% formalin or saline in preparation of a cell block to perform immunohistochemistry.

Compared with mediastinoscopy, EBUS-TBNA has the advantage that it is also able to routinely access retrotracheal mediastinal (station 3) and hilar lymph nodes (stations 10, 11, and 12) in addition to bilateral paratracheal and subcarinal nodes (stations 2, 4, and 7). Figure 1 shows the extent of accessible lymph nodes when using EBUS. In addition to pathologic nodes (those at that are FDG-avid or >1.0 cm), EBUS allows for broad sampling of normal nodes and fosters complete nodal staging. In fact, several studies suggest that patients with adenocarcinomas and CT/PET showing a normal mediastinum may be staged via EBUS-TBNA with all nodes larger than 5 mm being sampled (Herth et al. 2008b).

The false-negative rate of EBUS has been reported to be 15–28% (Cerfolio et al. 2010; Defranchi et al. 2010). A large meta-analysis of EBUS in lung cancer staging reviewed 365 publications; however, only ten were suitable for analysis. EBUS transbronchial needle aspiration biopsy had a pooled sensitivity of 88% (range 80–94%) and a specificity of nearly 100% (range 92–100%) (Adams et al. 2009). Notably 15–30% of patients had small cell lung cancer, and nodal involvement was near 70% (Adams et al. 2009). EBUS can be used for nodal staging of lung cancer, restaging the mediastinum after neoadjuvant therapy, assessment of isolated hilar or mediastinal lymphadenopathy, and sampling of perihilar parenchymal masses. The American College of Chest Physicians recommends 50 supervised procedures to achieve proficiency; however, there is evidence to suggest that thoracic surgeons can achieve proficiency after 10 supervised procedures (Groth et al. 2008).

4.3 Esophageal Ultrasound (EUS)

Esophageal ultrasound-guided fine needle aspiration (EUS-FNA) is a minimally invasive alternative technique for mediastinal staging of non-small cell lung cancer, and Access to mediastinal nodes is limited to left paratracheal (station 2L and 4L), subcarinal (station 7), paraesophageal (station 8), and inferior pulmonary ligament (station 9) lymph nodes (depicted in Fig. 1). EUS can visualize station 5 and 6 lymph nodes, but the feasibility of needle biopsy is limited to the lower part of station 5 with favorable anatomy. Advanced users have described a method to sample the para-aortic (station 6) lymph node without traversing the aorta (Liberman et al. 2012). EUS can also detect and biopsy metastatic (M1) disease in the adrenal glands and liver. Aside from thoracoscopy or thoracotomy, EUS is the only modality that can access N2 lymph nodes along the esophagus and inferior pulmonary ligament (station 8 and 9). Overall, the risks associated with EUS are minimal, with only several reports of mild bleeding and transient fever being reported and no deaths to date (Detterbeck et al. 2007).

EUS-FNA has been shown to be highly accurate in detecting mediastinal lymph node metastases with an overall diagnostic yield of 90%. A meta-analysis was performed to estimate the diagnostic accuracy of EUS-FNA for staging mediastinal lymph nodes (N2/N3 disease) in patients with lung cancer. Pooled meta-analysis of EUS staging of lung cancer demonstrated an 83% sensitivity (78–87%) and 97% specificity (96–98%). When analyzing EUS for radiographic abnormal lymph nodes seen on CT, the sensitivity = 90% and specificity = 97% (Micames et al. 2007). In another meta-analysis involving over 6500 patients, sensitivity of identifying N2/N3 was found to be 84% with a specificity of 99%; a false-negative rate was 19% and false-positive rate <1% (Detterbeck et al. 2007). Because of the insufficient negative predictive value, negative results with EUS-FNA in an enlarged lymph node should be verified by surgical staging (VATS, mediastinoscopy, or Chamberlain).

4.4 Anterior Mediastinotomy (Chamberlain Procedure)

This diagnostic procedure was first described by McNeill and Chamberlain in 1966 (McNeill and Chamberlain 1966) and is an outpatient procedure that can target enlarged prevascular (station 6) or aortopulmonary (station 5) lymph nodes in the setting of lung cancer or anterior mediastinal masses (as noted in Fig. 1). The procedure requires general anesthesia and a single lumen endotracheal tube. A 5 cm transverse incision is performed at the left sternal border over the second or third interspace, and careful dissection is carried out through the pectoralis muscle (Fig. 5). The mediastinum is entered, while the internal mammary artery and vein may be ligated or retracted depending on anatomy.

Potential pitfalls here are inadvertent biopsy of the left main pulmonary artery or aortic arch which may result in catastrophic hemorrhage, injury to phrenic or recurrent laryngeal nerve, pneumothorax, infection, and chylothorax. In a systemic review, the overall sensitivity of detecting N2/N3 disease via anterior mediastinotomy was found to be 87% in patients with left upper lobe tumors, and the false-negative rate was approximately 10% (Detterbeck et al. 2007). Adequate visualization is mandatory and if it cannot be achieved, thoracoscopy can be added through additional port incisions while intermittent ventilation is employed (Fig. 6).

Surgical Staging of Lung Cancer

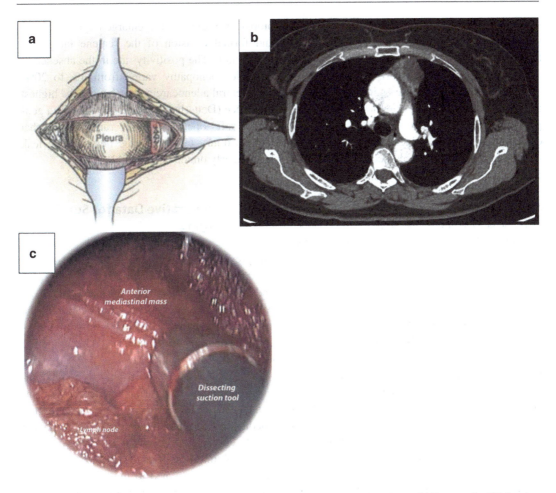

Fig. 6 Anterior mediastinotomy: (**a**) Transverse incision over the second costal cartilage. (**b**) Pt example: CT showing enlarged AP node and (**c**) Intraop findings via anterior mediastinotomy. (Origin M. Lanuti)

4.5 Thoracoscopy (VATS)

Video-assisted thoracoscopy (VATS) is another approach to stage of locally advanced lung cancer. VATS provides an opportunity to assess the hemithorax with the aid of a thoracoscope and affords access to stations 4, 7, 9, and 10 on the right chest and 5, 6, 7, 8, 9, and 10 on the left chest (Fig. 1). Unlike other previously noted procedures, VATS is frequently employed at the time of resection and can assess for pleural or pulmonary ipsilateral metastases and more accurately assess T-stage, particularly when the tumor abuts chest wall, vascular, or mediastinal structures. VATS is most commonly utilized to assess suspicious aortopulmonary (station 5) and para-aortic (station 6)

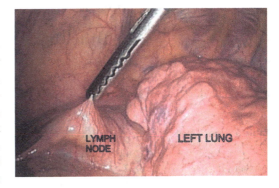

Fig. 7 Left VATS biopsy of aortopulmonary window node. (Origin M. Lanuti)

lymph nodes in the setting of a left upper lobe non-small cell lung cancer (Fig. 7). Complete assessment of station 5 and 6 lymph nodes in left upper lobe cancers has been given much debate as some data suggests that isolated involvement of these nodes does not impair survival (Landreneau et al. 1993; Roberts et al. 1999).

VATS is performed under general anesthesia and requires single lung ventilation. If no lung parenchymal biopsies are performed, same-day discharge is feasible. Diagnostic VATS is well tolerated with complications occurring in 2% of patients and no reported mortality (Detterbeck et al. 2007). For detection of N2 disease, test characteristics based on meta-analysis are as follows: sensitivity of ~75% (range 35–100%), a specificity of nearly 100%, false-negative rate of 15%, and false-positive rate of 0% (Detterbeck et al. 2007).

4.6 Supraclavicular (Scalene) Lymph Node Biopsy

Historically, scalene fat pad excision was the mainstay of nodal staging for lung cancer; however, this has been replaced by other procedures which allow more comprehensive assessment of the mediastinum. Supraclavicular lymph node biopsy is currently reserved for those patients with palpable disease and can provide an efficient approach to obtain tissue for both diagnosis and staging. Confirmation of node positive disease with this technique invokes at least pathologic TxN3 lung carcinoma (stage IIIB), in which case curative surgery is typically not recommended. Lymphadenopathy in this region can be approached via needle aspiration; however, a negative aspirate in a pathologically enlarged lymph node does not rule out disease. Excisional biopsy is preferred for enlarged lymph nodes, and formal excision of the scalene fat pad is uncommon. The positivity rate in the absence of palpable adenopathy varied from 3% to 20%, with central adenocarcinomas having the highest incidence (Detterbeck et al. 2007). This is a generally safe operation, with rare pitfalls that include injury to the phrenic nerve, chyle leak (particularly on the left), and bleeding.

4.7 Comparative Data for Surgical Staging

The previously noted staging approaches modalities are complimentary and may be performed under a single general anesthesia session. Application is typically based on location of the nodes in question (Table 5) and surgeon preference as there is little level 1 data comparing modalities.

To date, there have been only three randomized controlled clinical trials comparing conventional mediastinal nodal surgical staging (mediastinoscopy) of lung cancer to combined EBUS-TBNA and EUS-FNA. Two trials describe data involving more than 100 patients per study arm and were designed to implement mediastinoscopy as a follow-up modality to the EBUS/EUS arm if no nodal metastases were detected at needle aspiration biopsy (Sharples et al. 2012; Annema et al. 2010). In both of these randomized studies, thoracotomy with lymph node dissection was performed when there was no evidence of mediastinal tumor spread. Both studies demonstrated that the endosonographic modalities (EBUS/EUS) and mediastinoscopy were

Table 5 Lymph Node Stations accessibility by staging modality

Modality	Lymph Node Station										
	2	3	4R	4L	5,6	7	8	9	10	11	12
EBUS	x		x	x	x[a]	x			x	x	x
EUS	x			x	x	x	x	x			
Mediastinoscopy	x		x	x		x					
Extended mediastinoscopy	x		x	x	x	x					
Anterior mediastinotomy					x						
VATS		x	x	x	x	x	x	x	x	x	

[a]EBUS can access; however, not routine practice

complimentary and not mutually exclusive in the comprehensive evaluation of mediastinal lymph nodes. Endosonography (followed by surgical staging if negative) resulted in greater sensitivity and improved negative predictive values for establishing N2/N3 disease and fewer unnecessary thoracotomies. In a smaller study comparing EUS to mediastinoscopy, EUS was found to decrease the number of futile resections (Tournoy et al. 2008). It was, however, noted that mediastinoscopy was associated with a greater number of nodes sampled.

An interesting prospective trial evaluating test characteristics of EBUS-TBNA and mediastinoscopy involved 265 patients with biopsy proven lung cancer and suspicious nodes by imaging (Um et al. 2015). These patients underwent EBUS-TBNA ($n = 138$) or EBUS-TBNA followed by mediastinoscopy ($n = 127$); all patients with clear N2/N3 nodes then went on to have surgical resection with complete lymph node. Using lymph node dissection as "gold standard," the authors found that the sensitivity, specificity, accuracy, positive predictive value, and negative predictive value of EBUS-TBNA were 88%, 100%, 92.9%, 100%, and 85.2% versus 81.3%, 100%, 89%, 100%, and 79% for mediastinoscopy. Statistically significant differences ($p < 0.05$) in sensitivity, accuracy, and NPV were identified.

5 M-Stage Evaluation

The M-stage of a given presentation is determined by extrathoracic spread, with the brain, adrenals, bones, contralateral lung, and liver being among the most common locations (Table 1). Pleural and pericardial deposits also represent metastatic disease. CT, PET, or MRI are the primary vehicles for establishing metastatic involvement. If a diagnosis of lung cancer is already established based on the primary tumor or nodal involvement, a tissue diagnosis of suspicious extrathoracic lesions is typically not required. In dealing with lesions that have a less clear etiology, tissue should be obtained from the location that maximizes probability of success and minimizes risks of morbidity to the patient. Tissue may be obtained via CT-guided biopsy, excision biopsy, thoracentesis, VATS/laparoscopy, or pericardiocentesis.

CT-guided biopsy is among the most commonly utilized interventions and can be useful for obtaining tissue from bones, deep tissues, or viscera. Those lesions on the skin or subcutaneous tissue may be amenable to incision or excisional biopsy. These are appealing approaches given their safety profile and convenience as a day procedure. Thoracentesis is also an option for those patients with effusions and can establish a diagnosis of M1 disease in nearly 80% of those patients who have malignant pleural effusions (Rivera et al. 2007). In patients with cytologically negative effusions, VATS can establish pleural disease in 60–75% of patients, with a ~10% false-negative rate (De Giacomo et al. 1997). Pericardial fluid sampling is usually performed as a therapeutic maneuver for those patients with symptomatic effusions; however, it may provide evidence of M1 disease as well.

6 General Recommendations

Per current NCCN guideline, all patients with a confirmed or suspected diagnosis of lung cancer should undergo noninvasive staging with CT and PET (Non-Small Cell Lung Cancer: NCCN Evidence Blocks 2021). A full description of noninvasive imaging is beyond the scope of this discussion; however, we stress that the primary goal of PET is to identify locations of metastatic disease. Based on meta-analysis, PET has improved sensitivity (~75% vs. 50%) and similar specificity (approximately 75) as compared to traditional CT in identifying mediastinal lymph node metastases (Silvestri et al. 2007b). It is important to understand the primary limitations of PET which result in inaccuracies. False negatives arise most commonly in cases of micrometastatic nodal involvement, which escapes the sensitivity thresholds of current detection devices. In general, PET is unreliable identifying metabolic activity in nodes smaller than 8–10 mm. False positives arise when benign lesions display activity as is common for inflammatory (sarcoid, granuloma) or infectious processes. Despite limitations, PET performs well when evaluated in real-world scenarios and has a greater than 90% accuracy in identifying patients with N2/N3 disease in stage I lung cancer patients (Fernandez et al. 2015). False negatives were found only in patients with lesions measuring greater than 2.8 cm in this study.

Although PET may play a sufficient role for mediastinal staging in early-stage lung cancers located in the peripheral lung, surgical staging plays an important complimentary role in patients presenting with more advanced disease or tumors in central locations (Detterbeck et al. 2007). Invasive staging is recommended for all patients who present with suspicious mediastinal (N2/N3) node involvement, regardless of FDG uptake by PET. As noted in previous sections, the initial staging modality depends primarily on location of adenopathy and operator preference. EBUS-TBNA has become more common than mediastinoscopy in recent years; however, because sampling error exists with EBUS-TBNA (and EUS-TBNA) negative results of these modalities should prompt lymph node sampling with mediastinoscopy, Chamberlain, or VATS (Detterbeck et al. 2007; Um et al. 2015). Given higher risk of mediastinal involvement, mediastinal sampling should also be utilized for evaluation of patients with suspicious N1 lymph nodes or central tumors. Again, open lymph node sampling should be used to confirm endobronchial or pathologic results which do not correlate to imaging findings. For those patients with left upper lobe cancers in whom invasive mediastinal staging is indicated, sampling of the aortopulmonary window is warranted.

7 Conclusions

Complete and accurate staging of lung cancer patients is critical for proper triage and treatment assignment. Staging is often a multidisciplinary effort that incorporates both imaging and surgical procedures. These modalities are complimentary with each providing unique benefits and risks. Imaging and surgical staging procedures must be appreciated by members of the modern thoracic oncology team to maximize patient outcomes.

References

Adams K, Shah P, Lim E (2009) Test performance of EBUS and transbronchial needle aspiration biopsy for mediastinal staging in patients with lung cancer: systemic review and meta-analysis. Thorax 64:757–762

Adebibe M, Jarral O, Shipolini AR, McCormack DJ (2012) Does video-assisted mediastinoscopy have a better lymph node yield and safety profile than conventional mediastinoscopy? Interact Cardiovasc Thorac Surg 14(3):316–319

Annema JT, van Meerbeeck J, Rintoul RC, Dooms C, Deschepper E, Dekkers OM, De Leyn P, Braun J, Carroll NR, Praet M, de Ryck F, Vansteenkiste J, Vermassen F, Versteegh MI, Veseliç M, Nicholson AG, Rabe KF, Tournoy KG (2010) Mediastinoscopy vs endosonography for mediastinal nodal staging of lung cancer: a randomized trial. JAMA 304(20):2245–2252

Call S et al (2016) Video-assisted mediastinoscopic lymphadenectomy for staging non-small cell lung cancer. Ann Thorac Surg 101(4):1326–1333

Cangemi V et al (1996) Assessment of the accuracy of diagnostic chest CT scanning. Impact on lung cancer management. Int Surg 81(1):77–82

Carlens E (1959) Mediastinoscopy: a method for inspection and tissue biopsy in the superior mediastinum. Dis Chest 36:343–352

Cerfolio RJ, Bryant A, Eloubeidi MA, Frederick PA, Minnich DJ, Harbour KC, Dransfield MT (2010) The true false negative rates of esophageal and endobronchial ultrasound in the staging of mediastinal lymph nodes in patients with non-small cell lung cancer. Ann Thorac Surg 90(2):427–434

De Giacomo T et al (1997) Thoracoscopic staging of IIIB non-small cell lung cancer before neoadjuvant therapy. Ann Thorac Surg 64(5):1409–1411

Defranchi SA, Edell E, Daniels CE, Prakash UB, Swanson KL, Utz JP, Allen MS, Cassivi SD, Deschamps C, Nichols FC, Shen KR, Wigle DA (2010) Mediastinoscopy in patients with lung cancer and negative endobronchial ultrasound guided needle aspiration. Ann Thorac Surg 90(6):1753–1757

Deslauriers J et al (1976) Mediastinopleuroscopy: a new approach to the diagnosis of intrathoracic diseases. Ann Thorac Surg 22(3):265–269

Detterbeck FC (2018) The eighth edition TNM stage classification for lung cancer: what does it mean on main street? J Thorac Cardiovasc Surg 155(1):356–359

Detterbeck FC, Jantz M, Wallace M, Vansteenkiste J, Silvestri GA (2007) Invasive mediastinal staging of lung cancer; ACCP evidence based clinical practice guidelines (2nd edition). Chest 132(3):202S–220S

Detterbeck FC et al (2013) Executive summary: diagnosis and management of lung cancer, 3rd ed: American College of Chest Physicians evidence-based clinical practice guidelines. Chest 143(5 Suppl):7S–37S

Detterbeck FC et al (2017) The eighth edition lung cancer stage classification. Chest 151(1):193–203

Ergene G, Baysungur V, Okur E, Sevilgen G, Halezeroglu S (2012) Superiority of video-assisted to standard mediastinoscopy in non-small-cell lung cancer staging. Thorac Cardiovasc Surg 60(8):541–544

Fernandez FG et al (2015) Utility of mediastinoscopy in clinical stage I lung cancers at risk for occult mediastinal nodal metastases. J Thorac Cardiovasc Surg 149(1):35–41, 42.e1

Forde PM et al (2018) Neoadjuvant PD-1 blockade in resectable lung cancer. N Engl J Med 378(21):1976–1986

Groth SS, Whitson B, D'Cunha J, Andrade RS, Landis GH, Maddaus MA (2008) Endobronchial ultrasound-guided fine-needle aspiration of mediastinal lymph nodes: a single institution's early learning curve. Ann Thorac Surg 86:1104–1109

Hammoud ZT, Anderson RC, Meyers BF, Guthrie TJ, Roper CL, Cooper JD, Patterson GA (1999) The current role of mediastinoscopy in the evaluation of thoracic disease. J Thorac Cardiovasc Surg 118(5):894–899

Herth FJ, Annema J, Eberhardt R, Yasufuku K, Ernst A, Krasnik M, Rintoul RC (2008a) Endobronchial ultrasound with transbronchial needle aspiration for restaging the mediastinum in lung cancer. J Clin Oncol 26(20):3346–3350

Herth FJ, Eberhardt R, Krasnik M, Ernst A (2008b) Endobronchial ultrasound-guided transbronchial needle aspiration of lymph nodes in the radiologically and PET normal mediastinum in patients with lung cancer. Chest 133(4):887–891

Hurter T, Hanrath P (1992) Endobronchial sonography: feasibility and preliminary results. Thorax 47(7):565–567

Klenk C et al (2014) Ionising radiation-free whole-body MRI versus (18)F-fluorodeoxyglucose PET/CT scans for children and young adults with cancer: a prospective, non-randomised, single-centre study. Lancet Oncol 15(3):275–285

Krantz SB et al (2018) Invasive mediastinal staging for lung cancer by the Society of Thoracic Surgeons Database Participants. Ann Thorac Surg 106(4):1055–1062

Landreneau RJ et al (1993) Thoracoscopic mediastinal lymph node sampling: useful for mediastinal lymph node stations inaccessible by cervical mediastinoscopy. J Thorac Cardiovasc Surg 106(3):554–558

Lardinois D, Weder W, Hany TF, Kamel EM, Korom S, Seifert B, Von Schulthess GK, Steinert HC (2003) Staging of non-small-cell lung cancer with integrated positron-emission tomography and computed tomography. N Engl J Med 348(25):2500–2507

Lemaire A et al (2006) Nine-year single center experience with cervical mediastinoscopy: complications and false negative rate. Ann Thorac Surg 82(4):1185–1189. discussion 1189–1190

Liberman M, Duranceau A, Grunnenwald E, Thiffault V, Khereba M, Ferraro P (2012) Initial experience with a new technique of EUS access for biopsy of para-aortic (station 6) mediastinal lymph nodes with traversing the aorta. J Thorac Cardiovasc Surg 144(4):787–793

Little AG, Rusch V, Bonner JA, Gaspar LE, Green MR, Webb WR, Stewart AK (2005) Patterns of surgical care of lung cancer patients. Ann Thorac Surg 80(6):2051–2056

Manfredi R et al (1996) Accuracy of computed tomography and magnetic resonance imaging in staging bronchogenic carcinoma. MAGMA 4(3–4):257–262

McCloud TC, Bourgouin P, Greenberg RW, Kosiuk JP, Templeton PA, Shepard JO, Moore EH, Wain JC, Mathisen DJ, Grillo HC (1992) Bronchogenic carcinoma: analysis of staging in the mediastinum with CT by correlative lymph node mapping and sampling. Radiology 182:319–323

McNeill TM, Chamberlain JM (1966) Diagnostic anterior mediastinotomy. Ann Thorac Surg 2(4):532–539

Micames CG, McCrory D, Pavey DA, Jowell PS, Gress FG (2007) Endoscopic ultrasound guided fine-needle aspiration for non small cell lung cancer staging: a systematic review and meta-analysis. Chest 131(2):539–548

Mountain C (1986) A new international staging system for lung cancer. Chest 89(4):S225–S233

Non-Small Cell LUng Cancer: NCCN Evidence Blocks (2021). https://www.nccn.org/professionals/physician_gls/pdf/nscl_blocks.pdf

Ohno Y, Koyama H, Yoshikawa T et al (2011) N stage disease in patients with non-small cell lung cancer: efficacy of quantitative and qualitative assessment with STIR turbo spin-echo imaging, diffusion-weighted MR imaging, and fluorodeoxyglucose PET/CT. Radiology 261(2):605–615

Park BJ, Flores R, Downey RJ, Bains MS, Rusch VW (2003) Management of major hemorrhage during mediastinoscopy. J Thorac Cardiovasc Surg 126(3):726–731

Predina JD et al (2017) Intraoperative molecular imaging combined with positron emission tomography improves surgical management of peripheral malignant pulmonary nodules. Ann Surg 266(3):479–488

Reed CE, Harpole D, Posther KE, Woolson SL, Downey RJ, Meyers BF, Heelan RT, Horner MA, Jung SH, Silvestri GA, Siegal BA, Rusch VW (2003) Results of the American College of Surgeons Oncology Group Z0050 Trial: the utility of positron emission tomography in staging potentially operable non-small cell lung cancer. J Thorac Cardiovasc Surg 126(6):1943–1951

Rivera MP, Mehta AC, American College of Chest Physicians (2007) Initial diagnosis of lung cancer: ACCP evidence-based clinical practice guidelines (2nd edition). Chest 132(3 Suppl):131S–148S

Roberts JR, Wadsworth J (2007) Recurrent laryngeal nerve monitoring during mediastinoscopy: predictors of injury. Ann Thorac Surg 83(2):388–391

Roberts JR et al (1999) Prospective comparison of radiologic, thoracoscopic, and pathologic staging in patients with early non-small cell lung cancer. Ann Thorac Surg 68(4):1154–1158

Sebastian-Quetglas F et al (2003) Clinical value of video-assisted thoracoscopy for preoperative staging of non-small cell lung cancer. A prospective study of 105 patients. Lung Cancer 42(3):297–301

Sharples LD, Jackson C, Wheaton E, Griffith G, Annema JT, Dooms C, Tournoy KG, Deschepper E, Hughes V, Magee L, Buxton M, Rintoul RC (2012) Clinical effectiveness and cost-effectiveness of endobronchial and endoscopic ultrasound relative to surgical staging in potentially resectable lung cancer: results from the ASTER randomised controlled trial. Health Technol Assess 16(18):1–75

Silvestri GA, Gould M, Margolis ML, Tanoue LT, McCrory D, Toloza E, Detterbeck F (2007a) Noninvasive staging of non-small cell lung cancer: ACCP evidence based clinical practice guidelines (2nd edition). Chest 132(3):178S–201S

Silvestri GA et al (2007b) Noninvasive staging of non-small cell lung cancer: ACCP evidenced-based clinical practice guidelines (2nd edition). Chest 132(3 Suppl):178S–201S

Tournoy KG et al (2008) Endoscopic ultrasound reduces surgical mediastinal staging in lung cancer: a randomized trial. Am J Respir Crit Care Med 177(5):531–535

Turna A et al (2013) Video-assisted mediastinoscopic lymphadenectomy is associated with better survival than mediastinoscopy in patients with resected non-small cell lung cancer. J Thorac Cardiovasc Surg 146(4):774–780

Um SW et al (2015) Endobronchial ultrasound versus mediastinoscopy for mediastinal nodal staging of non-small-cell lung cancer. J Thorac Oncol 10(2):331–337

Varadarajulu S et al (2004) Accuracy of EUS in staging of T4 lung cancer. Gastrointest Endosc 59(3):345–348

Yasufuku K, Chiyo M, Sekine Y, Chhajed PN, Shibuya K, Iizasa T, Fujisawa T (2004) Real-time endobronchial ultrasound-guided transbronchial needle aspiration of mediastinal and hilar lymph nodes. Chest 126(1):122–128

Yuan M et al (2019) The emerging treatment landscape of targeted therapy in non-small-cell lung cancer. Signal Transduct Target Ther 4:61

Part III
Basic Treatment Considerations

Surgical Workup and Management of Early-Stage Lung Cancer

Stephanie H. Chang, Joshua Scheinerman, Jeffrey Jiang, Darian Paone, and Harvey Pass

Contents

1 Introduction 131
2 **Preoperative Assessment** 132
2.1 Staging 132
2.2 Imaging 132
2.3 Pulmonary Function Evaluation 133
2.4 Medical Clearance 134
2.5 Mediastinal Assessment 135
3 **Anatomy** 136
3.1 Pulmonary Segments 136
4 **Types of Surgical Resection** 136
4.1 Wedge Resections 136
4.2 Segmental Resection 137
4.3 Lobectomy 137
4.4 Pneumonectomy 137
4.5 Bilobectomy 138
4.6 Sleeve Lobectomy 138
4.7 Mediastinal Lymph Node Resection 138
5 **Surgical Resections for Suspected or Biopsy Proven Lung Cancer** 140
5.1 Suspected Lung Cancer Nodules 140
5.2 Stage I Disease 141
5.3 Stage II NSCLC 143
6 **Modalities for Surgical Resection** 144
6.1 Development of Minimally Invasive Thoracic Surgery 144
6.2 VATS 145
6.3 Robotic 146
6.4 VATS vs. Robotic 147
References 147

S. H. Chang (✉) · J. Scheinerman · J. Jiang · D. Paone · H. Pass
Department of Cardiothoracic Surgery, New York University Langone Health, New York, NY, USA
e-mail: stephanie.chang@nyulangone.org

1 Introduction

Lung cancer remains the leading cause of cancer-related deaths within the United States (National Cancer Institute Surveillance, Epidemiology, and End Results Program 2021a). Overall survival (OS) remains dismal at 21% at 5 years (National Cancer Institute Surveillance, Epidemiology, and End Results Program 2021b). Treatments for lung cancer include multiple modalities, including surgical resection, systemic treatment (chemotherapy or immunotherapy), and radiation, and depends on clinical staging. For early-stage lung cancers, stage I and II, surgery remains the preferred treatment and provides the best opportunity for curative intent. Surgical indications also extend to a portion of patients with stage IIIA disease (Lang-Lazdunski 2013) but this will not be discussed in this chapter.

The case for surgery stems largely from retrospective series in comparison to the natural history of early-stage cancer followed without therapy. Recent data demonstrates 5-year survival of 70–90% for stage I (Detterbeck et al. 2017), while historically untreated early lung cancers have 5-year survival of 6% (Raz et al. 2007). The goal of any operation should be complete resection of all tumor. Incomplete resection can lead to morbidity from the operation, delays chemoradiation, and provides no therapeutic benefit. This chapter will focus on the workup necessary for surgery and surgical management of non-small cell lung cancer (NSCLC) patients (84% of lung cancer)

(American Cancer Society 2021), with emphasis of adenocarcinoma and squamous cell carcinoma. Surgical management for patients with neuroendocrine cancers and small cell lung cancer (13% of lung cancer) (American Cancer Society 2021) will be mentioned briefly at the end of the chapter.

2 Preoperative Assessment

2.1 Staging

Clinical staging is critical in determining surgical candidacy for patients with lung cancer, since surgery is utilized for local control, and therefore not indicate as frontline treatment for many patients, and not for significantly advanced stage cancer. Lung cancer staging is based on the American Joint Commission on Cancer TNM staging system. T is based on characteristics of the primary tumor, N evaluates regional lymph nodes, and M describes distant metastasis (Table 1) (Detterbeck et al. 2017). The stage based on TNM is classified as seen in Table 2 (Detterbeck et al. 2017). Surgical resection can be indicated for patients with stage I, II, and IIIA disease and will be discussed later in the chapter. Clinical stage (based on imaging) is written as cTNM, pathologic staging (after resection) is pTNM, and pathologic stage after induction therapy is ypTNM.

2.2 Imaging

All patients with lung cancer should have a **chest computed tomography (CT) scan** within 3 months of surgical resection in order to appropriately assess the size and location of the lesion, as well as to assess for lymphadenopathy (National Comprehensive Cancer Network Clinical Practice Guidelines in Oncology 2021). Additionally, patients with suspected or biopsy proven non-small cell lung cancer should undergo a **positron emission tomography (PET) scan** (ideally as an integrated PET-CT) to characterize

Table 1 TNM definitions

	Definition
T	*Primary tumor characteristics*
Tx	Primary tumor cannot be assessed or the tumor is proven by malignant cells in sputum or bronchial washings but not seen on imaging or bronchoscopy
T0	No evidence of primary tumor
Tis	Carcinoma in situ
T1	Tumor ≤3 cm in greatest dimension, surrounded by lung or visceral pleura, without bronchoscopic evidence of invasion more proximal than the lobar bronchus
T1mi	Minimal invasive adenocarcinoma
T1a	Tumor ≤1 cm in greatest dimension
T1b	Tumor >1 cm and ≤2 cm in greatest dimension
T1c	Tumor >2 cm and ≤3 cm in greatest dimension
T2	Tumor >3 cm and ≤5 cm in greatest dimension OR
	Tumor with any of the following (T2a unless >4 cm and ≤5 cm): • Involves main bronchus but does not involve the carina • Invades visceral pleura • Associated with atelectasis or obstructive pneumonitis that extends to the hilar region
T2a	Tumor >3 cm and ≤4 cm in greatest dimension
T2b	Tumor >4 cm and ≤5 cm in greatest dimension
T3	Tumor >5 cm and ≤7 cm in greatest dimension OR
	Separate tumor in the same lobe as the primary OR
	Tumor that invades any of the following: • Chest wall (includes superior sulcus tumors) • Phrenic nerve • Parietal pericardium
T4	Tumor >7 cm in greatest dimension OR
	Separate tumor in a different ipsilateral (same side) lobe to that of the primary OR
	Tumor that invades any of the following: • Diaphragm • Mediastinum • Heart • Great vessels • Trachea • Recurrent laryngeal nerve • Esophagus • Vertebral body • Carina
N	*Regional lymph nodes*
Nx	Regional lymph nodes cannot be assessed

(continuved)

Table 1 (continued)

	Definition
N0	No regional lymph node metastasis
N1	Metastasis in ipsilateral peribronchial, hilar, or parenchymal lymph nodes, including involvement by direct extension
N2	Metastasis in subcarinal or ipsilateral mediastinal lymph nodes
N3	Metastasis in contralateral mediastinal or hilar lymph nodes, or any scalene or supraclavicular nodes
M	*Distant metastasis*
M0	No distant metastasis
M1	Distant metastasis
M1a	Separate tumor in a contralateral node OR Tumor with pleural or pericardial nodules OR Malignant pericardial or pleural effusion
M1b	Single extra thoracic metastasis in a single organ
M1c	Multiple extrathoracic metastases in one or several organs

Table 2 TNM staging

Stage	T	N	M
Occult carcinoma	Tx	N0	M0
0	Tis	N0	M0
IA1	T1mi	N0	M0
	T1a	N0	M0
IA2	T1b	N0	M0
IA3	T1c	N0	M0
IB	T2a	N0	M0
IIA	T2b	N0	M0
IIB	T1a–c	N1	M0
	T2a,b	N1	M0
	T3	N0	M0
IIIA	T1a–c	N2	M0
	T2a,b	N2	M0
	T3	N1	M0
	T4	N0–1	M0
IIIB	T1a–c	N3	M0
	T2a,b	N3	M0
	T3	N2	M0
	T4	N2	M0
IIIC	T3	N3	M0
	T4	N3	M0
IVA	Any T	Any N	M1a,b
IVB	Any T	Any N	M1c

the primary lesion and assess for hilar or mediastinal lymph node activity, which would warrant further workup (National Comprehensive Cancer Network Clinical Practice Guidelines in Oncology 2021). For patients with more advanced disease, particularly if for T3 or T4 disease or any clinical N1 or N2 disease, a brain magnetic resonance imaging (MRI) is necessary to complete staging and rule out metastatic disease prior to resection (National Comprehensive Cancer Network Clinical Practice Guidelines in Oncology 2021).

2.3 Pulmonary Function Evaluation

Pulmonary evaluation is required for both risk assessment and to estimate impact on postoperative pulmonary limitation. **Pulmonary function testing**, with an emphasis on **forced expiratory volume in 1 s (FEV1)** and **diffusion capacity for carbon monoxide (DLCO)**, is the cornerstone of evaluating lung function. Historically a predicted postoperative (ppo) value FEV1 and DLCO >40% was considered the cutoff for resection with acceptable risk of postoperative respiratory failure or long-term dyspnea and oxygen requirement (Brunelli 2010). More recent data tend to indicate this line can potentially be lowered to a predicted postoperative of 30%, based on other factors that evaluate patient function and exercise capacity (Fig. 1) (Brunelli et al. 2013). For patients with borderline ppoFEV1 or DLCO, a **quantitative perfusion (V/Q) scan** can be performed to more accurately assess ppoPFTs. If the resection region is minimally perfused, the effect on postoperative function may be minimal (Brunelli 2010; Lang-Lazdunski 2013). Additionally, for any patient who may require a pneumonectomy (resection of an entire lung), a V/Q scan is imperative to determine if the patient is a surgical candidate.

For patients who are in the borderline category of ppoPFTs, a functional test can be performed in the office. A **stair climb** assessment can be performed, with the target of a patient being able to climb stairs and gain a height of 22 m (Brunelli et al. 2013). However, measurement of stairs and number of flights that equals 22 m is highly variable between buildings. Thus, an easier measure-

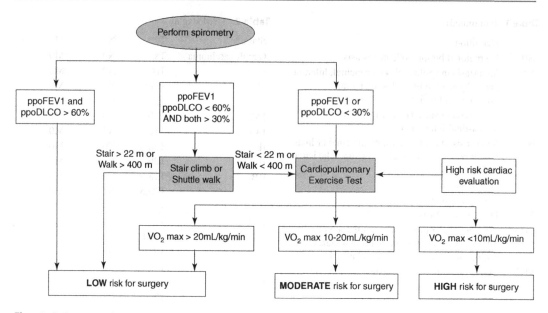

Fig. 1 Pulmonary function evaluation for surgery. Flowchart for evaluation of patients to stratify into low, moderate, or high risk for surgery. (Based on the guidelines published by the American College of Chest Physicians). *ppoDLCO* predicted postoperative diffusion capacity of carbon monoxide, *ppoFEV1* predicted postoperative forced expiratory volume in 1 s, *VO_2 max* maximal oxygen capacity, *mL* milliliter, *kg* kilogram, *min* minute

ment is a **shuttle walk** (walking back and forth down a hallway) distance of 400 m (Brunelli et al. 2013). In general, patient with the ability to meet the stair climb or shuttle walk test have good functional status and will tolerate lung resection.

Borderline patients (high cardiac risk, ppoFEV1 or ppoDLCO <30%, or inability to complete the stair climb or shuttle walk) should undergo further testing to maximal oxygen capacity (VO_2 max). VO_2 max is calculated from a **cardiopulmonary exercise test (CPET)** (Brunelli et al. 2013). A CPET is performed with the patient on a bicycle or treadmill with concurrent monitoring of lung and cardiac function. Those with VO_2 max >20 mL/kg/min are low risk for surgery, while those between 10 and 20 mL/kg/min are moderate risk for surgery. Patients with a VO_2 max <10 mL/kg/min are high risk for death and morbidity post resection and are not appropriate candidates for resection (Brunelli 2010). These patients should be referred to radiation oncology or interventional radiology to assess other forms of local therapy.

An **arterial blood gas (ABG)** is indicated for patients with intrinsic lung disease, such as chronic obstructive pulmonary disease (COPD). COPD patients often have elevated carbon dioxide, and a pre-resection pCO_2 > 45 mmHg is consistent with hypercarbia. Preoperative hypercarbia can be associated with increased operative risk and may preclude resection.

2.4 Medical Clearance

Preoperative workup also includes the history and evaluation of a patient's functional status. According to the American College of Cardiology/American Heart Association Guidelines, comorbidities and cardiac disease, history should be optimized prior to resection (Fleisher et al. 2014). All patients should have an **electrocardiogram (EKG)** prior to surgery. High cardiac risk patients may require further evaluation including **echocardiogram, stress test**, or **angiography** in consultation with a cardiologist (Fleisher et al. 2014). If an echocardiogram is performed, it is essential to assess the pulmonary artery (PA) pressure, as pulmonary hypertension increases surgical risk, and may be prohibitive at moderate to severe levels. All patients who are being considered for pneumonectomy should undergo an echocardiogram to assess PA pressures and right ventricle (RV) function, as RV function may deteriorate further after pneumonectomy.

Overall estimates of cardiac death or complication is around 1–5% and lung surgery is considered an intermediate risk operation. Patients with two or more risk factors require further workup and those with ischemic heart disease should be started on aspirin, statins, and B-blockers and continued through the perioperative period (Fleisher et al. 2007). If a patient needs a coronary intervention such as coronary artery bypass grafting or percutaneous coronary intervention, they should proceed with cardiac revascularization and delay pulmonary resection. After 6 weeks, the patient should be reevaluated for possible resection (Brunelli et al. 2013).

2.5 Mediastinal Assessment

While many early-stage patients do not need mediastinal assessment prior to surgery, there are characteristics associated with increased likelihood of nodal metastasis. Any lymphadenopathy (lymph node >1 cm in diameter) or PET positive lymph nodes should undergo staging (National Comprehensive Cancer Network Clinical Practice Guidelines in Oncology 2021). Additionally, clinical **stage II patients (T3+ disease or N1+ disease)** should have their mediastinal lymph nodes staged. For stage I patients, there is still a rate of occult N2 disease in 5% of patient (Meyers et al. 2006). **High-risk features of clinical stage I tumors** that may benefit from preoperative mediastinal assessment are **solid lesions, T2 tumors, central lesions**, and those with **elevated maximum standard uptake value (SUV_{max})** in the primary tumor (Lee et al. 2007).

In 284 cT1–2N0 patients who underwent surgery, N2 disease was found in >10% of patients with solid lesions (12.6% vs. 3.1% if there is a ground glass opacity component), T2 tumors (11.8% vs. 3.6% with T1), and central lesions (17.5% vs. 4.4% with peripheral lesions) (Gao et al. 2017). In a different study of 185 clinical stage I NSCLC patients who underwent resection, N1 and N2 disease occurred in 61.5% of central tumors, compared to 19.2% in peripheral lesions ($p = 0.002$) (Zhang et al. 2017). Finally, for patients with elevated maximum standard uptake value (SUV_{max}) in the primary tumor, there is a higher risk of nodal metastasis (Park et al. 2015). In the previously mentioned study of 185 clinical stage I NSCLC patients who underwent surgery, patients with pN0 had an SUV_{max} of 4.5 in the primary tumor, versus pN1 and N2 disease had an SUV_{max} of 7.8 ($p < 0.001$) (Zhang et al. 2017). A different study of 54 cT1–2N0 patients who were resected categorized patients into different risks for N2 disease based on tumor size and primary tumor SUV_{max}. Low risk (tumor ≤2.5 cm, $SUV_{max} \leq 4.35$) had a 4.3% rate of nodal metastasis, moderate risk (tumor ≤2.5 cm, $SUV_{max} > 4.35$ OR tumor >2.5 cm, $SUV_{max} \leq 4.35$) had a 22.7% rate, and high risk (tumor >2.5 cm, $SUV_{max} > 4.35$) had an 88.9% rate (Zhou et al. 2017). Thus, while no absolute cutoffs are used, high SUV_{max} may also be an indication for mediastinal staging.

Methods for staging include **endobronchial ultrasound (EBUS) with transbronchial biopsies** or mediastinoscopy. EBUS was developed in the 1990s, with an ultrasound probe at the end of a bronchoscope (Hürter and Hanrath 1992). The EBUS scope is inserted via the trachea and can be used to evaluate the paratracheal lymph nodes (stations 2 and 4), subcarinal lymph nodes (level 7), as well as the hilar (level 10), interlobar (level 11), and lobar (level 12) lymph nodes. After the lymph node is identified on ultrasound, a needle is inserted to obtain a biopsy for pathology. Currently, EBUS is the most common method for preoperative mediastinal assessment. The original gold standard for mediastinal assessment is **cervical mediastinoscopy**. In this method, a small incision is made above the sternal notch, and the incision is carried down to the pretracheal fascia. This plane is bluntly dissected, and a scope with a light source is inserted to visualize the plane (now with a fiberoptic camera at the end of the scope). This method allows for more tissue to be obtained than with an EBUS, but it is limited to paratracheal lymph nodes and subcarinal lymph nodes and occasionally to hilar nodes for more experienced surgeons. Cervical mediastinoscopy can be complicated by a higher rate of injury to the left recurrent laryngeal nerve or vascular injury requiring packing or immediate operative repair, compared to EBUS. Finally, a **Chamberlain procedure, or anterior mediastinoscopy**, can be performed to assess subaortic (level 5) and para-aortic (level 6) lymph nodes. In this procedure, a small incision is made in the second interspace, just left of the sternum, with care to avoid the left internal mammary artery and vein. The pleura is mobilized laterally to expose the level 5 and lymph nodes, which are then biopsied.

3 Anatomy

The right and left lung are each divided into lobes that are anatomically delineated by the presence of fissures. The **right lung** is the large lung and consists of three lobes: **upper, middle, and lower**. The major, or oblique fissure, separates the lower lobe from the upper and middle lobes. The middle and upper lobes are themselves separated by the minor, or horizontal fissure. The **left lung**, which is smaller due to the location of the heart toward the left pleural space, consists of two lobes: an **upper and lower lobe** separated by the major oblique fissure. The lungs are further divided into segments, described below. Of note, the left upper lobe consists of an apicoposterior and anterior component (which is equivalent to the right upper lobe) and the lingula (which corresponds to the right middle lobe). While many variants exist, the most common anatomy of the bronchus, artery, and vein is described (Nomori and Okada 2012).

3.1 Pulmonary Segments

The **right lung** consists of **ten segments**. The right upper lobe has three segments: apical (S1), posterior (S2), and anterior (S3). The right middle lobe has two segments: lateral (S4) and medial (S5). The right lower lobe has five segments: superior (S6), medial basilar (S7), anterior basilar (S8), lateral basilar (S9), and posterior basilar (S10).

The **left lung** consists of **eight segments**: The left upper lobe has four segments: apicoposterior (S1 + 2), anterior (S3), superior lingular (S4), and inferior lingular (S5). The left lower lobe has four segments: superior (S6), anteromedial basilar (S7 + 8), lateral basilar (S9), and posterobasilar (S10).

4 Types of Surgical Resection

Surgical resections are defined by two categories: anatomic versus nonanatomic resection and amount of tissue resected. Common surgeries are **wedge resection** (sublobar nonanatomic), **segmental resection** (sublobar anatomic), **lobectomy** (anatomic), and **pneumonectomy** (anatomic). Less common resections include **bilobectomy** (anatomic) and **sleeve resections** (anatomic).

4.1 Wedge Resections

A **wedge resection** is a **nonanatomic resection** with no formal division of segmental or lobar bronchi, pulmonary arteries, or pulmonary veins.

The resection is performed by resecting pulmonary parenchyma, with the extent of resection determined by the size and location of the lesion. Wedge resections are most common with peripheral lesions. The margin of the resection should be at least equal to the size of the lesion removed (National Comprehensive Cancer Network Clinical Practice Guidelines in Oncology 2021). For a 5 mm nodule, there should be at least a 5 mm margin, and for a 1.2 cm nodule, the margin should be 1.2 cm or greater.

4.2 Segmental Resection

A **segmental resection** is a **sublobar anatomic resection**, which is considered a parenchymal sparing procedure. However, it is very different from a wedge resection, as a segmentectomy is performed with an anatomic resection of bronchial and vascular anatomy, with removal of segmental (level 13) lymph nodes, as well as interlobar (level 11) and hilar (level 10) lymph nodes. Due to the formal division of structures in addition to improved lymphadenectomy along the segmental plane, a segmentectomy is considered to be a more appropriate oncologic procedure compared to a wedge resection. After the venous, bronchial, and pulmonary arterial structures are divided, the parenchyma is divided along the segmental plane. While traditionally the intersegment plane could be identified by inflating the residual segment, it is now common to use indocyanine green injection, either intravenously (Ferrari-Light et al. 2019) or via the divided segmental bronchus (Oh et al. 2013).

While each segment can be resected in isolation, the most common types of segmental resections are posterior segmentectomy (S2), superior segmentectomy (S6), basilar segmentectomy (S7–10), lingulectomy (S4, 5), and lingular sparing left upper lobectomy (S1–3). Each segment is performed with division of their respective bronchus, artery, and vein. For example, a superior segmental resection involves division of V6, A6, and B6.

4.3 Lobectomy

Lobectomy is an **anatomic resection of a lobe**, with division of the corresponding pulmonary artery, vein, and bronchus supplying the lobe, and includes removal of the relevant interlobar (level 11) and lobar (level 12) nodes. Interlobar nodes are found between the origins of the lobar bronchi, while the lobar nodes are located more peripherally adjacent to the lobar bronchi. Since all segments in the lobe are removed, the segmental (level 13) and subsegmental (level 14) lymph nodes will all be excised with the resection specimen. Due to division of the parenchyma along fissures, lobectomy is a larger resection with more parenchyma excised compared to segmentectomy but is also a more extensive oncologic resection. For central tumors close to the bifurcation of segmental structures, lobectomy may be necessary for complete resection of the tumor.

4.4 Pneumonectomy

Pneumonectomy is an **anatomic resection** of either the **entire right or left lung** with division of the associated broncho-vascular structures at the hilar level. Often, dissection of the central vascular structures is performed with division of the superior pulmonary vein, right or left PA, inferior pulmonary vein, and then right or left mainstem bronchus. It is important to have a short bronchial stump during the pneumonectomy.

Pneumonectomy is a much more morbid procedure compared to the others described in this section with a 3–8% postoperative mortality rate (Groth et al. 2015). Bronchopleural fistula (BPF), where the bronchus has a leak or dehiscence into the sterile pleural space, is a very challenging post-pneumonectomy complication (Groth et al. 2015). Risk factors for BPF include a long stump (>2 cm) (Groth et al. 2015), right-sided pneumonectomy (Mazzella et al. 2018), malnutrition (Mazzella et al. 2018), and preoperative radiation

(Groth et al. 2015). The rate of BPF can be as high as 11% (Groth et al. 2015), with a mortality rate up to 40%. Additionally, while pulmonary edema can occur after any type of pulmonary resection, postoperative pulmonary edema is much more likely after pneumonectomy, occurring in 3–5% of patients, with a greater than 50% mortality rate (Groth et al. 2015). Many other complications, including arrhythmias, acute respiratory distress syndrome, and pneumonia, can also occur and lead to significant morbidity or mortality.

4.5 Bilobectomy

Bilobectomy is less commonly performed anatomic resection. By definition, a bilobectomy is **resection of two lobes**, and **only applies to the right lung** (since a left-sided bilobectomy is a pneumonectomy). The two bilobectomies are either a right upper lobectomy with right middle lobectomy or a right middle lobectomy and right lower lobectomy. Indications for a bilobectomy are tumors that either cross the parenchymal fissure or have a central component requiring resection of two lobes to obtain a negative margin with complete excision of the tumor. A bilobectomy consisting of a right upper lobectomy and right lower lobectomy is not performed, since the right middle lobe is too small to fill the pleural space and is at high risk for torsion.

4.6 Sleeve Lobectomy

A **sleeve lobectomy** is resection of a lobe where part of the central airway or pulmonary artery is involved. The purpose of a sleeve lobectomy is to **remove the lobe with the cancer, as well as the affected airway or pulmonary artery**, in order to have a complete resection of the tumor. However, a sleeve lobectomy spares the remaining uninvolved lobe(s), which are then sewn back to the main bronchus or pulmonary artery. A "double sleeve" involved removing part of the main bronchi and main pulmonary artery, with the residual lobe being reimplanted to both.

4.7 Mediastinal Lymph Node Resection

Any suspected or proven lung cancer should have mediastinal lymph node sampling or dissection (National Comprehensive Cancer Network Clinical Practice Guidelines in Oncology 2021) to complete staging. Lymph nodes are classified based on anatomic descriptors (Rusch et al. 2009) with mediastinal (N2) lymph nodes consisting of level 1–9 lymph nodes. **Mediastinal lymph node sampling** (MLNS) involves the removal of one or more representative and/or macroscopically abnormal lymph nodes of a specific nodal station guided by preoperative or intraoperative findings (Lardinois et al. 2006; Keller et al. 2000). A systematic mediastinal lymph node sample should include **at a minimum three mediastinal nodal stations** and always the subcarinal stations for appropriate staging (National Comprehensive Cancer Network Clinical Practice Guidelines in Oncology 2021; Keller et al. 2000). Additionally, **a minimum of ten lymph nodes** (N1 and N2) should be removed in a MLNS, although this absolute number is a controversial point among thoracic surgeons. A **mediastinal lymph node dissection** (MLND) entails removing all of the lymphatic tissue of a given lymph node station within defined anatomic landmarks (Darling et al. 2011).

On the **right** side, the **mediastinal lymph node stations** for sampling or dissection are the **superior paratracheal (level 2R), inferior paratracheal (level 4R), subcarinal (level 7), paraesophageal (level 8), and inferior pulmonary ligament (level 9) lymph nodes**. Level 2R and 4R lymph nodes are bordered by the right lateral aspect of the trachea medially, mediastinal pleura laterally, the thoracic inlet superiorly, and the inferior border of the azygous vein inferiorly. The subcarinal space is bordered by the right and left mainstem bronchi laterally, carina superiorly, pericardium anteriorly, and esophagus posteriorly. Level 8 lymph nodes lie along the esophagus, inferior to the subcarinal space and extending down to the diaphragm. Level 9 lymph nodes are along or within the pulmonary ligament, extending from the inferior pulmonary vein to the diaphragm.

For **left**-sided lesions, the **mediastinal lymph node stations** for sampling or dissection are the **subaortic/aortopulmonary window (level 5), para-aortic (level 6), subcarinal (level 7), para-esophageal (level 8), and inferior pulmonary ligament (level 9) lymph nodes**. Level 5 lymph nodes are lateral to the ligamentum arteriosum and lie between the aortic arch and the left main pulmonary artery. Care must be taken during this dissection to not injure the recurrent laryngeal nerve, which courses next to this lymph node station. Level 6 lymph nodes are lateral to the ascending aorta and near the aortic arch. Care must be taken to not injure the phrenic nerve during this dissection. Level 7, 8, and 9 lymph nodes are in the same anatomic location bilaterally, with the left dissection fields the same as those described above. However, due to the longer left mainstem bronchus, the subcarinal space is a little more difficult to dissect out from the left side compared to the right.

Even with advancements in positron emission tomography and CT, pathologic upstaging occurs in up to 30% of patients (Suzuki et al. 2001).The importance of lymph node spread has been long established in the prognosis of lung cancer, and mediastinal spread conveys significantly worse prognosis. Advancements in imaging have allowed for more accurate clinical staging and better selection of appropriate operation for the lung cancer patient as well as essentially eliminating grossly incomplete resection or aborted thoracoscopy. R1 resections remain a possibility with micrometastasis at surgical margins or within subclinical lymph nodes and are unavoidable with current sensitivity of noninvasive staging. Controversy remains over the extent of lymph node dissection performed during lung resection, and there is significant variation with extent of lymph node resection between centers.

Because MLND can increase the lymph node harvest, it has been demonstrated to improve staging accuracy and therefore improve identification of occult N2 disease. This improvement in N staging can improve risk stratification and therefore increase detection of patients who may be candidates for adjuvant therapy (Ray et al. 2020). Additionally, the complete lymphadenectomy can remove micrometastasis and therefore maximize the possibility of a curative resection (Mokhles et al. 2017). However, the improvement in staging and micrometastasectomy has not consistently conferred an improvement in survival for early-stage NSCLC.

A large randomized controlled American College of Surgeons Oncology Group (ACOSOG) Z0030 trial showed that a thorough systematic sampling procedure provided equivalent survival to more formal mediastinal lymph node dissection in patients with early-stage NSCLC (Darling et al. 2011). A meta-analysis of four randomized controlled trials with complete data of local recurrence rates comparing MLND versus MLNS supported this finding (Huang et al. 2014). Additional findings included similar rates of local recurrence, distant metastasis, and complications between dissection and sampling (Mokhles et al. 2017). Notably, the ACOSOG Z0030 trial data was included in this meta-analysis. Concerns regarding generalizability of this trial and significant variations in lymph node dissections throughout community practices has led many to continue to encourage adherence to the routine use of mediastinal lymph node dissection (Riquet et al. 2014).

A more recent meta-analysis of randomized controlled trials of MLNS vs. MLND did demonstrate an absolute 7.6% risk reduction of death at 5 years with a complete mediastinal lymph node dissection (Mokhles et al. 2017). The authors, however, acknowledge an inability to determine whether the apparent survival benefit is due to the therapeutic effect of removing more nodes that are involved or of more accurate nodal staging resulting in an increase in the use of adjuvant treatment. This benefit is less clear in early-stage cancer or pure GGO lesions given their indolence and low propensity for spread and a number of randomized trials have shown equivalence (Huang et al. 2014). However, given the low risk of MLND, its potential for upstaging and survival benefit, our institution advocates for routing complete dissection. A current randomized trial between MLNS and MLND is still ongoing. The current STS and American College of Chest Physicians currently recommend lobectomy with complete lymph node dissection as "gold standard treatment" (Donington et al. 2012).

5 Surgical Resections for Suspected or Biopsy Proven Lung Cancer

The extent of surgical resection depends on the characteristics of the nodule, including if it is suspected or biopsy proven lung cancer, staging, and location of the tumor. Management of suspected lung cancer is different for ground glass opacity (GGO), multifocal disease, and solid nodules. Clinical stage I, II, and select IIIA NSCLC are often candidates for surgery, with staging, size and location of the nodule, and functional status of the patient. The goal for all surgical resection is complete excision of the malignancy. Resections can be classified as R0 (complete resection), R1 (microscopic residual tumor), or R2 (macroscopic residual tumor).

5.1 Suspected Lung Cancer Nodules

The implementation of low-dose helical CT for screening after the National Lung Cancer Screening Trial and NELSON trial demonstrated mortality benefit in high-risk patients has tilted the discovery of lung cancer toward early-stage disease (National Lung Screening Trial Research Team et al. 2011; de Koning et al. 2020). Over 1.6 million new incidental nodules are found annually and need further evaluation. A significant number of these are diagnostically ambiguous and range the spectrum of ground glass opacity (GGO) to part-solid and solid nodules. In the NELSON trial participants, 3.3% were found to have subsolid nodules, either pure or part-solid (Scholten et al. 2015). Ground glass opacities were first described in 1989 as "hazy CT densities" (Gamsu and Klein 1989). The current widely accepted definition by the Fleischer Society is a radiologic finding of a hazy opacity not obscuring the underlying pulmonary vessels or bronchi (Hansell et al. 2008). The definition was divided in 2002 to pure GGO and part-solid nodules where the solid component obscures underlying vascular and bronchial structure (Henschke et al. 2002; Hattori et al. 2017). Common methods of describing the solid portion include consolidation-to-tumor ratio (CTR) in lung windows or tumor disappearance ratio, the ratio of tumor size between mediastinal and lung windows (Zhang et al. 2020).

5.1.1 GGO and Part-Solid Lesions

While transient GGOs can represent a host of benign conditions, persistent lesions have a high likelihood of malignancy, ranging from 20% to 75% (Oh et al. 2007). The Early Lung Cancer Action Project (ELCAP) study reported 34% malignancy rate for pure GGOs and 63% for part-solid GGOs (Henschke et al. 1999). Despite having a high rate of malignancy, these are often indolent lesions with slow growth and low propensity for metastasis. As a significant number of GGOs will be transient, the Fleischner Society has put out recommendations for 3-month CT follow-up to confirm persistence and pure GGOs >5 mm to be followed with annual CT for 3 years. GGOs often have long volume-doubling time (VDT) with slow growth but have a high likelihood of being on the adenocarcinoma spectrum and being early-stage cancer. However, consistent growth of GGOs or changing characteristics, such as development of subsolid component, are concerning for early adenocarcinoma, warranting further investigation such as biopsy or resection. Part-solid tumors with increasing solid component or a solid component >6 mm are recommended for further workup and resection given their higher rate of malignancy (Naidich et al. 2013).

5.1.2 Multifocal GGO and Part-Solid Lesions

GGOs are also often multifocal, especially in the Asian population, and these lesions frequently have EGFR and K-ras mutations. Multifocal GGO or part-solid GGO disease represents roughly 5% of patients and presents a unique challenge, as these lesions likely represent multiple early-stage lesions on the adenocarcinoma spectrum. It is less likely that these are from intrapulmonary metastasis (Gazdar and Minna 2009). Indications for resection fall along the abovementioned criteria for pure or part-solid GGOs—once a lesion meets these criteria, biopsy or resection is indicated. Surgical treatment guidelines lack consensus, but we advocate for a localized wedge resection with MLND, due to the need to preserve pulmonary parenchyma in these patients that have a high likelihood of growth in other pure or part-solid GGOs. The remaining lesions should be closely followed on surveillance chest CTs.

With multifocal disease, localizing specific lesions may be particularly difficult, especially during minimally invasive resections. Localizing techniques, including ICG delivered via electromagnetic navigational bronchoscopy, have been invaluable at pinpointing tumors that have little solid component or that are deep to the visceral pleura or to distinguish between lesions (Abbas et al. 2017; Geraci et al. 2019). Novel modalities for bronchoscopy, including robotic platforms that merge electromagnetic navigation with video bronchoscopy, have also been reported efficacy at localizing peripheral lesions (Jiang et al. 2020).

5.1.3 Solid Tumors

Solid nodules are more concerning for malignancy and must first be differentiated from benign processes with a combination of CT, PET, and biopsy. For solid tumors, volume-doubling time (VDT) over 400 days is considered indolent and likely to be benign. Nodules that are followed on CT and PET with low VDTs require diagnosis and staging workup and will ultimately require an anatomic resection (McDonald et al. 2017). Non-biopsy proven suspicious clinical stage I NSCLC should be treated as stated in the next section.

5.2 Stage I Disease

Stage I NSCLC accounts for less than 20% of the cases and complete surgical resection is the mainstay of stage I NSCLC therapy. The gold standard operation for stage I disease is a lobectomy with MLND. During surgery, patients with a nonbiopsy proven peripheral lesion, a wedge resection may be performed with intraoperative frozen section to assess if the nodule is consistent with malignancy prior to an anatomic resection.

Small lesions less than 2 cm may be considered for a segmentectomy. Retrospective data supports oncologic equivalence. Early retrospective data evaluating segmentectomy ($n = 182$) versus lobectomy ($n = 246$) for stage I NSCLC showed similar disease-free recurrence and survival (Schuchert et al. 2007). However, they did note that a margin/tumor ratio <1 was associated with higher rates of recurrence (Schuchert et al. 2007). A 2014 Australian series by Landraneau et al. demonstrated no difference in 5-year recurrence rates or survival between clinical stage I segmentectomy or lobectomy patients (Landreneau et al. 2014). Yano et al. reported the experience of sublobar excisions of 28 Japanese institutions, noting 5-year 94% OS and 91% disease-free survival (DFS). Subgroup analysis demonstrated radiologically noninvasive (CTR <0.25) as a favorable prognostic indicator especially in cT1a disease (Yano et al. 2015). Tsutani et al. looked at 239 stage IA adenocarcinomas with CTR <50% and found no significant difference in 3-year DFS between lobectomy or any sublobar resection (96.4% lobectomy, 96.1% segmentectomy, 98.7% wedge) (Tsutani et al. 2014). Prospective, phase III, noncomparative data have shown similar high survival rates for sublobar resection in both JCOG0201 and JCOG0804. Both these studies also found CTR definitions of invasiveness <0.5 to delineate non-invasiveness and excellent prognosis with sublobar resection (Asamura et al. 2013; Aokage et al. 2017). Current NCCN guidelines recommend limited resection in disease meeting all the criteria of (1) stage IA, (2) maximum dimension <2 cm, (3) peripheral tumor location, and (4) CTR <50% (Ettinger et al. 2021). However, early reports of a prospective randomized clinical trial also demonstrate similar survival for patients who undergo segmentectomy compared to lobectomy for small peripheral nodules with CTR >0.5, indicating that the guidelines may change.

Segmentectomy is preferred over wedge resection, since wedge resections are nonanatomic and demonstrate higher rates of locoregional recurrence and worse 5-year survival in retrospective series of clinical stage I disease (Howington et al. 2013). Watanbe et al. found no difference in survival or locoregional recurrence, however, when limiting to stage IA GGOs with size <2 cm (Watanabe et al. 2005). However, this study was biased as wedge resection were performed on patients with less aggressive features on chest CT, and segmentectomy was for patients with higher risk findings on imaging (Watanabe et al. 2005). A meta-analysis demonstrated that for stage I NSCLC, segmentectomy was associated with improved survival compared to wedge resection, whereas for stage IA with tumor <2 cm, outcomes were comparable (Hou et al. 2016). However, all of these studies are limited by bias, as they are not randomized prospective controlled studies.

Only recently have randomized trials of lobectomy versus sublobar resections been reported. The two current studies are the Cancer and Leukemia Group B (CALGB) study 140,503 and the Japan Clinical Oncology Group (JCOG) study 0802. The CALGB study is a multicenter, international, noninferiority phase 3 clinical trial evaluating patients with peripheral clinical T1aN0M0, who are randomized into sublobar (wedge OR segmentectomy) or lobar resection (United States National Library of Medicine 2021). The primary endpoint is DFS, with final analysis still pending. However, earlier analysis on 697 patients demonstrated no difference in perioperative morbidity or mortality in these two groups (Altorki et al. 2018). The JCOG 0802 study randomized patients with clinical stage IA peripheral NSCLC or suspected nodule with a maximum tumor diameter of 2 cm, with 554 patients in the lobectomy arm and 552 in the segmentectomy arm (Asamura et al. 2021). Primary endpoints were OS, and secondary endpoints were DFS and local recurrence. For each arm, the CTR was 1.0 (solid lesions) in 51% of patients, and CTR was between 0.5 and 1.0 in an additional 35–37% of patients, with 90% of the lesions being adenocarcinoma, and a majority (82% in the lobectomy arm vs. 85% in the segmentectomy arm) having pathologic stage IA disease (Asamura et al. 2021). Five-year OS was 91.1% in the lobectomy arm and 94.3% in the segmentectomy arm ($p < 0.01$), while 5-year DFS was 87.9% in the lobectomy arm and 88% in the segmentectomy arm (p = NS) (Asamura et al. 2021).

5.2.1 Sublobar Resection in Medically Compromised Patients

Patients requiring lobectomy, but unable to tolerate the loss of pulmonary parenchyma, should be evaluated for sublobar resection. High-risk patients are identified on preoperative workup, as described earlier in this chapter (low ppoFEV1, ppoDLCO, low VO_2 max). Sublobar resection remains a possibility for cure but has a higher likelihood of recurrence. Mortality data is difficult to interpret as patients undergoing sublobar resection for medical compromise are inherently more at risk than healthier counterparts. A retrospective review of 784 patients by El-Sherif demonstrated higher rates of local recurrence in those undergoing wedge or segmentectomy for poor functional status (El-Sherif et al. 2006). A recent 2018 American College of Surgeons study of the National Cancer database propensity matched 325 patients between lobectomy and wedge/segmentectomy with similar 5-year OS, but 39% increased risk of recurrence (Subramanian et al. 2018). When only segmentectomies are considered, the recurrence rate is more favorable. Donahue et al. has reported 5-year survival of 79% in segmentectomy for high-risk patients and 35% recurrence (Donahue et al. 2012). Tumors smaller than 2 cm were also consistently found to have favorable long-term outcomes (Donahue et al. 2012). Sublobar resection has also been found to decrease perioperative complications in the elderly. In a multi-institutional study in China, >65 patients were found to have shorter operation time and less transfusion requirements, chest tube duration, and hospital stay (Zhang et al. 2019).

Margin guidelines suggest a 2 cm margin for tumors larger than 2 cm, or a ratio of margin:largest tumor diameter >1 (Howington et al. 2013), which is based on retrospective pathologic data. In Schuchert et al.'s report of 428 stage I tumors undergoing segmentectomy, 89% of local recurrences occurred in margins <2 cm and a higher local recurrence rate (25% vs. 6%) with ratios <1 in sublobar resections (Schuchert et al. 2007). Sublobar resection may be the only potential surgical cure in patients who are deemed high risk for surgery by cardiopulmonary reserve measurements. Similarly, for there high-risk patient, cryoablation (Moore et al. 2015) or stereotactic body radiation therapy (SBRT) (Shinde et al. 2018) may also play a role for small lesions in those medically unfit for any type of operation.

5.3 Stage II NSCLC

Stage II disease represents malignancies up to 7 cm, invading into chest wall, pericardium, phrenic nerve, involvement of the main bronchus without carina, or tumors less than 5 cm with N1 nodal metastasis. Surgery remains the standard of care after evaluation of resectability with complete disease removal. A full metastatic workup is required, including brain MRI, mediastinal lymph node staging, and resection planning for any involved chest wall structures.

Lobectomy remains the treatment of choice in single lobar large lesions with mediastinal lymph node dissection. T3 lesions that invade the chest wall should be resected en bloc with the involved chest wall, and the chest wall should be reconstructed depending on size of defect and location (Ettinger et al. 2021). Any cancers adherent or invading the secondary carina or mainstem bronchus will require a sleeve lobectomy, with reattachment of the residual lobe's bronchus to the mainstem bronchus. Additionally, any malignancy abutting or invading the right or left PA, or is adherent to the interlobar PA, can be removed with sleeve lobectomy and reconstruction of the pulmonary artery. In order to perform a PA sleeve or arterioplasty, central hilar control (clamping/occluding the right or left PA, superior pulmonary vein, and inferior pulmonary vein) is necessary to avoid significant blood loss. Tumors that cross the fissure may require either a bilobectomy, or a lobectomy and segmentectomy of the involved lung, depending on anatomy. Those involving both lobes on the left may require either a lobectomy and segmentectomy, or a pneumonectomy if the former is not possible. Central tumors not amenable to sleeve resection may require pneumonectomy to achieve an R0 resection. Stage II lung cancers require consideration of adjuvant therapy (Landreneau et al. 2014), which will be discussed in a different chapter.

Sleeve lobectomy is preferred over pneumonectomy if it is anatomically appropriate and if margin-negative resection can be achieved (Howington et al. 2013). In addition to decreased morbidity from surgery, as evidenced by the complications from pneumonectomy discussed previously in this chapter, sleeve lobectomy also preserves more lung function. Additionally, French study evaluated 1230 patients, which showed improved 5-year survival and decreased locoregional recurrence in the sleeve group as compared to the pneumonectomy group (Deslauriers et al. 2004).

6 Modalities for Surgical Resection

Current modalities for surgical resection include open surgery (thoracotomy) and minimally invasive surgery. Minimally invasive techniques for thoracic surgery include video-assisted thoracoscopic surgery (VATS) and robotic-assisted thoracoscopic surgery. Previously, a majority of lung cancer operations were performed via thoracotomy, though recent trends are toward VATS and robotic surgery (Krebs et al. 2020). There are many types of thoracotomies, though the most commonly performed for resection of NSCLC is a posterolateral thoracotomy, with division of the latissimus dorsi and sparing the serratus anterior. The thoracotomy is then created in the fifth interspace (between the fourth and fifth rib), and often one of the ribs is shingles to help with exposure and spreading the ribs. Less frequently, anterior thoracotomies in the fourth interspace (between the third and fourth rib) or a hemi-clamshell (division of the sternum down to the fourth intercostal space, with extension laterally into the fourth interspace) can be performed to help aid with exposure of anterior or mediastinal structures. This approach also allows for access to the heart, if needed.

6.1 Development of Minimally Invasive Thoracic Surgery

Since the first pneumonectomy performed for pulmonary malignancy back in 1933 by Graham, surgical therapy for lung cancer has rapidly and profoundly evolved. Fourteen year later, in 1947, Reinhoff published his experience with surgical therapy for lung cancer. This was the first report of lobectomy, with individually ligated vessels and bronchi, and all patients received surgery via thoracotomy (Rienhoff 1947). The 1950s and 1960s were marked by the idea of lung conservation with one report from Sommerwerck frequently treating early lung cancers with segmentectomy in 1970 (Kutschera 1984). The first stapling device was used in 1955, a novel method that is still used during pulmonary resection.

Interestingly, minimally invasive techniques to evaluate the chest developed earlier in the late 1800s. Swedish physicist Jacobaeus developed thoracoscopy for inspection of the pleural cavity using a candle as a light source. He even described using a second port and electrocautery to lyse adhesions (ADL and Cardoso 2012). Fast forward to the 1980s, the idea of VATS was incepted with the theoretical advantage of sparing rib spreading for postoperative pain improvement. However, the challenge of hilar structure control and mimicking the safe dissection of thoracotomy that was achieved over the last half-century would be an initial concern for surgeons. As time progressed, VATS become more and more of an accepted approach for lung cancer resection, with Lewis reporting on 100 VATS lobectomy patients in 1992 (Lewis et al. 1997). Later, McKenna popularized the classic, gold standard anterior-to-posterior approach of isolating the vein, artery, and then bronchus in his novel technique (McKenna 1994). Interest grew and technology progressed; however, skepticism about oncologic outcomes, safety of dissection, and cost was still prevalent among thoracic surgeons (ADL and Cardoso 2012). An initial RCT comparing muscle sparing thoracotomy to VATS lobectomy for early-stage NSCLC did not show more favorable results in these categories for the minimally invasive approach. However, techniques improved and surgeons had more practice; larger studies did indeed show an improvement in postoperative pain control, recovery time, length of stay, and post-op quality of life, while maintaining equivalent oncologic outcomes (ADL and Cardoso 2012; Mack et al. 1997; Sihoe 2014; Ghaly et al. 2016). In a 2016 retrospective study, Ghaly et al. demonstrated improved 5-year DFS and OS in VATS compared to thoracotomy in 193 segmentectomies performed for clinical stage I NSCLC over a 13-year period (Sihoe 2014). This data has been bolstered by several other large studies, including a 2009 JTCVS report by Rusch et al. showing similar 5-year survival in nearly 800 early-stage NSCLC patients undergoing

VATS vs. thoracotomy for resection (Flores et al. 2009).

The 2000s were marked by optimization of VATS technique as well as the rise of the da Vinci robotic platform by Intuitive Surgical. This system has been used in a variety of surgical fields with success including cardiac, general, urologic, colorectal, and gynecologic surgery. The benefits for oncology in general thoracic were only a natural progression. This concept allows for 3D vision, 10× optics, seated ergonomics for the operator, and wristed instruments that mock the movements of the human hands and fingers. Several studies have come out in support of this approach with respect to overall outcomes, including a 2020 retrospective propensity-matched analysis comparing VATS to the robotic approach. With more than 800 patients in the two groups, OS and cancer-specific mortality are similar (Sesti et al. 2020). With other purported attributes such as shorter hospital stay, less blood loss, reduced pain, and a lower 30-day mortality compared to thoracotomy, the robotic platform has grown to be a substantial piece of the armamentarium for the modern-day thoracic surgeon (Cao et al. 2012; Kent et al. 2014).

6.2 VATS

VATS is characterized by the avoidance of rib spreading, with one access incision less than 8 cm with two additional 5 mm port incisions. The patient is placed in lateral decubitus position with the operative side pointed toward the sky. It is important to both maximally flex the table at the level of the hips to open the rib spaces. Single lung ventilation is established prior to entry into the pleural spaced. The first port, typically camera port, is placed in the eighth intercostal space at the posterior axillary line. The second port is usually placed also in the eighth intercostal spaced, although this placement can vary one or two rib superior or inferior depending on where the lower lobe touches the diaphragm. This port is posterior, usually 4 cm from the spinous processes. After exposure of the superior pulmonary vein, the access port is created, usually 4 cm in length, at the level of this identified vein. This port is typically between the third and fifth intercostal space and is the most anterior port. As detailed above, the true advantages of the VATS approach lie in its decreased postoperative pain, time with chest tube drainage, and length of stay compared to traditional thoracotomy, while improving post-op quality of life and return to work with similar oncologic results (McKenna Jr et al. 1998; Gao et al. 2019).

Additionally, surgical resection for NSCLC can be performed through one-single port, known as uni-portal VATS. This approach offers violation of just a single rib space as well as a potential savings in postoperative pain. A 2013 study from Spain looked at 102 attempted uni-portal VATS lobectomies, with the incision at the fourth or fifth interspace, usually 5 cm in length. However, patients with upper lobectomies and extensive lymphadenectomy were found to have a higher rate of prolonged air leak or postoperative bleeding. The study cited two important factors in attempting uni-portal VATS: significant previous multiport VATS experience and familiarity with using the small anterior thoracotomy for open procedures. They also recommend doing several lower lobectomies before attempting upper lobe resection, as these tend to be more forgiving for the operator (Gonzalez-Rivas et al. 2013). Although this option has been proven to be safe and effective, most VATS are still performed with the multi-port technique, as this is technically easier and can significantly limit the postoperative pain associated with the traditional thoracotomy.

Centrally located NSCLC requiring sleeve lobectomy or pneumonectomy poses a unique challenge to the oncologic thoracic surgeon. The VATS technique can be applied to this type of resection, as many institutions have adopted this strategy for accomplishing their sleeve lobectomies and pneumonectomies (though with a high conversion-to-thoracotomy rate). One study from 2020 looked at surgical outcomes in NSLCC patients who underwent sleeve lobectomy using robotic, VATS, and traditional thoracotomy technique. After propensity matching, there was no difference in 90-day mortality or morbidity among the three groups (Qiu et al. 2020). Although more technically challenging than a conventional lobectomy, sleeve lobectomy can be done with the minimally invasive approach.

Pneumonectomy can be performed using a VATS technique. A single-center study looked at 107 pneumonectomies, 67 of which were performed via VATS (Battoo et al. 2014). There were similar rates of post-op complications, no major bleeding events, decreased 12-month pain scores, and a 16% conversion-to-thoracotomy rate. Several other studies have echoed these findings, including a 359-patient study that revealed a nearly 1 in 5 rate of conversion-to-thoracotomy (Yang et al. 2019). As with VATS sleeve lobectomy, successful completion of these extended types of resections often depend on the operator and the infrastructure that exists at their institution. Outcomes are best when performed by surgeons with significant VATS experience, at centers who have a considerable volume of patients that they have done extended pulmonary resections on in the past.

6.3 Robotic

Use of the robotic platform for pulmonary resection came to popularity in the 2000s. Unlike the VATS approach, the da Vinci robotic system involves two pieces of machinery to conduct the operation. The patient cart is a mobile piece of equipment that houses the four arms of the robot, allowing for a camera and three instruments controlled by the operator. The surgeon sits in a console, with foot pedals, finger/hand controls, and a 3D screen that is broadcast throughout the room. The surgeon has complete control of the behaviors of the camera and the three instruments. In addition, there is a bedside assistant who sets up the arms as indicated and has their own assistant port through which they can retract, suction, and retrieve intracorporeal materials as needed.

Current use of the DaVinci Xi system utilizes all four arms of the robot. At our institution, the four ports (one camera + 3 instrument ports) are placed in the eighth intercostal space, starting 4 cm anteriorly from the spinous processes. There should be roughly 8 cm between the remaining robotic ports with variation based on patient body habitus. We will make the anterior port a 12 mm stapling port, while the rest remain 8 mm ports. This stapling port is always the anteriormost port, except in the case of a right middle lobectomy, in which we place a second 12 mm stapling port for the third arm. The final utility port is the most inferior port placed just above the diaphragm in a manner to give the bedside assistant enough space away from the camera port. A 0° scope is used, though a 30° scope can be used if significant chest wall adhesions are present.

The implementation of robotic surgery has also extended to more complex thoracic surgeries including the sleeve lobectomy and pneumonectomy. As described above, sleeve resections are generally completed in the setting of centrally located NSCLC. The central-tumor location can impede a minimally invasive sleeve resection via a VATS approach if a need arises for approximation techniques to facilitate an anastomosis between distanced bronchial ends (Shanahan et al. 2019). The robotic platform, however, offers an advantage in depth perception and maneuverability that overcomes the technical constraints that have limited the use of VATS surgery in sleeve lobectomies. Given the recent integration of the robotic platform into advanced thoracic surgeries, long-term oncologic outcomes for robotic-assisted sleeve lobectomies are limited. However, several studies have demonstrated the safety and feasibility of the procedure, acceptable complication rates. Jiao et al. reported the largest series with 67 patients with no 90-day mortalities, few complications, and no conversions to open. Major complications included one anastomotic stricture, one chylothorax, and one stroke (Jiao et al. 2019). Another series showed no short-term mortality and minimal morbidity, and no patients with locoregional recurrence over a median 18-month follow-up (Geraci et al. 2020). Pan et al. had previously reported a similar series of 21 robotic sleeve resections with similar results, although with one 30-day mortality and marginally higher rates of complications (Pan et al. 2016).

The use of robot-assisted operations for pneumonectomy is feasible. However, data remains limited due to technical, safety, and oncologic concerns, restricting the ability to provide adequate data for comparative outcomes to VATS and open techniques. Descriptions of robotic pneumonectomies are limited to case studies in available literature.

6.4 VATS vs. Robotic

Comparison of VATS versus robotic is limited, with one study demonstrating OS and cancer-specific mortality are similar (Sesti et al. 2020). One propensity-matched cohort study of 2766 patients aged greater than 65 years old with resected NSCLC showed that robotic-assisted surgery was associated with lower complication rates compared with open thoracotomy and carried similar complication rates compared with VATS. While this study showing superiority of robotic surgery versus thoracotomy, they were unable to assess for any advance of robotic over VATS (Veluswamy et al. 2020). Further studies comparing the two modalities are necessary to further assess this question.

References

Abbas A, Kadakia S, Ambur V, Muro K, Kaiser L (2017) Intraoperative electromagnetic navigational bronchoscopic localization of small, deep, or subsolid pulmonary nodules. J Thorac Cardiovasc Surg 153(6):1581–1590

ADL S, Cardoso (eds) (2012) The evolution of VATS lobectomy. Topics in thoracic surgery. InTech, Shanghai, pp 181–210

Altorki NK, Wang X, Wigle D et al (2018) Perioperative mortality and morbidity after sublobar versus lobar resection for early-stage non-small-cell lung cancer: post-hoc analysis of an international, randomized, phase 3 trial (CALGB/Alliance 140503). Lancet Respir Med 6(12):915–924

American Cancer Society (2021) Cancer facts and figures 2021. https://www.cancer.org/content/dam/cancer-org/research/cancer-facts-and-statistics/annual-cancer-facts-and-figures/2021/cancer-facts-and-figures-2021.pdf. Accessed 15 Apr 2021

Aokage K, Saji H, Suzuki K et al (2017) A non-randomized confirmatory trial of segmentectomy for clinical T1N0 lung cancer with dominant ground glass opacity based on thin-section computed tomography (JCOG1211). Gen Thorac Cardiovasc Surg 65(5):267–272

Asamura H, Hishida T, Suzuki K et al (2013) Radiographically determined noninvasive adenocarcinoma of the lung: survival outcomes of Japan Clinical Oncology Group 0201. J Thorac Cardiovasc Surg 146(1):24–30

Asamura H, Okada M, Saji H et al (2021) Randomized trial of segmentectomy compared to lobectomy in small-sized peripheral non-small cell lung cancer (JCOG0802/WJOG4607L). In: American Association for Thoracic Surgery, 101st Annual Meeting; 2021 Apr 30–May 2; Virtual meeting. Abstract 163

Battoo A, Jahan A, Yang Z et al (2014) Thoracoscopic pneumonectomy: an 11-year experience. Chest 146(5):1300–1309

Brunelli A (2010) Risk assessment for pulmonary resection. Semin Thorac Cardiovasc Surg 22(1):2–13

Brunelli A, Kim AW, Berger KI, Addrizzo-Harris DJ (2013) Physiologic evaluation of the patient with lung cancer being considered for resectional surgery: diagnosis and management of lung cancer, 3rd ed: American College of Chest Physicians evidence-based clinical practice guidelines. Chest 143(5 Suppl):e166S–e190S

Cao C, Manganas C, Ang SC, Yan TD (2012) A systematic review and meta-analysis on pulmonary resections by robotic video-assisted thoracic surgery. Ann Cardiothorac Surg 1(1):3–10

Darling GE, Allen MS, Decker PA et al (2011) Randomized trial of mediastinal lymph node sampling versus complete lymphadenectomy during pulmonary resection in the patient with N0 or N1 (less than hilar) non-small cell carcinoma: results of the American College of Surgery Oncology Group Z0030 Trial. J Thorac Cardiovasc Surg 141(3):662–670

de Koning HJ, van der Aalst CM, de Jong PA et al (2020) Reduced lung-cancer mortality with volume CT screening in a randomized trial. N Engl J Med 382(6):503–513

Deslauriers J, Grégoire J, Jacques LF, Piraux M, Guojin L, Lacasse Y (2004) Sleeve lobectomy versus pneumonectomy for lung cancer: a comparative analysis of survival and sites or recurrences. Ann Thorac Surg 77:1152–1156

Detterbeck FC, Boffa DJ, Kim AW, Tanoue LT (2017) The eighth edition of lung cancer stage classification. Chest 151(1):193–203

Donahue JM, Morse CR, Wigle DA, Allen MS, Nichols FC, Shen KR et al (2012) Oncologic efficacy of anatomic segmentectomy in stage IA lung cancer patients with T1a tumors. Ann Thorac Surg 93(2):381–387

Donington J, Ferguson M, Mazzone P, Handy J Jr, Schuchert M, Fernando H et al (2012) American College of Chest Physicians and Society of Thoracic Surgeons consensus statement for evaluation and management for high-risk patients with stage I non-small cell lung cancer. Chest 142(6):1620–1635

El-Sherif A, Gooding WE, Santos R et al (2006) Outcomes of sublobar resection versus lobectomy for stage I non-small cell lung cancer: a 13-year analysis. Ann Thorac Surg 82(2):408–415

Ettinger DS, Wood DE, Aisner DL et al (2021) NCCN guidelines insights: non-small cell lung cancer, Version 2.2021. J Natl Compr Canc Netw 19(3):254–266

Ferrari-Light D, Geraci TC, Sasankan P, Cerfolio RJ (2019) The utility of near-infrared fluorescence and indocyanine green during robotic pulmonary resection. Front Surg 6:47

Fleisher LA, Beckman JA, Brown KA et al (2007) ACC/AHA 2007 guidelines on perioperative cardiovascular evaluation and care for noncardiac surgery: a report of the American College of Cardiology/American Heart Association Task Force on Practice Guidelines (Writing Committee to Revise the 2002 Guidelines on Perioperative Cardiovascular Evaluation for Noncardiac Surgery): developed in collaboration with the American Society of Echocardiography, American Society of Nuclear Cardiology, Heart Rhythm Society, Society of Cardiovascular Anesthesiologists, Society for Cardiovascular Angiography and Interventions, Society for Vascular Medicine and Biology, and Society for Vascular Surgery. Circulation 116(17):e418–e499

Fleisher LA, Fleischmann KE, Auerbach AD et al (2014) 2014 ACC/AHA guideline on perioperative cardiovascular evaluation and management of patients undergoing noncardiac surgery. Circulation 130:e278–e333

Flores RM, Park BJ, Dycoco J et al (2009) Lobectomy by video-assisted thoracic surgery (VATS) versus thoracotomy for lung cancer. J Thorac Cardiovasc Surg 138(1):11–18

Gamsu G, Klein JS (1989) High resolution computed tomography of diffuse lung disease. Clin Radiol 40(6):554–556

Gao SJ, Kim AW, Puchlaski JT et al (2017) Indications for invasive mediastinal staging in patients with early non-small cell lung cancer staged with PET-CT. Lung Cancer 109:36–41

Gao HJ, Jiang ZH, Gong L et al (2019) Video-assisted vs thoracotomy sleeve lobectomy for lung cancer: a propensity matched analysis. Ann Thorac Surg 108(4):1072–1079

Gazdar AF, Minna JD (2009) Multifocal lung cancers—clonality vs field cancerization and does it matter? J Natl Cancer Inst 101(8):541–543

Geraci TC, Ferrari-Light D, Kent A, Michaud G, Zervos M, Pass HI et al (2019) Technique, outcomes with navigational bronchoscopy using indocyanine green for robotic segmentectomy. Ann Thorac Surg 108(2):363–369

Geraci T, Ferrari-Light D, Wang S et al (2020) Robotic sleeve resection of the airway: outcomes and technical conduct using video vignettes. Ann Thorac Surg 110(1):236–240

Ghaly G, Kamel M, Nasar A et al (2016) Video-assisted thoracoscopic surgery is a safe and effective alternative to thoracotomy for anatomical segmentectomy in patients with clinical stage I non-small cell lung cancer. Ann Thorac Surg 101(2):465–472

Gonzalez-Rivas D, Paradela M, Fernandez R et al (2013) Uniportal video-assisted thoracoscopic lobectomy: two years of experience. Ann Thorac Surg 95(2):426–432

Groth SS, Burt BM, Sugarbaker DJ (2015) Management of complications after pneumonectomy. Thorac Surg Clin 25(3):335–348

Hansell DM, Bankier AA, MacMahon H, McLoud TC, Muller NL, Remy J (2008) Fleischner Society: glossary of terms for thoracic imaging. Radiology 246(3):697–722

Hattori A, Matsunaga T, Hayashi T, Takamochi K, Oh S, Suzuki K (2017) Prognostic impact of the findings on thin-section computed tomography in patients with subcentimeter non-small cell lung cancer. J Thorac Oncol 12(6):954–962

Henschke CI, McCauley DI, Yankelevitz DF et al (1999) Early Lung Cancer Action Project: overall design and findings from baseline screening. Lancet 354(9173):99–105

Henschke CI, Yankelevitz DF, Mirtcheva R et al (2002) CT screening for lung cancer: frequency and significance of part-solid and nonsolid nodules. AJR Am J Roentgenol 178(5):1053–1057

Hou B, Deng XF, Zhou D, Liu QX, Dai JG (2016) Segmentectomy versus wedge resection for the treatment of high-risk operable patients with stage I non-small cell lung cancer: a meta-analysis. Ther Adv Resp Dis 10(5):435–443

Howington JA, Blum MG, Chang AC, Balekian AA, Murthy SC (2013) Treatment of stage I and II non-small cell lung cancer: diagnosis and management of lung cancer, 3rd ed: American College of Chest Physicians evidence-based clinical practice guidelines. Chest 143(5 Suppl):e278S–e313S

Huang X, Wang J, Chen Q, Jiang J (2014) Mediastinal lymph node dissection versus mediastinal lymph node sampling for early stage non-small cell lung cancer: a systematic review and meta-analysis. PLoS One 9(10):e109979

Hürter T, Hanrath P (1992) Endobronchial sonography: feasibility and preliminary results. Thorax 47:565–567

Jiang J, Chang SH, Kent AJ, Geraci TC, Cerfolio RJ (2020) Current novel advances in bronchoscopy. Front Surg 7:596925. Epub 2020/12/12

Jiao W, Zhao Y, Qiu T, Xuan Y, Sun X, Qin Y et al (2019) Robotic bronchial sleeve lobectomy for central lung tumors: technique and outcome. Ann Thorac Surg 108:211–218

Keller SM, Adak S, Wagner H, Johnson DH (2000) Mediastinal lymph node dissection improves survival in patients with stages II and IIIa non-small cell lung cancer. Eastern Cooperative Oncology Group. Ann Thorac Surg 70(2):358–365

Kent M, Wang T, Whyte R, Curran T, Flores R, Gangadharan S (2014) Open, video-assisted thoracic surgery, and robotic lobectomy: review of a national database. Ann Thorac Surg 97(1):236–244

Krebs ED, Mehaffey JH, Sarosiek BM, Blank RS, Lau CL, Martin LW (2020) Is less really more? Reexamining video-assisted thoracoscopic versus open lobectomy in the setting of an enhanced recovery protocol. J Cardiovasc Thorac Surg 159(1):284–294

Kutschera W (1984) Segment resection for lung cancer. Thorac Cardiovasc Surg 32:102–104

Landreneau RJ, Normolle DP, Christie NA et al (2014) Recurrence and survival outcomes after anatomic segmentectomy versus lobectomy for clinical stage I non-small-cell lung cancer: a propensity-matched analysis. J Clin Oncol 32(23):2449–2455

Lang-Lazdunski L (2013) Surgery for nonsmall cell lung cancer. Eur Respir Rev 22(129):382–404

Lardinois D, De Leyn P, Van Schil P et al (2006) ESTS guidelines for intraoperative lymph node staging in non-small cell lung cancer. Eur J Cardiothorac Surg 30(5):787–792

Lee PC, Port JL, Korst RJ, Liss Y, Meherally, Altorki NK (2007) Risk factors for occult mediastinal metastases in clinical stage I non-small cell lung cancer. Ann Thorac Surg 84(1):177–181

Lewis RJ, Caccvale RJ, Sisler GE, Bocage JP, Mackenzie JW (1997) One hundred video-assisted thoracic surgical simultaneously stapled lobectomies without rib spreading. Ann Thorac Surg 63(5):1415–1421

Mack MJ, Scruggs GR, Kelly KM et al (1997) Video-assisted thoracic surgery: has technology found its place? Ann Thorac Surg 64:211–215

Mazzella A, Pardolesi A, Maisonneuve P et al (2018) Bronchopleural fistula after pneumonectomy: risk factors and management, focusing on open-window thoracostomy. Semin Thorac Cardiovasc Surg 30(1):104–113

McDonald F, De Waele M, Hendriks LE, Faivre-Finn C, Dingemans AC, Van Schil PE (2017) Management of stage I and II nonsmall cell lung cancer. Eur Respir J 49(1):1600764

McKenna RJ (1994) Lobectomy by video-assisted thoracic surgery with mediastinal node sampling for lung cancer. J Thorac Cardiovasc Surg 107:879–882

McKenna RJ Jr, Wolf RK, Brenner M, Fischel RJ, Wurnig P (1998) Is lobectomy by video-assisted thoracic surgery an adequate cancer operation? Ann Thorac Surg 66(6):1903–1908

Meyers BF, Hadded F, Siegel BA et al (2006) Cost-effectiveness of routine mediastinoscopy in computed tomography- and positron emission tomography-screened patients with stage I lung cancer. J Thorac Cardiovasc Surg 131(4):822–829

Mokhles S, Macbeth F, Treasure T et al (2017) Systematic lymphadenectomy versus sampling of ipsilateral mediastinal lymph-nodes during lobectomy for non-small-cell lung cancer: a systematic review of randomized trials and a meta-analysis. Eur J Cardiothorac Surg 51(6):1149–1156

Moore W, Talati R, Bhattacharji P, Bilfinger T (2015) Five-year survival after cryoablation of stage I non-small cell lung cancer in medically inoperable patients. J Vasc Interv Radiol 26:312–319

Naidich DP, Bankier AA, MacMahon H et al (2013) Recommendations for the management of subsolid pulmonary nodules detected at CT: a statement from the Fleischner Society. Radiology 266(1):304–317

National Cancer Institute Surveillance, Epidemiology, and End Results Program (2021a) Cancer stat facts: common cancer sites. https://seer.cancer.gov/statfacts/html/common.html. Accessed 15 Apr 2021

National Cancer Institute Surveillance, Epidemiology, and End Results Program (2021b) Cancer stat facts: lung and bronchus cancer. https://seer.cancer.gov/statfacts/html/lungb.html. Accessed 15 Apr 2021

National Comprehensive Cancer Network Clinical Practice Guidelines in Oncology (2021) Non-small cell lung cancer. V 4.2021, updated 3 Mar 2021. https://www.nccn.org/professionals/physician_gls/pdf/nscl.pdf. Accessed 15 Apr 2021

National Lung Screening Trial Research Team, Aberle DR, Adams AM, Berg CD et al (2011) Reduced lung-cancer mortality with low-dose computed tomographic screening. N Engl J Med 365(5):395–409

Nomori H, Okada M (2012) Illustrated anatomical segmentectomy for lung cancer. Springer, Tokyo

Oh JY, Kwon SY, Yoon HI et al (2007) Clinical significance of a solitary ground-glass opacity (GGO) lesion of the lung detected by chest CT. Lung Cancer 55(1):67–73

Oh S, Suzuki K, Miyasaka Y, Matsunaga T, Tsushima Y, Takamochi K (2013) New technique for lung segmentectomy using indocyanine green injection. Ann Thorac Surg 95:2188–2190

Pan X, Gu C, Wang R, Zhao H, Shi J, Chen H (2016) Initial experience of robotic sleeve resection for lung cancer patients. Ann Thorac Surg 102:1892–1897

Park SY, Yoon JK, Park KJ, Lee SJ (2015) Prediction of occult lymph node metastasis using volume-based PET parameters in small-sized peripheral non-small cell lung cancer. Cancer Imaging 15:21

Qiu T, Zhao Y, Xuan Y et al (2020) Robotic sleeve lobectomy for centrally located non-small cell lung cancer: a propensity score-weighted comparison with thoracoscopic and open surgery. J Thorac Cardiovasc Surg 160(3):838–846

Ray MA, Smeltzer MP, Faris NR, Osarogiagbon RU (2020) Survival after mediastinal node dissection, systematic sampling, or neither for early stage NSCLC. J Thorac Oncol 15(10):1670–1681

Raz DJ, Zell JA, Ou SH et al (2007) Natural history of stage I non-small cell lung cancer: implications for early detection. Chest 132:193–199

Rienhoff WF (1947) The present status of the surgical treatment of carcinoma of the lung. Ann Surg 125(5):541–564

Riquet M, Legras A, Mordant P et al (2014) Number of mediastinal lymph nodes in non-small cell lung cancer: a Gaussian curve, not a prognostic factor. Ann Thorac Surg 98(1):224–231

Rusch VW, Asamura H, Watanabe H et al (2009) The IASLC lung cancer staging project: a proposal for a new international lymph node map in the forthcoming seventh edition of the TNM classification for lung cancer. J Thorac Oncol 4(5):568–577

Scholten ET, de Jong PA, de Hoop B et al (2015) Towards a close computed tomography monitoring approach for screen detected subsolid pulmonary nodules? Eur Respir J 45(3):765–773

Schuchert MJ, Pettiford BL, Keeley S et al (2007) Anatomic segmentectomy in the treatment of stage I non-small cell lung cancer. Ann Thorac Surg 84(3):926–932

Sesti J, Langan RC, Bell J et al (2020) A comparative analysis of long-term survival of robotic versus thoracoscopic lobectomy. Ann Thorac Surg 110(4):1139–1146

Shanahan B, O'Sullivan KE, Redmond KC (2019) Robotic sleeve lobectomy recent advances. J Thorac Dis 11:1074–1075

Shinde A, Li R, Kim J, Salgia R, Hurria A, Amini A (2018) Stereotactic body radiation therapy (SBRT) for early-stage lung cancer in the elderly. Semin Oncol 45(4):210–219

Sihoe ADL (2014) The evolution of minimally invasive thoracic surgery: implications for the practice of uniportal thoracoscopic surgery. J Thorac Dis 6:S604–S617

Subramanian M, McMurry T, Meyers BF, Puri V, Kozower BD (2018) Long-term results for clinical stage IA lung cancer: comparing lobectomy and sublobar resection. Ann Thorac Surg 106(2):375–381

Suzuki K, Nagai K, Yoshida J, Nishimura M, Nishiwaki Y (2001) Predictors of lymph node and intrapulmonary metastasis in clinical stage IA non-small cell lung carcinoma. Ann Thorac Surg 72(2):352–356

Tsutani Y, Miyata Y, Nakayama H et al (2014) Appropriate sublobar resection choice for ground glass opacity-dominant clinical stage IA lung adenocarcinoma: wedge resection or segmentectomy. Chest 145(1):66–71

United States National Library of Medicine (2021) Comparison of different types of surgery in treating patients with stage IA non-small cell lung cancer. https://clinicaltrials.gov/ct2/show/NCT00499330. Accessed 4 May 2021

Veluswamy RR, Whittaker Brown SA et al (2020) Comparative effectiveness of robotic-assisted surgery for resectable lung cancer in older patients. Chest 157(5):1313–1321

Watanabe T, Okada A, Imakiire T, Koike T, Hirono T (2005) Intentional limited resection for small peripheral lung cancer based on intraoperative pathologic exploration. Jpn J Thorac Cardiovasc Surg 53(1):29–35

Yang CJ, Yendamuri S, Mayne NR et al (2019) The role of thoracoscopic pneumonectomy in the management of non-small cell lung cancer: a multicenter study. J Thorac Cardiovasc Surg 158(1):252–264

Yano M, Yoshida J, Koike T et al (2015) Survival of 1737 lobectomy-tolerable patients who underwent limited resection for cStage IA non-small-cell lung cancer. Eur J Cardiothorac Surg 47(1):135–142

Zhang S, Li S, Pei Y et al (2017) Impact of maximum standard uptake value of non-small cell lung cancer on detecting lymph node involvement in potential stereotactic body radiotherapy candidates. J Thorac Dis 9(4):1023–1031

Zhang Z, Feng H, Zhao H, Hu J, Liu L, Liu Y et al (2019) Sublobar resection is associated with better perioperative outcomes in elderly patients with clinical stage I non-small cell lung cancer: a multicenter retrospective cohort study. J Thorac Dis 11(5):1838–1848

Zhang Y, Fu F, Wen Z et al (2020) Segment location and ground glass opacity ratio reliably predict node-negative status in lung cancer. Ann Thorac Surg 109(4):1061–1068

Zhou X, Chen R, Huang G, Liu J (2017) Potential clinical value of PET/CT in predicting occult nodal metastasis in T1-T2N0M0 lung cancer patients staged by PET/CT. Oncotarget 8(47):82437–82445

Radiation Biology of Lung Cancer

Jose G. Bazan

Contents

1 **Radiobiologic Basis of Conventionally Fractionated Radiation Therapy** 152
1.1 DNA: The Critical Target for the Biologic Effects of Radiation Damage 152
1.2 The Linear–Quadratic (LQ) Model 152
1.3 The Four Rs of Radiobiology 153
1.4 Biologically Effective Dose 154

2 **Alternative Fractionation Schedules** 155
2.1 Hyperfractionated Radiation Therapy in Lung Cancer 155
2.2 Accelerated Fractionation Schedules in Lung Cancer 157
2.3 Hypofractionated Radiation Therapy in Lung Cancer 158
2.4 Clinical Applications of Moderately Hypofractionated Radiation Therapy 158
2.5 Clinical Applications of Stereotactic Ablative Radiotherapy for NSCLC 159

3 **Radiobiology of SABR** 160
3.1 Reexamining the Four "Rs" of Radiobiology in SABR 160
3.2 Dose Effect Models in SABR: Is the LQ Model Applicable 161
3.3 Effects of SABR: New Mechanisms of Cell Killing? 161

4 **Modification of Radiation Response** 162
4.1 Chemotherapy 162
4.2 Tumor Hypoxia 163
4.3 Immunotherapy with Radiation in NSCLC 164

5 **Flash Radiotherapy** 165

6 **Conclusion** 165

References 166

Abstract

Radiobiology is central to an understanding of the principles of radiotherapy today. In the early twentieth century, the use of large, single doses of radiation, or hypofractionation, declined as evidence mounted that these doses caused considerable damage to normal tissues. Based on radiobiology, treatments then shifted toward smaller daily doses over a period of several weeks as a way to reduce this damage yet still achieve tumor control. A paradigm shift toward hypofractionation occurred again in the early twenty-first century as advances in technology now enable high-dose radiation to more precisely target the tumor while minimizing the amount of normal tissues exposed. In this chapter, we explore the basic tenets of radiation biology in order to understand the rationale behind these vastly different approaches as they apply specifically to the treatment of lung cancer. We also examine ways to exploit the radiobiology of lung cancer by using various strategies with a focus on moderate hypofractionation, stereotactic ablative radiation therapy, and tumor hypoxia. We conclude with a discussion on the biology of combining immunotherapy with radiation in lung cancer.

J. G. Bazan (✉)
Department of Radiation Oncology,
City of Hope Comprehensive Cancer Center,
Duarte, CA, USA
e-mail: jbazan@coh.org

1 Radiobiologic Basis of Conventionally Fractionated Radiation Therapy

This section provides a review of the basic principles of radiobiology, including the mechanism of action of X-rays, the linear–quadratic (LQ) model of cell survival, and the four Rs of radiobiology. Taken together, these fundamentals help explain why radiation is most commonly delivered as a fractionated course over 5–6 weeks.

1.1 DNA: The Critical Target for the Biologic Effects of Radiation Damage

The biologic effects of radiation result principally from damage to a cell's deoxyribonucleic acid (DNA). The damage induced by radiation can be direct or indirect. Direct DNA damage occurs when the absorption of a photon by an atom releases an electron (a secondary electron) that then directly interacts with the DNA molecule. Indirect damage occurs when the secondary electron reacts with a water molecule to produce a free radical. It is the production of this free radical that leads to the DNA damage. Most of the DNA damage produced by the high-energy photons used in most medical linear accelerators is indirect damage (Hall and Giaccia 2012).

The types of DNA damage produced by radiation include base damage (more than 1000 lesions per cell per Gy), single-strand breaks (approximately 1000 per Gy), and double-strand breaks (approximately 20–40 per Gy) (Hall and Giaccia 2012). Among these lesions, DNA double-strand breaks correlate best with cell killing, because they can lead to certain chromosomal aberrations (dicentrics, rings, anaphase bridges) that are lethal to the cell. Lethality, from the perspective of radiation biology, means the loss of reproductive integrity of tumor clonogens; that is, the tumor cells may still be physically present or intact and may still be able to undergo a few cell divisions, but they are no longer able to form a colony of cells (Hall and Giaccia 2012).

1.2 The Linear–Quadratic (LQ) Model

Cell survival curves have a characteristic shape when plotted on a log-linear scale with radiation dose on the x-axis and the log of cell survival on the y-axis. At low doses, the curve tends to be straight (linear). As the dose increases, the curve bends over a region of several Gy—this region is often referred to as the shoulder of the survival curve. At very high doses, the curve tends to straighten out again (Hall and Giaccia 2012).

Many biophysical models have been proposed to mathematically capture this relationship between radiation dose and cell survival. A comprehensive review of all of these models is beyond the scope of this chapter but can be found in Hall and Giaccia (2012) and Brenner et al. (1998) The most commonly used model is the LQ model, which assumes that there are two components to cell killing, one that is proportional to the radiation dose and the other that is proportional to the square of the dose (Hall and Giaccia 2012). Cell survival in this model is represented by the following exponential function (Eq. 1):

$$S(D) = e^{-(\alpha D + \beta D^2)} \qquad (1)$$

where S is the fraction of cells surviving a dose, D, e is the mathematical constant approximately equal to 2.71828, and α and β are constants that represent the linear and quadratic components of cell killing, respectively. At dose $D = \dfrac{\alpha}{\beta}$, the contributions from the linear and quadratic components of cell killing are equal.

The LQ model is convenient in that it depends on only two parameters (α and β) and it is relatively easy to manipulate mathematically. However, there is also a biologic rationale for using this model. As mentioned earlier, DNA double-strand breaks are believed to be the primary mechanism leading to cell death. A single hit of radiation (one electron) can cause lethal injury by inducing breaks on two adjacent chromosomes (αD component). However, when two separate electrons cause the two chromosome breaks, cumulative injury can occur, and the probability of this occurrence is proportional to the square of the dose (βD^2) (Hall and Giaccia 2012).

1.3 The Four Rs of Radiobiology

The principles underlying fractionated radiotherapy can best be understood in terms of the classical four Rs of radiobiology: repair, reassortment, reoxygenation, and repopulation (Hall and Giaccia 2012).

1.3.1 Repair

Repair refers primarily to the ability of normal tissues to recover from sublethal DNA damage. Sublethal damage repair is the operational term for the increase in cell survival that is seen when a given radiation dose is split into two fractions separated by a time interval. Sublethal damage repair is simply the repair of DNA double-strand breaks (Hall and Giaccia 2012). In terms of the LQ model, tissues that have a greater capacity for DNA double-strand break repair have larger values for β and therefore a low $\frac{\alpha}{\beta}$ ratio. In contrast, most tumors and acutely responding tissues have a low capacity for repair and therefore a high $\frac{\alpha}{\beta}$ ratio.

1.3.2 Reassortment

Experiments have demonstrated that the most radiosensitive phases of the cell cycle are the M and G2 phases and the most radioresistant phase is the late S phase (Hall and Giaccia 2012). Reassortment is the principle that cells progress through the cell cycle during the interval between two doses of radiation. Cells that were not killed by the first dose of radiation were likely in a radioresistant phase of the cell cycle at that time. Between the first and second doses of radiation, these cells would have time to progress to the M or G2 phase and thus they would be more sensitive to the second dose of radiation.

1.3.3 Reoxygenation

The presence of oxygen within microseconds of radiation exposure is crucial for radiation-induced cell killing. Oxygen acts at the level of free radicals to effectively fix the radiation damage by inducing a permanent conformational change in the DNA molecule.

In the absence of oxygen (hypoxic conditions), as much as triple the amount of radiation may be needed to induce as much cell killing as would occur in the presence of oxygen (Hall and Giaccia 2012). Most tumors have areas of hypoxia. Hypoxia can be acute or chronic: acute hypoxia results from the temporary closing or blockage of a blood vessel; chronic hypoxia results from the limited diffusion distance (70 μm) of oxygen (Hall and Giaccia 2012).

In the late 1960s, van Putten and Kalman performed a set of experiments to determine the proportion of hypoxic cells in a transplantable sarcoma in a mouse model (Van Putten and Kallman 1968). They measured the proportion of hypoxic cells in the untreated tumor at 14%. They then administered five fractions of daily radiotherapy (1.9 Gy per fraction) to the tumor on Monday through Friday. The subsequent Monday, the hypoxic fraction was nearly the same, at 18%. They repeated the experiment except that they administered four fractions of 1.9 Gy each to the tumor on Monday through Thursday, and the hypoxic fraction measured on Friday was again constant at 14%.

These experiments provided some of the first evidence that reoxygenation occurs between deliveries of fractions of radiation. If reoxygenation did not occur, the proportion of hypoxic tumor cells would be expected to increase by the end of a fractionated course of treatment. Therefore, if enough time is allowed for reoxygenation to occur, the negative effects of hypoxia can be overcome.

1.3.4 Repopulation

Fractionation of radiation can lead to an increase in the surviving fraction of cancer cells if the interval between the two doses of radiation exceeds the length of the cell cycle time needed for the tumor cells to divide. Therefore, repopulation of tumor cells as a result of fractionation can be detrimental. In addition, treatment with any cytotoxic agent (e.g., chemotherapy drug or radiation) can trigger surviving tumor cells to divide faster than their normal cell cycle time or can reduce the number of cells lost; this phenomenon is known as accelerated repopulation (Fowler 1991). A high level of evidence supports this phenomenon in human tumors, including tumors of the lung and squamous cell carcinomas of the head and neck and the cervix. Because of this phenomenon, it is recommended that radiotherapy courses be completed without interruption.

1.3.5 Summary

The use of conventionally fractionated radiotherapy can now be understood in terms of the four Rs of radiobiology. Advantages of fractionation include reoxygenation of tumor cells to overcome hypoxia, reassortment of tumor cells into more sensitive phases of the cell cycle, and repair of sublethal damage in normal tissues to help reduce radiation toxicity. The main disadvantage of a fractionated course of radiation is that repopulation of tumor cells may occur, especially if the treatment course is prolonged beyond the expected time frame for completion.

1.4 Biologically Effective Dose

The biologically effective dose is a single dose value that can be used to compare the effectiveness of different fractionation schemes. This quantity is derived from the LQ model (Hall and Giaccia 2012). For a treatment schedule of n fractions each of size d, the first Eq. (1) can be rewritten as

$$S = e^{-n(\alpha d + \beta d^2)} \text{ or, alternatively, as } \frac{\ln S}{\alpha} = nd\left[1 + d/(\alpha/\beta)\right].$$

The quantity $\ln S$ is referred to as the biologically effective dose. When calculating the biologically effective dose for most tumors and tissues that respond acutely to radiation injury, the $\frac{\alpha}{\beta}$ ratio is usually set at 10 Gy; these tumors and tissues have a low capacity for repair, so the α term dominates the ratio. Late-responding tissues (e.g., the spinal cord) have a greater capacity for repair between fractions of radiation, so the β term dominates the $\frac{\alpha}{\beta}$ ratio. When calculating the biologically effective dose for late-respond tissues, $\frac{\alpha}{\beta} = 3$ Gy is the most common convention.

As an example, a common fractionation schedule used to treat non-small cell lung cancer (NSCLC) is 60 Gy in 30 fractions of 2 Gy each. Assuming $\frac{\alpha}{\beta} = 10$ for the tumor and $\frac{\alpha}{\beta} = 3$ for late-responding tissue, the biologically effective dose for this schedule would be given as

$$\text{BED}_{\text{tumor}} = (30 \text{ fractions})(2 \text{ Gy / fraction})\left(1 + \frac{2 \text{ Gy}}{10 \text{ Gy}}\right) = 72 \text{ Gy}_{10}.$$

$$\text{BED}_{\text{late-responding tissue}} = (30 \text{ fractions})(2 \text{ Gy / fraction})\left(1 + \frac{2 \text{ Gy}}{3 \text{ Gy}}\right) = 100 \text{ Gy}_{3}.$$

Alternatively, a fractionation schedule now used to treat patients who have a poor performance status or who are not candidates for concurrent chemotherapy is 60 Gy in 15 fractions of 4 Gy each. Again assuming $\frac{\alpha}{\beta} = 10$ for the tumor and $\frac{\alpha}{\beta} = 3$ for late-responding tissue, the biologically effective dose for this approach is

$$\text{BED}_{\text{tumor}} = (15\,\text{fractions})(4\,\text{Gy/fraction})\left(1 + \frac{4\,\text{Gy}}{10\,\text{Gy}}\right) = 84\,\text{Gy}_{10}.$$

$$\text{BED}_{\text{late-responding tissue}} = (15\,\text{fractions})(4\,\text{Gy/fraction})\left(1 + \frac{4\,\text{Gy}}{3\,\text{Gy}}\right) = 140\,\text{Gy}_{3}.$$

Even though the total dose was the same in both cases (60 Gy), the treatment schedule of 15 fractions of 4 Gy each has a higher tumor effective dose than the schedule of 30 fractions of 2 Gy each, but the 15-fraction schedule confers a higher risk to the late-responding tissue, such as the spinal cord if it is kept in the high-dose areas. The biologically effective dose is therefore a very useful tool that radiation oncologists often use when varying the fraction size from the standard 2 Gy per day. Note that this simple concept does not take into account other factors that affect the biologically effective dose, such as repopulation, reassortment, and reoxygenation. In addition, the applicability of the LQ model for estimating the biologically effective dose at larger doses per fraction is under debate, as will be discussed (Brown et al. 2013).

2 Alternative Fractionation Schedules

In 1980, the Radiation Therapy Oncology Group (RTOG) conducted a prospective randomized study of various radiation dose and fractionation schedules among patients with unresectable stage III lung cancer (Perez et al. 1980). Most of these patients were treated with conventional fractionation of 2 Gy per day to a dose of 40, 50, or 60 Gy. One group of patients received 40 Gy in a split-course fashion (20 Gy in 4 Gy per day over 5 days, 2-week rest period, 20 Gy in 4 Gy per day over 5 days). This trial showed a small benefit in local control for patients who received 50 Gy or 60 Gy compared with patients who received 40 Gy, although this benefit was no longer present after 2 years of follow-up. Nonetheless, this trial established 60 Gy given over 6 weeks as the optimal dose for stage III NSCLC.

Since that time, numerous approaches have been studied in an effort to improve the survival of individuals with locally advanced or early-stage unresectable lung cancer. Alternative fractionation schedules can be used as a means of improving outcomes without worsening toxicity.

2.1 Hyperfractionated Radiation Therapy in Lung Cancer

Hyperfractionation refers to giving an increased number of fractions but smaller fraction sizes (e.g., less than 1.8–2.0 Gy) to deliver a higher total dose over the same overall treatment time as with conventional fractionation CF (Hall and Giaccia 2012). Hyperfractionation is most commonly performed by delivering the radiation treatments two or three times per day, as opposed to once daily with convention fractionation. The final total dose delivered is often higher than the total dose administered on a conventional schedule. The overall goal of a hyperfractionated schedule is to achieve dose escalation and intensification while minimizing the likelihood of the late effects of radiotherapy.

The role of hyperfractionation in treating NSCLC has been studied extensively. One of the first cooperative group trials examining this question was RTOG 81-08 (Seydel et al. 1985). In this dose-finding and toxicity trial, all patients received 1.2 Gy twice daily (with 4–6 h between fractions) to a dose of 50.4 Gy, 60 Gy, 69.6 Gy, or 74.4 Gy. No treatment-related deaths occurred, and severe toxicity (pneumonitis, esophagitis, or pulmonary fibrosis) developed in only six patients (less than 9%). In the long-term update, the 5-year overall survival rate was 8.3% for patients who received 69.6 Gy, which compared favorably with the rate of 5.6% seen among patients who received 60 Gy with conventional fractionation in RTOG 78-11/79-17 (Cox et al. 1991).

In RTOG 83-11, 848 patients were randomly assigned to one of five arms: 60.0 Gy, 64.8 Gy, 69.6 Gy, 74.4 Gy, or 79.2 Gy (Cox et al. 1990). The fractionation schedule for all arms was 1.2 Gy twice daily separated by 4–8 h. No significant differences were found in early or late effects of radiotherapy across all the treatment arms. In addition, no significant differences were found in overall survival (60 Gy, 9.2 months; 64.8 Gy, 6.3 months; 69.6 Gy, 10.0 months; 74.4 Gy, 8.7 months; 79.2 Gy, 10.5 months). In a subgroup analysis of patients with favorable characteristics as defined by Cancer and Leukemia Group B criteria (Karnofsky Performance Status 70–100 and <6% weight loss), there was a significant dose response found for median overall survival among the three arms with lowest total dose, favoring the 69.6 Gy arm: 60 Gy, 10 months; 64.8 Gy, 7.8 months; and 69.6 Gy, 13.0 months ($p = 0.02$). No significant improvement in median overall survival occurred with dose escalation beyond 69.6 Gy in this trial.

The RTOG and Eastern Cooperative Oncology Group (ECOG) conducted an intergroup trial in which they performed a direct comparison of hyperfractionation and conventional fractionation in NSCLC. In RTOG 88-08/ECOG 4588, patients were randomly assigned to one of three arms: conventional fractionation to 60 Gy (2 Gy daily), hyperfractionation to 69.6 Gy (1.2 Gy twice daily), or induction chemotherapy followed by conventional fraction to 60 Gy (Sause et al. 1995). In this trial, induction chemotherapy was found to be superior to the treatments in the other two arms. In a direct comparison of patients who received hyperfractionation and patients who received conventional fractionation (without chemotherapy), no significant difference in median overall survival was found (12.3 vs. 11.4 months, respectively).

Fu et al. also conducted a phase III trial comparing conventional fractionation and hyperfractionation in NSCLC (Fu et al. 1994). In this trial, patients were randomly assigned to receive 63.9 ± 1.1 Gy CF (1.8–2.0 Gy daily) or 69.6 ± 2.1 Gy hyperfractionation (1.2 Gy twice daily). Toxicity and overall survival did not differ significantly between the two arms. In a subset analysis of patients with stages I–IIIA disease only, 2-year overall survival and local control were significantly superior in the hyperfractionation arm (32% vs. 6% and 28% vs. 13%, respectively; $p < 0.05$ for both).

In conclusion, although there is a strong radiobiologic rationale for a hyperfractionation approach, modest dose escalation (above 60 Gy) has not led to a convincing survival advantage in the randomized setting. Nonetheless, these trials were conducted at a time when computed tomography and three-dimensional planning were not widely available, thereby leading to large radiation-treatment fields often including elective node radiation. In addition, the accuracy of staging was limited, especially because of the lack of positron-emission tomography. With the technology available today and the unexpected initial results of RTOG 06-17 (to be discussed), radiation oncologists may now be able to fully exploit the expected radiobiologic advantages of hyperfractionation and other alternative fractionation regimens.

2.2 Accelerated Fractionation Schedules in Lung Cancer

Accelerated fractionation is defined as delivering the same total dose of radiation as in CF in a shorter overall treatment time by giving two or more fractions of radiation daily (Hall and Giaccia 2012). The rationale for using accelerated fractionation is to overcome repopulation of clonogenic tumor cells during fractionated radiotherapy, which should result in an increase in local control for a given total radiation dose. Practically speaking, pure accelerated fractionation (e.g., delivering 60 Gy in 2 Gy fractions over 3 weeks) is not possible because acute effects of radiation become limiting. As a result, accelerated fractionation schedules in the clinic must reduce the daily fraction size, introduce a predetermined rest period (split-course), or reduce the final total dose. Most accelerated fractionation schedules incorporate smaller fraction sizes given multiple times daily and are therefore hybrids of accelerated fractionation and hyperfractionation.

The Medical Research Council of London compared conventional fractionation with an accelerated fractionation regimen for patients with stage I–III or unresectable lung cancer (Saunders et al. 1997). Of these patients, 37% had stage I or II disease and 82% had tumors with squamous cell histology. In this trial, the accelerated fractionation regimen consisted of continuous hyperfractionated accelerated radiotherapy (CHART). CHART was delivered to a total dose of 54 Gy given in 1.5 Gy fractions three times per day (with a 6-h interfraction interval) over 12 consecutive days (including weekends). Patients in the conventional fractionation arm received 60 Gy in 30 fractions over 6 weeks. Despite the lower total dose, patients in the CHART arm had a significant reduction in the risk of death, with a hazard ratio of 0.76, which corresponded to an increase in 2-year overall survival of 9% (29% vs. 20%; $p = 0.004$) (Saunders et al. 1997). Patients in this arm had a similar relative risk reduction with respect to local disease progression, with a hazard ratio of 0.77. As indicated in a subsequent report on the trial, the results for overall survival and disease progression were maintained with longer follow-up (Saunders et al. 1999). As expected, short-term toxicity was worse in the CHART arm, with severe dysphagia occurring at a rate of 19% compared with 3% in the conventional fractionation arm. The rates of late toxicity were not different between the two arms.

More recently, ECOG 2597 compared conventional fractionation with accelerated fractionation radiation after induction chemotherapy (two cycles of carboplatin and paclitaxel) for patients with stage III lung cancer (Belani et al. 2005). Patients in the conventional fractionation arm received a total dose of 64 Gy (2 Gy daily). Patients in the accelerated fractionation arm received hyperfractionated accelerated radiotherapy (HART) to a total dose of 57.6 Gy in three daily fractions of 1.5 Gy (fraction 1), 1.8 Gy (fraction 2), and 1.5 Gy (fraction 3) given over 12 days. This trial was terminated early because of poor accrual. The median overall survival was numerically superior in the HART arm than in the conventional fractionation arm (20.3 vs. 14.9 months), but this difference did not reach significance. Overall acute grade 3 or higher toxicity did not differ between the two arms, although rates of esophagitis tended to be higher in the HART arm (25% vs. 18%). Although the results of this study are provocative, induction chemotherapy followed by radiotherapy is no longer the standard of care for this group of patients.

In a similar study, termed CHARTWEL (CHART weekend less), investigators compared conventional fractionation given as 66 Gy in 33 fractions over 6.5 weeks with the CHARTWEL regimen of 60 Gy in 1.5 Gy fractions three times per day over 2.5 weeks (Baumann et al. 2011). No difference in overall survival or local control was found for patients in either arm, but increased acute toxicity was found among patients in the CHARTWEL arm. However, in the subset of patients with more advanced cancer and among patients who received neoadjuvant chemotherapy, patients who received the CHARTWEL regimen had a significant local control advantage (p = 0.006–0.025 for more advanced cancer; p = 0.019 for neoadjuvant chemotherapy) (Baumann et al. 2011).

Overall, the results of accelerated fractionation regimens for treating lung cancer appear promising. Although the CHART data in particular appear to correspond well with the expected radiobiologic results of an accelerated fractionation schedule, the inclusion of a large percentage of patients with early-stage (stages I–II) cancer and the high percentage of patients with squamous cell histology make it hard to extrapolate the findings to current patients with locally advanced NSCLC among whom the proportion of squamous cell histology is declining. In addition, as a result of trials such as RTOG 94-10 (Curran Jr et al. 2011), the current standard of care for patients with locally advanced lung cancer is concurrent chemoradiation therapy. A CHART-type regimen may be a reasonable alternative for patients who are not candidates for chemotherapy, but additional studies are needed to test the effectiveness and tolerability of such a regimen in this patient population. A meta-analysis of individual data from 2000 patients treated in ten trials showed a significantly improved overall survival with modified fractionation (i.e., hyperfractionation or accelerated fractionation) for patients with nonmetastatic NSCLC (p = 0.009). For patients with small cell lung cancer (SCLC), a positive trend toward improved overall survival was found. As expected, dose intensification resulted in higher rates of acute esophageal toxicity (Mauguen et al. 2012).

2.3 Hypofractionated Radiation Therapy in Lung Cancer

The use of large once daily fraction sizes over a shorter number of treatments is termed hypofractionation. The daily fraction sizes are generally >3 Gy and the number of total treatments delivered is often in the range of 15–20 with hypofractionated radiation therapy. As discussed previously, NSCLC has a high α/β ratio (α/β = 10) and thereby shows a lower sensitivity to an increase in the daily fraction size. However, late-responding normal tissues (α/β = 3) have an increased sensitivity to an increase in the daily fraction size. Therefore, the radiobiological expectation is that hypofractionation will lower the therapeutic ratio between tumors and late-responding tissues and has the ability to cause significant late toxicities. For example, early studies of hypofractionated regimens in patients with breast cancer showed extremely high rates of brachial plexopathy (Powell et al. 1990). As a result, hypofractionated regimens fell out of favor for several decades due to these toxicities.

However, recent technological advances in tumor and normal tissue imaging coupled with significant improvements in radiation planning and delivery of external beam radiation with multileaf collimators and intensity-modulated radiation therapy enable radiation oncologists to conform the high-dose radiation to the target volume and spare adjacent normal tissues (De Los Santos et al. 2013; Nahum and Uzan 2012). These technological advances enable an improvement in the therapeutic ratio by increasing radiation dose to the tumor and reducing radiation dose and volume of normal tissue exposure. Stereotactic ablative radiation therapy (SABR), also known as stereotactic body radiation therapy (SBRT), is an extreme form of hypofractionation in patients with lung cancer in which doses on the order of 10–20 Gy per fraction are delivered over 1–5 fractions. Here, we will discuss modestly hypofractionated regimens (3–4 Gy per fraction to 45–60 Gy total dose) and SABR.

2.4 Clinical Applications of Moderately Hypofractionated Radiation Therapy

Moderately hypofractionated radiation schedules have been studies extensively in patients with early-stage NSCLC. These regimens included 48 Gy in 12 fractions, 55 Gy in 20 fractions, 60 Gy in 20 fractions, and 60 Gy in 15 fractions (Bonfili et al. 2010; Cheung et al. 2002; Din et al. 2013; Faria et al. 2006; Gauden et al. 1995;

Lester et al. 2004; Oh et al. 2013; Slotman et al. 1996; Soliman et al. 2011). Overall, these types of regimens have largely been replaced by SABR regimens for patients with early-stage NSCLC. The true clinical application of moderately hypofractionated radiation therapy is in patients with locally advanced disease (stage III), in patients not suitable for concurrent chemotherapy, or in patients with limited metastatic disease in which treating the primary disease in the lung and lymph nodes is felt to be important for local control.

In a small Italian trial of 30 patients with poor performance status, patients with locally advanced NSCLC received 60 Gy in 20 fractions without chemotherapy (Osti et al. 2013). This regimen was shown to have acceptable toxicity with only two patients experiencing grade 2 pneumonitis, one patient with grade 3 esophagitis, and one patient with grade 3 hematologic toxicity. Median OS for these patients with poor PS was 1 year.

A more recent phase I dose escalation trial studied a 15-fraction hypofractionated regimen in patients with stage III or stage IV NSCLC with poor PS. The three dose arms were 50 Gy (3.33 Gy/fraction, $N = 15$ patients), 55 Gy (3.67 Gy/fraction, $N = 21$ patients), and 60 Gy (4 Gy/fraction, $N = 19$ patients) (Westover et al. 2015). The maximum tolerated dose was not reached, so 60 Gy in 15 fractions was considered safe and effective. In terms of treatment-related toxicities, one patient in the 55 Gy group and one patient in the 60 Gy group developed grade ≥3 esophagitis, and there were 13 patients (5 in the 50 Gy group, 4 in the 55 Gy group, and 4 in the 60 Gy group) that developed grade ≥3 dyspnea, though only 2 were felt to be related to treatment. It is important to note that the 60 Gy in 15-fraction regimen for locally advanced NSCLC is safe but only in the modern era of radiation delivery where gross disease is well visualized on imaging and small margins are used for the target volumes, daily on-board image guidance, and strict normal tissue constraints. A phase III trial comparing 60 Gy in 15 fractions to 60 Gy in 30 fractions in stage III/IV patients with poor PS is currently ongoing (Iyengar et al. 2016).

A recent phase I trial of moderate hypofractionation in patients with stage III NSCLC was conducted by the Cancer and Leukemia Group B cooperative group in the setting of concurrent chemotherapy (Urbanic et al. 2018). In this study, the total radiation dose remained constant at 60 Gy, but there were four cohorts of patients with a decreasing number of fractions per cohort: 27 fractions (2.22 Gy/fraction), 24 fractions (2.5 Gy/fraction), 22 fractions (2.82 Gy/fraction), and 20 fractions (3 Gy/fraction). Patients received concurrent chemotherapy with weekly carboplatin + paclitaxel. A total of 22 patients were accrued and grade 5 toxicity occurred in 3 patients (1 in the 24-fraction and 2 in the 22-fraction arm). The maximum tolerated dose was deemed to be 60 Gy in 24 fractions with concurrent chemotherapy. These results are consistent with earlier phase II studies demonstrating that concurrent chemotherapy can be safely delivered with modestly hypofractionated radiation therapy in stage III NSCLC as long as the daily fraction size remains <3 Gy per fraction (Cho et al. 2009; Maguire et al. 2014).

2.5 Clinical Applications of Stereotactic Ablative Radiotherapy for NSCLC

SABR is an extreme form of hypofractionation. Just as with moderate hypofractionation, it was not until the development of precision, highly conformal image-guided radiation therapy with advanced delivery techniques that SABR regimens could be safely explored for extracranial indications such as early-stage NSCLC. SABR regimens for early-stage NSCLC deliver a high BED_{10} that is on the order of ≥100 Gy generally delivered in 1–5 fractions total over 1–2 weeks. With these regimens, long-term primary tumor control rates are consistently ≥90% (Singh et al. 2019; Timmerman et al. 2010; Videtic et al. 2015, 2019).

In the clinic, SABR has become the standard of care for early-stage NSCLC in medically inoperable patients (Brada et al. 2015; Vansteenkiste et al. 2014). The role of SABR for patients with medically inoperable disease is controversial and has been the subject of several prospective studies that closed early due to slow accrual (Chang et al. 2015; Deng et al. 2017; Timmerman et al. 2018) and remains the subject of ongoing clinical trials [NCT01753414, NCT02468024, NCT02984761, NCT02629458].

In terms of dose and fractionation, peripheral lung tumors are generally treated in 1 fraction (30–34 Gy × 1) or 3 fractions (18–20 Gy × 3) based on several prospective studies including RTOG 0236, RTOG 0915, and a multi-institutional randomized phase II study by Singh et al. (Singh et al. 2019; Timmerman et al. 2010; Videtic et al. 2015). Based on consensus guidelines, peripheral tumors that lie in close proximity to the chest wall are often treated with 4–5-fraction regimens (10 Gy × 5 or 12 Gy × 4) in order to minimize the risk of chest wall pain and rib fracture (Guckenberger et al. 2017).

Central lung tumors are those that are located within 2 cm of the proximal bronchial tree or immediately adjacent to the pleura covering the mediastinum or pericardium (Owen and Sio 2020). Ultracentral tumors are those that are within 1 cm of the proximal bronchial tree and are often adjacent to structures such as the esophagus, mediastinum, or great vessels (Owen and Sio 2020). An early phase II trial by Timmerman et al. demonstrated excessive severe toxicity, including death, in patients with centrally located tumors (defined as within 2 cm of the proximal bronchial tree) that received 60–66 Gy in three fractions (Timmerman et al. 2006). Due to toxicity, central and ultracentral tumors are often treated with lower doses per fraction and over a larger number of fractions compared to peripheral tumors in an effort to minimize the risk of toxicity. For example, RTOG 0813 was a phase I/II clinical trial that studied the safety of dose escalation for central tumors from 10 Gy × 5 fractions up to 12 Gy × 5 fractions (Bezjak et al. 2019). This study found that the maximum tolerated dose was 12 Gy × 5 fractions, resulting in an estimated 7% probability of dose-limiting toxicities and an overall 18% rate of grade ≥3 toxicities. In a separate prospective trial by Roach et al., a dose of 11 Gy × 5 was used and this resulted in a high rate of grade ≥3 toxicity of 43%. More protracted but still extremely hypofractionated course of 7–7.5 Gy × 8–10 fractions or 10–12.5 Gy × 4–5 fractions have been studied for central and ultracentral tumors with promising results in retrospective series (Chaudhuri et al. 2015; Haasbeek et al. 2011; Tekatli et al. 2015). Prospective trials are currently being conducted to find the optimal dose and fractionation for central/ultracentral tumors, such as the ongoing multicenter phase I dose escalation SUNSET study (Giuliani et al. 2018).

3 Radiobiology of SABR

The exceedingly high tumor control rates seen with SABR regimens in early-stage NSCLC leads many to question whether the four "Rs" of radiobiology adequately explain the tumor cell killing effects seen with SABR or whether different mechanisms of action may be at play with these large dose per fraction regimens (Brown et al. 2014; Brown and Koong 2008).

3.1 Reexamining the Four "Rs" of Radiobiology in SABR

As previously mentioned, the classical four "Rs" of radiobiology that form the basis of conventional fractionation are repair, redistribution, reoxygenation, and repopulation.

3.1.1 Repair in SABR
With conventional radiation, sublethal DNA damage repair in tumor cells will lead to reduced radiosensitivity. However, with the high doses per fraction used in SABR regimens, more necroptosis is induced than apoptosis, resulting in more lethal damage to the majority of tumor cells (Brown et al. 2014; Kreuzaler and Watson 2012; Wang et al. 2018).

3.1.2 Redistribution in SABR
Ablative doses on the order of 20 Gy or higher are associated with cell cycle block at all stages of the cell cycle (Qiu et al. 2020). Therefore,

there is no redistribution of tumor cells through the cell cycle since tumor cells in both the sensitive G2/M phases and insensitive phases of the cell cycle will be directly killed (Lewanski and Gullick 2001).

3.1.3 Reoxygenation in SABR

In SABR regimens, there may be less reoxygenation of initially hypoxic tumor cells given that the treatment courses are completed within 1–2 weeks. In addition, there may be persistent tumor hypoxia that results from vascular injury to the tumor microenvironment with SABR regimens (Kelada et al. 2018; Song et al. 2014). However, the doses used in SABR regimens may be high enough to ablate both hypoxic and oxygenated cells.

3.1.4 Repopulation in SABR

Repopulation of tumor cells is a concern with conventionally fractionated radiation regimens that last for several weeks. However, since SABR regimens are completed within 1–2 weeks, there is no time for tumor cell repopulation.

3.2 Dose Effect Models in SABR: Is the LQ Model Applicable

If we apply the LQ formalism to the fractionation schemes used in lung SABR, we can see that SABR delivers a large biologically effective dose (biologically effective dose in the equation) to the tumors. For example, one of the most commonly used schedules is 60 Gy given in three fractions of 20 Gy each. Using the assumption that $\alpha/\beta = 10$, the BED_{10} of this regimen is $BED_{10} = 60\ Gy\ (1 + 20/10) = 180\ Gy_{10}$. In order to achieve this same BED_{10} using conventional fractionation with 2 Gy per fraction, one would have to deliver a total dose of 150 Gy in 75 fractions. If these treatments were given once a day, it would take more than 15 weeks to complete the treatment course and efficacy would be lost because of repopulation. Simply put, one could argue that the success of SABR is due mostly to the delivery of very high doses of radiation to the tumor in a short time. On the other hand, loss of treatment efficacy may result from hypoxia-related radioresistance when large doses per fraction are used (Carlson et al. 2011).

Whether the LQ model appropriately applies to the high doses per fraction used in SABR is a subject of debate. Some investigators have argued that because the LQ model is continuously curving downward as the dose increases, this model actually overestimates clonogenic cell killing in the SABR dose ranges. This has led to the proposal for a piecemeal function for cell survival, termed the universal survival curve (Park et al. 2008). This function combines the LQ model for low doses per fraction and another model, known as the multitarget model (Elkind et al. 1967), for larger doses per fraction. These authors found that the fit for the survival curve of an NSCLC cell line (H460) up to more than 15 Gy per fraction was vastly improved using the universal survival curve rather than the LQ model, especially as the dose per fraction increased above 10 Gy (Park et al. 2008).

In summary, the four "Rs" of radiobiology seem to have little application to SABR regimens. Instead, the extreme hypofractionation used in SABR appears to induce direct cell death independent of these radiobiological principles. In addition, the LQ model does not adequately capture the cell kill effect seen with SABR. This has led to speculation as to whether new mechanisms of cell killing may be involved in SABR regimens (Brown studies).

3.3 Effects of SABR: New Mechanisms of Cell Killing?

As discussed earlier, the principles of classic radiobiology can be understood in terms of DNA double-strand break damage and the four Rs of radiobiology. However, this understanding has been driven in large part by experiments that used conventional fractionation (1.8–2 Gy per fraction). Despite the finding that the LQ model may overestimate cell killing in vitro (because the $\beta D2$ component predicts a continuously bending curve as the dose increases but experimental models are more consistent with a linear curve at these high doses), clinical studies have shown that the LQ model may actually underestimate tumor control by stereotactic radiosurgery and SABR (Kirkpatrick et al. 2008). Thus, several groups have hypothesized that mechanisms other than DNA double-strand breaks may be responsible for the enhanced effects of SABR.

One hypothesis is that the vascular endothelium is a unique target of the high-dose radiation used in SABR. More specifically, the hypothesis is that large, single fractions of radiation (>8–10 Gy) activate the acid sphingomyelinase pathway, ultimately resulting in the generation of ceramide, which stimulates endothelial cell apoptosis (Fuks and Kolesnick 2005; Garcia-Barros et al. 2003). Another hypothesis is that SABR doses of at least 10 Gy induce substantial vascular damage, disrupting the intratumoral microenvironment and thereby indirectly leading to tumor cell death (Park et al. 2012).

Another potential mechanism for the increased efficacy of SABR is that radiation creates a large amount of tumor antigens, which may augment the immune response (Lugade et al. 2005). Specifically, radiation may directly or indirectly activate inflammatory cytokines such as IL-1 and TNF-α that then lead to an increase in CD8+ T cells and a reduction of myeloid-derived suppressor cells (Filatenkov et al. 2015). As a result, there is an increase in immunogenic cell death which will continue to enhancing the immune response and recruitment of immune cells to the microenvironment (Bernstein et al. 2016).

Although these proposed mechanisms are intriguing and may well help to explain the excellent clinical results seen with SABR, some experts believe that SABR is successful because of the large biologically effective dose delivered to the tumor. A group of investigators pooled the data from nearly 2700 patients with medically inoperable stage I NSCLC who were treated with three-dimensional conformal radiotherapy or SABR (single-fraction or multifraction) (Brown et al. 2013). Using both the LQ model and the universal survival curve, they calculated the biologically effective dose for each patient. They then plotted the tumor control probability as a function of the BED and the results were consistent in that the tumor control probability increased as the biologically effective dose increased, regardless of which treatment patients received. At least for patients with stage I NSCLC, the results of this analysis indicated that different biologic mechanisms are not necessarily responsible for the success of SABR. The analysis does not, however, rule out the existence of these alternative or supplementary mechanisms.

4 Modification of Radiation Response

4.1 Chemotherapy

Conceptually, chemotherapy combined with radiotherapy has been explored to improve the therapeutic ratio. Chemotherapy may be integrated with radiotherapy in a variety of ways (Bentzen et al. 2007). In induction therapy, chemotherapy is given before local therapy (radiotherapy or surgery). This approach, which reduces the local tumor burden and addresses micrometastatic disease up-front, may be advantageous in that a reduced tumor size would result in smaller radiation treatment volumes, which could reduce acute and long-term toxicity. However, using induction chemotherapy followed by a course of radiotherapy extends the patient's overall treatment time. From a radiobiologic perspective, the extended treatment time could allow for accelerated repopulation in the primary tumor and thereby result in inferior outcomes.

Another approach is to give concurrent chemotherapy, that is, to deliver chemotherapy during the course of radiotherapy. With this approach, the overall treatment time is not extended because the definitive local and systemic therapies are given together. A disadvantage of this approach is that it often results in more acute toxicity, both local (i.e., radiation esophagitis) and systemic (i.e., myelosuppression). Concurrent chemoradiation therapy is currently a standard of care for patients with medically inoperable stage III NSCLC.

4.2 Tumor Hypoxia

As mentioned earlier, tumor hypoxia may reduce the efficacy of radiotherapy. Intraoperative measurement of tumor partial pressure of oxygen (pO_2) among patients undergoing resection of early-stage NSCLC demonstrated that tumor hypoxia existed to a certain degree in these tumors and correlated with higher expression of hypoxia-induced genes such as carbonic anhydrase IX (CAIX) (Le et al. 2006). In addition, tumor hypoxia and elevated expression of osteopontin correlated with worse prognosis in these patients. Therefore, investigators are interested in targeting hypoxia with radiotherapy in NSCLC. Two classes of drugs have been investigated to help overcome the detrimental effects of tumor hypoxia: hypoxic cell radiosensitizers and hypoxic cytotoxins.

4.2.1 Hypoxic Cell Radiosensitizers

In the 1960s, investigators began searching for compounds that mimic oxygen and that could therefore overcome chronic hypoxia by diffusing deep into the poorly vascularized portions of a tumor. These efforts led to the development of a class of drugs known as azoles, which have been extensively studied in the clinical setting. The results of earlier meta-analyses indicated that the benefit of using these agents (and other modifiers of hypoxia) is most pronounced for patients with head and neck cancers and less pronounced for patients with lung cancer (Overgaard 2007; Overgaard and Horsman 1996).

Investigators are showing a renewed interest in the azoles—for use in combination with single-fraction SABR (Brown et al. 2010). A potential shortcoming of single-fraction SABR from the perspective of classic radiobiology is that this treatment does not take advantage of tumor reoxygenation. Multifraction SABR regimens could potentially be converted to single-fraction regimens in combination with a hypoxic radiosensitizer. Clinical trials with patients with NSCLC are needed to fully address this question.

4.2.2 Hypoxic Cytotoxins

An alternative to radiosensitizing hypoxic tumor cells is to develop a compound that selectively targets hypoxic cells. One common hypoxic cytotoxin is mitomycin C, which is a component of chemotherapy regimens used to treat squamous cell carcinomas of the anal canal. This drug has also been used as part of chemotherapy regimens for NSCLC, but it is no longer in widespread use for this indication.

Another hypoxic cytotoxin, tirapazamine, has been prospectively studied in patients with locally advanced NSCLC and limited-stage SCLC in several trials (Le et al. 2004, 2009; Williamson et al. 2005). The results have been mixed. Two prospective nonrandomized trials examining tirapazamine added to concurrent chemoradiation therapy for patients with SCLC have had promising results (Le et al. 2004, 2009). However, among patients with NSCLC, adding tirapazamine to standard chemoradiation therapy did not improve survival but did result in increased toxicity (Williamson et al. 2005). At this time, modifying hypoxia by adding tirapazamine or other hypoxic cytotoxins is not routinely done for patients with lung cancer.

4.2.3 Future Directions in Hypoxia

The U.S. National Cancer Institute has recognized that in order to continue improving the therapeutic index of radiotherapy, the technologic innovations that have occurred in radiation oncology must be supplemented with biologic innovations such as new radiosensitizing agents (Lin et al. 2013). The National Cancer Institute recommends a series of steps to promote the rapid development of combined radiotherapy with targeted agents. However, appropriate preclinical models are needed to test the benefit of radiation combined with targeted therapy, especially agents targeting the tumor microenvironment or tumor hypoxia. One study has shown that the level of tumor oxygenation, as reflected by hypoxia imaging and the uptake of a hypoxic cell marker (pimonidazole), is highly dependent on the location of the xenograft tumor; the same tumor growing in the lungs showed considerably less hypoxia than it did growing subcutaneously. Moreover, the level of imaging hypoxia correlated well with tumor response to hypoxic cell cytotoxin (Graves et al. 2010). The results of studies like this one indicate that judicious selection of a preclinical model may improve the link between preclinical research and clinical practice.

4.3 Immunotherapy with Radiation in NSCLC

Immune checkpoint inhibitors (ICI) have changed the landscape of the management of many malignancies, including patients with NSCLC. For example, ICIs are now used in patients with stage IV NSCLC (Brahmer et al. 2015; Herbst et al. 2016; Vokes et al. 2018) and given as adjuvant consolidation systemic therapy in patients that have completed concurrent chemoradiation for stage III NSCLC (Antonia et al. 2018). An area of intense study in both the preclinical and clinical settings is the combination of SABR with ICIs. Interest in the approach of combining SABR with ICIs arose from a report nearly a decade ago in which Postow et al. showed that the administration of ipilimumab with SABR (9.5 Gy × 3 fractions) reversed required resistance to ipilimumab and also caused a disease response within the radiation field and outside of the radiation field (abscopal effect) (Postow et al. 2012).

4.3.1 Mechanism for Synergy of SABR + ICI

Radiation therapy can both augment and inhibit the immune response. Mechanisms of enhanced tumor-specific immunity include release of tumor-associated antigens from dying tumor cells, recruitment and activation of antigen-presenting cells, priming tumor-specific T cells, and inducing release of cytokines and chemokines (Walshaw et al. 2016; Xing et al. 2019). However, radiation may inhibit the immune response by depleting lymphocytes, which are highly sensitive to radiation, as well as by inducing immune suppressive cells (MDSCs, regulatory T cells) and inhibitory cytokines (TGF-β and IL-10) (Ishihara et al. 2017). Finding the right balance between harnessing the activating effects of radiation on the immune system while minimizing the inhibitor effects remains a major challenge which has led to the study of combining ICIs with radiation.

While the synergistic effect of ICIs with radiation has been seen in conventionally fractionated radiation therapy, it is more commonly reported in SABR regimens. For example, in a preclinical study of mice with murine melanoma, tumor-reactive T cells increased as the size of the radiation dose increased from 5 Gy × 1 fraction to 15 Gy × 1 fraction (Schaue et al. 2012). In another preclinical study, mice received anti-PD1 agent and were irradiated to the same BED but with two different regimens (11.5 Gy × 2 fractions versus 4 Gy × 9 fractions) (Lan et al. 2018). The group of mice that received 11.5 Gy × 2 had better tumor control and OS compared to those that received 4 Gy × 9 fractions. These examples show that SABR may enhance antitumor immunity.

4.3.2 Clinical Applications of SABR + ICI in NSCLC

Many clinical trials have been or are currently being conducted to study the efficacy of ICIs + SABR in NSCLC. A phase II randomized study of 76 patients with recurrent or metastatic NSCLC showed that the combination of SBRT + pembrolizumab resulted in a higher overall response rate compared to those that received pembrolizumab alone (36% vs. 18%) (Theelen et al. 2019). In 2019, Chicas-Sett et al. published a comprehensive review of the combination of SABR with ICIs in 1736 patients with metastatic NSCLC across 6 prospective studies and 12 retrospective studies. The study found local control rates of 71% and an impressively high abscopal response rate of 41% when SABR was combined with ICIs (Chicas-Sett et al. 2019). There are many ongoing studies of SABR + ICIs in advanced and early-stage NSCLC (NCT02599454, NCT03574220, NCT02599454, NCT03050554, NCT03383302, NCT03446911, NCT02904954, NCT0311097, NCT03924869,

NCT03833154, NCT03275597, NCT02492568, NCT03955198, NCT03867175).

The timing of ICI relative to SABR remains a clinical problem to be solved. ICIs may be given prior to SABR, after SABR, or with SABR. More and more evidence is accumulating that the optimal regimen may be SABR with concurrent ICI. For example, Pinnameneni et al. retrospectively reviewed outcomes of patients with metastatic NSCLC that receive nivolumab and SABR and found that patients that received nivolumab during SABR had better overall survival compared to those that received SABR followed by nivolumab (Pinnamaneni et al. 2017). In a series of 260 patients with brain metastases of different histologies, including NSCLC, Chen et al. found that patients that received SABR concurrent with ICI therapy had better overall survival compared to those that did not receive concurrent therapy (Chen et al. 2018). Similar results have been found in other studies (Lehrer et al. 2019; Samstein et al. 2017). While more prospective studies are clearly needed, it does appear at this time that the optimal sequencing is concurrent SABR with ICI.

The optimal dose and fractionation of SABR to be used with ICI remains another clinical dilemma. The BED of the SABR regimen appears to be an important metric for inducing the abscopal response. In a meta-analysis of preclinical models by Marconi et al., a SABR regimen with a BED_{10} of ≥ 60 Gy was associated with a 50% probability of generating an abscopal response (Marconi et al. 2017). Similarly, in a study utilizing the National Cancer Database, Foster et al. demonstrated that for patients receiving immunotherapy and SABR, a SABR regimen with $BED_{10} \geq 60$ Gy was associated with improved overall survival (Foster et al. 2019).

5 Flash Radiotherapy

Daily radiation treatments are generally delivered on the order of minutes (e.g., 2 Gy/min). FLASH radiation therapy delivers radiation at an ultrahigh dose rate, nearly instantaneously, on the order of 100 Gy/s (Montay-Gruel et al. 2018).

The unique potential of FLASH is the ability to achieve the same tumor control rate for a given dose of radiation but without damaging the surrounding normal tissues. In preclinical studies, FLASH has been shown to achieve the same tumor control efficacy while at the same time sparing normal tissue (Favaudon et al. 2014; Montay-Gruel et al. 2017). The significant differential effect of FLASH radiation therapy on tumors and normal tissues makes it an exciting treatment approach to translate to the clinic.

The first human patient was recently treated with FLASH (Bourhis et al. 2019). This patient had lymphoma involving the skin that had progressed after multiple prior treatments. A dose of 15 Gy was delivered in 90 ms to a skin tumor that measured 3.5 cm in diameter. At 3 weeks posttreatment, there was minimal skin irritation, and by 5 months posttreatment, the lesion had completely resolved without any damage to the surrounding skin. Clinical trials are currently under development to investigate FLASH radiation on a larger scale. If successful, this is the type of approach that could revolutionize radiation treatments in the coming decades, including for patients with NSCLC.

6 Conclusion

Radiotherapy remains a critical treatment modality for patients with lung cancer. Use of the fundamental principles of radiation biology has led to the development of novel radiation treatment approaches, including alternative fractionation schedules, combining immunotherapy with radiation, and SABR, and these approaches have had a substantial effect in the clinical setting. Nonetheless, unanswered questions remain that radiation biologists and clinicians working together can help translate into meaningful applications for patient care: Are there truly new mechanisms of cell death at play in SABR? Is the LQ model valid at the doses used in SABR? How can we best combine immunotherapy with radiation? Will FLASH radiotherapy revolutionize the treatment of NSCLC? The ultimate goal of answering these types of questions is to improve the outcomes for patients with lung cancer.

References

Antonia SJ et al (2018) Overall survival with durvalumab after chemoradiotherapy in stage III NSCLC. N Engl J Med 379:2342–2350

Baumann M et al (2011) Final results of the randomized phase III CHARTWEL-trial (ARO 97-1) comparing hyperfractionated-accelerated versus conventionally fractionated radiotherapy in non-small cell lung cancer (NSCLC). Radiother Oncol 100:76–85

Belani CP et al (2005) Phase III study of the Eastern Cooperative Oncology Group (ECOG 2597): induction chemotherapy followed by either standard thoracic radiotherapy or hyperfractionated accelerated radiotherapy for patients with unresectable stage IIIA and B non-small-cell lung cancer. J Clin Oncol 23:3760–3767

Bentzen SM, Harari PM, Bernier J (2007) Exploitable mechanisms for combining drugs with radiation: concepts, achievements and future directions. Nat Clin Pract Oncol 4:172–180

Bernstein MB, Krishnan S, Hodge JW, Chang JY (2016) Immunotherapy and stereotactic ablative radiotherapy (ISABR): a curative approach? Nat Rev Clin Oncol 13:516–524

Bezjak A et al (2019) Safety and efficacy of a five-fraction stereotactic body radiotherapy schedule for centrally located non-small-cell lung cancer: NRG Oncology/RTOG 0813 Trial. J Clin Oncol 37:1316–1325

Bonfili P et al (2010) Hypofractionated radical radiotherapy in elderly patients with medically inoperable stage I–II non-small-cell lung cancer. Lung Cancer 67:81–85

Bourhis J et al (2019) Treatment of a first patient with FLASH-radiotherapy. Radiother Oncol 139:18–22

Brada M, Pope A, Baumann M (2015) SABR in NSCLC—the beginning of the end or the end of the beginning? Radiother Oncol 114:135–137

Brahmer J et al (2015) Nivolumab versus docetaxel in advanced squamous-cell non-small-cell lung cancer. N Engl J Med 373:123–135

Brenner DJ, Hlatky LR, Hahnfeldt PJ, Huang Y, Sachs RK (1998) The linear-quadratic model and most other common radiobiological models result in similar predictions of time-dose relationships. Radiat Res 150:83–91

Brown JM, Koong AC (2008) High-dose single-fraction radiotherapy: exploiting a new biology? Int J Radiat Oncol Biol Phys 71:324–325

Brown JM, Diehn M, Loo BW Jr (2010) Stereotactic ablative radiotherapy should be combined with a hypoxic cell radiosensitizer. Int J Radiat Oncol Biol Phys 78:323–327

Brown JM, Brenner DJ, Carlson DJ (2013) Dose escalation, not "new biology," can account for the efficacy of stereotactic body radiation therapy with non-small cell lung cancer. Int J Radiat Oncol Biol Phys 85:1159–1160

Brown JM, Carlson DJ, Brenner DJ (2014) The tumor radiobiology of SRS and SBRT: are more than the 5 Rs involved? Int J Radiat Oncol Biol Phys 88:254–262

Carlson DJ, Keall PJ, Loo BW Jr, Chen ZJ, Brown JM (2011) Hypofractionation results in reduced tumor cell kill compared to conventional fractionation for tumors with regions of hypoxia. Int J Radiat Oncol Biol Phys 79:1188–1195

Chang JY et al (2015) Stereotactic ablative radiotherapy versus lobectomy for operable stage I non-small-cell lung cancer: a pooled analysis of two randomised trials. Lancet Oncol 16:630–637

Chaudhuri AA et al (2015) Stereotactic ablative radiotherapy (SABR) for treatment of central and ultra-central lung tumors. Lung Cancer 89:50–56

Chen LD et al (2018) Concurrent immune checkpoint inhibitors and stereotactic radiosurgery for brain metastases in non-small cell lung cancer, melanoma, and renal cell carcinoma. Int J Radiat Oncol 100:916–925

Cheung PC et al (2002) Accelerated hypofractionation for early-stage non-small-cell lung cancer. Int J Radiat Oncol Biol Phys 54:1014–1023

Chicas-Sett R et al (2019) Stereotactic ablative radiotherapy combined with immune checkpoint inhibitors reboots the immune response assisted by immunotherapy in metastatic lung cancer: a systematic review. Int J Mol Sci 20

Cho KH et al (2009) A Phase II study of synchronous three-dimensional conformal boost to the gross tumor volume for patients with unresectable Stage III non-small-cell lung cancer: results of Korean Radiation Oncology Group 0301 study. Int J Radiat Oncol Biol Phys 74:1397–1404

Cox JD et al (1990) A randomized phase I/II trial of hyperfractionated radiation therapy with total doses of 60.0 Gy to 79.2 Gy: possible survival benefit with greater than or equal to 69.6 Gy in favorable patients with Radiation Therapy Oncology Group stage III non-small-cell lung carcinoma: report of Radiation Therapy Oncology Group 83-11. J Clin Oncol 8:1543–1555

Cox JD et al (1991) Five-year survival after hyperfractionated radiation therapy for non-small-cell carcinoma of the lung (NSCCL): results of RTOG protocol 81-08. Am J Clin Oncol 14:280–284

Curran WJ Jr et al (2011) Sequential vs. concurrent chemoradiation for stage III non-small cell lung cancer: randomized phase III trial RTOG 9410. J Natl Cancer Inst 103:1452–1460

De Los Santos J et al (2013) Image guided radiation therapy (IGRT) technologies for radiation therapy localization and delivery. Int J Radiat Oncol Biol Phys 87:33–45

Deng HY et al (2017) Radiotherapy, lobectomy or sublobar resection? A meta-analysis of the choices for treating stage I non-small-cell lung cancer. Eur J Cardiothorac Surg 51:203–210

Din OS et al (2013) Accelerated hypo-fractionated radiotherapy for non small cell lung cancer: results from 4 UK centres. Radiother Oncol 109:8–12

Elkind MM, Whitmore GF, American Institute of Biological Sciences (1967) The radiobiology of cultured mammalian cells. Gordon and Breach, New York

Faria SL et al (2006) Absence of toxicity with hypofractionated 3-dimensional radiation therapy for inoperable, early stage non-small cell lung cancer. Radiat Oncol 1:42

Favaudon V et al (2014) Ultrahigh dose-rate FLASH irradiation increases the differential response between normal and tumor tissue in mice. Sci Transl Med 6:245ra293

Filatenkov A et al (2015) Ablative tumor radiation can change the tumor immune cell microenvironment to induce durable complete remissions. Clin Cancer Res 21:3727–3739

Foster CC et al (2019) Overall survival according to immunotherapy and radiation treatment for metastatic non-small-cell lung cancer: a National Cancer Database analysis. Radiat Oncol 14:18

Fowler JF (1991) Rapid repopulation in radiotherapy: a debate on mechanism. The phantom of tumor treatment—continually rapid proliferation unmasked. Radiother Oncol 22:156–158

Fu S, Jiang GL, Wang LJ (1994) [Hyperfractionated irradiation for non-small cell lung cancer (NSCLC)—a phase III clinical trial]. Zhonghua Zhong Za Zhi 16, 306–309

Fuks Z, Kolesnick R (2005) Engaging the vascular component of the tumor response. Cancer Cell 8:89–91

Garcia-Barros M et al (2003) Tumor response to radiotherapy regulated by endothelial cell apoptosis. Science 300:1155–1159

Gauden S, Ramsay J, Tripcony L (1995) The curative treatment by radiotherapy alone of stage I non-small cell carcinoma of the lung. Chest 108:1278–1282

Giuliani M et al (2018) SUNSET: stereotactic radiation for ultracentral non-small-cell lung cancer- a safety and efficacy trial. Clin Lung Cancer 19: e529–e532

Graves EE et al (2010) Hypoxia in models of lung cancer: implications for targeted therapeutics. Clin Cancer Res 16:4843–4852

Guckenberger M et al (2017) ESTRO ACROP consensus guideline on implementation and practice of stereotactic body radiotherapy for peripherally located early stage non-small cell lung cancer. Radiother Oncol 124:11–17

Haasbeek CJ, Lagerwaard FJ, Slotman BJ, Senan S (2011) Outcomes of stereotactic ablative radiotherapy for centrally located early-stage lung cancer. J Thorac Oncol 6:2036–2043

Hall EJ, Giaccia AJ (2012) Radiobiology for the radiologist. Wolters Kluwer Health/Lippincott Williams & Wilkins, Philadelphia

Herbst RS et al (2016) Pembrolizumab versus docetaxel for previously treated, PD-L1-positive, advanced non-small-cell lung cancer (KEYNOTE-010): a randomised controlled trial. Lancet 387:1540–1550

Ishihara D, Pop L, Takeshima T, Iyengar P, Hannan R (2017) Rationale and evidence to combine radiation therapy and immunotherapy for cancer treatment. Cancer Immunol Immunother 66:281–298

Iyengar P et al (2016) A phase III randomized study of image guided conventional (60 Gy/30 fx) versus accelerated, hypofractionated (60 Gy/15 fx) radiation for poor performance status stage II and III NSCLC patients-an interim analysis. Int J Radiat Oncol 96:E451–E451

Kelada OJ et al (2018) High single doses of radiation may induce elevated levels of hypoxia in early-stage non-small cell lung cancer tumors. Int J Radiat Oncol Biol Phys 102:174–183

Kirkpatrick JP, Meyer JJ, Marks LB (2008) The linear-quadratic model is inappropriate to model high dose per fraction effects in radiosurgery. Semin Radiat Oncol 18:240–243

Kreuzaler P, Watson CJ (2012) Killing a cancer: what are the alternatives? Nat Rev Cancer 12:411–424

Lan J et al (2018) Targeting myeloid-derived suppressor cells and programmed death ligand 1 confers therapeutic advantage of ablative hypofractionated radiation therapy compared with conventional fractionated radiation therapy. Int J Radiat Oncol Biol Phys 101:74–87

Le QT et al (2004) Phase I study of tirapazamine plus cisplatin/etoposide and concurrent thoracic radiotherapy in limited-stage small cell lung cancer (S0004): a Southwest Oncology Group study. Clin Cancer Res 10:5418–5424

Le QT et al (2006) An evaluation of tumor oxygenation and gene expression in patients with early stage non-small cell lung cancers. Clin Cancer Res 12:1507–1514

Le QT et al (2009) Phase II study of tirapazamine, cisplatin, and etoposide and concurrent thoracic radiotherapy for limited-stage small-cell lung cancer: SWOG 0222. J Clin Oncol 27:3014–3019

Lehrer EJ et al (2019) Treatment of brain metastases with stereotactic radiosurgery and immune checkpoint inhibitors: an international meta-analysis of individual patient data. Radiother Oncol 130:104–112

Lester JF, Macbeth FR, Brewster AE, Court JB, Iqbal N (2004) CT-planned accelerated hypofractionated radiotherapy in the radical treatment of non-small cell lung cancer. Lung Cancer 45:237–242

Lewanski CR, Gullick WJ (2001) Radiotherapy and cellular signalling. Lancet Oncol 2:366–370

Lin SH et al (2013) Opportunities and challenges in the era of molecularly targeted agents and radiation therapy. J Natl Cancer Inst 105:686–693

Lugade AA et al (2005) Local radiation therapy of B16 melanoma tumors increases the generation of tumor antigen-specific effector cells that traffic to the tumor. J Immunol 174:7516–7523

Maguire J et al (2014) SOCCAR: a randomised phase II trial comparing sequential versus concurrent chemotherapy and radical hypofractionated radiotherapy in patients with inoperable stage III Non-Small Cell Lung Cancer and good performance status. Eur J Cancer 50:2939–2949

Marconi R, Strolin S, Bossi G, Strigari L (2017) A meta-analysis of the abscopal effect in preclinical models: is the biologically effective dose a relevant physical trigger? PLoS One 12:e0171559

Mauguen A et al (2012) Hyperfractionated or accelerated radiotherapy in lung cancer: an individual patient data meta-analysis. J Clin Oncol 30:2788–2797

Montay-Gruel P et al (2017) Irradiation in a flash: unique sparing of memory in mice after whole brain irradiation with dose rates above 100Gy/s. Radiother Oncol 124:365–369

Montay-Gruel P et al (2018) X-rays can trigger the FLASH effect: ultra-high dose-rate synchrotron light source prevents normal brain injury after whole brain irradiation in mice. Radiother Oncol 129: 582–588

Nahum AE, Uzan J (2012) (Radio)biological optimization of external-beam radiotherapy. Comput Math Methods Med 2012:329214

Oh D, Ahn YC, Kim B, Pyo H (2013) Hypofractionated three-dimensional conformal radiation therapy alone for centrally located cT1-3N0 non-small-cell lung cancer. J Thorac Oncol 8:624–629

Osti MF et al (2013) Image guided hypofractionated 3-dimensional radiation therapy in patients with inoperable advanced stage non-small cell lung cancer. Int J Radiat Oncol Biol Phys 85:e157–e163

Overgaard J (2007) Hypoxic radiosensitization: adored and ignored. J Clin Oncol 25:4066–4074

Overgaard J, Horsman MR (1996) Modification of hypoxia-induced radioresistance in tumors by the use of oxygen and sensitizers. Semin Radiat Oncol 6:10–21

Owen D, Sio TT (2020) Stereotactic body radiotherapy (SBRT) for central and ultracentral node-negative lung tumors. J Thorac Dis 12:7024–7031

Park C, Papiez L, Zhang S, Story M, Timmerman RD (2008) Universal survival curve and single fraction equivalent dose: useful tools in understanding potency of ablative radiotherapy. Int J Radiat Oncol Biol Phys 70:847–852

Park HJ, Griffin RJ, Hui S, Levitt SH, Song CW (2012) Radiation-induced vascular damage in tumors: implications of vascular damage in ablative hypofractionated radiotherapy (SBRT and SRS). Radiat Res 177:311–327

Perez CA et al (1980) A prospective randomized study of various irradiation doses and fractionation schedules in the treatment of inoperable non-oat-cell carcinoma of the lung. Preliminary report by the Radiation Therapy Oncology Group. Cancer 45:2744–2753

Pinnamaneni R et al (2017) Sequence of stereotactic ablative radiotherapy and immune checkpoint blockade in the treatment of metastatic lung cancer. J Clin Oncol 35

Postow MA et al (2012) Immunologic correlates of the abscopal effect in a patient with melanoma. N Engl J Med 366:925–931

Powell S, Cooke J, Parsons C (1990) Radiation-induced brachial plexus injury: follow-up of two different fractionation schedules. Radiother Oncol 18:213–220

Qiu B, Aili A, Xue L, Jiang P, Wang J (2020) Advances in radiobiology of stereotactic ablative radiotherapy. Front Oncol 10:1165

Samstein R, Rimner A, Barker CA, Yamada Y (2017) Combined immune checkpoint blockade and radiation therapy: timing and dose fractionation associated with greatest survival duration among over 750 treated patients. Int J Radiat Oncol 99:S129–S130

Saunders M et al (1997) Continuous hyperfractionated accelerated radiotherapy (CHART) versus conventional radiotherapy in non-small-cell lung cancer: a randomised multicentre trial. CHART Steering Committee. Lancet 350:161–165

Saunders M et al (1999) Continuous, hyperfractionated, accelerated radiotherapy (CHART) versus conventional radiotherapy in non-small cell lung cancer: mature data from the randomised multicentre trial. CHART Steering committee. Radiother Oncol 52:137–148

Sause WT et al (1995) Radiation Therapy Oncology Group (RTOG) 88-08 and Eastern Cooperative Oncology Group (ECOG) 4588: preliminary results of a phase III trial in regionally advanced, unresectable non-small-cell lung cancer. J Natl Cancer Inst 87:198–205

Schaue D, Ratikan JA, Iwamoto KS, McBride WH (2012) Maximizing tumor immunity with fractionated radiation. Int J Radiat Oncol Biol Phys 83:1306–1310

Seydel HG et al (1985) Hyperfractionation in the radiation therapy of unresectable non-oat cell carcinoma of the lung: preliminary report of a RTOG Pilot Study. Int J Radiat Oncol Biol Phys 11:1841–1847

Singh AK et al (2019) One versus three fractions of stereotactic body radiation therapy for peripheral stage I to II non-small cell lung cancer: a randomized, multi-institution, phase 2 trial. Int J Radiat Oncol Biol Phys 105:752–759

Slotman BJ, Antonisse IE, Njo KH (1996) Limited field irradiation in early stage (T1–2N0) non-small cell lung cancer. Radiother Oncol 41:41–44

Soliman H et al (2011) Accelerated hypofractionated radiotherapy for early-stage non-small-cell lung cancer: long-term results. Int J Radiat Oncol Biol Phys 79:459–465

Song CW, Kim MS, Cho LC, Dusenbery K, Sperduto PW (2014) Radiobiological basis of SBRT and SRS. Int J Clin Oncol 19:570–578

Tekatli H, Senan S, Dahele M, Slotman BJ, Verbakel WF (2015) Stereotactic ablative radiotherapy (SABR) for central lung tumors: plan quality and long-term clinical outcomes. Radiother Oncol 117:64–70

Theelen W et al (2019) Effect of pembrolizumab after stereotactic body radiotherapy vs pembrolizumab alone on tumor response in patients with advanced non-small cell lung cancer: results of the PEMBRO-RT phase 2 randomized clinical trial. JAMA Oncol 5:1276–1282

Timmerman R et al (2006) Excessive toxicity when treating central tumors in a phase II study of stereotactic body radiation therapy for medically inoperable early-stage lung cancer. J Clin Oncol 24:4833–4839

Timmerman R et al (2010) Stereotactic body radiation therapy for inoperable early stage lung cancer. JAMA 303:1070–1076

Timmerman RD et al (2018) Stereotactic body radiation therapy for operable early-stage lung cancer: findings from the NRG Oncology RTOG 0618 Trial. JAMA Oncol 4:1263–1266

Urbanic JJ et al (2018) Phase 1 study of accelerated hypofractionated radiation therapy with concurrent chemotherapy for stage III non-small cell lung cancer: CALGB 31102 (Alliance). Int J Radiat Oncol Biol Phys 101:177–185

Van Putten LM, Kallman RF (1968) Oxygenation status of a transplantable tumor during fractionated radiation therapy. J Natl Cancer Inst 40:441–451

Vansteenkiste J et al (2014) 2nd ESMO Consensus Conference on Lung Cancer: early-stage non-small-cell lung cancer consensus on diagnosis, treatment and follow-up. Ann Oncol 25:1462–1474

Videtic GM et al (2015) A randomized phase 2 study comparing 2 stereotactic body radiation therapy schedules for medically inoperable patients with stage I peripheral non-small cell lung cancer: NRG Oncology RTOG 0915 (NCCTG N0927). Int J Radiat Oncol Biol Phys 93:757–764

Videtic GM et al (2019) Long-term follow-up on NRG Oncology RTOG 0915 (NCCTG N0927): a randomized phase 2 study comparing 2 stereotactic body radiation therapy schedules for medically inoperable patients with stage I peripheral non-small cell lung cancer. Int J Radiat Oncol Biol Phys 103:1077–1084

Vokes EE et al (2018) Nivolumab versus docetaxel in previously treated advanced non-small-cell lung cancer (CheckMate 017 and CheckMate 057): 3-year update and outcomes in patients with liver metastases. Ann Oncol 29:959–965

Walshaw RC, Honeychurch J, Illidge TM (2016) Stereotactic ablative radiotherapy and immunotherapy combinations: turning the future into systemic therapy? Br J Radiol 89:20160472

Wang HH et al (2018) Ablative hypofractionated radiation therapy enhances non-small cell lung cancer cell killing via preferential stimulation of necroptosis in vitro and in vivo. Int J Radiat Oncol Biol Phys 101:49–62

Westover KD et al (2015) Precision hypofractionated radiation therapy in poor performing patients with non-small cell lung cancer: phase 1 dose escalation trial. Int J Radiat Oncol Biol Phys 93:72–81

Williamson SK et al (2005) Phase III trial of paclitaxel plus carboplatin with or without tirapazamine in advanced non-small-cell lung cancer: Southwest Oncology Group Trial S0003. J Clin Oncol 23:9097–9104

Xing D, Siva S, Hanna GG (2019) The abscopal effect of stereotactic radiotherapy and immunotherapy: fool's gold or el dorado? Clin Oncol (R Coll Radiol) 31:432–443

Radiation Time, Dose, and Fractionation in the Treatment of Lung Cancer

David L. Billing and Andreas Rimner

Contents

1 **Non-Small Cell Lung Cancer** 172
1.1 Dose Escalation with Conventional Fractionation 172
1.2 Hyperfractionation and Acceleration 175
1.3 Moderate and Ultra-Hypofraction with Stereotactic Body Radiotherapy 176

2 **Small Cell Lung Cancer** 179
2.1 Concurrent Chemoradiation and Hyperfractionation 180
2.2 Hypofractionation and Stereotactic Body Radiotherapy 182

References 183

D. L. Billing · A. Rimner (✉)
Department of Radiation Oncology, Memorial Sloan Kettering Cancer Center, New York, NY, USA
e-mail: rimnera@mskcc.org

Abstract

Radiation therapy plays a vital role in the definitive management of early stage and locally advanced lung cancer. Local treatment failure is a primary cause of disease progression in lung cancer and improved local control has been associated with improved overall survival in both non-small cell (NSCLC) and small cell lung cancers (SCLC) (Arriagada et al. 1991; Machtay et al. 2012; Pignon et al. 1992). Delivery of radiation to the intrathoracic sites of disease is limited by the sensitivity of the surrounding non-neoplastic tissues, in particular the normal lung, esophagus, and heart. As such, substantial effort has been made to optimize radiation treatments to maximize tumor control while minimizing toxicity. Technological advancements have led to better imaging of tumors and organs at risk at the time of treatment planning and more precise delivery of therapeutic radiation. Other ways to improve the therapeutic ratio for lung radiotherapy include altering variables such as radiation dose, fractionation schedule, and time interval between treatments. This chapter will focus on the seminal trials that have established the standards for these factors in modern lung radiotherapy, specifically in the nonoperative management of early stage NSCLC (defined as stage I-IIB according to the American Joint Committee on Cancer staging system), locally advanced NSCLC (defined as stages IIIA-B according to the American Joint Committee on Cancer staging system), and limited stage SCLC (LS-SCLC, defined as disease limited to the ipsilateral hemithorax and regional lymph nodes).

1 Non-Small Cell Lung Cancer

Improved local control is associated with better overall survival in NSCLC (Machtay et al. 2012). The role of radiation in the definitive nonoperative management of both early stage and locally advanced NSCLC is well established. In an effort to improve local control, and by extension, survival, several trials have attempted to maximize the biologically effective dose to the tumor by altering dose and fractionation schedule to variable effect.

1.1 Dose Escalation with Conventional Fractionation

Conventionally fractionation radiation, defined as radiation treatments administered in 1.8–2.0 Gy fractions, typically given 5 days a week over the course of several weeks, is widely used in many cancers including NSCLC (see Table 1 for a summary of fractionation definitions used this chapter). Conventional fractionation has been used in the treatment of all stages of NSCLC, and at the time this chapter was written, remains a cornerstone for patients with unresectable or medically inoperable locally advanced disease (AJCC eighth edition stage IIB-III). Approximately 35% of NSCLC cases are diagnosed as locally advanced, with the majority of these being medically inoperable (Goldstraw et al. 2016).

The initial landmark study that established the benchmark for standard dose fractionation in NSCLC patients was conducted by the Radiation Therapy Oncology Group (RTOG) in the 1970s. In RTOG 7311, 365 patients with medically inoperable stage I/II or unresectable stage III NSCLC were treated with radiation alone in one of four fractionation schemes, three of which involved conventionally fractionated doses: 40 Gy in 20 fractions, 50 Gy in 25 fractions, and 60 Gy in 30 fractions. The fourth study arm involved administration of a higher dose per fraction (4.0 Gy per day given 5 days per week) given in a split course of two 20 Gy treatments administered each over 1 week, separated by a 2 week break for a total of 40 Gy in 10 fractions. Significantly, this study demonstrated superior local control at 3 years follow-up in the 60 Gy arm (65%), compared to the 50Gy (51%), 40 Gy (42%), and 40 Gy split course (47%) arms. The improvement in local control came at the expense of increased severe toxicity, occurring on the order of 5–10% (Perez et al. 1980). While initial results showed improved 3 years overall survival in the 50 Gy and 60 Gy arms, the survival benefit was no longer present on 5 years follow-up, primarily due to a high rate of distant metastases in all treatment arms, suggesting the need for more effective systemic therapy alongside radiation (Perez et al. 1987). Since this trial was published, chemotherapy and radiation have become the standard for medically inoperable or unresectable locally advanced NSCLC, and in particular concurrent chemotherapy and radiation have been shown to improve survival

Table 1 Fractionation definitions for lung cancer

Schedule	Dose per fraction (Gy)	No. fractions per week	Interval between fractions (h)	Total no. fractions	Duration of treatments (weeks)	Total dose (Gy)
Conventional	1.8–2.2	3–5	24	25–40	5–8	55–80
Hyper	1–1.5	10–21	4–12	↑	NC or ↓	NC or ↑
Moderate hypo	3–5	3–5	24–48	↓	↓	NC or ↓
Ultra hypo	>5	1–5	24–48	↓↓	↓↓	NC or ↓

↓ or ↑ indicate decreases or increases relative to values given for standard fractionation schedule; NC indicates no change

(Anne Aupérin et al. 2010; Curran et al. 2011). Nonetheless, RTOG 7301 established 60 Gy in 30 fractions as the standard dose for radiation treatment alone. This fractionation scheme has been used as the standard dose in subsequent lung cancer clinical trials of sequential and concurrent chemotherapy and radiation.

Given the poor long-term progression free and overall survival rates in RTOG 7301, it was hypothesized that dose escalation beyond 60Gy would provide further improvement in outcomes. Counterbalancing the desire to dose escalate radiotherapy were concerns over severe toxicity to healthy organs at risk (OARs), in particular the lung, esophagus, and heart. The advent of 3D conformal radiotherapy (3DCRT) involving CT based planning allowed for more accurate delivery of radiation as well as better understanding of the relationship of dose and organ volume treated to normal tissue toxicity. Dose-volume histograms allowed the development of volumetric dose parameters to more clearly define the risk of toxicity to OARs. An influential analysis of 99 NSCLC patients treated with definitive radiation showed the volume of lung receiving more than 20 Gy (V_{20}) was the single best predictor of radiation pneumonitis, with higher lung V_{20} resulting in a greater incidence severe toxicity (Graham et al. 1999). Lung V_{20} has since been established as a key dose constraint parameter and standard criterion for clinical trials of radiation treatments for thoracic malignancies. For a summary of the OAR dose constraints used in the major dose escalation trials discussed in this section see Table 2.

One such trial that tested the feasibility of dose escalation while utilizing lung V_{20} to constrain lung dose was RTOG 9311. This phase II trial, which included 177 patients with stage I-III inoperable NSCLC, stratified participants into two dose escalation groups, one in which V_{20} was <25% and a second where V_{20} was 25–36%. Group 1 underwent dose escalation with treatments that utilized 2.2 Gy fractions: 70.9 Gy, 77.4 Gy, 83.8 Gy, and 90.3 Gy. Similarly, the second V_{20} group was dose escalated to 70.9 and 77.4 Gy. The trial concluded that radiation doses could be safely escalated to 83.8 Gy if V_{20} was less than 25% and 77.4 Gy if V_{20} was between 25% and 36% (J. Bradley et al. 2005).

Other single institution phase I studies also addressed the feasibility of dose escalation in locally advanced or medically inoperable NSCLC. A trial of 104 patients at Memorial Sloan Kettering Cancer Center tested conventionally fractionated radiation doses from 70.2 Gy to 90 Gy. In this study, the maximum tolerated dose was determined to be 84 Gy, as patients assigned to the 90 Gy dose level experienced unacceptable pulmonary toxicity. Additionally, it was observed that patients who received 80 Gy or more had improved overall survival compared to those who received less than 80 Gy (Rosenzweig et al. 2005). Similarly, a phase I trial from the University of Michigan stratified patients by volume of normal lung irradiated followed by dose escalation with conventionally fractionated radiation. In this study, doses of up to 102.9 Gy were safely achieved in

Table 2 Constraints used in NSCLC dose escalation and hyperfractionation trials

Study	Expansions (cm)	Lung	Heart	Esophagus	Spinal cord
RTOG 7301	n/a	None	None	None	$D_{max} < 45$ Gy
RTOG 9311	PTV = GTV + 1.0	$V_{20} < 36\%$	None	None	None
CHARTWEL	PTV = GTV + 1–1.5	$V_{20} < 50\%$ $V_{30} < 35\%$	None	None	$D_{max} < 48$ Gy
RTOG 0617	CTV = ITV + 0.5–1.0 PTV = CTV 0.5–1.5	$V20 < 37\%$ $D_{mean} < 20$ Gy	$V_{60} < 33\%$ $V_{45} < 66\%$ $V_{40} < 100\%$	$D_{mean} < 34$ Gy	$D_{max} < 50.5$ Gy
RTOG 1106	CTV = ITV + ≥0.5 PTV = CTV + ≥0.5	$D_{mean} < 20$ Gy	Dmean <40 Gy V40 < 80% V60 < 30%	$D_{max} < 72$ $D_{mean} < 34$	$D_{max} < 50$ Gy

GTV gross tumor volume, *CTV* clinical target volume, *PTV* planning target volume, *ITV* internal target volume, D_{max} maximum dose, D_{mean} mean dose, V_x volume of tissue receiving X Gy patients with low volumes of irradiated normal lung (Hayman et al. 2001).

While concurrent chemotherapy was an exclusionary factor in RTOG 9311 and relatively few patients received concurrent chemotherapy in the MSKCC and University of Michigan dose escalation trials, RTOG 0117 was a Phase I/II trial of radiation dose escalation in conjunction with weekly carboplatin and paclitaxel. This study found that the maximum tolerated radiation dose with concurrent carboplatin/paclitaxel was 74 Gy in 37 fractions (Bradley et al. 2010), a treatment regimen that would be used as the experimental arm in the subsequent RTOG 0617 trial.

RTOG 0617 was a landmark trial that built on the promising data from RTOG 0117 and multiple institutional studies demonstrating promising local control and survival benefits with dose escalation using standard fractionation. This multicenter phase III trial accrued 544 patients with unresectable stage III NSCLC and utilized a two by two factorial design to randomize patients to standard dose radiation (60 Gy in 30 fractions) or high dose radiation (74 Gy in 37 fractions) with or without cetuximab. All patients were treated with concurrent carboplatin and paclitaxel. Somewhat surprisingly, the trial closed early due to the high dose radiation arm crossing the futility boundary. With a median follow-up of 22.9 months, the high dose radiation arm had decreased 2 year survival (45% vs 58%, $p = 0.03$) and a trend towards higher rates of local failure (38.6% vs 30.7%, $p = 0.13$) (Bradley et al. 2015). The significant difference in overall survival was maintained at 5 years favoring the standard dose arm (23% vs 32.1%, $p = 0.05$). There was also a trend towards worse local control in the escalated dose arm at 5 years (incidence 38.2% vs 45.7%, $p = 0.07$) (Bradley et al. 2020). There was no significant difference in the rates of grade 3+ pulmonary toxicity; however, there were significantly higher rates of grade 3+ esophagitis in the high dose arm (21% vs 7%). On multivariate analysis, increased risk of death was associated with higher radiation dose, higher PTV volume, esophagitis grade, and higher radiation doses to the heart (as represented by heart volume receiving greater than 5 Gy and greater than 30 Gy). This suggests that increased toxicity, particularly heart related toxicity, may be partly responsible for the inferior outcomes associated with higher dose radiation. Based on this trial, the standard fractionation regimen of 60 Gy in 30 fractions remains the standard of care for locally advanced NSCLC treated with chemotherapy in the USA.

RTOG 0617 highlights the continued challenge of balancing increasing radiation dose to the neoplastic tissue with toxicity. Many open questions still remain in regards to the optimal dose of conventionally fractionated radiation in locally advanced NSCLC. A large retrospective study using the National Cancer Database suggested a survival benefit at 66–70 Gy, but a plateau in benefit above 70 Gy (Brower et al. 2016), therefore it is possible that the optimal dose of conventionally fractionated radiation exists somewhere between 60 and 70 Gy. Additionally, many patients with locally advanced NSCLC patients are not candidates for chemotherapy based on comorbidities or performance status, and the optimal dose for radiation monotherapy in this subset of patients is also unclear. A retrospective analysis from Memorial Sloan Kettering Cancer Center of patients who received radiation monotherapy or sequential chemoradiation showed an overall survival and local control benefit with radiation doses above 66 Gy (Sonnick et al. 2018).

Boosts to the remaining sites of gross disease at the end of a treatment course, also known as adaptive radiotherapy, either with higher doses of conventionally fractionated or hypofractionated radiation is an emerging area of interest that has showed promise in multiple phase I/II trials, but await confirmation in larger multicenter randomized trials (Feddock et al. 2013; Higgins et al. 2017). RTOG 1106 is one such trial of adaptive radiotherapy that is currently awaiting data maturation at the time this chapter was written. Outside of standard fractionated radiotherapy, efforts to maximize tumor response and minimize normal tissue toxicity have continued through alterations in the dose per fraction and number of fractions, i.e., hyper- or hypofractionation.

1.2 Hyperfractionation and Acceleration

Hyperfractionated radiation is a smaller dose delivered per fraction (typically 1.2 to 1.6 Gy) over an increased number of total fractions in comparison to conventionally fractionated radiation. Accelerated radiation, or the delivery of radiation treatments over a shorter time course compared with conventionally fractionated radiation is often combined with hyperfractionated radiotherapy. Accelerated hyperfractionation may be more effective in treating rapidly dividing cancer cells by limiting the time for tumor repair and repopulation with surviving clonogens between fractions. At the same time, hyperfractionation may reduce the late toxicity experienced by normal tissues. On the other hand, accelerated hyperfractionation has the potential to worsen acute toxicity. Additionally, hyperfractionated radiation regimens can be inconvenient for the patient and place a greater demand on healthcare facilities and resources.

Early dose escalation studies with hyperfractionation, such as RTOG 8311, experimented with doses ranging from 60Gy to 79.2Gy, delivered as twice daily 1.2 Gy fractions separated by 4–6 h, 5 days a week. The 69.6 Gy arm of the study was found to have a survival benefit compared to lower dose arms with acceptable toxicity, No further survival benefit was observed with doses beyond 69.6 Gy. Additionally, comparison with historical controls of conventionally fractionated 60 Gy radiation suggested a survival benefit with the 69.6 Gy hyperfractionated regimen (Cox et al. 1990). However, the phase III RTOG 8808/ECOG 4588 trial, which included a conventionally fractionated 60 Gy arm and a hyperfractionated 69.6 Gy arm, failed to show any survival benefit with a hyperfractionated radiation course (Sause et al. 2000). Similarly, RTOG 9410 included a conventionally fractionated 60 Gy arm and a hyperfractionated 69.6 Gy arm, each treated with concurrent chemotherapy. With the caveat that the chemotherapy regimens in each arm were different, the conventionally fractionated arm had superior overall survival, but there was a trend towards improved local control in the hyperfractionated arm. Furthermore, there was significantly more grade 3 esophagitis with hyperfractionation, occurring in 45% of patients compared to 22% of patients receiving conventionally fractionated radiation (Curran et al. 2011).

While the trials discussed above deployed hyperfractionated regimens, they occurred over the same absolute time length as conventionally fractionated radiation, and as such were not accelerated. The largest study of accelerated hyperfractionated radiation took place in Europe in the late 1990s. This phase III trial randomized 563 patients with inoperable NSCLC to conventionally fractionated radiation in 60 Gy over 6 weeks or continuous hyperfractionated accelerated radiotherapy (CHART) in 54 Gy administered as 1.5 Gy fractions, three times a day, over 12 consecutive days. The CHART arm showed significantly improved overall survival at 2 and 3 years compared to the conventionally fractionated arm (2 years OS: 30% vs 21%, 3 years OS 20% vs 13%). There was a 21% reduction in the relative risk of local progression in the CHART arm. These benefits were more pronounced in squamous cell histology, which made up 81% of patients enrolled. However, there was a significant increase in severe dysphagia in the CHART arm, defined as patients who were reduced to fluid only intake as a result of symptoms (19% vs 3%) and a trend towards increased pneumonitis requiring treatment or hospitalization (Saunders et al. 1997, 1999).

Given that many radiation centers are closed on the weekends, a consecutive 12 day treatment course is often not feasible. Therefore, the CHARTWEL trial was a randomized phase III trial of CHART delivered as 60 Gy in 40 fractions three times a day, 5 days a week for 2.5 weeks (weekends off) compared with 66 Gy in 33 fractions delivered over 6.5 weeks. In contrast to the initial CHART trial, there was no significant difference in survival between the two arms at 2, 3, and 5 years. However, there were increased rates of dysphagia and radiographic pneumonitis in the hyperfractionated arm (Baumann et al. 2011).

While a meta-analysis of hyperfractionated radiation trials in NSCLC has suggested an overall survival benefit compared to standard fractionation (Mauguen et al. 2012), hyperfractionated radiation has fallen out of favor in the USA in recent years given the conflicting results and logistical difficulties compared to conventionally fractionated or hypofractionated treatment regimens. At the time this chapter was written, there are no major clinical trials of hyperfractionation in NSCLC underway.

1.3 Moderate and Ultra-Hypofraction with Stereotactic Body Radiotherapy

Hypofractionation is the delivery of larger radiation doses per fraction over fewer total radiation treatments (see Table 1). From a radiobiology standpoint, hypofractionation may allow for delivery of higher biologically effective doses (BED) to the tumor allowing for a higher chance of local control. Conversely, hypofractionation may result in increased late toxicity to normal tissues and allow for repopulation of tumor between fractions with radioresistance clonogens resulting in decreased local control (Cox 1985). From a patient standpoint, hypofractionation is more convenient as it reduces the total number of visits necessary to complete a given treatment, reduces the financial burden associated with long courses of radiation, and lessens demand on healthcare resources.

Advances in image guided technology, particularly the cone beam CT, combined with improved motion management (i.e., 4D CT scans and deep inspiratory breath hold), and radiation delivery techniques such as intensity modulated radiotherapy (IMRT) have allowed for more accurate delivery of radiation permitting smaller treatment margins and minimization of dose to the surrounding tissues. Thus, they have allowed delivery of higher doses per fraction without unacceptable increase in toxicities. Ultrahypofractionated radiation, also referred to as stereotactic body radiotherapy (SBRT), stereotactic ablative radiotherapy (SABR), and stereotactic radiosurgery (SRS), is a form of image guided radiation that utilizes high doses of radiation per fraction (>5Gy per fraction), frequently delivered over one to five fractions. Given that radiation toxicity increases with volume of tissue treated (Videtic et al. 2017), SBRT has achieved its best results in early stage lung cancer, in particular as definitive management of cT1 and T2 tumors where it is now standard of care for patients who are medically inoperable.

Early stage NSCLC, defined as stage I or II by the AJCC staging system, comprises approximately 30% of all lung cancer diagnoses (Groome et al. 2007). While surgery remains the primary treatment modality for early stage NSCLC, many patients are not surgical candidates due to age, medical comorbidities, preference, or tumor location. Population based studies demonstrate abysmal lung cancer specific survival without treatment even in the presence of significant medical comorbidities, highlighting the necessity of definitive clinical management for patients with early stage disease (Raz et al. 2007).

The feasibility and safety of the SBRT technique were established in the 1990s. In a phase I study that included patients with solitary lung tumors, excellent local control with minimal toxicity was demonstrated for doses ranging from 8 to 66 Gy given in 1 to 4 fractions (Blomgren et al. 1995). Similarly, a phase I study of 45 patients with primary or metastatic lung tumors tested doses of 30 to 75 Gy administered in 5 to 15 fractions. Of the 66 total lesions that received SBRT, only two experienced local progression with a median follow-up of 11 months (Uematsu et al. 1998). Furthermore, a retrospective analysis of Japanese trials of hypofractionated radiation regimens for early stage NSCLC suggested improved local control with BED >100 Gy assuming an alpha/beta ratio of 10 (Onishi et al. 2007), for comparison, the BED for standard the fractionation of 60 Gy in 30 fractions is 72 Gy.

Building on the above studies, the University of Indiana conducted a phase I dose escalation trial of SBRT in which 37 patients with medically inoperable stage I (cT1-T2) NSCLC were assigned to receive progressively higher doses of radiation in three fraction regimens beginning with 24 Gy in 3 fractions and increasing up to 60 Gy in three fractions (Timmerman et al. 2003). No local failures were observed in the patients receiving at least 18 Gy per fraction and the maximum tolerated dose was not reached. Similarly, a multi-institutional phase II study of SBRT for inoperable early stage NSCLC administered as 45 Gy in 3 fractions demonstrated a 3 year local control rate of >90% with minimal toxicity (Baumann et al. 2009). For a summary of the OAR dose constraints used in the major trials discussed in this section see Table 3.

However, a subsequent Phase II study of SBRT from the University of Indiana that assigned patients with T1 disease to 60 Gy in 3 fractions and those with T2 disease to 66 Gy in 3 fractions showed a significant increase in toxicity for centrally located tumors, defined as the gross tumor volume (GTV) falling within 2 cm of the proximal bronchial tree. Four of six treatment-related deaths were observed in the centrally located tumor subset, and about half of the patients experienced severe toxicity compared to 17% in patients with non-centrally located tumors (Timmerman et al. 2006). Several studies have confirmed the increase in toxicity with centrally located tumors, and at present, there are several fractionation schemes that have been shown to be safe and feasible including 60 Gy in 5 fractions (Bezjak et al. 2019), 60 Gy in 8 fractions (Haasbeek et al. 2011), 70 Gy in 10 fractions (Chang et al. 2014), and 60 Gy in 15 fractions. Early phase prospective studies to investigate optimal dosing of central tumors, such as SUNSET (NCT03306680), are underway at the time this chapter was written to help answer this open question in the field. For a more detailed discussion of SBRT in centrally located tumors, please see chap. 25.

Based on the encouraging results from the initial phase I dose escalation study, the RTOG 0236 study was the first multicenter Phase II trial of SBRT in North America. The trial enrolled 55 patients with medically inoperative cT1-T2 peripherally located tumors who then received a radiation dose of 54 Gy in 3 fractions, with treatments occurring at least 40 hours apart. The 3 years primary tumor control rate was 97.6% with only a single patient experiencing treatment failure. Treatment-related grade 3+ toxicity was observed in 16.1% of patients (Timmerman et al. 2010). Five years follow-up demonstrated durable primary tumor control at a rate of 92.7%. However, 5 year disease free survival was only 26%, owing to high rates of locoregional (31%) and distant (31%) recurrences. Five years rate of grade 3+ toxicity, primarily pulmonary or musculoskeletal was 30.9% with no grade 5 events (Timmerman et al. 2018a).

Other SBRT dose fractionation regimens including single dose treatments have been the subject of phase II prospective trials. The RTOG 0915 trial was a phase II study between 2009 and 2011 that randomized medically inoperable patients with peripheral cT1 or T2 N0M0 NSCLC to either radiation treatment with 34 Gy in 1

Table 3 Constraints used in NSCLC SBRT trials

Study	Lung	Trachea and bronchus	Heart	Esophagus	Spinal cord
RTOG 0236	$V_{20} < 10\%$	$D_{max} < 30$ Gy	$D_{max} < 30$ Gy	$D_{max} < 27$ Gy	$D_{max} < 18$ Gy
RTOG 0915[a]	$V_7 < 1{,}500$ cc $V_{7.5} < 1{,}000$ cc	$D_{max} < 20.2$ Gy	$D_{max} < 22$ Gy	$D_{max} < 15.4$ Gy	$D_{max} < 14$ Gy
SPACE[b]	None	None	None	None	$D_{max} < 21$ Gy
CHISEL[b]	$V_{20} < 15\%$	None	$D_{max} < 30$ Gy	$D_{max} < 27$ Gy	$D_{max} < 18$ Gy
RTOG 0813[c]	$V_{12.5} < 1{,}500$ cc $V_{13.5} < 1{,}000$ cc	$D_{max} < 18$ Gy	$D_{max} < 32$ Gy	$D_{max} < 27.5$	$D_{max} < 22.5$ Gy
SUNSET[d]	$D_{mean} < 12$ Gy	$D_{max} < 64$ Gy	$D_{max} < 64$ Gy	$D_{max} < 45$ Gy	$D_{max} < 32$ Gy

D_{max} maximum dose, D_{mean} mean dose, V_x volume of tissue receiving X Gy
[a]Dose constraints used for the single fraction arm
[b]Dose constraints used for the SBRT arm
[c]Trial of centrally located tumors
[d]Trial of ultra-centrally located tumors

fraction (BED = 150 Gy) or 48 Gy in 4 daily fractions (BED = 105 Gy). Consistent with previous SBRT trials, 5 years primary local control rates were high in both the 34 Gy (89.4%) and 48 Gy (93.2%) arms, whereas progression free survival was relatively low (19.1% vs 33.3%, not significant). There was no statistically significant difference in toxicity, with 2.6% of patients in the single fraction arm compared with 11.1% of patients in the 4 fraction arm experiencing grade 3+ toxicity (Videtic et al. 2019). Similarly, a single institution phase II study comparing 30Gy in 1 fraction with 60 Gy in 3 fractions showed no difference in progression free survival and grade 3+ toxicity (Singh et al. 2017). Hence, single fraction SBRT appears to be a safe and effective alternative fractionation for the treatment of patients with peripherally located stage I NSCLC.

Given the excellent local control rates and favorable toxicity profiles observed in phase II studies, SBRT has been rapidly adopted as standard of care for medically inoperable patients with stage I lung cancer. Historically, however, early stage lung cancer was treated with conventional fractionation. Retrospective studies suggested improvements in both local control and survival with SBRT compared to standard fractionation for early stage lung cancer (von Reibnitz et al. 2018). Recently, two randomized studies have compared standard fractionation with SBRT in a prospective fashion and have shown at least equal local control and toxicity. The Stereotactic Precision and Conventional radiotherapy Evaluation (SPACE) trial randomized medically inoperable peripheral T1-T2 NSCLC patients to SBRT with 66 Gy in 3 fractions delivered over 1 week or 3D conventional fractionated radiotherapy (3DCRT) with 70 Gy in 35 fractions over 7 weeks. Despite having a significantly higher number of patients with T2 tumors in the SBRT cohort, there was no significant difference in 3 years local control, progression free survival, and overall survival. There was a significant reduction in rates of esophagitis in the SBRT arm (8% vs 30% in 3DCRT, $p = 0.006$) and a trend towards reduced rates of pneumonitis (19% vs 34% in 3DCRT, $p = 0.26$). Furthermore, patients treated with 3DCRT reported significantly worse dyspnea, chest pain, and cough (Nyman et al. 2016). However, this trial has several limitations, including suboptimal staging and workup, as PET scan was optional and only 64% of enrolled patients had pathologic confirmation of lung cancer. As alluded to above, there was an imbalance in the baseline characteristics between groups, with a significantly higher number of T2 tumors and male patients in the SBRT group (T2, 47% vs 25% 3DCRT) and (male 45% vs 36% 3DCRT). Finally, there was a difference in the prescription dose constraints between arms possibly resulting in undercoverage of the target in the SBRT arm. Specifically, the protocol specified that the SBRT arm has 100% dose prescribed to the isocenter with the periphery of the planned target volume (PTV) required to receive more than 68% of the dose compared to the conventional fractionation arm which required the 95% isodose line to cover 95% of the PTV.

Another randomized trial of conventionally fractionated radiation vs. standard fractionation was the TROG 09.02 CHISEL study which was conducted in patients with medically inoperable peripheral cT1-T2 NSCLC. This three arm trial randomized patients to two SBRT treatment schedules delivered over the course of 2 weeks: 54 Gy in 3 fractions or 48Gy in 4 fractions if the tumor was less than 2 cm from the chest wall, or standard fractionation radiotherapy in 66 Gy in 33 fractions over 6.5 weeks. At median follow-up of 2 years, there were significantly fewer local progression events in the SBRT arm compared to the standard fractionation arm (hazard ratio 0.32, $p = 0.0077$). There was no significant difference between the SBRT arms and the standard fractionation arm in terms of grade 3+ toxicity (Ball et al. 2019). These prospective data are also supported by a retrospective study using the National Cancer Database to compare patients who received SBRT with those that received conventionally fractionated radiation. This analysis showed a significant overall survival benefit in patients that received SBRT (Haque et al. 2018). Taken together these trials support the use of SBRT as the standard therapy for patients with early stage NSCLC, as SBRT offers at least equivalent local control outcomes with less toxicity and the added benefit of increased patient convenience.

Given the larger treatment volumes required for radiotherapy of locally advanced NSCLC, ultrahypofractionated or SBRT regimens are generally not used due to safety concerns. However, moderately hypofractionated treatment regimens (i.e., 2.25–4 Gy per fraction, over 15–25 fractions see Table 1) are becoming increasingly being explored, made possible by highly conformal radiation techniques such as IMRT or proton therapy. Like ultrahypofractionated radiation, moderately hypofractionated radiation regimens are more convenient for the patient, reduce demand on healthcare facilities, and lower cost. A phase II study of moderately hypofractionated radiation, 60 Gy in 15 fractions that included patients with peripheral T1-T3N0M0 NSCLC showed a 2 years local control rate of 87.4% with relatively low rates of grade 3+ toxicity, demonstrating that this technique was feasible in patients with larger tumor size (Cheung et al. 2014). CALGB 31102 was a phase I study that investigated the toxicity of different moderately hypofractionated radiation regimens in locally advanced (stage III) NSCLC in combination with concurrent chemotherapy. In this study, patients were assigned to four separate 60Gy regimens: in 27, 24, 22, and 20 fractions. The maximum tolerated dose was found to be the 60 Gy in 24 fraction regimen, with further attempts at reduction of fraction number beyond 24 treatments resulting in unacceptable toxicity (Urbanic et al. 2018). A large retrospective study also suggests a hypofractionated approach may be feasible for patients who are not candidates for chemotherapy (Iocolano et al. 2020).

Other areas of active interest in NSCLC include combination of radiation with immunotherapy or targeted systemic therapies given the success of the PACIFIC trial, as it is currently poorly understood how these may impact radiation dose and fractionation. The PACIFIC trial was a phase III study of consolidative durvalumab after concurrent radiation and platinum based chemotherapy. This study demonstrated a significant increase in median progression free survival in the patients who received durvalumab (16.8 months vs 5.6 months placebo, $p < 0.001$) as well as an increase in median time to death or distant metastasis (23.2 months vs 14.6 months placebo, $p < 0.001$) (Antonia et al. 2017). At the time this chapter was written, further prospective trials examining both hypofractionated radiation and concurrent immunotherapy in locally advanced lung cancer are currently underway. This includes NRG-LU004 (NCT03801902) which is comparing concurrent durvalumab with radiation given as 60 Gy in 30 fractions or 60 Gy in 15 fractions, and PCG-LUN005, which is investigating the use of protons in hypofractionated radiation.

2 Small Cell Lung Cancer

Small cell lung cancer (SCLC) represents approximately 15% of lung cancer diagnoses but accounts for about 25% of lung cancer deaths. The number of SCLC cases has declined in many countries since the 1980s, largely due to a decrease in smoking rates. SCLC is associated with rapid cell doubling time and early distant spread. As such, the majority of SCLC cases are metastatic or advanced on diagnosis. Only about one-third of patients present as limited stage (LS-SCLC), defined by the Veteran Affairs Lung Group (VALG) as disease that is confined to one hemithorax (including hilar, mediastinal lymph nodes, and ipsilateral supraclavicular lymph nodes) that can be encompassed in a reasonable radiation portal. While the VALG staging system is still widely used due to its simplicity and usage in many clinical trials, TNM staging as defined by the International Association for the Study of Lung Cancer (IASLC) is now the preferred staging system for SCLC (Goldstraw et al. 2016). LS-SCLC corresponds to stage I-III by the TNM staging grouping system. The TNM system has been validated in large database studies for both clinically and surgically staged patients (Vallières et al. 2009; Shepherd et al. 2007), and has been shown to provide superior prognostic value (Micke et al. 2002; Wu et al. 2017). As observed in NSCLC, improved local control is associated with increased overall survival (Warde and Payne 1992). Until recently the majority of progress in clinical outcomes of patients with SCLC has been due to the addition of RT in different clinical scenarios, optimizing the timing of radiation with respect to chemotherapy, altered fractionation, and dose.

2.1 Concurrent Chemoradiation and Hyperfractionation

Given the rapid doubling time and early dissemination observed with SCLC, chemotherapy and radiation are the standard of care in the treatment of limited stage disease with curative intent. Additionally, patients with a favorable response to chemotherapy are typically offered prophylactic cranial irradiation (PCI) (Aupérin et al. 1999). Early clinical trials that compared surgery with radiation as initial treatment of LS-SCLC showed a survival benefit with radiation although long-term rates of overall survival were low in both arms (Fox and Scadding 1973). Additionally, high rates of local progression observed with chemotherapy alone underscored the need for a bimodality approach in the treatment of SCLC. A number of clinical trials then investigated the addition of thoracic radiation to various chemotherapy regimens before, during, or after chemotherapy. In 1992, two influential meta-analyses of such trials demonstrated benefits with this combined approach. In a meta-analysis of 11 randomized trials of 2,140 patients with LS-SCLC treated with chemotherapy with or without thoracic radiation, Pignon et al. found an absolute mortality benefit of 5.4% at 3 years with the addition of radiation (Pignon et al. 1992). Similarly, Warde and Payne found a 5% survival benefit and a local control benefit of 20% at 2 years in a meta-analysis of 11 randomized trials including 1911 patients with LS-SCLC (Warde and Payne 1992).

Furthermore, prospective trials have demonstrated benefits with concurrent chemoradiation, including the Japanese Clinical Oncology Group (JCOG) 9104 study. This was a phase III trial that compared sequential to concurrent radiotherapy. Both trial arms received 4 cycles of cisplatin and etoposide chemotherapy along with radiation to the pre-chemotherapy disease with 45 Gy in 30 fractions administered twice per day over the course of 3 weeks. Patients with a complete or near complete response were given PCI. The concurrent chemoradiation arm started radiation on day two of the first chemotherapy cycle, whereas the sequential arm began radiation after the fourth and final cycle. There was a trend towards improvement in median survival with concurrent chemoradiation (27.2 months vs 19.7 months with sequential), however this benefit was not statistically significant ($p = 0.097$). After adjustment for differences in prognostic factors between the two arms, the hazard ratio for death was observed to significantly decreased in the concurrent arm (HR 0.70, $p = 0.02$). Hematologic toxicity was significantly increased in the concurrent arm with 88% of patients experiencing grade 3+ leukopenia compared to 54% in the sequential arm. There was no significant difference in the rates of nonhematologic toxicity between groups (Takada et al. 2002). When combined with the data from the Intergroup 0096 trial (to be discussed below) which utilized concurrent chemotherapy and demonstrated favorable survival outcomes compared to historical controls (Turrisi et al. 1999), concurrent chemoradiation represents the standard of care in LS-SCLC patients with good performance status.

In vitro studies show that SCLC cell lines are highly sensitive to radiation (Carney et al. 1983). Therefore, it was theorized that smaller doses of radiation per fraction, i.e., hyperfractionation, would produce adequate tumor control while minimizing toxicity to normal tissues. Furthermore, given the rapid growth rate of SCLC, it was also hypothesized that accelerated fractionation in two daily treatments would prevent tumor repopulation between fractions. The landmark Intergroup 0096 trial compared conventionally fractionated radiation with accelerated hyperfractionated radiation in 417 patients with LS-SCLC receiving 4 cycles of concurrent cisplatin and etoposide. Patients with a complete response to chemoradiation were offered PCI. The conventionally fractionated arm was given 45 Gy in 25 daily fractions over the course of 5 weeks. The accelerated hyperfractionation arm was given 45 Gy in 30 twice daily fractions over the course of 3 weeks. Both arms initiated thoracic radiation during the first chemotherapy cycle. With 8 years of follow-up, there was a statistically significant increase in median survival with the accelerated hyperfractionated radiation (23 months vs 19 months with conventional fractionation, $p = 0.04$). There was no statistically significant difference in survival rates at 2 years (47% accelerated hyperfractionation vs 41% conventional fractionation), however longer follow-up revealed a survival benefit with the hyperfractionated regimen at 5 years (26% vs 16%, $p = 0.04$). There was a trend towards a lower cumulative rate of local failure with in the accelerated hyperfractionation arm but this was not statistically significant (36% vs 62%, $p = 0.06$). There was a higher rate of acute grade 3 esophagitis in the hyperfractionated arm (27% vs 11%) (Turrisi et al. 1999). For a summary of the OAR dose constraints used in the trials discussed in this section see Table 4. Based on the results of this trial, the 45 Gy in 30 twice daily fractions became the standard radiation dose for LS-SCLC.

One of the main criticisms of the Intergroup 0096 trial is that the conventionally fractionated arm delivered a lower biologically equivalent dose than the hyperfractionated arm. Since its publication, prospective trials using higher doses of conventionally fractionated regimens have been shown to be safe and feasible. The Cancer and Leukemia Group B (CALGB) 39808 study was a single arm phase II study that aimed to evaluate the safety and efficacy of a conventionally fractionated radiation regimen of 70 Gy in 35 fractions with concurrent cisplatin and etoposide for LS-SCLC. This trial demonstrated similar rates of toxicity, progression free survival, and overall survival to the accelerated hyperfractionated arm of the Intergroup 0096 (Bogart et al. 2004), suggesting that dose escalated conventionally fractionated radiation may be a viable alternative to twice daily hyperfractionated radiation.

To test this hypothesis, the CONVERT trial was a phase III randomized trial of accelerated hyperfractionated thoracic radiation (45 Gy in 30 twice daily fractions given over 3 weeks) compared to conventionally fractionated radiation (66 Gy in 33 daily fractions given over 6.5 weeks) in 574 LS-SCLC patients undergoing concurrent chemotherapy with cisplatin and etoposide. With a median of 4 years follow-up, there was no statistically significant difference between arms in median survival (30 months hyperfractionated vs 25 months conventionally fractionated, $p = 0.14$) or 2 years overall survival (56% hyperfractionated vs 51% conventionally fractionated). There was no difference in rates of grade 3+ pneumonitis or esophagitis between the arms, however, there was a statistically significant increase in the rate of grade 4 neutropenia in the hyperfractionation arm (49% vs 38% conventional fractionation, $p = 0.05$). Given that the trial was designed as a superiority trial to detect a 12% survival benefit in the conventionally fractionated arm rather

Table 4 Constraints used in SCLC trials

Study	Expansions (cm)	Lung	Heart	Esophagus	Spinal cord
Intergroup 0096	PTV = CTV + 1–1.5	None	None	None	None
JCOG 9104	PTV = GTV + 1.5	None	None	None	$D_{max} < 30$ Gy
Sun et al. (2013)	PTV = CTV + 1–1.5	$V_{20} < 35\%$ $D_{mean} < 20$ Gy	None	None	$D_{max} < 50$ Gy
CONVERT	CTV = GTV + 0.5 PTV = CTV + 1 CM	$V_{20} < 35\%$	$V45 < 30\%$	None	$D_{max} < 42$ Gy
CALGB 30610	PTV = CTV + 0.5–1	$V_{20} < 40\%$ $D_{mean} < 20$ Gy	$V_{60} < 33\%$ $V_{45} < 66\%$ $V_{40} < 100\%$	$D_{mean} < 34$ Gy	$D_{max} < 41$ Gy

GTV gross tumor volume, *CTV* clinical target volume, *PTV* planning target volume, *ITV* internal target volume, D_{max} maximum dose, D_{mean} mean dose, V_x volume of tissue receiving X Gy than a noninferiority trial to determine equivalence, the study authors concluded that twice daily accelerated hyperfractionation should remain the standard of care for LS-SCLC (Faivre-Finn et al. 2017). The CALGB 30610 study is a phase III study that has completed accrual at the time this chapter was written comparing 45Gy in 30 twice daily fractions with 70 Gy in 30 fractions based on the earlier phase II CALGB 39808 discussed above. This trial may help to clarify the optimal fractionation scheme in LS-SCLC, however at present, 45 Gy in 30 twice daily fractions remains standard of care for those patients with adequate functional status.

2.2 Hypofractionation and Stereotactic Body Radiotherapy

Hypofractionated regimens may be more convenient for the patients than twice daily hyperfractionated treatments and retrospective studies have suggested comparable outcomes (Zayed et al. 2020), however, few recent trials have explored hypofractionation in SCLC given its intrinsic high radiosensitivity and thus a lesser need for higher doses per fraction. On the other hand, hypofractionated regimens may allow for increased tumor repopulation given the high growth rates of SCLC. A phase II trial of 157 patients with LS-SCLC randomized patients to 45 Gy in 30 twice daily fractions or a hypofractionated regimen of 42 Gy in 15 daily fractions. There was no difference in median survival, progression free survival, overall survival at 1 year, or rates of grade 3+ toxicity. However, a significantly higher rate of patients in the twice daily arm achieved a complete response than the hypofractionated arm (33% vs 13%, $p = 0.003$) (Grønberg et al. 2016). At the time this chapter was written, there are no major trials investigating hypofractionated radiation regimens in LS-SCLC.

While most cases of SCLC are locally advanced at presentation, a small subset of patients present without evidence of nodal involvement. Advances in imaging technology have improved the capability to detect patients that are truly node negative. A retrospective analysis of 283 patients with LS-SCLC from Memorial Sloan Kettering Cancer Center showed superior survival, lower rates of distant and brain metastases in patients with node negative stage I and II SCLC (Wu et al. 2017). A large National Cancer Database study of patients with cT1-T2 N0 SCLC suggested a survival benefit with surgery plus adjuvant chemotherapy over concurrent chemotherapy and thoracic radiation (5 years overall survival 47.6% vs 29.8%, $p < 0.01$) (Yang et al. 2018). However, many patients with early stage node negative SCLC are medically inoperable. While these medically inoperable patients would be historically treated with concurrent chemotherapy and hyperfractionated radiation, there is increasing interest in utilizing SBRT given the encouraging local control and toxicity results observed in NSCLC. A database study of 2,107 patients with early stage lung cancer, of which 150 received SBRT plus chemotherapy with the remaining undergoing concurrent chemoradiation, suggested equivalent outcomes in terms of overall survival (Verma et al. 2019). Similarly, a multi-instutitional series of 74 patients with T1-T2 N0 SCLC treated with a median dose of 50 Gy in 5 fractions demonstrated excellent 3 years local control (96.1%) and disease free survival (64.4%) (Verma et al. 2017). Therefore, the use of SBRT in early stage SCLC is an active area of interest in the field of lung cancer radiation oncology.

Combining radiation with immunotherapy is also an emerging field. Based on the success of trials demonstrating survival benefits with immunotherapy in extensive stage small cell lung cancer (ES-SCLC) (Horn et al. 2018; Paz-Ares et al. 2019), it has been hypothesized that immunotherapy may also benefit patients with LS-SCLC. At present, it is unknown how immunotherapy will or should impact the dose and fractionation of thoracic radiotherapy. At the time this chapter was written, there are several ongoing clinical trials investigating immunotherapy and radiation on LS-SCLC, including NRG LU-005 (NCT 03811002) and ACHILES (NCT 03540420).

References

Antonia SJ, Villegas A, Daniel D, Vicente D, Murakami S, Hui R, Yokoi T et al (2017) Durvalumab after chemoradiotherapy in stage III non–small-cell lung cancer. N Engl J Med 377(20):1919–1929. https://doi.org/10.1056/NEJMoa1709937

Arriagada R, le Chevalier T, Quoix E, Ruffie P, de Cremoux H, Douillard J-Y, Tarayre M et al (1991) Astro plenary: effect of chemotherapy on locally advanced non-small cell lung carcinoma: a randomized study of 353 patients. Int J Radiat Oncol Biol Phys 20(6):1183–1190. https://doi.org/10.1016/0360-3016(91)90226-T

Aupérin A, Arriagada R, Pignon JP, Le Péchoux C, Gregor A, Stephens RJ, Kristjansen PE et al (1999) Prophylactic cranial irradiation for patients with small-cell lung cancer in complete remission. Prophylactic cranial irradiation overview collaborative group. N Engl J Med 341(7):476–484. https://doi.org/10.1056/NEJM199908123410703

Aupérin A, Le Péchoux C, Rolland E, Curran WJ, Furuse K, Fournel P, Belderbos J et al (2010) Meta-analysis of concomitant versus sequential Radiochemotherapy in locally advanced non-small-cell lung cancer. J Clin Oncol Off J Am Soc Clin Oncol 28(13):2181–2190. https://doi.org/10.1200/JCO.2009.26.2543

Ball D, Tao Mai G, Vinod S, Babington S, Ruben J, Kron T, Chesson B et al (2019) Stereotactic ablative radiotherapy versus standard radiotherapy in stage 1 non-small-cell lung cancer (TROG 09.02 CHISEL): a phase 3, open-label, randomised controlled trial. Lancet Oncol 20(4):494–503. https://doi.org/10.1016/S1470-2045(18)30896-9

Baumann P, Nyman J, Hoyer M, Wennberg B, Gagliardi G, Lax I, Drugge N et al (2009) Outcome in a prospective phase II trial of medically inoperable stage I non-small-cell lung cancer patients treated with stereotactic body radiotherapy. J Clin Oncol Off J Am Soc Clin Oncol 27(20):3290–3296. https://doi.org/10.1200/JCO.2008.21.5681

Baumann M, Herrmann T, Koch R, Matthiessen W, Appold S, Wahlers B, Kepka L et al (2011) Final results of the randomized phase III CHARTWEL-trial (ARO 97-1) comparing hyperfractionated-accelerated versus conventionally fractionated radiotherapy in non-small cell lung cancer (NSCLC). Radiother Oncol 100(1):76–85. https://doi.org/10.1016/j.radonc.2011.06.031

Bezjak A, Paulus R, Gaspar LE, Timmerman RD, Straube WL, Ryan WF, Garces YI et al (2019) Safety and efficacy of a five-fraction stereotactic body radiotherapy schedule for centrally located non–small-cell lung cancer: NRG oncology/RTOG 0813 trial. J Clin Oncol 37(15):1316–1325. https://doi.org/10.1200/JCO.18.00622

Blomgren H, Lax I, Näslund I, Svanström R (1995) Stereotactic high dose fraction radiation therapy of extracranial tumors using an accelerator. Clinical experience of the first thirty-one patients. Acta Oncol (Stockholm, Sweden) 34(6):861–870. https://doi.org/10.3109/02841869509127197

Bogart JA, Herndon JE, Lyss AP, Watson D, Miller AA, Lee ME, Turrisi AT, Green MR, Cancer and Leukemia Group B study 39808 (2004) 70 Gy thoracic radiotherapy is feasible concurrent with chemotherapy for limited-stage small-cell lung cancer: analysis of cancer and leukemia group B study 39808. Int J Radiat Oncol Biol Phys 59(2):460–468. https://doi.org/10.1016/j.ijrobp.2003.10.021

Bradley J, Graham MV, Winter K, Purdy JA, Komaki R, Roa WH, Ryu JK, Bosch W, Emami B (2005) Toxicity and outcome results of RTOG 9311: A phase I-II dose-escalation study using three-dimensional conformal radiotherapy in patients with inoperable non–small-cell lung carcinoma. Int J Radiat Oncol Biol Phys 61(2):318–328. https://doi.org/10.1016/j.ijrobp.2004.06.260

Bradley JD, Bae K, Graham MV, Byhardt R, Govindan R, Fowler J, Purdy JA, Michalski JM, Gore E, Choy H (2010) Primary analysis of the phase II component of a phase I/II dose intensification study using three-dimensional conformal radiation therapy and concurrent chemotherapy for patients with inoperable non–small-cell lung cancer: RTOG 0117. J Clin Oncol 28(14):2475–2480. https://doi.org/10.1200/JCO.2009.27.1205

Bradley JD, Paulus R, Komaki R, Masters G, Blumenschein G, Schild S, Bogart J et al (2015) Standard-dose versus high-dose conformal radiotherapy with concurrent and consolidation carboplatin plus paclitaxel with or without cetuximab for patients with stage IIIA or IIIB non-small-cell lung cancer (RTOG 0617): a randomised, two-by-two factorial phase 3 study. Lancet Oncol 16(2):187–199. https://doi.org/10.1016/S1470-2045(14)71207-0

Bradley JD, Hu C, Komaki RR, Masters GA, Blumenschein GR, Schild SE, Bogart JA et al (2020) Long-term results of NRG oncology RTOG 0617: standard- versus high-dose chemoradiotherapy with or without cetuximab for unresectable stage III non-small-cell lung cancer. J Clin Oncol Off J Am Soc Clin Oncol 38(7):706–714. https://doi.org/10.1200/JCO.19.01162

Brower JV, Amini A, Chen S, Hullett CR, Kimple RJ, Wojcieszynski AP, Bassetti M et al (2016) Improved survival with dose-escalated radiotherapy in stage III non-small-cell lung cancer: analysis of the national cancer database. Ann Oncol 27(10):1887–1894. https://doi.org/10.1093/annonc/mdw276

Carney DN, Mitchell JB, Kinsella TJ (1983) In vitro radiation and chemotherapy sensitivity of established cell lines of human small cell lung cancer and its large cell morphological variants. Cancer Res 43(6):2806–2811

Chang JY, Li Q-Q, Xu Q-Y, Allen PK, Rebueno N, Gomez DR, Balter P et al (2014) Stereotactic ablative radiation therapy for centrally located early stage or isolated parenchymal recurrences of non-small cell lung cancer: how to fly in a 'no fly zone'. Int J Radiat Oncol

Biol Phys 88(5):1120–1128. https://doi.org/10.1016/j.ijrobp.2014.01.022

Cheung P, Faria S, Ahmed S, Chabot P, Greenland J, Kurien E, Mohamed I et al (2014) Phase II study of accelerated hypofractionated three-dimensional conformal radiotherapy for stage T1-3 N0 M0 non-small cell lung cancer: NCIC CTG BR.25. J Natl Cancer Inst 106(8). https://doi.org/10.1093/jnci/dju164

Cox JD (1985) Large-dose fractionation. (hypofractionation). Cancer 55(S9):2105–2111. https://doi.org/10.1002/1097-0142(19850501)55:9+<2105::AID-CNCR2820551412>3.0.CO;2-T

Cox JD, Azarnia N, Byhardt RW, Shin KH, Emami B, Pajak TF (1990) A randomized phase I/ii trial of hyperfractionated radiation therapy with total doses of 60.0 Gy to 79.2 Gy: possible survival benefit with greater than or equal to 69.6 Gy in favorable patients with radiation therapy oncology group stage III non-small-cell lung carcinoma: report of radiation therapy oncology group 83-11. J Clin Oncol 8(9):1543–1555. https://doi.org/10.1200/JCO.1990.8.9.1543

Curran WJ, Paulus R, Langer CJ, Komaki R, Lee JS, Hauser S, Movsas B et al (2011) Sequential vs. concurrent chemoradiation for stage III non-small cell lung cancer: randomized phase III trial RTOG 9410. J Natl Cancer Inst 103(19):1452–1460. https://doi.org/10.1093/jnci/djr325

Faivre-Finn C, Snee M, Ashcroft L, Appel W, Barlesi F, Bhatnagar A, Bezjak A et al (2017) Concurrent once-daily versus twice-daily chemoradiotherapy in patients with limited-stage small-cell lung cancer (CONVERT): an open-label, phase 3, randomised, superiority trial. Lancet Oncol 18(8):1116–1125. https://doi.org/10.1016/S1470-2045(17)30318-2

Feddock J, Arnold SM, Shelton BJ, Sinha P, Conrad G, Chen L, Rinehart J, McGarry RC (2013) Stereotactic body radiation therapy can be used safely to boost residual disease in locally advanced non-small cell lung cancer: A prospective study. Int J Radiat Oncol Biol Phys 85(5):1325–1331. https://doi.org/10.1016/j.ijrobp.2012.11.011

Fox W, Scadding JG (1973) Medical research council comparative trial of surgery and radiotherapy for primary treatment of small-celled or oat-celled carcinoma of bronchus. Ten-year follow-up. Lancet (London, England) 2(7820):63–65. https://doi.org/10.1016/s0140-6736(73)93260-1

Goldstraw P, Chansky K, Crowley J, Rami-Porta R, Asamura H, Eberhardt WEE, Nicholson AG et al (2016) The IASLC lung cancer staging project: proposals for revision of the TNM stage groupings in the forthcoming (eighth) edition of the TNM classification for lung cancer. J Thorac Oncol 11(1):39–51. https://doi.org/10.1016/j.jtho.2015.09.009

Graham MV, Purdy JA, Emami B, Harms W, Bosch W, Lockett MA, Perez CA (1999) Clinical dose-volume histogram analysis for pneumonitis after 3D treatment for non-small cell lung cancer (NSCLC). Int J Radiat Oncol Biol Phys 45(2):323–329. https://doi.org/10.1016/s0360-3016(99)00183-2

Grønberg BH, Halvorsen TO, Fløtten Ø, Brustugun OT, Brunsvig PF, Aasebø U, Bremnes RM et al (2016) Randomized phase II trial comparing twice daily hyperfractionated with once daily hypofractionated thoracic radiotherapy in limited disease small cell lung cancer. Acta Oncol (Stockholm, Sweden) 55(5):591–597. https://doi.org/10.3109/0284186X.2015.1092584

Groome, Patti A., Vanessa Bolejack, John J. Crowley, Catherine Kennedy, Mark Krasnik, Leslie H. Sobin, Peter Goldstraw, et al. 2007. "The IASLC lung cancer staging project: validation of the proposals for revision of the T, N, and M descriptors and consequent stage groupings in the forthcoming (seventh) edition of the TNM classification of malignant tumours." J Thorac Oncol 2 (8): 694–705. https://doi.org/10.1097/JTO.0b013e31812d05d5

Haasbeek CJA, Lagerwaard FJ, Slotman BJ, Senan S (2011) Outcomes of stereotactic ablative radiotherapy for centrally located early-stage lung cancer. J Thorac Oncol 6(12):2036–2043. https://doi.org/10.1097/JTO.0b013e31822e71d8

Haque W, Verma V, Polamraju P, Andrew F, Brian Butler E, Teh BS (2018) Stereotactic body radiation therapy versus conventionally fractionated radiation therapy for early stage non-small cell lung cancer. Radiother Oncol 129(2):264–269. https://doi.org/10.1016/j.radonc.2018.07.008

Hayman JA, Martel MK, Ten Haken RK, Normolle DP, Todd RF, Littles JF, Sullivan MA, Possert PW, Turrisi AT, Lichter AS (2001) Dose escalation in non-small-cell lung cancer using three-dimensional conformal radiation therapy: update of a phase I trial. J Clin Oncol Off J Am Soc Clin Oncol 19(1):127–136. https://doi.org/10.1200/JCO.2001.19.1.127

Higgins KA, Pillai RN, Chen Z, Tian S, Zhang C, Patel P, Pakkala S et al (2017) Concomitant chemotherapy and radiotherapy with SBRT boost for unresectable stage III non–small cell lung cancer: a phase I study. J Thorac Oncol 12(11):1687–1695. https://doi.org/10.1016/j.jtho.2017.07.036

Horn L, Mansfield AS, Szczęsna A, Havel L, Krzakowski M, Hochmair MJ, Huemer F et al (2018) First-line atezolizumab plus chemotherapy in extensive-stage small-cell lung cancer. N Engl J Med 379(23):2220–2229. https://doi.org/10.1056/NEJMoa1809064

Iocolano M, Wild AT, Hannum M, Zhang Z, Simone CB, Gelblum D, Wu AJ, Rimner A, Shepherd AF (2020) Hypofractionated vs. conventional radiation therapy for stage III non-small cell lung cancer treated without chemotherapy. Acta Oncol (Stockholm, Sweden) 59(2):164–170. https://doi.org/10.1080/0284186X.2019.1675907

Machtay M, Bae K, Movsas B, Paulus R, Gore EM, Komaki R, Albain K, Sause WT, Curran WJ (2012) Higher biologically effective dose of radiotherapy is associated with improved outcomes for locally advanced non-small cell lung carcinoma treated with chemoradiation: an analysis of the radiation therapy oncology group. Int J Radiat Oncol Biol Phys 82(1):425–434. https://doi.org/10.1016/j.ijrobp.2010.09.004

Mauguen A, Le Péchoux C, Saunders MI, Schild SE, Turrisi AT, Baumann M, Sause WT et al (2012) Hyperfractionated or accelerated radiotherapy in lung cancer: an individual patient data meta-analysis. J Clin Oncol Off J Am Soc Clin Oncol 30(22):2788–2797. https://doi.org/10.1200/JCO.2012.41.6677

Micke P, Faldum A, Metz T, Beeh K-M, Bittinger F, Hengstler J-G, Buhl R (2002) Staging small cell lung cancer: veterans administration lung study group versus International Association for the Study of Lung Cancer—what limits limited disease? Lung Cancer (Amsterdam, Netherlands) 37(3):271–276. https://doi.org/10.1016/s0169-5002(02)00072-7

Nyman J, Hallqvist A, Lund J-Å, Brustugun O-T, Bergman B, Bergström P, Friesland S, Lewensohn R, Holmberg E, Lax I (2016) SPACE – A randomized study of SBRT vs conventional fractionated radiotherapy in medically inoperable stage I NSCLC. Radiother Oncol 121(1):1–8. https://doi.org/10.1016/j.radonc.2016.08.015

Onishi H, Shirato H, Nagata Y, Hiraoka M, Fujino M, Gomi K, Niibe Y et al (2007) Hypofractionated stereotactic radiotherapy (HypoFXSRT) for stage I non-small cell lung cancer: updated results of 257 patients in a Japanese multi-institutional study. J Thorac Oncol 2(7):S94–S100. https://doi.org/10.1097/JTO.0b013e318074de34

Paz-Ares L, Dvorkin M, Chen Y, Reinmuth N, Hotta K, Trukhin D, Statsenko G et al (2019) Durvalumab plus platinum–etoposide versus platinum–etoposide in first-line treatment of extensive-stage small-cell lung cancer (CASPIAN): A randomised, controlled, open-label, phase 3 trial. Lancet 394(10212):1929–1939. https://doi.org/10.1016/S0140-6736(19)32222-6

Perez CA, Stanley K, Rubin P, Kramer S, Brady L, Perez-Tamayo R, Brown GS, Concannon J, Rotman M, Seydel HG (1980) A prospective randomized study of various irradiation doses and fractionation schedules in the treatment of inoperable non-oat-cell carcinoma of the lung. Preliminary report by the radiation therapy oncology group. Cancer 45(11):2744–2753. https://doi.org/10.1002/1097-0142(19800601)45:11<2744::aid-cncr2820451108>3.0.co;2-u

Perez CA, Pajak TF, Rubin P, Simpson JR, Mohiuddin M, Brady LW, Perez-Tamayo R, Rotman M (1987) Long-term observations of the patterns of failure in patients with unresectable non-oat cell carcinoma of the lung treated with definitive radiotherapy. Report by the radiation therapy oncology group. Cancer 59(11):1874–1881. https://doi.org/10.1002/1097-0142(19870601)59:11<1874::aid-cncr2820591106>3.0.co;2-z

Pignon JP, Arriagada R, Ihde DC, Johnson DH, Perry MC, Souhami RL, Brodin O, Joss RA, Kies MS, Lebeau B (1992) A meta-analysis of thoracic radiotherapy for small-cell lung cancer. N Engl J Med 327(23):1618–1624. https://doi.org/10.1056/NEJM199212033272302

Raz DJ, Zell JA, Ignatius Ou S-H, Gandara DR, Anton-Culver H, Jablons DM (2007) Natural history of stage I non-small cell lung cancer: implications for early detection. Chest 132(1):193–199. https://doi.org/10.1378/chest.06-3096

Rosenzweig KE, Fox JL, Yorke E, Amols H, Jackson A, Rusch V, Kris MG, Ling CC, Leibel SA (2005) Results of a phase I dose-escalation study using three-dimensional conformal radiotherapy in the treatment of inoperable nonsmall cell lung carcinoma. Cancer 103(10):2118–2127. https://doi.org/10.1002/cncr.21007

Saunders M, Dische S, Barrett A, Harvey A, Gibson D, Parmar M (1997) Continuous hyperfractionated accelerated radiotherapy (CHART) versus conventional radiotherapy in non-small-cell lung cancer: a randomised multicentre trial. CHART steering committee. Lancet (London, England) 350(9072):161–165. https://doi.org/10.1016/s0140-6736(97)06305-8

Saunders M, Dische S, Barrett A, Harvey A, Griffiths G, Palmar M (1999) Continuous, hyperfractionated, accelerated radiotherapy (CHART) versus conventional radiotherapy in non-small-cell lung cancer: mature data from the randomised multicentre trial. CHART steering committee. Radiother Oncol 52(2):137–148. https://doi.org/10.1016/s0167-8140(99)00087-0

Sause W, Kolesar P, Taylor S, Johnson D, Livingston R, Komaki R, Emami B et al (2000) Final results of phase III trial in regionally advanced unresectable non-small cell lung cancer: radiation therapy oncology group, eastern cooperative oncology group, and southwest oncology group. Chest 117(2):358–364. https://doi.org/10.1378/chest.117.2.358

Shepherd FA, Crowley J, Van Houtte P, Postmus PE, Carney D, Chansky K, Shaikh Z, Goldstraw P, International Association for the Study of Lung Cancer International Staging Committee and Participating Institutions (2007) The International Association for the Study of Lung Cancer lung cancer staging project: proposals regarding the clinical staging of small cell lung cancer in the forthcoming (seventh) edition of the tumor, node, metastasis classification for lung cancer. J Thorac Oncol 2(12):1067–1077. https://doi.org/10.1097/JTO.0b013e31815bdc0d

Singh AK, Gomez Suescun JA, Stephans KL, Bogart JA, Lili T, Malhotra H, Videtic GM, Groman A (2017) A phase 2 randomized study of 2 stereotactic body radiation therapy regimens for medically inoperable patients with node-negative, peripheral non–small cell lung cancer. Int J Radiat Oncol Biol Phys 98(1):221–222. https://doi.org/10.1016/j.ijrobp.2017.01.040

Sonnick MA, Oro F, Yan B, Desai A, Wu AJ, Shi W, Zhang Z et al (2018) Identifying the optimal radiation dose in locally advanced non–small-cell lung cancer treated with definitive radiotherapy without concurrent chemotherapy. Clin Lung Cancer 19(1):e131–e140. https://doi.org/10.1016/j.cllc.2017.06.019

Sun J-M, Ahn YC, Choi EK, Ahn M-J, Ahn JS, Lee S-H, Lee DH et al (2013) Phase III trial of concurrent thoracic radiotherapy with either first- or third-cycle chemotherapy for limited-disease small-cell lung cancer†. Ann Oncol 24(8):2088–2092. https://doi.org/10.1093/annonc/mdt140

Takada M, Fukuoka M, Kawahara M, Sugiura T, Yokoyama A, Yokota S, Nishiwaki Y et al (2002) Phase III study of concurrent versus sequential thoracic radiotherapy in combination with cisplatin and etoposide for limited-stage small-cell lung cancer: results of the Japan clinical oncology group study 9104. J Clin Oncol Off J Am Soc Clin Oncol 20(14):3054–3060. https://doi.org/10.1200/JCO.2002.12.071

Timmerman R, Papiez L, McGarry R, Likes L, DesRosiers C, Frost S, Williams M (2003) Extracranial stereotactic radioablation: results of a phase I study in medically inoperable stage I non-small cell lung cancer. Chest 124(5):1946–1955. https://doi.org/10.1378/chest.124.5.1946

Timmerman R, McGarry R, Yiannoutsos C, Papiez L, Tudor K, DeLuca J, Ewing M et al (2006) Excessive toxicity when treating central tumors in a phase II study of stereotactic body radiation therapy for medically inoperable early-stage lung cancer. J Clin Oncol Off J Am Soc Clin Oncol 24(30):4833–4839. https://doi.org/10.1200/JCO.2006.07.5937

Timmerman R, Paulus R, Galvin J, Michalski J, Straube W, Bradley J, Fakiris A et al (2010) Stereotactic body radiation therapy for inoperable early stage lung cancer. JAMA 303(11):1070–1076. https://doi.org/10.1001/jama.2010.261

Timmerman RD, Hu C, Michalski JM, Bradley JC, Galvin J, Johnstone DW, Choy H (2018a) Long-term results of stereotactic body radiation therapy in medically inoperable stage I non–small cell lung cancer. JAMA Oncol 4(9):1287. https://doi.org/10.1001/jamaoncol.2018.1258

Turrisi AT, Kim K, Blum R, Sause WT, Livingston RB, Komaki R, Wagner H, Aisner S, Johnson DH (1999) Twice-daily compared with once-daily thoracic radiotherapy in limited small-cell lung cancer treated concurrently with cisplatin and etoposide. N Engl J Med 340(4):265–271. https://doi.org/10.1056/NEJM199901283400403

Uematsu M, Shioda A, Tahara K, Fukui T, Yamamoto F, Tsumatori G, Ozeki Y, Aoki T, Watanabe M, Kusano S (1998) Focal, high dose, and fractionated modified stereotactic radiation therapy for lung carcinoma patients: a preliminary experience. Cancer 82(6):1062–1070. https://doi.org/10.1002/(sici)1097-0142(19980315)82:6<1062::aid-cncr8>3.0.co;2-g

Urbanic JJ, Wang X, Bogart JA, Stinchcombe TE, Hodgson L, Schild SE, Bazhenova L, Hahn O, Salgia R, Vokes EE (2018) Phase 1 study of accelerated Hypofractionated radiation therapy with concurrent chemotherapy for stage III non-small cell lung cancer: CALGB 31102 (alliance). Int J Radiat Oncol Biol Phys 101(1):177–185. https://doi.org/10.1016/j.ijrobp.2018.01.046

Vallières E, Shepherd FA, Crowley J, Van Houtte P, Postmus PE, Carney D, Chansky K, Shaikh Z, Goldstraw P, International Association for the Study of Lung Cancer International Staging Committee and Participating Institutions (2009) The IASLC lung cancer staging project: proposals regarding the relevance of TNM in the pathologic staging of small cell lung cancer in the forthcoming (seventh) edition of the TNM classification for lung cancer. J Thorac Oncol 4(9):1049–1059. https://doi.org/10.1097/JTO.0b013e3181b27799

Verma V, Simone CB, Allen PK, Gajjar SR, Shah C, Zhen W, Harkenrider MM et al (2017) Multi-institutional experience of stereotactic ablative radiation therapy for stage I small cell lung cancer. Int J Radiat Oncol Biol Phys 97(2):362–371. https://doi.org/10.1016/j.ijrobp.2016.10.041

Verma V, Hasan S, Wegner RE, Abel S, Colonias A (2019) Stereotactic ablative radiation therapy versus conventionally fractionated radiation therapy for stage I small cell lung cancer. Radiother Oncol 131(February):145–149. https://doi.org/10.1016/j.radonc.2018.12.006

Videtic GMM, Donington J, Giuliani M, Heinzerling J, Karas TZ, Kelsey CR, Lally BE et al (2017) Stereotactic body radiation therapy for early-stage non-small cell lung cancer: executive summary of an ASTRO evidence-based guideline. Pract Radiat Oncol 7(5):295–301. https://doi.org/10.1016/j.prro.2017.04.014

Videtic GM, Paulus R, Singh AK, Chang JY, Parker W, Olivier KR, Timmerman RD et al (2019) Long term follow-up on NRG oncology RTOG 0915 (NCCTG N0927): A randomized phase II study comparing 2 stereotactic body radiation therapy schedules for medically inoperable patients with stage I peripheral non-small cell lung cancer. Int J Radiat Oncol Biol Phys 103(5):1077–1084. https://doi.org/10.1016/j.ijrobp.2018.11.051

von Reibnitz D, Shaikh F, Wu AJ, Treharne GC, Dick-Godfrey R, Foster A, Woo KM et al (2018) Stereotactic body radiation therapy (SBRT) improves local control and overall survival compared to conventionally fractionated radiation for stage I non-small cell lung cancer (NSCLC). Acta Oncol (Stockholm, Sweden) 57(11):1567–1573. https://doi.org/10.1080/0284186X.2018.1481292

Warde P, Payne D (1992) Does thoracic irradiation improve survival and local control in limited-stage small-cell carcinoma of the lung? A meta-analysis. J Clin Oncol Off J Am Soc Clin Oncol 10(6):890–895. https://doi.org/10.1200/JCO.1992.10.6.890

Wu AJ, Gillis A, Foster A, Woo K, Zhang Z, Gelblum DY, Downey RJ et al (2017) Patterns of failure in limited-stage small cell lung cancer: implications of TNM stage for prophylactic cranial irradiation. Radiother Oncol 125(1):130–135. https://doi.org/10.1016/j.radonc.2017.07.019

Yang C-FJ, Chan DY, Shah SA, Yerokun BA, Wang XF, D'Amico TA, Berry MF, Harpole DH (2018) Long-term survival after surgery compared with concurrent chemoradiation for node-negative small cell lung cancer. Ann Surg 268(6):1105–1112. https://doi.org/10.1097/SLA.0000000000002287

Zayed S, Chen H, Ali E, Rodrigues GB, Warner A, Palma DA, Louie AV (2020) Is there a role for hypofractionated thoracic radiation therapy in limited-stage small cell lung cancer? A propensity score matched analysis. Int J Radiat Oncol Biol Phys 108(3):575–586. https://doi.org/10.1016/j.ijrobp.2020.06.008

Optimizing Lung Cancer Radiotherapy Treatments Using Personalized Dose-Response Curves

Joseph O. Deasy, Jeho Jeong, Maria Thor, Aditya Apte, Andrew Jackson, Ishita Chen, Abraham Wu, and Andreas Rimner

Contents

1 Introduction 190
2 Tumor Response: A Very Short Summary of Important Radiobiological Mechanisms 191
3 An Energy Budget Compartment Model to Predict Tumor Control Probability 192
4 Accounting for Subclinical Disease Extension 196
5 General Considerations Regarding Correlations Between Dosimetric Predictors and Outcomes 198
6 Dose-Volume Predictors of Esophageal Toxicity 199
7 Dose-Volume Predictors of Radiation Pneumonitis 200
8 Heart Irradiation and Cardiotoxicity 202
9 Bronchial Radiation Toxicity 203
10 Putting the Pieces Together: Radiotherapy Planning Using Personalized Dose-Response Curves 204
11 Driving Planning Using the Generalized Equivalent Uniform Dose Function 206
12 Conclusion 207
References 208

Abstract

In this chapter we review the use of prediction models to personalize the physical parameters associated with lung cancer radiotherapy treatment planning, including the fractionation schedule. New models and data are continuing to emerge that support moving away from a one-size-fits-all, or one-size-fits-many approach. In most cases, radiotherapy for non-small lung cancer is a toxicity-limited treatment with still suboptimal tumor local control. We will discuss the dose-volume determinants, for important lung cancer radiotherapy endpoints, including esophagitis, pneumonitis, bronchial stenosis, and cardiotoxicity. We will discuss in detail tumor response and tumor local control modeling, and how to design a clinical trial to use personalized toxicity and tumor control curves to individualize

J. O. Deasy (✉) · J. Jeong · M. Thor · A. Apte · A. Jackson
Department of Medical Physics, Memorial Sloan Kettering Cancer Center, New York, NY, USA
e-mail: deasyj@mskcc.org

I. Chen · A. Wu · A. Rimner
Department of Radiation Oncology, Memorial Sloan Kettering Cancer Center, New York, NY, USA

dose and fractionation. The main point of this chapter is that a new clinical paradigm is emerging of using published and validated models to inform treatment decisions on a patient-specific basis.

1 Introduction

Remarkably, the current US standard radiotherapy regime for many non-small cell lung cancers (NSCLC) with suspected or positive lymph nodes (2 Gy × 30 weekday fractions) was established via a randomized clinical trial in 1974 by the RTOG (Cox et al. 1991), whereas hypofractionated methods for tumors without lymphatic spread have demonstrated superior control with intolerable toxicity only for central/ultracentral treatments (Chang and Timmerman 2007).

In this chapter, we take a holistic view of the critical physical factors that must be quantitatively balanced to achieve success in the treatment of NSCLC using radiotherapy. By success, we mean maximizing the likelihood that radiotherapy will eradicate gross disease, as well as suspected occult disease, while minimizing both acute severe toxicity and longer-term toxicity. What makes the successful delivery of lung cancer radiotherapy so difficult? Primarily, it is the complex interplay between dose-volume drivers of normal tissue toxicity and the dose-volume drivers of tumor control. *The interlocking and complicated nature of these challenges has impeded progress in optimizing lung cancer radiotherapy.* While this chapter focuses on the driving time-dose-volume determinants of local control, the entire process of effective treatment of lung cancer will also require other physics-driven improvements in image guidance and strategies to limit and/or account for breathing motion, which this chapter will not cover.

In the last 30 years, physics-and-engineering-driven advances in clinical radiotherapy include computerized linac control, multileaf collimators, high-resolution and fast CTs, MRIs for treatment simulations, FDG-PET for staging, treatment room MRI for target definition of the day, proton therapy for reduced integral dose, and treatment room cone-beam CT for setup. Most recently, deep learning/AI methods have been used to autocontour tumors and normal tissues. These approaches will continue to evolve and interact with scientific advances driven by biological or chemical modifiers, genomic biomarkers, immunotherapies, etc. Undoubtedly, physical methods can be greatly improved *by better utilizing the information they generate in the planning process*, both by improving predictive models relating time-dose-volume factors to toxicity and local control and by deploying the models in the clinic to improve therapy on a customized basis.

To introduce this paradigm, consider Fig. 1, which shows a set of modeled dose-response curves based on the treatment plan for a single patient, as a function of fractional dose scaled up or down, but with fixed fractionation and a fixed dose distribution. As shown here, dose escalation to a high rate of tumor control (say, 90%) would come at the cost of increased toxicity risk, as expected. Typically, the toxicity curves are shallow, as shown here, rather than the usual cartoon of therapeutic index that shows nearly parallel TCP and NTCP curves.

Lung tumors change over time, with relatively rapid changes in the microenvironment, in some cases leading to the resolution of hypoxia over a short time frame (i.e., 2–3 weeks), resulting in microenvironmental reoxygenation and tumor regression or erosion (Hill 2017; Riaz et al. 2017). Tumor changes, which can be predicted to some extent (Zhang et al. 2014, 2018; Seibert et al. 2007), can partially be accounted for at the beginning of a multiweek course of radiotherapy but also motivate monitoring and potential adaptation during a course of radiotherapy. New artificial intelligence (AI) driven technologies both make this emerging paradigm possible, while also increasing the accuracy of monitoring accumulated dose during a course of radiotherapy and allowing for more aggressive and tighter margins. Truly optimizing outcomes in lung cancer radiotherapy will thus require continuing advances in technology and response modeling. A critical issue has always been the reliability of the predictive models. Yet it seems reasonable to recognize that we are now long past the point of

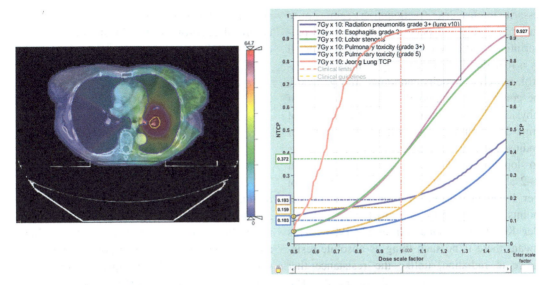

Fig. 1 An example of personalized dose-response curves based on a specific planning dose distribution. The response curves are tied closely to the details of the tumor shape and location. The "operating point" of the plan is a scale factor of 1.0, adjustable, which implies TCP and NTCP values projected onto the left axis. Using personalized dose-response curves, still within clinical protocols, would be a natural evolution beyond merely using population guideline dose-volume histogram goals and fixed fractionation regimens

having usable models that improve upon a "one-size-fits-all" approach (Allen Li et al. 2012; Deasy et al. 2015).

The Quantitative Analysis of Normal Tissue Effects in the Clinic, QUANTEC (2010), was a successful effort to propose treatment tolerance guidelines based on the massive amount of data that had resulted from the widespread adoption of 3-D treatment planning in the 1990s and 2000s (Marks et al. 2010a). Yet the QUANTEC reports often looked forward to a future era when the bewildering array of published clinical metrics (e.g., "mean dose less than 26 Gy") would be replaced by mathematical functions of greater generality and less bias (Bentzen et al. 2010). Although the growing availability of validated normal tissue complication probability (NTCP) models has allowed radiotherapy treatment planning systems to design "radiobiologically optimal" treatment plans, on a patient-specific basis, this largely has not happened, and one often sees declarations such as this one: "…it will always be necessary to rely on clinical trials for the final choice of a protocol" (Joiner and van der Kogel 2016).

In this chapter, we take the unapologetic position (as we have elsewhere (Deasy et al. 2015)) that (some) radiobiological models should be used clinically as decision support tools and surpass one-size-fits all approaches and cooperative group planning guidelines. We will emphasize models that have been fit to large datasets where possible. To address the overall problem of lung cancer radiotherapy, we will be selective; more complete reviews of the relevant literature have been published elsewhere (Brodin et al. 2018; Rancati and Fiorino 2019; Shrieve and Loeffler 2010; Werner-Wasik et al. 2010; Marks et al. 2010b).

2 Tumor Response: A Very Short Summary of Important Radiobiological Mechanisms

The ability to "fine-tune" or optimize dose distributions and fractionation regimes with respect to outcome probability models is a critical path toward improvement in radiotherapy. A validated TCP model can be used to identify unnecessarily intense dose-fractionation regimes or to more precisely and personally guide dose prescriptions and dose distribution optimization. It is a remarkable fact that long-term tumor control, as well as toxicity endpoints, may generally be considered sigmoidally shaped functions of physical factors, encapsulating the impact of time-dose-volume. The differences in tumor radiosensitivity are relatively modest, giving rise to slopes of dose-response (commonly) of about 1–2 absolute percent changes in tumor control per 1 percent change in dose at their steepest points (i.e., near 50% control) (Joiner and van der Kogel 2016; Okunieff et al. 1995). This means there is no such thing as absolute resistance to radiation, unlike the resistance that emerges in most drug-based treatments. The basic clinical radiobiology of lung tumors, as for other tumors, is known to be critically dependent on the presence (or absence) of hypoxia, which is protective against DNA damage (Overgaard 2011; Nahum et al. 2003; Donald Chapman and Nahum 2016). The proliferation of tumor cells during radiotherapy has also been recognized as detrimental. Withers and successive researchers recognized that when the overall treatment time of a radiotherapy protocol is too long (longer than a "kickoff time" of about 3–4 weeks), there is a corresponding loss of local control that is proportional to the treatment time prolonged past "kickoff" (Withers et al. 1988; Fowler 1991; Fowler and Lindstrom 1992). Apparently, tumors typically rid themselves of most hypoxic cells (they "reoxygenate"), several weeks into radiotherapy, due to tumor cell death during mitosis and the resultant mass experiences reduced competition for chemical resources. Although not proven, it appears that this reoxygenation then gives rise to the observed "kickoff" of loss of local control (Petersen et al. 2001). Another important factor is the association of glucose with an increasingly radioresistant phenotype, possibly due to an increase in reliance on glycolysis under hypoxic conditions (Dierckx and Van de Wiele 2008; Jeong and Deasy 2014). While each of these factors may differ in individual tumors, we capture these basic causal mechanisms in a dynamic mathematical cell state model which well-fits the clinical tumor control data across all fractionation regimes for early-stage lung cancer.

3 An Energy Budget Compartment Model to Predict Tumor Control Probability

The central problem of radiobiological modeling of tumor response is to model the relationship and tradeoffs between proliferative states and nonproliferative hypoxic states, both of which are fundamental to tumor response (Joiner and van der Kogel 2016). Our approach to consistently and effectively integrating these two phenomena is to introduce an "energy budget" that enforces a cellular competition for local chemical energy resources at each location within the tumor. The model is hence named the Energy Budget TCP model, or EB-TCP. The flux of chemical resources, in particular glucose and oxygen, locally extracted from the blood supply, differs throughout a tumor, and over time (Dewhirst and Secomb 2017; Lan et al. 2010; Dewhirst et al. 1998; Braun et al. 1999), due to the typically chaotic nature of the vasculature. This will contribute to the heterogeneity in response between patients and the shallowness of tumor dose-response.

Most efforts to model tumor response have searched for a low-dimensional formula with a few parameters that can be used to curve-fit fractionation results. Such efforts have only been partially successful as data fitting exercises, are subject to unexplained outliers, and have questionable mechanistic meaning (Shuryak et al. 2015). Integral equations have been used to account for known heterogeneities in radiosensitivity, for example, the "Marsden" model (Webb and Nahum 1993) that integrates over a radiosensitivity distribution or the model of Chapman and Nahum used to account for known heterogeneity in hypoxia status (Nahum et al. 2003). A few investigators have taken a true mechanistic modeling approach to better understand the longitudinal response to radiotherapy, usually based on differential equations (Prokopiou et al. 2015). Here we describe a flexible approach to modeling the evolution of tumor response that captures the dynamic interplay between proliferation and hypoxia.

As a starting point, we model tumors as though they consist of a single microscopically heterogeneous voxel of mixed cells competing for a limited and steady (time-averaged) supply of chemical resources.[1] At least for early-stage lung tumors, we will see that this appears to be an adequate assumption. Once we assume a local energy budget, then how do we deal with the incredibly complex tumor microenvironment? Our approach is to introduce a tumor cellular state-space model that models cells possibly changing states over time. The model uses the smallest number of defined compartments as possible, of clear radiobiological meaning, yet still reconcilable with the known drivers of tumor biology, including proliferation, hypoxia, and cell shedding (the cell loss factor) (Joiner and van der Kogel 2016).

State-space modeling, as opposed to a differential equation approach, has the flexibility needed to implement transition probability rules. The minimal model whose initial state is determined using the classical factors of the growth fraction, the cell loss factor, and the volume doubling time is a three-state (three-compartment) model, including (1) a Proliferating compartment (labeled the P-compartment) containing cells receiving adequate glucose and oxygen to move through the cell cycle toward reproduction, (2) an Intermediate compartment (labeled the I-compartment) of cells that receive adequate glucose to survive metabolically, but do not receive enough oxygen to proliferate (thus being hypoxic), and (3) a starving, extremely Hypoxic compartment (labeled the H-compartment), containing cells that lack oxygen as well as glucose, (Jeong et al. 2013). Figure 2 visually illustrates the concept. Modeling parameters, discussed in more detail elsewhere (Jeong and Deasy 2014; Jeong et al. 2017), are kept minimal by avoiding any attempt to model compartment membership by microscopic location. Cell damage due to radiation dose is modeled using the standard linear–quadratic description of cell kill based on one-track (alpha) vs. two-track (beta) damage. The impact of hypoxia is accounted for separately for the I-compartment and the H-compartment, through oxygen enhancement ratio (OER) dose modifying factors, as suggested by Carlson et al. (2006). Cell death is assumed to occur following failed mitosis, although multiple divisions are allowed before death. Senescence is not currently included. Tumor proliferation and cell death are computed in virtual 15-min slices, and cell compartment levels are updated accordingly. Modifications of radiosensitivity variation throughout the cell cycle are also introduced, which are important for single-fraction treatments. One key advantage of this energy budget model is the flexibility to model any given temporal fractionation scheme, and the resulting dynamic response profile over time. But the most important advantage of the model is that it well-describes the published local control data.

As shown in Fig. 3, the EB-TCP model well-fits data across the full fractionation regime for early-stage lung cancer, based on 38 published cohorts. A fit to other validation data cohorts is similarly good and is not shown. The resulting best fit parameters were alpha = 0.305/Gy and alpha/beta = 2.8 Gy, which are similar to values seen in the laboratory. The best fit oxygen enhancement ratio (OER) of the I-compartment cells was 1.7, which is not surprising for chronically (and possibly intermittently) hypoxic cells. These parameters differ from traditional values quoted for lung tumors (alpha/beta = 10 Gy), but this is not surprising as one implication of the successful modeling is that naked linear–quadratic modeling is a vast oversimplification of the underlying biological response process. Instead of a deus ex machina "kickoff" time effect—previously assumed to be a discontinuous and puzzling feature of clinical dose-response—reoxygenation comes naturally from integrating hypoxia with the process of proliferation. Over-fitting is not an issue given the small

---
[1] This assumption could ultimately be relaxed by using imaging information to seed the model parameters.

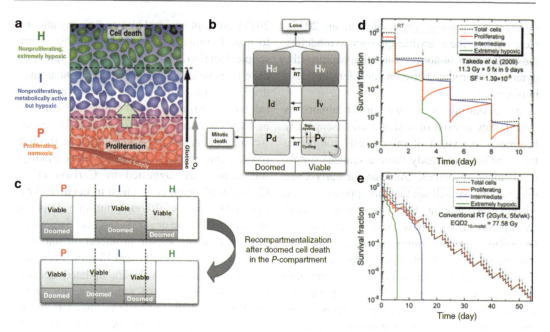

Fig. 2 The basics of the Energy Budget TCP (EB-TCP) compartmental model. (**a**) Cells either have enough oxygen and glucose to cycle (P-compartment), or they only have adequate glucose (I-compartment), or they are starving and extremely hypoxic (H-compartment). (**b**) During RT, only cycling cells die from radiation damage, through failed mitosis, (**c**) dead proliferating cells are replaced with I-compartment cells, (**d**) the level of survival of any time course of radiation is simulated in silico in 15-min time slices and then (**e**) matched to a conventionally fractionated but equal survival level treatment regime. (Reprinted with permission from Jeong et al. 2017)

number of parameters and large number of cohorts and patients:[2] the model describes the data very well as shown by the likelihood values in Fig. 3. To paraphrase George Box, this model is not correct, but it is definitely useful.

Radiobiological implications The EB-TCP model has several radiobiological implications. The results demonstrate that single-fraction outcomes are completely consistent with classical radiobiological principles as captured by the model; there is no need to invoke new mechanisms. This supports using the term "hypofractionated RT," instead of "stereotactic ablative radiotherapy." The model also implies that failures of hypofractionated radiotherapy regimes come predominantly from an extremely small fraction of hypoxic cells that happen to survive radiation randomly. For fractionation schedules longer than about 3 weeks, failure is primarily due to cells that were protected from early fractions by hypoxia and then reoxygenated. The issue of whether the L-Q model is really adequate at high doses per fraction is also relatively moot when considering the role of hypoxia as a dose modifier: dose is effectively cut by a factor of 1/OER, or about 0.6 of the nominal fractional dose. Thus, the part of the cell-survival curve normally identified as departing from the L-Q model (roughly >15 Gy) (Guerrero and Allen Li 2004) has little impact except for extremely large hypofractionated doses. In most cases it is the lower dose part of the cell-survival curve that describes hypoxic cell response. The model was also recently applied to carbon beam radiotherapy trial results, which were again well-fit (Jeong et al. 2020). In that case, the best fit alpha value was much higher than for photons, and there was little fraction repair, both results as expected from in vitro observations. Surprisingly, dose heterogeneity seems to be a mild factor in tumor

---

[2] The slope and saturation level of TCP was fixed prior to fitting for alpha, beta, TCD50, and the two OER values.

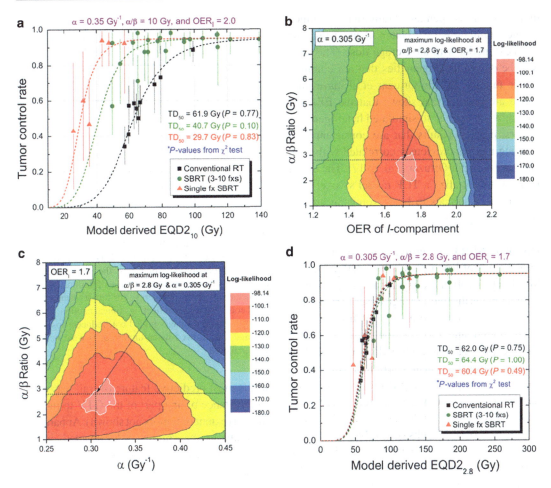

Fig. 3 Fitting of the EB-TCP data to early-stage, localized NSCLC cohorts (38 cohorts, 2701 patients). (**a**) Fits using assumed (L-Q) parameters, (**b**) and (**c**) show log-likelihood surfaces and 95% surface contours demonstrating small confidence intervals, and (**d**) final fits showing excellent fit across all fractionation regimes (also validated against a further 23 cohorts.) Alternative fractionation schedules can be compared using this model at TCP4RT.info. (Reprinted with permission from Jeong et al. 2017)

response, as the analysis used the average of the isodose level encompassing the tumor with the maximum dose. The EB-TCP model has been implemented in a web-interface at TCP4RT.info. We hasten to add that this online tool is meant to provide insight into protocol differences.[3]

Key clinical implications from this analysis for early-stage disease are that: (1) Local control is never expected to reach 100%—in fact, it seems to reach a maximum value of about 94–96%; (2) the model can be used to select fractionation schemes to reach a given TCP, with the optimal fractionation being near 90% TCP. The dose tradeoff against normal tissue damage becomes unfavorable above about 90% TCP, above which tumor response saturates while normal tissue dose damage continues to escalate.

Unfortunately, the problem of extending this successful TCP to account for dose heterogeneity remains unsolved. In unpublished work, we have found that simply treating each voxel of the

---

[3] It does not take the dose distribution into account in any way and is not meant to be used to guide individual patient management.

tumor as an independent "tumorlet"—a much smaller tumor—is no better than using the EB-TCP model with an average dose. This may well be due to heterogeneities that are common within tumors. Crispin-Ortuzar et al. have published an analysis that shows that the EB-TCP model, when applied to simulated heterogeneous tumors, predicts results that are consistent with imaging metrics previously correlated with poor outcome (Crispin-Ortuzar et al. 2017). The use of imaging to initialize a TCP model's voxel-wise parameters continues to be a promising area of active investigation.

Optimal SBRT fractionation regimes The implications of having a reliable TCP model for SBRT fractionation are significant. In particular, for treatments that require high doses to radiation-sensitive structures, the number of fractions can be increased and the fraction dose decreased while exploring how high a dose is needed to maintain a response near saturation. This is perhaps more favorable than previously appreciated due to the steady reoxygenation that occurs over a few weeks. For example, a schedule of 5 Gy in 12 fractions over 4 weeks (given M-W-F) is predicted to have a TCP = 0.91, whereas delivering the same fractionation over 3 weeks (all weekdays) gives 50% more avoidable failures: TCP = 0.86, due to a lack of reoxygenation (try this at TCP4RT.info). Preferring a larger number of fractions (6–10), rather than <5, is also a conclusion reached by Ruggieri et al. (2017), using a different kind of modeling that also accounts for hypoxia. We will return to the question of the optimal fractionation regime when we consider planning aspects, below.

Before leaving the topic of TCP, we want to acknowledge and emphasize that modeling itself can sometimes hide other factors that come into play clinically. Figure 4 shows a plot of isolated lung tumor GTVs (center-of-mass), projected onto transverse reference anatomy in the thorax (WUSTL data, 1991–2001). Red dots indicate treatment failures. The most predictive feature on a purely dosimetric basis was the volume receiving more than 55 Gy for standard fractionation,

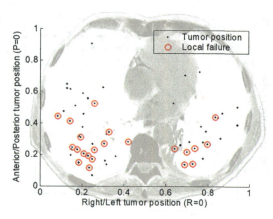

Fig. 4 Relative center-of-mass positions of lung tumor GTVs (WUSTL data, 1991–2001). Failure increased as tumors were closer to the spinal cord. The data ultimately had a simple dosimetric explanation: the volume receiving at least 55 Gy was most predictive of failure, and this parameter was lower on average for tumors nearer to the spinal cord, apparently reflecting clinical caution. In other words, in this pre-image-guided era, reduced dosimetric coverage was allowed when tumor edges were nearer to the spinal cord

but the most predictive feature overall was minimum distance of any part of the GTV to the spinal cord (extent of tumors not shown). Apparently, proximity to the spinal cord impacted overall plan aggressiveness, and this impacted local control rates (Hope et al. 2005).

4 Accounting for Subclinical Disease Extension

One of the most significant physical elements of radiotherapy treatment planning in lung (as well as elsewhere) is the choice of margin to adequately irradiate potential microscopic extensions of tumor cells that are too small to be imageable. According to the currently accepted ICRU philosophy (Morgan-Fletcher 2001; Purdy 2004), a clinical target volume, or CTV, is added as an expansion of the GTV for this purpose, although this is often omitted or smaller for SBRT treatments. Such margins, often chosen between 5 and 10 mm around the entire tumor for conventional fractionation, significantly increase the potential toxicity of the treatment, particularly for smaller targets treated with hypofractionation, and particularly if the high-dose volume abuts a dose-sensitive structure. An excellent recent overview of subclinical extension is given by Apolle et al. (2017), who state that "After immense improvements in GTV definition and the derivation of institution-dependent PTV margins, the CTV is now the least well-understood piece of the target volume concept."

Where do these margin numbers come from? There are few strong sources of data regarding subclinical extension. Even for imageable spiculations, precise identification and contouring is imprecise, and the GTV delineation is often not so much an outline as it is a net to catch an irregular tumor border. In addition to spiculations, tumor extension can be in the form of blobs or islands (possibly unconnected to the central lesion). The problem is made even more difficult by the need to quantify extensions, both in distance and in numbers of cells.

Early work quantifying subclinical extension includes that of Chao et al. (2003), who reviewed existing publications and concluded that subclinical extension could often be described using an exponential falloff. Several more recent reports have attempted to quantify extension of subclinical extension. Grills et al. (2007) examined 35 lung cases pathologically and found that the mean per-case maximal microscopic extension distance was 7.2 mm, was systematically smaller for higher nuclear grade tumors, and a margin of 9 mm would cover 90% of microscopic extensions. A report on adequacy of surgical margins by Kara et al. concluded that a margin of 1.5 cm from the macroscopic tumor edge would result in clear margins for 93% of cases (Kara et al. 2000). Giraud et al., addressing radiotherapy planning specifically, concluded that a margin of 8 mm for adenocarcinoma or 6 mm for squamous cell carcinoma could cover 95% of subclinical disease (Giraud et al. 2000).

An under-discussed issue is that most contouring does not attempt to closely follow a tumor edge and effectively bags together disease, capturing some of the subclinical extension. Another important issue, raised by Stroom et al., is how CTVs should be combined with other geometrical uncertainties to form the final margin added to the GTV. Stroom et al. argue that CTV margins should not be added together linearly with other uncertainties (that comprise the PTV), but quadratically. This may seem like an obscure point, but the motivation is clear: it would have a significant impact on reducing the use of overly aggressive margins. The motivation is twofold: effectively, subclinical disease acts like a shift in the GTV margin, similar to a systematic geometric shift over the course of a treatment, but is uncorrelated from the other geometrical sources of setup imprecision. In addition, subclinical extension does not occur equally around a tumor but at largest extent is localized. It therefore acts like an uncorrelated shift of the GTV and should therefore be treated as another quadratic term.

The most detailed analysis of the impact of subclinical disease extension on TCP to date has been performed by Siedschalg et al. (2011), who sampled from distributions of microscopic cells in a statistically reasonable way and used cell kill relationships to model the potential impact. They show that if there is no margin outside the GTV whatsoever, then this would be expected to have about a 10% impact on SBRT results. This may explain the saturation effect of our TCP modeling, which shows a saturation at about 94% for most cohorts even at high doses. They therefore advocate for a specific addition of a margin even in SBRT to account for subclinical disease extension.

The use of imaging features to identify tumors at high risk of significant subclinical extension has been underutilized as an approach for personalizing dose planning. Salgeuro et al. found that radiomic image features extracted from CT scans could be correlated to local subclinical disease extension from matched pathology (Salguero et al. 2013). Using such a prediction model based on a few CT imaging features, RT patients with a high risk of microscopic disease extension failed locally at a significantly higher rate than those with a low predicted microscopic disease extension. Predicting the potential risk of microscopic disease extension has thus been demonstrated as a promising avenue of research that could further guide personalized dose planning. They conclude, "In patients with a high risk of MDE [microscopic disease extension] it may be advisable to enforce this expansion or to define a CTV around the GTV that is given at least a minimum dose." This approach was further investigated by van Loon et al. (2012), who examined both FDG-PET and CT factors to predict microscopic extension. On multivariate modeling, tumor volume and mean CT Hounsfield tumor intensities were selected over SUVmax. In a study looking at only FDG-PET features, Meng et al. correlated maximum subclinical disease extension with FDG-PET characteristics and showed that extension correlated positively with SUVmax. They suggested that "…margins of 1.93 mm, 3.90 mm, and 9.60 mm for SUVmax ≤5, 5–10, and >10 added to the gross tumor volume would be adequate to cover 95% of ME [microscopic extension]" (Meng et al. 2012).

Bortfeld and colleagues have been studying how to account for subclinical disease directly in the treatment planning optimization process (Shusharina et al. 2018). Their interesting proposal is to treat the problem probabilistically. This would have many advantages, in particular, the optimizer could choose to introduce protective coldspots that overlap with critical anatomy in cases where the impact on local control probability is low enough. As Apolle et al. conclude: "Since cell density decreases toward the target edge, the dose delivered to these regions can also be reduced without relinquishing tumor control. This can, in turn, facilitate normal tissue sparing or central isotoxic dose escalation."

5 General Considerations Regarding Correlations Between Dosimetric Predictors and Outcomes

We cover the dosimetric predictors of toxicity because they can often be altered, on a protocol or even patient-by-patient basis, potentially with negligible impact on TCP. As Schanne et al. say "Dosimetric parameters remain the most reliable predictors of pulmonary and esophageal toxicity and are also factors that are feasible to modify without the risk of adverse events or reduced efficacy of the treatment" (Schanne et al. 2019).

The literature on dose-volume correlates of toxicity is fraught with uncertainties (Bentzen et al. 2010; Deasy and Muren 2014). In particular, correlations between different dose-volume parameters for single-institution studies are nearly unavoidable due to institutionally consistent approaches to beam field arrangements and even more importantly *the imprint of dose prescriptions*. If the typical prescription is 60 Gy, then $V65$ and $V70$ are much less likely to correlate with local control than $V55$, and *this has nothing to do with radiobiology*. Not surprisingly, a very wide range of dosimetric parameters have been identified as "best correlated" to a given toxicity endpoint for individual datasets. It follows that having the highest correlation to an endpoint in a given dataset does not imply the best generalizability to other cohorts at other institutions. Vx for local control also has poor statistical distribution characteristics, often being zero, and poor radiobiological justification (*Is it plausible that x Gy is such an important dose?*). More robust metrics include Dx, the minimum dose to the hottest $x\%$ volume. In our view, however, MOHx, defined as the mean of the hottest $x\%$ of volume, and gEUD, the generalized equivalent uniform dose, are superior metrics, as they represent averages over different parts of the DVH, and do not try to pick out a suspiciously specific dose threshold. We also find from experience that MOHx often generates higher univariate correlations than Vx or Dx (Thor et al. 2020). In addition, MOHx and gEUD are convex (Clark et al. 2008; Choi and Deasy 2002), which is a technical mathematical characteristic that makes treatment plan optimization much easier, whereas Vx and Dx are not convex and are difficult, though not impossible, to deal with in treatment plan optimization. Determining correlation vs. causation is made all the more difficult as institutional treatment planning guidelines are nearly guaranteed to impact resulting plan parameters which are allowed to vary, and which are purposefully held steady. Underlying biology may be inherently more sensitive to a given part of the dose-volume histogram curve, but if that part of the curve is consistently held to similar DVH loads, then the impact of that dose range will not present as significant on a statistical outcomes analysis. This issue is made even more difficult as such institutional guidelines are seldom reported in outcomes analyses.

6 Dose-Volume Predictors of Esophageal Toxicity

Severe esophagitis often involves extreme discomfort and pain, difficulty eating, and may lead to treatment interruption detrimental to disease control. Heavy dose loading of the esophagus during lung cancer RT is known to cause morbidity through two main mechanisms: (1) confluent esophagitis over relatively large patches due to destruction of rapid turnover epithelial cells lining the inner esophageal wall, and the subsequent regeneration of epithelium (if radiation kill of basal cells is not too extensive) in the first few months following RT, with severe symptoms subsiding in a few weeks following RT (Shrieve and Loeffler 2010). This mechanism, the main source of esophageal toxicity for conventional fractionation, reaches a peak during a course of RT, typically in 2–6 weeks, with earlier peaks for higher dose per week regimes (Werner-Wasik et al. 2010). (2) For hypofractionated regimes, high doses due to PTV overlap with the esophagus can lead to esophageal stricture or fistula, and total severe toxicity may be more a function of "hot spot" dose characteristics (maximum dose, maximum dose averaged over 1 cc, and the like) (Schanne et al. 2019).

We first discuss confluent esophagitis, which is more commonly observed for conventional fractionation schemes. For severe acute esophagitis, regarding DVH predictors, the central question is whether mean dose really captures the dosimetric risk, or if risk is more closely related to the high-dose region of the DVH. For conventional fractionation, mean dose appears to be well correlated with severe acute esophagitis. Prior to QUANTEC, two studies using the gEUD model indicated results similar to mean dose (or mean square dose) as a predictor (Chapet et al. 2005; Belderbos et al. 2005). A recent post-QUANTEC systematic review by Brodin et al. introduced a useful "relevance score" based on key criteria considering patient numbers, study design, radiotherapy relevance, and quality of the modeling approach (Brodin et al. 2018). The highest scored studies identified mean dose as a key predictor. Huang et al. reported an analysis based on RTOG 93-11 data supplemented with Washington University data, resulting in a logistic function of (0.069 × mean esophagus dose + 1.50 × ConChemo − 3.13) to predict symptomatic acute esophagitis (Huang et al. 2012). The usefulness of mean dose was again confirmed by the clinical experience of Yorke et al. (2021): after implementing more stringent attempts to reduce the esophageal mean dose in routine planning at MSK ("…encourage treatment planners to achieve a MED close to 21 Gy while still permitting MED to go up to the previous guideline of 34 Gy in difficult cases."), a subsequent drop in severe acute esophagitis (48–38%) was observed, precisely consistent with the model of Huang et al. The Huang model was subsequently tested in two other datasets (Thor et al. 2019a; Huang et al. 2017) and found to give useful predictions, although the calibration was moderately worse.

Because acute esophagitis occurs during a course of radiotherapy, and peak symptom intensity occurs sooner for more dose per week, it is logical that time factors would be important and that dose per week would impact the risk and intensity of esophagitis. This and other factors were tested in a model by Dehing-Oberije et al., who found that age, gender, WHO performance status, mean esophageal dose, maximum esophageal dose, and overall treatment time were all significant and could be validated on multiple datasets (Oberije et al. 2015).

Hallqvist et al.'s (2018) reported on a trial that was terminated early due to high toxicity and poor survival in the high-dose arm, escalated to 84 Gy by adding an additional 2 Gy fraction each week compared to a lower dose 68 Gy regimen in 34 fractions. Three fatalities, among the 18 high-dose patients, resulted due to post-RT esophageal fistulas as confirmed by autopsy; all fistulas were located in the high-dose regions. Management solutions may include using more fractions or employing more precise target imaging and setup procedures to maximize falloff along the PTV-esophagus border. In contrast, the mean esophagus dose can be altered via beam/beamlet weighting and is more controllable via treatment plan optimization, although here again more precise setup pays in terms of tissue avoidance. We will return to this issue when we discuss treatment planning below.

The idea that esophagitis may be avoided if at least some of the circumference is spared and given a low dose has been given credibility by the recent results of Kamran et al., who report no cases of severe acute esophagitis (RTOG Grade 3+) when proton therapy patients are carefully planned to avoid delivering high dose to the esophagus wall contralateral to the target volume (Kamran et al. 2021). The importance of the higher-dose part of the DVH is apparent in data regarding hypofractionated radiotherapy, where high-dose parameters more frequently emerge (Schanne et al. 2019; Stephans et al. 2014; Wu et al. 2014). The hottest part of the dose distribution for normal tissues almost always occurs in the target margins.

7 Dose-Volume Predictors of Radiation Pneumonitis

Radiation-induced pneumonitis (denoted RP) is an episodic, inflammatory syndrome that typically reaches a peak 3–8 months after radiotherapy and is characterized by fever, dyspnea, and a cough (Small and Woloschak 2006). RP is a dose-limiting complication and in unusual cases can be fatal. A related morbidity is chronic loss of lung function due to fibrosis following radiation damage (Giuranno et al. 2019). Preexisting lung comorbidities are known to increase the risk of RP. At the time of QUANTEC, the only established pneumonitis predictors were mean lung dose, the commonly used $V20$, and a strong indication that inferior lung position resulted in increased toxicity risk (Marks et al. 2010b; Seppenwoolde et al. 2000; Hope et al. 2006). In all cases, the predictive models had relatively shallow dose-response curves.

Preclinical studies from Groningen showed that combined irradiation of rat hearts and lungs impacted the development of RP: "We confirmed that the tolerance dose for early lung function damage depends not only on the lung region that is irradiated but also that concomitant irradiation of the heart severely reduces the tolerance of the lung" (van Luijk et al. 2005). In a later study they concluded that (van Luijk et al. 2007): "The detrimental effect of dose to the heart on the incidence of [loss of lung function] can be described by a dose dependent decrease in functional reserve of the lung." Other groups, including ours, then started looking for the potential impact of heart irradiation in clinical data. Indeed, we found that heart parameters were frequently selected in bootstrapped multivariate models correlated with RP (Huang et al. 2011), as shown in Fig. 5. "The most significant univariate variables were heart-related, such as heart $V65$ (percent volume receiving at least 65 Gy) (Spearman Rs = 0.245, $p < 0.001$). The best-performing logistic regression model included heart $D10$ (minimum dose to the hottest 10% of the heart), lung $D35$, and maximum lung dose (Spearman Rs = 0.268, $p < 0.0001$)." A later analysis breaking the dataset into cardiac substructures showed that heart variables were even more predictive of RP, with left atrium variables ($D10$, $D20$) dominating lung variables (Huang et al. 2013). Using a separate dataset but from the same institution (WUSTL) again showed that heart dose-volume variables (including $V40$, $D20$, $D30$) were better correlated with RP than lung variables ($D20$ was the best) (Deasy et al. 2012). An analysis published in a later analysis of 258 patients treated at MSKCC showed that heart $D45$ was frequently selected on bootstrap multivariate modeling (von Reibnitz et al. 2019). An analysis of RP risk following RT for mesothelioma in 103 patients found strong heart dose-volume predictors; mean lung dose in contrast was not predictive. An analysis of RP risk following RT for mesothelioma also found strong heart dose-volume predictors; mean lung dose was not predictive (Yorke et al. 2017). In a large group of postoperative RT patients ($N = 243$) relatively low-dose thresholds were important for lung and heart on univariate

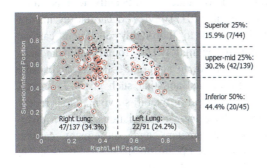
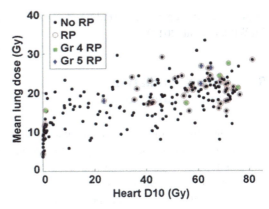

Fig. 5 Complicating factors in radiation pneumonitis. (Left) WUSTL data of GTVs projected onto reference anatomy showing that the rate of RP (red circles) increases as the GTV center of mass is more inferior (Bradley et al. 2007). (Right) WUSTL data showing a role for heart irradiation in RP: RP increases more strongly as heart $D10$ increases independent of lung mean dose. (Reprinted with permission from Huang et al. 2011). We emphasize that a generally valid description of RP causal factors still eludes us and needs more research

analysis (total lung $V4$ and $D75$; heart $V16$ and $D60$) (Shepherd et al. 2021).

However, a detailed analysis by Tucker et al. using a large single-institution dataset investigated many two-parameter models and showed that several models using either lung parameters or mixed heart and lung parameters had similar performance metrics but that heart variables did not have a strong impact. In another large study, Wisjman et al. (2017) included radiation dose to the cardiac atria and ventricles but did not show that whole-heart or heart substructure related DVH variables were important in the prediction of radiation pneumonitis. Likewise, in another comparison of multiple published models using a new MSKCC dataset, only a model with mean lung dose and refit clinical risk factors of pulmonary comorbidity and increasing age was judged as passing validation (Thor et al. 2019a). None of these models has high discrimination. It appears that we are still far from completely understanding dose-volume risk factors for RP.

Focusing on the late effect of lung fibrosis seen in Hodgkin's lymphoma radiotherapy patients, Cella et al. identified a key role for heart irradiation (Cella et al. 2015). Surprisingly, they found that the risk of late lung fibrosis was driven as much or more by heart dose-volume parameters. In particular, the best predictor of late fibrosis was heart $V30$, with minor contributions by lung-related parameters.

Interstitial lung disease is a particularly important pulmonary comorbidity, which can be evaluated via an FDG-PET scans (Li et al. 2018), thereby providing a quantitative risk predictor. FDG-PET at baseline and the uptake of FDG-PET during RT have been shown to be predictors of RP (McCurdy et al. 2012; Castillo et al. 2014; Petit et al. 2011). Inferior location within the lungs still appears to be relevant to the prediction of RP. This was one of the key factors picked up by Bradley et al. and was also a risk factor identified in the voxel-wise analysis of Palma et al. (2019) but was not seen in another large dataset (Vinogradskiy et al. 2012). Future models need to further validate any role of anatomic location.

In summary, knowledge is still unsettled regarding the role of heart dose-volume variables in pneumonitis, as well as dose location in the lungs. Differences in reports could be due to institutional differences in treatment planning guidelines, fractionation schemes, beam arrangements, etc. More research is clearly needed to clarify these issues, preferably using interinstitutional datasets to reduce treatment procedure bias, and to produce more predictive models. Simple modeling methods are seemingly unable to make much more progress on this problem, which likely will require machine learning and/or spatial mapping approaches (Palma et al. 2019; McWilliam et al. 2017).

8 Heart Irradiation and Cardiotoxicity

Perhaps no topic in radiotherapy lung cancer has been as surprising as the emerging appreciation of cardiotoxicity as a common and deadly side effect of thoracic radiotherapy. The field was shaken from its dogmatic slumbers by the randomized Phase III trial RTOG 0617, which showed definitively that 74 Gy treatments, in 2 Gy/weekday fractions, were leading to early mortality compared to 60 Gy treatments with the same fractionation (Bradley et al. 2015). Early dosimetric analysis indicated that some heart-related dosimetric variables were related to this increased mortality. Thor et al. published a detailed dosimetric analysis showing definitively that heart-related dose-volume factors were drivers of limited overall survival, as shown in Fig. 6, although a true spatial identification of the cause was not addressable (Thor et al. 2020). Other reports have added significantly to this story. Dess et al. (2017) reviewed cardiac events for 125 patients to thoroughly document cardiac events following RT. They found that mean heart dose was predictive of grade 3 and greater cardiac toxicity events, and that such grade 3+ events were predictive of overall survival. Other recent reports have shown associations between dose-volume parameters and subsequent cardiac abnormalities (Wang et al. 2017; Speirs et al. 2017; Hotca et al. 2019).

The most detailed spatial analysis to date has been conducted by the Manchester group, who mapped dose distributions to a single representative anatomy for $N = 1101$ patients (McWilliam et al. 2017). Their analysis seems to implicate the base of the heart as a key risk region. As for any single-institution dataset, however, some caution is in order.

The most causally informative analysis to date may be the retrospective review by Atkins et al. (2021), of 701 Harvard patients, to determine the relationship between cardiac substructure irradiation parameters, major adverse cardiac events, and all-cause mortality. Several predictors were

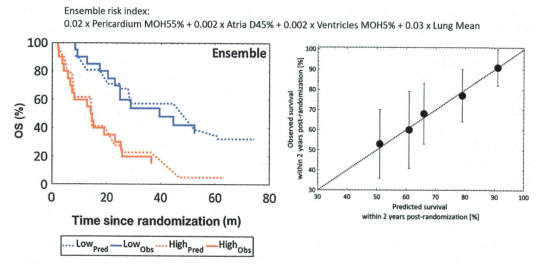

Fig. 6 Dose-volume drivers of risk of early mortality in the Phase III trial RTOG 0617 (Thor et al. 2020). (Left) validation of riskiest 1/6 and safest 1/6 of patients in set-aside validation dataset. The predicted split has excellent agreement with data at all time points. The C-index for the complete validation dataset was $C = 0.89$. (Right) Calibration against the validation dataset was excellent and demonstrates the magnitude of the problem: this is a treatment-caused effect. (Figures used with permission)

identified. Adjusting for other risk factors, treatment plans with left ascending coronary artery $V15$ Gy $> 10\%$ implied increased risk of major cardiac events (HR = 14) as well as mortality (HR = 1.6). It is particularly significant that dosimetric predictors could be tied both to a credible causal mechanism (cardiotoxicity) and to increased mortality. In a related preclinical study, radiation damage to mouse hearts was compared between irradiation of the base, middle, or apex, and it was shown that base irradiation caused the most heart damage (Ghita et al. 2020). In an analysis of heart valve dysfunction following thoracic irradiation for Hodgkin's lymphoma (seen in 30% of patients), it was found that a predictive dosimetric model optimally included both heart- and lung-related terms (Cella et al. 2014), with larger lung volumes (independent of dose) being protective and high heart maximum doses being riskier.

The impact of thoracic irradiation on the immune system is another underexplored topic (Contreras et al. 2018; Thor et al. 2019b). In particular, the potential impact of irradiation of blood as it is repeatedly exposed to radiation during traversals of the cardiovascular system is relatively unknown. A motivating factor is the potential impact of even relatively low-dose irradiation on circulating lymphocytes, which are known to be a very strong biomarker of mortality across many cancer sites (Lambin et al. 2020). The very steep risk separation seen by Thor et al. in the analysis of RTOG 0617 data (Thor et al. 2020), for example, seems to support the idea that cardiotoxicity may not be the entire story, and other mechanisms may also be at work. Avoiding blood irradiation in general is relatively difficult in treatment planning (as represented, for example, by the mean dose to the pericardium), particularly if central lymph nodes need to be irradiated. In contrast, if most cardiotoxicity comes from radiation dose to the region of the left ascending coronary artery/left atrium, then it would be relatively straightforward to implement this region as a strong avoidance structure using AI autocontouring.

9 Bronchial Radiation Toxicity

Early experience of SBRT, often conducted with extremely high equivalent dose values, demonstrated high risks of severe toxicity and death when high-dose regions overlapped with central structures, such as the main branches of the bronchial tree (Timmerman et al. 2014). Irradiation of the central bronchial branches comes with a risk of bleeding, which can range in severity from manageable to fatal (Haseltine et al. 2016). Irradiated bronchial branches often stenose, partially or completely, due to local radiation damage, within a year.

Miller et al. (2005) reported that bronchial stenosis could be observed even in dose-escalated external beam patients, with stenosis of approximately 4% at 74 Gy rising to 25% for patients given approximately 86 Gy in twice weekday fractions of 1.6 Gy. Karlsson et al. (2013) retrospectively analyzed the relationship between atelectasis and the highest dose to the central bronchii for 64 SBRT patients (2–5 fractions of 4–20 Gy). They found a clear increase in radiographic atelectasis based on maximum doses to bronchial volumes (defined as the minimum dose within a 0.1 cc cube.) An LQ-based EQD of 147, assuming alpha/beta = 3 Gy, resulted in an optimal threshold of higher risk.

Careful work by Kazemzadeh et al. (2018) is informative regarding risk of stenosis as a function of local dose and the size of the bronchial branches. Their results indicating a steep bronchial dose-diameter effect: stenosis collapse becomes relatively common above an isotoxic threshold line defined approximately by 45 Gy for 2.5 mm diameter (small bronchii), and 65 Gy to bronchii of 7.5 mm. They clearly demonstrate, as one might expect, that smaller branches stenose at lower doses compared to larger branches that only stenose at larger doses.

Duijm et al. (2016) carefully computed doses to bronchial subregions for patients receiving 50 Gy in five fractions and concluded that stenosis becomes radiographically evident at Dmax > 55 Gy for mid-bronchi or >65 Gy for main stem bronchi, a result that is roughly consistent with what Kazemzadeh et al. saw. Tekalti et al. (2018) pooled hypofractionated lung cancer treatment data from two centers to examine predictors of toxicity. They showed that any overlap between the PTV and trachea or main stem bronchus, or any bronchial volume receiving more than 130 Gy dose, computed in 2 Gy equivalent fractions assuming alpha/beta = 3, was a strong risk factor for toxicity. Hence, it is clear that any attempt to optimize SBRT for lung including central and ultracentral treatments needs to consider the quantitative risk of bronchial stenosis. A quantitative model of bronchial toxicity dose-response would be critical in guiding the safe use of SBRT for central and ultracentral lesions.

10 Putting the Pieces Together: Radiotherapy Planning Using Personalized Dose-Response Curves

As noted at the top of the chapter, current radiotherapy practice for lung cancer takes a generally depersonalized approach to dose and fractionation protocols: patients who look similar regarding basic clinical features typically get the same or very similar dose prescriptions. Given the recent quantitative modeling results described here, we can go beyond such a "one-size-fits-all" paradigm. AAPM Taskgroup 166 (Allen Li et al. 2012) proposed that "...the dose–volume criteria, which are merely surrogate measures of biological responses, should be replaced by biological indices in order for the treatment process to more closely reflect clinical goals of radiotherapy." Along the same lines, to quote Nahum and Uzan (2012): "...if today's sophisticated imaging, treatment planning and radiation-delivery techniques, and tomorrow's genome-based patient biology are to be translated into maximum clinical benefit then the stipulation of a fixed dose to the target volume in today's treatment protocols must be replaced by individualized doses, and, in certain situations, individualized fractionation." Given these advancements, it is now reasonable to revisit this area. As Pizarro and Hernandez remark (2017): "RT treatment schedules can be optimized on a patient-by-patient basis through radiobiological analysis."

Nahum and Uzan have usefully described a scale of increasing sophistication in radiobiological optimization: Level I individualizes prescription dose on an isotoxic (i.e., iso-NTCP) basis; Level II individualizes prescription dose and also the number of fractions on an isotoxic basis; Level III uses radiobiological functions such as gEUD, TCP, or NTCP as direct objective functions in IMRT planning; Level IV is informed by imaging information, for example, by using high FDG-PET regions to guide a boost; finally, Level V uses other personalized biological information, such as radiosensitivity biomarkers based on an assay or genomic profiling. This chapter primarily contemplates Levels I–IV, and in this section we focus on the use of radiobiological functions, or closely correlated dose-volume surrogates, to drive treatment planning.

Nahum and Uzan describe their experience with UK protocols to personalize lung tumor prescriptions to maximize tumor control at a given isotoxicity, using their BioSuite software system. Figure 7, taken from Nahum and Uzan (2012), schematically illustrates personalized TCP and NTCP dose-response curves and the potential advantage of using them to prescribe treatments. They are "personalized" because they are based on treatment planning dose distribution data for a particular patient. The two arrows on the "Tumor Dose" axis indicate two different "isotoxic" prescription doses, both denoted Dpr, that are associated with different NTCP curves corresponding to large overlap or small overlap between the tissue at risk and the target volume. The TCP curve predicts a difference in TCP from ≈45% to ≈90% between these two very different clinical situations.

In Fig. 8, also from Nahum and Uzan (2012), toxicity predictions are shown for radiation pneumonitis and severe esophagitis, for two treatment plans on the same patient case, when the prescription dose is selected to be isoeffective for tumor response. The drop in severe esophagitis is driven by the L-Q correction for smaller fractions,

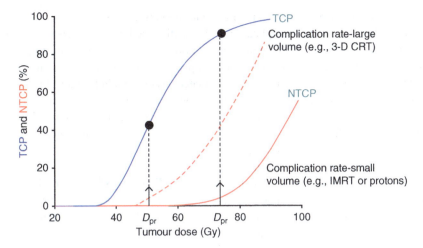

Fig. 7 Illustration of the potential impact of using personalized dose-response curves to guide treatments, from Nahum and Uzan (2012). Here, two different "isotoxic" prescription doses, both denoted Dpr, are associated with illustrative cases which correspond to "large volume" and "small volume" overlap of the high-dose region and the organ at risk. These are very different clinical situations, leading to different NTCP curves, and response curves could be used to inform clinical decisions. (Open-source license)

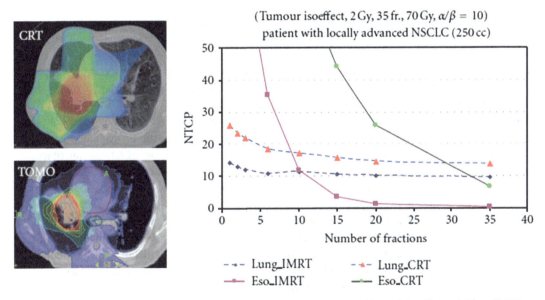

Fig. 8 This figure, from Nahum and Uzan (2012), compares predicted NTCP values, for 3D-CRT and tomotherapy dose distributions shown on the left, at tumor isoeffective doses (according to the L-Q model). Note that esophagitis appears with a stronger fractionation sensitivity than pneumonitis toxicity (denoted Lung_IMRT or Lung_CRT). This type of planning comparison can help choose an optimal fractionation regime for a given patient. (Open-source license)

whereas RP is not known to have a similar fractionation sensitivity. Clearly, optimal fraction selection depends on the details of the dose distribution and is therefore quite patient specific.

Recently, Pizaro and Hernandez (2017) proposed a practical procedure for selecting a dose and fractionation plan on an individualized basis by using radiobiological principles. As a prelude, we define P+ as the probability of achieving tumor control without a major complication, computed as TCP × (1 − NTCP), assuming as usual no radiosensitivity correlations between the endpoints. Begin by generating an initial dose distribution using a target biologically equivalent dose (BED). Next, consider multiple fractionation regimes assuming the same precomputed dose distribution. For each fractionation regime, we can find an optimal fraction dose scaling factor, used to multiply the base treatment plan dose distribution, that will maximize the value of P+. This is a Level II radiobiological optimization process on the scale defined by Nahum and Uzan.

We have been working toward a similar process for ultracentral lung tumors. The interface we constructed was partially shown in Fig. 1. We envision a practical process whereby: (1) a few candidate fractionation regimes are considered in parallel, (2) candidate treatment plans are produced based primarily on dose-volume guidelines for each fractionation scheme, and (3) based on scaling the dose distribution up or down, we first try to find the most hypofractionated (fewest fraction) regime that results in 90% TCP without violating NTCP limits. This may be feasible, for example, if the tumor is spatially isolated from sensitive structures, or impossible, for example, if the tumor abuts dose-sensitive structures such as the esophagus. If the resulting NTCP is too high for any important endpoints, then there is no one-size-fits-all approach. In that case, the physician (and possibly the patient), informed by the tradeoffs between the TCP curve and the NTCP curves, will make a decision. Our premise here is that the shape of these personalized dose-response curves, and the inherent tradeoffs encapsulated therein, should inform the clinical decision.

To make radiobiological planning easier when comparing different fractionation regimes, Schell et al. (2010) point out the advantages of comparing treatment plans using so-called effective dose histograms, whereby each voxel is converted to the dose equivalent if given in a standard number of fractions (e.g., 30). This makes histograms comparable, despite potentially different numbers of delivery fractions. To illustrate, they present an analysis of prostate planning. Due to the intensified cell kill at higher fractional doses, hypofractionation is strongly preferred and the impact on sparing normal tissues can be estimated. They conclude that: "biological models allow the quantitative comparison of different fractionation schemes shedding light on various schemes that are used in clinical practice."

11 Driving Planning Using the Generalized Equivalent Uniform Dose Function

The generalized equivalent uniform dose (gEUD) and equivalent formulations (Kutcher et al. 1991) were used early on to analyze DVHs. The gEUD is attractive mathematically, being a convex function (Choi and Deasy 2002), thereby avoiding multiple local minima, and it has an attractive radiobiological interpretation, according to the tuning parameter, "a" (see Fig. 9). The gEUD function effectively averages over the DVH curve, thus avoiding placing too much emphasis on preselected cut points. Many authors have supported the use of gEUD in optimized planning (Wu et al. 2003). Both the Pinnacle system (Philips) and the Raystation system (Raysearch) currently support using gEUD as an objective function. Another function with attractive computational and radiobiological application is MOHx, the mean of the hottest x%, pronounced "mow." This function, technically known as a mean-tail-dose function (Bortfeld et al. 2008), is convex, meaning it will not lead to suboptimal local trapping in the optimization process (Clark et al. 2008).

The use of full-blown prediction models to drive planning improvements is still in the startup phase in radiotherapy. Possibly the first systematic use of radiobiological optimization is the report from Christianen et al. (2016), on a clinical trial to test the value of optimizing to reduce the predicted risk of late swallowing toxicity in head and neck cancer patients treated with IMRT. In a remarkable success, rates of dysphagia at 6 months post-RT were reduced at a level exactly predicted by the modeling (27.5% reduced to

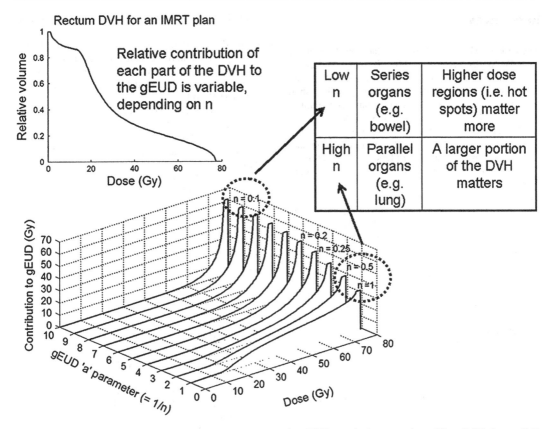

Fig. 9 How does the generalized equivalent uniform dose (gEUD) function work? The gEUD function has a single parameter that determines the part of the DVH curve that is given the most weight. This parameter (confusingly) is either written as "*a*" or "*n*," where $a = 1/n$. When "*a*" is 1, the gEUD equals the mean dose. When "*a*" is larger ("*n*" is <1), the gEUD preferentially weights the high-dose part of the DVH, as shown. (Reprinted with permission from Marks et al. 2010a)

22.6%). Other emerging uses of prediction models for planning include approaches for selecting patients who are likely to benefit from proton therapy (Rwigema et al. 2019; Langendijk et al. 2018).

12 Conclusion

Our goal in this short chapter has been to emphasize emerging knowledge in lung cancer radiotherapy that could be used to implement clinical protocols to select treatments based on predictive models and the resulting personalized dose-response curves. Such an approach furthermore has the virtue of being inexpensive once validated predictive models and planning tools become widely commercially available. At the same time, this review has highlighted multiple areas where continued research could reduce uncertainty and increase the power of the resulting predictive models. Emerging paradigms of immunotherapies and targeted agents, for example, will likely require extensive study of the impact on the models discussed here.

Acknowledgments We gratefully acknowledge funding support from the US NIH (R01CA198121, R01CA085181) and Varian Corporation. Many colleagues have contributed to ideas and results emphasized in this chapter, including Jeffrey Bradley, Clifford Robinson, Andrew Hope, Patricia Lindsay, James Alaly, Gita Suneja, Andrew Fontanella, Mireia Crispin-Ortuzar, Vanessa Clark, Paras Tiwari, Yao Xie, Yixin Chen, Ellen Huang, and Allen Nahum.

References

Allen Li X, Alber M, Deasy JO, Jackson A, Ken Jee K-W, Marks LB, Martel MK, Mayo C, Moiseenko V, Nahum AE et al (2012) The use and QA of biologically related models for treatment planning: short report of the TG-166 of the therapy physics committee of the AAPM. Med Phys 39(3):1386–1409

Apolle R, Rehm M, Bortfeld T, Baumann M, Troost EGC (2017) The clinical target volume in lung, head-and-neck, and esophageal cancer: lessons from pathological measurement and recurrence analysis. Clin Transl Radiat Oncol 3:1–8

Atkins KM, Chaunzwa TL, Lamba N, Bitterman DS, Rawal B, Bredfeldt J, Williams CL, Kozono DE, Baldini EH, Nohria A, Hoffmann U, Aerts HJW, Mak RH (2021) Association of left anterior descending coronary artery radiation dose with major adverse cardiac events and mortality in patients with non–small cell lung cancer. JAMA Oncol 7(2):206–219

Belderbos J, Heemsbergen W, Hoogeman M, Pengel K, Rossi M, Lebesque J (2005) Acute esophageal toxicity in non-small cell lung cancer patients after high dose conformal radiotherapy. Radiother Oncol 75(2):157–164

Bentzen SM, Constine LS, Deasy JO, Eisbruch A, Jackson A, Marks LB, Ten Haken RK, Yorke ED (2010) Quantitative Analyses of Normal Tissue Effects in the Clinic (QUANTEC): an introduction to the scientific issues. Int J Radiat Oncol Biol Phys 76(3 Suppl):S3–S9

Bortfeld T, Craft D, Dempsey JF, Halabi T, Romeijn HE (2008) Evaluating target cold spots by the use of tail EUDs. Int J Radiat Oncol Biol Phys 71(3):880–889

Bradley JD, Hope A, El Naqa I, Apte A, Lindsay PE, Bosch W, Matthews J, Sause W, Graham MV, Deasy JO, RTOG (2007) A nomogram to predict radiation pneumonitis, derived from a combined analysis of RTOG 9311 and institutional data. Int J Radiat Oncol Biol Phys 69(4):985–992

Bradley JD, Paulus R, Komaki R, Masters G, Blumenschein G, Schild S, Bogart J, Hu C, Forster K, Magliocco A, Kavadi V, Garces YI, Narayan S, Iyengar P, Robinson C, Wynn RB, Koprowski C, Meng J, Beitler J, Gaur R, Curran W Jr, Choy H (2015) Standard-dose versus high-dose conformal radiotherapy with concurrent and consolidation carboplatin plus paclitaxel with or without cetuximab for patients with stage IIIA or IIIB non-small-cell lung cancer (RTOG 0617): a randomised, two-by-two factorial phase 3 study. Lancet Oncol 16(2):187–199

Braun RD, Lanzen JL, Dewhirst MW (1999) Fourier analysis of fluctuations of oxygen tension and blood flow in R3230Ac tumors and muscle in rats. Am J Physiol Heart Circ Physiol 277(2):H551–H568

Brodin NP, Kabarriti R, Garg MK, Guha C, Tomé WA (2018) Systematic review of normal tissue complication models relevant to standard fractionation radiation therapy of the head and neck region published after the QUANTEC reports. Int J Radiat Oncol Biol Phys 100(2):391–407

Carlson DJ, Stewart RD, Semenenko VA (2006) Effects of oxygen on intrinsic radiation sensitivity: a test of the relationship between aerobic and hypoxic linear-quadratic (LQ) model parameters. Med Phys 33(9):3105–3115

Castillo R, Pham N, Ansari S, Meshkov D, Castillo S, Li M, Olanrewaju A, Hobbs B, Castillo E, Guerrero T (2014) Pre-radiotherapy FDG PET predicts radiation pneumonitis in lung cancer. Radiat Oncol 9:74

Cella L, Palma G, Deasy JO, Oh JH, Liuzzi R, D'Avino V, Conson M, Pugliese N, Picardi M, Salvatore M, Pacelli R (2014) Complication probability models for radiation-induced heart valvular dysfunction: do heart-lung interactions play a role? PLoS One 9(10):e111753

Cella L, D'Avino V, Palma G, Conson M, Liuzzi R, Picardi M, Pressello MC, Boboc GI, Battistini R, Donato V, Pacelli R (2015) Modeling the risk of radiation-induced lung fibrosis: irradiated heart tissue is as important as irradiated lung. Radiother Oncol 117(1):36–43

Chang BK, Timmerman RD (2007) Stereotactic body radiation therapy: a comprehensive review. Am J Clin Oncol 30(6):637–644

Chao KSC, Blanco AI, Dempsey JF (2003) A conceptual model integrating spatial information to assess target volume coverage for IMRT treatment planning. Int J Radiat Oncol Biol Phys 56(5):1438–1449

Chapet O, Kong F-M, Lee JS, Hayman JA, Ten Haken RK (2005) Normal tissue complication probability modeling for acute esophagitis in patients treated with conformal radiation therapy for non-small cell lung cancer. Radiother Oncol 77(2):176–181

Cox JD, Azarnia N, Byhardt RW, Shin KH, Emami B, Perez CA (1991) N2 (clinical) non-small cell carcinoma of the lung: prospective trials of radiation therapy with total doses 60 Gy by the radiation therapy oncology group. Int J Radiat Oncol Biol Phys 20(1):7–12

Hill RP (2017) The changing paradigm of tumour response to irradiation. Br J Radiol 90(1069):20160474

Riaz N, Sherman EJ, Katabi N, Leeman JE, Higginson DS, Boyle J, Singh B, Morris LG, Wong RJ, Tsai CJ, Schupak K, Gelblum DY, McBride SM, Hatzoglou V, Baxi SS, Pfister DG, Dave A, Humm J, Schöder H, Lee NY (2017) A personalized approach using hypoxia resolution to guide curative-intent radiation dose-reduction to 30 Gy: a novel de-escalation paradigm for HPV-associated oropharynx cancers (OPC). J Clin Oncol 35(15_Suppl):6076

Zhang P, Yorke E, Hu Y-C, Mageras G, Rimner A, Deasy JO (2014) Predictive treatment management: incorporating a predictive tumor response model into robust prospective treatment planning for non-small cell lung cancer. Int J Radiat Oncol Biol Phys 88(2):446–452

Seibert RM, Ramsey CR, Hines JW, Kupelian PA, Langen KM, Meeks SL, Scaperoth DD (2007) A model for predicting lung cancer response to therapy. Int J Radiat Oncol Biol Phys 67(2):601–609

Zhang P, Yorke E, Mageras G, Rimner A, Sonke J-J, Deasy JO (2018) Validating a predictive atlas of tumor shrinkage for adaptive radiotherapy of locally advanced lung cancer. Int J Radiat Oncol Biol Phys. https://doi.org/10.1016/j.ijrobp.2018.05.056

Deasy JO, Mayo CS, Orton CG (2015) Treatment planning evaluation and optimization should be biologically and not dose/volume based. Med Phys 42(6):2753–2756

Marks LB, Yorke ED, Jackson A, Ten Haken RK, Constine LS, Eisbruch A, Bentzen SM, Nam J, Deasy JO (2010a) Use of normal tissue complication probability models in the clinic. Int J Radiat Oncol Biol Phys 76(3 Suppl):S10–S19

Joiner MC, van der Kogel A (2016) Basic clinical radiobiology, 5th edn. CRC Press, Boca Raton, FL. 384 p

Rancati T, Fiorino C (2019) Modelling radiotherapy side effects: practical applications for planning optimisation. CRC Press, Boca Raton, FL. 494 p

Shrieve DC, Loeffler JS (2010) Human radiation injury. Lippincott Williams & Wilkins, Philadelphia. 533 p

Werner-Wasik M, Yorke E, Deasy J, Nam J, Marks LB (2010) Radiation dose-volume effects in the esophagus. Int J Radiat Oncol Biol Phys 76(3 Suppl):S86–S93

Marks LB, Bentzen SM, Deasy JO (2010b) Radiation dose–volume effects in the lung. Int J Radiat Oncol Biol Phys. http://www.redjournal.org/article/S0360-3016(09)03293-3/abstract

Okunieff P, Morgan D, Niemierko A, Suit HD (1995) Radiation dose-response of human tumors. Int J Radiat Oncol Biol Phys 32(4):1227–1237

Overgaard J (2011) Hypoxic modification of radiotherapy in squamous cell carcinoma of the head and neck—a systematic review and meta-analysis. Radiother Oncol 100(1):22–32

Nahum AE, Movsas B, Horwitz EM, Stobbe CC, Chapman JD (2003) Incorporating clinical measurements of hypoxia into tumor local control modeling of prostate cancer: implications for the α/β ratio. Int J Radiat Oncol Biol Phys 57(2):391–401

Donald Chapman J, Nahum AE (2016) Radiotherapy treatment planning: linear-quadratic radiobiology. CRC Press, Boca Raton, FL. 190 p

Withers HR, Taylor JM, Maciejewski B (1988) The hazard of accelerated tumor clonogen repopulation during radiotherapy. Acta Oncol 27(2):131–146

Fowler JF (1991) The phantom of tumor treatment-continually rapid proliferation unmasked. Radiother Oncol 22(3):156–158

Fowler JF, Lindstrom MJ (1992) Loss of local control with prolongation in radiotherapy. Int J Radiat Oncol Biol Phys 23(2):457–467

Petersen C, Zips D, Krause M, Schöne K, Eicheler W, Hoinkis C, Thames HD, Baumann M (2001) Repopulation of FaDu human squamous cell carcinoma during fractionated radiotherapy correlates with reoxygenation. Int J Radiat Oncol Biol Phys 51(2):483–493

Dierckx RA, Van de Wiele C (2008) FDG uptake, a surrogate of tumour hypoxia? Eur J Nucl Med Mol Imaging 35(8):1544–1549

Jeong J, Deasy JO (2014) Modeling the relationship between fluorodeoxyglucose uptake and tumor radioresistance as a function of the tumor microenvironment. Comput Math Methods Med 2014:847162

Dewhirst MW, Secomb TW (2017) Transport of drugs from blood vessels to tumour tissue. Nat Rev Cancer 17(12):738–750

Lan L, Izatt JA, Dewhirst MW (2010) Longitudinal optical imaging of tumor metabolism and hemodynamics. J Biomed Opt. https://doi.org/10.1117/1.3285584.short

Dewhirst MW, Braun RD, Lanzen JL (1998) Temporal changes in PO_2 of R3230AC tumors in Fischer-344 rats. Int J Radiat Oncol Biol Phys 42(4):723–726

Shuryak I, Carlson DJ, Brown JM, Brenner DJ (2015) High-dose and fractionation effects in stereotactic radiation therapy: analysis of tumor control data from 2965 patients. Radiother Oncol 115(3):327–334

Webb S, Nahum AE (1993) A model for calculating tumour control probability in radiotherapy including the effects of inhomogeneous distributions of dose and clonogenic cell density. Phys Med Biol 38(6):653–666

Prokopiou S, Moros EG, Poleszczuk J, Caudell J, Torres-Roca JF, Latifi K, Lee JK, Myerson R, Harrison LB, Enderling H (2015) A proliferation saturation index to predict radiation response and personalize radiotherapy fractionation. Radiat Oncol 10:159

Jeong J, Shoghi KI, Deasy JO (2013) Modelling the interplay between hypoxia and proliferation in radiotherapy tumour response. Phys Med Biol 58(14):4897–4919

Jeong J, Oh JH, Sonke J-J, Belderbos J, Bradley JD, Fontanella AN, Rao SS, Deasy JO (2017) Modeling the cellular response of lung cancer to radiation therapy for a broad range of fractionation schedules. Clin Cancer Res 23(18):5469–5479

Guerrero M, Allen Li X (2004) Extending the linear–quadratic model for large fraction doses pertinent to stereotactic radiotherapy. Phys Med Biol 49(20):4825

Jeong J, Taasti VT, Jackson A, Deasy JO (2020) The relative biological effectiveness of carbon ion radiation therapy for early stage lung cancer. Radiother Oncol. https://doi.org/10.1016/j.radonc.2020.09.027

Crispin-Ortuzar M, Jeong J, Fontanella AN, Deasy JO (2017) A radiobiological model of radiotherapy response and its correlation with prognostic imaging variables. Phys Med Biol 62(7):2658–2674

Ruggieri R, Stavrev P, Naccarato S, Stavreva N, Alongi F, Nahum AE (2017) Optimal dose and fraction number in SBRT of lung tumours: a radiobiological analysis. Phys Med 44:188–195

Hope AJ, Lindsay PE, El Naqa I, Bradley JD, Vivic M, Deasy JO (2005) Clinical, dosimetric, and location-related factors to predict local control in non-small cell lung cancer. Int J Radiat Oncol Biol Phys 63:S231

Morgan-Fletcher SL (2001) Prescribing, recording and reporting photon beam therapy (Supplement to ICRU Report 50), ICRU Report 62. ICRU, pp. ix+52, 1999

(ICRU Bethesda, MD) $65.00 ISBN 0-913394-61-0. BJR Suppl 74(879):294

Purdy JA (2004) Current ICRU definitions of volumes: limitations and future directions. Semin Radiat Oncol 14(1):27–40

Grills IS, Fitch DL, Goldstein NS, Yan D, Chmielewski GW, Welsh RJ, Kestin LL (2007) Clinicopathologic analysis of microscopic extension in lung adenocarcinoma: defining clinical target volume for radiotherapy. Int J Radiat Oncol Biol Phys 69(2):334–341

Kara M, Sak SD, Orhan D, Yavuzer S (2000) Changing patterns of lung cancer; (3/4 in.) 1.9 cm; still a safe length for bronchial resection margin? Lung Cancer 30(3):161–168

Giraud P, Antoine M, Larrouy A, Milleron B, Callard P, De Rycke Y, Carette M-F, Rosenwald J-C, Cosset J-M, Housset M, Touboul E (2000) Evaluation of microscopic tumor extension in non–small-cell lung cancer for three-dimensional conformal radiotherapy planning. Int J Radiat Oncol Biol Phys 48(4):1015–1024

Siedschlag C, Boersma L, van Loon J, Rossi M, van Baardwijk A, Gilhuijs K, Stroom J (2011) The impact of microscopic disease on the tumor control probability in non-small-cell lung cancer. Radiother Oncol 100(3):344–350

Salguero FJ, Belderbos JSA, Rossi MMG, Blaauwgeers JLG, Stroom J, Sonke J-J (2013) Microscopic disease extensions as a risk factor for loco-regional recurrence of NSCLC after SBRT. Radiother Oncol 109(1):26–31

van Loon J, Siedschlag C, Stroom J, Blauwgeers H, van Suylen R-J, Knegjens J, Rossi M, van Baardwijk A, Boersma L, Klomp H et al (2012) Microscopic disease extension in three dimensions for non–small-cell lung cancer: development of a prediction model using pathology-validated positron emission tomography and computed tomography features. Int J Radiat Oncol Biol Phys 82(1):448–456

Meng X, Sun X, Mu D, Xing L, Ma L, Zhang B, Zhao S, Yang G, Kong F-MS, Yu J (2012) Noninvasive evaluation of microscopic tumor extensions using standardized uptake value and metabolic tumor volume in non-small-cell lung cancer. Int J Radiat Oncol Biol Phys 82(2):960–966

Shusharina N, Craft D, Chen Y-L, Shih H, Bortfeld T (2018) The clinical target distribution: a probabilistic alternative to the clinical target volume. Phys Med Biol 63(15):155001

Schanne D, Unkelbach J, Guckenberger M (2019) Lungs and esophagus. Modelling radiotherapy side effects: practical applications for planning optimisation. CRC Press, Boca Raton, FL, p 243

Deasy JO, Muren LP (2014) Advancing our quantitative understanding of radiotherapy normal tissue morbidity. Acta Oncol 53(5):577–579

Thor M, Deasy JO, Hu C, Gore E, Bar-Ad V, Robinson C, Wheatley M, Oh JH, Bogart J, Garces YI, Kavadi VS, Narayan S, Iyengar P, Witt JS, Welsh JW, Koprowski CD, Larner JM, Xiao Y, Bradley J (2020) Modeling the impact of cardio-pulmonary irradiation on overall survival in NRG Oncology trial RTOG 0617.

Clin Cancer Res. https://doi.org/10.1158/1078-0432.CCR-19-2627

Clark VH, Chen Y, Wilkens J, Alaly JR, Zakaryan K, Deasy JO (2008) IMRT treatment planning for prostate cancer using prioritized prescription optimization and mean-tail-dose functions. Linear Algebra Appl 428(5–6):1345–1364

Choi B, Deasy JO (2002) The generalized equivalent uniform dose function as a basis for intensity-modulated treatment planning. Phys Med Biol 47(20):3579–3589

Huang EX, Bradley JD, El Naqa I, Hope AJ, Lindsay PE, Bosch WR, Matthews JW, Sause WT, Graham MV, Deasy JO (2012) Modeling the risk of radiation-induced acute esophagitis for combined Washington University and RTOG trial 93-11 lung cancer patients. Int J Radiat Oncol Biol Phys 82(5):1674–1679

Yorke ED, Thor M, Gelblum DY, Gomez DR, Rimner A, Shaverdian N, Shepherd AF, Simone CB II, Wu A, McKnight D, Jackson A (2021) Treatment planning and outcomes effects of reducing the preferred mean esophagus dose for conventionally fractionated non-small cell lung cancer radiotherapy. J Appl Clin Med Phys 22(2):42–48

Thor M, Deasy J, Iyer A, Bendau E, Fontanella A, Apte A, Yorke E, Rimner A, Jackson A (2019a) Toward personalized dose-prescription in locally advanced non-small cell lung cancer: validation of published normal tissue complication probability models. Radiother Oncol 138:45–51

Huang EX, Robinson CG, Molotievschi A, Bradley JD, Deasy JO, Oh JH (2017) Independent test of a model to predict severe acute esophagitis. Adv Radiat Oncol 2(1):37–43

Oberije C, De Ruysscher D, Houben R, van de Heuvel M, Uyterlinde W, Deasy JO, Belderbos J, Dingemans A-MC, Rimner A, Din S, Lambin P (2015) A validated prediction model for overall survival from stage III non-small cell lung cancer: toward survival prediction for individual patients. Int J Radiat Oncol Biol Phys 92(4):935–944

Hallqvist A, Bergström S, Björkestrand H, Svärd A-M, Ekman S, Lundin E, Holmberg E, Johansson M, Friesland S, Nyman J (2018) Dose escalation to 84 Gy with concurrent chemotherapy in stage III NSCLC appears excessively toxic: results from a prematurely terminated randomized phase II trial. Lung Cancer 122:180–186

Kamran SC, Yeap BY, Ulysse CA, Cronin C, Bowes CL, Durgin B, Gainor JF, Khandekar MJ, Tansky JY, Keane FK et al (2021) Assessment of a contralateral esophagus-sparing technique in locally advanced lung cancer treated with high-dose chemoradiation: a phase 1 nonrandomized clinical trial. JAMA Oncol. https://jamanetwork.com/journals/jamaoncology/article-abstract/2778095

Stephans KL, Djemil T, Diaconu C, Reddy CA, Xia P, Woody NM, Greskovich J, Makkar V, Videtic GMM (2014) Esophageal dose tolerance to hypofractionated stereotactic body radiation therapy: risk factors for late toxicity. Int J Radiat Oncol Biol Phys 90(1):197–202

Wu AJ, Williams E, Modh A, Foster A, Yorke E, Rimner A, Jackson A (2014) Dosimetric predictors of esophageal toxicity after stereotactic body radiotherapy for central lung tumors. Radiother Oncol 112(2):267–271

Small W, Woloschak GE (2006) Radiation toxicity: a practical medical guide. Springer Science & Business Media, New York. 187 p

Giuranno L, Ient J, De Ruysscher D, Vooijs MA (2019) Radiation-induced lung injury (RILI). Front Oncol 9:877

Seppenwoolde Y, Muller SH, Theuws JCM, Baas P, Belderbos JSA, Boersma LJ, Lebesque JV (2000) Radiation dose-effect relations and local recovery in perfusion for patients with non–small-cell lung cancer. Int J Radiat Oncol Biol Phys 47(3):681–690

Hope AJ, Lindsay PE, El Naqa I, Alaly JR, Vicic M, Bradley JD, Deasy JO (2006) Modeling radiation pneumonitis risk with clinical, dosimetric, and spatial parameters. Int J Radiat Oncol Biol Phys 65(1):112–124

Huang EX, Hope AJ, Lindsay PE, Trovo M, El Naqa I, Deasy JO, Bradley JD (2011) Heart irradiation as a risk factor for radiation pneumonitis. Acta Oncol 50(1):51–60

van Luijk P, Novakova-Jiresova A, Faber H, Schippers JM, Kampinga HH, Meertens H, Coppes RP (2005) Radiation damage to the heart enhances early radiation-induced lung function loss. Cancer Res 65(15):6509–6511

van Luijk P, Faber H, Meertens H, Schippers JM, Langendijk JA, Brandenburg S, Kampinga HH, Coppes RP (2007) The impact of heart irradiation on dose–volume effects in the rat lung. Int J Radiat Oncol Biol Phys 69(2):552–559

Huang E, Folkert M, Bradley J, Apte A, Deasy J (2013) TU-G-108-02: left atrium dose-volume parameters predict for clinically significant radiation pneumonitis. Med Phys 40(6Part27):453

Deasy J, Robinson C, Huang E, Molotievschi A, Bradley J (2012) Independent test of a model to predict radiation pneumonitis after definitive radiation therapy for locally advanced non-small cell lung cancer: heart irradiation is (again) a statistically significant risk factor. Int J Radiat Oncol Biol Phys 84(3):S32

von Reibnitz D, Yorke ED, Oh JH, Apte AP, Yang J, Pham H, Thor M, Wu AJ, Fleisher M, Gelb E, Deasy JO, Rimner A (2019) Serum alpha-2-macroglobulin as an intrinsic radioprotective factor in patients undergoing thoracic radiation therapy. bioRXiv. https://doi.org/10.1101/656090

Yorke ED, Jackson A, Kuo LC, Ojo A, Panchoo K, Adusumilli P, Zauderer MG, Rusch VW, Shepherd A, Rimner A (2017) Heart dosimetry is correlated with risk of radiation pneumonitis after lung-sparing hemithoracic pleural intensity modulated radiation therapy for malignant pleural mesothelioma. Int J Radiat Oncol Biol Phys 99(1):61–69

Shepherd AF, Iocolano M, Leeman J, Imber BS, Wild AT, Offin M, Chaft JE, Huang J, Rimner A, Wu AJ, Gelblum DY, Shaverdian N, Simone CB II, Gomez DR, Yorke ED, Jackson A (2021) Clinical and dosimetric predictors of radiation pneumonitis in patients with non-small cell lung cancer undergoing postoperative radiation therapy. Pract Radiat Oncol 11(1):e52–e62

Wijsman R, Dankers FJ, Troost EGC, Hoffmann AL, van der Heijden EH, de Geus-Oei L-F, Bussink J (2017) Inclusion of incidental radiation dose to the cardiac atria and ventricles does not improve the prediction of radiation pneumonitis in advanced-stage non-small cell lung cancer patients treated with intensity modulated radiation therapy. Int J Radiat Oncol Biol Phys 99(2):434–441

Li F, Zhou Z, Wu A, Cai Y, Wu H, Chen M, Liang S (2018) Preexisting radiological interstitial lung abnormalities are a risk factor for severe radiation pneumonitis in patients with small-cell lung cancer after thoracic radiation therapy. Radiat Oncol 13(1):82

McCurdy MR, Castillo R, Martinez J, Al Hallack MN, Lichter J, Zouain N, Guerrero T (2012) [18F]-FDG uptake dose–response correlates with radiation pneumonitis in lung cancer patients. Radiother Oncol 104(1):52–57

Petit SF, van Elmpt WJC, Oberije CJG, Vegt E, Dingemans A-MC, Lambin P, Dekker AL, De Ruyscher D (2011) [18F] fluorodeoxyglucose uptake patterns in lung before radiotherapy identify areas more susceptible to radiation-induced lung toxicity in non-small-cell lung cancer patients. Int J Radiat Oncol Biol Phys 81(3):698–705

Palma G, Monti S, Xu T, Scifoni E, Yang P, Hahn SM, Durante M, Mohan R, Liao Z, Cella L (2019) Spatial dose patterns associated with radiation pneumonitis in a randomized trial comparing intensity-modulated radiation therapy with passive scattering proton therapy for locally advanced non-small cell lung cancer. Int J Radiat Oncol Biol Phys. https://www.sciencedirect.com/science/article/pii/S0360301619302743

Vinogradskiy Y, Tucker SL, Liao Z, Martel MK (2012) Investigation of the relationship between gross tumor volume location and pneumonitis rates using a large clinical database of non-small-cell lung cancer patients. Int J Radiat Oncol Biol Phys 82(5):1650–1658

McWilliam A, Kennedy J, Hodgson C, Vasquez Osorio E, Faivre-Finn C, van Herk M (2017) Radiation dose to heart base linked with poorer survival in lung cancer patients. Eur J Cancer 85:106–113

Dess RT, Sun Y, Matuszak MM, Sun G, Soni PD, Bazzi L, Murthy VL, Hearn JWD, Kong F-M, Kalemkerian GP, Hayman JA, Ten Haken RK, Lawrence TS, Schipper MJ, Jolly S (2017) Cardiac events after radiation therapy: combined analysis of prospective multicenter trials for locally advanced non-small-cell lung cancer. J Clin Oncol 35(13):1395–1402

Wang K, Pearlstein KA, Patchett ND, Deal AM, Mavroidis P, Jensen BC, Lipner MB, Zagar TM, Wang Y, Lee CB, Eblan MJ, Rosenman JG, Socinski MA, Stinchcombe TE, Marks LB (2017) Heart dosimetric analysis of three types of cardiac toxicity in patients treated on dose-escalation trials for Stage III non-small-cell lung cancer. Radiother Oncol 125(2):293–300

Speirs CK, DeWees TA, Rehman S, Molotievschi A, Velez MA, Mullen D, Fergus S, Trovo M, Bradley JD, Robinson CG (2017) Heart dose is an independent dosimetric predictor of overall survival in locally advanced non–small cell lung cancer. J Thorac Oncol 12(2):293–301

Hotca A, Thor M, Deasy JO, Rimner A (2019) Dose to the cardio-pulmonary system and treatment-induced electrocardiogram abnormalities in locally advanced non-small cell lung cancer. Clin Transl Radiat Oncol 19:96–102

Ghita M, Gill EK, Walls GM, Edgar KS, McMahon SJ, Osorio EV, Bergom C, Grieve DJ, Watson CJ, McWilliam A, Aznar M, van Herk M, Williams KJ, Butterworth KT (2020) Cardiac sub-volume targeting demonstrates regional radiosensitivity in the mouse heart. Radiother Oncol 152:216–221

Contreras JA, Lin AJ, Weiner A, Speirs C, Samson P, Mullen D, Campian J, Bradley J, Roach M, Robinson C (2018) Cardiac dose is associated with immunosuppression and poor survival in locally advanced non-small cell lung cancer. Radiother Oncol 128(3):498–504

Thor M, Montovano M, Hotca A, Luo L, Jackson A, Wu AJ, Deasy JO, Rimner A (2019b) Are unsatisfactory outcomes after concurrent chemoradiotherapy for locally advanced non-small cell lung cancer due to treatment-related immunosuppression? Radiother Oncol. https://doi.org/10.1016/j.radonc.2019.07.016

Lambin P, Lieverse RIY, Eckert F, Marcus D, Oberije C, van der Wiel AMA, Guha C, Dubois LJ, Deasy JO (2020) Lymphocyte-sparing radiotherapy: the rationale for protecting lymphocyte-rich organs when combining radiotherapy with immunotherapy. Semin Radiat Oncol 30(2):187–193

Timmerman RD, Herman J, Cho LC (2014) Emergence of stereotactic body radiation therapy and its impact on current and future clinical practice. J Clin Oncol 32(26):2847–2854

Haseltine JM, Rimner A, Gelblum DY, Modh A, Rosenzweig KE, Jackson A, Yorke ED, Wu AJ (2016) Fatal complications after stereotactic body radiation therapy for central lung tumors abutting the proximal bronchial tree. Pract Radiat Oncol 6(2):e27–e33

Miller KL, Shafman TD, Anscher MS, Zhou S-M, Clough RW, Garst JL, Crawford J, Rosenman J, Socinski MA, Blackstock W, Sibley GS, Marks LB (2005) Bronchial stenosis: an underreported complication of high-dose external beam radiotherapy for lung cancer? Int J Radiat Oncol Biol Phys 61(1):64–69

Karlsson K, Nyman J, Baumann P, Wersäll P, Drugge N, Gagliardi G, Johansson K-A, Persson J-O, Rutkowska E, Tullgren O, Lax I (2013) Retrospective cohort study of bronchial doses and radiation-induced atelectasis after stereotactic body radiation therapy of lung tumors located close to the bronchial tree. Int J Radiat Oncol Biol Phys 87(3):590–595

Kazemzadeh N, Modiri A, Samanta S, Yan Y, Bland R, Rozario T, Wibowo H, Iyengar P, Ahn C, Timmerman R, Sawant A (2018) Virtual bronchoscopy-guided treatment planning to map and mitigate radiation-induced airway injury in lung SAbR. Int J Radiat Oncol Biol Phys 102(1):210–218

Duijm M, Schillemans W, Aerts JG, Heijmen B, Nuyttens JJ (2016) Dose and volume of the irradiated main bronchi and related side effects in the treatment of central lung tumors with stereotactic radiotherapy. Semin Radiat Oncol 26(2):140–148

Tekatli H, Duijm M, Oomen-de Hoop E, Verbakel W, Schillemans W, Slotman BJ, Nuyttens JJ, Senan S (2018) Normal tissue complication probability modeling of pulmonary toxicity after stereotactic and hypofractionated radiation therapy for central lung tumors. Int J Radiat Oncol Biol Phys 100(3):738–747

Nahum AE, Uzan J (2012) (Radio)biological optimization of external-beam radiotherapy. Comput Math Methods Med. https://www.hindawi.com/journals/cmmm/2012/329214/abs/

Pizarro F, Hernández A (2017) Optimization of radiotherapy fractionation schedules based on radiobiological functions. Br J Radiol 90(1079):20170400

Schell S, Wilkens JJ, Oelfke U (2010) Radiobiological effect based treatment plan optimization with the linear quadratic model. Z Med Phys 20(3):188–196

Kutcher GJ, Burman C, Brewster L, Goitein M, Mohan R (1991) Histogram reduction method for calculating complication probabilities for three-dimensional treatment planning evaluations. Int J Radiat Oncol Biol Phys 21(1):137–146

Wu Q, Djajaputra D, Wu Y, Zhou J, Liu HH, Mohan R (2003) Intensity-modulated radiotherapy optimization with gEUD-guided dose–volume objectives. Phys Med Biol 48(3):279

Christianen MEMC, van der Schaaf A, van der Laan HP, Verdonck-de Leeuw IM, Doornaert P, Chouvalova O, Steenbakkers RJHM, Leemans CR, Oosting SF, van der Laan BFAM, Roodenburg JLN, Slotman BJ, Bijl HP, Langendijk JA (2016) Swallowing sparing intensity modulated radiotherapy (SW-IMRT) in head and neck cancer: clinical validation according to the model-based approach. Radiother Oncol 118(2):298–303

Rwigema J-CM, Langendijk JA, Paul van der Laan H, Lukens JN, Swisher-McClure SD, Lin A (2019) A model-based approach to predict short-term toxicity benefits with proton therapy for oropharyngeal cancer. Int J Radiat Oncol Biol Phys 104(3):553–562

Langendijk JA, Boersma LJ, Rasch CRN, van Vulpen M, Reitsma JB, van der Schaaf A, Schuit E (2018) Clinical trial strategies to compare protons with photons. Semin Radiat Oncol 28(2):79–87

Tumor Motion Control

Hiroki Shirato, Shinichi Shimizu, Hiroshi Taguchi, Seishin Takao, Naoki Miyamoto, and Taeko Matsuura

Contents

1 Overview 214
2 **Anatomical Concerns in Tumor Motion** 215
2.1 Physiological Conditions 215
2.2 Pathological Conditions 217
3 **Tumor Motion Control Process and Risk Management** 218
4 **Treatment Preparation and 4D Planning** 218
4.1 Imaging 218
4.2 The Safety Margin Approach 218
4.3 The Robust Approach 221
5 **Tumor Motion Control Maneuvers** 222
5.1 Relaxed Steady Breathing 222
5.2 Stereotactic Body Frames and Compression Plates 222
5.3 Deep Inspiration Breath Holding (DIBH) 222
5.4 Active Breathing Control (ABC) 223
6 **Adaptive External Beam Radiotherapy Systems (AEBRS) for Intrafractional Movements of Target Volumes** 223
6.1 General Concept 223
6.2 Beam Gating Using External Surrogate Markers 225
6.3 Beam Gating Using Internal Fiducial Markers 226
6.4 Beam Tracking 226
7 **Fiducial Markers** 228
8 **Setup of Patients** 228
9 **Delivery of the Beam** 228
9.1 Interplay Effects 228
9.2 Intrafractional Baseline Shift/Drift 229
9.3 Real-Time-Image Gated Proton Beam Therapy (RGPT) 230
10 **Clinical Studies** 232
11 **Concluding Remarks** 232
References 232

H. Shirato (✉)
Faculty of Medicine, Hokkaido University, Sapporo, Japan
e-mail: shirato@med.hokudai.ac.jp; hshirato@gmail.com

S. Shimizu
Faculty of Medicine, Osaka University, Osaka, Japan

H. Taguchi
Hokkaido University Hospital, Sapporo, Japan

S. Takao · N. Miyamoto · T. Matsuura
Faculty of Engineering, Hokkaido University, Sapporo, Japan

Abstract

Lung tumors in the thorax move by respiration during radiotherapy. Four-dimensional computed tomography (4DCT) and patient-dependent determination of margins for tumor motion are strongly recommended in the treatment planning of high-dose external beam therapy, such as stereotactic body radiotherapy (SBRT) for lung cancers. As tumor motion control maneuvers, relaxed steady breathing, a stereotactic body frame and compression plate, deep inspiration breath holding, and active breathing control have been introduced. Meanwhile, it has become obvious that the respiratory motion of lung tumors is different in different patients, on different days, and at different times in the same patient. To accommodate this, daily online imaging and soft tissue setup are now recommended. Three-dimensional image-guided radiotherapy (3D IGRT) is increasingly used with or without internal fiducial markers. Broader application of the 3D IGRT as the minimum requirement is proposed to replace 2D IGRT by experts. Adaptive external beam radiotherapy systems (AEBRS) for intrafractionally moving target volumes, such as beam gating and beam tracking, have been developed to improve the reproducibility of tumor motion control. The superiority of 4DCT planning in clinical outcomes has been suggested in a randomized trial of SBRT for early-stage lung cancer.

1 Overview

Intrathoracic tumors may move several centimeters with respiratory motion, and improvements in anatomical and temporal accuracy about tumor motion have been an important subject in radiotherapy. If the patient is rigid and moves regularly like a plastic phantom, the spatial coordinates of the patient with a moving tumor can be exactly registered to the coordinates of the treatment room in every setup. The patient with the tumor is, however, soft (not rigid) and moves voluntarily or involuntarily in time and space. Therefore, the registration of the coordinates of the patient to the treatment room is not simple. Four-dimensional radiotherapy (4DRT) as a new concept has been proposed to accommodate the temporal changes in anatomy (Shirato et al. 1998).

Meanwhile, time-resolved four-dimensional computed tomography (4DCT) has been widely introduced in radiation treatment planning (RTP) for lung cancers to reduce the uncertainties in the planning target volume (PTV) due to tumor motion. Tumor motion control maneuvering, such as relaxed steady breathing, a stereotactic body frame and compression plate, deep inspiration breath holding, and active breath control with/without audiovisual feedback, has been utilized for lung cancers (Cole et al. 2014). It has become obvious that the respiratory motion of the lung tumor can change from patient to patient, day to day, and temporally in the same patient (Shirato et al. 2006). Considering this, daily online imaging and soft tissue setup procedures are now recommended in addition to 4DCT planning and patient-dependent determination of margins for tumor motion irrespective of the technology for tumor motion control in high-dose, high-precision radiotherapy for lung cancer (De Ruysscher et al. 2017). Real-time 3D IGRT is recommended by experts in this field as the next critical step in external beam radiotherapy to replace 2D IGRT (Keall et al. 2018; Molitoris et al. 2018).

The adaptive external beam radiotherapy system (AEBRS) for intrafractionally moving target volumes, which combine external beam radiotherapy equipment and devices to detect tumor motion during irradiation, has been developed to improve the effectiveness and reproducibility of tumor control maneuvers. Beam gating using external surrogates, beam gating using real-time internal imaging, and beam tracking have been commercially available for photon and particle beam therapy. Scientific knowledge of lung tumor motion and control measures in external beam radiotherapy has advanced dramatically in the recent 20 years (Shimizu et al. 2000; Seppenwoolde et al. 2002; Knybel et al. 2016).

A phase 3 randomized clinical trial (RCT) has been able to show the clinical benefit of SBRT on local control and survival of patients with stage 1 non-small cell lung cancer in which 4DCT was used to determine the PTV (Ball et al. 2019). The authors pointed out that considerations of tumor motion are important since no benefit of the SBRT was observed in another RCT in which 4DCT had not been used in most of the patients (Nyman et al. 2016).

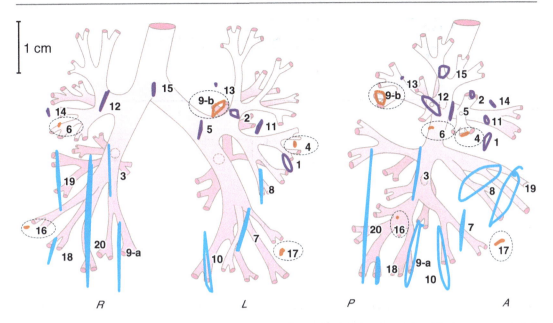

Fig. 1 Orthogonal projections of the trajectories of the 21 tumors on (left) the coronal (LR-CC) and (right) the sagittal (AP-CC) plane. The tumors are displayed at the approximate position, based on the localization. Tumors that were in close contact with bones are circled. (Reproduced from Seppenwoolde et al. Int J Radiat Oncol Biol Phys, 2002, with permission)

2 Anatomical Concerns in Tumor Motion

2.1 Physiological Conditions

Inspiration requires contraction of the diaphragm and the external intercostal muscles located between the ribs. Contraction of the diaphragm makes the diaphragm move downward and increases the craniocaudal (CC) dimensions of the thoracic cavity, resulting in pulmonary expansion (Wade 1954). The external intercostal muscles contract to elevate the lower ribs and push the sternum outward, increasing the anteroposterior (AP) dimensions of the thoracic cavity. The total of the resistance of healthy lungs is so small that the respiratory muscles need to generate low-magnitude pressure or force to overcome the flow resistance of the lungs. Expiration is normally passive because of the elastic recoil. Considering these physiological conditions is essential to understand why the tumors in the lower lobe have larger amplitudes in the CC direction than those in the upper lobe and why tumors in the anterior lung tend to move with hysteresis in free breathing (Seppenwoolde et al. 2002) (Fig. 1). The respiratory motion can change with the biochemical condition (CO_2 concentration, exercise), body position (standing, supine), abdominal contents (food intake, constipation), and emotional condition (anxiety, relaxation). The main respiratory muscles are under both voluntary and involuntary (automatic) control. A large interfractional difference in the amplitude of lung tumors and intrafractional gradual baseline shift/drift in the same patient can be attributed to these factors (Shirato et al. 2006; Takao et al. 2016). The absolute amplitudes of the lung tumor motion in the right-left (RL), CC, and AP directions were 8.2 ± 6.5 mm (mean ± standard deviation (SD)), 10.7 ± 8.6 mm, and 8.8 ± 7.0 mm, respectively, which have been estimated from the trajectory of a fiducial marker near the tumor in 60 treatments of 21 patients (Shirato et al. 2006). Figure 2 shows that the absolute amplitude of the marker varied considerably from patient to patient and at different treatment days for the same patient. It is consistent with the recent clinical observations of intra- and interfractional motion variation in

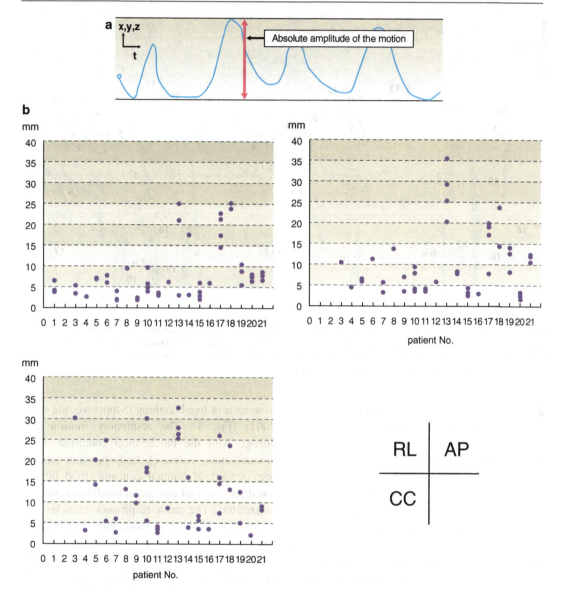

Fig. 2 (**a**) Absolute amplitude determined from the time signal of the tumor motion in *x*, *y*, and *z* directions. The absolute amplitudes of marker movements were defined as the distance between the maximum and minimum coordinates along each of the axes (*x*, *y*, and *z*) in each log file. (**b**) The absolute amplitudes of the trajectories in right-left (RL), craniocaudal (CC), and anteroposterior (AP) directions for 60 treatment days in 21 patients. (Reproduced from Shirato et al. Int J Radiat Oncol Biol Phys, 2006, with permission)

MR-guided lung SBRT by Thomas et al. where they found large interfractional changes in amplitude (Thomas et al. 2018). Figure 3 shows the maximum, median, and minimum speeds of the marker (log scale) estimated from the change in fiducial marker position. The maximum marker speed exceeded 33 mm/s in 10 (16%) of the 60 treatments with the highest speed at 94 mm/s. These findings must be taken into account in tumor motion control in radiotherapy.

The physiological differences between free breathing and voluntary expiration should be considered when the breath-holding technique is used for tumor motion control. Involuntary control arises from the brain stem and spinal cord and voluntary control arises from the motor and

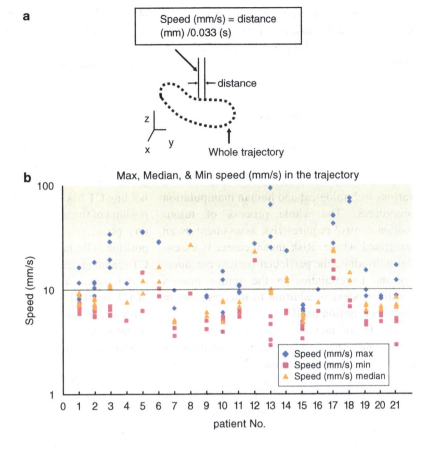

Fig. 3 (a) Speed of the marker determined from the trajectory of the marker. (b) The maximum, minimum, and median speeds of the marker for 60 treatment days in 21 patients are plotted in long scale. (Reproduced from Shirato et al. Int J Radiat Oncol Biol Phys, 2006, with permission)

premotor cortex of the brain. In voluntary expiration, the external intercostal muscles contract and pull the rib cage downward, and the abdominal muscles assist by pulling the rib cage down and increasing abdominal pressure which forces the diaphragm up.

Lung tumors near the cardiac or aortic wall and mediastinal lymph nodes move due to the heart beat with an amplitude of 1–4 mm, usually less than the respiratory motion (Seppenwoolde et al. 2002; Schmidt et al. 2016). Schmidt et al. investigated the three-dimensional (3D) trajectory of fiducial markers implanted in mediastinal LNs. The intrafractional motion of the LNs has an amplitude of 2.1 ± 0.5 (mean ± SD) mm in the LR direction, 7.3 ± 2.6 mm in the CC direction, and 3.3 ± 1.3 mm in the AP direction. The cardiac motion ranges were 1.3 ± 0.7 mm in the LR direction, 1.3 ± 0.6 mm in the CC direction, and 2.3 ± 1.5 mm in the AP direction.

2.2 Pathological Conditions

Respiratory motion of lung tumors depends on the pathological changes in the lung tissue. In chronic obstructive lung diseases, the lung is hyperinflated to overcome the increased flow resistance, and the diaphragm operates at a positional disadvantage to its proper function, and there is a larger demand on the intercostal muscles to assist in respiration. Patients with interstitial fibrosis suffer from frequent drawing of breath and shortness of breath with small amplitudes affecting the lung tumor motion (Onodera et al. 2011). The lung tumor motion can also be altered by attachment of the tumor to rigid structures, pleural adhesion after pleuritis, thoracic surgery, a history of thoracic irradiation, diabetes mellitus, hypothyroidism, asthma, inflammation of lung tissue, medication, chest pain, malnutrition, disuse atrophy, and muscle fatigue. The respiratory function test was not simply related to the craniocaudal amplitude of the motion of the fiducial marker near lung tumors (Onimaru et al. 2005).

3 Tumor Motion Control Process and Risk Management

Most tumor motion control solutions involve various technological and human manipulation procedures. The whole process of tumor motion control requires risk assessment as an integrated whole. Risk management is essential to irradiate the particular patient considering the uncertainties in the tumor motion control process in addition to uncertainties in the tumor motion itself.

The tumor motion control process can be divided into phases: (1) assessment of the total extent of the possible motion; (2) selection of a tumor motion control method; (3) placement of fiducial markers if required; (4) 4D imaging for the treatment planning; (5) 4D treatment planning considering potential tumor shifts, rotation, and deformation; (6) setup and pretreatment verification of the tumor position; (7) real-time monitoring of the tumor motion; (8) delivery of the radiotherapy; and (9) posttreatment verification of the tumor motion. Any failure or intentional simplification in these phases of the process can be a cause of irradiation hazards including underdosage of the target and overdosage of critical structures. The tumor motion control process often integrates multiple pieces of equipment and software from different vendors so that information flow and hazardous situations should be analyzed by the responsible organizations including with the vendors. Each institution should perform risk assessments about their own tumor motion control process using methods such as failure mode and effect analysis and also risk fishbone diagrams. If risk reduction is required, the person who is in charge of the radiotherapy department should establish risk management plans to reduce the risk to acceptable levels.

4 Treatment Preparation and 4D Planning

4.1 Imaging

To obtain information of three-dimensional tumor motion, fluoroscopy, slow CT, breath-holding CT, and 4DCT have been used. Slow CT has been found useful to establish the gross 3D tumor position but CT images may be blurred by the tumor motion during the scanning. Breath-holding CT has been found useful to observe the position of the target volume at a specific respiratory phase as a "snapshot" and as a result the position of the target volume at the breath-holding CT scanning may not be the same as the position of the target in daily treatment. The time-resolved 4DCT or 4D PET/CT has been widely used to estimate the tumor motion in lung cancer in recent years and introduced in the RTP for lung cancers to reduce the uncertainty due to tumor motion.

Liu et al. (2007) have used 4DCT to assess the lung tumor motion and have shown that the principal component of the tumor motion was in the CC direction with only 10.8% of tumors moving >1.0 cm. However, Harada et al. have shown that 4DCT may underestimate the maximum amplitude of tumors during the actual delivery of irradiation (Harada et al. 2016). The mean differences in the amplitude detected by 4DCT and fluoroscopic real-time tumor tracking (RTRT) were 5.7 ± 8.0 mm, 12.5 ± 16.7 mm, and 6.8 ± 8.5 mm in the RL, CC, and AP directions, respectively, in the lower lobe in the Harada et al. study. The 4DCT also offers a "snapshot" of motion due to breathing for the brief period of time on a specific day, and the uncertainties in tumor location observed here are to be considered in the treatment planning using 4DCT (Shirato et al. 2006; Thomas et al. 2018).

4.2 The Safety Margin Approach

The safety margin approach has been widely used with 4DCT to mitigate the effect of uncertainties in tumor motion in photon treatment plans. Various approaches have been reported to determine PTV for moving lung tumors: typically, the internal target volume (ITV; encompassing the entire tumor excursion in one breathing cycle), mid-position approach (MidP; irradiation at the geometric time-weighted mean tumor position), and gated treatment (gating; irradiation to a restricted portion of the respiratory cycle) (Fig. 4). Wolthaus et al. (2008) have shown that the ITV method resulted in a significantly larger PTV than conventional CT scanning in free breathing; the relative volume change (%) was $6 \pm 5\%$ (mean ± standard deviation) in off-line (on body anatomy) correction protocols and $33 \pm 20\%$ in online (on tumor) correction protocols. Using the MidP approach, the relative volume change (%) was $-9 \pm 9\%$ in off-line correction and $0 \pm 0\%$ in online correction. The relative volume change (%) was the smallest in gating: $-11 \pm 11\%$ in off-line correction and $-4 \pm 6\%$ in online correction.

Ezhil et al. have proposed patient-specific internal gross tumor volumes (IGTV) for lung cancer using 4DCT. The $IGTV_{AllPhases}$ is defined to be the envelope of respiratory motion of the gross tumor volume (GTV) contours from, for example, all of ten respiratory phases (Ezhil et al. 2009).

The safety margin approach for photon therapy cannot be simply extended to particle beam therapy such as proton or carbon beam therapy. Different approaches are mandatory because of the steep falloff in dose distribution and range uncertainties in particle beam therapy. Interfractional anatomical changes may result in serious dose distortions due to density variations along the beam path. Misalignment of the proton beam with the patient can cause significant cold or hotspots within the target volume in the presence of tissue heterogeneities, such as dense bone, pneumothorax (free air), or skin surface irregularities along the beam path.

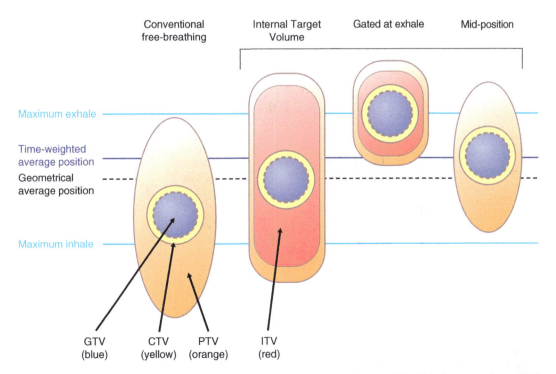

Fig. 4 Schematic overview of different treatment planning concepts: conventional free breathing, internal target volume (ITV), gating (at exhale), and mid-position. *GTV* gross tumor volume, *CTV* clinical target volume, *PTV* planning target volume. (Reprint from Wolthaus et al. Int J Radiat Oncol Biol Phys 2008 with permission)

Park et al. have proposed using the beam-specific PTV (bsPTV) approach to reduce the uncertainties in proton beam therapy (Park et al. 2012). In the bsPTV method, systematic range uncertainties were accounted for by adding distal margins and proximal margins for each ray trace from the beam source to the distal and proximal surfaces of CTV. The bsPTV also adds margins to account for a possible range of errors due to misalignments. The resulting bsPTV closely conformed to conventional PTV in photon therapy except for the area where the operation for range uncertainties had the greatest impact. Park et al. have reported that the minimum coverage to the CTV dropped from 99% to 67% using conventional PTV but from 99% to 94% using the bsPTV suggesting a better robustness in treatment planning using bsPTV. If we use a large internal margin for the intrafractional organ motion with lung cancer, the physical shape of the bsPTV may become very different from the PTV in photon therapy (Fig. 5). Four-dimensional CT is shown to be useful to reduce the overestimation of the distal margins illustrated in Fig. 5 (Lin et al. 2015). The benefit of gating with lung cancer is apparent to reduce the size of the bsPTV

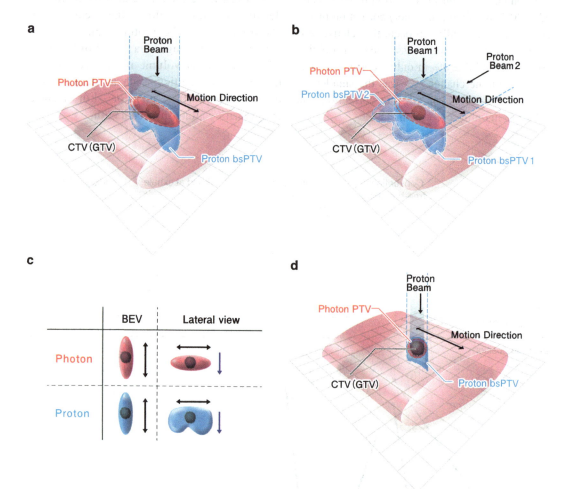

Fig. 5 The conceptual comparison between bsPTV in proton beam therapy and PTV in photon therapy. (**a**) A three-dimensional (3D) illustration of the proton bsPTV and photon PTV when a beam is coming vertically to a CTV (GTV) which is moving perpendicular to the beam angle. (**b**) A 3D illustration of the comparison for two rectangular beams. (**c**) Beam's eye view (BED) and lateral views of the PTV in photon therapy and bsPTV in proton therapy for the CTV (GTV). (**d**) A 3D illustration of the proton bsPTV in gated proton therapy

(Fig. 5). The bsPTV approach presents limitations since it cannot be used in multi-beam, simultaneously optimized particle beam plans, such as in intensity-modulated proton therapy (IMPT).

4.3 The Robust Approach

The safety margin approach to dealing with uncertainties due to tumor motion is often overconservative and unavoidably increases the radiation exposure of normal tissue. However, if we assume a fixed pattern of organ motion from the 4DCT, ignore the fact that tumor motion may change day by day, and use tight margins for the tumor motion, substantial cold spots will appear in the CTV. The robust approach has been introduced to account for uncertainties in the averaged tumor motion detected by 4DCT (Chan et al. 2006). Without assuming an unchanging tumor motion, the uncertainties in tumor motion may be considered to account for and to determine the treatment parameters and dose distribution. The uncertainty in tumor motion prediction (i.e., the error bars for the average tumor location at each phase of a respiration cycle) was calculated from the data of an internal fiducial marker or an external surrogate marker with the actual patient or with population data from past patients (Fig. 6).

The robustness in uncertainties of tumor motion in this approach compared to the safety margin approach is suggested in Fig. 7 (Chan et al. 2006).

Heath et al. (2009) compared two robust approaches with a safety margin approach, MidP, in a simulation study of IMRT for lung cancers and found that the robust approaches tended to spare the organs at risk with similar target coverages. The robust approach can be expected to be especially useful in IMPT planning for lung cancers where the uncertainties considered are not only in the tumor motion and setup but also in the range of a particle beam and in the relative biological effectiveness (RBE) (Unkelbach et al. 2007; Fredriksson 2012; Unkelbach and Paganetti 2018). Various methods such as "composite worst-case method," "probabilistic approach," and "voxel-wise worst-case method" have been reported to represent the effect of these uncertainties (Unkelbach and Paganetti 2018; Yock et al. 2019). Fredriksson (2012) has reported that the utilization of more "information" than is conventionally considered in the optimization can lead to robust target coverage and lower OAR doses than the safety margin approach. These metrics have been incorporated into the treatment planning of IMPT in clinical studies (Liu et al. 2012) and are now installed in RTP systems commercially available. It is important to remember

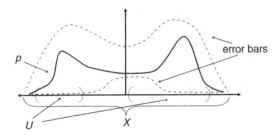

Fig. 6 A visualization of the model of uncertainty in a robust approach. The model consists of a "nominal" probability mass function (pmf), p, surrounded by upper and lower "error bars." X is defined as the domain of the nominal pmf and error bars. U is defined as "uncertainty region". (reprinted from Chan et al. Phys Med Biol, 2006, with permission)

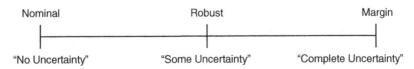

Fig. 7 A visualization of the continuum of robustness. "Nominal" represents "no uncertainty," and the "Margin" represents "complete uncertainty." "Robust" represents the flexibility of the robust approach. (Reprinted from Chan et al. Phys Med Biol, 2006, with permission)

that the predictability of the robust approach depends on the "information" utilized in the optimization but more studies are required to fully elucidate its clinical safety and effectiveness.

5 Tumor Motion Control Maneuvers

5.1 Relaxed Steady Breathing

A stable and reproducible patient position during all imaging procedures and treatment is essential for high-dose high-precision radiotherapy with lung cancer (De Ruysscher et al. 2017). From this consideration, relaxed steady respiration, free breathing without conscious intervention, is the most advantageous although it is vulnerable to any change in the tumor motion from those in the predictions made by the plan. Recently, there has been research into the efficacy of free-breathing respiratory motion predictions based on machine learning algorithms. The long short-term memory neural networks were developed to predict the respiratory motion of external surrogate signals on the patient surface (Lin et al. 2019a). A super-learner model was proposed to use clinical data and non-4D diagnostic CT image data reducing the work involved in recording 4DCT for the planning (Lin et al. 2019b). However, these studies are still immature and not ready to be used for the prediction of lung tumor motion in free breathing.

5.2 Stereotactic Body Frames and Compression Plates

Lax et al. (1994) have reported that a stereotactic body frame with a compression plate was useful to restrict the diaphragmatic movements to 5–10 mm. Patients are forced to maintain a shallow breath by the compression of the diaphragm by abdominal pressure. Compression plates on the patient abdomen have been used to restrict the motion of the diaphragm by maintaining a shallow breath with the device commercially available. Many clinical outcomes of SBRT have been reported from institutions where the technique was used. Using stereotactic body frame with a compression plate may be useful in selected patients but negative effects have also been observed in patients having used this approach (Bengua et al. 2010). Under the abdominal compression patients are likely to breathe using the intercostal muscles so that interfractional deviations of the target position may be larger than those in free breathing. Similarly, the use of a cradle or evacuated cushion, and abdominal compression is also not adequate for a precise setup without image guidance (Grills et al. 2008; Bissonnette et al. 2009). Since it is not always effective and sometimes results in effects that are contrary to the expected results, external body fixation and abdominal compression without image guidance for the soft tissue have become insufficient. In the EORTC recommendations, it is stated that SBRT can be safely delivered without rigid immobilization devices (De Ruysscher et al. 2017).

5.3 Deep Inspiration Breath Holding (DIBH)

Irradiation at the end of inspiration has been considered the logical tumor motion control to reduce the irradiated volume of normal lung tissue arising from high-dose irradiated volumes. Deep inspiration breath-holding (DIBH) techniques involve verbally coaching the patient to repeatedly perform the same reproducible deep inspiration level throughout the various phases of the treatment planning and delivery. The DIBH maneuver begins with the patient in quiet tidal breathing, followed by a slow deep inspiration, slow deep expiration, then another slow deep inspiration to the maximal inspiration level, and then holding the breath (the breath hold). During this process, a spirometer monitors the patient respiration level and audiovisual feedback may also be used. Hanley et al. (1999) have reported that the DJBH maneuver was highly reproducible, with intra-breath-hold reproducibility of 1.0 ± 0.9 mm and inter-breath-hold reproducibility of 2.5 ± 1.6 mm. The Henley et al. report suggested that the volume of the lungs exposed to more than 25 Gy can be reduced by 30% compared to free-breathing plans, while respiration gating can reduce the volume by 18%. Josipovic et al. have shown that the DIBH using visual feedback is highly reproducible for simple targets such as a peripheral tumor mass with no mediastinal involvement, or a mediastinal mass without separation between the primary tumors and the involved lymph nodes (Josipovic et al. 2016).

5.4 Active Breathing Control (ABC)

Wong et al. (1999) have introduced the approach of active breathing control. The patient's breathing is monitored continuously and at a preset lung volume during either inspiration or expiration, the airflow of the patient is temporarily blocked, thereby immobilizing the breathing motion. The duration of the ABC is that which is comfortably maintained by each individual patient. The ABC procedure was well tolerated in the 12 patients in Wong et al.'s study suggesting that ABC provides a simple means to minimize breathing motion. A commercially available ABC apparatus consists of a breathing tube with a mouthpiece and filter, connected to a digital volume transducer and pickup assembly and a balloon valve that can be inflated to halt respiration. The goal of the device is to induce reproducible breath holds at the same lung volume, during and across sessions, whether this may be radiotherapy delivery, CT, or PET examinations. Kaza et al. (2017) took advantage of a recently available MR-compatible ABC device to investigate the reproducibility of breath-held lung volumes under ABC control while avoiding ionizing radiation exposure. Overall, lung volumes controlled by the ABC devices agreed better than with self-controlled breath holds, as suggested by the average ABC variation of 1.8% of the measured lung volumes (99 mL), compared to the 4.1% (226 mL) variability observed on average with self-sustained breath holding.

In EORTC recommendations, DIBH and ABC are categorized as interventions to reduce tumor motion which may be useful in selected patients (De Ruysscher et al. 2017).

6 Adaptive External Beam Radiotherapy Systems (AEBRS) for Intrafractional Movements of Target Volumes

6.1 General Concept

The reproducibility of tumor motion control processes depends on patient conditions, coaching, and additional factors. External beam radiotherapy equipment can be combined with the tumor motion detection equipment in automatic beam adaptation to tumor motion.

Beam adaptation expresses changes in beam-on timing, beam direction, or absorbed dose distributions, according to the received (planned) treatment parameters (IEC, TR62926). An adaptive external beam radiotherapy system (AEBRS) for intrafractionally moving target volumes is the system that monitors patient anatomy or physiology and based on the monitored information allows changes to treatment parameters during the course of the radiotherapy. Beam gating and beam tracking are included in beam adaptation provided that they are used to change the absorbed dose distribution. In the ESTRO recommendations, the gating and tracking may be of value in a small subgroup of patients subject to large tumor motions (De Ruysscher et al. 2017).

The AEBRS is increasingly important to deliver prescribed doses to intrafractionally moving target volumes. The AEBRS consists of three components: external beam equipment (EBE), motion detection equipment (MDE), and a motion coordinating function (MCF) as shown in Fig. 8. The MCF is the function that adapts treatment parameters according to the parameters provided by the MDE.

There are many different types of MDE, used to monitor intrafractional organ motion; these include airflow meters, strain gauges, infrared sensors, magnetic field sensors, X-ray-based image

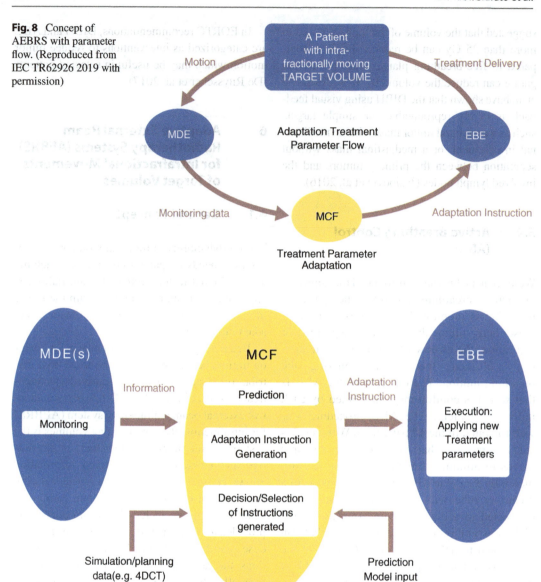

Fig. 8 Concept of AEBRS with parameter flow. (Reproduced from IEC TR62926 2019 with permission)

Fig. 9 Functions and information flow of an AEBRS. (Reproduced from IEC TR62926, 2019, with permission)

guidance such as fluoroscopy, ultrasound equipment, magnetic resonance imaging equipment, and positron emission tomographs. The MRI-linac (Elekta and ViewRay Inc., Cleveland, OH) has been developed for AEBRS using MRI as the MDE.

In AEBRS, intrafraction monitoring of the target volume position and shape using the MDE, a controlled and accurate coordination of the MDE and EBE is crucial to correctly apply the treatment parameter changes. An MCF ensures that motion information is appropriately linked to the 4D treatment plan, selects treatment parameters, and sends proper adaptation instructions to the EBE. The EBE can include electron accelerators generating the therapeutic X-ray beam, proton beam generators, or carbon beam generators. There are many possible combinations of MDE, EBE, and MCF and the MCF itself can be installed as a part of an MDE and EBE, or as a separate piece of equipment (Figs. 9 and 10).

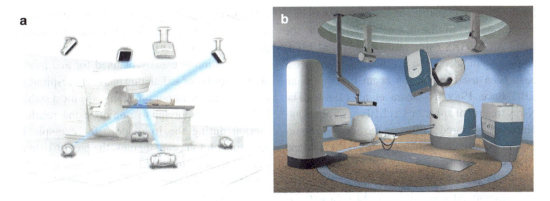

Fig. 10 Examples of AEBRS. (**a**) SyncTraX for gated radiotherapy with internal fiducial marker. (**b**) Cyberknife for tracking radiotherapy

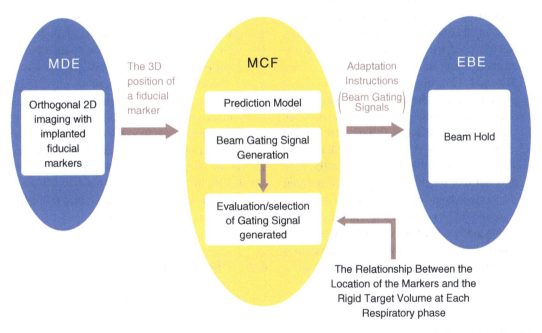

Fig. 11 Bean gating system for intrafractionally moving target volumes. (Reproduced from IEC TR62926, 2019, with permission)

Human operation will be required in the various phases of the whole process.

6.2 Beam Gating Using External Surrogate Markers

Figure 11 shows an example of a reference model of a beam gating system. As shown, it consists of the MDE, EBE, and MCF. The MDE monitors the target volume motion and provides the information to the MCF. The "prediction" sub-function of the MCF integrates information into its in-built compensation model. The "adaptation instruction generation" sub-function generates the beam hold instructions to the decision/selection sub-function. The MCF decision functions verify this output against the pretreatment established simulation data and select the appropriate gates to be provided as an adaptation instruction for the EBE. The adaptation instructions can be a simple signal to the gating interface of the EBE. An AEBRS using airflow meters as MDE and gating in adaptation instructions in the MCF have been used for proton beam therapy as an EBE since 1989 by Ohara et al. (1989). The X-ray treatment apparatus as EBE has been combined with infrared sensors on the abdominal surface (Varian) or strain gauges (Elekta and ANZAI) as MDE. The amplitude and the phase of signals from the MDE are compared with the pretreatment established threshold data and the signal is sent to the gating interface of the EBE.

However, the correlation of the internal lung tumor motion with external surrogate indicators of respiration has been reported to be poor (Hoisak et al. 2004). If an abdominal surface marker was used, the mean amplitude- and phase-based gating beam-to-beam variation was as high as 37% and 42% from the previous treatment beam, respectively (Berbeco et al. 2005). The residual motion (95th percentile) was between 0.7 and 5.8 mm, 0.8 and 6.0 mm, and 0.9 and 6.2 mm for the 20%, 30%, and 40% duty cycle windows, respectively. Berbeco et al. (2005) have pointed out that treatment margins that account for the motion should be individualized and daily imaging should be performed in gated radiotherapy using surface markers. The latency from the detection of the motion to the actual irradiation is also an important issue to ensure not to irradiate the patient at the wrong respiratory phase.

6.3 Beam Gating Using Internal Fiducial Markers

An AEBRS is where room- or gantry-mounted X-ray images are connected to an EBE, enabling fluoroscopic imaging of internal fiducial markers near the tumor from multiple angles, and by 3D measurements of the marker position in real time, here every 0.033 s (Shirato et al. 1999; Shimizu et al. 2014). The gating window for the marker has been generated before treatment using 4DCT to irradiate the lung cancer only when the marker position is within ±2.0 mm from the planned position for the RL, CC, and AP directions (Shirato et al. 2000). In the MCF, the "beam hold instruction" is generated when the 3D maker position is outside the gating window. Lung cancer irradiation is usually planned for and irradiated at the end-of-exhalation phase in a respiratory cycle where the tumor position is the most stable. When it is important to minimize the residual motion during the irradiation, for example in scanning proton beam therapy, the precise data of trajectory of an internal fiducial marker is useful for four-dimensional dose assessment in conjugation with 4DCT images and the scanning beam data in AEBRS (Kanehira et al. 2017) (Fig. 12). The physician and/or physicists can determine the type of fiducial marker, the size of the gating window, and the frequency and exposure of the fluoroscopic monitoring (Miyamoto et al. 2019). The table position can be corrected when baseline shift/drift becomes apparent during the delivery of irradiation. The EBE can be any X-ray generator, proton beam, or carbon beam. Several innovations exploring the RTRT concept have been developed in the recent 10 years: SyncTraX (a new RTRT system which can be connected to the Varian TrueBeam, Shimadzu, Kyoto, Japan) for the X-ray generator, Probeat-RT (Hitachi, Tokyo, Japan) proton beam, and Hybeat (Hitachi, Tokyo, Japan) for carbon beams.

6.4 Beam Tracking

To change the relative beam direction to the target, allowances for irradiation and related equipment movements in EBE are made according to beam adaptation instructions in beam tracking (Fig. 13). Cyberknife (Accuray Inc., Sunnyvale, CA) and VERO (BrainLab, Munich, Germany, and Mitsubishi Heavy Industries, Yokohama, Japan) have been classified as AEBRS when beam tracking is used for intrafractionally moving targets. Using an external surrogate and infrared sensor as the MDE1 and intermittent fluoroscopic imaging of the internal fiducial markers as MDE2, a correlation model provides real-time updates of the target volume orientation in MCF. In the MCF, the 3D position of the target volume is calculated with the prediction model

Tumor Motion Control

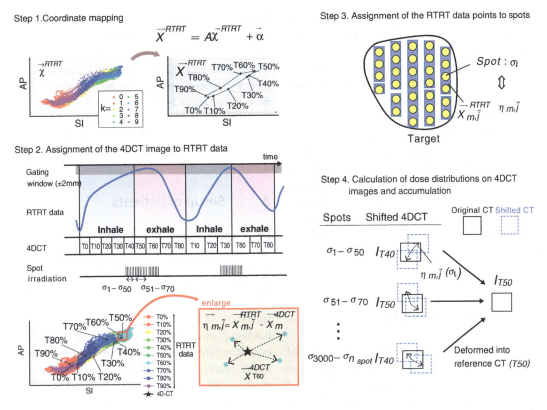

Fig. 12 An example of study workflow for the four-dimensional dose calculation. *RTRT* real-time tumor-tracking radiation therapy. Step 1: Coordinate mapping from the trajectory of an internal fiducial marker. Step 2: Assignment of the 4DCT image to RTRT data. Step 3: Assignment of the RTRT data points to spots. Step 4: Calculation of dose distributions on 4DCT images and accumulation. (Reprinted from Kanehira et al. Int J Radiat Oncol Biol Phys, 2017, with permission)

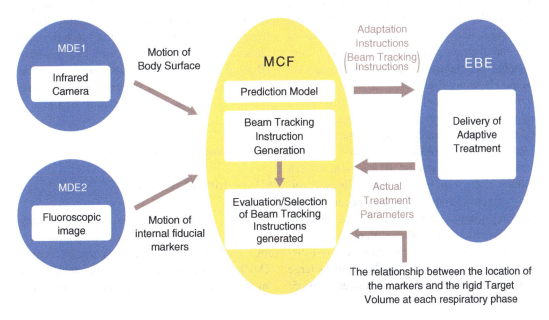

Fig. 13 Beam tracking system for intrafractionally moving target volumes. (Modified from IEC TR62926, 2019, with permission)

accounting for the latency, and beam adaptation instructions are generated. The EBE uses beam adaptation instructions from the MCF to determine new treatment parameters. Hoogeman et al. (2009) have reported the standard deviations describing intrafraction variations around the whole-fraction mean error of 0.2–1.9 mm for the CC, 0.1–1.9 mm for the LR, and 0.2–2.5 mm for the AP directions using Cyberknife. The variation in prediction errors caused by time delays of about 100 ms increased with the respiration motion amplitude. The intrafractional baseline shift can be accommodated for by frequent updating of the correlation model, enabling a considerable reduction in unnecessary irradiation of normal lung tissue.

7 Fiducial Markers

Internal metallic fiducial markers can be detected by X-ray fluoroscopy. Fiducial markers have been used for real-time monitoring, tracking, and real-time-image gating of lung tumor positions in radiotherapy. Transbronchial implantation technology for RTRT was reported in 2002 (Harada et al. 2002). The fixation rate was 76–89% from the start to the end of SBRT and 68–70% at the last follow-up (Imura et al. 2005; Anantham et al. 2007; Harley et al. 2019). The transbronchial fiberscopic implantation method is improved with the fixation rate above 90% using new recently commercially available navigation devices (Bowling et al. 2019). Baker et al. in the Netherlands have reported that the success rate of endovascular coil placement into subsegmental pulmonary artery branches near tumors via the femoral vein was 99.8% with grade 3 cardiac arrhythmia in one patient (0.2%) out of 416 patients. There were higher rates of clinically relevant complications such as pneumothorax requiring hospital admission and chest tubes in 13% in transthoracic marker placements.

Interfractional marker-to-tumor centroid displacement is significant when the tumor is large or the treatment time is long (Imura et al. 2005; Roman et al. 2012). Affected mediastinal lymph nodes (LNs) are often included in the radiotherapy target but the motion of LN in the mediastinum can be significantly different from that with primary tumors, and appropriate margins for LN need to be determined separately from those for the primary tumor. Volumetric imaging, not fiducial markers, is expected to overcome these problems.

8 Setup of Patients

Daily online imaging and soft tissue setup are now recommended in high-dose, high-precision radiotherapy for lung cancer in the ESTRO guidelines (De Ruysscher et al. 2017). The setup using soft tissue or fiducial markers requires consideration of the trajectory of the motion, interfractional changes relative to the surrounding bone structure, rotation/deformation of the tumor, and displacement of the fiducial markers (Shirato et al. 2006). Four-dimensional cone beam CT (4D CBCT) has been shown to be useful to measure and correct the time-weighted mean tumor position in SBRT for lung cancer (Sonke et al. 2009). The ESTRO recommendation is to use 4D CBCT for the daily setup in SBRT (De Ruysscher et al. 2017). Two fluoroscopic X-rays on the treatment room or on the gantry of a proton beam therapy system and fiducial markers near the lung cancer have been shown to be useful for the daily 4D setup registering the motion trajectory of the fiducial marker without increases in setup time (Shirato et al. 2006; Yoshimura et al. 2020).

9 Delivery of the Beam

9.1 Interplay Effects

In IMRT, volumetric modulated arc therapy (VMAT), beam scanning proton or carbon therapy, and intensity-modulated particle therapy (IMPT), a narrow beam with a diameter much smaller than the mass of the lung cancer is used.

Low-dose spots of the accumulated dose in the target volume and high-dose spots outside of the target volume can easily be generated by the tumor motion, a phenomenon commonly ascribed to the so-called interplay effect. Jakobi et al. (2018) have analyzed the interplay effect of beam scanning proton therapy in free breathing and found serious underdosages to the target volume for tumor motion >5 mm. Grassberger et al. (2013) suggested a serious deterioration from 87.0% to 2.7% in the 2-year local control rate when the interplay effect is not accounted for single- or hypofractionated lung cancer treatment with the beam scanning proton beam therapy.

A fractionated treatment protocol can reduce the impact of interplay effects using robust optimization in simulation studies (Li et al. 2014; Inoue et al. 2016). Conventional fractionation is recommended to reduce the interplay effect through statistical averaging, showing that the interplay effect is a problem when hypofractionation is used for lung cancer. Grassberger et al. (2013) showed that a large spot size is important to minimize interplay effects of spot scanning proton beam therapy for lung cancer. Although the large spot size is significantly robust toward motion, it also increases the dose to the normal parts of the lungs considerably due to the broader lateral penumbra. Layered rescanning can mitigate the interplay effect for lung cancer patients treated with scanning proton therapy through statistical averaging (Grassberger et al. 2015). Other measures to reduce the interplay effect are very similar to those described for tumor motion control: 4D planning, breath holding, gating, and tracking.

9.2 Intrafractional Baseline Shift/Drift

Mainly because of muscle relaxation or shallow breathing, it is well known that intrafractional baseline shift/drift of the lung tumor position occurs during the delivery of the therapeutic beam. The incidence of intrafractional baseline shift/drift exceeding 3.0 mm was <10% within 5 min of the start of the treatment and the incidence of baseline shift/drift rose gradually with the shift/drift along the CC axis, reaching approximately 40% for the middle and lower lung fields at 20 min (Takao et al. 2016) (Fig. 14). A baseline shift/drift exceeding 5.0 mm had occurred in 24.8% of cases at 20 min. For the upper lung field, approximately 15% of the markers were subject to shift/drift of 3.0 mm or more at 20 min.

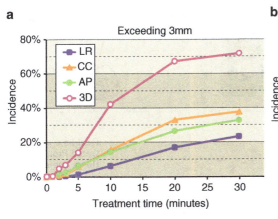
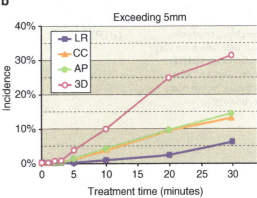
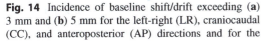

Fig. 14 Incidence of baseline shift/drift exceeding (**a**) 3 mm and (**b**) 5 mm for the left-right (LR), craniocaudal (CC), and anteroposterior (AP) directions and for the square root of sum of 3 directions (3D). (Reproduced from Takao et al. Int J Radiat Oncol Biol Phys, 2016, with permission)

Degradation of the dose coverage in SBRT and that of dose homogeneity in IMRT and IMPT may occur when the treatment time is long. Real-time tumor monitoring and frequent realignments of the table position using the RTRT system concept are helpful to compensate for the changes in dose coverage due to baseline shift/drift (Takao et al. 2016).

9.3 Real-Time-Image Gated Proton Beam Therapy (RGPT)

It is reported that gating, using a duty cycle of 30% at the end of the exhalation phase, can mitigate the interplay effect for lung cancer patients treated with scanning proton therapy reported in a simulation study (Grassberger et al. 2015). However, it is well known from much experience in photon therapy that gated radiotherapy using external surrogate markers is not always sufficiently reliable to reduce the impact of interplay effects and intrafractional baseline shifts in hypofractionated schedules.

Real-time-image gated proton beam therapy (RGPT) systems have been developed to reduce the interplay effects where the scanning beam is gated to irradiate a moving target only when the fiducial marker near the target is within a gating window using two sets of X-ray fluoroscopes mounted at right angles on the 360° gantry (Fig. 15) (Matsuura et al. 2013). The concept of RGPT is similar to the RTRT system but RGPT is more complicated since a synchrotron is used (Fujii et al. 2017). New technologies such as multiple gating beam delivery systems (Yamada et al. 2016) and a short-range applicator (Matsuura et al. 2016) were introduced to ensure that there is no prolonging of the treatment time. The appropriate size of the gating window was found to be ±2 mm to be able to minimize the interplay effect without prolonging the treatment time (Kanehira et al. 2017) (Fig. 14). It is notable that the actual beam delivery time is much shorter than the time for the precise setup of the patients both with and without RGPT (Fig. 16) (Yoshimura et al. 2020). The mean total treatment processing time in the treatment room (from the time when the patient enters the treatment room to the time when the patient exits the treatment room) was 34.1 ± 2.3 min when RGPT is used. It should also be noted that the beam is continuously *ON* throughout the respiration cycle if the amplitude of the fiducial marker is less than 4 mm (−2 to 2 mm) in each direction and stayed in the gating window in

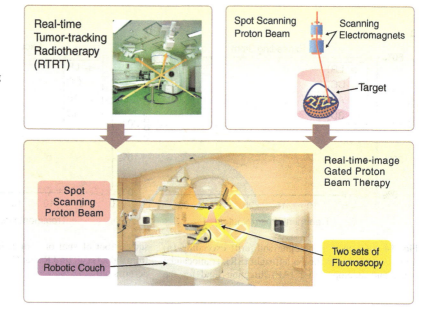

Fig. 15 Real-time-image gated proton beam therapy (RGPT) system which has been developed combining real-time tumor-tracking radiotherapy (RTRT) technology and spot scanning proton beam technology

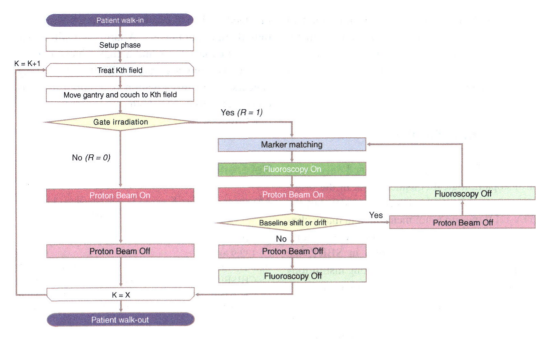

Fig. 16 Flowchart of the RGPT in one treatment session with X treatment fields. K is the index number of the treatment field and R represents the usage of the gating function. (Reproduced from Yoshimura et al. J Appl Clin Med Phys, 2020, with permission)

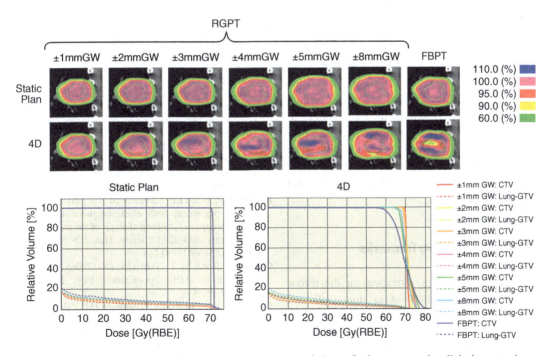

Fig. 17 An example of dose distributions (upper) and dose-volume histograms (lower) for the static plan and four-dimensional simulations for real-time-image gated proton beam therapy (RGPT) plans with gating window (GW) = ±1–8 mm and free-breathing proton therapy (FBPT) for one patient. The range of motion on 4DCT was 1.9 (left-right), 7.3 (craniocaudal), and 2.9 (anteroposterior) mm. In the upper graphs, clinical target volume (CTV) and internal CTV are delineated in green and dark green, respectively, and dose values are scaled by the prescription dose of 70 Gy (relative biological effectiveness). (Reproduced from Kanehira, et al. Int J Radiat Oncol Biol Phys, 2017, with permission)

RTRT and RGPT (Fig. 17). The amplitude of the fiducial marker is often less than 4 mm for lung cancers at the upper lung field but the marker is still useful to reduce the interfractional setup error.

10 Clinical Studies

The GTV-CTV margin is determined only based on histopathological considerations in the original definition in ICRU report 83 (2010) but the GTV-CTV margin is not mentioned in many clinical studies on SBRT. Since a notable ambiguity still exists in GTV-CTV margin in SBRT, the resultant PTV can be different among institutions even when the same ITV margin is used. A guideline should fix this problem.

Many devices for tumor motion control are installed in hospitals worldwide. However, any superiority of the tumor motion control to conventional radiotherapy for lung cancer is not certain yet in terms of clinical outcomes. Most clinical studies on tumor motion control are retrospective or single-arm prospective studies.

A phase III randomized clinical trial (RCT) has been able to show the clinical benefit of SBRT on local control and survival of patients with stage 1 non-small cell lung cancer in which 4DCT was used to determine the PTV (Ball et al. 2019). The authors there pointed out the importance of the considerations of tumor motion since no benefit of the SBRT was observed in another RCT in which 4DCT had not been used (Nyman et al. 2016).

11 Concluding Remarks

There have been many advances in the tumor motion control for early-stage non-small cell lung cancers. However, it is still difficult to perform precise 4DRT for large tumors and tumors of complex morphology. We can measure the motion at multiple positions in the patient in real time but encounter mathematical difficulties when the difficulty is due to the number of objects involved in the calculations to select the optimal radiotherapy parameters. A large gap still exists between expectations and actual achievement in the precise and accurate 4DRT for these lung cancers. More investigation is required to overcome the large gap both by researchers and practitioners.

References

Anantham D, Feller-Kopman D, Shanmugham LN et al (2007) Electromagnetic navigation bronchoscopy-guided fiducial placement for robotic stereotactic radiosurgery of lung tumors: a feasibility study. Chest 132:930–935

Ball D, Mai GT, Vinod S et al (2019) TROG 09.02 CHISEL investigators. Stereotactic ablative radiotherapy versus standard radiotherapy in stage 1 non-small-cell lung cancer (TROG 09.02 CHISEL): a phase 3, open-label, randomised controlled trial. Lancet Oncol 20:494–503

Bengua G, Ishikawa M, Sutherland K et al (2010) Evaluation of the effectiveness of the stereotactic body frame in reducing respiratory intrafractional organ motion using the real-time tumor-tracking radiotherapy system. Int J Radiat Oncol Biol Phys 77:630–636

Berbeco RI, Nishioka S, Shirato H, Chen GT, Jiang SB (2005) Residual motion of lung tumours in gated radiotherapy with external respiratory surrogates. Phys Med Biol 50:3655–3667

Bissonnette JP, Franks KN, Purdie TG et al (2009) Quantifying interfraction and intrafraction tumor motion in lung stereotactic body radiotherapy using respiration-correlated cone beam computed tomography. Int J Radiat Oncol Biol Phys 75:688–695

Bouilhol G, Ayadi M, Rit S et al (2013) Is abdominal compression useful in lung stereotactic body radiation therapy? A 4DCT and dosimetric lobe-dependent study. Phys Med 29:333–340

Bowling MR, Folch EE, Khandhar SJ et al (2019) Fiducial marker placement with electromagnetic navigation bronchoscopy: a subgroup analysis of the prospective, multicenter NAVIGATE study. Ther Adv Respir Dis 2019:1753466619841234

Chan TC, Bortfeld T, Tsitsiklis JN (2006) A robust approach to IMRT optimization. Phys Med Biol 51:2567–2583

Cole AJ, Hanna GG, Jain S, O'Sullivan JM (2014) Motion management for radical radiotherapy in non-small cell lung cancer. Clin Oncol (R Coll Radiol) 26:67–80

De Ruysscher D, Faivre-Finn C, Moeller D et al (2017) Lung Group and the Radiation Oncology Group of the European Organization for Research and Treatment of Cancer (EORTC). European Organization for Research and Treatment of Cancer (EORTC) recommendations for planning and delivery of high-dose, high precision radiotherapy for lung cancer. Radiother Oncol 124:1–10

Ezhil M, Vedam S, Balter P et al (2009) Determination of patient-specific internal gross tumor volumes for lung cancer using four-dimensional computed tomography. Radiat Oncol 4:4. https://doi.org/10.1186/1748-717X-4-4

Fredriksson A (2012) A characterization of robust radiation therapy treatment planning methods-from expected value to worst case optimization. Med Phys 39:5169–5181

Fujii Y, Matsuura T, Matsuzaki Y, et al (2017) U.S. Patent 20200054897A1

Grassberger C, Dowdell S, Lomax A et al (2013) Motion interplay as a function of patient parameters and spot size in spot scanning proton therapy for lung cancer. Int J Radiat Oncol Biol Phys 86:380–386

Grassberger C, Dowdell S, Sharp G, Paganetti H (2015) Motion mitigation for lung cancer patients treated with active scanning proton therapy. Med Phys 42:2462–2469

Grills IS, Hugo G, Kestin LL et al (2008) Image-guided radiotherapy via daily online cone-beam CT substantially reduces margin requirements for stereotactic lung radiotherapy. Int J Radiat Oncol Biol Phys 70:1045–1056

Hanley J, Debois MM, Mah D et al (1999) Deep inspiration breath-hold technique for lung tumors: the potential value of target immobilization and reduced lung density in dose escalation. Int J Radiat Oncol Biol Phys 45:603–611

Harada T, Shirato H, Ogura S et al (2002) Real-time tumor-tracking radiation therapy for lung carcinoma by the aid of insertion of a gold marker using bronchofiberscopy. Cancer 95:1720–1727

Harada K, Katoh N, Suzuki R et al (2016) Evaluation of the motion of lung tumors during stereotactic body radiation therapy (SBRT) with four-dimensional computed tomography (4DCT) using real-time tumor-tracking radiotherapy system (RTRT). Phys Med 32:305–311

Harley DP, Krimsky WS, Sarkar S, Highfield D, Aygun C, Gurses B (2019) Fiducial marker placement using endobronchial ultrasound and navigational bronchoscopy for stereotactic radiosurgery: an alternative strategy. Ann Thorac Surg 89:368–373

Heath E, Unkelbach J, Oelfke U (2009) Incorporating uncertainties in respiratory motion into 4D treatment plan optimization. Med Phys 36:3059–3071

Hoisak JD, Sixel KE, Tirona R, Cheung PC, Pignol JP (2004) Correlation of lung tumor motion with external surrogate indicators of respiration. Int J Radiat Oncol Biol Phys 60:1298–1306

Hoogeman M, Prévost JB, Nuyttens J, Pöll J, Levendag P, Heijmen B (2009) Clinical accuracy of the respiratory tumor tracking system of the cyberknife: assessment by analysis of log files. Int J Radiat Oncol Biol Phys 74:297–303

ICRU (2010) Prescribing, recording, and reporting intensity-modulated photon-beam therapy (IMRT) ICRU report 83. International Commission on Radiation Units and Measurements, Bethesda, MD

Imura M, Yamazaki K, Shirato H et al (2005) Insertion and fixation of fiducial markers for setup and tracking of lung tumors in radiotherapy. Int J Radiat Oncol Biol Phys 63:1442–1447

Inoue T, Widder J, van Dijk LV et al (2016) Limited impact of setup and range uncertainties, breathing motion, and interplay effects in robustly optimized intensity modulated proton therapy for stage III non-small cell lung cancer. Int J Radiat Oncol Biol Phys 96:661–669

International Electrotechnical Commission (2019) Medical electrical system – guidelines for sage integration and operation of adaptive external-beam radiotherapy systems for real-time adaptive radiotherapy. IEC Technical Report 62926 Edition 1.0

Jakobi A, Perrin R, Knopf A, Richter C (2018) Feasibility of proton pencil beam scanning treatment of free-breathing lung cancer patients. Acta Oncol 57:203–210

Josipovic M, Persson GF, Dueck J et al (2016) Geometric uncertainties in voluntary deep inspiration breath hold radiotherapy for locally advanced lung cancer. Radiother Oncol 118:510–514

Kanehira T, Matsuura T, Takao S et al (2017) Impact of real-time image gating on spot scanning proton therapy for lung tumors: a simulation study. Int J Radiat Oncol Biol Phys 97:173–181

Kaza E, Dunlop A, Panek R et al (2017) Lung volume reproducibility under ABC control and self-sustained breath-holding. J Appl Clin Med Phys 18:154–162

Keall PJ, Nguyen DT, O'Brien R et al (2018) Review of real-time 3-dimensional image guided radiation therapy on standard-equipped cancer radiation therapy systems: are we at the tipping point for the era of real-time radiation therapy? Int J Radiat Oncol Biol Phys 102:922–931

Knybel L, Cvek J, Molenda L, Stieberova N, Feltl D (2016) Analysis of lung tumor motion in a large sample: patterns and factors influencing precise delineation of internal target volume. Int J Radiat Oncol Biol Phys 96:751–758

Lax I, Blomgren H, Näslund I, Svanström R (1994) Stereotactic radiotherapy of malignancies in the abdomen. Methodological aspects. Acta Oncol 33:677–683

Li Y, Kardar L, Li X, Li H et al (2014) On the interplay effects with proton scanning beams in stage III lung cancer. Med Phys 41:021721

Lin L, Kang M, Huang S et al (2015) Beam-specific planning target volumes incorporating 4D CT for pencil beam scanning proton therapy of thoracic tumors. J Appl Clin Med Phys 16:5678

Lin H, Shi C, Wang B, Chan MF, Tang X, Ji W (2019a) Towards real-time respiratory motion prediction based on long short-term memory neural networks. Phys Med Biol 64:085010

Lin H, Zou W, Li T, Feigenberg SJ, Teo BK, Dong L (2019b) A super-learner model for tumor motion prediction and management in radiation therapy: development and feasibility evaluation. Sci Rep 9:14868

Liu HH, Balter P, Tutt T et al (2007) Assessing respiration-induced tumor motion and internal target volume using four-dimensional computed tomography for radiotherapy of lung cancer. Int J Radiat Oncol Biol Phys 68:531–540

Liu W, Zhang X, Li Y, Mohan R (2012) Robust optimization of intensity modulated proton therapy. Med Phys 39:1079–1091

Matsuura T, Miyamoto N, Shimizu S et al (2013) Integration of a real-time tumor monitoring system into gated proton spot-scanning beam therapy: an initial phantom study using patient tumor trajectory data. Med Phys 40:071729

Matsuura T, Fujii Y, Takao S et al (2016) Development and evaluation of a short-range applicator for treating superficial moving tumors with respiratory-gated spot-scanning proton therapy using real-time image guidance. Phys Med Biol 61:1515–1531

Miyamoto N, Maeda K, Abo D et al (2019) Quantitative evaluation of image recognition performance of fiducial markers in real-time tumor-tracking radiation therapy. Phys Med 65:33–39

Molitoris JK, Diwanji T, Snider JW III et al (2018) Advances in the use of motion management and image guidance in radiation therapy treatment for lung cancer. J Thorac Dis 10(Suppl 21):S2437–S2450

Nyman J, Hallqvist A, Lund JÅ et al (2016) SPACE - a randomized study of SBRT vs conventional fractionated radiotherapy in medically inoperable stage I NSCLC. Radiother Oncol 121:1–8

Ohara K, Okumura T, Akisada M et al (1989) Irradiation synchronized with respiration gate. Int J Radiat Oncol Biol Phys 17:853–857

Onimaru R, Shirato H, Fujino M et al (2005) The effect of tumor location and respiratory function on tumor movement estimated by real-time tracking radiotherapy (RTRT) system. Int J Radiat Oncol Biol Phys 63:164–169

Onodera Y, Nishioka N, Yasuda K et al (2011) Relationship between diseased lung tissues on computed tomography and motion of fiducial marker near lung cancer. Int J Radiat Oncol Biol Phys 79:1408–1413

Park PC, Zhu XR, Lee AK et al (2012) A beam-specific planning target volume (PTV) design for proton therapy to account for setup and range uncertainties. Int J Radiat Oncol Biol Phys 82:e329–e336

Roman NO, Shepherd W, Mukhopadhyay N, Hugo GD, Weiss E (2012) Interfractional positional variability of fiducial markers and primary tumors in locally advanced non-small-cell lung cancer during audiovisual biofeedback radiotherapy. Int J Radiat Oncol Biol Phys 83:1566–1572

Schmidt ML, Hoffmann L, Knap MM et al (2016) Cardiac and respiration induced motion of mediastinal lymph node targets in lung cancer patients throughout the radiotherapy treatment course. Radiother Oncol 121:52–58

Seppenwoolde Y, Shirato H, Kitamura K et al (2002) Precise and real-time measurement of 3D tumor motion in lung due to breathing and heartbeat, measured during radiotherapy. Int J Radiat Oncol Biol Phys 53:822–834

Shimizu S, Shirato H, Kagei K et al (2000) Impact of respiratory movement on the computed tomographic images of small lung tumors in three-dimensional (3D) radiotherapy. Int J Radiat Oncol Biol Phys 46:1127–1133

Shimizu S, Miyamoto N, Matsuura T et al (2014) A proton beam therapy system dedicated to spot-scanning increases accuracy with moving tumors by real-time imaging and gating and reduces equipment size. PLoS One 9:e94971

Shirato H, Shimizu S, Bo X et al (1998) Four-dimensional (4-D) treatment planning integrating respiratory phases and three-dimensional (3D) movement of lung and liver tumors using high-speed computed tomography (CT) and magnetic resonance imaging (MRI). In: Lemke HU, Inamura K, Farman A (eds) CAR '98. Elsevier, Amsterdam, pp 265–270

Shirato H, Shimizu S, Shimizu T, Nishioka T, Miyasaka K (1999) Real-time tumour-tracking radiotherapy. Lancet 353:1331–1332

Shirato H, Shimizu S, Kitamura K et al (2000) Four-dimensional treatment planning and fluoroscopic real-time tumor tracking radiotherapy for moving tumor. Int J Radiat Oncol Biol Phys 48:435–442

Shirato H, Suzuki K, Sharp GC et al (2006) Speed and amplitude of lung tumor motion precisely detected in four-dimensional setup and in real-time tumor-tracking radiotherapy. Int J Radiat Oncol Biol Phys 64:1229–1236

Sonke JJ, Rossi M, Wolthaus J, van Herk M, Damen E, Belderbos J (2009) Frameless stereotactic body radiotherapy for lung cancer using four-dimensional cone beam CT guidance. Int J Radiat Oncol Biol Phys 74:567–574

Takao S, Miyamoto N, Matsuura T et al (2016) Intrafractional baseline shift or drift of lung tumor motion during gated radiation therapy with a real-time tumor-tracking system. Int J Radiat Oncol Biol Phys 94:172–180

Thomas DH, Santhanam A, Kishan AU et al (2018) Initial clinical observations of intra- and interfractional motion variation in MR-guided lung SBRT. Br J Radiol 91:20170522

Unkelbach J, Paganetti H (2018) Robust proton treatment planning: physical and biological optimization. Semin Radiat Oncol 28:88–96

Unkelbach J, Chan TC, Bortfeld T (2007) Accounting for range uncertainties in the optimization of intensity modulated proton therapy. Phys Med Biol 52:2755–2773

Wade OL (1954) Movements of the thoracic cage and diaphragm in respiration. J Physiol 124:193–212

Wolthaus JW, Sonke JJ, van Herk M et al (2008) Comparison of different strategies to use four-dimensional computed tomography in treatment planning for lung cancer patients. Int J Radiat Oncol Biol Phys 70:1229–1238

Wong JW, Sharpe MB, Jaffray DA et al (1999) The use of active breathing control (ABC) to reduce margin for breathing motion. Int J Radiat Oncol Biol Phys 44:911–919

Yamada T, Miyamoto N, Matsuura T et al (2016) Optimization and evaluation of multiple gating beam delivery in a synchrotron-based proton beam scanning system using a real-time imaging technique. Phys Med 32:932–937

Yock AD, Mohan R, Flampouri S et al (2019) Robustness analysis for external beam radiation therapy treatment plans: describing uncertainty scenarios and reporting their dosimetric consequences. Pract Radiat Oncol 9:200–207

Yoshimura T, Shimizu S, Hashimoto T et al (2020) Analysis of treatment process time for real-time-image gated-spot-scanning proton-beam therapy (RGPT) system. J Appl Clin Med Phys 21:38–49

PET and PET/CT in Treatment Planning

Michael MacManus, Sarah Everitt, and Rodney J. Hicks

Contents

1 Introduction.. 237
2 Selecting Patients Who Are Candidates for Curative-Intent RT with 18F-FDG-PET.. 239
3 Local Extent of Disease................................. 240
4 Nodal Extent of Disease................................ 241
5 Distant Metastasis....................................... 242
6 Importance of Up-to-Date PET/CT Imaging in Radiotherapy Planning.............. 244
6.1 Using PET/CT for Target Volume Definition in Lung Cancer.................................... 244
7 The Process of Tumor Contouring on PET/CT.. 245
7.1 Targeting Tumor Subvolumes and Adapting Treatment to Response.................... 247
8 Normal Tissue Imaging in Treatment Planning.. 248
9 Conclusions... 249
References... 249

M. MacManus (✉) · S. Everitt
Department of Radiation Oncology, Peter MacCallum Cancer Centre, Melbourne, VIC, Australia

The Sir Peter MacCallum Department of Oncology, The University of Melbourne, Melbourne, VIC, Australia
e-mail: michael.macmanus@petermac.org

R. J. Hicks
The Sir Peter MacCallum Department of Oncology, The University of Melbourne, Melbourne, VIC, Australia

Department of Cancer Imaging, Peter MacCallum Cancer Centre, Melbourne, VIC, Australia

1 Introduction

Positron emission tomography/computed tomography (PET/CT) imaging now plays a fundamental role in treatment planning for patients with lung cancer, particularly for those who are candidates for potentially curative radiation therapy (RT) (Akhurst et al. 2015; De Ruysscher et al. 2010). ^{18}F-Fluorodeoxyglucose (^{18}F-FDG) remains the most widely used PET radiopharmaceutical in oncology and FDG-PET has proven to be the most accurate whole-body imaging modality for staging lung cancer since almost all types are highly metabolically active. This results in high contrast between FDG uptake in tumor and most surrounding normal tissues (apart from the central nervous system and urinary tract) facilitating lesion detection throughout the body including primary, nodal, and metastatic sites (MacManus et al. 2001). With dissemination of hybrid PET/CT scanners, the information provided by PET is complemented by detailed structural information from a contemporaneous CT component, but further complementary imaging using specialized CT protocols or magnetic resonance imaging (MRI) can provide additional correlative information to improve diagnostic certainty. Serial imaging provides unique insights in the evolution of cancers both structurally and metabolically in response to treatment and PET/CT has thus become an important diagnostic tool in therapeutic response assessment and restaging of suspected relapse.

In the context of radiation oncology, ^{18}F-FDG-PET plays a central role for target volume definition for locoregionally advanced disease, ensuring all areas of gross tumor are covered, while excluding as much normal tissue with a low probability of containing disease as possible (Konert et al. 2015). Stereotactic ablative radiation therapy (SABR) (Murray et al. 2017) is becoming more widely used for treating small primary lung tumors and oligometastases (Figs. 1 and 2) with curative intent but the smaller treatment volumes involved mandate even more precise target delineation in order to prevent local failure. PET plays an important role in selecting patients for this treatment. Complementing the increasing success of systemic therapies in advanced lung cancer, particularly including molecularly targeted therapies for cancers with specific oncogenic driver mutations (Dingemans et al. 2011), and, more broadly, immunotherapies for smoking-related disease that tends to have a high mutational burden, itself a predictor of benefit (Havel et al. 2019), newer indications for RT as a salvage or combination therapy are emerging. These include management of oligopersistent or oligoprogressive disease. Whole-body imaging with PET/CT is vital in selecting patients for RT and assisting in targeting disease that

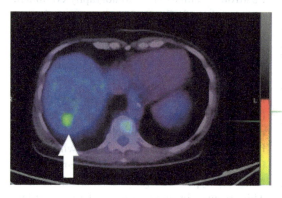
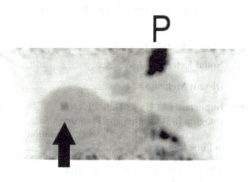

Fig. 1 Fused staging 4D FDG-PET/CT images (left panel) and maximum intensity projection images (right panel) from a patient with locally advanced primary adenocarcinoma of lung (indicated by "P") and a solitary liver metastasis

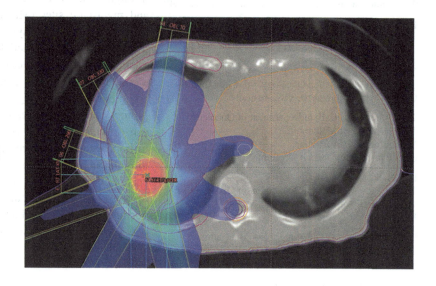

Fig. 2 Treatment plan for stereotactic ablative radiotherapy (SABR) to a synchronous PET-detected solitary liver metastasis. The primary tumor was treated with curative-intent chemoradiation. The liver lesion was not apparent on CT imaging

structural imaging modalities are unable to visualize clearly.

Most of the published literature on the use of PET in lung cancer RT planning relates to non-small cell lung cancer (NSCLC) where its value is clearly established. The available literature for small cell lung cancer (SCLC) is much sparser, because this histology is less common than NSCLC, is usually advanced at presentation and urgent systemic therapy is often deemed necessary and may compete with the logistics required for obtaining a baseline PET/CT. Nevertheless, because it is usually highly ^{18}F-FDG-avid, PET/CT is likely to be just as useful in target volume definition in limited-stage SCLC as it is in NSCLC, where similar anatomical and physiological considerations apply (Le Pechoux et al. 2020). Additionally, the higher a priori likelihood of metastatic disease in SCLC than NSCLC makes more sensitive systemic staging of value in identifying cases that are extensive rather than limited, with consequent prognostic and therapeutic implications.

This chapter will primarily review the role of PET scanning in RT planning in lung cancer, with an emphasis of locoregionally advanced NSCLC imaged with ^{18}F-FDG-PET. The value of PET in patients treated with SABR for localized, oligometastatic disease (Siva et al. 2015a) will also be briefly considered. There is increasing interest in the use of tracers other than ^{18}F-FDG to provide staging and biological information, including markers of proliferation and hypoxia, and there could be a role for these novel pharmaceuticals in RT planning in future. We will therefore briefly discus some of the most promising of these nonmetabolic tracers.

2 Selecting Patients Who Are Candidates for Curative-Intent RT with ^{18}F-FDG-PET

Whole-body staging with ^{18}F-FDG-PET is invaluable for identifying patients with NSCLC who are suitable for either curative-intent treatment with surgery, or RT, or chemoRT (Mac Manus et al. 2001; Gregory et al. 2012). Being more sensitive for the detection of metastatic disease than CT, PET can also detect previously unsuspected advanced disease, appropriately diverting such patients to systemic or palliative treatment options. In patients who on preceding evaluation are considered likely to be candidates for RT, staging PET/CT scan acquisition methodology can be adapted to simultaneously allow target volume definition by using RT planning setups including a flat palette and laser positioning (MacManus et al. 2009). This reduces the duplication of tests and can expedite treatment delivery with attendant cost savings and possibility of better outcomes given the predisposition of NSCLC for relatively rapid progression (Everitt et al. 2013). Because of the dual purposes of the staging PET scan, its twin roles of staging and target volume definition are inextricably entwined and must be considered together (Akhurst et al. 2015). Acquisition of PET/CT images in a position suitable for RT planning can help save time and increase efficiency.

While surgery is generally the preferred treatment for stage I and II NSCLC, patients considered unfit for surgery due to comorbidities such as lung or heart disease are increasingly being managed with curative-intent RT. In noncentral stage I NSCLC, SABR is usually considered superior to conventional RT, based especially on the CHISEL randomized trial that confirmed significant advantages in overall survival and local disease control for SABR (Ball et al. 2019). SABR is also associated with preservation of good quality of life (Nestle et al. 2020a).

Selected patients with stage III NSCLC, who have a good performance status and safely encompassable disease, are now commonly managed with curative-intent platinum-based chemoradiation. The failure of the RTOG 0617 study to show a survival advantage with higher dose RT (Eaton et al. 2016; Chun et al. 2017) has meant that the most widely used evidence-based treatment in curative-intent treatment of locoregionally advanced NSCLC is a combination of 60–66 Gy of conventionally fractionated RT with concurrent platinum-based chemotherapy. The PACIFIC trial has further refined this de facto standard of care by reporting a significant survival improvement for stage III patients who received adjuvant immune checkpoint blockade immunotherapy with durvalumab after chemoradiation, compared to patients who received placebo (Antonia et al. 2017, 2018). Thus, adjuvant immune checkpoint therapy for patients who have not progressed after chemoradiation is standard practice at many centers.

The incremental value of PET staging is greatest in patients who are already known to have more advanced disease (i.e., the rates of upstaging are much higher in patients with apparent stage III disease on CT staging than in those with apparent stage I). While PET commonly shows unexpected distant metastases in apparent stage III disease, it does so relatively less commonly in apparent stage I disease. While nodal staging may be revised by PET in patients in all stages, the likelihood of distant disease beyond the anatomically planned treatment volume increases from early to more advanced disease. The major advantage of PET imaging in nodal staging is its ability to detect metastasis in nonenlarged mediastinal and hilar nodes. This has implications not only for choosing the correct stage grouping and treatment modality (surgery vs. RT vs. palliation) but for target volume definition (whether a particular nodal station should receive high-dose irradiation or not), with downstream effects on lung or esophageal toxicity risk. The increasing use of endoscopic ultrasound-guided biopsies (EBUS) of hilar and mediastinal nodes to further interrogate nodes identified on PET as potentially being positive but possibly inflammatory, or likely negative but adjacent to an involved field making microscopic disease below the levels of PET detectability more likely, has meant that previously unattainable levels of accuracy can be attained in locoregional staging. Recognizing that nodal staging only becomes relevant if locoregional cure is feasible, there are significant advantages in using ^{18}F-FDG PET/CT prior to EBUS to obviate its need if distant metastases are detected or to guide representative sites for target EBUS examination if not (Kalade et al. 2008).

Local, nodal, and systemic staging with PET will be considered in more detail as they relate to target volume definition.

3 Local Extent of Disease

Multimodality imaging is becoming increasingly widely used to determine the local extent of disease in nonsurgical cases, particularly extension into adjacent tissues. For example, CT and MRI imaging can complement each other in the assessment of bony and soft tissue extent of disease in patients with superior sulcus tumors (Metcalfe et al. 2013). PET scanning can also provide valuable information concerning the local extent of disease in these and other cases. ^{18}F-FDG-PET can show bony invasion and soft tissue extensions that are not apparent on CT and can help clarify the nature of regions of equivocal soft tissue abnormality on MRI.

One of the most significant contributions of ^{18}F-FDG-PET is the identification of the boundary between atelectactic lung and contiguous tumor. On a standard RT planning CT scan, tumor and collapsed lung usually appear to be of the same density and often cannot readily be distinguished. Intravenous contrast may improve the contrast between tumor and normal tissues on planning CT scans, but usually this is insufficient to confidently delineate tumor in the presence of adjacent atelectasis. In this setting, ^{18}F-FDG-PET is of great value (Mac Manus et al. 2001; Nestle et al. 1999) and can usually demonstrate a clear boundary between tumor and collapsed lung. Despite the lower resolution of PET compared to CT, contouring of the tumor is usually feasible and the volume of non-tumor-containing lung needlessly exposed to high-dose radiation can often be greatly reduced. Expansion of collapsed lung during the course of radiotherapy may significantly alter the anatomical relations of tumor and require adaption of the treatment plan. Although it is relatively uncommon to perform ^{18}F-FDG PET/CT during the course of RT, significant alteration in the regional anatomy may warrant this to ensure adequate targeting of disease.

Another common contouring problem in lung cancer is the presence of nodules and adjacent to the primary tumor. Such lesions may be nonmalignant or may represent tumor satellite nodules. ^{18}F-FDG avidity in nodules of similar intensity to the primary tumor (Gould et al. 2001), after allowing for the size of these nodules according to the principles of partial-volume effect, would argue in favor of inclusion of such lesions in the target volume (Herder et al. 2004) and bland lesions without ^{18}F-FDG uptake can generally be safely excluded if the primary is itself ^{18}F-FDG-avid. In patients with large target volumes, inclusion or exclusion of additional tumor sites can make the difference between curative-intent versus palliative-intent therapies because of organ-at-risk constraints. It is generally impossible to use multiple biopsies to assess all potential local disease extensions. For this reason, imaging must be relied upon in a majority of cases and the most accurate available imaging should always be used. This generally means that ^{18}F-FDG-PET should be a key part of the multimodality imaging workup, although MRI generally remains indispensable for assessing chest wall and neural axis involvement.

Another element of intrathoracic disease extension is pleural extension, either directly along the chest wall or as discrete pleural metastases that may be impossible to appreciate on CT imaging, especially if the patient has a reactive effusion or benign pleural plaques. In these cases, ^{18}F-FDG PET can help clarify the target volume if the extension is direct. Alternatively, ^{18}F-FDG may suggest a more palliative approach if there are discrete pleural metastases because the entire pleural surface would then be considered at risk. It should be noted that prior talc pleurodesis can severely compromise such assessment due to the establishment of inflammatory talc granulomas that are highly ^{18}F-FDG-avid (Murray et al. 1997). Close correlation to identify radiopaque talc deposits on noncontrast CT with focal ^{18}F-FDG uptake is required to differentiate these from active disease.

In patients with ^{18}F-FDG-avid tumors that are unsafe to biopsy, for example, in cases where there is severe emphysema or large bullae (Louie et al. 2014), the characteristic radiological and metabolic characteristics of the lesion as imaged on ^{18}F-FDG PET/CT can provide sufficient confidence in the diagnosis of lung cancer for local radiotherapy to be delivered, either as conventional fractionated therapy or SABR. The latter is particularly attractive in cases of severe parenchymal lung disease due to lower toxicity despite high local control rates.

4 Nodal Extent of Disease

Because CT-based (as with most other structural imaging-based) nodal staging criteria in lung cancer are dependent solely on nodal dimensions (Glazer et al. 1984), inaccuracies are encountered frequently due to the presence of tumor in small (short axis <1 cm) nodes and by the high prevalence of large reactive but nonmalignant nodes in patients with lung cancer. Lymph nodes with short axis transverse diameters >1 cm are considered to be positive (Glazer et al. 1984). Textural analysis can help make the assessment a little more accurate (Andersen et al. 2016).

One of the best documented advances in lung cancer imaging achieved by PET and PET/CT is the very significant improvement in the accuracy of staging nodal disease in the thorax. An early meta-analysis that compared stand-alone PET-based and CT-based staging indicated convincingly that ^{18}F-FDG PET assessment was much more accurate than CT ($p < 0.001$) (Gould et al. 2003). For CT, median sensitivity and specificity were only 61% and 79%, respectively, whereas for PET-based staging sensitivity and specificity increased to 85% and 90%, respectively. PET was more sensitive but less specific when lymph nodes were enlarged (median sensitivity, 100%, median specificity, 78%) compared to the situation when normal-sized nodes (sensitivity, 82%, specificity, 93%, $p = 0.002$) were present.

With modern scanners, ^{18}F-FDG PET/CT-based nodal staging has again been shown to be both more accurate and more cost-effective than CT-based staging (Sogaard et al. 2011). The accuracy of nodal staging can be increased by mediastinoscopy in selected cases (Videtic et al. 2008). A major advance in intrathoracic nodal staging has been the increasing availability of endoscopic ultrasound-guided biopsy of accessible intrathoracic nodes (EBUS). EBUS (Steinfort et al. 2013, 2016), when combined with ^{18}F-FDG PET/CT information, is playing an increasing role in helping define the nodal target volume in patients treated with RT. This technique allows the direct interrogation of accessible nodes and can detect low-volume metastasis in small ^{18}F-FDG-negative nodes. This technique may also aid in the exclusion of nodes that are enlarged but do not contain cancer or have ^{18}F-FDG uptake due to other pathologies such as tuberculosis or sarcoid-like granuloma. There is increasing evidence that nodal mapping with EBUS in addition to PET/CT can significantly refine the nodal target volume to include sites of active nodal disease while excluding negative nodes (Steinfort et al. 2016).

5 Distant Metastasis

Historically, the identification of distant metastasis in a lung cancer patient has almost always marked a transition from curative-intent to palliative-intent therapy. Before the advent of ^{18}F-FDG-PET, the identification of distant extracranial metastases was unreliable, compromised by the low sensitivity and limited specificity of the standard diagnostic CT scan of the chest and upper abdomen ± radionuclide bone scanning leading to many patients being treated curatively only to fail early at distant sites, and others to be denied potentially curative treatment. The ability of ^{18}F-FDG PET to detect metastasis in distant lymph nodes as well as adrenal, liver, lung, bone, pleura, and soft tissues has transformed our ability to perform systemic staging. In a situation where a collection of different staging investigations of varying sensitivity and sensitivity would have been performed in each patient, a single more accurate test can now replace these and provide a more comprehensive evaluation.

The frequent identification of unsuspected metastatic disease in NSCLC has been one of the major benefits of ^{18}F-FDG PET imaging (MacManus et al. 2001). With more comprehensive imaging of systemic metastases, it has become clearer that not all stage IV patients have the same prognosis. The importance of both the number and location of metastases is explicitly acknowledged in the eighth edition of the staging manual, in large part because of increased accuracy in systemic staging (Goldstraw et al. 2016). Patients with M1a disease have metastasis confined to lung, which may be solitary, and patients with M1b disease have a single extrathoracic metastasis. The increasing recognition of oligometastatic disease as a relatively favorable intermediate stage between localized and widespread disease has led to increasing use of local therapies such as SABR (Siva et al. 2015a; Chang et al. 2017) or surgery to remove or ablate limited metastatic disease. Patients with locoregionally advanced disease plus a single synchronous brain metastasis can experience long-term survival with a combination of radical chemoradiation to the thoracic disease and surgery and/or stereotactic radiosurgery to the brain disease. For this treatment to be successful, all intrathoracic disease must be accurately delineated and irradiated to high dose and systemic nonbrain metastases should be excluded by ^{18}F-FDG PET. Single distant nonbrain metastases may also be treated by SABR in patients with otherwise locoregionally advanced disease (Fig. 3) and they can also experience long-term progression-free survival after radical chemoradiation (Fig. 4) to thoracic disease and SABR or surgery to the site of metastasis. In these cases, ^{18}F-FDG PET plays a key role not only in RT planning for the intrathoracic disease but also in identifying and localizing soli-

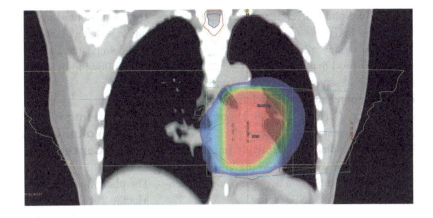

Fig. 3 Curative-intent thoracic chemoradiation plan (60 Gy in 30 fractions) for a patient with a locally advanced lung cancer and synchronous solitary hepatic metastasis. The liver metastasis was treated with SABR

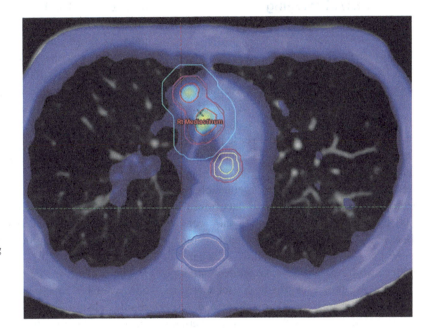

Fig. 4 Treatment planning FDG-PET/CT scan showing nodal target volumes in a patient with stage III NSCLC. The gross tumor volume (GTV) of FDG-avid nodes is indicated in red and the planning target volume (PTV) in blue. The nearby esophagus is circled in yellow and a conformal avoidance volume is delineated in red to assist in limiting the dose to this structure in the treatment planning process

tary (or oligo) metastases outside the CNS, and PET may also assist in RT planning ablation of solitary or oligometastases in such cases.

The ability of SABR to safely eradicate solitary adrenal metastasis has been complemented by the superior ability of ^{18}F-FDG PET to more accurately characterize the nature of adrenal enlargement (Yun et al. 2001) but PET can also detect tumor in nonenlarged adrenals. Similarly, in patients with solitary bone metastasis, PET/CT is extremely valuable both in lesion detection (Bury et al. 1998) and in radiotherapy planning. Liver metastases are often undetectable on CT imaging because they typically have similar CT density to normal liver parenchyma but are often well imaged on ^{18}F-FDG PET/CT (Grassetto et al. 2010). Solitary liver metastases may also be suitable for SABR.

Despite its key role in systemic staging, it is well understood that the high uptake of glucose makes the assessment of brain metastasis by ^{18}F-FDG PET unreliable and MRI is preferred for CNS staging (Seute et al. 2008; Hjorthaug et al. 2015). Interestingly, the PET tracer ^{18}F-fluorothymidine can effectively image proliferating brain metastasis due to the low uptake of this tracer in normal brain tissue and could potentially play a role in CNS staging.

6 Importance of Up-to-Date PET/CT Imaging in Radiotherapy Planning

It has been reported by several groups that NSCLC may progress rapidly between baseline staging PET/CT and subsequent treatment planning PET/CT imaging (Everitt et al. 2013; Lin et al. 2011). In several studies, approximately 30% of patients experienced disease progression that was sufficient to change treatment from curative to palliative intent, and palliatively treated patients experienced predictably poor survival. In a pooled analysis of data from >180 patients from five international centers, Bissonnette and colleagues reported that "longer intervals between imaging and treatment in patients with NSCLC were associated with high rates disease progression with consequent risks of geographic miss in RT planning and futile treatment in patients with M1 disease. Patients with more extensive initial nodal involvement and those with adenocarcinoma had the highest rates of stage migration. Dedicated RT planning PET/CT imaging is recommended, especially if >3 weeks have elapsed after initial staging" (Bissonnette et al. 2021). It has been conservatively recommended that PET/CT imaging should be repeated for planning purposes if more than 8 weeks elapses between initial staging scans and the onset of RT. However, as in the paper by Bissonnette and colleagues, we believe that this recommendation is too lax, given that disease progression within 2 weeks is relatively common. Accordingly, the practice at our institution is that a planning scan that is >3 weeks old will be repeated and RT initiated as soon as practical following this scan.

6.1 Using PET/CT for Target Volume Definition in Lung Cancer

The planning target volume (PTV) (Gregoire and Mackie 2011) is a region of tissue, defined by the radiation oncologist, that is intended to be irradiated to a defined dose within predefined minimum and maximum limits (e.g., prescribed dose ± 5%). The PTV, as a minimum, should include all sites of gross tumor, including the primary site and involved nodes, with margins applied to encompass likely microscopic disease extensions and further margins to allow for uncertainties in setup and physiological movement (Fig. 3). Intrathoracic tumors can move significantly due to the effects respiration and the cardiac cycle. This motion must be taken account of in the treatment planning process, for example, by increasing the target volume to cover the tumor in all parts of the movement cycle, by minimizing movement, as with deep inspiration breath hold (DIBH) techniques or by delivering the treatment in a particular part of the respiratory cycle ("gating").

For radiotherapy target volume definition, the best available imaging modality or modalities should always be used. For locoregionally advanced NSCLC, the most suitable imaging modality for target volume delineation is a recently acquired set of ^{18}F-FDG PET-CT images, supplemented in selected cases by MRI scanning or high-quality contrast-enhanced CT. PET/CT scanners dedicated to radiotherapy planning have increasingly been installed in cancer centers with lung cancer being the most common indication for this applied technology. Ideally, PET/CT images used for treatment planning should be acquired with careful patient immobilisation, ideally with the use of identical patient positioning lasers and other aids as are standard in the linear accelerator suite. The PET imaging suite therefore becomes part of the radiotherapy QA chain in such cases (Konert et al. 2015).

When the PET/CT images are imported into the RT planning system, the first task, leading to eventual creation of the PTV, is the definition of the gross tumor volume (GTV) as visualized on the scan, using a pointing device such as a mouse, a process known as "contouring." Although this process considers the anatomical boundaries when clearly demarcated, various techniques have been developed for "segmentation" of the ^{18}F-FDG PET abnormality that can automate and be more reproducible than manual contouring (Zhuang et al. 2019). This GTV can be expanded to take account of movement to generate an internal target volume or ITV. A further expansion to include suspected microscopic extension is generally used to generate a clinical target volume (CTV). In NSCLC, an expansion of the primary tumor GTV or ITV by 5–7 mm is commonly used to define the CTV, based on data from histopathological analysis of resected lung cancers. The CTV may then be expanded to produce the final PTV.

The ^{18}F-FDG PET component of a standard PET-CT scan, because of its relatively long acquisition time, can provide useful information on the average position of tumor sites. With activity integrated over time, blurring of activity at the extremes of motion do not contribute significantly to apparent GTV. Accordingly, the metabolic tumor volume is immediately applicable for GTV definition when imported into the planning system. A limitation of a standard 3D PET/CT acquisition is freezing of tumor motion on the CT component of the scan due to its near instantaneous acquisition speed. This commonly leads to difficulties in image reconstruction due to inappropriate attenuation correction and misinterpretation regarding anatomical correlates in patients with tumors that have extensive excursion with respiration, especially for those located near the diaphragm. Acquisition of a 4D CT scan on the radiotherapy simulator, subsequently fused with the planning PET scan, helps provide valuable additional information for tumor contouring that solves some of the problems encountered with 3D CT acquisitions. A more ideal account of tumor movement, especially for lesions not clearly visualized on the CT component of the scan, can be gained from a 4D-PET/CT acquisition (Chirindel et al. 2015; Callahan et al. 2014; Sindoni et al. 2016) in which both the CT and PET acquisitions are gated to respiratory motion (Callahan et al. 2011). 4D PET can also be used to facilitate gated therapy in which the treatment beam is only turned on when the tumor is in a particular part of the respiratory cycle, thereby reducing the exposure of normal tissues.

The use of PET and PET/CT for (Nestle et al. 1999) contouring primary tumors and grossly involved lymph nodes (De Ruysscher et al. 2005a) is likely to be associated with increased accuracy of tumor definition and is certainly associated with significantly greater interobserver reproducibility (Caldwell et al. 2001) compared to contouring with CT alone.

7 The Process of Tumor Contouring on PET/CT

There are practical difficulties to be overcome when using PET/CT images for defining target volumes in lung cancer. The PET images themselves have "soft" boundaries and require considerable benchmarking work to establish the optimum windowing and level settings to give the most accurate representation of the tumor. Typical accompanying 3D CT images from the planning PET/CT acquisition have sharp edges but are acquired at a single point in the respiratory cycle and may not be perfectly registered with the PET scan. There can be significant variation between observers in determining the tumor boundary using PET unless an exhaustive and rigorous contouring protocol is followed. In 2016, the International Atomic Energy Agency (IAEA) published an expert report in order to provide "best practice and evidence-based recommendations for the use of ^{18}F-FDG PET/CT for the purposes of radiotherapy target volume delineation (TVD) for curative-intent treatment of non-small cell lung cancer" (Konert et al. 2015). The report concluded that "appropriately timed and technically adequate PET/CT imaging is an essential component in the radiotherapy treatment planning process for lung cancer." The definition of "technically adequate" included that the scan was acquired under optimum conditions for radiotherapy, ideally with the assistance of specially trained staff. The report recognized that further research was essential in the fields of 4D PET/CT imaging and automated tumor volume definition techniques. The report also provided specific guidance on the interpretation of PET/CT for imaging and contouring tumors, concluding that, with the current state of knowledge, a visual contouring approach by an expert observer was more appropriate than an automated contouring method. Although promising work was continuing on machine learning and other techniques that could help increase reproducibility, none of the available methods was in itself sufficient to replace the human observer completely and that, at the time of publication, all automated contouring techniques required human editing.

A major contribution to knowledge of the use of PET/CT in treatment planning in lung cancer was made by Nestle and colleagues who conducted the only relevant randomized trial in the area. This trial helped answer the question "can we rely on PET/CT data for radiation treatment planning in lung cancer?" They conducted a "multicenter, open-label, randomized, controlled trial (PET-Plan) in 24 centers in Austria, Germany, and Switzerland" in patients with locally advanced non-small cell lung cancer suitable for chemoradiotherapy. They hoped to determine if "target volume reduction is feasible and effective compared with conventional planning in the context of radical chemoradiotherapy," comparing treatment volumes that were an expansion of the PET volumes, compared to "standard" PET- and CT-based RT planning with elective nodal irradiation. As would be expected, the PET-alone volumes were smaller than the standard volumes. At a median follow-up of 29 months, the risk of locoregional progression in the ^{18}F-FDG PET-based target group was actually lower than that in the conventional target group (14% vs. 29% at 1 year) (Nestle et al. 2020b). Surprisingly, early esophageal and later lung toxicities were similar in the two arms. This trial confirms what had already become a virtual standard of care around the world, with replacement of historic elective nodal irradiation target volume definition protocols with more conformal PET-based volumes. A limiting factor in this study was that all patients had PET information available, and this study really compared two ways of incorporating the data into the treatment planning process.

Although a visual approach to contouring of PET-based tumor volumes is widely used (Werner-Wasik et al. 2012), various auto-segmentation methods have been developed to help define the tumor volume as a stand-alone technique or to serve as a baseline for editing by a visual contouring (Hatt et al. 2017) method. As in the experimental arm of the Nestle PET Plan study, at most international centers, target volume definition in NSCLC commences with GTV definition (De Ruysscher et al. 2005b). In a pilot trial that preceded the PET-Plan trial (Fleckenstein et al. 2011) autocontour was used as the starting point for tumor contouring and this was modified for the trial itself. Use of an automated system could potentially bring more standardization to the evaluation of mediastinal nodes (Nestle et al. 2015).

A report by the American Association of Physicists in Medicine (AAPM) summarized the most promising autocontouring or segmentation methods and concluded that no single method was available that could give good results in all circumstances (Hatt et al. 2017). Although of potential value, auto-segmentation should always be subject to human editing (MacManus et al. 2009; Doll et al. 2014). One approach as used in RTOG clinical trials is to define an initial ^{18}F-FDG PET tumor volume, for subsequent human editing, using automated thresholding at 1.5 times the mediastinum blood pool followed by manual editing (Mahasittiwat et al. 2013).

When SABR is given for small primary or metastatic lung cancers, the lesions are typically surrounded by aerated lung and are usually well visualized on CT. A 4D-CT scan can adequately delineate the extent of motion with respiration, especially important for lesions near the diaphragm (De Ruysscher et al. 2010; Brandner et al. 2017). A 3D-PET scan can sometimes provide additional useful information but the primary role of ^{18}F-FDGPET/CT in this setting is to exclude macroscopic nodal involvement. The potential value of 4D PET information in treatment planning for SABR is being explored in the phase II LungTech trial (Adebahr et al. 2015; Lambrecht et al. 2016) which will recruit 150 patients from 23 EORTC centers in eight countries.

Although there are no randomized data concerning the use or nonuse of three-dimensional imaging with CT scanning for selecting patients or defining radiotherapy treatment volumes in lung cancer, the very powerful evidence that does exist for the superior accuracy of CT compared to plain radiographs or tomograms, including a strong suggestion of improved survival (Chen et al. 2011), would render any protocol that deliberately randomized patients to a two-dimensional imaging approach unethical. Despite the absence of randomized data, CT planning was universally adopted. Similarly, with respect to the use of PET in RT planning for lung cancer, equipoise no longer exists. In stage IIIA NSCLC, 5-year overall survival of >30% is no longer unusual in patients selected for treatment using PET (Mac Manus et al. 2013), and in the immunotherapy era survival has improved even further. The superior outcomes of the PACIFIC trial were seen in patients who had PET staging and who had target volume definition assisted by PET (Antonia et al. 2018). It would now be considered unethical to not use PET, when available for staging lung cancer, or to ignore evidence of previously occult disease, if detected by ^{18}F-FDG PET, when planning treatment volumes, in the absence of strong evidence for a competing superior imaging modality.

7.1 Targeting Tumor Subvolumes and Adapting Treatment to Response

Historically, a key aim of RT planning in NSCLC has been to deliver a uniform and essentially equal dose of radiation to all regions of gross tumor, regardless of biology or interim response to therapy. However, it has long been suggested that some regions of tumor may be more or less radiosensitive than others and that RT dose should be delivered in a more nuanced way, with more dose going to more resistant regions of tumor. The idea of selectively targeting tumor subvolumes for differential radiation doses has been described as "dose painting" (Bentzen 2005) and this has proved to be controversial (Hall 2005). It has long been known that hypoxic cells are more radioresistant than oxygenated cells (Deschner and Gray 1959) and that bioreductive metabolism in hypoxic tumor regions can cause the accumulation of PET hypoxia tracers (Bollineni et al. 2012a). Both ^{18}F-misonadazole (F-MISO) and ^{18}F-fluoroazomycin arabinoside (FAZA) (Bollineni et al. 2013) have been used to image patients with NSCLC. A greater degree of tumor hypoxia is almost certainly a negative prognostic factor, conferring both radioresistance (Deschner and Gray 1959) and a higher risk of metastasis.

The use of PET, including 4D PET, to identify tumor regions, potentially suitable for dose painting, has been explored (Bollineni et al. 2013). In a pilot study, Vera and colleagues explored the dynamics of ^{18}F-MISO, ^{18}F-FDG, and ^{18}F-FLT PET/CT scans in a small cohort, comparing baseline and 46 Gy scans. Proliferation and metabolism declined to a greater degree than imageable hypoxia (Vera et al. 2011). A further small study showed differences in ^{18}F-MISO PET scans acquired before, during, and after RT (Koh et al. 1995). Trinkaus and colleagues showed that persistence of ^{18}FAZA-PET was associated with poorer outcomes (Trinkaus et al. 2013). Preliminary planning studies have indeed explored dose painting of hypoxic regions using different tracers (Even et al. 2015), but no evidence yet exists that this can actually improve outcomes in lung cancer.

FAZA and F-Miso PET scans often have low tumor-to-background ratios and often fail to image lung tumors. Novel hypoxia tracers that may have superior characteristics are being explored. One of the more promising alternative hypoxia imaging agents is [^{64}Cu] [Cu-diacetyl-bis(N(4)-methylthiosemicarbazone)], abbreviated to Cu ATSM (Liu et al. 2020), which may ultimately have superior imaging characteristics to FAZA or Miso but uses a radioisotope that is more difficult to work with than ^{18}F. Hypoxia targeting with RT remains a tantalizing prospect, but it is still unclear that this is a stable characteristic of tumors that can be effectively targeted at the macroscopic level by dose painting with radiotherapy.

Imaging during the course of fractionated RT with cone beam CT has become routine and it is clear that tumors change in volume and location during a treatment course (Yan et al. 2005; Li et al. 2007; Hugo et al. 2007). The observation that tumor dimensions change and the possibility that tumor biology also changes during RT have encouraged the concept of response-adapted therapy. Changes in ^{18}F-FDG uptake detected by PET occur much more rapidly than changes in volume detected by CT and we also know that ^{18}F-FDG PET is superior to CT for estimating survival (Mac Manus et al. 2003) and relapse distribution (Mac Manus et al. 2005).

Researchers have been exploring the use of PET during RT to create "response-adapted" treatment plans that modify RT delivery based on the location and volume of intense residual tumor tracer uptake. This resource-intensive approach has been explored in a number of academic centers (Jaffray et al. 2002, 1999; Nielsen et al. 2009; Sorcini and Tilikidis 2006). In the PET boost trial, the baseline PET scan was used to explore the feasibility of boosting high ^{18}F-FDG uptake regions to a higher dose (van Elmpt et al. 2012). Kong and colleagues took this concept into the realms of response-adapted therapy, having previously demonstrated that tumors have often shrunk in volume and have reduced FDG uptake after 45 Gy. They conducted a phase 2 clinical trial in 42 patients with stage II to stage III NSCLC and reported that delivery of an escalated radiation dose to FDG-avid tumor detected by mid-treatment was possible and may be associated with favorable local disease control (Kong et al. 2017). The role of adaptive PET-based dose escalation is being pursued in NRG-RTOG 1106/ACRIN 6697, a randomized exploring the feasibility and safety of performing adaptive radiotherapy (RT) escalation in patients with locally advanced non-small cell lung cancer (NSCLC). It is expected that there will be a 1% improvement in local disease control with each 1 Gy of dose escalation. The most appropriate time points for imaging and replanning remain uncertain (van Baardwijk et al. 2007). The range of potential dose escalation can potentially be very wide: for example, range of 30–102 Gy (mean, 58 Gy) was reported in a small cohort (Feng et al. 2009) with PET/CT response-adapted therapy.

While ^{18}F-FDG can be used for interim response assessment based on glucose uptake in tumors, uptake in normal tissues, including lung, can lead to difficulties in scan interpretation (Bollineni et al. 2012b; Mac Manus et al. 2011). There is significant potential for other PET tracers that image physiological processes such as proliferation. In a prospective study of 60 patients imaged with both ^{18}F-FDG and ^{18}F-FLT PET/CT scans at baseline and at weeks 2 and 4 of chemoRT (Everitt et al. 2014), Everitt and colleagues unexpectedly discovered that stable disease detected on a week 2 FLT PET/CT was linked to superior progression-free and overall survival compared to partial or complete FLT uptake reduction (Ball et al. 2017), suggesting that cell cycle arrest in S-phase, which is associated high ^{18}F-FLT uptake, early during RT may be an important precursor to radiation-induced cell death. However, interim FLT did not appear to be so promising for response-adapted therapy due to the low level of FLT uptake seen in a high proportion of patients as treatment progressed.

8 Normal Tissue Imaging in Treatment Planning

Radiation-induced lung toxicity is a common dose-limiting effect of RT in NSCLC (Mah et al. 1987; Boersma et al. 1996), which has classic clinical and radiological features

(Yankelevitz et al. 1994; Ogasawara et al. 2002). Radiation-induced pneumonitis can be visualized on PET scans due to uptake of ^{18}F-FDG in lungs and pleura. PET imaging may even identify pneumonitis before symptoms are reported by patients (Mac Manus et al. 2011). Esophageal toxicity can also be identified on serial ^{18}F-FDG PET due to increased glucose uptake corresponding to the organ (Mac Manus et al. 2011; Hicks et al. 2004; Guerrero et al. 2007; Hart et al. 2008; Abdulla et al. 2014; McCurdy et al. 2013, 2012) which is dose related (Guerrero et al. 2007).

Lung tissue is often of variable quality in lung cancer patients due to coexistent pulmonary disease associated with heavy tobacco use. Some regions of lung are more "high functioning" than others and have superior ventilation and perfusion. In RT treatment planning, it would be attractive to spare "high-functioning" lung from radiation and where possible "dump" radiation dose in areas of low-functioning lung to preserve lung function in patients treated with curative-intent RT. PET can be used to show the geographic distribution of ventilation with gallium-68-labeled nanoparticles (Galligas) and perfusion with macroaggregated albumin (MAA) (Siva et al. 2014). Preliminary studies have reported early reductions in lung perfusion on ^{68}Ga-MAA PET that precede changes in ventilation or radiographic changes of pneumonitis (Siva et al. 2015b). PET tracers that show lung function have the potential to inform radiotherapy planning, allowing planners to spare normal lung tissue, either based on baseline scans or on scans performed during treatment that can take account of dynamic changes in ventilation and perfusion (Siva et al. 2015c). Based on preliminary studies, Bucknell and colleagues studies have published a protocol in which 20 stage III NSCLC chemoradiation patients will undergo "ventilation and perfusion PET/CT to identify highly functioning lung volumes and avoidance of these using VMAT planning" (Bucknell et al. 2020). Patients will receive a dose of 69 Gy, compared to the standard institutional dose of 60 Gy.

9 Conclusions

It is now hard to conceive of effectively managing lung cancer patients using RT without having timely access to ^{18}F-FDG PET/CT for selection, target volume definition, and monitoring. Nevertheless, optimal integration of this information into current treatment paradigms continues to evolve on the basis of ongoing research, improved instrumentation, more sophisticated image analysis, and greater understanding of the biological drivers of disease progression and response. As treatment combinations become more complex, potentially more toxic, and certainly more expensive, the cost implications of incorporating PET/CT into the evaluation process will be increasingly offset by the savings accrued in avoiding futile treatments or abandoning ineffective therapy before toxicity or disease progression obviates institution of alternative management options.

Our experience suggests that a close working relationship between imaging specialists and radiation oncologists is both vital to the success of integrating molecular imaging techniques into routine clinical practice of thoracic RT and rewarding intellectually for both groups. We need to work together to further advance practices and further engage the broader molecular imaging field which involves exciting developments in radiochemistry, physics, and image analysis techniques including radiomics and artificial intelligence. Although not discussed herein, the next opportunity and challenge will be the incorporation of genomic predictors of radiation response and interrogation of the tumor immune environment in real time.

References

Abdulla S, Salavati A, Saboury B, Basu S, Torigian DA, Alavi A (2014) Quantitative assessment of global lung inflammation following radiation therapy using FDG PET/CT: a pilot study. Eur J Nucl Med Mol Imaging 41(2):350–356

Adebahr S, Collette S, Shash E, Lambrecht M, Le Pechoux C, Faivre-Finn C et al (2015) LungTech, an EORTC Phase II trial of stereotactic body radiotherapy for centrally located lung tumours: a clinical perspective. Br J Radiol 88(1051):20150036

Akhurst T, MacManus M, Hicks RJ (2015) Lung cancer. PET Clin 10(2):147–158

Andersen MB, Harders SW, Ganeshan B, Thygesen J, Torp Madsen HH, Rasmussen F (2016) CT texture analysis can help differentiate between malignant and benign lymph nodes in the mediastinum in patients suspected for lung cancer. Acta Radiol 57(6):669–676

Antonia SJ, Villegas A, Daniel D, Vicente D, Murakami S, Hui R et al (2017) Durvalumab after chemoradiotherapy in stage III non-small-cell lung cancer. N Engl J Med 377(20):1919–1929

Antonia SJ, Villegas A, Daniel D, Vicente D, Murakami S, Hui R et al (2018) Overall survival with durvalumab after chemoradiotherapy in stage III NSCLC. N Engl J Med 379(24):2342–2350

van Baardwijk A, Bosmans G, Dekker A, van Kroonenburgh M, Boersma L, Wanders S et al (2007) Time trends in the maximal uptake of FDG on PET scan during thoracic radiotherapy. A prospective study in locally advanced non-small cell lung cancer (NSCLC) patients. Radiother Oncol 82(2):145–152

Ball D, Everitt S, Hicks R, Callahan J, Herschtal A, Kron T et al (2017) Serial FDG and FLT PET/CT during curative-intent chemo-radiotherapy for NSCLC impacts patient management and may predict clinical outcomes. J Thorac Oncol 12(1):S420

Ball D, Mai GT, Vinod S, Babington S, Ruben J, Kron T et al (2019) Stereotactic ablative radiotherapy versus standard radiotherapy in stage 1 non-small-cell lung cancer (TROG 09.02 CHISEL): a phase 3, open-label, randomised controlled trial. Lancet Oncol 20(4):494–503

Bentzen SM (2005) Theragnostic imaging for radiation oncology: dose-painting by numbers. Lancet Oncol 6(2):112–117

Bissonnette JP, Sun A, Grills IS, Almahariq MF, Geiger G, Vogel W et al (2021) Non-small cell lung cancer stage migration as a function of wait times from diagnostic imaging: a pooled analysis from five international centres. Lung Cancer 155:136–143

Boersma LJ, Damen EM, de Boer RW, Muller SH, Valdes Olmos RA, van Zandwijk N et al (1996) Recovery of overall and local lung function loss 18 months after irradiation for malignant lymphoma. J Clin Oncol 14(5):1431–1441

Bollineni VR, Wiegman EM, Pruim J, Groen HJ, Langendijk JA (2012a) Hypoxia imaging using Positron Emission Tomography in non-small cell lung cancer: implications for radiotherapy. Cancer Treat Rev 38(8):1027–1032

Bollineni VR, Widder J, Pruim J, Langendijk JA, Wiegman EM (2012b) Residual (1)(8)F-FDG-PET uptake 12 weeks after stereotactic ablative radiotherapy for stage I non-small-cell lung cancer predicts local control. Int J Radiat Oncol Biol Phys 83(4):e551–e555

Bollineni VR, Kerner GS, Pruim J, Steenbakkers RJ, Wiegman EM, Koole MJ et al (2013) PET imaging of tumor hypoxia using 18F-fluoroazomycin arabinoside in stage III-IV non-small cell lung cancer patients. J Nucl Med 54(8):1175–1180

Brandner ED, Chetty IJ, Giaddui TG, Xiao Y, Huq MS (2017) Motion management strategies and technical issues associated with stereotactic body radiotherapy of thoracic and upper abdominal tumors: a review from NRG oncology. Med Phys 44:2595

Bucknell N, Hardcastle N, Jackson P, Hofman M, Callahan J, Eu P et al (2020) Single-arm prospective interventional study assessing feasibility of using gallium-68 ventilation and perfusion PET/CT to avoid functional lung in patients with stage III non-small cell lung cancer. BMJ Open 10(12):e042465

Bury T, Barreto A, Daenen F, Barthelemy N, Ghaye B, Rigo P (1998) Fluorine-18 deoxyglucose positron emission tomography for the detection of bone metastases in patients with non-small cell lung cancer. Eur J Nucl Med 25(9):1244–1247

Caldwell CB, Mah K, Ung YC, Danjoux CE, Balogh JM, Ganguli SN et al (2001) Observer variation in contouring gross tumor volume in patients with poorly defined non-small-cell lung tumors on CT: the impact of 18FDG-hybrid PET fusion. Int J Radiat Oncol Biol Phys 51(4):923–931

Callahan J, Kron T, Schneider-Kolsky M, Hicks RJ (2011) The clinical significance and management of lesion motion due to respiration during PET/CT scanning. Cancer Imaging 11:224–236

Callahan J, Kron T, Siva S, Simoens N, Edgar A, Everitt S et al (2014) Geographic miss of lung tumours due to respiratory motion: a comparison of 3D vs 4D PET/CT defined target volumes. Radiat Oncol 9:291

Chang JH, Gandhidasan S, Finnigan R, Whalley D, Nair R, Herschtal A et al (2017) Stereotactic ablative body radiotherapy for the treatment of spinal oligometastases. Clin Oncol 29:e119

Chen AB, Neville BA, Sher DJ, Chen K, Schrag D (2011) Survival outcomes after radiation therapy for stage III non-small-cell lung cancer after adoption of computed tomography-based simulation. J Clin Oncol 29(17):2305–2311

Chirindel A, Adebahr S, Schuster D, Schimek-Jasch T, Schanne DH, Nemer U et al (2015) Impact of 4D-(18) FDG-PET/CT imaging on target volume delineation in SBRT patients with central versus peripheral lung tumors. Multi-reader comparative study. Radiother Oncol 115(3):335–341

Chun SG, Hu C, Choy H, Komaki RU, Timmerman RD, Schild SE et al (2017) Impact of intensity-modulated radiation therapy technique for locally advanced non-small-cell lung cancer: a secondary analysis of the NRG oncology RTOG 0617 randomized clinical trial. J Clin Oncol 35(1):56–62

De Ruysscher D, Wanders S, van Haren E, Hochstenbag M, Geeraedts W, Utama I et al (2005a) Selective mediastinal node irradiation based on FDG-PET scan data in patients with non-small-cell lung cancer: a prospective clinical study. Int J Radiat Oncol Biol Phys 62(4):988–994

De Ruysscher D, Wanders S, Minken A, Lumens A, Schiffelers J, Stultiens C et al (2005b) Effects of radiotherapy planning with a dedicated combined PET-CT-simulator of patients with non-small cell lung cancer on dose limiting normal tissues and radiation dose-escalation: a planning study. Radiother Oncol 77(1):5–10

De Ruysscher D, Faivre-Finn C, Nestle U, Hurkmans CW, Le Pechoux C, Price A et al (2010) European Organisation for Research and Treatment of Cancer recommendations for planning and delivery of high-dose, high-precision radiotherapy for lung cancer. J Clin Oncol 28(36):5301–5310

Deschner EE, Gray LH (1959) Influence of oxygen tension on x-ray-induced chromosomal damage in Ehrlich ascites tumor cells irradiated in vitro and in vivo. Radiat Res 11(1):115–146

Dingemans AM, de Langen AJ, van den Boogaart V, Marcus JT, Backes WH, Scholtens HT et al (2011) First-line erlotinib and bevacizumab in patients with locally advanced and/or metastatic non-small-cell lung cancer: a phase II study including molecular imaging. Ann Oncol 22(3):559–566

Doll C, Duncker-Rohr V, Rucker G, Mix M, MacManus M, De Ruysscher D et al (2014) Influence of experience and qualification on PET-based target volume delineation. When there is no expert-ask your colleague. Strahlenther Onkol 190(6):555–562

Eaton BR, Pugh SL, Bradley JD, Masters G, Kavadi VS, Narayan S et al (2016) Institutional enrollment and survival among NSCLC patients receiving chemoradiation: NRG oncology radiation therapy oncology group (RTOG) 0617. J Natl Cancer Inst 108(9):djw034

van Elmpt W, De Ruysscher D, van der Salm A, Lakeman A, van der Stoep J, Emans D et al (2012) The PET-boost randomised phase II dose-escalation trial in non-small cell lung cancer. Radiother Oncol 104(1):67–71

Even AJ, van der Stoep J, Zegers CM, Reymen B, Troost EG, Lambin P et al (2015) PET-based dose painting in non-small cell lung cancer: comparing uniform dose escalation with boosting hypoxic and metabolically active sub-volumes. Radiother Oncol 116(2):281–286

Everitt S, Plumridge N, Herschtal A, Bressel M, Ball D, Callahan J et al (2013) The impact of time between staging PET/CT and definitive chemo-radiation on target volumes and survival in patients with non-small cell lung cancer. Radiother Oncol 106(3):288–291

Everitt SJ, Ball DL, Hicks RJ, Callahan J, Plumridge N, Collins M et al (2014) Differential (18)F-FDG and (18)F-FLT uptake on serial PET/CT imaging before and during definitive chemoradiation for non-small cell lung cancer. J Nucl Med 55(7):1069–1074

Feng M, Kong FM, Gross M, Fernando S, Hayman JA, Ten Haken RK (2009) Using fluorodeoxyglucose positron emission tomography to assess tumor volume during radiotherapy for non-small-cell lung cancer and its potential impact on adaptive dose escalation and normal tissue sparing. Int J Radiat Oncol Biol Phys 73(4):1228–1234

Fleckenstein J, Hellwig D, Kremp S, Grgic A, Groschel A, Kirsch CM et al (2011) F-18-FDG-PET confined radiotherapy of locally advanced NSCLC with concomitant chemotherapy: results of the PET-PLAN pilot trial. Int J Radiat Oncol Biol Phys 81(4):e283–e289

Glazer GM, Orringer MB, Gross BH, Quint LE (1984) The mediastinum in non-small cell lung cancer: CT-surgical correlation. AJR Am J Roentgenol 142(6):1101–1105

Goldstraw P, Chansky K, Crowley J, Rami-Porta R, Asamura H, Eberhardt WE et al (2016) The IASLC lung cancer staging project: proposals for revision of the TNM stage groupings in the forthcoming (Eighth) edition of the TNM classification for lung cancer. J Thorac Oncol 11(1):39–51

Gould MK, Maclean CC, Kuschner WG, Rydzak CE, Owens DK (2001) Accuracy of positron emission tomography for diagnosis of pulmonary nodules and mass lesions: a meta-analysis. JAMA 285(7):914–924

Gould MK, Kuschner WG, Rydzak CE, Maclean CC, Demas AN, Shigemitsu H et al (2003) Test performance of positron emission tomography and computed tomography for mediastinal staging in patients with non-small-cell lung cancer: a meta-analysis. Ann Intern Med 139(11):879–892

Grassetto G, Fornasiero A, Bonciarelli G, Banti E, Rampin L, Marzola MC et al (2010) Additional value of FDG-PET/CT in management of "solitary" liver metastases: preliminary results of a prospective multicenter study. Mol Imaging Biol 12(2):139–144

Gregoire V, Mackie TR (2011) State of the art on dose prescription, reporting and recording in Intensity-Modulated Radiation Therapy (ICRU report No. 83). Cancer Radiother 15(6–7):555–559

Gregory DL, Hicks RJ, Hogg A, Binns DS, Shum PL, Milner A et al (2012) Effect of PET/CT on management of patients with non-small cell lung cancer: results of a prospective study with 5-year survival data. J Nucl Med 53(7):1007–1015

Guerrero T, Johnson V, Hart J, Pan T, Khan M, Luo D et al (2007) Radiation pneumonitis: local dose versus [18F]-fluorodeoxyglucose uptake response in irradiated lung. Int J Radiat Oncol Biol Phys 68(4):1030–1035

Hall EJ (2005) Dose-painting by numbers: a feasible approach? Lancet Oncol 6(2):66

Hart JP, McCurdy MR, Ezhil M, Wei W, Khan M, Luo D et al (2008) Radiation pneumonitis: correlation of toxicity with pulmonary metabolic radiation response. Int J Radiat Oncol Biol Phys 71(4):967–971

Hatt M, Lee JA, Schmidtlein CR, Naqa IE, Caldwell C, De Bernardi E et al (2017) Classification and evaluation strategies of auto-segmentation approaches for PET: report of AAPM task group No. 211. Med Phys 44:e1

Havel JJ, Chowell D, Chan TA (2019) The evolving landscape of biomarkers for checkpoint inhibitor immunotherapy. Nat Rev Cancer 19(3):133–150

Herder GJ, Golding RP, Hoekstra OS, Comans EF, Teule GJ, Postmus PE et al (2004) The performance of (18)

F-fluorodeoxyglucose positron emission tomography in small solitary pulmonary nodules. Eur J Nucl Med Mol Imaging 31(9):1231–1236

Hicks RJ, Mac Manus MP, Matthews JP, Hogg A, Binns D, Rischin D et al (2004) Early FDG-PET imaging after radical radiotherapy for non-small-cell lung cancer: inflammatory changes in normal tissues correlate with tumor response and do not confound therapeutic response evaluation. Int J Radiat Oncol Biol Phys 60(2):412–418

Hjorthaug K, Hojbjerg JA, Knap MM, Tietze A, Haraldsen A, Zacho HD et al (2015) Accuracy of 18F-FDG PET-CT in triaging lung cancer patients with suspected brain metastases for MRI. Nucl Med Commun 36(11):1084–1090

Hugo GD, Yan D, Liang J (2007) Population and patient-specific target margins for 4D adaptive radiotherapy to account for intra- and inter-fraction variation in lung tumour position. Phys Med Biol 52(1):257–274

Jaffray DA, Drake DG, Moreau M, Martinez AA, Wong JW (1999) A radiographic and tomographic imaging system integrated into a medical linear accelerator for localization of bone and soft-tissue targets. Int J Radiat Oncol Biol Phys 45(3):773–789

Jaffray DA, Siewerdsen JH, Wong JW, Martinez AA (2002) Flat-panel cone-beam computed tomography for image-guided radiation therapy. Int J Radiat Oncol Biol Phys 53(5):1337–1349

Kalade AV, Eddie Lau WF, Conron M, Wright GM, Desmond PV, Hicks RJ et al (2008) Endoscopic ultrasound-guided fine-needle aspiration when combined with positron emission tomography improves specificity and overall diagnostic accuracy in unexplained mediastinal lymphadenopathy and staging of non-small-cell lung cancer. Intern Med J 38(11):837–844

Koh WJ, Bergman KS, Rasey JS, Peterson LM, Evans ML, Graham MM et al (1995) Evaluation of oxygenation status during fractionated radiotherapy in human nonsmall cell lung cancers using [F-18]fluoromisonidazole positron emission tomography. Int J Radiat Oncol Biol Phys 33(2):391–398

Konert T, Vogel W, MacManus MP, Nestle U, Belderbos J, Gregoire V et al (2015) PET/CT imaging for target volume delineation in curative intent radiotherapy of non-small cell lung cancer: IAEA consensus report 2014. Radiother Oncol 116(1):27–34

Kong FM, Ten Haken RK, Schipper M, Frey KA, Hayman J, Gross M et al (2017) Effect of midtreatment PET/CT-adapted radiation therapy with concurrent chemotherapy in patients with locally advanced non-small-cell lung cancer: a phase 2 clinical trial. JAMA Oncol 3(10):1358–1365

Lambrecht M, Melidis C, Sonke JJ, Adebahr S, Boellaard R, Verheij M et al (2016) Lungtech, a phase II EORTC trial of SBRT for centrally located lung tumours - a clinical physics perspective. Radiat Oncol 11:7

Le Pechoux C, Faivre-Finn C, Ramella S, McDonald F, Manapov F, Putora PM et al (2020) ESTRO ACROP guidelines for target volume definition in the thoracic radiation treatment of small cell lung cancer. Radiother Oncol 152:89–95

Li XA, Qi XS, Pitterle M, Kalakota K, Mueller K, Erickson BA et al (2007) Interfractional variations in patient setup and anatomic change assessed by daily computed tomography. Int J Radiat Oncol Biol Phys 68(2):581–591

Lin P, Koh ES, Lin M, Vinod SK, Ho-Shon I, Yap J et al (2011) Diagnostic and staging impact of radiotherapy planning FDG-PET-CT in non-small-cell lung cancer. Radiother Oncol 101(2):284–290

Liu T, Karlsen M, Karlberg AM, Redalen KR (2020) Hypoxia imaging and theranostic potential of [(64)Cu][Cu(ATSM)] and ionic Cu(II) salts: a review of current evidence and discussion of the retention mechanisms. EJNMMI Res 10(1):33

Louie AV, Senan S, Patel P, Ferket BS, Lagerwaard FJ, Rodrigues GB et al (2014) When is a biopsy-proven diagnosis necessary before stereotactic ablative radiotherapy for lung cancer?: a decision analysis. Chest 146(4):1021–1028

Mac Manus MP, Hicks RJ, Ball DL, Kalff V, Matthews JP, Salminen E et al (2001) F-18 fluorodeoxyglucose positron emission tomography staging in radical radiotherapy candidates with nonsmall cell lung carcinoma: powerful correlation with survival and high impact on treatment. Cancer 92(4):886–895

Mac Manus MP, Hicks RJ, Matthews JP, McKenzie A, Rischin D, Salminen EK et al (2003) Positron emission tomography is superior to computed tomography scanning for response-assessment after radical radiotherapy or chemoradiotherapy in patients with non-small-cell lung cancer. J Clin Oncol 21(7):1285–1292

Mac Manus MP, Hicks RJ, Matthews JP, Wirth A, Rischin D, Ball DL (2005) Metabolic (FDG-PET) response after radical radiotherapy/chemoradiotherapy for non-small cell lung cancer correlates with patterns of failure. Lung Cancer 49(1):95–108

Mac Manus MP, Ding Z, Hogg A, Herschtal A, Binns D, Ball DL et al (2011) Association between pulmonary uptake of fluorodeoxyglucose detected by positron emission tomography scanning after radiation therapy for non-small-cell lung cancer and radiation pneumonitis. Int J Radiat Oncol Biol Phys 80(5):1365–1371

Mac Manus MP, Everitt S, Bayne M, Ball D, Plumridge N, Binns D et al (2013) The use of fused PET/CT images for patient selection and radical radiotherapy target volume definition in patients with non-small cell lung cancer: results of a prospective study with mature survival data. Radiother Oncol 106(3):292–298

MacManus MP, Hicks RJ, Matthews JP, Hogg A, McKenzie AF, Wirth A et al (2001) High rate of detection of unsuspected distant metastases by pet in apparent stage III non-small-cell lung cancer: implications for radical radiation therapy. Int J Radiat Oncol Biol Phys 50(2):287–293

MacManus M, Nestle U, Rosenzweig KE, Carrio I, Messa C, Belohlavek O et al (2009) Use of PET and PET/CT for radiation therapy planning: IAEA expert report 2006-2007. Radiother Oncol 91(1):85–94

Mah K, Van Dyk J, Keane T, Poon PY (1987) Acute radiation-induced pulmonary damage: a clinical study on the response to fractionated radiation therapy. Int J Radiat Oncol Biol Phys 13(2):179–188

Mahasittiwat P, Yuan S, Xie C, Ritter T, Cao Y, Ten Haken RK et al (2013) Metabolic tumor volume on pet reduced more than gross tumor volume on CT during radiotherapy in patients with non-small cell lung cancer treated with 3DCRT or SBRT. J Radiat Oncol 2(2):191–202

McCurdy MR, Castillo R, Martinez J, Al Hallack MN, Lichter J, Zouain N et al (2012) [18F]-FDG uptake dose-response correlates with radiation pneumonitis in lung cancer patients. Radiother Oncol 104(1):52–57

McCurdy M, Bergsma DP, Hyun E, Kim T, Choi E, Castillo R et al (2013) The role of lung lobes in radiation pneumonitis and radiation-induced inflammation in the lung: a retrospective study. J Radiat Oncol 2(2):203–208

Metcalfe P, Liney GP, Holloway L, Walker A, Barton M, Delaney GP et al (2013) The potential for an enhanced role for MRI in radiation-therapy treatment planning. Technol Cancer Res Treat 12(5):429–446

Murray JG, Erasmus JJ, Bahtiarian EA, Goodman PC (1997) Talc pleurodesis simulating pleural metastases on 18F-fluorodeoxyglucose positron emission tomography. AJR Am J Roentgenol 168(2):359–360

Murray P, Franks K, Hanna GG (2017) A systematic review of outcomes following stereotactic ablative radiotherapy in the treatment of early-stage primary lung cancer. Br J Radiol 90(1071):20160732

Nestle U, Walter K, Schmidt S, Licht N, Nieder C, Motaref B et al (1999) 18F-deoxyglucose positron emission tomography (FDG-PET) for the planning of radiotherapy in lung cancer: high impact in patients with atelectasis. Int J Radiat Oncol Biol Phys 44(3):593–597

Nestle U, Rischke HC, Eschmann SM, Holl G, Tosch M, Miederer M et al (2015) Improved inter-observer agreement of an expert review panel in an oncology treatment trial--insights from a structured interventional process. Eur J Cancer 51(17):2525–2533

Nestle U, Adebahr S, Kaier K, Gkika E, Schimek-Jasch T, Hechtner M et al (2020a) Quality of life after pulmonary stereotactic fractionated radiotherapy (SBRT): results of the phase II STRIPE trial. Radiother Oncol 148:82–88

Nestle U, Schimek-Jasch T, Kremp S, Schaefer-Schuler A, Mix M, Kusters A et al (2020b) Imaging-based target volume reduction in chemoradiotherapy for locally advanced non-small-cell lung cancer (PET-Plan): a multicentre, open-label, randomised, controlled trial. Lancet Oncol 21(4):581–592

Nielsen M, Bertelsen A, Westberg J, Jensen HR, Brink C (2009) Cone beam CT evaluation of patient set-up accuracy as a QA tool. Acta Oncol 48(2):271–276

Ogasawara N, Suga K, Karino Y, Matsunaga N (2002) Perfusion characteristics of radiation-injured lung on Gd-DTPA-enhanced dynamic magnetic resonance imaging. Invest Radiol 37(8):448–457

Seute T, Leffers P, ten Velde GP, Twijnstra A (2008) Detection of brain metastases from small cell lung cancer: consequences of changing imaging techniques (CT versus MRI). Cancer 112(8):1827–1834

Sindoni A, Minutoli F, Pontoriero A, Iati G, Baldari S, Pergolizzi S (2016) Usefulness of four dimensional (4D) PET/CT imaging in the evaluation of thoracic lesions and in radiotherapy planning: review of the literature. Lung Cancer 96:78–86

Siva S, Callahan J, Kron T, Martin OA, MacManus MP, Ball DL et al (2014) A prospective observational study of Gallium-68 ventilation and perfusion PET/CT during and after radiotherapy in patients with non-small cell lung cancer. BMC Cancer 14:740

Siva S, Senan S, Ball D (2015a) Ablative therapies for lung metastases: a need to acknowledge the efficacy and toxicity of stereotactic ablative body radiotherapy. Ann Oncol 26(10):2196

Siva S, Hardcastle N, Kron T, Bressel M, Callahan J, MacManus MP et al (2015b) Ventilation/perfusion positron emission tomography-based assessment of radiation injury to lung. Int J Radiat Oncol Biol Phys 93(2):408–417

Siva S, Thomas R, Callahan J, Hardcastle N, Pham D, Kron T et al (2015c) High-resolution pulmonary ventilation and perfusion PET/CT allows for functionally adapted intensity modulated radiotherapy in lung cancer. Radiother Oncol 115(2):157–162

Sogaard R, Fischer BM, Mortensen J, Hojgaard L, Lassen U (2011) Preoperative staging of lung cancer with PET/CT: cost-effectiveness evaluation alongside a randomized controlled trial. Eur J Nucl Med Mol Imaging 38(5):802–809

Sorcini B, Tilikidis A (2006) Clinical application of image-guided radiotherapy, IGRT (on the Varian OBI platform). Cancer Radiother 10(5):252–257

Steinfort DP, Liew D, Irving LB (2013) Radial probe EBUS versus CT-guided needle biopsy for evaluation of peripheral pulmonary lesions: an economic analysis. Eur Respir J 41(3):539–547

Steinfort DP, Siva S, Leong TL, Rose M, Herath D, Antippa P et al (2016) Systematic endobronchial ultrasound-guided mediastinal staging versus positron emission tomography for comprehensive mediastinal staging in NSCLC before radical radiotherapy of non-small cell lung cancer: a pilot study. Medicine 95(8):e2488

Trinkaus ME, Blum R, Rischin D, Callahan J, Bressel M, Segard T et al (2013) Imaging of hypoxia with (18) F-FAZA PET in patients with locally advanced non-small cell lung cancer treated with definitive chemoradiotherapy. J Med Imaging Radiat Oncol 57(4):475–481

Vera P, Bohn P, Edet-Sanson A, Salles A, Hapdey S, Gardin I et al (2011) Simultaneous positron emission tomography (PET) assessment of metabolism with (1)(8)F-fluoro-2-deoxy-d-glucose (FDG), proliferation with (1)(8)F-fluoro-thymidine (FLT), and hypoxia with (1)(8)fluoro-misonidazole (F-miso) before and during radiotherapy in patients with non-small-cell lung cancer (NSCLC): a pilot study. Radiother Oncol 98(1):109–116

Videtic GM, Rice TW, Murthy S, Suh JH, Saxton JP, Adelstein DJ et al (2008) Utility of positron emission tomography compared with mediastinoscopy for delineating involved lymph nodes in stage III lung cancer: insights for radiotherapy planning from a surgical cohort. Int J Radiat Oncol Biol Phys 72(3):702–706

Werner-Wasik M, Nelson AD, Choi W, Arai Y, Faulhaber PF, Kang P et al (2012) What is the best way to contour lung tumors on PET scans? Multiobserver validation of a gradient-based method using a NSCLC digital PET phantom. Int J Radiat Oncol Biol Phys 82(3):1164–1171

Yan D, Lockman D, Martinez A, Wong J, Brabbins D, Vicini F et al (2005) Computed tomography guided management of interfractional patient variation. Semin Radiat Oncol 15(3):168–179

Yankelevitz DF, Henschke CI, Batata M, Kim YS, Chu F (1994) Lung cancer: evaluation with MR imaging during and after irradiation. J Thorac Imaging 9(1):41–46

Yun M, Kim W, Alnafisi N, Lacorte L, Jang S, Alavi A (2001) 18F-FDG PET in characterizing adrenal lesions detected on CT or MRI. J Nucl Med 42(12):1795–1799

Zhuang M, Garcia DV, Kramer GM, Frings V, Smit EF, Dierckx R et al (2019) Variability and repeatability of quantitative uptake metrics in (18)F-FDG PET/CT of non-small cell lung cancer: impact of segmentation method, uptake interval, and reconstruction protocol. J Nucl Med 60(5):600–607

Target Volume Delineation in Non-small Cell Lung Cancer

Jessica W. Lee, Haijun Song, Matthew J. Boyer, and Joseph K. Salama

Contents

1 Introduction 255
2 CT Simulation 256
3 Respiratory Motion Management 257
4 PET and MRI 259
5 Target Volume Delineation 260
5.1 Gross Tumor Volume (GTV) 260
5.2 Clinical Target Volume (CTV) 261
5.3 Planning Target Volume (PTV) 262
6 Stereotactic Body Radiation Therapy (SBRT) 263
7 Moderately Hypofractionated RT 264
8 Preoperative and Postoperative RT 264
9 Palliative RT 266
10 Conclusion 267

References 267

J. W. Lee · H. Song · M. J. Boyer · J. K. Salama (✉)
Department of Radiation Oncology,
Durham, NC, USA

Radiation Oncology Clinical Service, Durham VA Health System, Durham, NC, USA
e-mail: joseph.salama@duke.edu

1 Introduction

Radiation therapy (RT) is an established treatment for all stages of non-small cell lung cancer (NSCLC), from definitive RT for early-stage disease to palliative RT for advanced and metastatic disease. Identifying the appropriate RT target for each patient starts at the time of consultation, where the radiation oncologist synthesizes the patient's history, physical exam, imaging, and pathology with evidence-based treatment paradigms. When RT is recommended, the treatment planning workflow starts with a three-dimensional (and now often a four-dimensional) computed tomography (CT) simulation, which has largely supplanted two-dimensional treatment planning. Following CT simulation, the radiation oncologist delineates target volumes and organs at risk, defines planning objectives, and then engages in an iterative process of plan optimization and plan evaluation, culminating in image-guided radiation therapy (IGRT). These steps are intertwined; for instance, the reproducibility of patient setup and the type of image guidance used are reflected in the target volume margins. The steps may also vary based on the treatment intent and technique, with different workflows for stereotactic body radiation therapy (SBRT) for early-stage (or oligometastatic) disease, three-dimensional conformal radiation therapy (3D CRT) or intensity-modulated radiation therapy (IMRT) for locoregionally advanced disease, and palliative RT for symptomatic metastatic disease.

This chapter delves into the steps involved in target volume delineation for NSCLC, starting with CT simulation, which can involve respiratory motion management and incorporation of diagnostic imaging. Target volumes for the most common clinical scenarios are then considered in turn, for conventionally fractionated RT, stereotactic body radiation therapy (SBRT), moderately hypofractionated RT, preoperative and postoperative RT, and palliative RT.

2 CT Simulation

Prior to CT simulation, the anatomic location, technique (e.g., SBRT, moderately hypofractionated or conventionally fractionated 3D CRT or IMRT), and treatment intent (e.g., curative or palliative) should be identified as best as possible, as these factors influence the selection of immobilization devices, scan range, use of and type of intravenous contrast, respiratory motion assessment and management, and other aspects of the simulation procedure. For instance, custom immobilization and respiratory motion management may be needed for an outpatient receiving curative-intent SBRT for NSCLC close to the diaphragm, but not necessary for an inpatient receiving palliative RT for a central tumor causing hemoptysis. Though most of the discussion below concerns curative-intent RT, considerations for palliative RT will also be discussed in a separate section.

Patient positioning and immobilization during CT simulation are critical, as the reproducibility of the patient, and therefore the reproducibility of the target volume, is intrinsically linked to the accuracy and precision of treatment delivery. In general, patients should be positioned supine with their arms up, to maximize the number of possible radiation beam angles for treatment. For targets located near the lung apex and supraclavicular fossa, positioning the arms at the sides of the patient may be advantageous for targeting appropriately. The ideal immobilization technique should be comfortable for the patient, should be inexpensive, should maintain its shape during treatment, and should not interfere with CT simulation, image guidance during RT, or RT delivery itself. A standard wing board with grip handles for the hands can be useful for keeping arms overhead in a reproducible position and may be sufficient for conventionally fractionated 3D CRT. For conventionally fractionated IMRT or especially SBRT, custom immobilization of the torso may be needed to minimize setup variation. Polyurethane foam (e.g., Alpha Cradle® by Smithers Medical Products, North Canton, OH, USA), vacuum bags (e.g., Vac-Lok™ by CIVCO, Orange City, IA, USA, and BlueBAG BodyFIX® by Elekta, Stockholm, Sweden), or thermoplastic masks (e.g., Multifix™ by CIVCO, Orange City, IA, USA) can be molded to fit the patient at the time of CT simulation to keep the torso and arms in a reproducible position.

The CT scan range should encompass the anticipated target volume and organs at risk (OARs) including the bilateral lungs, which typically requires a scan from the neck to the mid-abdomen. Specifically, the cricoid cartilage through the entire liver volume has been recommended by clinical trial protocols (Bradley et al. 2015). For axial slice thickness, 3 mm is typically sufficient. Recent SBRT trial protocols such as Radiation Therapy Oncology Group (RTOG) 0236 and RTOG 0813 for early-stage disease recommend ≤3 mm in the region of the tumor, while conventionally fractionated trial protocols such as RTOG 0617 for stage III disease recommend 3 mm in the region of the tumor and 8–10 mm elsewhere (Bradley et al. 2015; Timmerman et al. 2010; Bezjak et al. 2019). Postoperative trial protocols such as the Lung Adjuvant Radiotherapy Trial (Lung ART, discussed below) recommend a maximal thickness of 5 mm through the entire thorax (Spoelstra et al. 2010).

Intravenous (IV) contrast is helpful in curative-intent RT to visualize the gross primary tumor, especially gross nodal disease, and to distinguish disease from mediastinal structures or atelectasis. IV contrast is also useful in postoperative RT to visualize residual disease and vascular boundaries for anatomic lymph node stations. Similarly, oral contrast may be useful for distinguishing disease in close proximity to the esophagus. Recent SBRT trial protocols require or recommend IV contrast if a diagnostic CT has not been performed within the last 8 weeks (Timmerman et al. 2010; Bezjak et al. 2019; Videtic et al. 2015). IV contrast is also recommended in recent protocols employing conventionally fractionated RT for definitive treatment of stage III disease or in the postoperative setting (Bradley et al. 2015; Spoelstra et al. 2010). In practice, IV contrast is generally not necessary for visualization of peripheral primary tumors prior to SBRT. These tumors are usually easily distinguished from aerated lung parenchyma, and some SBRT trial protocols do not specifically recommend or require IV contrast (Hurkmans et al. 2009).

Apart from respiratory motion assessment and management and incorporation of diagnostic imaging, which are discussed in detail below, other considerations during CT simulation for NSCLC include the use of radiopaque skin markers and nothing by mouth (NPO) instructions. Skin markers can be helpful in rare cases of skin involvement or more commonly in palliative RT to mark the sites of pain. Keeping patients NPO prior to treatment may be useful in rare instances of altered anatomy (e.g., hiatal hernia), where a left lower lobe lung tumor is unexpectedly close to the stomach.

3 Respiratory Motion Management

While patient immobilization methods can reduce variation in daily patient setup, even the most precise patient position cannot account for internal lung tumor motion during the respiratory cycle. Broadly, strategies for respiratory motion management include motion encompassment, abdominal compression, breath hold, respiratory gating, and real-time tumor tracking (Molitoris et al. 2018).

In motion encompassment, four-dimensional (4D) CTs are acquired over time to capture the range of lung tumor motion. One commonly used method is to link respiratory amplitude to CT acquisition in real time. CT images are captured throughout at least one respiratory cycle and then retrospectively binned into different respiratory phases (e.g., peak inhalation, mid-inhalation, peak exhalation). This reconstructed 4D CT can be viewed as a movie in some treatment planning systems. Different CT datasets can also be derived from this 4D CT, such as the maximum-intensity projection (MIP) and average-intensity projection datasets, which represent the maximum and mean Hounsfield unit of each voxel during the different respiratory phases. The MIP is particularly useful, more so than the average scan, for encompassing tumor motion during target delineation, given the typically stark visual difference in density between the tumor and surrounding lung parenchyma (Bradley et al. 2006). Figure 1 shows how tumor volume on the MIP dataset includes the range of tumor motion, in contrast to tumor volume on the average scan. However, care must be taken for tumors close to the liver or other structures of similar intensity, which can obscure the tumor on a MIP dataset. Other methods include acquiring CTs only at maximum inhalation and maximum exhalation and acquiring slow CTs. By using a slow gantry rotation speed (e.g., 4 s/revolution) that is equal to or greater than the length of an average respiratory cycle, slow CTs can also capture tumor motion throughout the respiratory cycle (Lagerwaard et al. 2001). Motion encompassment, as opposed to other techniques such as abdominal compression or breath hold, has the advantage of delivering RT while the patient is freely breathing, which may be helpful for reduc-

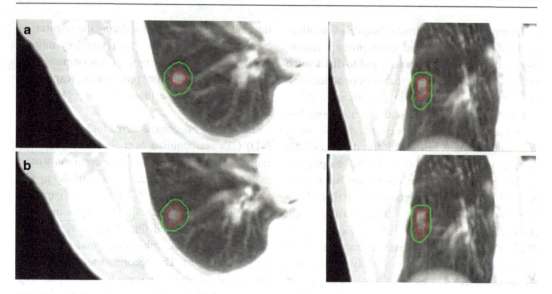

Fig. 1 (a) Axial and coronal average scan derived from a 4D CT simulation with average GTV (red) and final PTV (green) delineated. (b) Axial and coronal MIP scan derived from the same 4D CT simulation with MIP GTV (red) and same final PTV (green) delineated. Compared to the average scan, the MIP GTV better encompasses the superior-inferior motion of this tumor with respiration

ing treatment time and for patients with poor pulmonary function who may find the limitations of respiratory motion management uncomfortable. However, there are disadvantages to this technique. One disadvantage is that the patient's breathing pattern during simulation is assumed to be the same as during treatment. This is often but not always the case, and if not, target volumes may not encompass tumors. Additionally, another disadvantage to motion encompassment is that more normal lung tissue may be included in target volumes. Thus, when tumor motion is above a certain threshold on the initial 4D CT, typically >1 cm in any direction, alternative measures to reduce respiratory motion may be considered, such as breath hold or respiratory gating.

Limiting respiratory motion during CT simulation can be achieved through abdominal compression or breath hold. Abdominal compression limits diaphragmatic excursion and may be especially useful for lower lobe tumors close to the diaphragm. Commercially available abdominal compression systems include a flat abdominal compression plate (e.g., BodyFIX® Diaphragm Control by Elekta in Stockholm, Sweden) or a vacuum-based abdominal wrap (e.g., BodyFIX® dual-vacuum technology by Elekta in Stockholm, Sweden). A retrospective comparison of these two systems found that both reduce superior-inferior and overall respiratory motion compared to free breathing techniques, though the abdominal compression plate was faster to set up and more comfortable for patients (Han et al. 2010). Limiting respiratory motion can also be achieved through inhalation or exhalation breath hold, ideally with a system to synchronize breath hold with CT acquisition and treatment delivery. For example, the Active Breathing Coordinator™ by Elekta (Stockholm, Sweden) has patients breathe solely through a mouthpiece that is connected to a flow valve, preventing additional air movement during treatment than was used at simulation and ensuring reproducible inspiratory or expiratory breath-hold volumes. This technique may also be paused by the patient at any time based on his or her comfort (Wong et al. 1999). For lung tumors, deep inspiratory breath hold is typically used as this reduces lung tissue density, resulting in increased lung tissue sparing (Rosenzweig et al. 2000; Hanley et al. 1999).

In respiratory gating, external or internal landmarks are used to track respiratory or tumor motion in real time, and the treatment beam is on only at specified phases of the respiratory cycle. External methods include the real-time position management (RPM) system by Varian (Palo Alto, CA, USA), which uses external infrared reflective markers placed on the chest or abdomen that are tracked by video camera, generating a respiratory waveform. This infrared camera system is also used for 4D CT and breath-hold methods discussed previously. Another alternative is to place radiopaque (typically gold) fiducials in or near the tumor, which are visible to imaging and typically do not migrate (Willoughby et al. 2006). While respiratory gating can allow for patients to breath freely during treatment turning the beam on in the appropriate respiratory cycle phase, treatment times are typically longer than with other techniques. This is an important consideration especially when delivering high monitor unit treatments like SBRT.

Fiducials placed in or near the tumor can also be used for real-time intrafraction tumor tracking. Fiducial position can be synchronized with beam aperture, typically with multileaf collimator (MLC) tracking on a standard linear accelerator or with robotic arm tracking in the CyberKnife® system (Sunnyvale, CA, USA). As placement of fiducials can be associated with pneumothorax, fiducial-free tracking systems have also been developed. One fiducial-free technique is to match the intensity of live orthogonal X-ray images obtained during treatment with the digitally reconstructed radiographs from the CT simulation (Bibault et al. 2012). Real-time intrafraction tracking has also been explored in magnetic resonance (MR) linear accelerators, typically also using MLC tracking. Tracking with MR linear accelerators is also noninvasive and does not add ionizing radiation exposure to the patient, though the magnetic field can cause slight dose distortions that need to be accounted for during treatment planning and delivery (Menten et al. 2016).

4 PET and MRI

In addition to obtaining a CT simulation, ideally with respiratory motion management, additional imaging modalities such as 2-deoxy-2-[^{18}F]fluoro-D-glucose (FDG) positron emission tomography (PET) and less commonly MRI can be incorporated to guide target volume delineation. PET is the standard of care for staging NSCLC and should typically be available for visual reference or registration to the CT simulation. Registration of diagnostic imaging may be limited due to differences in patient position and respiration. Where available, PET and MRI can also be acquired in the treatment position along with the CT simulation. PET is especially useful for distinguishing primary tumor from atelectasis or other consolidations and for identifying metabolically active disease in lymph nodes, as shown in Fig. 2, all of which can affect target volume delineation. In RTOG 0515, a phase II study of 47 patients with NSCLC where either CT alone or a fused PET/CT was used to derive target volumes, PET/CT altered nodal volumes in 51% of patients (Bradley et al. 2012). A recent staging PET is also critical for accurate target delineation. The European Society for Therapeutic Radiology and Oncology (ESTRO) consensus guidelines suggest that the interval between staging PET and CT simulation should be <3 weeks (Nestle et al. 2018). A retrospective of 47 PET scans repeated within 120 days of the initial staging PET found that 51% showed new nodal or metastatic disease at a median of 42 days. If the repeat PET was obtained at a shorter interval of 20 days, the rate of upstaging was lower at 17% (Geiger et al. 2014). If induction chemotherapy is planned, then the initial staging PET will be used to guide postchemotherapy volumes.

In addition to PET imaging, pathologic mediastinal evaluation is also the standard of care to improve staging accuracy, though it may be omit-

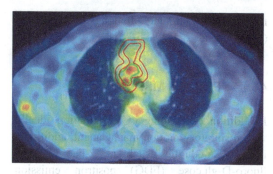

Fig. 2 Axial PET/CT fused to CT simulation demonstrating hypermetabolic (solid red) stage III NSCLC, with overlying nodal GTV contours (green line) and PTV (red line)
PET/CT, positron emission tomography-computed tomography; NSCLC, non-small cell lung cancer; GTV, gross tumor volume

ted for peripheral T1–T2 tumors. Mediastinal evaluation may be performed with endobronchial or esophageal ultrasound or mediastinoscopy. In a prospective trial of PET staging, 14% of patients without CT or PET evidence of N2 disease were found to have pathologically involved mediastinal nodes, most commonly in the posterior mediastinum (Cerfolio et al. 2005). Lymph nodes found to be involved on PET or by pathologic mediastinal evaluation should be included in the nodal gross tumor volume (GTV). Conversely, lymph nodes that are not involved by either PET or pathologic evaluation can be safely excluded. The same study found that in CT-enlarged lymph nodes that are negative by PET, EBUS further reduces the false-negative rate from 13% to 3% (Peeters et al. 2016).

Magnetic resonance imaging (MRI) is typically not used in routine thoracic staging of NSCLC, though its soft tissue visualization is useful for assessing superior sulcus, chest wall, or paraspinal tumors and for characterization of brachial plexus or spinal cord involvement (Bainbridge et al. 2017).

Recent studies have investigated the use of MRI for lung cancer screening and staging, and while MRI does have benefits including the absence of radiation exposure and avoiding the logistics related to radiotracers for PET, challenges include low proton density in the lungs leading to reduced signal-to-noise ratio as well as artifacts due to air-tissue interfaces in the lung and patient or cardiopulmonary motion (Sim et al. 2020).

5 Target Volume Delineation

Target volume delineation on the CT simulation dataset incorporates diagnostic imaging, pathology, and patient setup and treatment delivery considerations. The International Commission on Radiation Units and Measurements (ICRU) reports provide standardized information on prescribing and reporting radiation to target volumes and organs at risk. ICRU report No. 83 describes target volumes in the era of IMRT (Gregoire and Mackie 2011). The standard target volumes are the gross tumor volume (GTV), which is the gross extent and location of malignant disease; the clinical target volume (CTV), which is the GTV plus subclinical malignant disease (either by direct extension or occult nodal disease); and the planning target volume (PTV), which is the CTV plus geometric uncertainty from internal organ motion and external setup variation.

The GTV, CTV, and PTV are each discussed below, in the context of conventionally fractionated RT, which is standardly used for medically inoperable, locally advanced NSCLC. Special considerations and modifications for stereotactic body radiation therapy (SBRT) in early-stage NSCLC, moderately hypofractionated RT, preoperative and postoperative RT, and palliative RT are then reviewed separately.

5.1 Gross Tumor Volume (GTV)

Primary gross tumor volume (GTV) in the lung parenchyma should be contoured on preset lung windows, e.g., width range of 1500–2000 HU and level range of −700 to −500 HU; these presets may vary across different vendors (Bankier et al. 2017). If the primary tumor is invading the mediastinum or chest wall, preset mediastinal windows, e.g., width range of 350–400 HU and level range of 30–70 HU, can also be used to identify tumor (Bankier et al. 2017). Mediastinal windows can also be useful to exclude vessels and atelectasis. The nodal GTV should be contoured on preset mediastinal windows and should include nodes involved either by PET or by pathological staging. A SUV maximum of >2.5 is typically used as a cutoff for involved nodes on PET (Hellwig et al. 2007). Figure 2 shows an example of nodal GTV contours guided by PET. If PET and pathological staging cannot be obtained, then a short-axis measurement >1 cm is commonly used for involved nodes on CT (Staples et al. 1988). Separate primary and nodal GTV structures can be used, as the subsequent CTV expansions for each of these may be different. The addition of IV contrast and PET registration can also be helpful in distinguishing tumor from normal structures, which is discussed in detail in the simulation section above.

While GTV delineation appears straightforward, there is variation across radiation oncologists and radiologists (Giraud et al. 2002; Steenbakkers et al. 2005, 2006). In addition to delineating GTV on the preset windows above, firstly in the axial plane, these studies found that inspecting volumes on the coronal and sagittal planes reduced interphysician variation (Steenbakkers et al. 2005). Incorporating a PET scan can also reduce variation, with one study reporting that three-dimensional variation was 1.0 cm on CT alone and decreased to 0.4 cm with the addition of a PET scan (Steenbakkers et al. 2006). In general, the most common source of variation tends to be in areas with atelectasis of normal lung parenchyma, which should not be included in the GTV. Other regions of uncertainty can occur near the pulmonary vessels, azygous vein, and supraclavicular fossa, where understanding of radiologic anatomy is critical. Esophagus and blood vessels are also sometimes confused for pathologically involved nodes. Lastly, another area of uncertainty is in variable treatment of spicules of the primary tumor. It is not clear whether these spicules should be included in the GTV, though one strategy is to at least ensure that they are within the CTV (Bowden et al. 2002). One study also found that junior physicians and diagnostic radiologists tend to delineate smaller volumes than senior physicians and radiation oncologists (Giraud et al. 2002).

For motion encompassment on a 4D CT simulation, the GTV should also be contoured on the MIP image set, as shown in Fig. 1. The GTVs reflecting tumor motion throughout the respiratory cycle are combined to form the internal GTV (IGTV) and used for further CTV and PTV expansions. Alternatively, the CTV can be modified based on the 4D CT dataset, and the CTVs reflecting tumor motion can be combined to form an internal target volume (ITV).

5.2 Clinical Target Volume (CTV)

The clinical target volume (CTV) is typically a 5–10 mm expansion from the primary tumor GTV or IGTV to include microscopic tumor extension, with some guidelines recommending 5–8 mm (Nestle et al. 2018). These expansions can be traced back to studies of pathologic microscopic extension. One study found that a 5 mm margin around grossly visible tumor covers 80% of microscopic extension for adenocarcinomas (ACC) and 91% for squamous cell carcinoma (SCC) (Giraud et al. 2000). To cover 95% of microscopic disease, margins of 8 and 6 mm would be needed for ACC and SCC, respectively (Giraud et al. 2000). Another study of adenocarcinoma suggested that microscopic disease beyond grossly visible tumor may be higher for low-grade disease, owing to higher rates of adenocarcinoma in situ or lepidic growth (Grills et al. 2007). A summary of studies examining microscopic extension and the corresponding margins needed is shown in

Table 1 Clinicopathologic studies comparing microscopic extension (ME) to imaging

Study	N	Inflated	PET	Microscopic extension	Margin around GTV needed to cover ME
Giraud et al. (2000)	70	Yes	No	ACC: Mean ME 2.69 mm SCC: Mean ME 1.48 mm	ACC: 8 mm to cover 95% of ME SCC: 6 mm to cover 95% of ME
Li et al. (2003)	43	No	No	ACC: Mean ME 2.18 mm SCC: Mean ME 1.33 mm	ACC: 7 mm to cover 95% of ME SCC: 5 mm to cover 95% of ME
Grills et al. (2007)	35, ACC only	No	No	Mean ME 7.2 mm, higher ME for lower grade tumors	9 mm on CT lung windows to cover ME in 90% of cases
van Loon et al. (2012)	34	Yes	Yes	50% of cases with any ME	26 mm to cover ME in 90% of cases
Chan et al. (2001)	5	Unknown	No	0, found that microscopic extension was ≤GTV on CT in 5/5 patients	

Table 1. In conventionally fractionated treatment, the nodal CTV expansion is typically equal to or smaller than primary GTV expansion, up to 5–8 mm, though increased margin can be considered for nodes ≥20 mm, as the incidence of extracapsular extension (ECE) increases with larger lymph node size (Yuan et al. 2007). Another alternative method is to designate the involved lymph node station as the CTV. In general, the CTV should be trimmed around natural anatomic boundaries where microscopic disease extension is not expected, such as vertebral bodies, ribs, heart, esophagus, and great vessels.

Elective nodal irradiation is generally not indicated in patients receiving definitive radiation therapy, as multiple prospective and retrospective trials have shown that the rates of isolated nodal progression are low in initially uninvolved lymph node stations (Kepka and Socha 2015). For instance, in a retrospective series from Memorial Sloan Kettering from 2001 of patients treated with 3D CRT, target volumes included CT-enlarged or pathologically involved nodes (PET was not utilized in this study) and the 2-year actuarial rate of elective nodal progression was 7.6% (Rosenzweig et al. 2001). In the PET era, a prospective phase I/II study from Maastricht included patients staged with PET and treated with 3D CRT, and 1/44 patients developed an isolated nodal progression, for a crude rate of 2.3% (De Ruysscher et al. 2005). In a retrospective study from Maastricht of patients staged with PET and treated with intensity-modulated radiation therapy (IMRT), the 2-year actuarial risk for isolated nodal progression was of 2.4% (Martinussen et al. 2016). Similarly, in RTOG 0515, only 1/47 patients developed an elective nodal progression for a crude rate of 2% (Bradley et al. 2012). Thus, selective nodal radiation with either 3D CRT or IMRT is reasonable and associated with low rates of elective nodal progression. A systematic review suggested that elective nodal progression was overall low in patients staged with either CT alone or PET/CT at 6.3% (Kepka and Socha 2015). A summary of prospective studies of elective nodal progression rates following PET-guided volume delineation is adapted from this systemic review and shown in Table 2 (Kepka and Socha 2015). Isolated nodal progression rates are reported where available.

5.3 Planning Target Volume (PTV)

The planning target volume (PTV) accounts for variations in internal tumor motion, e.g., respiratory motion, and external patient setup. As the PTV reflects geometric uncertainty, not subclinical disease, it is generally not trimmed at anatomic boundaries, unlike the CTV. In RTOG 0617, for a 4D CT with breath hold or respiratory gating, a PTV expansion of at least

Table 2 Prospective studies of elective nodal progression (ENP) following PET in NSCLC

Study	N	ENP %	RT	Stage	Median follow-up (months)
Lao et al. (2014)	156	12.2	SBRT 24–60 Gy/1–10 fractions	I	20
Fakiris et al. (2009)	70	8.6	SBRT 60–66 Gy/3 fractions	I	50.2
Ricardi et al. (2010)	62	12.9	SBRT 45 Gy/3 fractions	I	28
Hoopes et al. (2007)	57	10.5	SBRT dose escalation 24–72 Gy/3 fractions	I	42.5
Timmerman et al. (2010)	55	3.6	SBRT 54 Gy/3 fractions	I	34.4
Bral et al. (2011)	40	5	SBRT 60 Gy/3–4 fractions	T1-T3N0	16
Van Baardwijk et al. (2012)	137	4.4	Hyperfractionated accelerated 51–69 Gy in 1.5 Gy BID to 45 Gy and then 2 Gy QD with induction carboplatin/gemcitabine and concurrent cisplatin/vinorelbine or cisplatin/etoposide	III	30.9
Belderbos et al. (2006)	65	3.1	Dose escalation 49.5–94.5 Gy in 2.25 Gy/fraction; 18% induction CHT	I–III	17
Kolodziejczyk et al. (2012)	50	6	52 Gy/13 fractions or 66 Gy/30 fractions for T1–T3N0, or 58.8 Gy/21 fractions for stage III with or without induction chemotherapy	I–III	32
Bradley et al. (2012)	47	2	≥60 Gy conventionally fractionated with or without induction chemotherapy	II–III	12.9
De Ruysscher et al. (2005)	44	2.3	61.2 Gy/34 fractions or 64.8 Gy/36 fractions	I–III	16
Fleckenstein et al. (2011)	23	4.3	66.6–73.8 Gy with concurrent chemotherapy	II–III	27.2
Tada et al. (2012)	22	4.5	Hyperfractionated dose escalation 54–72 Gy in 1.5 Gy BID with concurrent carboplatin/paclitaxel	III	Not specified
Chen et al. (2013)	10	0	Median 60 Gy with induction carboplatin/paclitaxel and concurrent paclitaxel	III	33.6

1.0 cm superior-inferior and 0.5 cm in the axial plane is recommended. For a 4D CT used with an ITV approach, i.e., using a CTV structure that incorporates tumor position across the respiratory cycle, at least a 1.0 cm uniform expansion is recommended. In the absence of a 4D CT, expansions of at least 1.5 cm superior-inferior and 1.0 cm in the axial plane are recommended (Bradley et al. 2015). In practice, reproducibility of external patient setup varies across physicians and institutions, due to factors such as custom immobilization and onboard imaging to verify tumor location, and different PTV margins may be used in practice.

6 Stereotactic Body Radiation Therapy (SBRT)

SBRT is used in patients with early-stage NSCLC who either are medically inoperable and/or decline surgery. General practice parameters on SBRT have been outlined by the American College of Radiology (ACR) and American Society for Radiation Oncology (ASTRO) (Chao et al. 2020). SBRT involves higher radiation doses per fraction with total treatment delivered in five fractions or less with rapid dose falloff outside the target. Compared to conventionally fractionated RT, each SBRT fraction requires a higher degree of precision and accuracy, which is accomplished with a frame-based or frameless three-dimensional coordinate system. For example, in NSCLC, frameless localization is ideally performed with a cone beam CT (CBCT) acquired with each SBRT fraction. Accurate targeting is achieved by matching to a structure that is fixed in relation to the tumor, such as a fiducial marker or bony landmark, or to the tumor itself.

Incorporation of diagnostic imaging, custom patient immobilization, and respiratory motion management, which are discussed above in the simulation section, are generally needed to facilitate precise and accurate SBRT delivery. Target delineation of the GTV is similar as described in the GTV section, though reduced CTV and PTV expansions are used. As the target in SBRT is the tumor itself and not necessarily suspected microscopic extension, zero GTV-to-CTV expansion is typically used, as recommended in multiple protocols including RTOG 0236, 0915, and 0813. As setup variation should be reduced with image-guided stereotactic localization, smaller PTV expansions can be used as well. In the absence of a 4D CT, a GTV-to-PTV expansion of 1.0 cm superior-inferior and 0.5 cm in the axial plane is recommended (Timmerman et al. 2010). With a 4D CT simulation and an ITV that incorporates respiratory motion, a uniform ITV-to-PTV expansion of 0.5 cm is recommended (Videtic et al. 2015). SBRT delivery also requires strict QA protocols, which are beyond the scope of this chapter (Chao et al. 2020). As discussed above, daily image guidance is a standard part of SBRT procedures to ensure that the tumor falls within the PTV on each fraction.

Highly precise and accurate hypofractionated RT in greater than five fractions has also been described, such as 60 Gy in eight fractions for centrally located, early-stage NSCLC by Haasbeek et al. (Haasbeek et al. 2011). In this study, 4D CT was performed on all patients and a motion-encompassing ITV was generated using the MIP dataset. A uniform 3 mm ITV-to-PTV expansion was used, with dose prescribed to the 80% isodose line. This initial published experience used orthogonal X-rays for localization, as CBCT was not yet available. This treatment regimen with the aforementioned planning constraints had high rates of treated tumor control and limited toxicity (De Ruysscher et al. 2005).

7 Moderately Hypofractionated RT

In patients with locoregionally advanced disease who are not suitable for curative-intent concurrent cytotoxic chemotherapy and radiation, moderately hypofractionated RT with or without sequential chemotherapy is an alternative. Simulation and target volume delineation for these patients are much the same as in conventionally fractionated RT. For example, a phase 1 dose escalation trial by Westover et al. demonstrated the feasibility of 60 Gy in 15 fractions alone in 55 patients with stage II–IV or recurrent NSCLC and poor performance status (Westover et al. 2015). In this trial, patients were immobilized with either standard or custom devices, and daily image guidance with fluoroscopy, X-rays, or CBCT was used. Primary and nodal GTV delineation was similar to the guidelines discussed above in the GTV section, with no elective nodal irradiation. CTV and PTV expansions were also similar to those used in conventionally fractionated RT, with a 5–10 mm GTV-to-CTV expansion and a 5–10 mm CTV-to-PTV expansion. Hypofractionated RT was generally well tolerated in these patients, and the maximally tolerated dose was not reached, though local control could not be estimated as the median overall survival of these patients was 6 months (Westover et al. 2015).

8 Preoperative and Postoperative RT

Compared to the target volumes used in definitive RT, target volumes may differ following induction chemotherapy and especially following surgery, where the gross disease has been resected. In general, pretreatment diagnostic imaging is useful in providing guidance as to where microscopic disease may still reside. In postoperative RT, the operative report and surgical pathology findings are similarly useful for identifying the areas at risk of disease recurrence. For example, Fig. 3 shows an example of a postoperative volume in a patient who had a positive margin following pneumonectomy.

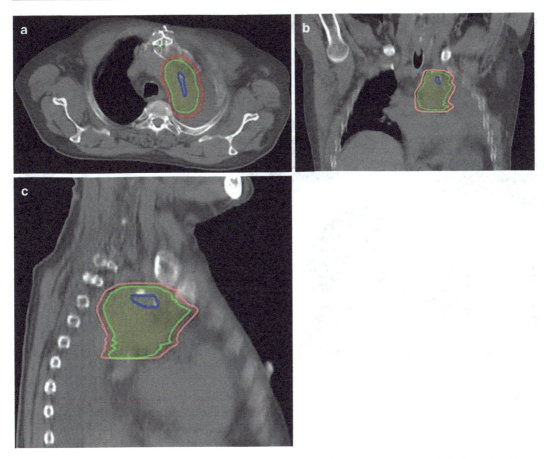

Fig. 3 (a) Axial CT demonstrating postoperative target volumes in a postpneumonectomy patient with positive margins, with GTV (blue), CTV (green), and PTV (red) contours. (b) Coronal and (c) sagittal views also shown CT, computed tomography; GTV, gross tumor volume; CTV, clinical target volume; PTV, planning target volume

Preoperative RT with concurrent chemotherapy, radical surgical resection, and adjuvant chemotherapy is the standard of care for superior sulcus tumors, as established by the Southwest Oncology Group 9416 trial (Rusch et al. 2007). This phase II trial included superior sulcus tumors with Pancoast syndrome or invasion of the chest wall, spine, or subclavian vasculature. MRI of the thoracic spine and brachial plexus was recommended but not required, and this trial predated the routine use of PET imaging. The radiation target consisted of the primary tumor and ipsilateral supraclavicular region and received conventionally fractionated 45 Gy with chemotherapy. Figure 4 shows volumes in a patient with a superior sulcus adenocarcinoma.

Apart from superior sulcus tumors, the use of preoperative RT is debated. The phase III German Lung Cancer Cooperative Group trial, which accrued through 2003, found no progression-free survival benefit with preoperative chemoRT vs. preoperative chemotherapy and postoperative RT, though preoperative RT did increase mediastinal downstaging and pathologic response (Thomas et al. 2008). CT-based planning was required, and the radiation target in the preoperative RT arm was the primary tumor with a 1.5 cm margin and the ipsilateral hilum and ipsilateral mediastinum with a 0.5–1 cm margin.

The use of postoperative RT in patients with pathologic N2 disease is also controversial. While a retrospective analysis of patients enrolled

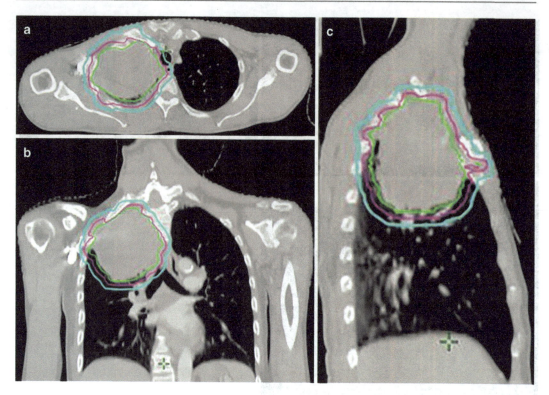

Fig. 4 (**a**) Axial CT demonstrating a large superior sulcus tumor with GTV (green), CTV (magenta), and PTV (cyan) contours. (**b**) Coronal and (**c**) sagittal views also shown CT, computed tomography; GTV, gross tumor volume; CTV, clinical target volume; PTV, planning target volume

on the Adjuvant Navelbine International Trialist Association (ANITA) trial suggested a survival benefit in pN2 disease, a recent presentation of the phase III Lung Adjuvant Radiotherapy Trial (Lung ART) at the 2020 European Society for Medical Oncology reported no disease-free survival benefit, with the final publication pending (Douillard et al. 2008; Le Pechoux et al. 2020). Postoperative CTVs can also vary considerably between radiation oncologists, up to threefold among expert thoracic radiation oncologists (Spoelstra et al. 2010). One approach is to include the pathologically involved lymph node stations, ipsilateral hilar lymph node station (station 10), intervening lymph nodes, and one lymph node station above and below the involved nodes. The Lung ART protocol has specific recommendations for each involved lymph node station in the setting of mediastinal radiation for pathologic N2 disease (Spoelstra et al. 2010). In this protocol, the postoperative CTV includes the resected lymph nodes, bronchial stump, ipsilateral hilar lymph node station (station 10), mediastinal pleura extending to the tumor bed, subcarinal lymph nodes (station 7), and lower paratracheal lymph nodes (station 4). Inclusion of subaortic and para-aortic lymph nodes (stations 5 and 6) is also recommended for left-sided tumors.

9 Palliative RT

Palliative RT can be effective for symptomatic relief of NSCLC in patients with locoregionally advanced or metastatic disease, or those otherwise ineligible for curative-intent therapy. Palliative RT is especially useful for hemoptysis, pain, and dyspnea, and to a lesser degree for cough (Sundstrom et al. 2004). The workflow for palliative RT differs from that of conventionally fractionated RT in several ways. The time from consultation to treatment delivery may be shorter in palliative RT, in order to provide more rapid relief of symptoms, and the prescribed doses are typically lower. Custom immobilization is typically not needed, and the delineated target should only include symptomatic disease, rather than all of the disease present in the thorax. In palliative RT clinical trials, parallel opposed fields were designed usually with a 1.5–2 cm margin on the desired target disease, dose was prescribed to midplane, and the length of spinal cord length within the fields was restricted to <12–16 cm, depending on the dose prescribed (Sundstrom et al. 2004; Bezjak et al. 2002). A similar approach is used in the era of CT-based planning, where a limited number of fields may be designed to encompass symptomatic thoracic disease with a 1.5–2 cm margin to allow for internal motion and setup error while avoiding the spinal cord and other organs at risk.

10 Conclusion

Defining the radiation target in NSCLC begins at the time of consultation and CT simulation. Incorporating a diagnostic PET scan, which is the standard of care for staging NSCLC, can be helpful in distinguishing primary and nodal disease (GTV). At CT simulation, addition of IV contrast is also useful for identifying enhancing gross disease, and custom patient immobilization may be used to minimize external variations in patient setup. Respiratory motion management accounts for internal variation in lung tumor position during the respiratory cycle, and may include motion encompassment, abdominal compression, breath hold, respiratory gating, or real-time tumor tracking. Primary and nodal GTVs are then delineated on the CT simulation dataset; routine inclusion of elective nodal stations is not recommended. GTV-to-CTV expansions are 5–8 mm to include microscopic disease. Pathologic studies show that up to 7–8 mm or 5–6 mm is needed in adenocarcinoma and squamous cell carcinoma, respectively, to include 95% of microscopic extension for the primary tumor. CTV-to-PTV expansions are also typically 5–10 mm, depending on the expected reproducibility of tumor position.

Target delineation in NSCLC also depends heavily on the clinical context. Compared to conventionally fractionated RT for locally advanced NSCLC, SBRT for early-stage disease requires higher precision and accuracy, which may be accomplished with custom immobilization, respiratory motion management, and daily CBCT image guidance. With this level of reproducibility, smaller GTV-to-PTV margins of 5–10 mm total are used. In conventionally fractionated postoperative RT, the consensus for CTV delineation is not as clear, with considerable variation between radiation oncologists, though generally the postoperative CTV at least includes the pathologically involved lymph node stations, bronchial stump, ipsilateral hilar nodes, and subcarinal nodes. In palliative RT where lower doses are employed, only symptomatic disease is included, and 1.5–2 cm to the block edge is typically sufficient to account for internal target motion and daily setup variation.

References

Bainbridge H et al (2017) Magnetic resonance imaging in precision radiation therapy for lung cancer. Transl Lung Cancer Res 6(6):689–707

Bankier AA et al (2017) Recommendations for measuring pulmonary nodules at CT: a statement from the Fleischner Society. Radiology 285(2):584–600

Belderbos JS et al (2006) Final results of a phase I/II dose escalation trial in non-small-cell lung cancer using three-dimensional conformal radiotherapy. Int J Radiat Oncol Biol Phys 66(1):126–134

Bezjak A et al (2002) Randomized phase III trial of single versus fractionated thoracic radiation in the palliation of patients with lung cancer (NCIC CTG SC.15). Int J Radiat Oncol Biol Phys 54(3):719–728

Bezjak A et al (2019) Safety and efficacy of a five-fraction stereotactic body radiotherapy schedule for centrally located non-small-cell lung cancer: NRG Oncology/RTOG 0813 Trial. J Clin Oncol 37(15):1316–1325

Bibault JE et al (2012) Image-guided robotic stereotactic radiation therapy with fiducial-free tumor tracking for lung cancer. Radiat Oncol 7:102

Bowden P et al (2002) Measurement of lung tumor volumes using three-dimensional computer planning software. Int J Radiat Oncol Biol Phys 53(3):566–573

Bradley JD et al (2006) Comparison of helical, maximum intensity projection (MIP), and averaged intensity (AI)

4D CT imaging for stereotactic body radiation therapy (SBRT) planning in lung cancer. Radiother Oncol 81(3):264–268

Bradley J et al (2012) A phase II comparative study of gross tumor volume definition with or without PET/CT fusion in dosimetric planning for non-small-cell lung cancer (NSCLC): primary analysis of Radiation Therapy Oncology Group (RTOG) 0515. Int J Radiat Oncol Biol Phys 82(1):435–441. e1

Bradley JD et al (2015) Standard-dose versus high-dose conformal radiotherapy with concurrent and consolidation carboplatin plus paclitaxel with or without cetuximab for patients with stage IIIA or IIIB non-small-cell lung cancer (RTOG 0617): a randomised, two-by-two factorial phase 3 study. Lancet Oncol 16(2):187–199

Bral S et al (2011) Prospective, risk-adapted strategy of stereotactic body radiotherapy for early-stage non-small-cell lung cancer: results of a phase II trial. Int J Radiat Oncol Biol Phys 80(5):1343–1349

Cerfolio RJ et al (2005) Improving the inaccuracies of clinical staging of patients with NSCLC: a prospective trial. Ann Thorac Surg 80(4):1207–1213. discussion 1213-4

Chan R et al (2001) Computed tomographic-pathologic correlation of gross tumor volume and clinical target volume in non-small cell lung cancer: a pilot experience. Arch Pathol Lab Med 125(11):1469–1472

Chao ST et al (2020) ACR-ASTRO practice parameter for the performance of stereotactic body radiation therapy. Am J Clin Oncol 43(8):545–552

Chen M et al (2013) Involved-field radiotherapy versus elective nodal irradiation in combination with concurrent chemotherapy for locally advanced non-small cell lung cancer: a prospective randomized study. Biomed Res Int 2013:371819

De Ruysscher D et al (2005) Selective mediastinal node irradiation based on FDG-PET scan data in patients with non-small-cell lung cancer: a prospective clinical study. Int J Radiat Oncol Biol Phys 62(4):988–994

Douillard JY et al (2008) Impact of postoperative radiation therapy on survival in patients with complete resection and stage I, II, or IIIA non-small-cell lung cancer treated with adjuvant chemotherapy: the adjuvant Navelbine international Trialist Association (ANITA) randomized trial. Int J Radiat Oncol Biol Phys 72(3):695–701

Fakiris AJ et al (2009) Stereotactic body radiation therapy for early-stage non-small-cell lung carcinoma: four-year results of a prospective phase II study. Int J Radiat Oncol Biol Phys 75(3):677–682

Fleckenstein J et al (2011) F-18-FDG-PET confined radiotherapy of locally advanced NSCLC with concomitant chemotherapy: results of the PET-PLAN pilot trial. Int J Radiat Oncol Biol Phys 81(4):e283–e289

Geiger GA et al (2014) Stage migration in planning PET/CT scans in patients due to receive radiotherapy for non-small-cell lung cancer. Clin Lung Cancer 15(1):79–85

Giraud P et al (2000) Evaluation of microscopic tumor extension in non-small-cell lung cancer for three-dimensional conformal radiotherapy planning. Int J Radiat Oncol Biol Phys 48(4):1015–1024

Giraud P et al (2002) Conformal radiotherapy for lung cancer: different delineation of the gross tumor volume (GTV) by radiologists and radiation oncologists. Radiother Oncol 62(1):27–36

Gregoire V, Mackie TR (2011) State of the art on dose prescription, reporting and recording in intensity-modulated radiation therapy (ICRU report no. 83). Cancer Radiother 15(6–7):555–559

Grills IS et al (2007) Clinicopathologic analysis of microscopic extension in lung adenocarcinoma: defining clinical target volume for radiotherapy. Int J Radiat Oncol Biol Phys 69(2):334–341

Haasbeek CJ et al (2011) Outcomes of stereotactic ablative radiotherapy for centrally located early-stage lung cancer. J Thorac Oncol 6(12):2036–2043

Han K et al (2010) A comparison of two immobilization systems for stereotactic body radiation therapy of lung tumors. Radiother Oncol 95(1):103–108

Hanley J et al (1999) Deep inspiration breath-hold technique for lung tumors: the potential value of target immobilization and reduced lung density in dose escalation. Int J Radiat Oncol Biol Phys 45(3):603–611

Hellwig D et al (2007) 18F-FDG PET for mediastinal staging of lung cancer: which SUV threshold makes sense? J Nucl Med 48(11):1761–1766

Hoopes DJ et al (2007) FDG-PET and stereotactic body radiotherapy (SBRT) for stage I non-small-cell lung cancer. Lung Cancer 56(2):229–234

Hurkmans CW et al (2009) Recommendations for implementing stereotactic radiotherapy in peripheral stage IA non-small cell lung cancer: report from the quality assurance working party of the randomised phase III ROSEL study. Radiat Oncol 4:1

Kepka L, Socha J (2015) PET-CT use and the occurrence of elective nodal failure in involved field radiotherapy for non-small cell lung cancer: a systematic review. Radiother Oncol 115(2):151–156

Kolodziejczyk M et al (2012) Incidence of isolated nodal failure in non-small cell lung cancer patients included in a prospective study of the value of PET-CT. Radiother Oncol 104(1):58–61

Lagerwaard FJ et al (2001) Multiple "slow" CT scans for incorporating lung tumor mobility in radiotherapy planning. Int J Radiat Oncol Biol Phys 51(4):932–937

Lao L et al (2014) Incidental prophylactic nodal irradiation and patterns of nodal relapse in inoperable early stage NSCLC patients treated with SBRT: a case-matched analysis. Int J Radiat Oncol Biol Phys 90(1):209–215

Le Pechoux C, Pourel N, Barlesi F, Faivre-Finn C, Lerouge D, Zalcman G, Antoni D, Lamezec B, Nestle U, Boisselier P, Thillays F, Paumier A, Dansin E, Peignaux K, Madelaine J, Pichon E, Larrouy A, Riesterer O, Lavole A, Bardet A (2020) An international randomized trial, comparing post-operative conformal radiotherapy (PORT) to no PORT, in patients with completely resected non-small cell lung cancer (NSCLC) and mediastinal N2 involvement: primary end-point analysis of LungART (IFCT-0503, UK NCRI, SAKK) NCT00410683. Ann Oncol 31(S4):S1178

Li WL et al (2003) A comparative study on radiology and pathology target volume in non-small-cell lung cancer. Zhonghua Zhong Liu Za Zhi 25(6):566–568

Martinussen HM et al (2016) Is selective nodal irradiation in non-small cell lung cancer still safe when using IMRT? Results of a prospective cohort study. Radiother Oncol 121(2):322–327

Menten MJ et al (2016) Lung stereotactic body radiotherapy with an MR-linac - quantifying the impact of the magnetic field and real-time tumor tracking. Radiother Oncol 119(3):461–466

Molitoris JK et al (2018) Advances in the use of motion management and image guidance in radiation therapy treatment for lung cancer. J Thorac Dis 10(Suppl. 21):S2437–S2450

Nestle U et al (2018) ESTRO ACROP guidelines for target volume definition in the treatment of locally advanced non-small cell lung cancer. Radiother Oncol 127(1):1–5

Peeters ST et al (2016) Selective mediastinal node irradiation in non-small cell lung cancer in the IMRT/VMAT era: how to use E(B)US-NA information in addition to PET-CT for delineation? Radiother Oncol 120(2):273–278

Ricardi U et al (2010) Stereotactic body radiation therapy for early stage non-small cell lung cancer: results of a prospective trial. Lung Cancer 68(1):72–77

Rosenzweig KE et al (2000) The deep inspiration breath-hold technique in the treatment of inoperable non-small-cell lung cancer. Int J Radiat Oncol Biol Phys 48(1):81–87

Rosenzweig KE et al (2001) Elective nodal irradiation in the treatment of non-small-cell lung cancer with three-dimensional conformal radiation therapy. Int J Radiat Oncol Biol Phys 50(3):681–685

Rusch VW et al (2007) Induction chemoradiation and surgical resection for superior sulcus non-small-cell lung carcinomas: long-term results of Southwest Oncology Group Trial 9416 (Intergroup Trial 0160). J Clin Oncol 25(3):313–318

Sim AJ et al (2020) A review of the role of MRI in diagnosis and treatment of early stage lung cancer. Clin Transl Radiat Oncol 24:16–22

Spoelstra FO et al (2010) Variations in target volume definition for postoperative radiotherapy in stage III non-small-cell lung cancer: analysis of an international contouring study. Int J Radiat Oncol Biol Phys 76(4):1106–1113

Staples CA et al (1988) Mediastinal nodes in bronchogenic carcinoma: comparison between CT and mediastinoscopy. Radiology 167(2):367–372

Steenbakkers RJ et al (2005) Observer variation in target volume delineation of lung cancer related to radiation oncologist-computer interaction: a 'Big Brother' evaluation. Radiother Oncol 77(2):182–190

Steenbakkers RJ et al (2006) Reduction of observer variation using matched CT-PET for lung cancer delineation: a three-dimensional analysis. Int J Radiat Oncol Biol Phys 64(2):435–448

Sundstrom S et al (2004) Hypofractionated palliative radiotherapy (17 Gy per two fractions) in advanced non-small-cell lung carcinoma is comparable to standard fractionation for symptom control and survival: a national phase III trial. J Clin Oncol 22(5):801–810

Tada T et al (2012) A phase I study of chemoradiotherapy with use of involved-field conformal radiotherapy and accelerated hyperfractionation for stage III non-small cell lung cancer: WJTOG 3305. Int J Radiat Oncol Biol Phys 83(1):327–331

Thomas M et al (2008) Effect of preoperative chemoradiation in addition to preoperative chemotherapy: a randomised trial in stage III non-small-cell lung cancer. Lancet Oncol 9(7):636–648

Timmerman R et al (2010) Stereotactic body radiation therapy for inoperable early stage lung cancer. JAMA 303(11):1070–1076

van Baardwijk A et al (2012) Mature results of a phase II trial on individualised accelerated radiotherapy based on normal tissue constraints in concurrent chemoradiation for stage III non-small cell lung cancer. Eur J Cancer 48(15):2339–2346

van Loon J et al (2012) Microscopic disease extension in three dimensions for non-small-cell lung cancer: development of a prediction model using pathology-validated positron emission tomography and computed tomography features. Int J Radiat Oncol Biol Phys 82(1):448–456

Videtic GM et al (2015) A randomized phase 2 study comparing 2 stereotactic body radiation therapy schedules for medically inoperable patients with stage I peripheral non-small cell lung cancer: NRG Oncology RTOG 0915 (NCCTG N0927). Int J Radiat Oncol Biol Phys 93(4):757–764

Westover KD et al (2015) Precision hypofractionated radiation therapy in poor performing patients with non-small cell lung cancer: phase 1 dose escalation trial. Int J Radiat Oncol Biol Phys 93(1):72–81

Willoughby TR et al (2006) Evaluation of an infrared camera and X-ray system using implanted fiducials in patients with lung tumors for gated radiation therapy. Int J Radiat Oncol Biol Phys 66(2):568–575

Wong JW et al (1999) The use of active breathing control (ABC) to reduce margin for breathing motion. Int J Radiat Oncol Biol Phys 44(4):911–919

Yuan S et al (2007) Determining optimal clinical target volume margins on the basis of microscopic extracapsular extension of metastatic nodes in patients with non-small-cell lung cancer. Int J Radiat Oncol Biol Phys 67(3):727–734

The Radiation Target in Small Cell Lung

Gregory M. M. Videtic

Contents

1 Overview of RT in SCLC 271
2 Historical Perspectives on Lung Cancer Target Definition 273
3 SCLC Target Definition and the Impact of CHT 274
4 SCLC Target Definition and the Regional Lymph Nodes 277
5 SCLC Target Definition and FDG-PET 278
6 SCLC Target Definition in Extensive Disease 279
7 Conclusions 280
References 280

Abstract

The historic target for treating small cell lung cancer with curative radiation was simply defined by what could be "safely" encompassed within a single (hemi-thoracic) "portal" drawn on a chest X-ray film. Six decades of advances in radiologic and nuclear medicine imaging have led to a revision of this classically defined target to one that more accurately reflects the true extent of actual disease. Accuracy in target definition has been matched to advances in technology for radiotherapy (RT) planning and delivery so that current treatment approaches are more likely to result in optimal cancer control while minimizing normal tissue irradiation and treatment-related side effects. This chapter will review historic trials and ongoing studies to provide a comprehensive understanding on the evolution of the RT target in small cell lung cancer.

1 Overview of RT in SCLC

Thoracic RT (TRT) is an integral component in the standard management of patients presenting with small cell lung cancer (SCLC). Its role in improving outcomes when treating limited stage disease (LS-SCLC) has been confirmed in numerous randomized clinical trials and in

G. M. M. Videtic (✉)
Department of Radiation Oncology, Taussig Cancer Institute, Cleveland Clinic, Cleveland, OH, USA
e-mail: videtig@ccf.org

subsequent meta-analyses (Cooper and Spiro 2006; Lee et al. 2006; Faivre-Finn et al. 2005a; Faivre-Finn et al. 2005b; Socinski and Bogart 2007; Curran Jr 2001; De Ruysscher and Vansteenkiste 2000). The addition of TRT to combination chemotherapy (CHT) significantly reduces the risk of loco-regional failure (Bleehen et al. 1983; Bunn Jr et al. 1987; Mira et al. 1982; Perez et al. 1984; Perry et al. 1987a), and two meta-analyses have shown an absolute long-term survival gain of 5% (Pignon et al. 1992; Warde and Payne 1992). The role of TRT in extensive stage disease (ES-SCLC) is well established for palliation of local symptoms. Its role in improving overall survival (OS) in selected advanced disease patients is controversial. In 1997, Jeremic et al. published results of a phase III study of ES-SCLC patients given induction CHT who were then randomized to either TRT with concurrent low-dose daily CHT or to CHT alone. The 5-year survival rate of those receiving TRT versus those not receiving was 9.1% vs. 3.7%, respectively, and was statistically significant (Jeremic et al. 1999). In 2015, Slotman et al. (Slotman et al. 2015) published their phase III study of TRT given after prophylactic cranial irradiation (PCI) compared to PCI alone for ES-SCLC patients with response after 4–6 cycles of CHT. Their primary endpoint of improved OS at 1 year with TRT was not met although 2-year survival and local control were improved. RTOG 0937 was a randomized phase II study comparing PCI after CHT alone to PCI after CHT followed by consolidative TRT and/or a limited number of partially responding distant metastases. It did not show an improvement in OS by the addition of TRT (Gore et al. 2017). The addition of TRT is therefore not considered standard of care for extensive disease at this time given its inconsistent benefit for OS.

Curative radiotherapy (RT) for SCLC also includes PCI, which is considered routine in the treatment of LS-SCLC, since it produces a ~50% reduction in the rate of developing brain metastases and an absolute improvement in OS of approximately 5% (Auperin et al. 1999). In a phase III trial of ES-SLCLC patients who had responded to 4–6 cycles of CHT, the addition of PCI improved OS and prevented development of symptomatic brain disease compared to routine follow up (Slotman et al. 2007). In response to this finding of improved survival, Takahashi and colleagues conducted a phase III trial in which ES-SCLC patients who had undergone brain imaging following palliative CHT were randomized either to PCI or to routine brain MRI monitoring. The study did not show any difference in terms of OS between the two arms although the brain failure rate in the PCI arm was lower (Takahashi et al. 2017). *The role of PCI in ES-SCLC remains controversial because of its unclear impact on survival.*

The timing and total dose of TRT to deliver have historically been active areas of investigation and subjects of much debate but the majority of clinicians no longer consider these controversial questions. In the setting of LS-SCLC, the bulk of published evidence supports early (cycle 1 or 2) versus late initiation of TRT with concurrent CHT because of its favorable impact on survival. Early TRT start is the model adopted in contemporary trials (Samson et al. 2007; Fried et al. 2004; Huncharek and McGarry 2004; Jeremic 2006; Turrisi 3rd et al. 1999; Faivre-Finn et al. 2017). Regarding total dose, the standard of care for the treatment of LS-SCLC is 45 Gy given as twice daily (BID) fractions of 1.5 Gy for a total of 30 fractions over 3 weeks. Initially demonstrated to be superior to a once-daily fractionation schedule in the landmark phase III Intergroup 0096 study (Turrisi 3rd et al. 1999), this dose/fractionation schedule was re-confirmed as the standard of care by the results of the CONVERT (Concurrent ONce daily VErsus twice daily RT) phase III trial in which patients were randomized to either 45 Gy/1.5 Gy BID in 30 fractions or to 66 Gy in 33 once-daily fractions, both starting with the second cycle of CHT (Faivre-Finn et al. 2017). Another phase III trial has investigated dose escalation (70 Gy/2 Gy once-daily versus 45 Gy/1.5 Gy BID), with the final results from CALGB 30610/RTOG 0538 pending (Anon n.d.-a).

In step with other RT parameters, those underlying SCLC target definition have also evolved over the last decades. The purpose of the present chapter is therefore to review the current concepts that inform the practice for delineating the appropriate volumes for treatment.

2 Historical Perspectives on Lung Cancer Target Definition

In principle, when planning curative RT for lung cancer (whether non-small cell lung cancer (NSCLC) or SCLC) the target volume of tissue irradiated to a high-dose should only encompass the entire tumor and any microscopic extension of disease, and be kept as small as possible to minimize damage to normal tissues. From the 1960s to the 1990s, lung cancer treatment volumes were designed with limited visualization of disease. In other words, clinicians crafted treatment "portals" using anatomic landmarks that would encompass the parenchymal lung tumor as well as overtly involved lymph nodes (LNs) as detected on chest radiographs (viz., their only source of diagnostic imaging). In addition, these portals had to include regional nodes considered at risk in the mediastinum and the bilateral hilar and supraclavicular (SCF) nodal basins. This was because all the regional LNs, even if apparently clinically uninvolved, needed to be irradiated in order to treat potential microscopic lung cancer spread, since imaging-based definition of disease extent was crude. The target that resulted from this approach invariably caused fairly large volumes of the chest to be irradiated by relatively static, "formulaic" TRT field arrangements such as opposed anterior–posterior fields, followed by a boost to involved tumor and nodes using oblique fields sparing the spinal cord (Videtic et al. 2008a).

From the 1990s onwards, a rapid evolution in radiologic imaging allowed clinicians to move away from the limitations of the chest radiograph to highly sophisticated means of tumor definition and identification, whether by computed tomography (CT) scan of the chest or by fluorodeoxyglucose (FDG)-positron emission tomography (PET) imaging (FDG-PET) (Senan and De Ruysscher 2005; Aristei et al. 2010). This enhanced ability to define disease through imaging was complemented by parallel developments in bronchoscopy and ultrasound techniques for assessment of the mediastinum. Endobronchial ultrasound (EBUS) guided needle aspiration and/or esophageal endoscopic ultrasound (EUS) with guided fine-needle aspiration (FNA) are now often utilized to more precisely characterize involvement of mediastinal LNs (Murakami et al. 2014).

This enhanced understanding of nodal involvement has had a particular impact on the issue of prophylactic mediastinal (regional) lymph node (MLN) irradiation in LS-SCLC as part of TRT. As noted above, radiation oncologists historically defined the lung cancer portal so that there was comprehensive inclusion of all MLN stations irrespective of disease status ("elective nodal irradiation" [ENI]) (Emami 1996) and this was especially true because the distinction between primary tumor and mediastinal disease was difficult to establish on radiographs, or because the disease often appeared as a conglomerate, relatively indistinct central tumor mass surrounding normal structures (Videtic et al. 2008a). With a better understanding of the true extent of disease, it became more appropriate then for clinicians to treat gross disease only, i.e., the primary tumor and involved nodes only, or "non-ENI" approach.

Refinements in identifying the SCLC target were matched by standardization of RT practice regarding dose reporting, target definitions, and normal structure labeling, as presented in updates from the International Commission on Radiation Units and Measurements (International Commission on Radiation Units and Measurements 1993; International Commission on Radiation Units and Measurements 1999). Terms such as gross tumor volume (GTV) indicating detectable or visible disease; clinical target volume (CTV), containing the GTV with sufficient margins to account for subclinical disease extension; and planning target volume (PTV), a geometrical parameter obtained by adding adequate margins around the CTV to account for uncertainties linked to set-up errors and organ motion, are now routinely assigned to structures during RT target delineation. Accurate accounting for organ-motion-associated geometric uncertainties and daily set-up errors has also become feasible and sophisticated. An internal target volume (ITV) reflecting potential tumor displacements in space can be regularly defined and lead to minimizing PTV expansions for motion. Enhanced means of verification imaging before and during RT delivery are now accomplished by sophisticated means of image-guided RT (IGRT) systems. IGRT may permit real time adjustment of RT as needed on the basis of response according to therapy-induced tumor changes (Lozano Ruiz et al. 2020). With this historical perspective in mind, Table 1 provides a reference list of completed or ongoing clinical trials over the last 35 years and documents their evolving approaches to target delineation in LS-SCLC.

3 SCLC Target Definition and the Impact of CHT

One of the earliest questions relative to defining the optimal treatment volume for SCLC was related to the effect of pre-TRT CHT on the size of the tumor. Tumor shrinkage that can rapidly occur with as little as one CHT cycle prompted the question of what would then be considered the appropriate TRT target to be treated, i.e., the pre-CHT or the post-CHT volume visible on imaging. The first prospective trial to address this question, SWOG 7924, was carried out by the Southwest Oncology Group (SWOG) and its results were published in 1987 (Kies et al. 1987). This phase III trial involved 466 patients and had a complex randomization schema based on response to CHT: patients with a partial response or stable disease after 4 cycles of CHT (non-platinum based) were randomized to RT fields based on either the pre- or the post-CHT volume of disease. No statistical differences in survival or recurrence patterns were noted as a function of volume treated. Complete responders had local recurrence rates of 50% with RT, and 72% without RT, and partial responders or those with stable disease had local recurrence rates of 32% for pre-CHT volumes vs. 28% for post-CHT volumes. Since local failure did not increase using post-CHT volumes, they were judged appropriate for target delineation. The details of the portals used in this protocol are relevant. As stated by the authors, the volume as determined from a chest x-ray included: the primary tumor, the surrounding abnormal lung, the low supraclavicular area, "which gave a very large portal in some patients" (Kies et al. 1987). In the pre-CHT arm, the X-ray was taken before the induction CHT; in the reduced-field arm, the post-induction X-ray served for planning.

In the decades following this landmark SWOG study, only retrospective analyses continued to be published addressing the pre- vs. post-CHT targeting question for LS-SCLC, with the majority suggesting that a post-CHT target was appropriate at the time of planning (Perez et al. 1981; Mira and Livingston 1980; Liengswangwong et al. 1994; Tada et al. 1998; White et al. 1982; Arriagada et al. 1991; Brodin et al. 1990). It is only recently that the only other prospective study exploring this question has been published, almost 35 years after SWOG 7924. In 2020, Hu et al. (Hu et al. 2020) reported the results of their randomized study of using a pre-CHT versus a post-CHT target in treating LS-SCLC. Unlike the SWOG study, this trial was conducted in the era of modern RT planning, including access to PET and use of 3D conformal techniques. After 2 cycles of etoposide and cisplatin, patients were randomized to receive either TRT to the post-CHT (study arm) or to the pre-CHT tumor volume (control arm). TRT consisted of 45 Gy/1.5 Gy BID. The control arm GTV included the primary tumor (GTV-T) as determined prior to treatment along with all positive pre-CHT LNs (GTV-N) (LNs in the mediastinum with a greatest dimension ≥ 1 cm, or LNs with positive tumor cell sampling, or an F-18 fluoro-2-deoxyglucose standard uptake value ≥ 2.5 on PET/CT at initial

Table 1 Target volume definitions from completed and ongoing prospective studies in SCLC

Publication year	Author/title (ref.)	Study type	Planning/delivery	RT start with CHT cycle	Overall target definition
Ongoing	NRG LU007 "RAPTOR" (Anon n.d.-c)	Phase II/III	3D/IMRT/IGRT		Post-CHT GTV then ITV; CTV = ITV + 0.5 cm then adjusted to eliminate OARs overlap; PTV = CTV + 0.5 cm
Ongoing	NRG LU005 (Anon n.d.-b)	Phase II/III	3D/IMRT	With cycle 2	Post-CHT GTV then ITV; CTV = ITV + 0.5 cm then adjusted to OARs; PTV = CTV + 0.5 cm
Completed, not published	CALGB 30610/RTOG 0538 (Anon n.d.-a)	Phase III	3D/IMRT	With cycle 1 or 2	1. GTV by CT, and PET if available 2. ITV for motion 3. CTV1-GTV + ipsilateral hilum; CTV2-revised; GTV after CHT; otherwise no ENI 4. PTV 1 and 2- non-ITV or ITV based margins, between 15 and 5 mm, respectively
2020	Hu et al. (2020)	Phase III	3D/IMRT	With cycle 3: 1. Pre-CHT volume 2. Post-CHT volume	1. Pre-CHT GTV: Primary tumor and involved nodes (by PET and CT); CTV = pre-CHT GTV + 0.8 cm 2. Post-CHT GTV: Residual tumor and nodes at simulation; CTV = post-CHT + 0.8 cm 3. No ENI but involved nodal basins covered pre- and post-CHT, even if CR
2017	EORTC-CONVERT (Faivre-Finn et al. 2017)	Phase III	3D	With cycle 2	1. GTV by CT, and PET if available 2. CTV = GTV + 5 mm 3. PTV = 10 mm sup/inf; 8 mm lat 4. No ENI
2010	van Loon et al. (2010a)	Phase II	3D	Post-CHT (median of 18 days)	1. GTV and PTV defined by PET and CT 2. If induction CHT, post-CHT volume considered GTV of primary tumor but for MLNs, pre-CHT used 3. If PET negative in mdstnm and CT positive, mdstnm not included in GTV. 4. Margin from GTV to CTV = 5 mm, from CTV to PTV = 5 mm for MLNs and 10 mm for primary 5. No ENI
2007	Schild et al. (2007)	Phase II	2D	Post-CHT cycle 4/5 of 6	Split course: Cycle 4- primary tumor with ipsilateral hilar, mediastinal, and SCF nodes; cycle 5-cone-down to "reduced" mdstnm and only involved SCF
2006	Spiro et al. (2006)	Phase III	2D	Pre-CHT	Arms 1, 2: Primary tumor with margin + entire mdstnm; SCF if involved
2006	Baas et al. (2006a)	Phase II	3D	After cycle 1 CHT	Primary tumor + all clinical and radiological involved lymph nodes with a short-axis diameter of ≥1 cm

(continued)

Table 1 (continued)

Publication year	Author/title (ref.)	Study type	Planning/delivery	RT start with CHT cycle	Overall target definition
2006	De Ruysscher et al. (2006a)	Phase II	3D	CT during the first cycle of CHT	GTV = primary tumor and MLNs with a short-axis diameter of ≥1 cm PTV = GTV + margin
2004	Bogart et al. (2004)	Phase II	2D or 3D	After cycle 2 CHT	GTV = pos- induction lung tumor and involved MLN (pre- and post-CHT) CTV1 [to 44 Gy] = GTV + ipsilateral non-involved MLNs + margin CTV2 [to 70 Gy] = GTV + ipsilateral hilum
2002	Takada et al. (2002)	Phase III	Not specified	Pre-CHT	Arm 1: RT with CHT cycle 1- primary disease with margin, ipsilateral hilum, entire mdstnm, SCF if involved Arm 2: RT after 4 cycles CHT- "pretreatment tumor volume"
2001	Skarlos et al. (2001)	Randomized phase II	2D	Pre-CHT	Arm 1: To 30 Gy- primary tumor + entire mdstnm + bilateral hila; SCF if involved To 45 Gy- primary tumor Arm 2- "initial tumor volume"
1999	Turrisi et al. (1999)	Phase III	2D	Pre-CHT	Primary tumor, bilateral mediastinal and ipsilateral hilar lymph nodes; SCF only if involved; specifically: "Inferior border … 5 cm below the carina or to a level including ipsilateral hilar structures, whichever was lower"
1997	Jeremic et al. (1997)	Phase III	2D	Pre-CHT	Arm 1: Primary tumor, ipsilateral hilum, entire mdstnm; SCF only if involved Arm 2: Initial tumor volume
1997	Work et al. (1997)	Phase III	2D (rare 3D)	Pre-CHT	Primary tumor, ipsilateral hilum, entire mdstnm; SCF only if involved
1993	Murray et al. (1993)	Phase III	2D ("CT-planning not mandatory")	Pre-CHT	Arms 1, 2: Primary tumor with margin + entire mdstnm; SCF if involved
1987	Perry et al. (1987b)	Phase III	2D	Pre-CHT	Arms 1, 2: To 40Gy-primary tumor with margin + entire mdstnm; bilateral hila, bilateral SCF; Boost to 50 Gy- residual disease on a mid-course CXR
1987	Kies et al. (1987)	Phase III	2D	Arm "wide-field": Pre-CHT Arm "reduced field": Post-CHT	Primary tumor, "abnormal appearing lung", mdstnm, "low" SCF
1981	Perez et al. (1981)	Phase III	2D	Pre-CHT	Arms 1, 2: Primary tumor with margin + entire mdstnm; bilateral hila, bilateral SCF

CT computed tomography, *PTV* planning target volume, *GTV* gross tumor volume, *CTV* clinical target volume, *ITV* internal target volume, *CHT* chemotherapy, *MLN* mediastinal lymph node, *RT* radiotherapy, *SCF* supraclavicular fossa, *mdstnm* mediastinum, *ENI* elective nodal irradiation, *3D* three-dimensional conformal radiotherapy, *IMRT* intensity modulated radiotherapy, *IGRT* image-guided radiotherapy, *OARs* organs at risk staging). For patients who were randomized to irradiation of the post-CHT volumes, the clinical target volume-tumor (CTV-T) included the post-CHT residual GTV-T with a margin of 0.8 cm. For patients who were randomized to the control arm (i.e., irradiation of the pre-CHT primary tumor extent), the CTV-T included the pre-CHT GTV-T with a margin of 0.8 cm. The clinical target volume-LN (CTV-N) contained the positive pre-CHT LN regions. The pre-CHT GTV-T volumes were contoured on simulation CT images by referring to corresponding diagnostic CT images obtained before induction CHT. Hu et al. found that use of the post-CHT target for treatment planning was not associated with increased rates of local failure or changes in OS and thus confirmed the SWOG 7924 results for the modern era.

With reference to recent trials and the timing of TRT relative to CHT, all patients enrolled on CONVERT (Faivre-Finn et al. 2017) started their RT with the second cycle of cisplatin/etoposide, independent of their TRT dose randomization. In the CALGB 30610/RTOG 0538 study (Anon n.d.-a), patients on either TRT arm were permitted to start with either cycle 1 or cycle 2 of CHT. In addition, there were planned volume reductions in the target at a specified dose level [44 Gy] in the two conventionally fractionated arms. This adapted target accounted for tumor response to the combination of chemoRT delivered to that dose level. Since this study remains unpublished, there is no data on the effect, if any, of these targets adaptations on outcomes. For patients enrolled to NRG LU005 (Anon n.d.-b) which is randomizing LS-SCLC patients to concurrent chemoRT ± immunotherapy, TRT starts with cycle 2 independent of the TRT dose/fractionation schedule selected. Therefore, except for a cohort of patients on RTOG 0538, all current trials studies assume planning based on the post-CHT volume after 1 cycle of CHT.

For patients deemed not suited to concurrent chemoRT, it may be appropriate to deliver TRT sequentially, following the completion of CHT. This may arise especially when patient factors such as impaired pulmonary function introduce unacceptable risk of TRT-related toxicity. In the scenario where RT would follow full course CHT, it would possible to observe a complete response (CR) to CHT. In other words, the primary lung tumor and involved LNs would essentially have disappeared as targets. Given the awareness that use of TRT is still required for optimal local control, following the model of SWOG 7924 (Kies et al. 1987), the treatment target would essentially consist of a CTV that covered the known involved mediastinal nodal basins and to treat this zone to full dose, but not include the previously involved lung field.

4 SCLC Target Definition and the Regional Lymph Nodes

As noted earlier, historic progress in imaging lung cancer led to a move away from prophylactic irradiation of uninvolved regional LNs in the mediastinum, or ENI. That said, the early shift in clinical practice away from ENI towards targets limited to disease-bearing areas only was essentially empiric and not prompted by prospective trials. Studies specifically addressing ENI issues are therefore relatively recent. The first clinical study to date directly addressing the issue of ENI in SCLC was a phase II trial published by De Ruysscher et al. in 2006 (De Ruysscher et al. 2006b). The authors explicitly wished to evaluate the patterns of recurrence when ENI was omitted in patients with LS-SCLC. Twenty-seven patients received TRT to 45 Gy/30 fractions (1.5 Gy twice daily) concurrent with carboplatin and etoposide (CbE). Only the primary tumor and the positive nodal areas on the pretreatment CT scan were irradiated. A PET scan was not performed. After a median time of 18 months post-RT, 7 patients developed a local recurrence. Three patients (11%) developed an isolated nodal failure, all of them in the ipsilateral SCF. The authors concluded that the sample size limited their results, but cautioned that omission of ENI on the basis of CT scans in patients with LS-SCLC resulted in a higher than expected rate of isolated nodal failures in the ipsilateral SCF. In the 2006 Phase II study by Baas et al., the TRT target volume for irradiation was planned to start within 1 week after the start of the second cycle of CHT and included the primary tumor and all clinical and radiologically involved lymph nodes with a short-axis diameter of >1 cm; this was termed "involved field irradiation" (Baas et al. 2006b). A PET scan was not performed. The authors reported an in-field recurrence rate of 24%. Out-of-field failures were only seen in 2 patients. Belderbos et al. (Belderbos et al. 2007) compared the failure patterns in this work by Baas et al. (Baas et al. 2006b) with those of De Ruysscher study (De Ruysscher et al. 2006b) and noted that isolated SCF failures were seen in both studies. Since it had been reported that routine ultrasound of the supraclavicular area has improved the clinical (CT) staging of SCLC patients (van Overhagen et al. 2004), Belderbos et al. (Belderbos et al. 2007) suggested that this test be incorporated in the assessment of LS-SCLC in whom non-ENI RT fields are being contemplated. Van Loon et al. (van Loon et al. 2008) provided results from a planning study incorporating FDG-PET in the TRT planning for target definition and reported 24% of treatment plans were changed compared to CT-based planning, with both increases and decreases in GTV observed. Subsequently, van Loon and her colleagues published results from a series of 60 patients treated with concurrent CHT and hyperfractionated TRT [45 Gy], with PET scan-based selective nodal irradiation (van Loon et al. 2010b). They observed a low rate of isolated nodal failures (3%). This was in contrast with the findings from their aforementioned study of CT-based selective nodal irradiation, which resulted in a higher percentage of isolated nodal failures (11%) (De Ruysscher et al. 2006b). A retrospective study from the USA by Watkins et al. of 52 patients treated with hyperfractionated TRT starting at CHT cycle 1 or 2 and with involved MLNs defined by CT and/or PET criteria, showed that involved-field TRT did not appear to have an adverse impact on anticipated patterns of failure or survival (Watkins et al. 2010).

Considering contemporary phase III trials, the CONVERT trial (Anon n.d.-c) explicitly stated that the clinical target not involve an ENI approach. The GTV was to be defined as only identifiable lung tumor and involved LNs (defined on CT as nodes>1 cm in short-axis). From that volume, the CTV would be expanded from the GTV isotropically with a 0.5 cm margin. In CALGB 30610/RTOG 0538 (Anon n.d.-a), comprehensive ENI was modified to a selective inclusion of at-risk non-involved LNs. Elective treatment of the supraclavicular fossae was explicitly forbidden, however inclusion of the tumor's ipsilateral hilum was mandated in all cases and elective inclusion of specified mediastinal LNs was detailed as a function of tumor location. In the currently accruing NRG LU005 trial (Faivre-Finn et al. 2005a), the protocol explicitly states that the GTV contoured should reflect the tumor seen on the planning CT simulation scan and not a larger pre-CHT volume.

In 2020, Farrell et al. (Farrell et al. 2020) reported the results of an online survey conducted to determine the current patterns of practice in the USA regarding ENI in the treatment of LS-SCLC. Survey invitations were sent to 6,954 e-mail addresses of radiation oncologists, with analyzable responses received from a total of 309 respondents. They found that nearly two-thirds (64%) of respondents did not recommend ENI for patients with LS-SCLC. The authors noted that this recommendation was different than what had been found in earlier surveys where ENI was considered standard. They commented that this shift in routine practice paralleled the movement away from ENI being employed in modern clinical trials such as CONVERT. The latter trial's results have in fact demonstrated that omitting ENI does not compromise local control.

5 SCLC Target Definition and FDG-PET

When considering the role of PET in SCLC target delineation, there are insights to be gained from how PET was introduced into TRT planning of NSCLC, since this has been a much more active area of investigation. For NSCLC, PET has been shown to have a higher sensitivity, specificity, and accuracy for detecting tumor involvement in MLNs than CT imaging (van Baardwijk et al. 2006). However, the gold standard for confirming extent of MLN metastases in NSCLC has conventionally been by physical visualization and sampling of nodes, as during mediastinoscopy or EBUS (Rusch 2005). There have been rare studies looking at validating PET-defined nodal targets in RT planning for NSCLC against the pathologic standard (Videtic et al. 2008b). For SCLC, although EBUS has been employed to stage the mediastinum (Wada et al. 2010), there have been no studies that have looked at confirming PET-derived target delineation against a pathologic standard validation when it applies to TRT planning.

There are a number of publications reporting on the utility of PET in the staging of SCLC that have value with respect to RT planning. Bradley et al. (Bradley et al. 2004) prospectively performed PET scanning on 24 patients determined by conventional staging to have LS-SCLC. PET identified unsuspected regional nodal metastases in 6 (25%) of 24 patients compared with CT: 1 patient with N1 disease on CT was found to have N2 disease by PET; 5 patients with clinical N2 disease on CT were found to have N3 disease. As in other studies, none of the PET findings was confirmed histologically. The RT plan, however, was significantly altered to include the PET-positive/CT-negative nodes within the high-dose region in each of these patients. In a retrospective study by Kamel et al. (Kamel et al. 2003), PET scans had an impact on RT in 8 patients (19%). In 5 patients (12%), PET scans resulted in a change of RT field and volume after identifying additional active tumor foci, which were not identified by the conventional staging methods. In 5 patients with limited disease, PET detected additional metastatic foci: ipsilateral pulmonary metastasis ($n = 1$) and contralateral mediastinal ($n = 1$), contralateral supraclavicular ($n = 2$), and contralateral cervical ($n = 1$) lymph node metastases. Sager et al. (Sager et al. 2019) summarized the utility of FDG-PET for planning SCLC by stating that integrated PET/CT "assists in the designation of RT portals with its high accuracy to detect intrathoracic tumor and nodal disease."

In the realm of clinical trials, it is interesting to note that for the recently published phase III CONVERT trial, PET for TRT planning was not mandated, since at the time of the trial's design, there was not a consensus on the application of this modality in the management of SCLC. That said, in the protocol itself, it was noted that if PET scans have been used for staging, then the GTV was required to include any PET-positive LNs. Recently, the CONVERT investigators published the results of an exploratory analysis of the impact of PET staging on the overall outcomes from this trial. Remarkably, Manoharan et al. (Manoharan et al. 2019) have showed that survival outcomes were not significantly different in patients staged with or without ^{18}F-FDG PET/CT. Although this was not correlated with the quality of TRT delivered, this finding suggests the need for further validation on PET's role in LS-SCLC when it comes to TRT target design.

6 SCLC Target Definition in Extensive Disease

Since most clinicians consider the primary role of TRT in ES-SCLC to be palliative, target delineation for patients presenting with thoracic symptoms will be always individualized based on disease extent and clinical need. With relevance to ES-SCLC, it is possible to extrapolate from the results of a recent retrospective study that looked at the impact of target volume size in palliative RT for a cohort of NSCLC patients and analyzed the OS stratified for clinical and planning target volume (CTV and PTV) size (Nieder et al. 2021). The authors found that target volume size was not significantly associated with survival. Clinicians therefore need to be mindful not to underestimate the fields required to appropriately palliate patients with large tumor burdens, as can be seen with ES-SCLC.

In contrast to its conventional palliative role in ES-SCLC, evidence from the late 1990s suggested a potential positive impact of TRT on OS. Jeremic et al. (Jeremic et al. 1999) reported a near tripling of 5-year OS in favorable ES-SCLC patients who had been randomized to the addition of TRT to standard CHT. In that study, accelerated hyperfractionated RT [54 Gy/36 fractions

BID in 18 treatment days] and concurrent low-dose daily CHT were instituted after three induction cycles of cisplatin-etoposide and compared with CHT alone. PCI was offered to responders in both groups. The target volume in the TRT group included all gross disease and the ipsilateral hilum with a 2-cm margin and the entire mediastinum with a 1-cm margin. Both SCF were routinely irradiated. TRT improved local control and survival and there was no difference between combined RT-CHT and CHT alone group in terms of broncho-pulmonary toxicity. Notwithstanding the findings of this study, this approach to care in ES-SCLC was not broadly adopted into practice.

Renewed interest in exploring possible OS benefits of TRT in ES-SCLC became widespread after a 2015 publication looking at the role of chest RT after CHT and PCI. Slotman et al. (Slotman et al. 2015) conducted a phase III trial looking at the impact on OS of adding TRT after PCI compared to PCI alone for ESCLC patients who showed any response after 4–6 cycles of CHT. The TRT consisted of 30 Gy in 10 fractions using conventional field set-ups. The PTV included the post-CHT volume with a 15 mm margin to account for microscopic disease and set-up errors. Hilar and mediastinal nodal stations that were considered involved pre-CHT were always included, even in case of full response. Although the primary endpoint of this study, improvement in OS at 1 year by the addition of TRT, was not met, secondary endpoints of local control as well as 2-year OS were improved and this has prompted some clinicians to administer TRT in selected favorable patients. In a similar domain, RTOG 0937 was a randomized phase II study comparing PCI alone to PCI and consolidative RT to the chest and to a limited number of partially responding distant metastases. Unfortunately, its results did not show any improvement in OS in the experimental arm by the addition of RT (Gore et al. 2017).

In light of the recent addition of immunotherapy to the standard systemic management of ES-SCLC because it produces improved OS, the role of TRT remains unclear. In the phase III trial that proved the benefit of atezoluzimab when added to standard palliative CHT, the use of "consolidation" TRT was expressly forbidden (Horn et al. 2018). NRG LU007 is a recently initiated prospective phase II/III trial comparing atezolizumab + RT to maintenance atezolizumab alone for patients with ES-SCLC, after 4–6 cycles of etoposide/platinum doublet plus atezolizumab [RAPTOR trial] (Anon n.d.-c). Like RTOG 0937, the experimental arm will consist of consolidative RT to the chest and to a limited number of partially responding distant metastases, up to 5 isocenters in total. Targeting details for the thoracic component of this trial are in Table 1.

7 Conclusions

Defining the appropriate target when treating a SCLC patient with RT has evolved substantially over the past three decades in parallel with advancements in diagnostic imaging. The ability to more accurately define the extent of disease has allowed for more precise target definition. This has had applications both to limited and extensive stages of disease. Along with a better understanding of where the cancer is, better tools at delivering radiation have meant that for the dose of radiation delivered, there is increased chance for improved cancer control and limiting normal tissue toxicity. Better outcomes from RT in managing SCLC are more achievable now than ever. As immunotherapy plays an increasingly prominent role in the treatment of SCLC, how it interacts and enhances the efficacy of RT will remain an active area of investigation. Ongoing randomized clinical trials should provide the most up-to-date evidence to guide radiation oncologists in optimal planning of RT delivery to the tumor.

References

Anon (n.d.-a). https://clinicaltrials.gov/ct2/show/NCT00632853

Anon (n.d.-b). https://clinicaltrials.gov/ct2/show/NCT03811002?term=LU005&draw=2&rank=1

Anon (n.d.-c). https://clinicaltrials.gov/ct2/show/NCT04402788?term=LU007&draw=1&rank=1

Aristei C, Falcinelli L, Palumbo B, Tarducci R (2010) PET and PET-CT in radiation treatment planning for lung cancer. Expert Rev Anticancer Ther 10:571–584

Arriagada R, Pellae-Cosset B, Ladron de Guevara JC, el Bakry H, Benna F, Martin M, de Cremoux H, Baldeyrou P, Cerrina ML, Le Chevalier T (1991) Alternating radiotherapy and chemotherapy schedules in limited small cell lung cancer: analysis of local chest recurrences. Radiother Oncol 20:91–98

Auperin A, Arriagada R, Pignon JP, Le Pechoux C, Gregor A, Stephens RJ et al (1999) Prophylactic cranial irradiation for patients with small-cell lung cancer in complete remission. Prophylactic cranial irradiation overview collaborative group. N Engl J Med 341:476–484

Baas P, Belderbos JS, Senan S, Kwa HB, van Bochove A, van Tinteren H, Burgers JA, van Meerbeeck JP (2006a) Concurrent chemotherapy (carboplatin, paclitaxel, etoposide) and involved-field radiotherapy in limited stage small cell lung cancer: a Dutch multicenter phase II study. Br J Cancer 94:625–630

Baas P, Belderbos JS, Senan S, Kwa HB, van Bochove A, van Tinteren H, Burgers JA, van Meerbeeck JP (2006b) Concurrent chemotherapy (carboplatin, paclitaxel, etoposide) and involved-field radiotherapy in limited stage small cell lung cancer: a Dutch multicenter phase II study. Br J Cancer 94:625–630

Belderbos J, Baas P, Senan S (2007) Reply: patterns of nodal recurrence after omission of elective nodal irradiation for limited-stage small-cell lung cancer. Br J Cancer 97:276

Bleehen NM, Bunn PA, Cox JD, Dombernowsky P, Fox RM, Høst H, Joss R, White JE, Wittes RE (1983) Role of radiation therapy in small cell anaplastic carcinoma of the lung. Cancer Treat Rep 67:11–19

Bogart JA, Herndon JE 2nd, Lyss AP, Watson D, Miller AA, Lee ME, Turrisi AT, Green MR, Cancer and Leukemia Group B study 39808 (2004) 70 Gy thoracic radiotherapy is feasible concurrent with chemotherapy for limited-stage small-cell lung cancer: analysis of cancer and leukemia group B study 39808. Int J Radiat Oncol Biol Phys 59:460–468

Bradley JD, Dehdashti F, Mintun MA, Govindan R, Trinkaus K, Siegel BA (2004) Positron emission tomography in limited-stage small-cell lung cancer: a prospective study. J Clin Oncol 22:3248–3254

Brodin O, Rikner G, Steinholtz L, Nou E (1990) Local failure in patients treated with radiotherapy and multidrug chemotherapy for small cell lung cancer. Acta Oncol 29:739–746

Bunn PA Jr, Lichter AS, Makuch RW, Cohen MH, Veach SR, Matthews MJ, Anderson AJ, Edison M, Glatstein E, Minna JD et al (1987) Chemotherapy alone or chemotherapy with chest radiation therapy in limited stage small cell lung cancer. A prospective, randomized trial. Ann Intern Med 106:655–662

Cooper S, Spiro SG (2006) Small cell lung cancer: treatment review. Respirology 11:241–248

Curran WJ Jr (2001) Therapy of limited stage small cell lung cancer. Cancer Treat Res 105:229–252

De Ruysscher D, Vansteenkiste J (2000) Chest radiotherapy in limited-stage small cell lung cancer: facts, questions, prospects. Radiother Oncol 55:1–9

De Ruysscher D, Bremer RH, Koppe F, Wanders S, van Haren E, Hochstenbag M, Geeraedts W, Pitz C, Simons J, ten Velde G, Dohmen J, Snoep G, Boersma L, Verschueren T, van Baardwijk A, Dehing C, Pijls M, Minken A, Lambin P (2006a) Omission of elective node irradiation on basis of CT-scans in patients with limited disease small cell lung cancer: a phase II trial. Radiother Oncol 80:307–312

De Ruysscher D, Bremer RH, Koppe F, Wanders S, van Haren E, Hochstenbag M, Geeraedts W, Pitz C, Simons J, ten Velde G, Dohmen J, Snoep G, Boersma L, Verschueren T, van Baardwijk A, Dehing C, Pijls M, Minken A, Lambin P (2006b) Omission of elective node irradiation on basis of CT-scans in patients with limited disease small cell lung cancer: a phase II trial. Radiother Oncol 80:307–312

Emami B (1996) Three-dimensional conformal radiation therapy in bronchogenic carcinoma. Semin Radiat Oncol 6:92–97

Faivre-Finn C, Lee LW, Lorigan P, West C, Thatcher N (2005a) Thoracic radiotherapy for limited-stage small-cell lung cancer: controversies and future developments. Clin Oncol (R Coll Radiol) 17:591–598

Faivre-Finn C, Lorigan P, West C, Thatcher N (2005b) Thoracic radiation therapy for limited-stage small-cell lung cancer: unanswered questions. Clin Lung Cancer 7:23–29

Faivre-Finn C, Snee M, Ashcroft L, Appel W, Barlesi F, Bhatnagar A, Bezjak A, Cardenal F, Fournel P, Harden S, Le Pechoux C, McMenemin R, Mohammed N, O'Brien M, Pantarotto J, Surmont V, Van Meerbeeck JP, Woll PJ, Lorigan P, Blackhall F, CONVERT Study Team (2017) Concurrent once-daily versus twice-daily chemoradiotherapy in patients with limited-stage small-cell lung cancer (CONVERT): an open-label, phase 3, randomised, superiority trial. Lancet Oncol 18:1116–1125

Farrell MJ, Yahya JB, Degnin C, Chen Y, Holland JM, Henderson MA, Jaboin JJ, Harkenrider MM, Thomas CR Jr, Mitin T (2020) Elective nodal irradiation for limited-stage small-cell lung cancer: survey of US radiation oncologists on practice patterns. Clin Lung Cancer 21:443–449

Fried DB, Morris DE, Poole C, Rosenman JG, Halle JS, Detterbeck FC, Hensing TA, Socinski MA (2004) Systematic review evaluating the timing of thoracic radiation therapy in combined modality therapy for limited-stage small-cell lung cancer. J Clin Oncol 22:4785–4793

Gore EM, Hu C, Sun AY, Grimm DF, Ramalingam SS, Dunlap NE, Higgins KA, Werner-Wasik M, Allen AM, Iyengar P, Videtic GMM, Hales RK, McGarry RC, Urbanic JJ, Pu AT, Johnstone CA, Stieber VW, Paulus R, Bradley JD (2017) Randomized phase II study comparing prophylactic cranial irradiation alone to prophylactic cranial irradiation and consolidative extracranial irradiation for extensive-disease small cell lung cancer (ED SCLC): NRG oncology RTOG 0937. J Thorac Oncol 12:1561–1570

Horn L, Mansfield AS, Szczęsna A, Havel L, Krzakowski M, Hochmair MJ, Huemer F, Losonczy G, Johnson ML, Nishio M, Reck M, Mok T, Lam S, Shames DS, Liu J, Ding B, Lopez-Chavez A, Kabbinavar F, Lin W, Sandler A, Liu SV, IMpower133 Study Group (2018) First-line atezolizumab plus chemotherapy in extensive-stage small-cell lung cancer. N Engl J Med 379:2220–2229

Hu X, Bao Y, Xu YJ, Zhu HN, Liu JS, Zhang L, Guo Y, Jin Y, Wang J, Ma HL, Xu XL, Song ZB, Tang HR, Peng F, Fang M, Kong Y, Chen MY, Dong BQ, Zhu L, Yu C, Yu XM, Hong W, Fan Y, Zhang YP, Chen PC, Zhao Q, Jiang YH, Zhou XM, Chen QX, Sun WY, Mao WM, Chen M (2020) Final report of a prospective randomized study on thoracic radiotherapy target volume for limited-stage small cell lung cancer with radiation dosimetric analyses. Cancer 126:840–849

Huncharek M, McGarry R (2004) A meta-analysis of the timing of chest irradiation in the combined modality treatment of limited-stage small cell lung cancer. Oncologist 9:6665–6672

International Commission on Radiation Units and Measurements (1993) ICRU Report 50: Prescribing, Recording, and Reporting Photon Beam Therapy. International Commission in Radiation Unit and Measurements, Bethesda, MD

International Commission on Radiation Units and Measurements (1999) ICRU Report 62: Prescribing, Recording, and Reporting Photon Beam Therapy (Supplement to ICRU Report 50). International Commission in Radiation Unit and Measurements, Bethesda, MD

Jeremic B (2006) Timing of concurrent radiotherapy and chemotherapy in limited-disease small-cell lung cancer: meta-analysis of meta-analyses. Int J Radiat Oncol Biol Phys 64:981–982

Jeremic B, Shibamoto Y, Acimovic L, Milisavljevic S (1997) Initial versus delayed accelerated hyperfractionated radiation therapy and concurrent chemotherapy in limited small-cell lung cancer: a randomized study. J Clin Oncol 15:893–900

Jeremic B, Shibamoto Y, Nikolic N, Milicic B, Milisavljevic S, Dagovic A, Aleksandrovic J, Radosavljevic-Asic G (1999) Role of radiation therapy in the combined-modality treatment of patients with extensive disease small-cell lung cancer: a randomized study. J Clin Oncol 17:2092–2099

Kamel EM, Zwahlen D, Wyss MT, Stumpe KD, von Schulthess GK, Steinert HC (2003) Whole-body (18) F-FDG PET improves the management of patients with small cell lung cancer. J Nucl Med 44:1911–1917

Kies MS, Mira JG, Crowley JJ, Chen TT, Pazdur R, Grozea PN, Rivkin SE, Coltman CA Jr, Ward JH, Livingston RB (1987) Multimodal therapy for limited small-cell lung cancer: a randomized study of induction combination chemotherapy with or without thoracic radiation in complete responders; and with wide-field versus reduced-field radiation in partial responders: a southwest oncology group study. J Clin Oncol 5:592–600

Lee CB, Morris DE, Fried DB et al (2006) Current and evolving treatment options for limited stage small cell lung cancer. Curr Opin Oncol 18:162–172

Liengswangwong V, Bonner JA, Shaw EG, Foote RL, Frytak S, Eagan RT, Jett JR, Richardson RL, Creagan ET, Su JQ (1994) Limited-stage small-cell lung cancer: patterns of intrathoracic recurrence and the implications for thoracic radiotherapy. J Clin Oncol 12:496–502

Lozano Ruiz FJ, Ileana Pérez Álvarez S, Poitevin Chacón MA, Maldonado Magos F, Prudencio RR, Cabrera Miranda L, Arrieta O (2020) The importance of image guided radiotherapy in small cell lung cancer: case report and review of literature. Rep Pract Oncol Radiother 25:146–149

Manoharan P, Salem A, Mistry H, Gornall M, Harden S, Julyan P, Locke I, McAleese J, McMenemin R, Mohammed N, Snee M, Woods S, Westwood T, Faivre-Finn C (2019) ^{18}F-fludeoxyglucose PET/CT in SCLC: analysis of the CONVERT randomized controlled trial. J Thorac Oncol 14:1296–1305

Mira JG, Livingston RB (1980) Evaluation and radiotherapy implications of chest relapse patterns in small cell lung carcinoma treated with radiotherapy-chemotherapy: study of 34 cases and review of the literature. Cancer 46:2557–2565

Mira JG, Livingston RB, Moore TN, Chen T, Batley F, Bogardus CR Jr, Considine B Jr, Mansfield CM, Schlosser J, Seydel HG (1982) Influence of chest radiotherapy in frequency and patterns of chest relapse in disseminated small cell lung carcinoma. A Southwest Oncology Group Study. Cancer 50:1266–1272

Murakami Y, Oki M, Saka H, Kitagawa C, Kogure Y, Ryuge M, Tsuboi R, Oka S, Nakahata M, Funahashi Y, Hori K, Ise Y, Ichihara S, Moritani S (2014) Endobronchial ultrasound-guided transbronchial needle aspiration in the diagnosis of small cell lung cancer. Respir Investig 52:173–178

Murray N, Coy P, Pater JL, Hodson I, Arnold A, Zee BC, Payne D, Kostashuk EC, Evans WK, Dixon P et al (1993) Importance of timing for thoracic irradiation in the combined modality treatment of limited-stage small-cell lung cancer. The National Cancer Institute of Canada Clinical Trials Group. J Clin Oncol 11:336–344

Nieder C, Imingen KS, Mannsaker B, Yobuta R (2021) Palliative thoracic radiotherapy for non-small cell lung cancer: is there any impact of target volume size on survival? Anticancer Res 41:355–358

Perez CA, Krauss S, Bartolucci AA, Durant JR, Lowenbraun S, Salter MM, Storaalsi J, Kellermeyer R, Comas F (1981) Thoracic and elective brain irradiation with concomitant or delayed multiagent chemotherapy in the treatment of localized small cell carcinoma of the lung: a randomized prospective study by the southeastern cancer study group. Cancer 47:2407–2413

Perez CA, Einhorn L, Oldham RK, Greco FA, Cohen HJ, Silberman H, Krauss S, Hornback N, Comas F, Omura G et al (1984) Randomized trial of radiotherapy to the thorax in limited small-cell carcinoma of the lung treated with multiagent chemotherapy and elective brain irradiation: a preliminary report. J Clin Oncol 2:1200–1208

Perry MC, Eaton WL, Propert KJ, Ware JH, Zimmer B, Chahinian AP, Skarin A, Carey RW, Kreisman H, Faulkner C et al (1987a) Chemotherapy with or without radiation therapy in limited small-cell carcinoma of the lung. N Engl J Med 316:912–918

Perry MC, Eaton WL, Propert KJ, Ware JH, Zimmer B, Chahinian AP, Skarin A, Carey RW, Kreisman H, Faulkner C et al (1987b) Chemotherapy with or without radiation therapy in limited small-cell carcinoma of the lung. N Engl J Med 316:912–918

Pignon JP, Arriagada R, Ihde DC, Johnson DH, Perry MC, Souhami RL, Brodin O, Joss RA, Kies MS, Lebeau B et al (1992) A meta-analysis of thoracic radiotherapy for small-cell lung cancer. N Engl J Med 327:1618–1624

Rusch VW (2005) Mediastinoscopy: an endangered species? J Clin Oncol 23:8283–8285

Sager O, Dincoglan F, Demiral S, Uysal B, Gamsiz H, Elcim Y, Gundem E, Dirican B, Beyzadeoglu M (2019) Utility of molecular imaging with 2-deoxy-2-[fluorine-18] fluoro-D-glucose positron emission tomography (18F-FDG PET) for small cell lung cancer (SCLC): a radiation oncology perspective. Curr Radiopharm 12:4–10

Samson DJ, Seidenfeld J, Simon GR, Turrisi AT 3rd, Bonnell C, Ziegler KM, Aronson N, American College of Chest Physicians (2007) Evidence for management of small cell lung cancer: ACCP evidence-based clinical practice guidelines (2nd edition). Chest 132(3 Suppl):314S–323S

Schild SE, Bonner JA, Hillman S, Kozelsky TF, Vigliotti AP, Marks RS, Graham DL, Soori GS, Kugler JW, Tenglin RC, Wender DB, Adjei A (2007) Results of a phase II study of high-dose thoracic radiation therapy with concurrent cisplatin and etoposide in limited-stage small-cell lung cancer (NCCTG 95-20-53). J Clin Oncol 25:3124–3129

Senan S, De Ruysscher D (2005) Critical review of PET-CT for radiotherapy planning in lung cancer. Crit Rev Oncol Hematol 56:345–351

Skarlos DV, Samantas E, Briassoulis E, Panoussaki E, Pavlidis N, Kalofonos HP, Kardamakis D, Tsiakopoulos E, Kosmidis P, Tsavdaridis D, Tzitzikas J, Tsekeris P, Kouvatseas G, Zamboglou N, Fountzilas G (2001) Randomized comparison of early versus late hyperfractionated thoracic irradiation concurrently with chemotherapy in limited disease small-cell lung cancer: a randomized phase II study of the Hellenic cooperative oncology group (HeCOG). Ann Oncol 12:1231–1238

Slotman B, Faivre-Finn C, Kramer G, Rankin E, Snee M, Hatton M, Postmus P, Collette L, Musat E, Senan S, Group (2007) Prophylactic cranial irradiation in extensive small-cell lung cancer. N Engl J Med 357:664–672

Slotman BJ, van Tinteren H, Praag JO, Knegjens JL, El Sharouni SY, Hatton M, Keijser A, Faivre-Finn C, Senan (2015) Use of thoracic radiotherapy for extensive stage small-cell lung cancer: a phase 3 randomised controlled trial. Lancet 385:36–42

Socinski MA, Bogart JA (2007) Limited-stage small-cell lung cancer: the current status of combined-modality therapy. J Clin Oncol 25:4137–4145

Spiro SG, James LE, Rudd RM, Trask CW, Tobias JS, Snee M, Gilligan D, Murray PA, Ruiz de Elvira MC, O'Donnell KM, Gower NH, Harper PG, Hackshaw AK, London Lung Cancer Group (2006) Early compared with late radiotherapy in combined modality treatment for limited disease small-cell lung cancer: a London Lung Cancer Group multicenter randomized clinical trial and meta-analysis. J Clin Oncol 24:3823–3830

Tada T, Minakuchi K, Koda M, Masuda N, Matsui K, Kawase I, Nakajima T, Nishioka M, Fukuoka M, Kozuka T (1998) Limited-stage small cell lung cancer: local failure after chemotherapy and radiation therapy. Radiology 208:511–515

Takada M, Fukuoka M, Kawahara M, Sugiura T, Yokoyama A, Yokota S, Nishiwaki Y, Watanabe K, Noda K, Tamura T, Fukuda H, Saijo N (2002) Phase III study of concurrent versus sequential thoracic radiotherapy in combination with cisplatin and etoposide for limited-stage small-cell lung cancer: results of the Japan clinical oncology group study 9104. J Clin Oncol 20:3054–3060

Takahashi T, Yamanaka T, Seto T, Harada H, Nokihara H, Saka H, Nishio M, Kaneda H, Takayama K, Ishimoto O, Takeda K, Yoshioka H, Tachihara M, Sakai H, Goto K, Yamamoto N (2017) Prophylactic cranial irradiation versus observation in patients with extensive-disease small-cell lung cancer: a multicentre, randomised, open-label, phase 3 trial. Lancet Oncol 18:663–671

Turrisi AT 3rd, Kim K, Blum R, Sause WT, Livingston RB, Komaki R, Wagner H, Aisner S, Johnson DH (1999) Twice-daily compared with once-daily thoracic radiotherapy in limited small-cell lung cancer treated concurrently with cisplatin and etoposide. N Engl J Med 340:265–2671

van Baardwijk A, Baumert BG, Bosmans G, van Kroonenburgh M, Stroobants S, Gregoire V, Lambin P, De Ruysscher D (2006) The current status of FDG-PET in tumour volume definition in radiotherapy treatment planning. Cancer Treat Rev 32:245–260

van Loon J, Offermann C, Bosmans G, Wanders R, Dekker A, Borger J, Oellers M, Dingemans AM, van Baardwijk A, Teule J, Snoep G, Hochstenbag M, Houben R, Lambin P, De Ruysscher D (2008) 18FDG-PET based radiation planning of mediastinal lymph nodes in limited disease small cell lung cancer changes radiotherapy fields: a planning study. Radiother Oncol 87:49–54 van Loon J, De Ruysscher D, Wanders R, Boersma L, Simons J, Oellers M, Dingemans AM, Hochstenbag M, Bootsma G, Geraedts W, Pitz C, Teule J, Rhami A, Thimister W, Snoep G, Dehing-Oberije C, Lambin P (2010a) Selective nodal irradiation on basis of (18) FDG-PET scans in limited-disease small-cell lung cancer: a prospective study. Int J Radiat Oncol Biol Phys 77:329–336

van Loon J, De Ruysscher D, Wanders R, Boersma L, Simons J, Oellers M, Dingemans AM, Hochstenbag M, Bootsma G, Geraedts W, Pitz C, Teule J, Rhami A, Thimister W, Snoep G, Dehing-Oberije C, Lambin P (2010b) Selective nodal irradiation on basis of (18) FDG-PET scans in limited-disease small-cell lung cancer: a prospective study. Int J Radiat Oncol Biol Phys 77:329–336

van Overhagen H, Brakel K, Heijenbrok MW, van Kasteren JH, van de Moosdijk CN, Roldaan AC, van Gils AP, Hansen BE (2004) Metastases in supraclavicular lymph nodes in lung cancer: assessment with palpation, US, and CT. Radiology 232:75–80

Videtic GM, Belderbos JS, Spring Kong FM, Kepka L, Martel MK, Jeremic B (2008a) Report from the International Atomic Energy Agency (IAEA) consultants' meeting on elective nodal irradiation in lung cancer: small-cell lung cancer (SCLC). Int J Radiat Oncol Biol Phys 72:327–334

Videtic GM, Rice TW, Murthy S, Suh JH, Saxton JP, Adelstein DJ, Mekhail TM (2008b) Utility of positron emission tomography compared with mediastinoscopy for delineating involved lymph nodes in stage III lung cancer: insights for radiotherapy planning from a surgical cohort. Int J Radiat Oncol Biol Phys 72:702–706

Wada H, Nakajima T, Yasufuku K, Fujiwara T, Yoshida S, Suzuki M, Shibuya K, Hiroshima K, Nakatani Y, Yoshino I (2010) Lymph node staging by endobronchial ultrasound-guided transbronchial needle aspiration in patients with small cell lung cancer. Ann Thorac Surg 90:229–234

Warde P, Payne D (1992) Does thoracic irradiation improve survival and local control in limited-stage small- carcinoma of the lung? A meta-analysis. J Clin Oncol 10:890–895

Watkins JM, Wahlquist AE, Zauls AJ, Shirai K, Garrett-Mayer E, Aguero EG, Silvestri GA, Sherman CA, Sharma AK (2010) Involved-field radiotherapy with concurrent chemotherapy for limited-stage small-cell lung cancer: disease control, patterns of failure and survival. J Med Imaging Radiat Oncol 54:483–489

White JE, Chen T, McCracken J, Kennedy P, Seydel HG, Hartman G, Mira J, Khan M, Durrance FY, Skinner O (1982) The influence of radiation therapy quality control on survival, response and sites of relapse in oat cell carcinoma of the lung: preliminary report of a southwest oncology group study. Cancer 50:1084–1090

Work E, Nielsen OS, Bentzen SM, Fode K, Palshof T (1997) Randomized study of initial versus late chest irradiation combined with chemotherapy in limited-stage small-cell lung cancer. Aarhus lung cancer group. J Clin Oncol 15:3030–3037

Radiation Sensitizers

Mansi K. Aparnathi, Sami Ul Haq, Zishan Allibhai, Benjamin H. Lok, and Anthony M. Brade

Contents

1 **Radiation Sensitizers** 286
2 **Oxygen** 288
2.1 Hyperbaric Oxygen 288
2.2 Carbogen 288
2.3 Efaproxiral 289
2.4 Red Blood Cell Transfusion 289
2.5 Erythropoietin 289
3 **Targeting Hypoxic Cells** 290
3.1 Hypoxic Cell Radiosensitizers 290
3.2 Bioreductive Drugs, Hypoxic Cell Cytotoxins, Reactive Oxygen Species Modulators 291
4 **Boron Neutron Capture Theory (BNCT)** 292
5 **DNA Repair Inhibitors** 292
5.1 Targeting Cell Signaling Pathways 292
5.2 PARP Inhibitors 294
5.3 Epigenetic Radiosensitizers 295
6 **Apoptosis-Modulating Agents** 296
6.1 BCL2 Inhibitors 296
6.2 Cyclooxygenase (COX)-2 Inhibitors ... 296
7 **Conclusion** 297
References 297

Mansi K. Aparnathi and Sami Ul Haq contributed equally with all other contributors.

M. K. Aparnathi
Radiation Medicine Program,
Princess Margaret Cancer Centre/University Health Network, Toronto, ON, Canada

Abstract

Discovery of effective radiosensitization strategies that improve the therapeutic ratio for patients with lung cancer has been a goal of researchers and an area of vigorous investiga-

S. U. Haq
Institute of Medical Science,
University of Toronto, Toronto, ON, Canada

Z. Allibhai
Department of Radiation Oncology,
Southlake Regional Health Centre,
Newmarket, ON, Canada

Department of Radiation Oncology,
University of Toronto, Toronto, ON, Canada

B. H. Lok (✉)
Radiation Medicine Program,
Princess Margaret Cancer Centre/University Health Network, Toronto, ON, Canada

Institute of Medical Science,
University of Toronto, Toronto, ON, Canada

Department of Radiation Oncology, University of Toronto, Toronto, ON, Canada

Department of Medical Biophysics, University of Toronto, Toronto, ON, Canada
e-mail: benjamin.lok@rmp.uhn.ca

A. M. Brade (✉)
Department of Radiation Oncology,
University of Toronto, Toronto, ON, Canada

Department of Radiation Oncology,
Peel Regional Cancer Centre,
Credit Valley Hospital, Trillium Health Partners,
Mississauga, ON, Canada
e-mail: Anthony.brade@thp.ca

tion for the past several decades. A pure radiosensitizer is a drug, a modality of therapy, or an intervention that, on its own, lacks direct antitumor activity but enhances the cytotoxicity of radiotherapy when employed in combination. In this chapter we outline the previous and ongoing attempts to radiosensitize lung cancers through improved tumor oxygenation, augmentation of the effectiveness of radiotherapy in hypoxic tumor cells, and use of drugs that modulate with DNA repair and apoptosis. To date, no pure radiosensitization strategy has established itself in standard practice but the current research suggests that this field continues to hold great promise for the improvement of outcome in patients with lung cancer.

1 Radiation Sensitizers

Although radiotherapy has traditionally played a major role in the treatment of non-small cell lung cancers (NSCLC), its effectiveness had been limited by an unfavorable therapeutic ratio, whereby it is challenging to deliver optimal doses of radiation to tumors without excessive normal tissue toxicity.

Recently, a number of technological advances in both imaging and radiation delivery have further improved our ability to spare normal tissue. A further approach to enhancing the therapeutic ratio is to selectively increase the radiosensitivity of the target tumor. The advantages of this approach are potentially significant given that the presumed radioresistance of NSCLC has long been a major obstacle to the efficacy of RT.

A pure radiosensitizer is a drug, a modality of therapy, or an intervention that on its own lacks direct antitumor activity but enhances the cytotoxicity of radiotherapy when employed in combination. Many chemotherapeutic agents (e.g., platins, taxanes, and topoisomerase modulators) enhance the cytotoxicity of radiotherapy when the two modalities are combined but, as they generally effect some degree of antitumor activity when administered as single agents, are therefore not considered pure radiosensitizers. Similarly, newer classes of drugs have been developed to exploit tumor-specific mutations or target-specific molecular based alterations within the tumor or its microenvironment. Some of these also augment the efficacy of radiotherapy and have single agent efficacy against lung cancer and are thus not pure radiosensitizers. Chapters Bauman and Edelman 2022; Farris MK et al. 2022; and He K et al. 2022 in this text detail molecularly targeted drugs and combinations of radiotherapy with chemotherapy or immunotherapy in lung cancer, respectively. This chapter focuses on radiosensitizing strategies and their potential relevance to the treatment of lung cancer (Fig. 1).

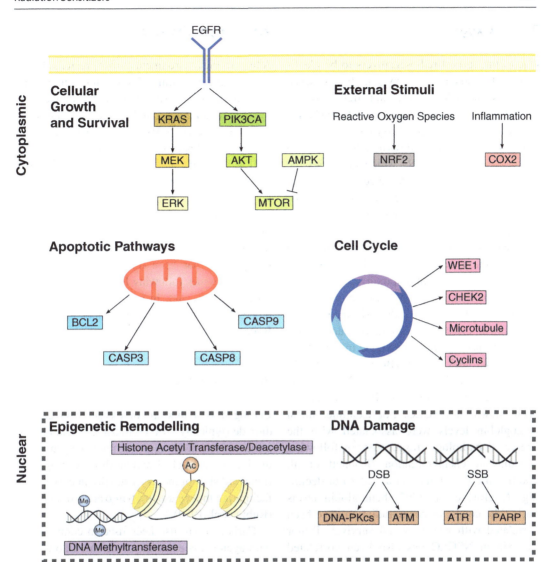

Fig. 1 Potential cellular targets to radiosensitize lung tumor cells. The figure highlights a number of proteins that mediate (1) cellular growth and survival, (2) apoptosis, (3) cell cycle, and (4) external stimuli responses that can be targeted to improve radiosensitivity. It also highlights several nuclear proteins involved in (1) epigenetic remodeling and (2) DNA damage repair pathways that can also be targeted to radiosensitize lung tumors. Abbreviations: *EGFR* epidermal growth factor receptor; *KRAS* Kirsten rat sarcoma viral proto-oncogene; *MEK* mitogen-activated protein kinase kinase 1 (*MAP2K1*); *ERK* mitogen-activated protein kinase 1 (*MAPK1*); *PIK3CA* phosphatidylinositol-4,5-bisphosphate 3-kinase catalytic subunit alpha; *AKT* AKT serine/threonine kinase 1 (*AKT1*); *AMPK* protein kinase AMP-activated catalytic subunit alpha 2 (*PRKAA2*); *MTOR* mechanistic target of rapamycin kinase; *NRF2* nuclear factor, erythroid 2 like 2 (*NFE2L2*); *COX2* prostaglandin-endoperoxide synthase 2 (*PTGS2*); *BCL2* BCL2 apoptosis regulator; *CASP3* caspase 3; *CASP8* caspase 8; *CASP9* caspase 9; *WEE1* WEE1 G2 checkpoint kinase; *CHEK2* checkpoint kinase 2; *DNA-PKcs* protein kinase, DNA-activated, catalytic subunit (*PRKDC*); *ATM* ataxia telangiectasia mutated; *ATR* ataxia telangiectasia and Rad3-related protein; *PARP* poly(ADP-ribose) polymerase 1 (*PARP1*)

2 Oxygen

One of the earliest radiosensitizers to be identified and studied was oxygen. Its presence increases the yield, variety, and lifetime of the radical species formed secondary to tumor/tissue irradiation. The impact of oxygen on radiation effect is mathematically described by the oxygen enhancement ratio (OER) which quantifies the relative dose required to produce a certain biologic effect under hypoxic conditions versus that required to achieve the same effect in aerated conditions.

The presence of a hypoxic cell subpopulation is a common feature of solid tumors, and although the extent of hypoxia varies widely from tumor to tumor and within tumors, it contributes significantly to radioresistance. While the clinical effect of hypoxia on cancer outcomes has been best demonstrated in the setting of head and neck cancers (Becker et al. 1998), cervical cancer (Höckel et al. 1993), and soft-tissue sarcomas (Brizel et al. 1996), it has also been shown in NSCLC. For example, mean hemoglobin levels were associated with the degree of pathologic response seen following neoadjuvant chemoradiation (Robnett et al. 2002) while low (Laurie et al. 2006) or declining (MacRae et al. 2002) hemoglobin levels during the course of chemoradiation have been correlated with worse overall survival. Tumor hypoxia in NSCLC has also been correlated with an increased incidence of distant metastasis and poorer overall prognosis (Eschmann et al. 2005). Hypoxia has been demonstrated to trigger the downregulation of key DNA repair pathways, leading to genetic instability. Thus, tumor hypoxia is a key driver of metastatic spread and treatment resistance (Brizel et al. 1996; Brown and Giaccia 1998).

Considerable effort has been focused on discovering interventions by which tumor hypoxia can be reduced. These have included artificial means of increasing hemoglobin oxygenation levels as well as measures to optimize the hemoglobin levels themselves.

2.1 Hyperbaric Oxygen

A hyperbaric environment allows greater solubility of oxygen within plasma and hemoglobin saturation, thus maximizing oxygen delivery to hypoxic tumor cells. Randomized trials studying hyperbaric oxygen (HBO) conducted in patients with head and neck cancer (Henk et al. 1977) as well as cervical cancer (Watson et al. 1978) had shown improvements in local control and/or survival. Furthermore, there exist several logistical issues in both the availability and administration of HBO during a standard course of fractionated radiotherapy. As a result, the role of HBO in clinical practice has been limited to the repair of damaged tissues following RT where it has been shown to limit and, in some cases, reverse the process of radiation damage (Bennett et al. 2005; Bui et al. 2004).

2.2 Carbogen

Carbogen is a mixture of oxygen and carbon dioxide (typically 95% O_2 to 5% CO_2) and it has a theoretical advantage over pure oxygen since the increased level of carbon dioxide triggers a rightward shift of the oxyhemoglobin curve, thus facilitating the release of O_2 into areas of hypoxia (Rubin et al. 1979).

Carbogen has also been used in combination with agents that enhance tumor blood flow, e.g., nicotinamide, thus providing a synergistic effect. This combination of agents was studied in a phase II trial from the Netherlands which found that the use of ARCON (accelerated radiotherapy with carbogen and nicotinamide) yielded high control rates in laryngeal cancer (Kaanders et al. 1998). While data regarding late toxicity and outcomes is not yet mature, the subsequent phase III study comparing ARCON versus accelerated radiation only demonstrated a mild increase in confluent mucositis (Janssens et al. 2012). This is consistent with results from a phase III study in locally advanced bladder cancer where the addition of ARCON to RT improved both local control and overall survival without significantly increasing late morbidity (Hoskin et al. 2010).

In regard to lung cancer, a similar phase I/II study was launched in Switzerland to investigate the effects of adding carbogen and/or nicotinamide to accelerated radiation for locally advanced NSCLC stage IIIA or IIIB. There was no difference in radiologic response or time to progression between the three groups, and no increase in radiotherapy-related adverse events. However, a significant proportion of patients in the two groups that received nicotinamide developed significant ($\geq$G2) emesis which was shown to adversely affect their quality of life (Bernier et al. 1999); thus this strategy is unlikely to be pursued further in this disease.

2.3 Efaproxiral

Efaproxiral (RSR-13) is an allosteric effector of hemoglobin which enhances its oxygen-carrying capacity, effectively increasing the delivery of oxygen to otherwise hypoxic regions. Phase I and II studies demonstrated that this compound is safe and effective in improving tumor oxygenation and potentiating radiation effect. The REACH (radiation-enhancing allosteric compounds of hypoxic brain metastases) trial was a phase III study designed to evaluate the addition of efaproxiral to whole-brain radiotherapy in patients with brain metastasis (Suh et al. 2006). No difference in overall survival was found for the entire group, over half of whom had metastatic NSCLC. An unplanned subset analysis did however show that in the subset of patients with metastatic breast cancer (20% of patients), the addition of efaproxiral improved survival as well as quality of life (Scott et al. 2007).

A phase II trial was designed to test the efficacy and safety of efaproxiral given concurrently with radiation following induction chemotherapy for locally advanced NSCLC. This combination yielded an overall response rate of 75% and a very encouraging median survival of 20.6 months, while the rates of severe toxicity were relatively low (Choy et al. 2005). These encouraging results prompted the proposal of a phase III study; however, this trial was never launched (Choy, personal correspondence).

2.4 Red Blood Cell Transfusion

Transfusion represents a potentially direct means of improving oxygen delivery to tumors in anemic patients. An important study evaluating transfusion to counter anemia was undertaken in cervical cancer patients at Princess Margaret Hospital. This trial suggested that transfusions might improve outcomes in patients who were anemic while undergoing definitive radiotherapy (Fyles et al. 1998). The role of potentially confounding variables in this study is however unclear, and the relationship between hemoglobin levels and treatment outcome is indeed a complex one.

The systemic administration of hemoglobin vesicle (HbV), which serves as an artificial oxygen carrier, represents a recently developed alternative to red cell transfusion. Animal studies of HbV have demonstrated that it increases oxygen tension within tumor tissue and that this positively affects the tumor's response to radiation (Yamamoto et al. 2009). This was the first study to test tumor oxygenation using a liposome-type artificial oxygen carrier, and further studies are anticipated.

2.5 Erythropoietin

Erythropoietin (EPO) is a glycoprotein hormone that controls erythropoiesis through its interactions with the erythropoietin receptor (EPOR) found on bone marrow stem cells. Human recombinant erythropoietin (and similar exogenous agents) represents another method by which hemoglobin levels may be increased, and a number of trials have studied the effect of EPO in the management of anemic cancer patients. Although encouraging results were found in anemic lung cancer patients undergoing chemotherapy (Vansteenkiste et al. 2002), subsequent trials in breast and head and neck cancer patients actually suggested that these agents worsened outcomes (Henke et al. 2003; Leyland-Jones 2003). A subsequent meta-analysis of 9353 patients from 53 studies studying the effects of epoetin or darbepoetin demonstrated an increased risk of thromboembolic events as well as increased mortality from the use of these agents (Bohlius et al. 2009).

3 Targeting Hypoxic Cells

3.1 Hypoxic Cell Radiosensitizers

Hypoxic cell radiosensitizers are compounds with strong electron affinity that mimic the radiosensitizing effect of oxygen by virtue of their ability to "fix" damage produced by free radicals. As with oxygen, their strong electron affinity can fix radiation damage. Analogous to the aforementioned OER metric, the efficacy of a hypoxic cell radiosensitizer is expressed numerically as a sensitizer enhancement ratio (SER).

Misonidazole, a nitroimidazole compound, exhibits high electron affinity, induces the formation of free radicals, and depletes radioprotective thiols, thereby sensitizing hypoxic cells to the cytotoxic effects of ionizing radiation (Knight et al. 1979). It was found to be a potent radiosensitizer of cells in culture, activity which was subsequently confirmed in animal studies. However, in the clinical setting, it caused severe, dose-limiting peripheral neuropathy. Newer generation nitroimidazole compounds such as etanidazole and pimonidazole were subsequently developed to improve the pharmacokinetic profile of this class of drugs and reduce toxicity. Unfortunately, their SERs were also reduced and the two large phase III trials studying etanidazole in locally advanced head and neck carcinomas did not yield any improvements in outcome over conventionally fractionated radiation alone (Lee et al. 1995; Eschwège et al. 1997).

Several other promising pathways have also been explored in preclinical models. The SGK1 pathway, involved in unsaturated fatty acid uptake, has been shown to be important in radiosensitization (Matschke et al. 2016). Radioresistant adenocarcinoma cell lines treated with an SGK1 inhibitor demonstrated the dependence of hypoxic tumor cells on unsaturated fatty acid uptake, highlighting SGK1 as a possible target. In this study, inhibition of SGK1 then resulted in radiosensitizing of cells (Matschke et al. 2016). Another in vitro study, using niclosamide as a HIF1A and VEGF signaling inhibitor, demonstrated radiosensitivity by increasing apoptosis (Xiang et al. 2017). Inhibition of VEGF and STAT3 also led to radiosensitivity by inducing G2/M arrest (Hu et al. 2019). Similarly, inflammation mediators such as plasminogen activator inhibitor-1 (PAI1/SERPINE1) have also shown promise. PAI1 has been observed to be secreted by hypoxic radioresistant cells in a paracrine manner to signal radiosensitive cells (Kang et al. 2016). PAI1 made NSCLC cell lines radioresistant by activating the AKT/ERK/Snail pathway highlighting yet another pathway of interest (Kang et al. 2016). Similarly, modulating the mTOR/Akt/PI3K pathway can also lead to the development of radioresistance in hypoxic lung tumors (Zhang et al. 2019a). In hypoxic tumor cell populations, the DNA-dependent protein kinase (DNAPK) can also be potentially important in making cells radioresistant. A study observed that inhibiting DNAPK in combination with carbon ion irradiation was especially effective in radiosensitizing and subsequent targeted killing of such cell populations (Klein et al. 2017). The autophagy pathway is similarly shown to be important in radiosensitivity. Hypoxia-induced autophagy has been shown to mediate radioresistance through c-Jun-mediated Beclin1 expression, making Beclin1 a viable target (Schilling et al. 2012).

Hypoxic tumor cell populations are especially deficient in homologous repair (HR). This can be leveraged by using PARP inhibitors as these can exhibit contextual synthetic lethal effects (Chan et al. 2010). In NSCLC cell lines and PDX models, the PARP inhibitor olaparib has been shown to radiosensitize hypoxic regions in the tumor in

PDX models, leading to increased hypoxic tumor population death due to increased number of unrepaired DNA DSBs. However, this radiosensitization was not observed in well-oxygenated regions of the tumor (Jiang et al. 2016). Similar activity was seen in other studies (Fok et al. 2019), where inhibiting DNAPK, implicated in hypoxia, and treatment with olaparib led to greater genomic instability and increased apoptosis. These studies highlight a potential role for treating hypoxic tumor populations using PARP inhibitors. The use of PARP inhibitors in nonhypoxic tumor cell is described in a subsequent section (DNA repair inhibitors: PARP inhibitors, Sect. 5.2).

Many other targets such as miRNA miR-155 (Babar et al. 2011), lysyl oxidase (Gong et al. 2016), and heat-shock protein 90 (Schilling et al. 2012) have shown potential as radiosensitizers in cell line studies whereas properties like the redux ratio of FAD/(NADH and FAD) can be used to monitor radiosensitivity (Lee et al. 2018).

Several of these pathways have been examined in clinical trials without much success. Nitroglycerin, a muscle relaxant, was tested in a phase II study of 42 stage IB-IV NSCLC patients receiving chemoradiotherapy. Nitroglycerin was used to reduce hypoxia in lung tumor cells to radiosensitize the cells; however, no improvement in 2-year overall survival or reduction in hypoxia was noted (Reymen et al. 2020). Another clinical trial has examined buparlisib, a PI3K inhibitor, in a phase I study in advanced NSCLC patients receiving thoracic radiotherapy. No toxicity was noted when buparlisib dose was escalated in this phase I study suggesting that the compound could be used in phase II clinical trials to determine its radiosensitization potential (McGowan et al. 2019).

3.2 Bioreductive Drugs, Hypoxic Cell Cytotoxins, Reactive Oxygen Species Modulators

Bioreductive drugs are agents that undergo metabolic reduction to generate cytotoxic radical species. This process is facilitated by bioreductive enzymes and lower oxygen conditions present in tumors compared to normal tissues. While it should be mentioned that bioreductive drugs are not radiosensitizers per se, they do however act in a complementary fashion with radiation by selectively targeting and killing hypoxic cells that would otherwise be radioresistant. The most well studied of these compounds is tirapazamine, and early lab studies suggested a supra-additive effect when combined with ionizing radiation (Wilson et al. 1996). Unfortunately, efforts to use this compound in clinical trials have been hampered by unpleasant side effects associated with this agent such as nausea and muscle cramping. Furthermore, adding tirapazamine to chemoradiation in the phase III TROG 02.02/HeadSTART trial and phase II SWOG study for patients with locally advanced head and neck carcinoma and limited-disease SCLC, respectively, did not demonstrate improved overall survival (Rischin et al. 2010).

Other agents have also been examined for their utility as bioreductive drugs in lung cancer. β-Lapachone (a.k.a. ARQ761), a antineoplastic quinone, undergoes a robust, futile redox cycle in cancer cells with high levels of NQO1 (NAD(P)H:quinone oxidoreductase 1) producing massive amounts of reactive oxygen species (ROS) including hydrogen peroxide (H_2O_2). Administration of ARQ761 after IR treatment hyperactivates PARP, lowers NAD+/ATP levels, and increases DSB and the inability to repair DNA damage confers radiosensitivity upon NSCLC cell lines and orthotopic and subcutaneous PDXs, without affecting normal tissue. This selectivity is achieved due to overexpression of NQO1 in NSCLC (Motea et al. 2020). NSCLC with KEAP1 mutation expresses high levels of NRF2 (NFE2L2), protecting cells against oxidative stress and xenobiotics. NRF2 expression and binding activity are further increased by IR. A screen for radiosensitizers (8000 compounds) in cells with mutated KEAP1 identified IM3829 as a potential radiosensitizer that induces apoptosis mediated by increased ROS accumulation and caspase 3 and PARP cleavage. Further validation was done in NSCLC cell lines and xenograft models (Lee et al. 2012).

4 Boron Neutron Capture Theory (BNCT)

BNCT is another potentially viable radiosensitizing strategy. Essentially, BNCT utilizes a stable boron-10 isotope that is preferentially taken up by cancerous cells. These boron-10 atoms can be irradiated with a neutron beam which releases an α particle (helium-4) and recoiling lithium-7 nuclei. BNCT had been investigated in treating malignant gliomas and HNCs as it allowed for sparing of adjacent critical structures.

In the past decade, several studies have examined BNCT for usage in lung cancer. One such study examined the feasibility of using BNCT for two specific NSCLC patient cases, and laid out a framework for treating lung lesions (Farías et al. 2014). In the same year, a multinational group used the Oak Ridge National Laboratory's irradiation model to conduct Monte Carlo calculations of simulated lung tumors that showed healthy lung tissue sparing (Krstic et al. 2014). Preclinical work using EML4-ALK mice engrafted with A549 cells, and with MCF-7-derived lung metastases, showed that lung lesions were effectively treated with BNCT. In this study, the boron compounds were encased in a novel LDL nanoparticle carrier while minimal healthy tissue toxicity was observed. This was seen in another in vivo study (Trivillin et al. 2019) where lung metastases were effectively treated with BNCT and increased survival in rats by 45%. More clinical data from a major consortium in Argentina examined toxicity profiles of lung metastases in sheep models with favorable results observed (Farías et al. 2015). Finally, another study examined irradiation models to calculate lung tumor depth (shallow/deep), again finding BNCT suitable for lung lesion treatment (Yu et al. 2017). Overall, preclinical studies and simulated irradiation models suggest BNCT to be feasible for use in lung cancer, particularly for lung metastases (Suzuki 2020).

5 DNA Repair Inhibitors

Radiation therapy functions through its ability to damage DNA, directly or indirectly. One mechanism of therapeutic resistance therefore is the ability of cancer cells to identify and repair DNA damage. The use of pharmacological agents that can inhibit DNA repair pathways in cancer cells has the potential to counter the phenomenon of therapeutic resistance, thus enhancing the cytotoxicity of radiation. Important DNA repair pathways include homologous recombination repair (HRR), nonhomologous end joining (NHEJ), base excision repair (BER), nucleotide excision repair (NER), mismatch repair (MMR), and translesion DNA synthesis (TLS) (Helleday et al. 2008).

The development of novel agents that can inhibit or modulate these pathways is an area of intense ongoing study. For example, the first phase I platform study sponsored by the University of Leeds and funded by the Cancer Research UK has been recently designed for the safety assessment of multiple novel drug-RT combinations in LA-NSCLC to inform how inhibitors of the DNA damage response (DDR) such as PARP, ATR, Wee1, ATM, and DNAPK can be combined with radical RT (60 Gy delivered in 2 Gy once-daily fractions) in NSCLC patients unfit for concurrent CRT (Walls et al. 2020).

Many other cell signaling pathways that may be relevant in radiosensitization are still being investigated using preclinical models. In this section, we outline some of the major classes of drugs that modulate DNA repair.

5.1 Targeting Cell Signaling Pathways

NSCLC often displays amplification of EGFR (Ohsaki et al. 2000) which activates the phosphatidylinositol 3-kinase (PI3K)/AKT pathway as well as the KRAS-Raf-Mek-ERK signaling cascade, both of which induce radioresistance through the promotion of DNA repair. The mitogen-activated protein (MAP) kinase cascade is involved in cancer cell proliferation, survival, and metastases, thus playing an important role in the progression and maintenance of cancer (Shannon et al. 2009). This pathway (which is often upregulated in tumors) is activated following exposure to ionizing radiation, and can modulate DNA DSB repair. Inhibition of these cell signaling pathways can affect DNA repair pathways to enhance the radiosensitivity of lung cancer cells and it is elaborated below.

5.1.1 EGFR Inhibition

Under hypoxic conditions, NSCLC cells harbored a greater number of stalled replication forks and decreased fork velocity, enhancing their radiosensitivity. Within an altered DNA damage response of hypoxic NSCLC cells, mutant EGFR expression or EGFR blockade demonstrates synthetic lethality sensitizing the cells to IR (Saki et al. 2017). Gefitinib, an EGFR inhibitor, radiosensitizes NSCLC cells by inhibiting ATM activity and therefore inducing mitotic cell death (Park et al. 2010). Erlotinib, icotinib, and cetuximab have been shown to downregulate NHEJ repair of DSBs with erlotinib interfering with signaling through both AKT and MAPK but cetuximab functioning through MAPK in human NSCLC cell lines (Kriegs et al. 2010). Icotinib (EGFR-TKI) radiosensitized H1650 cells by inhibiting EGFR activation via phosphorylation and blocking AKT, ERK1/2 (Zhang et al. 2018). HS-10182, an EGFR tyrosine kinase inhibitor, selectively radiosensitized NSCLC cells with T790M mutation. As compared to A549 cells with wild-type EGFR, H1975 cells with mutated EGFR when co-treated with HS-10182 and IR show increased levels of cleaved caspase-3, -8 and -9, increased PARP cleavage, significant increase in DNAPKcs, persistent DNA damage as observed by greater number of γH2AX foci, inability to repair DNA damage induced by IR due to suppressed expression of RAD50, and higher apoptosis (Chen et al. 2018).

5.1.2 AKT Inhibition

Modulation of the mTOR/AKT/PI3K pathway is important in the development of radioresistance in hypoxic lung tumors (Zhang et al. 2019a). Paeonol, a natural compound, significantly delayed tumor growth in vivo when combined with IR by inhibiting activation of the PI3K/AKT pathway and downregulation of COX2 (elaborated in Sect. 6.2—Cyclooxygenase (COX)-2 Inhibitors) and survivin, thereby augmenting radiation-induced apoptosis (Lei et al. 2013).

Resveratrol radiosensitizes NSCLC cells by inhibition of p-AKT and p-MTOR, increased p-p53 and p-CHK2, increased DNA-DSBs, and induced nonapoptotic senescence (Luo et al. 2013). Statins such as simvastatin and lovastatin that are primarily used as anticholesterol agents have also been shown to inhibit ATK pathway, activate AMPK pathway, and downregulate DNAPKcs, and have thereby shown to inhibit growth in both NSCLC (Bellini et al. 2003) and SCLC (Khanzada et al. 2006) when co-treated with IR.

5.1.3 ATM Inhibition

ATM inhibitor (ATMi) AZD0156 radiosensitizes NSCLC cells and PDXs by abrogating radiation-induced ATM signaling (Riches et al. 2020). In lung, gastric, and breast cancer cell lines in vitro and in triple-negative breast cancer xenograft models, AZD0156 can impede the repair of DNA damage induced by PARP inhibitor (PARPi, olaparib), resulting in elevated DNA double-strand break signaling, cell cycle arrest, and apoptosis, and demonstrates synergistic effect with IR (Riches et al. 2020). Clinically achievable metformin doses inhibit the growth of NSCLC cells and tumor when co-treated with IR via an ATM-AMPK-dependent pathway (Storozhuk et al. 2013).

Decreased expression of IGF-1R leads to improved radiosensitivity of squamous cell carcinoma (SCC), and the underlying mechanism may be associated with the decreased expression of proteins involved in ATM/H2AX/53BP1 DNA damage repair and the HIF-1α/MMP-9 hypoxic pathway, which results in the induction of apoptosis and increased radiosensitivity. IGF1R may represent a novel approach for lung SCC radiation treatment (Liu et al. 2018).

5.1.4 Mitogen-Activated Protein (MAP) Kinase Inhibition

In vivo study of AZD6244 in NSCLC demonstrated an impressive SER of 3.38 (Chung et al. 2009). In a high-throughput viability screen of 1040 compounds with IR in NSCLC cell line H1299, niclosamide was identified as a potent radiosensitizer. Cells when co-treated with niclosamide and ROS generator such as IR/H_2O_2 showed more phosphorylation of p38 MAPK and c-Jun axis leading to radio and H_2O_2 sensitization (Lee et al. 2014). Overexpression of transducer of erbB2.1 (TOB1) recombinant protein in NSCLC cell line NCI-H1975 when exposed to IR-activated MAPK/ERK pathway phosphorylated p53 leading to reduced G2/M arrest, high gH2AX, and reduced clonogenic cell survival. Knockdown of TOB1 in A549 cells made the cells radioresistant, indicating that TOB1 is a potential modulator of radiosensitivity in NSCLC (Sun et al. 2013) and may be exploited therapeutically.

5.1.5 MEK Inhibition

MAPK/ERK pathway which is often overactive in some cancers can be therapeutically targeted using MEK inhibitors. KRAS mutation in NSCLC H460 constitutively activates downstream KRAS-RAF-MEK-ERK signaling cascade. A drug screen for radiosensitizers with Custom Clinical Collection (146 compounds) in H460 shows PARP inhibitors as top hits, followed by inhibitors of pathways downstream of "mutant KRAS" (PI3K, AKT, mTOR, MEK1/2). MEK1/2 inhibitor trametinib selectively sensitized KRAS mutant lung cancer cells to IR (Lin et al. 2014). In a recent study, selective radiosensitization of KRAS mutant cells protected by CHK1 was achieved by proton irradiation, leading to slow fork progression and preferential fork stalling (Al Zubaidi et al. 2021).

5.2 PARP Inhibitors

PARP is a nuclear enzyme that plays an important role in sensing and repairing DNA damage via the modification of a number of key proteins, particularly those involved in single-strand-break repair via BER (Ménissier De Murcia et al. 1997; Dantzer et al. 2000). With continuous PARP inhibition, single-strand breaks are converted to double-strand breaks, and thus PARP inhibitors demonstrate synthetic lethality in tumors that are reliant on NHEJ and BER (such as those affected by BRCA1 or BRCA2 mutations) (Chalmers et al. 2010).

Preclinical studies of PARP inhibitors in lung cancer models have been encouraging (Albert et al. 2007). NSCLC cell lines, Calu-6 and A549 and Calu-6 PDX, radiosensitized with combination treatment of olaparib and IR (Senra et al. 2011). PARP (olaparib) and RAD51 (B02) inhibitors were able to radiosensitize pancreatic and lung cancer cell lines by persistent DNA damage, delayed apoptosis, prolonged cell cycle arrest, and senescence upon proton irradiation. Concentration of each drug was chosen such that they do not elicit cytotoxicity by themselves but sensitize the cells to radiation and can be used as pure radiosensitizers (Wéra et al. 2019). In SCLC, talazoparib radiosensitized multiple cell lines and PDX models with PARP trapping potency correlating with SCLC radiosensitization (Laird et al. 2018). KRAS mutant subset NSCLC on exposure to IR shows increased DNA damage and replication stress. Nucleotide exhaustion by WEE1 inhibitor (AZD1775) and PARP trapping by olaparib lead to inhibition DDR, persistent DNA damage, and collapsed replication fork ultimately leading to radiosensitization (Parsels et al. 2018). LT626 effectively radiosensitized lung and pancreatic cancers in vitro and PDX with increased expression of γH2AX and 53BP1 foci and upregulated expression of phosphorylated ATM, ATR, and their respective kinases (Hastak et al. 2017). HO3089 radiosensitized various cancer cells mediated by various MAPK pathways. Radiosensitization of U251 glioblastoma and A549 NSCLC was mediated by ERK1/2 and JNK/SAPK and in murine 4T1 breast cancer cell line it was mediated by p38. HO3089 radiosensitizes via proapoptotic processes where p53 plays a crucial role. Since MAPKs work in synergy with HO3089 to manifest radiosensitization, inhibition of MAPKs reversed the radiosensitization effect of PARPi (Hocsak et al. 2014). Niraparib (MK-4827) radiosensitizes human lung, breast, and prostate cancer cell lines by inhibiting base excision repair (Bridges et al. 2014). MK-4827 strongly enhances the response of human lung and breast cancer xenografts to radiation regardless of p53 status (Wang et al. 2012).

Several clinical trials are underway to exploit radiosensitizing potential of PARP inhibitors in lung patients. A study to define the maximal tolerated dose (MTD) of olaparib in combination with high-dose radiotherapy with or without daily-dose cisplatin in locally advanced NSCLC is in progress at the Netherlands Cancer Institute (NCT01562210). A phase I dose-escalating study for determining MTD of talazoparib and evaluating the safety of combining talazoparib and low-dose consolidative thoracic radiotherapy for small cell lung cancer (SCLC) patients is underway at the Princess Margaret Cancer Center, University Health Network, Toronto (NCT04170946). A similar trial is ongoing at the Memorial Sloan Kettering Cancer Center, NY, to test the safety of olaparib, combined with radiation therapy for participants with SCLC (NCT03532880). Another randomized multi-arm trial is being undertaken evaluating the safety and efficacy of thoracic radiation therapy followed by durvalumab either as monotherapy or in combination with tremelimumab or olaparib in participants with extensive-stage SCLC (ES-SCLC; NCT03923270).

5.3 Epigenetic Radiosensitizers

To analyze the mechanism of epigenetic control of radiosensitivity, the CpG methylation profiles of radiosensitive H460 and radioresistant H1299 human NSCLC cell lines were analyzed using microarray profiling. Differentially methylated gene (DMG) analysis showed that CpG regions of 747 genes were hypermethylated and 344 genes were hypomethylated in radioresistant cell line H1299 (Kim et al. 2010). Further study of these genes might give an insight into the underlying mechanisms that could potentially be exploited therapeutically.

Overexpression of **DNA methyl transferases (DNMTs)** is commonly seen in NSCLC leading to aberrant methylation patterns. Treatment of cells with 5-AZA, a DNMT inhibitor, induces an NHEJ defect mediated through Ku80 depletion, which potently sensitizes tumor to RT-induced DNA damage, leading to cytotoxicity (Abbotts et al. 2019).

Histone deacetylases (HDAC) modulate the acetylation status of histones, thus affecting the gene transcription. HDAC1 and HDAC2 are often upregulated in NSCLC and their expression is positively correlated with pTNM staging and poor prognosis and negatively correlated with differentiation and apoptotic index (Han et al. 2012). HDAC overactivity has been associated with tumorigenesis, presumably through transcriptional repression of tumor suppressor genes (Zhang et al. 2004). The HDAC inhibitor (HDACi) class of agents have been shown to suppress the ability of cancer cells to repair DSBs in response to ionizing radiation (Marks et al. 2000). Studies evaluating different HDACi have demonstrated that co-treatment with these agents increases the radiosensitivity in NSCLC cells (Zhang et al. 2009; Geng et al. 2006; Cuneo et al. 2007). Vorinostat, a first-generation HDACi, radiosensitized NSCLC cells via suppression of caspase-8 inhibitor, FLIP (McLaughlin et al. 2016), or by increased acetylation of p53 at lysine 382 and simultaneous decrease in the expression of c-myc (Seo et al. 2011). A pan-HDAC inhibitor, abexinostat, radiosensitized two NSCLC cell lines and PDX by increasing radiation-induced caspase-dependent apoptosis, persistent DNA double-strand breaks, and decreased DNA damage signaling and repair (Rivera et al. 2017). Pretreatment of NSCLC cells with HDAC inhibitors trichostatin A and SK-7041 led to abrogation of G2/M arrest and sensitized the cells to IR (Kim et al. 2013). A novel HDAC inhibitor, NDACI054, sensitizes human lung, colorectal, head and neck, and pancreatic cancer cells to radiotherapy in 3D ECM cultures. Combination-treated cells demonstrated high γH2AX/p53BP1-positive foci, slightly elevated levels of caspase-3, and PARP1 cleavage with significant cytotoxicity (Hehlgans et al. 2013). A dose escalation study of vorinostat in combination with palliative radiotherapy for patients with NSCLC is currently being carried out at Yale University (NCT00821951). Ongoing and future studies will help to determine whether this promising strategy is clinically relevant.

Histone acetyltransferase (HAT) works in conjunction with HDAC to regulate transcription. Interestingly, some studies have shown that HAT inhibitors may also have potent radiosensitizing effects (Bandyopadhyay et al. 2009). Knockdown of an oncogene, hMOF, a H4K16 HAT, increased in vitro the sensitizer enhancement ratio (SER), downregulated the expression of p-ATM and RAD51, and sensitized the cells to IR (Li et al. 2019). When exposed to radiation, miR-4497 silences MED13L which can trigger dismantling of mediator complex leading to reduced recruitment of acetyltransferase P300 to chromatin, reduced H3K27Ac signal, inhibition of oncogene PRKCA, and radiosensitizing of lung cancer cells to IR (Zhang et al. 2020). C646, a HAT p300 inhibitor, in combination with IR enhanced mitotic catastrophe in NSCLC cells (A549, H460, and H157) through the abrogation of G2 checkpoint maintenance (Oike et al. 2014).

6 Apoptosis-Modulating Agents

6.1 BCL2 Inhibitors

BCL2 and its family of genes are involved in regulating pro/antiapoptotic pathways. While the relative importance of apoptosis (as opposed to mitotic catastrophe) in radiation-induced cytotoxicity in solid tumors is debatable, preclinical evidence suggests that modulating apoptotic pathways can be a viable radiosensitization strategy in lung cancer. Preclinical studies suggest that targeting BCL2 proteins sensitizes cells to radiation. Typically, cells treated with BCL2 inhibitors show increased apoptotic cell fractions (Nolte et al. 2018; Moretti et al. 2010; Park et al. 2004). In NSCLC studies, increased superoxide/ROS formation (Nolte et al. 2018) and increased caspase-3 and p62 are observed (Kim et al. 2009a). Overexpression of the regulator of G-protein signaling 5 reduces the survival rate and enhances the radiation response of human lung cancer cells by increasing PARP cleavage, low pro-caspase-3/9, high BAK, low BCL2, and high BAX ultimately leading to apoptotic cell death (Xu et al. 2015).

Delphinidin, an antioxidant, radiosensitizes NSCLC by autophagy-mediated apoptosis by two pathways: one, by inhibiting the phosphorylation of PI3K, AKT, and mTOR, suppressing mTOR pathway, and the other, by phosphorylation of MAPK-JNK leading to activation of JNK pathway, BCL2/BCLXl phosphorylation, dissociation of the BCL2:beclin-1 complex, and release of cytochrome C leading to activation of caspase-9 and caspase-3 that regulate the cascades of autophagy and apoptosis (Kang et al. 2020). Luteolin radiosensitizes NSCLC cells by enhancing apoptotic cell death through activation of a p38/ROS/caspase cascade, downregulation of BCL2, activation of caspase-3, -8, and -9, and phosphorylation of p38 MAPK leading to ROS accumulation and apoptosis. Sensitization is independent of p53 and PTEN expression. NCI-H460 and -H1299 NSCLC cells were radiosensitized by luteolin in vitro and growth of NCI-H460 PDX in vivo was delayed by 21.8 days in the combination therapy group (Cho et al. 2015). Huachansu, containing cardiac glycosides, enhances radiosensitivity of human NSCLC cells with wild-type p53 (H460 and A549), but has no effect on H1299 (p53 null) cells. HCS prolonged γH2AX foci, increased cleaved caspase-3 and cleaved PARP, reduced BCL2, lowered p53 protein levels, and increased apoptosis (Wang et al. 2011). Radioresistance in NSCLC has been observed through stabilization of HIF-1alpha (Wang et al. 2019). Similarly, in SCLC, inhibiting BCL2 radiosensitizes cells with the induction of the NF-kappa B pathway and caspase-3/8/9 (Loriot et al. 2014). However, BCL2 inhibitors have shown no effect on clinical outcomes in SCLC patients (Rudin et al. 2008).

6.2 Cyclooxygenase (COX)-2 Inhibitors

COX2 mediates prostaglandin synthesis in response to various stimuli such as inflammation and exposure to carcinogens. This enzyme has been found to be upregulated in many tumors including cancer of the lung (Komaki et al. 2004) where it serves to inhibit apoptosis and modulate cell proliferation (Diederich et al. 2010). Several preclinical models and phase I studies have demonstrated that COX2 inhibitors and other nonsteroidal anti-inflammatory drugs (NSAIDs) increase radiosensitivity of tumors without significantly increasing toxicity. Nimesulide-treated NSCLC cell lines demonstrate radiosensitivity in xenograft models through the caspase-8/Bid pathway resulting in increased apoptosis (Kim et al. 2009b). Celecoxib has also been examined in vitro. NSCLC cell lines treated with celecoxib are radiosensitized by downregulation of Akt/mTOR pathway (Zhang et al. 2019b) and induced G0/G1 arrest (Han et al. 2017; Sun et al. 2017). Further examination in cell lines indicates that celecoxib radiosensitizes by disrupting chromosomal architecture near COX2 gene, decreasing expression by inhibiting p65 nuclear translocation (Sun et al. 2018). In NSCLC, COX2 expression is indicative of radiosensitivity (Yang et al. 2013). Unfortunately, clinical trials indicate that COX2 inhibitors do not improve clinical outcomes in lung cancer (Bi et al. 2019; Mutter et al. 2009).

7 Conclusion

In conclusion, to date, no clear benefit has been established for pure radiosensitization strategies in lung cancer. Many novel approaches in this field have shown recent promise, however. The ability to selectively enhance the radiosensitivity of tumor cells continues to hold appeal, particularly when combined with recent technological advances that enable the delivery of radiation with increased accuracy and precision. Along with improvements in cytotoxic chemotherapy, targeted agents, and immunotherapy this field remains a potentially fruitful area of research in the quest to further increase the therapeutic ratio and improve outcome in patients with lung cancer.

References

Abbotts R, Topper MJ, Biondi C et al (2019) DNA methyltransferase inhibitors induce a BRCAness phenotype that sensitizes NSCLC to PARP inhibitor and ionizing radiation. Proc Natl Acad Sci U S A 116:22609–22618. https://doi.org/10.1073/pnas.1903765116

Al Zubaidi T, Gehrisch OHF, Genois MM et al (2021) Targeting the DNA replication stress phenotype of KRAS mutant cancer cells. Sci Rep 11(1):3656. https://doi.org/10.1038/s41598-021-83142-y

Albert JM, Cao C, Kwang WK et al (2007) Inhibition of poly(ADP-ribose) polymerase enhances cell death and improves tumor growth delay in irradiated lung cancer models. Clin Cancer Res 13:3033–3042. https://doi.org/10.1158/1078-0432.CCR-06-2872

Babar IA, Czochor J, Steinmetz A et al (2011) Inhibition of hypoxia-induced miR-155 radiosensitizes hypoxic lung cancer cells. Cancer Biol Ther 12:908–914. https://doi.org/10.4161/cbt.12.10.17681

Bandyopadhyay K, Banères JL, Martin A et al (2009) Spermidinyl-CoA-based HAT inhibitors block DNA repair and provide cancer-specific chemo- and radio-sensitization. Cell Cycle 8:2779–2788. https://doi.org/10.4161/cc.8.17.9416

Bauman JR, Edelman MJ (2022) Targeted therapies in non-small cell lung cancer. Med Radiol Radiat Oncol. https://doi.org/10.1007/174_2022_312

Becker A, Hänsgen G, Blocking M et al (1998) Oxygenation of squamous cell carcinoma of the head and neck: comparison of primary tumors, neck node metastases, and normal tissue. Int J Radiat Oncol Biol Phys 42:35–41. https://doi.org/10.1016/S0360-3016(98)00182-5

Bellini MJ, Polo MP, De Alaniz MJT, De Bravo MG (2003) Effect of simvastatin on the uptake and metabolic conversion of palmitic, dihomo-γ-linoleic and α-linolenic acids in A549 cells. Prostaglandins Leukot Essent Fatty Acids 69:351–357. https://doi.org/10.1016/S0952-3278(03)00149-2

Bennett MH, Feldmeier J, Hampson N et al (2005) Hyperbaric oxygen therapy for late radiation tissue injury. Cochrane Database Syst Rev 2016(4):CD005005. https://doi.org/10.1002/14651858.CD005005.pub2

Bernier J, Denekamp J, Rojas A et al (1999) ARCON: accelerated radiotherapy with carbogen and nicotinamide in non-small cell lung cancer: a phase I/II study by the EORTC. Radiother Oncol 52:149–156. https://doi.org/10.1016/S0167-8140(99)00106-1

Bi N, Liang J, Zhou Z et al (2019) Effect of concurrent chemoradiation with celecoxib vs concurrent chemoradiation alone on survival among patients with non-small cell lung cancer with and without cyclooxygenase 2 genetic variants: a phase 2 randomized clinical trial. JAMA Netw Open 2:e1918070. https://doi.org/10.1001/jamanetworkopen.2019.18070

Bohlius J, Schmidlin K, Brillant C et al (2009) Recombinant human erythropoiesis-stimulating agents and mortality in patients with cancer: a meta-analysis of randomised trials. Lancet 373:1532–1542. https://doi.org/10.1016/S0140-6736(09)60502-X

Bridges KA, Toniatti C, Buser CA et al (2014) Niraparib (MK-4827), a novel poly(ADP-ribose) polymerase inhibitor, radiosensitizes human lung and breast cancer cells. Oncotarget 5:5076–5086. https://doi.org/10.18632/oncotarget.2083

Brizel DM, Scully SP, Harrelson JM et al (1996) Tumor oxygenation predicts for the likelihood of distant metastases in human soft tissue sarcoma. Cancer Res 56:941–943

Brown JM, Giaccia AJ (1998) The unique physiology of solid tumors: opportunities (and problems) for cancer therapy. Cancer Res 58:1408–1416

Bui QC, Lieber M, Withers HR et al (2004) The efficacy of hyperbaric oxygen therapy in the treatment of radiation-induced late side effects. Int J Radiat Oncol Biol Phys 60:871–878. https://doi.org/10.1016/j.ijrobp.2004.04.019

Chalmers AJ, Lakshman M, Chan N, Bristow RG (2010) Poly(ADP-ribose) polymerase inhibition as a model for synthetic lethality in developing radiation oncology targets. Semin Radiat Oncol 20:274–281. https://doi.org/10.1016/j.semradonc.2010.06.001

Chan N, Pires IM, Bencokova Z et al (2010) Contextual synthetic lethality of cancer cell kill based on the tumor microenvironment. Cancer Res 70:8045–8054. https://doi.org/10.1158/0008-5472.CAN-10-2352

Chen Y, Wang Y, Zhao L et al (2018) EGFR tyrosine kinase inhibitor HS-10182 increases radiation sensitivity in non-small cell lung cancers with EGFR T790M mutation. Cancer Biol Med 15:39–51. https://doi.org/10.20892/j.issn.2095-3941.2017.0118

Cho HJ, Ahn KC, Choi JY et al (2015) Luteolin acts as a radiosensitizer in non-small cell lung cancer cells by enhancing apoptotic cell death through activation of a p38/ROS/caspase cascade. Int J Oncol 46:1149–1158. https://doi.org/10.3892/ijo.2015.2831

Choy H, Nabid A, Stea B et al (2005) Phase II multicenter study of induction chemotherapy followed by concurrent efaproxiral (RSR13) and thoracic radiotherapy for patients with locally advanced non-small-cell lung cancer. J Clin Oncol 23:5918–5928. https://doi.org/10.1200/JCO.2005.08.011

Chung EJ, Brown AP, Asano H et al (2009) In vitro and in vivo radiosensitization with AZD6244 (ARRY-142886), an inhibitor of mitogen-activated protein kinase/extracellular signal-regulated kinase 1/2 kinase. Clin Cancer Res 15:3050–3057. https://doi.org/10.1158/1078-0432.CCR-08-2954

Cuneo KC, Fu A, Osusky K et al (2007) Histone deacetylase inhibitor NVP-LAQ824 sensitizes human non-small cell lung cancer to the cytotoxic effects of ionizing radiation. Anticancer Drugs 18:793–800. https://doi.org/10.1097/CAD.0b013e3280b10d57

Dantzer F, De La Rubia G, Ménissier-De Murcia J et al (2000) Base excision repair is impaired in mammalian cells lacking poly(ADP-ribose) polymerase-1. Biochemistry 39:7559–7569. https://doi.org/10.1021/bi0003442

Diederich M, Sobolewski C, Cerella C et al (2010) The role of cyclooxygenase-2 in cell proliferation and cell death in human malignancies. Int J Cell Biol 2010:215158. https://doi.org/10.1155/2010/215158

Eschmann S, Paulsen F, Reimold M et al (2005) Prognostic impact of hypoxia imaging with before radiotherapy. Radiochemistry 46:253–260

Eschwège F, Sancho-Garnier H, Chassagne D (1997) Results of a European randomized trial of etanidazole combined with radiotherapy in head and neck carcinomas. Int J Radiat Oncol Biol Phys 39:275–281. https://doi.org/10.1016/s0360-3016(97)00327-1

Farías RO, Bortolussi S, Menéndez PR, González SJ (2014) Exploring Boron Neutron Capture Therapy for non-small cell lung cancer. Phys Med 30:888–897. https://doi.org/10.1016/j.ejmp.2014.07.342

Farías RO, Garabalino MA, Ferraris S et al (2015) Toward a clinical application of ex situ boron neutron capture therapy for lung tumors at the RA-3 reactor in Argentina. Med Phys 42:4161–4173. https://doi.org/10.1118/1.4922158

Farris MK, Steber C, Helis C, Blackstock W (2022) Combined radiotherapy and chemotherapy: theoretical considerations and biological premises. Med Radiol Radiat Oncol. https://doi.org/10.1007/174_2022_314

Fok JHL, Ramos-Montoya A, Vazquez-Chantada M et al (2019) AZD7648 is a potent and selective DNA-PK inhibitor that enhances radiation, chemotherapy and olaparib activity. Nat Commun 10:1–15. https://doi.org/10.1038/s41467-019-12836-9

Fyles AW, Milosevic M, Wong R et al (1998) Oxygenation predicts radiation response and survival in patients with cervix cancer. Radiother Oncol 48:149–156. https://doi.org/10.1016/S0167-8140(98)00044-9

Geng L, Cuneo KC, Fu A et al (2006) Histone deacetylase (HDAC) inhibitor LBH589 increases duration of γ-H2AX foci and confines HDAC4 to the cytoplasm in irradiated non-small cell lung cancer. Cancer Res 66:11298–11304. https://doi.org/10.1158/0008-5472.CAN-06-0049

Gong C, Gu R, Jin H et al (2016) Lysyl oxidase mediates hypoxia-induced radioresistance in non-small cell lung cancer A549 cells. Exp Biol Med 241:387–395. https://doi.org/10.1177/1535370215609694

Han Y, Zhang Y, Yang L-h et al (2012) X-radiation inhibits histone deacetylase 1 and 2, upregulates Axin expression and induces apoptosis in non-small cell lung cancer. Radiat Oncol 7:1. https://doi.org/10.1186/1748-717X-7-183

Han ZQ, Liao H, Shi F et al (2017) Inhibition of cyclooxygenase-2 sensitizes lung cancer cells to radiation-induced apoptosis. Oncol Lett 14:5959–5965. https://doi.org/10.3892/ol.2017.6940

Hastak K, Bhutra S, Parry R, Ford JM (2017) Poly (ADP-ribose) polymerase inhibitor, an effective radiosensitizer in lung and pancreatic cancers. Oncotarget 8:26344–26355. https://doi.org/10.18632/oncotarget.15464

He K, Selek U, Barsoumian HB et al (2022) Mechanisms of action of radiotherapy and immunotherapy in lung cancer: Implications for clinical practice. Med Radiol Radiat Oncol. https://doi.org/10.1007/174_2022_315

Hehlgans S, Storch K, Lange I, Cordes N (2013) The novel HDAC inhibitor NDACI054 sensitizes human cancer cells to radiotherapy. Radiother Oncol 109:126–132. https://doi.org/10.1016/j.radonc.2013.08.023

Helleday T, Petermann E, Lundin C et al (2008) DNA repair pathways as targets for cancer therapy. Nat Rev Cancer 8:193–204. https://doi.org/10.1038/nrc2342

Henk JM, Kunkler PB, Smith CW (1977) RADIOTHERAPY AND HYPERBARIC OXYGEN IN HEAD AND NECK CANCER final report of first controlled clinical trial. Lancet 2:101–103. https://doi.org/10.1016/s0140-6736(77)90116-7

Henke M, Laszig R, Rübe C et al (2003) Erythropoietin to treat head and neck cancer patients with anaemia undergoing radiotherapy: randomised, double-blind, placebo-controlled trial. Lancet (London, England) 362:1255–1260. https://doi.org/10.1016/S0140-6736(03)14567-9

Höckel M, Knoop C, Schlenger K et al (1993) Intratumoral pO2 predicts survival in advanced cancer of the uterine cervix. Radiother Oncol 26:45–50. https://doi.org/10.1016/0167-8140(93)90025-4

Hocsak E, Cseh A, Szabo A et al (2014) PARP inhibitor attenuated colony formation can be restored by MAP kinase inhibitors in different irradiated cancer cell lines. Int J Radiat Biol 90:1152–1161. https://doi.org/10.3109/09553002.2014.934927

Hoskin PJ, Rojas AM, Bentzen SM, Saunders MI (2010) Radiotherapy with concurrent carbogen and nicotinamide in bladder carcinoma. J Clin Oncol 28:4912–4918. https://doi.org/10.1200/JCO.2010.28.4950

Hu C, Zhuang W, Qiao Y et al (2019) Effects of combined inhibition of STAT3 and VEGFR2 pathways on the radiosensitivity of non-small-cell lung cancer cells. Onco Targets Ther 12:933–944. https://doi.org/10.2147/OTT.S186559

Janssens GO, Terhaard CH, Doornaert PA et al (2012) Acute toxicity profile and compliance to accelerated radiotherapy plus carbogen and nicotinamide for clinical stage T2-4 laryngeal cancer: results of a phase III randomized trial. Int J Radiat Oncol Biol Phys 82:532–538. https://doi.org/10.1016/j.ijrobp.2010.11.045

Jiang Y, Verbiest T, Devery AM et al (2016) Hypoxia potentiates the radiation-sensitizing effect of olaparib in human non-small cell lung cancer xenografts by contextual synthetic lethality. Int J Radiat Oncol Biol Phys 95:772–781. https://doi.org/10.1016/j.ijrobp.2016.01.035

Kaanders JHAM, Pop LAM, Marres HAM et al (1998) Accelerated radiotherapy with carbogen and nicotinamide (ARCON) for laryngeal cancer. Radiother Oncol 48:115–122. https://doi.org/10.1016/S0167-8140(98)00043-7

Kang JH, Kim W, Kwon TW et al (2016) Plasminogen activator inhibitor-1 enhances radioresistance and aggressiveness of non-small cell lung cancer cells. Oncotarget 7:23961–23974. https://doi.org/10.18632/oncotarget.8208

Kang SH, Bak DH, Chung BY et al (2020) Delphinidin enhances radio-therapeutic effects via autophagy induction and JNK/MAPK pathway activation in non-small cell lung cancer. Korean J Physiol Pharmacol 24:413–422. https://doi.org/10.4196/kjpp.2020.24.5.413

Khanzada UK, Pardo OE, Meier C et al (2006) Potent inhibition of small-cell lung cancer cell growth by simvastatin reveals selective functions of Ras isoforms in growth factor signalling. Oncogene 25:877–887. https://doi.org/10.1038/sj.onc.1209117

Kim KW, Moretti L, Mitchell LR et al (2009a) Combined Bcl-2/mammalian target of rapamycin inhibition leads to enhanced radiosensitization via induction of apoptosis and autophagy in non-small cell lung tumor xenograft model. Clin Cancer Res 15:6096–6105. https://doi.org/10.1158/1078-0432.CCR-09-0589

Kim BM, Won J, Maeng KA et al (2009b) Nimesulide, a selective COX-2 inhibitor, acts synergistically with ionizing radiation against A549 human lung cancer cells through the activation of caspase-8 and caspase-3. Int J Oncol 34:1467–1473

Kim EH, Park AK, Dong SM et al (2010) Global analysis of CpG methylation reveals epigenetic control of the radiosensitivity in lung cancer cell lines. Oncogene 29:4725–4731. https://doi.org/10.1038/onc.2010.223

Kim JH, Kim IH, Shin JH et al (2013) Sequence-dependent radiosensitization of histone deacetylase inhibitors trichostatin A and SK-7041. Cancer Res Treat 45:334–342. https://doi.org/10.4143/crt.2013.45.4.334

Klein C, Dokic I, Mairani A et al (2017) Overcoming hypoxia-induced tumor radioresistance in non-small cell lung cancer by targeting DNA-dependent protein kinase in combination with carbon ion irradiation. Radiat Oncol 12:1–8. https://doi.org/10.1186/s13014-017-0939-0

Knight RC, Rowley DA, Skolimowski I, Edwards DI (1979) Mechanism of action of nitroimidazole antimicrobial and antitumour radiosensitizing drugs: effects of reduced misonidazole on DNA. Int J Radiat Biol 36:367–377. https://doi.org/10.1080/09553007914551151

Komaki R, Liao Z, Milas L (2004) Improvement strategies for molecular targeting: cyclooxygenase-2 inhibitors as radiosensitizers for non-small cell lung cancer. Semin Oncol 31:47–53. https://doi.org/10.1053/j.seminoncol.2003.12.014

Kriegs M, Kasten-Pisula U, Rieckmann T et al (2010) The epidermal growth factor receptor modulates DNA double-strand break repair by regulating non-homologous end-joining. DNA Repair (Amst) 9:889–897. https://doi.org/10.1016/j.dnarep.2010.05.005

Krstic D, Markovic VM, Jovanovic Z et al (2014) Monte Carlo calculations of lung dose in ORNL phantom for boron neutron capture therapy. Radiat Prot Dosimetry 161:269–273. https://doi.org/10.1093/rpd/nct365

Laird JH, Lok BH, Ma J et al (2018) Talazoparib is a potent radiosensitizer in small cell lung cancer cell lines and xenografts. Clin Cancer Res 24:5143–5152. https://doi.org/10.1158/1078-0432.CCR-18-0401

Laurie SA, Jeyabalan N, Nicholas G et al (2006) Association between anemia arising during therapy and outcomes of chemoradiation for limited small-cell lung cancer. J Thorac Oncol 1:146–151. https://doi.org/10.1016/s1556-0864(15)31530-6

Lee DJ, Cosmatos D, Marcial VA et al (1995) Results of an RTOG phase III trial (RTOG 85-27) comparing radiotherapy plus etanidazole with radiotherapy alone for locally advanced head and neck carcinomas. Int J Radiat Oncol Biol Phys 32:567–576. https://doi.org/10.1016/0360-3016(95)00150-W

Lee S, Lim M-J, Kim M-H et al (2012) An effective strategy for increasing the radiosensitivity of human lung cancer cells by blocking Nrf2-dependent antioxidant responses. Free Radic Biol Med 53:807–816. https://doi.org/10.1016/j.freeradbiomed.2012.05.038

Lee S-l-o, Son AR, Ahn J, Song JY (2014) Niclosamide enhances ROS-mediated cell death through c-Jun activation. Biomed Pharmacother 68:619–624. https://doi.org/10.1016/j.biopha.2014.03.018

Lee DE, Alhallak K, Jenkins SV et al (2018) A radiosensitizing inhibitor of HIF-1 alters the optical redox state of human lung cancer cells in vitro. Sci Rep 8:1–10. https://doi.org/10.1038/s41598-018-27262-y

Lei Y, Li HX, Sen JW et al (2013) The radiosensitizing effect of Paeonol on lung adenocarcinoma by augmentation of radiation-induced apoptosis and inhibition of the PI3K/Akt pathway. Int J Radiat Biol 89:1079–1086. https://doi.org/10.3109/09553002.2013.825058

Leyland-Jones B (2003) Reflection and reaction breast cancer trial with erythropoietin terminated unexpectedly. Lancet 4:459–460

Li N, Tian G-W, Tang L-R, Li G (2019) hMOF reduction enhances radiosensitivity through the homologous recombination pathway in non-small-cell lung cancer. Onco Targets Ther 12:3065–3075. https://doi.org/10.2147/ott.s192568

Lin SH, Zhang J, Giri U et al (2014) A high content clonogenic survival drug screen identifies MEK inhibitors as potent radiation sensitizers for KRAS mutant non-small-cell lung cancer. J Thorac Oncol 9:965–973. https://doi.org/10.1097/JTO.0000000000000199

Liu X, Chen H, Xu X et al (2018) Insulin-like growth factor-1 receptor knockdown enhances radiosensitivity via the HIF-1α pathway and attenuates ATM/H2AX/53BP1 DNA repair activation in human lung squamous carcinoma cells. Oncol Lett 16:1332–1340. https://doi.org/10.3892/ol.2018.8705

Loriot Y, Mordant P, Dugue D et al (2014) Radiosensitization by a novel Bcl-2 and Bcl-XL inhibitor S44563 in small-cell lung cancer. Cell Death Dis 5:1–13. https://doi.org/10.1038/cddis.2014.365

Luo H, Wang L, Schulte BA et al (2013) Resveratrol enhances ionizing radiation-induced premature senescence in lung cancer cells. Int J Oncol 43:1999–2006. https://doi.org/10.3892/ijo.2013.2141

MacRae R, Shyr Y, Johnson D, Choy H (2002) Declining hemoglobin during chemoradiotherapy for locally advanced non-small cell lung cancer is significant. Radiother Oncol 64:37–40. https://doi.org/10.1016/S0167-8140(02)00151-2

Marks PA, Richon VM, Rifkind RA (2000) Histone deacetylase inhibitors: inducers of differentiation or apoptosis of transformed cells. J Natl Cancer Inst 92:1210–1216. https://doi.org/10.1093/jnci/92.15.1210

Matschke J, Wiebeck E, Hurst S et al (2016) Role of SGK1 for fatty acid uptake, cell survival and radioresistance of NCI-H460 lung cancer cells exposed to acute or chronic cycling severe hypoxia. Radiat Oncol 11:1–12. https://doi.org/10.1186/s13014-016-0647-1

McGowan DR, Skwarski M, Bradley KM et al (2019) Buparlisib with thoracic radiotherapy and its effect on tumour hypoxia: a phase I study in patients with advanced non-small cell lung carcinoma. Eur J Cancer 113:87–95. https://doi.org/10.1016/j.ejca.2019.03.015

McLaughlin KA, Nemeth Z, Bradley CA et al (2016) FLIP: a targetable mediator of resistance to radiation in non-small cell lung cancer. Mol Cancer Ther 15:2432–2441. https://doi.org/10.1158/1535-7163.MCT-16-0211

Ménissier De Murcia J, Niedergang C, Trucco C et al (1997) Requirement of poly(ADP-ribose) polymerase in recovery from DNA damage in mice and in cells. Proc Natl Acad Sci U S A 94:7303–7307. https://doi.org/10.1073/pnas.94.14.7303

Moretti L, Li B, Kim KW et al (2010) AT-101, a Pan-Bcl-2 inhibitor, leads to radiosensitization of non-small cell lung cancer. J Thorac Oncol 5:680–687. https://doi.org/10.1097/JTO.0b013e3181d6e08e

Motea EA, Huang X, Singh N et al (2020) NQO1-dependent, tumor-selective radiosensitization of non-small cell lung cancers. Clin Cancer Res 25:2601–2609. https://doi.org/10.1158/1078-0432.CCR-18-2560

Mutter R, Lu B, Carbone DP et al (2009) A phase II study of celecoxib in combination with paclitaxel, carboplatin, and radiotherapy for patients with inoperable stage IIIA/B non-small cell lung cancer. Clin Cancer Res 15:2158–2165. https://doi.org/10.1158/1078-0432.CCR-08-0629

Nolte EM, Joubert AM, Lakier R et al (2018) Exposure of breast and lung cancer cells to a novel estrone analog prior to radiation enhances Bcl-2-mediated cell death. Int J Mol Sci 19:2887. https://doi.org/10.3390/ijms19102887

Ohsaki Y, Tanno S, Fujita Y et al (2000) Epidermal growth factor receptor expression correlates with poor prognosis in non-small cell lung cancer patients with p53 overexpression. Oncol Rep 7:603–607. https://doi.org/10.3892/or.7.3.603

Oike T, Komachi M, Ogiwara H et al (2014) C646, a selective small molecule inhibitor of histone acetyltransferase p300, radiosensitizes lung cancer cells by enhancing mitotic catastrophe. Radiother Oncol 111:222–227. https://doi.org/10.1016/j.radonc.2014.03.015

Park JK, Chung YM, Kim BG et al (2004) N′-(phenyl-2-yl-methylene)-hydrazine carbodithioic acid methyl ester enhances radiation-induced cell death by targeting Bcl-2 against human lung carcinoma cells. Mol Cancer Ther 3:403–407

Park SY, Kim YM, Pyo H (2010) Gefitinib radiosensitizes non-small cell lung cancer cells through inhibition of ataxia telangiectasia mutated. Mol Cancer 9:1–12. https://doi.org/10.1186/1476-4598-9-222

Parsels LA, Karnak D, Parsels JD et al (2018) PARP1 trapping and DNA replication stress enhance radiosensitization with combined WEE1 and PARP inhibitors. Mol Cancer Res 16:222–232. https://doi.org/10.1158/1541-7786.MCR-17-0455

Reymen BJT, van Gisbergen MW, Even AJG et al (2020) Nitroglycerin as a radiosensitizer in non-small cell lung cancer: results of a prospective imaging-based phase II trial. Clin Transl Radiat Oncol 21:49–55. https://doi.org/10.1016/j.ctro.2019.12.002

Riches LC, Trinidad AG, Hughes G et al (2020) Pharmacology of the ATM inhibitor AZD0156: potentiation of irradiation and olaparib responses preclinically. Mol Cancer Ther 19:13–25. https://doi.org/10.1158/1535-7163.MCT-18-1394

Rischin D, Peters LJ, O'Sullivan B et al (2010) Tirapazamine, cisplatin, and radiation versus cisplatin and radiation for advanced squamous cell carcinoma of the head and neck (TROG 02.02, headstart): a phase III trial of the Trans-Tasman Radiation Oncology Group. J Clin Oncol 28:2989–2995. https://doi.org/10.1200/JCO.2009.27.4449

Rivera S, Leteur C, Mégnin F et al (2017) Time dependent modulation of tumor radiosensitivity by a pan HDAC inhibitor: abexinostat. Oncotarget 8:56210–56227. https://doi.org/10.18632/oncotarget.14813

Robnett TJ, Machtay M, Hahn SM et al (2002) Pathological response to preoperative chemoradiation worsens with anemia in non-small cell lung cancer patients. Cancer J 8:263–267. https://doi.org/10.1097/00130404-200205000-00010

Rubin P, Hanley J, Keys HM et al (1979) Carbogen breathing during radiation therapy—the radiation therapy oncology group study. Int J Radiat Oncol Biol Phys 5:1963–1970. https://doi.org/10.1016/0360-3016(79)90946-5

Rudin CM, Salgia R, Wang X et al (2008) Randomized phase II study of carboplatin and etoposide with or without the bcl-2 antisense oligonucleotide oblimersen for extensive-stage small-cell lung cancer: CALGB 30103. J Clin Oncol 26:870–876. https://doi.org/10.1200/JCO.2007.14.3461

Saki M, Makino H, Javvadi P et al (2017) EGFR mutations compromise hypoxia-associated radiation resistance through impaired replication fork-associated DNA damage repair. Mol Cancer Res 15:1503–1516. https://doi.org/10.1158/1541-7786.MCR-17-0136

Schilling D, Bayer C, Li W et al (2012) Radiosensitization of normoxic and hypoxic H1339 lung tumor cells by heat shock protein 90 inhibition is independent of hypoxia inducible factor-1α. PLoS One 7:1–11. https://doi.org/10.1371/journal.pone.0031110

Scott C, Suh J, Stea B et al (2007) Improved survival, quality of life, and quality-adjusted survival in breast cancer patients treated with efaproxiral (Efaproxyn) plus whole-brain radiation therapy for brain metastases. Am J Clin Oncol 30:580–587. https://doi.org/10.1097/COC.0b013e3180653c0d

Senra JM, Telfer BA, Cherry KE et al (2011) Inhibition of PARP-1 by olaparib (AZD2281) increases the radiosensitivity of a lung tumor xenograft. Mol Cancer Ther 10:1949–1958. https://doi.org/10.1158/1535-7163.MCT-11-0278

Seo SK, Jin HO, Woo SH et al (2011) Histone deacetylase inhibitors sensitize human non-small cell lung cancer cells to ionizing radiation through acetyl p53-mediated c-myc down-regulation. J Thorac Oncol 6:1313–1319. https://doi.org/10.1097/JTO.0b013e318220caff

Shannon AM, Telfer BA, Smith PD et al (2009) The mitogen-activated protein/extracellular signal-regulated kinase kinase 1/2 inhibitor AZD6244 (ARRY-142886) enhances the radiation responsiveness of lung and colorectal tumor xenografts. Clin Cancer Res 15:6619–6629. https://doi.org/10.1158/1078-0432.CCR-08-2958

Storozhuk Y, Hopmans SN, Sanli T et al (2013) Metformin inhibits growth and enhances radiation response of non-small cell lung cancer (NSCLC) through ATM and AMPK. Br J Cancer 108:2021–2032. https://doi.org/10.1038/bjc.2013.187

Suh JH, Stea B, Nabid A et al (2006) Phase III study of efaproxiral as an adjunct to whole-brain radiation therapy for brain metastases. J Clin Oncol 24:106–114. https://doi.org/10.1200/JCO.2004.00.1768

Sun KK, Zhong N, Yang Y et al (2013) Enhanced radiosensitivity of NSCLC cells by transducer of erbB2.1 (TOB1) through modulation of the MAPK/ERK pathway. Oncol Rep 29:2385–2391. https://doi.org/10.3892/or.2013.2403

Sun J, Liu N-B, Zhuang H-Q et al (2017) Celecoxib-erlotinib combination treatment enhances radiosensitivity in A549 human lung cancer cell. Cancer Biomark 19:45–50. https://doi.org/10.3233/CBM-160323

Sun Y, Dai H, Chen S et al (2018) Disruption of chromosomal architecture of cox2 locus sensitizes lung cancer cells to radiotherapy. Mol Ther 26:2456–2465. https://doi.org/10.1016/j.ymthe.2018.08.002

Suzuki M (2020) Boron neutron capture therapy (BNCT): a unique role in radiotherapy with a view to entering the accelerator-based BNCT era. Int J Clin Oncol 25:43–50. https://doi.org/10.1007/s10147-019-01480-4

Trivillin VA, Serrano A, Garabalino MA et al (2019) Translational boron neutron capture therapy (BNCT) studies for the treatment of tumors in lung. Int J Radiat Biol 95:646–654. https://doi.org/10.1080/09553002.2019.1564080

Vansteenkiste J, Pirker R, Massuti B et al (2002) Double-blind, placebo-controlled, randomized phase III trial of darbepoetin alfa in lung cancer patients receiving chemotherapy. J Natl Cancer Inst 94:1211–1220. https://doi.org/10.1093/jnci/94.16.1211

Walls GM, Oughton JB, Chalmers AJ et al (2020) CONCORDE: a phase I platform study of novel agents in combination with conventional radiotherapy in non-small-cell lung cancer. Clin Transl Radiat Oncol 25:61–66. https://doi.org/10.1016/j.ctro.2020.09.006

Wang L, Raju U, Milas L et al (2011) Huachansu, containing cardiac glycosides, enhances radiosensitivity of human lung cancer cells. Anticancer Res 31:2141–2148

Wang L, Mason KA, Ang KK et al (2012) MK-4827, a PARP-1/-2 inhibitor, strongly enhances response of human lung and breast cancer xenografts to radiation. Invest New Drugs 30:2113–2120. https://doi.org/10.1007/s10637-011-9770-x

Wang G, Xiao L, Wang F et al (2019) Hypoxia inducible factor-1α/B-cell lymphoma 2 signaling impacts radiosensitivity of H1299 non-small cell lung cancer cells in a normoxic environment. Radiat Environ Biophys 58:439–448. https://doi.org/10.1007/s00411-019-00802-4

Watson ER, Halnan KE, Dische S et al (1978) Hyperbaric oxygen and radiotherapy: a Medical Research Council trial in carcinoma of the cervix. Br J Radiol 51:879–887. https://doi.org/10.1259/0007-1285-51-611-879

Wéra AC, Lobbens A, Stoyanov M et al (2019) Radiation-induced synthetic lethality: combination of poly(ADP-ribose) polymerase and RAD51 inhibitors to sensitize cells to proton irradiation. Cell Cycle 18:1770–1783. https://doi.org/10.1080/15384101.2019.1632640

Wilson WR, Denny WA, Pullen SM et al (1996) Tertiary amine N-oxides as bioreductive drugs: DACA N-oxide, nitracrine N-oxide and AQ4N. Br J Cancer 27:S43–S47

Xiang M, Chen Z, Yang D et al (2017) Niclosamide enhances the antitumor effects of radiation by inhibiting the hypoxia-inducible factor-1α/vascular endothelial growth factor signaling pathway in human lung cancer cells. Oncol Lett 14:1933–1938. https://doi.org/10.3892/ol.2017.6372

Xu Z, Zuo Y, Wang J et al (2015) Overexpression of the regulator of G-protein signaling 5 reduces the survival rate and enhances the radiation response of human lung cancer cells. Oncol Rep 33:2899–2907. https://doi.org/10.3892/or.2015.3917

Yamamoto M, Izumi Y, Horinouchi H et al (2009) Systemic administration of hemoglobin vesicle elevates tumor tissue oxygen tension and modifies tumor response to irradiation. J Surg Res 151:48–54. https://doi.org/10.1016/j.jss.2007.12.770

Yang HJ, Kim N, Seong KM et al (2013) Investigation of radiation-induced transcriptome profile of radioresistant non-small cell lung cancer A549 cells using RNA-seq. PLoS One 8:e59319. https://doi.org/10.1371/journal.pone.0059319

Yu H, Tang X, Shu D et al (2017) Influence of neutron sources and 10B concentration on boron neutron capture therapy for shallow and deeper non-small cell lung cancer. Health Phys 112:258–265. https://doi.org/10.1097/HP.0000000000000601

Zhang Y, Adachi M, Zhao X et al (2004) Histone deacetylase inhibitors FK228, N-(2-aminophenyl)-4-[N-(pyridin-3-yl-methoxycarbonyl)amino-methyl] benzamide and m-carboxycinnamic acid bis-hydroxamide augment radiation-induced cell death in gastrointestinal adenocarcinoma cells. Int J Cancer 110:301–308. https://doi.org/10.1002/ijc.20117

Zhang F, Zhang T, Teng ZH et al (2009) Sensitization to γ-irradiation-induced cell cycle arrest and apoptosis by the histone deacetylase inhibitor trichostatin A in non-small cell lung cancer (NSCLC) cells. Cancer Biol Ther 8:823–831. https://doi.org/10.4161/cbt.8.9.8143

Zhang S, Fu Y, Wang D, Wang J (2018) Icotinib enhances lung cancer cell radiosensitivity in vitro and in vivo by inhibiting MAPK/ERK and AKT activation. Clin Exp Pharmacol Physiol 45:969–977. https://doi.org/10.1111/1440-1681.12966

Zhang F, Fan B, Mao L (2019a) Radiosensitizing effects of Cyclocarya paliurus polysaccharide on hypoxic A549 and H520 human non-small cell lung carcinoma cells. Int J Mol Med 44:1233–1242. https://doi.org/10.3892/ijmm.2019.4289

Zhang P, He D, Song E et al (2019b) Celecoxib enhances the sensitivity of nonsmall-cell lung cancer cells to radiation-induced apoptosis through downregulation of the Akt/mTOR signaling pathway and COX-2 expression. PLoS One 14:1–15. https://doi.org/10.1371/journal.pone.0223760

Zhang N, Song Y, Xu Y et al (2020) MED13L integrates mediator-regulated epigenetic control into lung cancer radiosensitivity. Theranostics 10:9378–9394. https://doi.org/10.7150/thno.48247

Radioprotectors in the Management of Lung Cancer

Zhongxing Liao, Ting Xu, and Ritsuko Komaki

Contents

1 Introduction 303
2 **Strategies for Radioprotection and Mitigation** 305
2.1 Free Radical Scavengers: Thiol 305
2.2 DNA Repair 306
2.3 Redox Homeostasis: Manganese Superoxide Dismutase 307
2.4 Anti-Inflammatory Agents 311
2.5 Cytokines 312
3 **Summary** 315
References 315

1 Introduction

Radiation therapy has become increasingly important in the management of lung cancer at all stages. However, radiotherapy, given alone or with concurrent chemo- and immunotherapy, can have severe adverse effects on critical organs that are often in the path of the radiation beam depending on the location of the tumor. Immune checkpoint inhibitor therapy also has its own adverse effects that include inflammation of the lung (interstitial pneumonitis) and heart (myocarditis, pericarditis). In the randomized phase III PACIFIC clinical trial (Antonia et al. 2018) of lung cancer treated with concurrent chemoradiation therapy to be followed by durvalumab or placebo, only patients who did not develop symptomatic toxicity after the chemoradiation were randomized, which excluded at least 35–40% patients from the potential benefits of checkpoint inhibitor therapy because of concern over severe adverse sequelae. The ability to counteract the toxic effects of radiation, chemotherapy, and immune checkpoint inhibitors in their various combinations is imperative if treatment is to be curative without compromising quality of life.

The physiological and biological effects of ionizing radiation include damage to DNA, proteins, and lipid membranes, correspondingly leading to cell dysfunction or cell death, within both the tumor and the surrounding normal tissue. Physiologically, ionizing-radiation effects can be categorized as either direct or indirect. Direct effects include the sublethal or lethal injury from ionizing radiation induced by single- or double-strand breaks in DNA within cellular nuclei, and indirect effects are those characterized by interactions between the radiation and other molecules. The dominant indirect effects of radiation come from its interaction with water molecules, which produces reactive oxygen species (ROS) and reactive nitrogen species (Téoule 1987). The term "ROS" is a collective one that includes both free oxygen radicals, such as the superoxide ($O_2^{\bullet-}$), hydroxyl ($OH^\bullet$), peroxyl ($RO_2^\bullet$), and hydroperoxyl

Z. Liao (✉) · T. Xu
Department of Radiation Oncology, The University of Texas MD Anderson Cancer Center, Houston, TX, USA
e-mail: zliao@mdanderson.org

R. Komaki
Department of Radiation Oncology, Baylor College of Medicine, Houston, TX, USA

($HO_2^•$) radicals, and some nonradical oxidizing agents, such as hydrogen peroxide (H_2O_2). Reactive nitrogen species include mainly nitric oxide ($NO^•$) and peroxynitrite ($ONOO^-$) (Dertinger and Jung 1970). The free radicals produced by ionizing radiation can also induce "bystander effects," that is, biological responses in cells outside the path of the radiation beam, which create an environment of increased genetic instability that indirectly damages DNA and other cellular components. Radiation can also trigger cell death through a variety of mechanisms including apoptosis, mitotic catastrophe, necrosis, necroptosis, autophagy, and senescence depending on cell type (Sia et al. 2020). The irradiated cells can release cytokines, chemokines, and damage- (or danger-) associated molecular pattern molecules (DAMPs), which stimulate local and complex systemic responses in unirradiated cells. DAMPs can be recognized by macrophages and lymphocytes, which triggers several signaling pathways involved in inflammation, DNA repair, and reduction/oxidation (redox) metabolism (Yang et al. 2015). These processes are associated not only with increased production of free radicals but also with increased levels of several cytokines and chemokines, including tumor necrosis factor-alpha (TNF-α), tumor growth factor-beta (TGF-β), and the interleukins IL-1, IL-4, IL-6, IL-8, and IL-13, among others (Schaue et al. 2012). These effects can suppress antioxidant defenses in cells, leading to DNA breaks and cell death (Schaue et al. 2012). Moreover, radiation has effects on the human innate immune system via pattern recognition receptors (especially the Toll-like receptor [TLR]) to induce more inflammation and to give dendritic cells the ability to present antigens to components of the adaptive immune system in the lymph nodes and spleen (Keshavarz et al. 2021).

The cascade of events induced by irradiation and the affected signaling pathways can prompt both acute (acute inflammation) and late (fibrosis) adverse events that could be considered potential targets for normal tissue injury prevention and mitigation. Virtually all tissues and organs (e.g., heart, lung, esophagus, bone marrow, lymphatic system, skin) are at risk, including cells that have specific organ functions (e.g., pneumocytes, cardiomyocytes, lymphocytes), the supporting stroma (fibroblasts), and the vasculature. The main categories of radioprotectants and mitigators are those that (1) scavenge free radicals; (2) promote DNA repair; (3) maintain redox homeostasis; (4) modulate immune response and inflammatory cytokines; (5) inhibit apoptosis; and (6) restore functional cells (e.g., stem cell therapy) (Fig. 1).

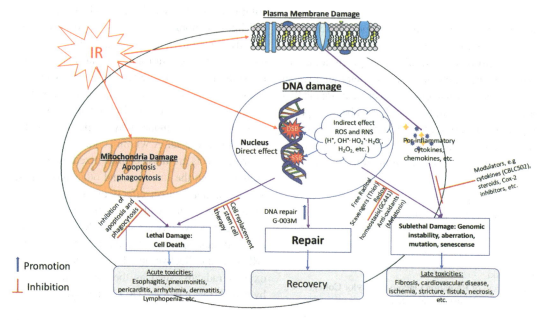

Fig. 1 Schematic illustration of mechanisms of radiation injury and targets for protection and mitigation. *IR* ionizing radiation

2 Strategies for Radioprotection and Mitigation

2.1 Free Radical Scavengers: Thiol

These events and reactions are tightly interconnected with one another and can affect downstream signaling pathways.

The protective capacity of thiol-containing compounds against normal tissue damage from radiation has been recognized for over half a century. The most effective compounds are those with a sulfhydryl, -SH, group at one terminus and a strong basic function, an amino group, at the other terminus. The general structure of these aminothiols is $H_2N(CH_2)_xNH(CH_2)_ySH$ (Andreassen et al. 2003); among these, phosphorothioates (such as WR-2721 [amifostine], WR-3689, WR-151327) are the most effective and least toxic. Thiols and their anions rapidly bind to free radicals such as OH and prevent them from reacting with cellular DNA. This type of protection from DNA damage by scavenging free radicals is oxygen dependent (Travis 1984). Another mode of protection occurs via H-atom donation (the fixation-repair model). Thiols compete with oxygen for radiation-induced DNA radicals. DNA radicals are "fixed" (not repaired) by reacting with oxygen, and potentially harmful hydroxyperoxides may be generated. However, DNA radicals can be chemically repaired when they react with thiols by donation of hydrogen (Durand and Olive 1989). Further, intracellular oxygen can be depleted as a result of thiol oxidation (Durand and Olive 1989), which would decrease the rate of oxygen-mediated DNA damage repair. Finally, thiols induce DNA packaging that may decrease the accessibility of DNA sites to radiolytic attack. This mechanism may be oxygen independent and may explain the protection from densely ionizing radiation such as neutrons (Savoye et al. 1997).

Amifostine (WR-2721) is a prodrug that is hydrolyzed by alkaline phosphatases that are enriched in normal tissues to form the active cytoprotective free thiol metabolite WR-1065 (Millán 2006). In preclinical setting, amifostine undergoes preferential rapid uptake into normal tissues but has negligible or slower uptake into tumor tissues. Although normal tissues actively concentrate amifostine against the concentration gradient, solid tumors generally absorb amifostine passively (Yuhas et al. 1980). This selectivity results, in part, from differences in pH and alkaline phosphatase at the level of the capillary endothelium, both being higher in normal tissues than in tumors (Rasey et al. 1986). The acidic tumor microenvironment inhibits the alkaline phosphatase necessary for uptake and conversion of amifostine to the active protective thiol WR-1065 (Calabro-Jones et al. 1985), a condition absent in normal tissues. Once inside the cell, WR-1065 acts as a scavenger of oxygen free radicals (Marzatico et al. 2000), which are reduced under the hypoxic conditions commonly present in solid tumors. Amifostine may also be less available to tumors because of defects in their vascular networks. A large body of preclinical data indicate that amifostine preferentially protects most normal tissues (including the lung), probably in a dose-dependent manner (Ormsby et al. 2014), from the effects of DNA-damaging agents such as radiation. In addition to interacting with radiation, amifostine has independent antimetastatic and antiangiogenic activities (Grdina et al. 2002; Giannopoulou and Papadimitriou 2003).

Clinically, amifostine has been one of the most extensively investigated thiols as a protector for various types of cancer therapies. Its therapeutic indications are neutropenia-related fever and infection induced by antitumor chemotherapeutics like alkylators (e.g., cyclophosphamide) and platinum-containing agents (e.g., cisplatin) (Calabro-Jones et al. 1985; Purdie et al. 1983). It is the only radioprotector that has been approved by the US Food and Drug Administration for reducing xerostomia in patients undergoing radiotherapy for head and neck cancer (Nicolatou-Galitis et al. 2013). However, a recent report of a phase III randomized trial of head and neck cancer failed to show any protective effect from intravenous pretreatment with amifostine on the incidence of grade ≥2 acute or late xerostomia, and other types of toxicity tended to be *more* severe with amifostine (Lee et al. 2019). In lung cancer studies, amifostine reduced the incidence of pneumonitis, lung fibrosis, and esophagitis in patients undergoing radiation therapy without compromising antitumor efficacy (Antonadou et al. 2001; Movsas et al. 2007) and reduced the incidence and severity of acute esophageal, pulmonary, and hematologic toxicity resulting from concurrent cisplatin-based chemotherapy and radiotherapy without effect on survival (Komaki et al. 2004). Hypotension was the most common adverse effect in that and previous studies, occurring in 65% of patients (Komaki et al. 2004). However, in an early report of RTOG 98-01, another phase III randomized study, amifostine did not reduce the rates of severe esophagitis (Movsas et al. 2005), even though an updated report of patient-reported outcomes suggested a possible advantage from amifostine in terms of less pain and swallowing symptoms (Movsas et al. 2007).

Unfortunately, the alkaline phosphatases that hydrolyze amifostine are ubiquitous in the endothelium, which may be responsible for some undesirable side effects in the autonomic nervous system. Because the serum concentration necessary for a radioprotective effect is quite close to the minimum concentration for toxic effects, the routine clinical use of intravenous amifostine has not gained popularity because of its association with severe nausea, hypotension, and malaise. Recently, alternative routes of delivery for amifostine have attracted research interest (Molkentine et al. 2019). Because the entire intestinal tract, especially the duodenum and jejunum, is enriched with intestinal alkaline phosphatases (Van Dongen et al. 1977), some have hypothesized that giving amifostine orally before radiation might activate those intestinal enzymes and hydrolyze amifostine to its active metabolite (Molkentine et al. 2019). Presumably this enterally activated form of amifostine would accumulate in high concentrations in the intestines and provide localized radioprotection with potentially fewer systemic side effects, which would be particularly useful during radiation therapy for pancreatic cancer, because the duodenum and jejunum are dose-limiting structures. Molkentine and colleagues showed that oral amifostine was well tolerated and effective in protecting against otherwise lethal doses of ablative radiation directed to the upper abdomen. Further, the level of accumulated WR-1065 was found to be significantly higher in the gastrointestinal tract than in the plasma, liver, or tumors (Molkentine et al. 2019). Another group is exploring the topical application of a new thermogel formulation loaded with the active thiol metabolite of amifostine (Clémenson et al. 2019). This thermogel, called CPh-1014, polymerizes at body temperature; its formulation and adhesive properties enable easy, direct application of amifostine thiol to mucocutaneous areas. These investigators found that topical application of CPh-1014 in in vivo mouse models reduced radiation-induced DNA damage in mucocutaneous tissues and reduced the severity of mucositis and dermatitis. This cytoprotective effect was confirmed by a decrease in number of DNA double-strand breaks in the irradiated epithelium. Notably, CPh-1014 did not affect the effectiveness of radiation therapy against tumors grafted at submucosal and subcutaneous sites. Moreover, topical application of CPh-1014 did not induce hypotension in dogs, unlike intravenous administration of amifostine (Clémenson et al. 2019).

Collectively, these studies point to new directions to explore the safe and effective use of amifostine as a clinical radioprotector, after the timing and route of application (e.g., intravenous, oral, or topical) are established more concretely.

2.2 DNA Repair

DNA, given its vulnerability to radiation-induced damage, is considered the prime target that initiates cell death, meaning that repair of DNA could represent an important mechanism of radiation protection. Radiation causes cell death when the cells cannot repair the damage (Hu et al. 2016). Cells have different types of repair mechanisms, such as base and nucleotide excision repair, mismatch repair, homologous recombination, and nonhomologous end joining, to restore genomic integrity and ensure cell survival (Hu et al. 2016). The response to DNA damage is complex; in one mechanism, the DNA damage sensor protein ATM activates NF-kB and subsequently activates DNA repair by homologous recombination (Fang et al. 2014). NF-kB also interacts with CtIP complexes and promotes the stabilization of BRCA1, thereby contributing to homologous recombination (Volcic et al. 2012). Another protein that determines how tumor cells repair DNA damage is nuclear factor erythroid 2-like 2 (Nrf2) (Jayakumar et al. 2015). Therefore, the oxidation/reduction state of cells and signaling proteins directly or indirectly participates in the restoration of DNA.

Podophyllotoxin is a ligan with antioxidant activity that directly targets DNA topoisomerase-2α (Zhang et al. 1992) as well as two components of tubulin, the alpha-4A chain (Screpanti et al. 2010) and the tubulin-β chain (Wolff et al. 1991). Podophyllotoxin participates in mitotic arrest and rejoining of DNA strand breaks (Wolff et al. 1991) as well as the enzymatic activation of cytochromes P450-2C19 and P450-3A4, both important in the NADPH-dependent electron transport pathway (Preissner et al. 2010). The radioprotective effect of podophyllotoxin has been tested in combination with rutin (Dutta et al. 2018), a flavonoid involved in free radical scavenging via targeting the steroidogenic enzyme AKR1C3 (Aldo-keto reductase family 1 member C3) and activating cytochromes P450-2C8, P450-2C9, P450-2D6, and P450-3A4, which subsequently regulate metabolic processes, cell proliferation, and death. This podophyllotoxin and rutin combination is referred to as G-003M (Yashavarddhan et al. 2017). In silico, in vitro, and in vivo studies demonstrated that G-003M mediated DNA repair via regulation of IR-induced ROS formation, membrane lipid peroxidation, nonprotein thiol glutathione (GSH) depletion, mitochondrial membrane potential (MMP) alteration, and oxidative damage to DNA; through regulation of proapoptotic (p53, Puma, Bax, Bak, Caspase-3, and Caspase-7) and antiapoptotic proteins (Bcl-2 and Bcl-xl), and through induction in the master redox regulator, Nrf-2, and its several downstream target proteins (Nqo-1, Ho-1, Gst, and Txnrd-1) through negative regulation of Keap-1. Mice pretreated with G-003M had shown significant recovery to CD3, CD19, and Gr-1 cell surface marker in mice bone marrow and spleen, which otherwise was significantly declined following irradiation (Singh et al. 2017). G-003M protected radiation-induced injury to intestinal stem cells via its effects on the Wnt pathway and minimized acute inflammation by restricting the infiltration of immune cells into the intestinal venules (Kalita et al. 2019). Finally, G-003M minimized pneumonitis and fibrosis induced by total thoracic irradiation in a mouse model by reducing ROS and nitric oxide levels; reducing cell death; reducing lung permeability; and reducing lung levels of IL-6, TNF-α, and TGF-β1, as well as extending survival (Verma et al. 2017). Because radiation-induced lymphopenia, pneumonitis, and fibrosis are well-known adverse events after concurrent chemoradiation for lung cancer, especially when immune checkpoint inhibitors are used, G-003M may be worth exploring as a countermeasure against radiation-induced lymphocytic, hemopoietic, and lung toxicity.

2.3 Redox Homeostasis: Manganese Superoxide Dismutase

ROS generated under physiological conditions are essential signaling molecules in cell processes ranging from proliferation to apoptosis. However, when generated under nonphysiological, stress-related conditions, such as during radiation or chemotherapy, ROS become toxic to both tumor cells and the surrounding normal tissue (Sarsour et al. 2009). The cytotoxicity of cancer therapies causes changes in mitochondrial metabolism that lead to formation of several ROS, including superoxide ($O_2^{\bullet-}$). Physiological levels of $O_2^{\bullet-}$ are generated during metabolic respiration and by the activity of cytochrome p450 enzyme isoforms, α-ketoglutarate dehydrogenase, glycerol-3-phosphate dehydrogenase, and NADPH-dependent oxidases (Handy and Loscalzo 2012). Stress induced by exposure to doxorubicin or radiation (Azzam et al. 2012; Sisakht et al. 2020) leads to more $O_2^{\bullet-}$ being generated. Manganese superoxide dismutase (MnSOD) is a ubiquitous metalloenzyme located within the mitochondria that is essential for the survival of all aerobic organisms, from bacteria to humans. One of nature's most efficient catalysts, MnSOD protects the redox machinery in the mitochondria from the superoxide radicals produced during normal respiration. In many pathologic conditions, such as inflammation caused by radiation-induced free radical damage, superoxide is abundantly produced and may overwhelm the cell's ability to efficiently remove it, thereby leading to tissue injury. The antioxidant activity of MnSOD inactivates superoxide and converts $O_2^{\bullet-}$ to hydrogen peroxide (H_2O_2), which is then converted to H_2O and O_2 by peroxidases. During radiation and chemotherapy, the cooperation between SOD enzymes and various antioxidant enzymes (e.g., catalases, glutathione peroxidase, peroxiredoxin reductase) catalyzes free radicals. If the peroxidases are not in balance, the ROS will result in oxidative damage.

Three major therapeutic approaches have been tested: MnSOD given as a drug; MnSOD gene therapy; and MnSOD as small-molecule mimics. Each approach is discussed briefly in the following sections.

2.3.1 MnSOD as a Drug

Early studies showed that systemic administration of SOD could prevent radiation injury and that the use of liposomal copper/zinc recombinant superoxide dismutase (Cu/ZnSOD) and manganese superoxide dismutase (MnSOD) could reduce preexisting radiation-induced fibrosis (Delanian et al. 1994; Lefaix et al. 1996). The activity of SOD given before radiation has generally been attributed to its radical scavenging effects, whereas the effects of SOD given after radiation are most likely related to its anti-inflammatory or immunostimulatory properties (Grdina et al. 2009; Mapuskar et al. 2019). Although MnSOD has shown promising results, practical issues arise from its short half-life (6 min) due to rapid renal clearance (Turrens et al. 1984). Protein engineering to increase the longevity of MnSOD may overcome these issues (Borrelli et al. 2009). An alternative method for increasing the half-life of MnSOD is delivery via liposomes, which extends the half-life to 4 h (Turrens et al. 1984).

2.3.2 MnSOD as Gene Therapy

Another approach to addressing the problem of short half-life of MnSOD is to induce the expression of genes that increase MnSOD production within cells in the tissue to be protected. Both in vitro and in vivo studies with mice have shown that MnSOD overexpression by vector delivery leads to significant toxicity for tumor cells and radioprotective properties for healthy cells (Ough et al. 2004; Yang et al. 2002), probably because healthy cells can remove H_2O_2 produced by dismutase enzymes by catalases and peroxidases, but tumor cells cannot. Even though a few early studies demonstrated some potential in radioprotection in animal studies (Petkau et al. 1978; Eastgate et al. 1993; Chen et al. 2017), the need to induce gene expression in vivo underscores the technologic challenges of this approach.

The use of liposomal plasmid preparations of MnSOD is another approach being tested in clinical trials to prevent esophagitis during chemoradiation therapy for NSCLC. One such phase I trial dose escalation study involved giving patients an MnSOD transgene in a plasmid within a liposome (MnSOD PL) orally and showed no significant toxicity, and the recommended dose for the phase II trial was 30 mg (Tarhini et al.

2011). The phase II study, begun in 2005 and estimated for completion in December 2020 (NCT00618917), is to examine the efficacy of MnSOD PL by assessing the incidence of grade 3 or 4 esophagitis and the clinical response to chemoradiation therapy.

The gene therapy approach to delivering agents specifically to targeted tissues is not limited to MnSOD but has high potential for a wide array of agents, including both cytotoxic and radioprotective agents. In its current forms, gene therapy can deliver DNA and other therapeutic nucleic acid materials such as small interfering RNA, antisense oligonucleotides, or microRNA. However, gene therapy has not gained wide clinical acceptance because of early reports of severe immunologic and carcinogenic side effects, poor target-cell specificity, inability to transfer large genes, and its high cost. Nonviral vectors, in particular nanocarriers, are being evaluated instead and may provide a new avenue for MnSOD gene therapy.

2.3.3 MnSOD as Small-Molecule Mimics

2.3.3.1 Manganese Porphyrins

To date, the most promising small-molecule mimics of MnSOD are the Mn porphyrins (MnPs), which structurally resemble the iron-containing heme group. MnPs are attractive because they are not antigenic, they are stable, they can penetrate subcellular membranes, they can scavenge other ROS such as peroxynitrites (Gauter-Fleckenstein et al. 2008), and they can be modified to optimize their effectiveness. MnPs react not only with superoxide but also with numerous small and large reactive oxygen, nitrogen, and sulfur species (Batinic-Haberle and Spasojevic 2019). MnPs have catalase- and glutathione peroxidase-like activities, peroxynitrite-reducing activity, and the ability to oxidize ascorbate (Ferrer-Sueta et al. 1999). MnPs can act as both antioxidants (reducing $O_2^{\cdot -}$ to H_2O_2) and pro-oxidants (oxidizing $O_2^{\cdot -}$ to O_2). If H_2O_2 is maintained at less than nM levels, as is the case in normal cells, the catalysis of $O_2^{\cdot -}$ dismutation results in antioxidant therapeutic effects. MnPs protected gastrointestinal crypt cells, rectum, bladder, and salivary glands from gamma radiation, X-ray radiation, and proton beam irradiation, either delivered in one large localized dose or in smaller fractionated doses, and either given before radiation exposure and continued afterward, or in some cases given *after* radiation exposure (Cline et al. 2018; Shrishrimal et al. 2017; Kosmacek et al. 2016).

The mechanisms by which MnPs protect cells from radiation rely on three major pathways: (1) regulate the immune response and inhibit inflammation by reducing the ability of NF-kB to bind to DNA through oxidation of the p50 subunit of NF-kB (and perhaps the p65 subunit as well); the oxidized p50 no longer binds to DNA, making NF-kB inactive and unable to transcribe pro-inflammatory genes in macrophages (Tse et al. 2004); (2) inhibit fibrosis via TGF-β/SMAD signaling by suppressing active TGF-β, reducing the expression of TGFbRII, and reducing the phosphorylation of SMAD2 and SMAD3; and (3) activates cytoprotective proteins such as the transcription factor NRF2 and promotes binding to ARE (antioxidant response element), which enhances the expression of antioxidant and cytoprotective genes (Zhao et al. 2017). The three major signaling pathways (NF-kB, TGF-β, and NRF2) are all regulated through the oxidation of key cysteines of redox-sensitive proteins (Batinic-Haberle et al. 2018). Cross talk between the pathways could also result in amplification of the changes induced by MnP treatment. However, more work is needed to fully understand how MnPs protect normal cells from radiation damage.

Two MnP mimetics, MnTE–2–PyP5+ and MnTnBuOE–2–PyP5+ (Gauter-Fleckenstein et al. 2014), have shown promising results with regard to protecting healthy cells during radiotherapy (Bruni et al. 2018). A third-generation, cationic, lipophilic, Mn- and porphyrin-based mimetic of human SOD2 is BMX-001 (Leu et al. 2017), which has been shown to have radioprotective effects on white matter in the brain while acting as a tumor radiosensitizer (Leu et al. 2017). Two related MnPs, Mn(III) *meso*-tetrakis(*N*-ethylpyridinium-2-yl)porphyrin (MnTE-2-PyP5+5+; BMX-010; AEOL10113) and Mn(III) *meso*-tetrakis (*Nn*-butoxyethylpyridinium-2-yl) porphyrin (MnTnBuOE-2-PyP5+5+; BMX-001001 [BioMimetix, Englewood, CO, USA]), are now being tested in five phase II clinical trials (Batinic-Haberle and Spasojevic 2019). The radioprotective effects of BMX-001 are being tested in clinical trials NCT03386500 (for patients with recently diagnosed anal cancer), NCT03608020 (for patients with multiple brain metastases), NCT02990468 (for patients with head and neck cancer), and NCT02655601 (for patients with high-grade glioma treated with concurrent radiation therapy and temozolomide).

2.3.3.2 GC4419

GC4419 (Galera Therapeutics, St. Louis, MO) is a selective small-molecule SOD mimic, which acts as both a protector and a mitigator of radiation-induced superoxide damage. GC4419 can rapidly and specifically convert $O_2^{\cdot-}$ to hydrogen peroxide (H_2O_2), arresting the initiation of that cascade without affecting tumor control (El-Mahdy et al. 2020).

In one preclinical study of lung fibrosis, a single treatment with GC4419 before a 54-Gy, single-dose focal irradiation of murine lung tissue reduced fibrotic density at 24 weeks. Further, daily doses of GC4419 after irradiation further reduced lung fibrosis, the extent of which varied according to the time of delivery. To address the possibility of tumor (rather than normal tissue) radioprotection, animals with H1299, A549, and HCC827 lung tumor xenografts were given GC4419 30 min before the tumors were irradiated with a single 18 Gy dose, followed by four additional daily doses of GC4419. Tumor growth was significantly delayed, and subsequent tumor cure assays showed that GC4419 enhanced the efficacy of radiation by a factor of 1.67. Moreover, dose enhancement by GC4419 was driven by the size of the dose per fraction. If the dose fractionation scheme is altered to include the biologically equivalent dose schedules of daily 2-Gy fractions for 16 days, daily 4.98-Gy fractions for 5 days, daily 7.3-Gy fractions for 3 days, or daily 9.9-Gy fractions for 2 days, the radiation-enhancing properties of GC4419 were more pronounced as the dose per fraction increases (Story et al. 2018; Sishc et al. 2020). The hypothesis from these results was that GC4419 was generating cytotoxic levels of hydrogen peroxide during the superoxide dismutation process (Sishc et al. 2020).

In a phase Ib trial (Anderson et al. 2016) followed by a randomized phase IIb study (Anderson et al. 2019), GC4419 reduced the incidence and duration of severe oral mucositis (grade 4) in patients with head and neck cancer compared with placebo in a dose-dependent fashion. A phase III trial (ROMAN; ClinicalTrials.gov identifier NCT03689712) of GC4419 is currently underway, with results reported in abstract form (Holmlund et al. 2020). Another trial currently ongoing is exploring the radioprotective effects of MnP in patients with late-stage glioma treated with concurrent radiotherapy and temozolomide (Stankovic et al. 2020). Both MnPs and Mn macrocycles are also being assessed as radioprotectors in head and neck cancer. A different SOD mimic, mangafodipir, is being studied as a protector against oxaliplatin neurotoxicity and other side effects of FOLFOX6 (Karlsson et al. 2017); an analog of this agent, calmangafodipir, is being studied in combination with FOLFOX6 for patients with advanced metastatic colorectal cancer; this latter trial (NCT01619423) completed enrollment in 2018.

In summary, the formation of reactive oxygen and nitrogen species creates oxidative stress, which triggers cell death and normal tissue injury in cancer therapy-induced toxicities, thus establishing the theory of using MnSOD to reduce the oxidative stress. An enhanced understanding of the key role of redox signaling pathways in cell biology, supported by abundant preclinical data on the action MnSOD compounds on redox signaling pathways, is necessary to translate these important findings to clinical use. This in turn will depend on diverse, highly synergistic multidisciplinary approaches.

2.4 Anti-Inflammatory Agents

2.4.1 Prostanoids, COX-2, and COX-2 Inhibitors

In response to physiological signals, stress, or injury (including radiation injury), cells produce prostanoids (prostaglandins and thromboxanes), a family of diverse, highly biologically active lipids derived from the enzymatic metabolism of arachidonic acid by cyclo-oxygenase (COX)-1 or COX-2. COX-1 is ubiquitous in normal tissues and is responsible for prostanoid production in those tissues; the prostanoids in turn have numerous functions in maintaining physiological homeostasis. In contrast, COX-2 is an inducible enzyme involved in prostaglandin production in pathologic states, particularly inflammatory processes and cancer. COX-2 can be induced by inflammatory cytokines (such as TNF-a, IL-1b, and platelet growth factors), oncogenes, growth factors, and hypoxia. Prostanoids, particularly prostaglandin E_2 (PGE_2), participate in the pathogenesis of various pathologic states such as inflammation. PGE_2 activates mononuclear cells (e.g., macrophages) and mediates the typical symptoms of inflammation through its vasodilatory action; this vasodilation augments the edema caused by substances that increase vascular permeability such as histamine. PGE_2 is also involved in the development of erythema and heat at the site of inflammation. Radiation-induced lung injury prompts the development of inflammatory tissue reactions, characterized by the production of abundant PGE_2, other prostaglandins, and pro-inflammatory cytokines. Because different prostanoids have complementary or antagonistic activities, the final biological effect on tissues depends on the balance of similar and opposing actions of the prostanoids involved.

Production of PGE_2 and other pro-inflammatory prostanoids can be suppressed by nonsteroidal anti-inflammatory drugs (NSAIDs), which inhibit both isoforms of COX enzyme, or by selective COX-2 inhibitors. Because selective COX-2 inhibitors do not inhibit prostanoid production in normal tissues, they are less toxic than the more commonly used NSAIDs. Interestingly, both prostanoids and their inhibitors have been reported to have radioprotective effects on normal tissues. For example, exogenous administration of PGE_2, other prostaglandins, or prostaglandin analogs to mice before irradiation has been shown to protect hematopoietic tissue, jejunal mucosa, dermis, and testis (Milas and Hanson 1995). Although the radioprotective abilities of the different prostaglandins vary widely, the prostaglandin analog misoprostol is among the most effective. Paradoxically, using NSAIDs to inhibit prostaglandins has also been shown to protect many tissues, including the lung, against radiation injury (Mohsen et al. 2018). The NSAID indomethacin reportedly protected mouse lung from radiation damage, but the protection was limited to the early pneumonitis phase of injury, and this COX-2 inhibitor did not confer significant protection from radiation-induced pneumonitis when the drug was administered a few days before and after lung irradiation (Milas et al. 1992). Subsequent experiments with a selective COX-2 inhibitor, celecoxib, suggested that giving the inhibitor during the development phase of acute pneumonitis may reduce the latency or severity of lung injury (Hunter et al. 2013). COX-2 inhibitors have also shown therapeutic benefit by enhancing tumor radioresponse in animal models (Mohsen et al. 2018), but no such benefit was observed in the CALGB 30801-Alliance phase III prospective randomized trial of patients treated for NSCLC (Edelman et al. 2014).

2.4.2 Corticosteroids and Immune Suppressants

Corticosteroids are highly potent anti-inflammatory agents that downregulate the inflammatory response and form the basis of treatment for established radiation-induced normal tissue injury, specifically radiation necrosis after cranial irradiation and pneumonitis after thoracic radiation therapy (Kalman et al. 2017). Steroids inhibit the production of all prostanoids because, in addition to their ability to inhibit COX enzymes, they prevent the release of arachidonic acid from membrane phospholipids by stimulating the generation and secretion of lipocortins (Barnes 1998). In one study, giving steroids at the time of irradiation protected rats from lung interstitial edema and delayed or suppressed radiation-induced alveolitis, but did not affect the development of pulmonary fibrosis (Ward et al. 1993). Although using steroids prophylactically has been examined, to date it has not been associated with reduced pulmonary or cerebral injury (Ruben et al. 2006).

2.5 Cytokines

Cytokines are small molecules consisting of proteins, peptides, or glycoproteins that are produced as soluble factors by a variety of distinct cells, including all cells of the immune system as well as endothelial, epithelial, and stromal cells (Vacchelli et al. 2012). Cytokines are involved in nearly every response to immune, inflammatory, and infectious stimuli. Ionizing radiation induces a cascade of tissue responses mediated by different pro-inflammatory cytokines, such as TNF-α, IL-1, IL-6, and TGF-β (Lierova et al. 2018). Many of the intricate mechanisms of communication events within and between cells after exposure to radiation can be targets for radioprotection (Lierova et al. 2018).

2.5.1 Toll-Like Receptor Agonists

The TLRs include a family of type I transmembrane receptors, which are characterized by an extracellular leucine-rich repeat domain and an intracellular Toll/IL-1 receptor domain (Smith et al. 2018). Interactions between the leucine-rich repeat domain and DAMPs lead to binding of the Toll/IL-1 receptor domain to cytoplasmic proteins and propagation of signaling in cells that results in the activation of several downstream networks, including the NF-κB, c-Jun N-terminal kinase, and p38 MAP kinase pathways (Liu et al. 2018; Vidya et al. 2018). Although these axes can regulate the expression of inflammatory cytokines, they are also responsible for the expression of antiapoptotic and proliferative genes. The ability of TLRs to distinguish "self" from "nonself" antigens is crucial to innate immunity; however, deregulation of TLR signaling induces inflammatory responses and the development of human cancers, the latter by enhancing proliferation and angiogenesis and also by providing cancer cells an opportunity to escape the immune system. TLR modulators have included both antagonists and agonists; considerable preclinical research on TLR agonists has led to some such agents to be tested in clinical trials for their antitumor and radioprotective properties, as described below (Keshavarz et al. 2021).

TLR agonists activate innate immunity and initiate long-lasting adaptive immunity by stimulating cytotoxic lymphocytes and natural killer cells and by inducing the maturation of dendritic cells, so presumably these agents could enhance the sensitivity of tumor cells to radiation and immunotherapies (Iribarren et al. 2016). Indeed, one such agent, CBLB502 (entolimod), a TLR5 agonist derived from *Salmonella* flagellin, has been shown to induce radioprotective activity without reducing tumor radiosensitivity (Burdelya et al. 2008). Two groups of investigators found that CBLB502 reduced the severity and duration of radiation-induced thrombocytopenia and neutropenia in mice and rhesus monkeys, and did so by promoting the regeneration of cells in small intestine, spleen, thymus, bone marrow, and the male reproductive system (Burdelya et al. 2008; Krivokrysenko et al. 2010); and increased the survival of animals after total-body irradiation (Krivokrysenko et al. 2015; Bai et al. 2018).

In another series of experiments, activation of TLRs by intestinal microflora in mice decreased radiation-induced DNA damage via activating the expression of genes associated with DNA repair, including *Irg1* (immune-responsiveness gene 1), *Gadd45b* (growth arrest and DNA damage-inducible 45 beta), *Sod2* (superoxide dismutase 2), and *Rad21*, all of which have important roles in radioprotection (Chen et al. 2014). CBLB502 is currently in phase I clinical trials for head and neck cancer and for locally advanced or metastatic solid tumors (Keshavarz et al. 2021).

Another TLR agonist, KMRC011, is a modified version of CBLB502 manufactured by the Korea Institute of Industrial Technology. KMRC011 was created by selectively removing 34 amino acid residues from CBLB502 with a ubiquitin-specific protease (UBP1) to avoid an immune response (Kim et al. 2019). KMRC011 significantly improved survival rate of mice (relative to control) after 11 Gy of total-body irradiation; this effect was found to result from stimulating cell proliferation and anti-apoptosis and depended on the dosage and number of treatments with KMRC011 (Kim et al. 2019). Like CBLB502, KMRC011 also increased the expression of genes related to DNA repair, such as *Rad21*, *Gadd45b*, *Sod2*, and *Irg1*, while downregulating NF-κB p65 in the small intestine of lethally irradiated mice, suggesting that KMRC011-induced regulation of NF-κB signaling was at least partially responsible for its radioprotective activity (Kim et al. 2019). KMRC011 also induced the expression of G-CSF, IL-6, IFN-γ, TNF-α, and IP-10 (interferon-inducible protein 10), peak values of which depended on the route of administration. These investigators concluded that these cytokines could be used as biomarkers to evaluate the clinical effectiveness of KMRC011 (Kim et al. 2019).

In summary, preclinical and early clinical findings regarding the use of TLR5 agonists as radioprotectants have been encouraging (Keshavarz et al. 2021). Although these agents have yet to be tested in lung cancer, TLR agonists would seem to be attractive radioprotectors during lung cancer treatment, because concurrent chemoradiation is known to suppress bone marrow and induce lymphopenia, an adverse event that negatively affects survival. The ability of CBLB502 to mobilize hematopoietic and endothelial progenitor cells from bone marrow to the peripheral blood to counteract radiation injury may be worth exploring in conjunction with standard fractionation, hypofractionation, and ablative dose fractionation for lung cancer (Singh and Seed 2020).

2.5.2 Interleukin-1

IL-1 is the prototypical inflammatory cytokine; it is central to the inflammatory response in that it drives IL-6 signaling, which is activated in response to tissue injury (Dinarello 2011). Increased IL-1 levels have also been found in the heart and lungs after exposure to ionizing radiation (Rubin et al. 1995; Krüse et al. 2001). In experimental animal models, IL-1 induced the expression of genes associated with inflammasome biology in whole-transcriptome analysis of irradiated arteries; reduced mRNA levels of the inflammatory cytokines Ccl2 and Ccl5 and expression of the class II major histocompatibility antigen I-A^b; and induced systolic and diastolic dysfunction (Christersdottir et al. 2019). Blockade of IL-1 with anakinra, a recombinant human IL-1 receptor antagonist, or canakinumab, a human monoclonal IL-1 receptor antagonist, provided cardioprotection and improved left ventricular remodeling and function after acute myocardial infarction or doxorubicin-induced injury in mice (Zhu et al. 2010). Treatment with anakinra was also found to preserve the contractile reserve of the left ventricle and systolic function in mice after radiation to 14–20 Gy, although IL-1 blockade did not rescue the mice from severe myocardial and pericardial fibrosis or premature death after high-dose radiation (i.e., 20 Gy) (Christersdottir et al. 2019; Groarke et al. 2015).

Anakinra was approved by the US Food and Drug Administration for the treatment of rheumatoid arthritis in 2001 (Dinarello et al. 2012). Studies of atherosclerosis and atherothrombosis have also shown that IL-1 blockade can have cardioprotective effects by reducing apoptosis and minimizing the size of the myocardial infarct (Abbate et al. 2012). On the other hand, Novartis's CANTOS phase III trial of canakinumab, an anti-IL-1 therapy targeting IL-1β that is overexpressed in solid tumors including lung, showed that doses of 150 mg every 3 months led to significant reductions in high-sensitivity C-reactive protein and IL-6 levels (relative to placebo), with no significant reduction in lipid levels (from baseline), and a lower rate of recurrent cardiovascular events independent of lipid-level lowering (ClinicalTrials.gov ID NCT01327846) (Ridker et al. 2018). Another phase III trial, CANOPY-A, is being undertaken to evaluate the efficacy and safety of adjuvant canakinumab versus placebo in patients with surgically resected NSCLC (Garon et al. 2019). This trial (NCT03447769) is enrolling adult patients with completely resected stages II–IIIBNSCLC who have completed standard-of-care adjuvant treatments, including cisplatin-based chemotherapy and mediastinal radiation therapy (if applicable). Approximately 1500 patients will be randomized 1:1 to receive canakinumab (200 mg s.c., every 3 weeks) or placebo (s.c., every 3 weeks) for 18 cycles or until disease recurrence, unacceptable toxicity, treatment discontinuation, death, or loss to follow-up. The primary objective is disease-free survival; secondary objectives include overall survival, lung cancer-specific survival, safety, pharmacokinetics and immunogenicity of canakinumab, and patient-reported outcomes.

In summary, use of IL-1 receptor blockade is an attractive possibility for radioprotection in lung cancer treatment, although its timing in relation to cancer treatment requires clarification and more information is needed on the pathogenesis of radiation-induced cardiomyopathy.

2.5.3 Interleukin-6

IL-6 is a pleiotropic, pro-inflammatory cytokine that mediates the acute phase response to infection and injury; it stimulates the growth and differentiation of B and T lymphocytes to drive leukocyte trafficking and activation, and it induces the production of acute phase proteins by hepatocytes (Tanaka et al. 2014). IL-6 is synthesized by a variety of cells in the lung parenchyma, including alveolar macrophages, lung fibroblasts, and type II pneumocytes (Fleckenstein et al. 2007), and increased levels of circulating IL-6 may predict radiation pneumonitis (Chen et al. 2001). IL-6 is part of a highly complex and interrelated feedback system; it is also produced by mononuclear phagocytes, T cells, B cells, hepatocytes, and bone marrow cells (Rose-John et al. 2006). Secretion of IL-6 by mononuclear phagocytes and T cells leads to increases in acute phase proteins, such as C-reactive protein. IL-6 promotes T-cell proliferation and differentiation, B-cell differentiation and survival, and plasma cell production of IgG, IgA, and IgM. IL-6 is also expressed by cells of the cardiovascular system, including endothelial cells, vascular smooth muscle cells, and ischemic cardiac myocytes (Kanda and Takahashi 2004). Elevated circulating IL-6 levels have been observed in a variety of cardiovascular diseases, and excessive production of IL-6 can further exacerbate myocardial injury (Raymond et al. 2001). IL-6 is also expressed in response to cytokines such as IL-1, IL-17A, and TNF-α; moreover, IL-6 and IL-17A, produced primarily by T helper 17 cells [Th17], can trigger a positive feedback loop that amplifies IL-6 expression, and IL-6, combined with TGF-β, leads to the differentiation of naïve $CD4^+$ T cells into Th17 cells, which then produce IL-17A, IL-17F, IL-21, granulocyte-macrophage colony-stimulating factor (GM-CSF), IL-10, and IL-22. Finally, IL-6 primes Th17 cell development, whereas IL-1β and IL-23 lead to Th17-cell maturation and expansion (Hirahara et al. 2010).

Clinically, tocilizumab, a humanized monoclonal antibody that blocks IL-6 receptor signaling, has been approved in more than 100 countries worldwide for the treatment of rheumatoid arthritis, juvenile idiopathic arthritis, Castleman disease and Takayasu arteritis (Tanaka et al. 2014; Takeuchi et al. 2017), giant cell arteritis (Stone et al. 2017), and severe chimeric antigen receptor (CAR) T-cell-induced cytokine release syndrome (Le et al. 2018). Most recently, tocilizumab has been used to treat severe coronavirus disease 2019 (COVID-19) (Liu et al. 2020; Zhang et al. 2020), and a propensity-matched study of its safety and efficacy in patients with COVID-19 showed that its use was associated with better overall survival relative to controls (hazard ratio [HR] 0.499, $p = 0.035$) but with longer hospital stays (HR 1.658, $p = 0.019$), mainly because of biochemical, respiratory, and infectious adverse events (Rossotti et al. 2020). Clinical trials are ongoing to examine the effectiveness of tocilizumab in acute and chronic inflammatory diseases, including diabetes and systemic lupus erythematosus. However, clinical use of anti-IL-6 as a radioprotector in lung cancer is still in the concept stage, and considerable work remains to be done.

Although numerous cytokines have been tested in combination with other drugs in trials that also involved radiation, no reliable reports have been published that specifically address the effects of cytokines as radiomitigators. Detailed descriptions of medical countermeasures for radiation are provided in a comprehensive review by Singh and colleagues, which is updated annually (Singh and Seed 2020).

3 Summary

Having a multifaceted, mechanistic understanding of the biological and physiological effects of ionizing radiation is essential for the effective development of suitable and appropriately customized radiation countermeasure agents. To date, free radical scavenging has been the best studied means of radioprotection; DNA repair, modulation of the innate immune response and inflammatory cytokines, and stem cell replacement therapy (not described in this chapter) are emerging as potentially effective strategies. A holistic, multimechanistic approach will be necessary to achieve optimal radiation protection strategies for use during radiotherapy for cancer.

Acknowledgment The authors are in debt to Christine Wogan for her editorial expertise in the development of this chapter.

References

Abbate A, Van Tassell BW, Biondi-Zoccai GGL (2012) Blocking interleukin-1 as a novel therapeutic strategy for secondary prevention of cardiovascular events. BioDrugs 26:217–233

Andreassen CN, Grau C, Lindegaard JC (2003) Chemical radioprotection: a critical review of amifostine as a cytoprotector in radiotherapy. Semin Radiat Oncol 13(1):62–72

Anderson CM et al (2016) Phase Ib trial of superoxide (SO) dismutase (SOD) mimetic GC4419 to reduce chemoradiotherapy (CRT)-induced oral mucositis (OM) in patients (pts) with oral cavity or oropharyngeal carcinoma (OCC). J Clin Oncol 34: 10120–10120

Anderson CM et al (2019) Phase IIb, randomized, double-blind trial of GC4419 versus placebo to reduce severe oral mucositis due to concurrent radiotherapy and cisplatin for head and neck cancer. J Clin Oncol 37:3256–3265

Antonadou D et al (2001) Randomized phase III trial of radiation treatment ± amifostine in patients with advanced-stage lung cancer. Int J Radia Oncol Biol Phys 51:915–922

Antonia SJ et al (2018) Overall survival with durvalumab after chemoradiotherapy in stage III NSCLC. N Engl J Med 379:2342–2350

Azzam EI, Jay-Gerin J-P, Pain D (2012) Ionizing radiation-induced metabolic oxidative stress and prolonged cell injury. Cancer Lett 327:48–60

Bai H et al (2018) CBLB502, a toll-like receptor 5 agonist, offers protection against radiation-induced male reproductive system damage in mice†. Biol Reprod 100:281–291

Barnes PJ (1998) Anti-inflammatory actions of glucocorticoids: molecular mechanisms. Clin Sci 94:557–572

Batinic-Haberle I, Spasojevic I (2019) 25 years of development of Mn porphyrins — from mimics of superoxide dismutase enzymes to thiol signaling to clinical trials: the story of our life in the USA. J Porphyr Phthalocyanines 23:1326–1335

Batinic-Haberle I, Tovmasyan A, Spasojevic I (2018) Mn porphyrin-based redox-active drugs: differential effects as cancer therapeutics and protectors of normal tissue against oxidative injury. Antioxid Redox Signal 29:1691–1724

Borrelli A et al (2009) A recombinant MnSOD is radioprotective for normal cells and radiosensitizing for tumor cells. Free Radic Biol Med 46:110–116

Bruni A et al (2018) BMX-001, a novel redox-active metalloporphyrin, improves islet function and engraftment in a murine transplant model. Am J Transplant 18:1879–1889

Burdelya LG et al (2008) An agonist of toll-like receptor 5 has radioprotective activity in mouse and primate models. Science 320:226–230

Calabro-Jones PM, Fahey RC, Smoluk GD, Ward JF (1985) Alkaline phosphatase promotes radioprotection and accumulation of WR-1065 in V79-171 cells incubated in medium containing WR-2721. Int J Radiat Biol Relat Stud Phys Chem Med 47:23–27

Chen Y, Rubin P, Williams J, Hernady E, Smudzin T, Okunieff P (2001) Circulating IL-6 as a predictor of radiation pneumonitis. Int J Radiat Oncol Biol Phys 49:641–648

Chen H et al (2014) Activation of toll-like receptors by intestinal microflora reduces radiation-induced DNA damage in mice. Mutat Res 774:22–28

Chen HX et al (2017) Manganese superoxide dismutase gene-modified mesenchymal stem cells attenuate acute radiation-induced lung injury. Hum Gene Ther 28:523–532

Christersdottir T et al (2019) Prevention of radiotherapy-induced arterial inflammation by interleukin-1 blockade. Eur Heart J 40:2495–2503

Clémenson C et al (2019) Preventing radiation-induced injury by topical application of an amifostine metabolite-loaded thermogel. Int J Radia Oncol Biol Phys 104:1141–1152

Cline JM et al (2018) Post-irradiation treatment with a superoxide dismutase mimic, MnTnHex-2-PyP5+, mitigates radiation injury in the lungs of non-human primates after whole-thorax exposure to ionizing radiation. Antioxidants 7:40

Delanian S et al (1994) Successful treatment of radiation-induced fibrosis using liposomal CuZn superoxide dismutase: clinical trial. Radiother Oncol 32:12–20

Dertinger H, Jung H (1970) Direct and indirect actions of radiation. In: Molecular radiation biology. Springer, New York, NY, pp 70–90

Dinarello CA (2011) Interleukin-1 in the pathogenesis and treatment of inflammatory diseases. Blood 117:3720–3732

Dinarello CA, Simon A, van der Meer JWM (2012) Treating inflammation by blocking interleukin-1 in a broad spectrum of diseases. Nat Rev Drug Discov 11:633–652

Durand RE, Olive PL (1989) Radiosensitisation and radioprotection by BSO and WR-2721: the role of oxygenation. Br J Cancer 60:517–522

Dutta A, Gupta ML, Verma S (2018) Podophyllotoxin and rutin in combination prevents oxidative stress mediated cell death and advances revival of mice gastrointestinal following lethal radiation injury. Free Radic Res 52:103–117

Eastgate J et al (1993) A role for manganese superoxide dismutase in radioprotection of hematopoietic stem cells by interleukin-1. Blood 81:639–646

Edelman MJ et al (2014) Abstract CT238: phase III randomized, placebo controlled trial of COX-2 inhibition in addition to standard chemotherapy for advanced non-small cell lung cancer (NSCLC): CALGB 30801 (Alliance). Cancer Res 74:CT238-CT238

El-Mahdy MA et al (2020) The novel SOD mimetic GC4419 increases cancer cell killing with sensitization to ionizing radiation while protecting normal cells. Free Radic Biol Med 160:630–642

Fang L et al (2014) ATM regulates NF-κB-dependent immediate-early genes via RelA Ser 276 phosphorylation coupled to CDK9 promoter recruitment. Nucleic Acids Res 42:8416–8432

Ferrer-Sueta G, Batinić-Haberle I, Spasojević I, Fridovich I, Radi R (1999) Catalytic scavenging of peroxynitrite by isomeric Mn(III) N-methylpyridylporphyrins in the presence of reductants. Chem Res Toxicol 12:442–449

Fleckenstein K et al (2007) Using biological markers to predict risk of radiation injury. Semin Radiat Oncol 17:89–98

Garon EB et al (2019) CANOPY-A: a phase III study of canakinumab as adjuvant therapy in patients with surgically resected non-small cell lung cancer (NSCLC). J Clin Oncol 37:TPS8570-TPS8570

Gauter-Fleckenstein B et al (2008) Comparison of two Mn porphyrin-based mimics of superoxide dismutase in pulmonary radioprotection. Free Radic Biol Med 44:982–989

Gauter-Fleckenstein B et al (2014) Robust rat pulmonary radioprotection by a lipophilic Mn N-alkylpyridylporphyrin, MnTnHex-2-PyP(5+). Redox Biol 2:400–410

Giannopoulou E, Papadimitriou E (2003) Amifostine has antiangiogenic properties in vitro by changing the redox status of human endothelial cells. Free Radic Res 37:1191–1199

Grdina DJ, Murley JS, Kataoka Y (2002) Radioprotectants: current status and new directions. Oncology 63(Suppl 2):2–10

Grdina DJ et al (2009) Amifostine induces antioxidant enzymatic activities in normal tissues and a transplantable tumor that can affect radiation response. Int J Radia Oncol Biol Phys 73:886–896

Groarke JD et al (2015) Abnormal exercise response in long-term survivors of hodgkin lymphoma treated with thoracic irradiation: evidence of cardiac autonomic dysfunction and impact on outcomes. J Am Coll Cardiol 65:573–583

Handy DE, Loscalzo J (2012) Redox regulation of mitochondrial function. Antioxid Redox Signal 16:1323–1367

Hirahara K et al (2010) Signal transduction pathways and transcriptional regulation in Th17 cell differentiation. Cytokine Growth Factor Rev 21:425–434

Holmlund J et al (2020) ROMAN: reduction in oral mucositis with avasopasem manganese (GC4419)–phase III trial in patients receiving chemoradiotherapy for locally advanced, nonmetastatic head and neck cancer. J Clin Oncol 38:TPS6596-TPS6596

Hu B et al (2016) The DNA-sensing AIM2 inflammasome controls radiation-induced cell death and tissue injury. Science 354:765–768

Hunter NR et al (2013) Mitigation and treatment of radiation-induced thoracic injury with a cyclooxygenase-2 inhibitor, celecoxib. Int J Radia Oncol Biol Phys 85:472–476

Iribarren K et al (2016) Trial watch: immunostimulation with toll-like receptor agonists in cancer therapy. Oncoimmunology 5:e1088631

Jayakumar S, Pal D, Sandur SK (2015) Nrf2 facilitates repair of radiation induced DNA damage through homologous recombination repair pathway in a ROS independent manner in cancer cells. Mutat Res 779:33–45

Kalita B, Ranjan R, Gupta ML (2019) Combination treatment of podophyllotoxin and rutin promotes mouse Lgr5 + ve intestinal stem cells survival against lethal radiation injury through Wnt signaling. Apoptosis 24:326–340

Kalman NS, Zhao SS, Anscher MS, Urdaneta AI (2017) Current status of targeted radioprotection and radiation injury mitigation and treatment agents: a critical review of the literature. Int J Radia Oncol Biol Phys 98:662–682

Kanda T, Takahashi T (2004) Interleukin-6 and cardiovascular diseases. Jpn Heart J 45:183–193

Karlsson JOG, Andersson RG, Jynge P (2017) Mangafodipir a selective cytoprotectant - with special reference to oxaliplatin and its association to chemotherapy-induced peripheral neuropathy (CIPN). Transl Oncol 10:641–649

Keshavarz A et al (2021) Toll-like receptors (TLRs) in cancer; with an extensive focus on TLR agonists and antagonists. IUBMB Life 73:10–25

Kim J-Y et al (2019) Radioprotective effect of newly synthesized toll-like receptor 5 agonist, KMRC011, in mice exposed to total-body irradiation. J Radiat Res 60:432–441

Komaki R et al (2004) Effects of amifostine on acute toxicity from concurrent chemotherapy and radiotherapy for inoperable non–small-cell lung cancer: report of a randomized comparative trial. Int J Radia Oncol Biol Phys 58:1369–1377

Kosmacek EA, Chatterjee A, Tong Q, Lin C, Oberley-Deegan RE (2016) MnTnBuOE-2-PyP protects normal colorectal fibroblasts from radiation damage and simultaneously enhances radio/chemotherapeutic killing of colorectal cancer cells. Oncotarget 7:34532

Krivokrysenko V, Toshov I, Gleiberman A, Gudkov A, Feinstein E (2010) Single injection of novel medical radiation countermeasure CBLB502 rescues nonhuman primates within broad time window after lethal irradiation. In: 56th Annual Meeting of the Radiation Research Society, Maui, Hawaii

Krivokrysenko VI et al (2015) The toll-like receptor 5 agonist entolimod mitigates lethal acute radiation syndrome in non-human primates. PLoS One 10:e0135388

Krüse JJCM et al (2001) Structural changes in the auricles of the rat heart after local ionizing irradiation. Radiother Oncol 58:303–311

Le RQ et al (2018) FDA approval summary: tocilizumab for treatment of chimeric antigen receptor T cell-induced severe or life-threatening cytokine release syndrome. Oncologist 23:943

Lee MG, Freeman AR, Roos DE, Milner AD, Borg MF (2019) Randomized double-blind trial of amifostine versus placebo for radiation-induced xerostomia in patients with head and neck cancer. J Med Imaging Radiat Oncol 63:142–150

Lefaix J-L et al (1996) Successful treatment of radiation-induced fibrosis using CuZn-SOD and Mn-SOD: an experimental study. Int J Radia Oncol Biol Phys 35:305–312

Leu D et al (2017) CNS bioavailability and radiation protection of normal hippocampal neurogenesis by a lipophilic Mn porphyrin-based superoxide dismutase mimic, MnTnBuOE-2-PyP5+. Redox Biol 12:864–871

Lierova A et al (2018) Cytokines and radiation-induced pulmonary injuries. J Radiat Res 59:709–753

Liu Z et al (2018) Toll-like receptors and radiation protection. Eur Rev Med Pharmacol Sci 22:31–39

Liu B, Li M, Zhou Z, Guan X, Xiang Y (2020) Can we use interleukin-6 (IL-6) blockade for coronavirus disease 2019 (COVID-19)-induced cytokine release syndrome (CRS)? J Autoimmun 111:102452

Mapuskar KA et al (2019) Utilizing superoxide dismutase mimetics to enhance radiation therapy response while protecting normal tissues. Semin Radiat Oncol 29:72–80

Marzatico F et al (2000) In vitro antioxidant properties of amifostine (WR-2721, Ethyol). Cancer Chemother Pharmacol 45:172–176

Milas L, Hanson W (1995) Eicosanoids and radiation. Eur J Cancer 31:1580–1585

Milas L et al (1992) Radiation protection against early and late effects of ionizing irradiation by the prostaglandin inhibitor indomethacin. Adv Space Res 12:265–271

Millán JL (2006) Alkaline phosphatases. Purinergic Signal 2:335

Mohsen C et al (2018) COX-2 in radiotherapy: a potential target for radioprotection and radiosensitization. Curr Mol Pharmacol 11:173–183

Molkentine JM et al (2019) Enteral activation of WR-2721 mediates radioprotection and improved survival from lethal fractionated radiation. Sci Rep 9:1949

Movsas B et al (2005) Randomized trial of amifostine in locally advanced non–small-cell lung cancer patients receiving chemotherapy and hyperfractionated radiation: radiation therapy oncology group trial 98-01. J Clin Oncol 23:2145–2154

Movsas B et al (2007) Randomized trial of amifostine in locally advanced non–small cell lung cancer (NSCLC) patients receiving chemotherapy and hyperfractionated radiation (HRT): long-term survival results of Radiation Therapy Oncology Group (RTOG) 9801. J Clin Oncol 25:7529–7529

Nicolatou-Galitis O et al (2013) Systematic review of amifostine for the management of oral mucositis in cancer patients. Support Care Cancer 21:357–364

Ormsby RJ et al (2014) Protection from radiation-induced apoptosis by the radioprotector amifostine (WR-2721) is radiation dose dependent. Cell Biol Toxicol 30:55–66

Ough M et al (2004) Inhibition of cell growth by overexpression of manganese superoxide dismutase (MnSOD) in human pancreatic carcinoma. Free Radic Res 38:1223–1233

Petkau A, Chelack WS, Pleskach SD (1978) Protection by superoxide dismutase of white blood cells in X-irradiated mice. Life Sci 22:867–881

Preissner S et al (2010) SuperCYP: a comprehensive database on Cytochrome P450 enzymes including a tool for analysis of CYP-drug interactions. Nucleic Acids Res 38:D237–D243

Purdie JW, Inhaber ER, Schneider H, Labelle JL (1983) Interaction of cultured mammalian cells with WR-2721 and its thiol, WR-1065: implications for mechanisms of radioprotection. Int J Radiat Biol Relat Stud Phys Chem Med 43:517–527

Rasey JS, Krohn KA, Menard TW, Spence AM (1986) Comparative biodistribution and radioprotection studies with three radioprotective drugs in mouse tumors. Int J Radia Oncol Biol Phys 12:1487–1490

Raymond RJ, Dehmer GJ, Theoharides TC, Deliargyris EN (2001) Elevated interleukin-6 levels in patients with asymptomatic left ventricular systolic dysfunction. Am Heart J 141:435–438

Ridker PM et al (2018) Relationship of C-reactive protein reduction to cardiovascular event reduction following treatment with canakinumab: a secondary analysis from the CANTOS randomised controlled trial. Lancet 391:319–328

Rose-John S, Scheller J, Elson G, Jones SA (2006) Interleukin-6 biology is coordinated by membrane-bound and soluble receptors: role in inflammation and cancer. J Leukoc Biol 80:227–236

Rossotti R et al (2020) Safety and efficacy of anti-il6-receptor tocilizumab use in severe and critical patients affected by coronavirus disease 2019: a comparative analysis. J Infect 81:e11–e17

Ruben JD et al (2006) Cerebral radiation necrosis: incidence, outcomes, and risk factors with emphasis on radiation parameters and chemotherapy. Int J Radiat Oncol Biol Phys 65:499–508

Rubin P, Johnston CJ, Williams JP, McDonald S, Finkelstein JN (1995) A perpetual cascade of cytokines postirradiation leads to pulmonary fibrosis. Int J Radia Oncol Biol Phys 33:99–109

Sarsour EH, Kumar MG, Chaudhuri L, Kalen AL, Goswami PC (2009) Redox control of the cell cycle in health and disease. Antioxid Redox Signal 11:2985–3011

Savoye C, Swenberg C, Hugot S, Sy D, Sabattier R, Charlier M, Spotheim-Maurizot M (1997) Thiol WR-1065 and disulphide WR-33278, two metabolites of the drug Ethyol (WR-2721), protect DNA against fast neutroninduced strand breakage. Int J Radiat Biol 71:193–202

Schaue D, Kachikwu EL, McBride WH (2012) Cytokines in radiobiological responses: a review. Radiat Res 178:505–523., 519

Screpanti E et al (2010) A screen for kinetochore-microtubule interaction inhibitors identifies novel antitubulin compounds. PLoS One 5:e11603

Shrishrimal S, Kosmacek EA, Chatterjee A, Tyson MJ, Oberley-Deegan RE (2017) The SOD mimic, MnTE-2-PyP, protects from chronic fibrosis and inflammation in irradiated normal pelvic tissues. Antioxidants 6:87

Sia J, Szmyd R, Hau E, Gee HE (2020) Molecular mechanisms of radiation-induced cancer cell death: a primer. Front Cell Dev Biol 8:41

Singh VK, Seed TM (2020) Pharmacological management of ionizing radiation injuries: current and prospective agents and targeted organ systems. Expert Opin Pharmacother 21:317–337

Singh A et al (2017) Podophyllotoxin and rutin modulates ionizing radiation-induced oxidative stress and apoptotic cell death in mice bone marrow and spleen. Front Immunol 8:183

Sisakht M et al (2020) The role of radiation induced oxidative stress as a regulator of radio-adaptive responses. Int J Radiat Biol 96:561–576

Sishc BJ et al (2020) The superoxide dismutase mimetic GC4419 enhances tumor killing when combined with stereotactic ablative radiation. bioRxiv:2020.2003.2010.984443

Smith M et al (2018) Trial watch: toll-like receptor agonists in cancer immunotherapy. Oncoimmunology 7:e1526250

Stankovic JSK, Selakovic D, Mihailovic V, Rosic G (2020) Antioxidant supplementation in the treatment of neurotoxicity induced by platinum-based chemotherapeutics—a review. Int J Mol Sci 21:7753

Stone JH et al (2017) Trial of tocilizumab in giant-cell arteritis. N Engl J Med 377:317–328

Story MD et al (2018) The radioprotector GC4419 ameliorates radiation induced lung fibrosis while enhancing the response of non-small cell lung cancer tumors to high dose per fraction radiation exposures. Int J Radia Oncol Biol Phys 102:S187

Takeuchi T et al (2017) Sirukumab for rheumatoid arthritis: the phase III SIRROUND-D study. Ann Rheum Dis 76:2001–2008

Tanaka T, Narazaki M, Kishimoto T (2014) IL-6 in inflammation, immunity, and disease. Cold Spring Harb Perspect Biol 6:a016295

Tarhini AA et al (2011) A phase I study of concurrent chemotherapy (paclitaxel and carboplatin) and thoracic radiotherapy with swallowed manganese superoxide dismutase plasmid liposome protection in patients with locally advanced stage III non-small-cell lung cancer. Hum Gene Ther 22:336–342

Téoule R (1987) Radiation-induced DNA damage and its repair. Int J Radiat Biol Relat Stud Phys Chem Med 51:573–589

Travis EL (1984) The oxygen dependence of protection by aminothiols: implications for normal tissues and solid tumors. Int J Radia Oncol Biol Phys 10:1495–1501

Tse HM, Milton MJ, Piganelli JD (2004) Mechanistic analysis of the immunomodulatory effects of a catalytic antioxidant on antigen-presenting cells: implication for their use in targeting oxidation–reduction reactions in innate immunity. Free Radic Biol Med 36:233–247

Turrens JF, Crapo JD, Freeman BA (1984) Protection against oxygen toxicity by intravenous injection of liposome-entrapped catalase and superoxide dismutase. J Clin Invest 73:87–95

Vacchelli E et al (2012) Trial watch. Oncoimmunology 1:493–506

Van Dongen J, Kooyman J, Visser W, Holt S, Galjaard H (1977) The effect of increased crypt cell proliferation on the activity and subcellular localization of esterases and alkaline phosphatase in the rat small intestine. Histochem J 9:61–75

Verma S et al (2017) A combination of podophyllotoxin and rutin alleviates radiation-induced pneumonitis and fibrosis through modulation of lung inflammation in mice. Front Immunol 8:658

Vidya MK et al (2018) Toll-like receptors: significance, ligands, signaling pathways, and functions in mammals. Int Rev Immunol 37:20–36

Volcic M et al (2012) NF-κB regulates DNA double-strand break repair in conjunction with BRCA1–CtIP complexes. Nucleic Acids Res 40:181–195

Ward HE, Kemsley L, Davies L, Holecek M, Berend N (1993) The effect of steroids on radiation-induced lung disease in the rat. Radiat Res 136:22–28

Wolff J, Knipling L, Cahnmann H, Palumbo G (1991) Direct photoaffinity labeling of tubulin with colchicine. Proc Natl Acad Sci 88:2820–2824

Yang JQ et al (2002) v-Ha-ras mitogenic signaling through superoxide and derived reactive oxygen species. Mol Carcinog 33:206–218

Yang H et al (2015) MD-2 is required for disulfide HMGB1-dependent TLR4 signaling. J Exp Med 212:5–14

Yashavarddhan MH et al (2017) Targeting DNA repair through podophyllotoxin and rutin formulation in hematopoietic radioprotection: an in silico, in vitro, and in vivo study. Front Pharmacol 8:750

Yuhas JM, Spellman JM, Culo F (1980) The role of WR-2721 in radiotherapy and/or chemotherapy. Cancer Clin Trials 3:211–216

Zhang Y-L et al (1992) Antitumor agents, 130. novel 4β-arylamino derivatives of 3', 4'-didemethoxy-3', 4'-dioxo-4-deoxypodophyllotoxin as potent inhibitors of human DNA topoisomerase II. J Nat Prod 55:1100–1111

Zhang W et al (2020) The use of anti-inflammatory drugs in the treatment of people with severe coronavirus disease 2019 (COVID-19): the perspectives of clinical immunologists from China. Clin Immunol 214:108393

Zhao Y et al (2017) A novel redox regulator, MnTnBuOE-2-PyP5+, enhances normal hematopoietic stem/progenitor cell function. Redox Biol 12:129–138

Zhu J et al (2010) Recombinant human interleukin-1 receptor antagonist protects mice against acute doxorubicin-induced cardiotoxicity. Eur J Pharmacol 643:247–253

Chemotherapy for Lung Cancer

Mariam Alexander, Elaine Shum, Aditi Singh, and Balazs Halmos

Contents

1	Introduction..	322
2	**Chemotherapy in Early-Stage, Resectable Non-small Cell Lung Cancer**........................	323
2.1	Adjuvant Chemotherapy...................................	323
2.2	Neoadjuvant Systemic Therapy........................	327
2.3	Adjuvant Targeted Therapy..............................	329
3	**Chemotherapy in Locally Advanced, Unresectable NSCLC**...	329
4	**Metastatic Setting in NSCLC**............................	330
4.1	First Line: Combination with Immunotherapy...	331
4.2	Second-Line and Beyond..................................	334
5	**Role of Chemotherapy in Tumors with Driver Mutations/Targeted Therapy**....	335
6	**Combinations with Angiogenesis Inhibitors**..	336
7	**Antibody-Drug Conjugates**.............................	338
8	**Small Cell Lung Cancer**....................................	338
9	**Conclusion**...	340
References..		340

M. Alexander
Hollings Cancer Center, Medical University of South Carolina, Charleston, SC, USA

E. Shum
Perlmutter Cancer Center, New York University Langone Health, New York, NY, USA

A. Singh
Division of Hematology/Oncology, Department of Medicine, University of Pennsylvania, Philadelphia, PA, USA

B. Halmos (✉)
Department of Oncology, Montefiore Medical Center/Albert Einstein College of Medicine, Bronx, NY, USA
e-mail: bahalmos@montefiore.org

Abstract

Platinum-based chemotherapy has been the mainstay of treatment for metastatic non-small cell lung cancer (NSCLC) since the early 1990s. Over the last decade, there has been a revolution of treatment options in the realm of molecularly targeted therapy and immunotherapy. Although these advances have transformed the landscape of lung cancer therapy, cytotoxic chemotherapy continues to be an essential component of lung cancer treatment. Extensive evidence has demonstrated the clinical benefit of chemotherapy, either alone or in combination with other modalities, on survival and quality of life of patients with early-stage, locally advanced and advanced non-small cell lung cancer and constitutes the mainstay of therapy for small cell lung cancer. Chemotherapy also remains the standard of care in patients that have progressed after other agents and will continue to be a fundamental means of lung cancer management now in novel delivery formats as a key component of antibody-drug conjugates.

This chapter will discuss the history, current role of chemotherapy, and specific considerations for its clinical application in the era of personalized medicine.

1 Introduction

Lung cancer is the second most common cancer and the leading cause of cancer death in the United States with approximately 247,270 new cases of lung cancer that occurred in 2020 (American Cancer Society 2020). Lung cancer results in more deaths than breast cancer, prostate cancer, colorectal cancer, and leukemia combined in men greater than 40 years old and women greater than 60 years old. The past decade has seen a revolution of new advances in the management of NSCLC with remarkable progress in screening, diagnosis, and treatment. Recent advances in systemic treatment have been driven primarily by the development of molecularly targeted therapeutics and immune checkpoint inhibitors (ICIs), both of which have transformed this field with significantly improved patient outcomes (Pakkala and Ramalingam 2018; Marrone et al. 2016). However, despite these major changes in lung cancer management, the majority of patients with lung cancer still requires platinum-based chemotherapy during their optimal therapy, and moreover chemotherapy often remains the preferred second line of treatment after failure of molecular driver targeting agents and immunotherapy. Figure 1 provides a timeline of the landmark trials in the history of chemotherapy-based treatment in non-small cell lung cancer.

The advent of chemotherapy dates back to 1948 when Karnofsky et al. reported on the activity of nitrogen mustard in bronchogenic carcinoma (Karnofsky 1948). It was another 40 years before chemotherapy was shown to improve survival compared to best supportive care. The median overall survival of metastatic lung cancer prior to chemotherapy was a mere 2–4 months with best supportive care alone. The benefits of early generation chemotherapeutic agents, including methotrexate and doxorubicin, were modest (Rockswold et al. 1970). It was only in the 1980s and 1990s, with the introduction of platinum, taxanes, vinorelbine, and gemcitabine, when a survival benefit was seen. The 1995 Non-Small Cell Lung Cancer Collaborative group demonstrated that platinum-based chemotherapy

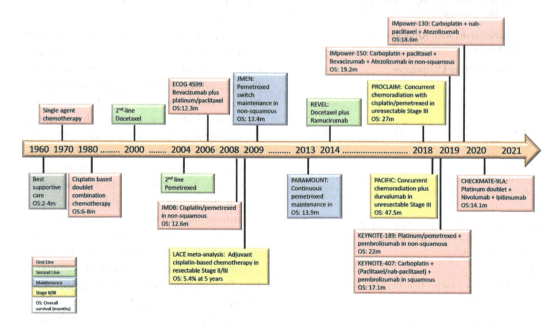

Fig. 1 Landmark trials in the history of chemotherapy-based treatment in non-small cell lung cancer

significantly improved overall survival (OS) over best supportive care (15% vs. 5% OS in 1 year) (Non-small Cell Lung Cancer Collaborative Group 1995). In addition, platinum doublets showed superior efficacy over non-platinum-based regimens or single-agent therapy (D'Addario et al. 2005). Based on this, combinations of platinum were recommended as the new generation of agents for the first-line treatment of advanced NSCLC and the pivotal ECOG1594 study demonstrated equivalence of multiple doublets incorporating carboplatin-based regimens with more novel agents yielding better tolerated treatment regimens (Schiller et al. 2002). In the early 2000s, the novel antifolate agent pemetrexed was introduced as a new chemotherapeutic agent first as a second-line agent (Hanna et al. 2004). Later pemetrexed demonstrated superior clinical benefit in nonsquamous histology over a gemcitabine-based regimen (Scagliotti et al. 2008), which showed that histology does matter in the treatment of lung cancer (Scagliotti et al. 2012; Rossi et al. 2018). Pemetrexed was then shown to have clinical benefit as a maintenance therapy significantly improving the median OS of patients with nonsquamous NSCLC (Ciuleanu et al. 2009). The mid-2000s and early 2010s heralded the development of antiangiogenic drugs such as bevacizumab and ramucirumab as well as drug delivery systems such as nanoparticle albumin-bound paclitaxel (nab-paclitaxel) as valid agents for lung cancer treatment (Adrianzen Herrera et al. 2019). Table 1 outlines the key chemotherapeutic agents currently in use for the treatment of this devastating disease.

2 Chemotherapy in Early-Stage, Resectable Non-small Cell Lung Cancer

2.1 Adjuvant Chemotherapy

Despite surgical resection, patients with early-stage lung cancer can still develop recurrence. The rates of recurrence are dependent on stage and other prognostic factors. As a result, the use of adjuvant chemotherapy with platinum-based regimens is generally recommended for patients with stages II and III and selected stage IB lung cancers based on several studies. The International Adjuvant Lung Cancer Trial (IALT) trial included 1867 patients that were randomized to cisplatin-based doublet chemotherapy or observation. The survival rate at 5 years was 45% with chemotherapy versus 40% with observation showing a statistically significant, albeit modest, overall survival benefit with the use of adjuvant chemotherapy (HR 0.86, 95% CI 0.76–0.98, $p < 0.03$) (Arriagada et al. 2004).

The regimen of cisplatin and vinorelbine for postoperative chemotherapy was explored in the NCIC CTG JBR.10 (Winton et al. 2005) and ANITA trials (Douillard et al. 2006) (Table 2). The JBR.10 trial investigated the role of adjuvant chemotherapy in patients with pathologic stage IB and II disease. The study included 482 patients comparing the use of vinorelbine plus cisplatin versus observation alone. Overall survival (OS) was found to be 94 months in the chemotherapy group versus 73 months in the observation group (HR 0.69, $p = 0.04$). An update in 2010 with a median follow-up of 9.3 years continued to show a survival advantage in the chemotherapy group, although only in patients with stage II NSCLC (median survival 6.8 vs. 3.6 years for patients on observation, $p = 0.01$). The ANITA trial enrolled 840 patients with stage IB-IIIA NSCLC and compared the use of postoperative vinorelbine plus cisplatin versus observation (Douillard et al. 2006). This important study showed a median survival of 65.7 months in the chemotherapy group compared to 43.7 months in the observation group ($p = 0.017$).

The Lung Adjuvant Cisplatin Evaluation (LACE) study was a meta-analysis that pooled patients from five large phase III adjuvant chemotherapy trials and found a 5.4% survival benefit of cisplatin-based adjuvant chemotherapy compared to observation supporting what had previously been reported (Pignon et al. 2008). When analyzed based on stage of disease, it demonstrated that patients with stage I disease derived no benefit from chemotherapy, whereas stage II and III disease did see a significant effect on survival.

Table 1 Key chemotherapeutic agents currently in use for the treatment of lung cancer

Class	Group	Mechanism/biology	Agent	Common side effects	Unique aspects	Common use
DNA-targeting agents	Platinum drugs DNA crosslinks	Higher sensitivity in cells with impaired DNA repair (BRCA, ERCC1)	Cisplatin (CDDP)	Myelotoxicity, high emetogenicity	Oto/Nephro/neurotoxicity Needs aggressive fluids and antiemetic support. Platinum hypersensitivity	Adjuvant therapy for NSCLC Concurrent chemoradiation (preferred in LSCLC)
			Carboplatin	More severe myelotoxicity than CDDP	Purely renally excreted, dosed based on Calvert formula	Concurrent chemoradiation for stage III NSCLC Carboplatin-based doublets for first-line advanced NSCLC ES-SCLC
	DNA-modifying agents	DNA alkylation	Cyclophosphamide	Myelotoxicity, hemorrhagic cystitis, secondary malignancies		Rarely used in ES-SCLC
		DNA alkylation/methylation on N7 or O-6 of guanines, repaired by MGMT	Temozolomide	Myelotoxicity, immune suppression	CNS penetration	Rarely used in ES-SCLC, CNS metastases
	Nucleoside analog	Integrates into DNA strand, masked chain termination	Gemcitabine	Mild myelotoxicity, prominent thrombocytopenia	Radiation recall Increased risk of XRT pulmonary toxicity	In squamous cell NSCLC in platinum-based doublet as adjuvant or single agent as second/third line in advanced NSCLC
	Antimetabolites	Folate antagonist blocking the activity of TS, GRFT and GRFT	Pemetrexed	Myelotoxicity, fluid retention, skin rash	Requires folic acid/B12 supplementation Not recommended with GFR <45 Not to be used in squamous histology	Platinum-based doublets Maintenance therapy Second-line therapy for nonsquamous NSCLC Mesothelioma
	DNA transcription targeting agent	Covalent binding of minor groove of DNA, changes in DNA transcription	Lurbinectedin	Myelotoxicity, GI side effects	Marine derived agent	Second/third-line ES-SCLC

Chemotherapy for Lung Cancer

Class	Group	Mechanism/biology	Agent	Common side effects	Unique aspects	Common use
Topoisomerase inhibitors	Topo I inhibitors	Blocks topo-I which relieves torsional strain in DNA by single-strand breaks	Topotecan	Myelotoxicity, GI side effects	Available both iv and oral	Second-line ES-SCLC
			Irinotecan	Myelotoxicity, severe diarrhea	Active metabolite SN-38 Toxicities dependent on activity of UGT1A1 enzyme	Second- and beyond-line ES-SCLC Liposomal formulation in development for SCLC
	Topo II inhibitors	Block topo II impairing DNA relegation resulting in DNA breaks	Etoposide	Myelotoxicity, GI toxicities, BL changes, secondary AML	Consider use of G-CSF support	In combination with CDDP/carboplatin for stage III NSCLC and ES-SCLC
			Doxorubicin	Myelotoxicity, cardiotoxicity, vesicant	Also alternate mechanisms of action	Rarely used in second/third-line ES-SCLC
Microtubule-targeting agents	Microtubule-inhibiting agents	Block beta-tubulin polymerization and thereby disrupt microtubule assembly impairing cell division/motility/trafficking	Vincristine	Neuropathy, myelotoxicity, vesicant	Dose needs to be capped to avoid severe neurotoxicity	Rarely used in second/third-line ES-SCLC
			Vinorelbine	Neuropathy, myelotoxicity, vesicant	Central line preferred	Platinum-based doublet in adjuvant therapy for NSCLC
	Microtubule-stabilizing agents	Stabilize GDP-bound tubulin thereby inhibiting depolymerization leading to mitotic inhibition	Paclitaxel	Neuropathy, myelotoxicity, hypersensitivity reactions	Needs to be solubilized in Cremaphor which leads to HS reactions Severe neuropathy precludes use with CDDP Requires steroid and antihistamine premedications	Carboplatin-based doublets for stage III NSCLC, first-line advanced NSCLC Second/third-line ES-SCLC
			Nab-paclitaxel	Neuropathy, myelotoxicity	Nanoalbumin-bound paclitaxel Drastically reduces risk of HS reactions No need for steroid premedications	Carboplatin-based doublets As single agent in second-line and beyond NSCLC
			Docetaxel	Myelotoxicity, GI side effects, neuropathy	Formulated in polysorbate 80 Requires steroid premedications	Platinum-based doublets for adjuvant NSCLC, second-line advanced NSCLC

CDDP cisplatin (cis-diamminedichloro-platinum), *TS* thymidylate synthase, *DHFR* dihydrofolate reductase, *GRFT* glycinamide ribonucleotide formyltransferase, *HS* hypersensitivity reactions

Table 2 Adjuvant trials

Trial	Stage	Regimen	Results
International adjuvant lung cancer trial (IALT) (Arriagada et al. 2004)	I–III (1986 AJCC classification)	Cisplatin-based doublet vs. observation	5-Years OS: 44.5% vs. 40.4% (HR 0.86, $p < 0.03$)
JBR.10 (Winton et al. 2005)	IB–II	Cisplatin/vinorelbine vs. observation	Median OS: 94 vs. 73 months (HR 0.69, $p = 0.04$)
ANITA (Douillard et al. 2006)	IB–IIIA (1986 AJCC classification)	Cisplatin/vinorelbine vs. observation	Median PFS: 36.3 vs. 20.7 months (HR 0.80, $p = 0.017$) Median OS: 65.7 vs. 43.7 months (HR 0.80, $p = 0.017$)
PEARLS/KEYNOTE-091 (Paz-Ares et al. 2022)	IB-IIIA (7th ed AJCC)	Pembrolizumab versus Placebo after adjuvant chemotherapy	Median DFS: 53.6 vs 42.0 months (HR: 0.76, $p = 0.0014$) OS 18 month rate: 91.7% vs 91.3% (HR 0.87; $p = 0.17$)
IMpower-010 (Felip et al. 2021) *FDA Approved for PD-L1 ≥ 1%*	II–IIIA (7th ed AJCC)	Atezolizumab versus BSC after adjuvant chemotherapy	Median DFS: not-reached vs. 35.3 months (HR 0.66, $p = 0.004$)

OS overall survival, *PFS* progression-free survival, *BSC* Best supportive care

While these studies mostly focused on the benefit of cisplatin and vinorelbine, the potential toxicities of vinorelbine make it less favorable for use. These toxicities include peripheral neuropathy and myelosuppression, and as a vesicant, it requires central intravenous access. The LACE meta-analysis did not favor one regimen over the other, but commonly for nonsquamous histology, cisplatin and pemetrexed is used, and for squamous histology, cisplatin with gemcitabine, docetaxel, or vinorelbine is recommended. The TREAT study compared the use of cisplatin and pemetrexed versus cisplatin and vinorelbine as adjuvant therapy in patients with stages IB-III nonsquamous lung cancer. The trial showed that cisplatin and pemetrexed was less toxic, and that overall survival was similar between the two regimens (Kreuter et al. 2013).

The CALGB 9633 study specifically explored adjuvant chemotherapy in patients with stage IB NSCLC using carboplatin and paclitaxel and while it did not find a survival advantage as it was underpowered to do so, a trend toward benefit was noted. An exploratory analysis of patients who had tumors >4 cm in diameter and received adjuvant chemotherapy did yield a survival difference (HR 0.69, 95% CI 0.48–0.99) (Strauss et al. 2008). Therefore, while less evidence-based, in patients who are reasonable candidates for adjuvant chemotherapy but are not candidates for cisplatin (e.g., kidney or hearing dysfunction), carboplatin-based doublets are viewed as acceptable.

The ECOG 1505 trial explored the use of bevacizumab in combination with adjuvant chemotherapy (Wakelee et al. 2016). The chemotherapy regimens included in this trial all used a cisplatin backbone with investigator's choice of either vinorelbine, docetaxel, gemcitabine (squamous) or pemetrexed (nonsquamous). Patients were randomized to receive chemotherapy alone or bevacizumab with adjuvant chemotherapy with bevacizumab continued for up to a year. The study did not find an improvement in median OS with the addition of bevacizumab (86 months with bevacizumab versus not reached, HR 0.99, 95% CI 0.82–1.19) and also reported increased grade 3–5 toxicities (Wakelee et al. 2016). Although the trial did not see the benefit of adding bevacizumab, it did provide noteworthy data with regard to the use of the four different chemotherapy regimens and did not find any differences in OS or disease-free survival (DFS) among them. As expected, vinorelbine was associated with more neutropenia and gemcitabine was associated with more thrombocytopenia. This study supports the standard of care use of cisplatin and pemetrexed for nonsquamous histology and cisplatin and gemcitabine for squamous histology, and all four chemotherapy regimens are listed as preferred regimens by NCCN guidelines for both adjuvant and neoadjuvant use.

Given the modest benefits of adjuvant chemotherapy, there is a clear need for additional adjuvant therapy strategies. IMpower010 is a Phase III open-label, randomized trial comparing the use of atezolizumab versus best supportive care in patients with stage IB-IIIA NSCLC as adjuvant therapy after surgery and chemotherapy. There was an improvement in DFS in patients with Stage II-IIIA with a PD-L1 expression of ≥ 1% (DFS: NR vs 25.3 months; HR 0.66, 95% CI 0.50-0.88) leading to its FDA approval in October 2021 (Felip et al. 2021). The Adjuvant Nivolumab in Resected Lung Cancers (ANVIL) trial, as part of the ALCHEMIST adjuvant trials, is a randomized phase III trial which enrolled patients to receive adjuvant nivolumab for up to a year or undergo observation following surgical resection and standard adjuvant chemotherapy with or without radiation (NCT02595944). This trial has completed accrual and results are eagerly awaited. A recently opened follow-up study in the ALCHEMIST umbrella protocol now is evaluating the use of checkpoint inhibitor therapy concurrent with adjuvant chemotherapy versus chemotherapy alone (NCT04267848). Additional phase III adjuvant studies using pembrolizumab and durvalumab are also being pursued (NCT02504372, NCT02273375).

2.2 Neoadjuvant Systemic Therapy

Administration of neoadjuvant chemotherapy is often considered with patients with resectable stage IIIA disease, usually with single station N2 involvement, tumors with chest wall invasion, and superior sulcus tumors (with concurrent radiation). The use of neoadjuvant chemotherapy has several advantages as opposed to administering adjuvant chemotherapy, such as increased therapeutic compliance, potential for downstaging, and early treatment of micrometastatic disease. Prolonged recovery from surgery can also impact a patient's ability to tolerate systemic therapy. In addition, neoadjuvant chemotherapy allows for analysis of the posttreatment effects on the primary tumor.

The use of neoadjuvant chemotherapy has been studied since the early 1990s (Rosell et al. 1994) and a meta-analysis explored the overall benefits for all histologic classes of NSCLC for selected patients including 13 randomized control trials showing that OS was significantly improved in patients receiving neoadjuvant chemotherapy compared to surgery alone (HR = 0.84, 95% CI 0.77–0.92, p = 0.0001) (Song et al. 2010). Another meta-analysis looked at 32 randomized trials, comparing 22 adjuvant trials with 10 neoadjuvant trials, and found no difference in OS or DFS between the two groups (Lim et al. 2009).

A phase III study exploring neoadjuvant chemotherapy with cisplatin and gemcitabine for stages IB to IIIA randomized patients to receive either three preoperative cycles of gemcitabine and cisplatin every 3 weeks followed by surgery, or surgery alone. In this study, 129 patients were randomly assigned to the chemotherapy plus surgery group, and 127 patients received at least one dose of chemotherapy. The study closed early but did find a significant survival benefit for patients with stages IIB and IIIA who received neoadjuvant chemotherapy (HR 0.63, 95% CI 0.43–0.92, p = 0.02) (Scagliotti et al. 2012).

Given the success of immune checkpoint inhibition in metastatic disease, several studies have explored the use of immunotherapy in early-stage disease (Table 3). The use of single agent nivolumab in the neoadjuvant setting was demonstrated in a small pilot study of 21 patients. In this study, the patients received two cycles of nivolumab preoperatively. The study found that 45% of patients had a major pathologic response (MPR) and no surgical delays related to immunotherapy (Forde et al. 2018). The NEOSTAR study is a phase 2 randomized clinical trial with two neoadjuvant treatment arms: nivolumab monotherapy and nivolumab and ipilimumab (Cascone et al. 2021). Forty-four patients were on the

Table 3 Neoadjuvant immunotherapy trials

Trial	Stage	Regimen	Results
Forde et al. (2018)	I–IIIA (7th ed AJCC)	Nivolumab × 2 cycles	MPR 45%
Shu et al. (2020)	IB–IIIA (7th ed AJCC)	Carboplatin/nab-paclitaxel + Atezolizumab	MPR 57% pCR 33%
NADIM (Provencio et al. 2020)	IIIA (7th ed AJCC)	Carboplatin/paclitaxel + Nivolumab	MPR 83% pCR 63% 2-Years PFS: 77.1% (95% CI 59.9–87.7)
NEOSTAR (Cascone et al. 2021)	I–IIIA (7th ed AJCC)	Nivolumab (D1, 15, 29) or Nivolumab (D1, 15, 29)/ipilimumab (D1)	Nivolumab: MPR 22%, pCR 10% Nivolumab/ipilimumab: MPR 38%, pCR 38%
CheckMate-816 (Forde et al. 2022) *FDA Approved*	IB–IIIA (7th ed AJCC)	Nivolumab + Platinum-doublet chemotherapy versus Platinum-doublet chemotherapy (Phase 3 Randomized trial)	EFS 31.6 months vs. 20.8 months (HR 0.63, 0.43-0.91, $p = 0.005$) pCR: 24% versus 2.2% (OR: 13.94, 3.49-55.75, $p < 0.001$)

MPR major pathological response, *pCR* pathological complete response, *EFS* Event-Free Survival, *pCR* pathologic complete response, *OR* odds ratio

study, of which 41 received neoadjuvant immunotherapy. The overall MPR for the study in the intention-to-treat population which included the 23 patients who received neoadjuvant nivolumab was 22% (CI 7–44%) and for the 21 patients who received neoadjuvant nivolumab and ipilimumab was 38% (CI 18–62%, $p = 0.235$). Of the 44 patients, 37 underwent surgical resection on study with a 24% MPR rate in the nivolumab arm versus 50% in the nivolumab and ipilimumab arm ($p = 0.098$). There were also more pathological complete responses (pCR) in the nivolumab and ipilimumab group at 38% (CI 18–62%) versus 10% who received nivolumab alone. Of the five patients (1 in nivolumab arm, 4 in nivolumab and ipilimumab arm) who did not undergo surgical resection, none were determined to be related to treatment-related adverse events (TRAEs). Two patients underwent surgical resection off trial, one of whom had a TRAE of grade 3 diarrhea/colitis after one dose of nivolumab and ipilimumab and so their treatment was changed to neoadjuvant chemotherapy (Cascone et al. 2021).

Combining chemotherapy and immunotherapy then started gaining interest. A phase II study enrolled 30 patients with resectable early-stage NSCLC and explored the addition of neoadjuvant atezolizumab in combination with carboplatin and nab-paclitaxel. In this study, 17 of 30 (57%) patients had a MPR and 10 of 30 (33%) patients had a pCR (Shu et al. 2020). The NADIM study, a single-arm phase II trial conducted in Spain enrolled 46 patients with resectable stage IIIA NSCLC who received neoadjuvant carboplatin and paclitaxel plus nivolumab for three cycles prior to surgery, followed by adjuvant nivolumab monotherapy for up to a year. At 24 months, PFS was 77.1% (95% CI 59.9–87.7). Forty-one of the 46 patients went on to have surgery, of which 83% had a MPR and 63% had a pCR. Although 93% of patients had treatment-related adverse events during neoadjuvant therapy, none of the adverse events reported led to surgery delay or death (Provencio et al. 2020). The randomized Phase II NADIM II trial using this neoadjuvant chemoimmunotherapy regimen versus chemotherapy alone is ongoing (NCT03838159).

These studies paved the way for the practice changing Phase III trial, Checkmate-816 (Forde et al. 2022). In this trial, patients with resectable Stage IB (≥4 cm)-IIIA NSCLC were randomized to receive nivolumab plus platinum-doublet chemotherapy versus chemotherapy alone for 3 cycles. The median event-free survival (EFS) was 31.6 months in the combination versus 20.8 months with chemotherapy alone (HR 0.63, 95% CI 0.43-0.91). The pathologic complete response rate was 24% when nivolumab was added versus 2.2% with chemotherapy alone (95% CI 0.6-5.6). These impres-

Table 4 Ongoing phase III neoadjuvant chemotherapy and immunotherapy trials

Trial	Stage	N	Treatment arms	Primary endpoint
CHECKMATE-816 (NCT02998528)	IB–IIIA	350	1. Platinum doublet + Nivolumab 2. Platinum doublet 3. Nivolumab + Ipilimumab (closed)	MPR, EFS
KEYNOTE-671 (NCT03423643)	IIB–IIIA	786	1. Platinum doublet + Pembrolizumab 2. Platinum doublet	EFS, OS
IMpower030 (NCT03456063)	II–IIIB	374	1. Platinum doublet + Atezolizumab 2. Platinum doublet	MPR, EFS
AEGEAN (NCT03800134)	IIA–IIIB	300	1. Platinum doublet + Durvalumab 2. Platinum doublet	MPR

MPR major pathological response, *EFS* event-free survival, *OS* overall survival

sive results led to the FDA approval of this combination regardless of PD-L1 expression in March 2022. Several other phase III neoadjuvant studies using immunotherapy combined with chemotherapy are currently ongoing (Table 4).

Neoadjuvant chemotherapy and radiation have also been extensively studied and demonstrate generally a higher rate of pathological responses; however, they are also associated with increased toxicity including surgical morbidity and mortality counterbalancing the benefits. The pivotal Intergroup study did not demonstrate a survival benefit for trimodality therapy over definitive chemoradiotherapy leading to lessening use of this approach (Albain et al. 2009). Given the heightened interest at present in the potential abscopal effect of radiotherapy facilitating immunotherapy responses, novel clinical study approaches are integrating subtotal doses of radiation into neoadjuvant treatment regimens (NCT02904954).

2.3 Adjuvant Targeted Therapy

The use of targeted therapy in the adjuvant setting has been of great interest but without high-level positive data or specific guideline recommendations until recently. The recently reported positive Phase III ADAURA trial included 682 patients with resected stage IB to IIIA NSCLC and EGFR exon 19 deletion or L858R mutations and randomized them to receive osimertinib or placebo for 3 years (Wu et al. 2020). In patients with stage II and IIIA NSCLC, the disease-free survival was 90% in the osimertinib group and 44% in the placebo group with a HR of 0.17 (99% CI 0.11–0.26, $p < 0.001$). The study was stopped 2 years early and the study was unblinded on study level given the evidence of efficacy. Most patients did receive adjuvant chemotherapy, but not all. Despite this, the benefit of adjuvant osimertinib was seen in both predefined subgroups, such as in stages IB versus II/III. OS data is not yet mature. Recently the FDA-approved adjuvant osimertinib for patients with resectable NSCLC and it is also endorsed by NCCN guidelines. A word of caution is that regardless of the recommendation for osimertinib, adjuvant chemotherapy should continue to be offered as appropriate given its known OS benefits. Future studies might address whether adjuvant chemotherapy could be omitted in certain patient subsets.

Exploration of tyrosine kinase inhibitors in the adjuvant setting for the other known driver mutations in NSCLC are ongoing, such as the ALCHEMIST trial with adjuvant crizotinib (NCT02201992) and the ALINA trial with adjuvant alectinib (NCT03456076) for ALK-positive NSCLC.

3 Chemotherapy in Locally Advanced, Unresectable NSCLC

Locally advanced, unresectable lung cancers have generally been managed with chemotherapy in combination with radiotherapy since the early 1980s. Randomized studies have shown an OS benefit with the addition of chemotherapy to radiation therapy (Dillman et al. 1990; Le Chevalier et al. 1991). The sequencing of these modalities has been debated but several studies have found that concurrent chemoradiation is more efficacious compared to sequential chemoradiation and this topic will be reviewed in detail in another chapter (Curran et al. 2011; Furuse et al. 1999; Aupérin et al. 2010; Belani et al. 2005; Liang et al. 2017; Atagi et al. 2012; Senan et al. 2016). The randomized phase III PACIFIC trial was the most practice-changing study of the last few decades for unresectable stage III NSCLC (Antonia et al. 2017, 2018). This study compared the consolidation use of the anti-PD-L1 antibody, durvalumab 10 mg/kg every 2 weeks versus placebo in patients with locally advanced, unresectable NSCLC. Patients could not have progressed after two or more cycles of concurrent chemoradiation and consolidation durvalumab was started between 1 and 42 days after completion of chemoradiation. Neoadjuvant chemotherapy was allowed but consolidation chemotherapy was not. Updated results have shown that the PFS was 17.2 months with durvalumab and 5.6 months for placebo (HR 0.51, 95% CI 0.41–0.63). In addition, the 3-year OS was not reached with durvalumab versus 29.1 months with placebo (HR 0.69, 95% CI 0.55–0.86) demonstrating a very substantial 10% or so overall survival benefit establishing this regimen as the current standard of care against which all new regimens will need to be measured (Gray et al. 2020). All platinum-based doublet chemotherapy regimens were permitted in this protocol with most patients receiving a platinum-etoposide or carboplatin-paclitaxel regimen. A large number of new studies are now founded upon this new standard of care regimen assessing the additional benefits of novel agents or defining sequencing questions integrated around a PACIFIC regimen backbone (Puri et al. 2020).

4 Metastatic Setting in NSCLC

General Principles
While the last 15 years have seen a drastic transformation in the management of advanced NSCLC with the introduction of targeted therapeutics for molecularly defined subsets of patients and checkpoint inhibitors guided by PD-L1 TPS score testing, conventional chemotherapy does remain a key element of cancer care for a significant majority of patients. Upfront optimal therapy for advanced NSCLC today requires careful biomarker testing—ideally using an NGS-based platform to be able to identify the largest number of patients eligible for the upfront use of targeted therapies such as EGFR/ALK/ROS1 where the level of evidence for frontline use is strongest. In addition, testing for other actionable alterations such as B-Raf V600E, MET exon 14 skipping, RET, NTRK fusions, and ErbB2 alterations open up active treatment choices or at least experimental options (Sharma et al. 2017). Lastly, with the emergence of K-ras G12C targeting agents, testing for K-ras alterations is also emerging as a key element of proper biomarker testing (Hong et al. 2020). ctDNA platforms facilitate the timely completion of such testing, and its use is validated both in the upfront biomarker testing of patients with advanced NSCLC and at the time of acquired resistance on targeted agents (Aggarwal et al. 2020, 2021). In the majority of NSCLC patients without an actionable alteration, the next key question needs to address candidacy for single-agent immunotherapy typically by performing PD-L1 immunohistochemistry testing, most commonly using the 22c3 antibody and TPS scoring (Mino-Kenudson et al. 2021). About a third of all patients with advanced NSCLC will fall into a high positive category (>50% TPS score) where single-agent immunotherapy is a prudent choice, although some patients (e.g., symptomatic/large tumor bulk) might still benefit from chemotherapy and immunotherapy combinations given their higher response rate (Alexander et al. 2020). Ultimately, at least half of the patients diagnosed with advanced NSCLC will not be good candidates for targeted therapy or single-agent immunotherapy. These patients generally are treated with combination chemotherapy and immunotherapy with histology-directed chemotherapy regimens (Kim and Halmos 2020).

Systemic chemotherapy alone today is rarely used in the frontline setting in the management of advanced NSCLC either mostly in patients who

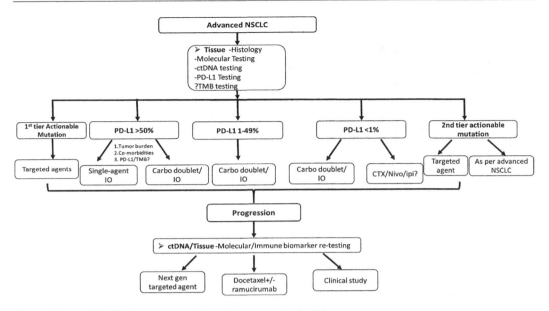

Fig. 2 Advanced NSCLC treatment paradigm without a molecular driver

are not candidates for immunotherapy (e.g., severe autoimmune disease or post-organ transplant), have progressed on prior immunotherapy (e.g., as given during management of locally advanced disease), or have a particular lung cancer subtype that is not viewed to likely benefit from immunotherapy. Figure 2 summarizes the general management schema of patients with advanced NSCLC.

Maintenance chemotherapy following initial four to six cycles of combination chemotherapy has been commonly utilized in patients with non-squamous tumors based on the results of the PARAMOUNT study demonstrating modest but significant overall survival benefits and now along with maintenance immunotherapy (Minami and Kijima 2015; Garon et al. 2021). Generally, no maintenance therapy is used in patients with other histologies, such as squamous or small cell lung cancers.

Antiangiogenic agents, such as the anti-VEGF monoclonal antibody, bevacizumab, and the VEGFR2 targeting monoclonal antibody, ramucirumab, have been approved due to modest added benefits alongside frontline chemotherapy for nonsquamous (Soria et al. 2013) and second-line chemotherapy for both squamous and nonsquamous NSCLC, respectively (Reck et al. 2018).

4.1 First Line: Combination with Immunotherapy

Immune checkpoint inhibitors (ICIs) have dramatically reshaped the therapeutic landscape of various solid tumor malignancies, including advanced NSCLC and SCLC (Hanna et al. 2020). The immune checkpoint pathway involving the receptor, programmed cell death-1 (PD-1) and its ligands programmed cell death-ligand 1 (PD-L1) and programmed cell death-ligand 2 (PD-L2) has proved to be particularly impactful. Two anti-PD-1 agents, pembrolizumab and nivolumab, and three anti-PD-L1 agents, atezolizumab, durvalumab, and cemiplimab, have FDA indications for the treatment of NSCLC or SCLC with multiple other agents under development. Immunotherapy is now an established part of routine care for the overwhelming majority of patients diagnosed with locally advanced and advanced lung cancer (Table 5). Pembrolizumab, a humanized monoclonal IgG4 anti-PD-L1 antibody, was one of the first agents to show efficacy in multiple clinical contexts initially approved based on the KEYNOTE-010 study (Herbst et al. 2016). Soon following first-line indications were granted for the treatment of metastatic NSCLC as a single agent initially in patients with tumors

Table 5 Current FDA-approved chemoimmunotherapy regimens for metastatic non-small cell lung cancer in the first-line setting

Pivotal study	Patient population	Intervention	Comparator arm	Primary outcome: OS/PFS in months (hazard ratio, 95% CI)	Toxicities	Reference
KEYNOTE-189	Nonsquamous; EGFR and ALK negative	Pemetrexed-platinum + Pembrolizumab followed by maintenance Pemetrexed + Pembrolizumab	Pemetrexed-platinum + followed by maintenance Pemetrexed	OS: 22 vs. 10.7 (HR: 0.56, 0.45–0.70) PFS: 9 vs. 4.9 (HR 0.48, 0.40–0.58)	Fatigue, nausea, decreased appetite, rash, vomiting, cough, dyspnea, pyrexia, diarrhea/constipation	Gadgeel et al. (2020)
KEYNOTE-407	Squamous	Carboplatin + (paclitaxel or nab-paclitaxel) + Pembrolizumab	Carboplatin + (paclitaxel or nab-paclitaxel)	OS: 17.1 vs. 11.6 (HR 0.71, 0.58–0.88) PFS: 8.0 vs. 5.1 (HR 0.57, 0.47–0.69)	Fatigue, nausea, decreased appetite, rash, vomiting, cough, dyspnea, pyrexia, diarrhea/constipation, alopecia, peripheral neuropathy	Paz-Ares et al. (2020)
IMpower-150	Nonsquamous; EGFR and ALK negative	Carboplatin + paclitaxel + bevacizumab + Atezolizumab	Carboplatin + paclitaxel bevacizumab	OS: 19.2 vs. 14.7 (HR: 0.78, 0.64–0.96) PFS: 8.5 vs. 7.0 (HR: 0.71, 0.59–0.85)	Rash, hepatitis, hypothyroidism, hyperthyroidism, pneumonitis, colitis	Reck et al. (2019)
Impower-130	Nonsquamous; EGFR and ALK negative	Carboplatin + nab-paclitaxel + Atezolizumab	Carboplatin+ nab-paclitaxel	OS: 18.6 vs. 13.9 (HR 0.80, 0.64–0.99) PFS: 7.2 vs. 6.5 (HR 0.75, 0.63–0.91)	Fatigue/asthenia, nausea, alopecia, constipation, diarrhea	West et al. (2019)
CHECKMATE-9LA	Any histology; EGFR and ALK negative	Platinum doublet (histology specific) + Nivolumab + Ipilimumab	Platinum doublet (histology specific)	OS: 14.1 vs. 10.7 (HR 0.69, 0.55–0.87) PFS: 6.8 vs. 5 (HR 0.70, 0.57–0.86)	Fatigue, arthralgias, nausea, diarrhea, rash	Paz-Ares et al. (2021)

PFS progression-free survival, *OS* overall survival, *HR* hazard rate

with high PD-L1 expression (defined originally as a tumor proportion score [TPS] ≥50% and subsequently widened based on the results of KEYNOTE-042 for TPS ≥1% and no EGFR or ALK genomic tumor aberrations) (Langer et al. 2016; Mok et al. 2019). Although some patients with NSCLC achieve long-term survival with immune checkpoint inhibitor therapy, many experience early disease progression indicating that the patient population is heterogeneous. Preclinical data suggest that chemotherapy can mediate immunologic effects and possibly have a synergistic antitumor effect via so-called immunogenic cell death, which led to the design of studies combining ICI with chemotherapy (Emens and Middleton 2015). The need to expand the patient population who benefit from long-term disease control with immunotherapy has underlined the importance of chemotherapy as a crucial therapeutic modality in lung cancer.

Preclinical data indicated that chemotherapy can modulate tumors to be more susceptible to ICI by releasing tumor-specific antigens, upregulating major histocompatibility complex expression, increasing the cytotoxic lymphocyte to regulatory T-cell ratio and inhibiting myeloid-derived suppressor cells (Ramakrishnan and Gabrilovich 2013). The first trial to show a possible additive or synergistic effect of the combination was KEYNOTE-021G, a phase 2 randomized study that suggested superiority of the combination of chemotherapy and ICI in previously untreated metastatic nonsquamous NSCLC without EGFR or ALK genomic aberrations, irrespective of PD-L1 expression (Langer et al. 2016). When pembrolizumab was added to a combination of carboplatin and pemetrexed, the ORR was 55% compared to 29% with chemotherapy alone. PFS was also significantly higher at 13 months compared to 6 months (HR 0.53). The Phase 3 KEYNOTE-189 trial then confirmed this benefit. In KEYNOTE-189, patients with nonsquamous NSCLC regardless of PD-L1 TPS received cisplatin or carboplatin plus pemetrexed in combination with pembrolizumab or placebo, followed by pemetrexed and pembrolizumab or placebo maintenance therapy. Overall survival was superior in the chemoimmunotherapy group for all subgroups of TPS: TPS <1% (HR 0.59, 95% CI 0.38–092), TPS 1–49% (HR 0.55, 95% CI 0.34–0.90), and TPS ≥50% (HR 0.42, CI 0.26–0.68) (Gandhi et al. 2018).

Similar results were seen with KEYNOTE-407 that studied treatment-naïve, advanced squamous NSCLC without an EGFR or ALK target (Paz-Ares et al. 2018). Patients were randomized to chemotherapy, carboplatin and paclitaxel/nab-paclitaxel with either pembrolizumab or placebo. The median OS with pembrolizumab compared to chemotherapy alone was higher with the addition of pembrolizumab: median OS 15.9 months (95% CI 13.2-not reached), compared to chemotherapy and placebo, median OS 11.3 months (95% CI 9.5–14.8) (Paz-Ares et al. 2018). Patients with PD-L1 <1% by TPS also had improved OS, HR 0.61 (95% CI 0.38–0.98) (Paz-Ares et al. 2018).

In a recent pooled analysis of the three trials indicated above, patients with PD-L1 negative tumors had improved survival with the addition of pembrolizumab to chemotherapy compared to chemotherapy alone indicating a synergy between these agents regardless of PD-L1 expression (Borghaei et al. 2020).

Combination of atezolizumab, a PD-L1 inhibitor, with chemotherapy also showed benefit in multiple trials. IMpower150 demonstrated improved survival of chemoimmunotherapy in treatment-naïve patients with advanced nonsquamous NSCLC. Patients who received combination atezolizumab, bevacizumab, carboplatin, and paclitaxel (ABCP) had a superior median OS of 19.2 months, compared to bevacizumab, carboplatin, and paclitaxel alone (BCP) with a median OS of 14.7 months, HR 0.78 (95% CI 0.64–0.96) (Socinski et al. 2018a). The improved PFS of ABCP was observed in all PD-L1 groups, including patients with PD-L1 expression less than 1% in the tumor cells and/or tumor infiltrating cells, HR 0.77 (95% CI 0.61–0.99), but the OS benefit was not statistically significant among the PD-L1 negative group (HR 0.82, 95% CI 0.62–1.08) (Socinski et al. 2018a, b). Another study incorporating atezolizumab in the frontline setting was IMpower130, where the addition to carboplatin and nab-paclitaxel improved both

PFS and OS (18.6 vs. 13.9 months, HR 0.79) (West et al. 2019). In the squamous population, IMpower131 randomized PD-L1 unselected patients with advanced, squamous NSCLC to chemotherapy with carboplatin and nab-paclitaxel with or without the addition of atezolizumab (Jotte et al. 2020). At a median follow-up of 17 months, the combination of atezolizumab and chemotherapy resulted in an improved PFS (6.3 vs. 5.6 months; HR 0.7) compared to chemotherapy alone.

Another therapeutic strategy employed in the first-line setting is harnessing the complementary mechanism of two distinct immunotherapy drugs, which has worked well in advanced melanoma. Dual CTLA-4 and PD-1 blockade simultaneously modulates the early T-cell priming phase in lymphoid organs and the effector phase of activated T cells at the tumor site (Robert 2020). CHECKMATE-9LA randomized patients with advanced NSCLC that were treatment naïve to combination immunotherapy with nivolumab plus the CTLA-4 inhibitor, ipilimumab, and two cycles of platinum-doublet chemotherapy versus platinum-doublet chemotherapy (Reck et al. 2020). Regardless of PD-L1 expression, the median OS was 14.1 months in the combination versus 10.7 months in chemotherapy alone (HR 0.69, 0.55–0.87). Despite a short median follow-up of 13.2 months, the efficacy of the combination with a low rate of early disease progression was clearly seen. While this regimen has gained FDA approval, it remains unclear whether any particular subsets of patients would benefit more from this approach versus the more widely used regimen of chemotherapy with single-agent immunotherapy. Further studies are awaited to address this important question.

When patients have tumors with high PD-L1 expression (TPS >50%), immunotherapy as monotherapy or immunotherapy combination (PD-L1 and CTLA-4 inhibitors) has shown efficacy over chemotherapy alone based on multiple pivotal trials such as KEYNOTE-024, KEYNOTE-042, and CHECKMATE-227 which will be discussed elsewhere (Mok et al. 2019; Carbone et al. 2017; Reck et al. 2019; Hellmann et al. 2018). A meta-analysis of five randomized trials indirectly compared the combination of pembrolizumab with chemotherapy to pembrolizumab alone (Zhou et al. 2019) and found that the combination had superior overall response rates and PFS (HR 0.55, 95% CI 0.32–0.97), but not OS (HR 0.76, 0.51–1.14). This suggests that the combination may be beneficial in a subset of patients that are identified as early rapid progressors, despite high PD-L1 expression. Studies are currently ongoing to better address baseline prognostic and predictive biomarkers to best optimize use. Pivotal studies such as INSIGNA/EA5163 are underway to assess whether first-line pembrolizumab monotherapy followed by pemetrexed and carboplatin with or without pembrolizumab after disease progression is superior to first-line pembrolizumab, pemetrexed, and carboplatin followed by pembrolizumab and pemetrexed maintenance in patients with metastatic nonsquamous PD-L1-positive NSCLC.

4.2 Second-Line and Beyond

When patients have progressive disease after first-line therapy and do not have any specific new molecular targets and remain candidates for treatment, there are a number of chemotherapy options available (Table 5). The efficacy of docetaxel in the second-line setting was demonstrated in a phase 3 trial of 373 patients with advanced NSCLC who had previously failed platinum-containing chemotherapy and were randomized to receive docetaxel versus a control regimen of vinorelbine or ifosfamide (Fossella et al. 2000). Patients who received docetaxel had a longer time to progression, an improved PFS, and a greater 1-year survival (32% vs. 19%, $p = 0.025$). Prior exposure to paclitaxel did not decrease the likelihood of response or survival. Weekly administration of the drug results in slightly decreased hematological toxicities without compromising efficacy (Gridelli et al. 2004).

Pemetrexed was shown to be superior as compared to docetaxel for patients with nonsquamous histology in the second-line setting. In a phase 3 trial of 571 patients with recurrent NSCLC randomly assigned to docetaxel or pemetrexed, the median OS was significantly better in patients with nonsquamous tumors (9.3 vs. 8.0 months, HR 0.78) but worse in patients with squamous tumors (6.2 vs. 7.4 months, HR1.56) (Hanna et al. 2004). There was significantly decreased incidence of neutropenic fever in the pemetrexed arm (Pujol et al. 2007). Both pemetrexed and docetaxel can be well tolerated in older patients with appropriate dosing and scheduling adjustments. Survival was similar in patients older than 70 years compared to younger patients in both pemetrexed (9.5 vs. 7.8 months) and docetaxel (7.7 vs. 8.0 months) (Weiss et al. 2006). As pemetrexed generally is now used in the frontline setting in platinum-based doublet combinations, its use in the second-line setting has been more limited.

Another option for patients who have progressed on first-line therapies is gemcitabine. In a randomized study of 300 NSCLC patients who have progressed on prior chemotherapies, gemcitabine improved quality of life within the first 2 months of treatment compared to supportive care alone (Anderson et al. 2000). However, there was no difference in tumor response or OS. There were however increased cases of flu-like symptoms and hair loss (Emens and Middleton 2015).

In patients that have been stable off therapy, it is reasonable to retreat with a previously used chemotherapeutic agent. In a retrospective study, patients who were retreated with the same initial regimen had improved response rates when compared to second-line docetaxel after a median interval off treatment of 5 months (Nagano et al. 2010). The median OS for the retreatment group was 17 months compared to 9 months with docetaxel (ORR 29% vs. 8%).

5 Role of Chemotherapy in Tumors with Driver Mutations/Targeted Therapy

Targeted therapies are credited with significant changes in outcomes for patients with mutations such as EGFR and ALK over the last decade (Ramalingam et al. 2020; Mok et al. 2020). These agents routinely demonstrate significantly improved response rates, extended PFS, and better tolerability when compared to intravenous chemotherapeutic agents and currently are recommended frontline therapies. However, relapse eventually occurs in all individuals with oncogene-driven advanced cancers, and while in certain contexts, next-generation agents or combination targeted therapies can be offered dependent on documented resistance mechanisms, at one point for most patients conventional chemotherapy-based strategies will be the most prudent and generally have quite robust activity.

Historical studies assessing concomitant administration of targeted agents with chemotherapy have yielded mixed results thus far (Sirotnak et al. 2000; Giaccone et al. 2004; Herbst et al. 2005; Gatzemeier et al. 2007). Most of the early efforts to incorporate targeted agents into the treatment of NSCLC concentrated on patients with advanced metastatic disease without biomarker selection. However, recent biomarker-selected clinical trials have led to promising results paving the way for future practice-changing studies.

The FASTACT-2 trial combined chemotherapy with erlotinib in an intercalated combination (erlotinib 150 mg/day day 15–28 of cycle) (Wu et al. 2013). There was an improvement in PFS (16.8 vs. 6.9 months, HR 0.25) and OS (31.4 vs. 20.6 months, HR 0.48) over chemotherapy alone in EGFR-mutated patients with similar toxicity profile in both groups.

Subsequently, two phase III clinical trials studied the combination of TKIs with chemotherapy in patients with EGFR-mutated tumors. The phase III NEJ009 trial combining chemotherapy (pemetrexed and carboplatin) with gefitinib in EGFR-mutated NSCLC showed improvements in OS and PFS (Hosomi et al. 2020). Patients were randomly assigned to gefitinib monotherapy or a combination of chemotherapy with gefitinib in the first-line setting. The combination had improved PFS (21 versus 12 months, HR 0.49) and OS (51 vs. 39 months, HR 0.72). However, there were significantly more toxicities observed in the combination. Another phase III trial with a similar trial design to the one above also showed significantly prolonged PFS and OS in patients where chemotherapy was added to gefitinib (PFS 16 vs. 8 months, HR 0.51; OS NR vs. 17 months, HR 0.45). Similar to the prior study, the combination led to increased grade 3 toxicities (Noronha et al. 2020a).

The Phase II OPAL study assessing the use of frontline third-generation EGFR TKI, osimertinib in combination with platinum-based chemotherapy thus far has shown that the combination is well tolerated (Morita et al. 2020). The followup to assess efficacy is ongoing and will provide information regarding the safety and preliminary efficacy of treatment for the highly anticipated FLAURA2 study. The phase 3 FLAURA 2 study (NCT04035486) will randomize patients to either osimertinib alone or osimertinib with pemetrexed and platinum chemotherapy. The results of this study are eagerly awaited as it may affect the future first-line treatment paradigm for EGFR-mutated NSCLC.

6 Combinations with Angiogenesis Inhibitors

Tumor angiogenesis is another therapeutic target in NSCLC and angiogenesis inhibitors are primarily used in the metastatic setting. Two monoclonal antibodies that block the function of VEGF-A or its receptor VEGFR-2 are currently approved by the US FDA in advanced NSCLC (Wang et al. 2017).

Bevacizumab is a humanized monoclonal antibody targeting VEGF-A that has been shown to improve overall response rate (ORR), and prolong PFS and OS when combined with platinum based-chemotherapy in the first-line setting in patients with advanced nonsquamous NSCLC (Soria et al. 2013). In a meta-analysis of four phase II/III clinical trials including 2194 patients with advanced NSCLC, bevacizumab in combination with chemotherapy significantly prolonged OS (HR 0.90; 95% confidence interval [CI] 0.81, 0.99; $p = 0.03$) and PFS (0.72; 95% CI 0.66, 0.79; $p < 0.001$) compared to chemotherapy alone. A significant increase in grade ≥ 3 proteinuria, hypertension, hemorrhagic events, and neutropenia was noted in the bevacizumab group (Soria et al. 2013) and prior studies indicated a high risk of such complications in patients with squamous cell NSCLC; therefore, bevacizumab should not be used in that context.

In patients treated with induction chemotherapy with or without bevacizumab without disease progression, maintenance bevacizumab, alone or in combination with chemotherapy, has also been studied, although with increased toxicity and a lack of overall survival benefit with the combination regimen (Ramalingam et al. 2019; Seto et al. 2020). Chemotherapy with bevacizumab has largely been replaced with immunotherapy alone, or in combination with chemotherapy in treatment-naive patients with advanced NSCLC (Gadgeel et al. 2020; Paz-Ares et al. 2020; Reck et al. 2016; Herbst et al. 2020).

Some hints of significant activity in combination with immunotherapy come from the IMpower150 trial which evaluated the combination of platinum-based doublet chemotherapy plus bevacizumab with different combinations of the PD-L1 inhibitor, atezolizumab. The study randomly assigned 1202 patients with advanced nonsquamous NSCLC to receive chemotherapy (carboplatin-paclitaxel) either in combination with bevacizumab (BCP), with atezolizumab (ACP), or with bevacizumab-atezolizumab (ABCP) in the first-line setting (Socinski et al. 2018a). An improvement in PFS (8.3 versus 6.8 months; HR 0.62, 95% CI 0.52–0.74) and OS (19.2 versus 14.7 months; HR 0.78, 95% CI 0.64–0.96) was observed in the EGFR/ALK wild-type (ITT population) subset of patients receiving ABCP compared to the BCP group. Higher rates of toxicity were also observed in the ABCP group. Interestingly, the benefit observed was also noted in the 14% of patients with EGFR- or ALK-mutant disease which suggests activity of angiogenic inhibition in this patient population. Moreover, in subsequent analysis, the median PFS and median OS were similar between ACP and BCP arms additionally suggesting notable activity to the antiangiogenic agent (Socinski et al. 2019). The median PFS was 5.4 months in patients with liver metastasis in both groups (HR 0.81, 95% CI 0.55–1.21). In patients without liver metastasis, median PFS was 6.9 months in the ACP group versus 7 months in the BCP group (HR 0.9, 95% CI 0.77–1.06). The median OS was 8.9 versus 9.4 months in ACP versus BCP groups with liver metastasis (HR 0.87, 95% CI 0.57–1.32). In patients without liver metastasis, median OS was 21 versus 17 months in ACP versus BCP groups (HR 0.84, 95% CI 0.68–1.04).

Bevacizumab has also been evaluated in the second- and third-line settings, where currently limited therapeutic options exist. An open-label trial randomized 166 patients with advanced NSCLC treated with one or two prior lines of therapy to receive either paclitaxel-bevacizumab or docetaxel (Cortot et al. 2020). Both median PFS (5.4 versus 3.9 months; HR 0.61, 95% CI 0.44–0.86 $p = 0.005$) and ORR improvement were noted in the combination group with no significant difference in OS or toxicity, although crossover occurred in 21 of 55 (38.2%) docetaxel-treated patients.

Ramucirumab has demonstrated an OS improvement when combined with docetaxel in the second-line setting (Table 6). In the REVEL trial, 1253 patients with NSCLC (including 26% with squamous cell carcinoma) who had progressed on initial platinum-based therapy were randomly assigned to docetaxel with or without ramucirumab (Garon et al. 2014). Patients in the combination group had longer median PFS (4.5 versus 3 months; HR 0.76, 95% CI 0.68–0.86) as well as OS (10.5 versus 9.1 months; HR 0.86, 95% CI 0.75–0.98). The observed incidence of grade 3 or 4 toxicity was also increased in the ramucirumab group (79% versus 72%), particularly the rate of bleeding (26.5% versus 12.9%).

Angiogenesis inhibitors have also been studied in combination with EGFR TKIs in EGFR-mutant NSCLC. Most trials have evaluated first-generation EGFR TKIs like erlotinib in combination with bevacizumab or ramucirumab and have shown an improvement in PFS when compared to TKI alone (PMID: 30975627, 25175099, 31591063). The combination of the third-generation EGFR TKI, osimertinib, and bevacizumab is also under active investigation (Yu et al. 2020), as well as osimertinib in combination with ramucirumab (NCT03909334).

Table 6 Guideline-recommended chemotherapy regimens for metastatic non-small cell lung cancer in the second-line setting

Drug	Patient population	Intervention/ comparator arm	Key outcome	Toxicities	Reference
Pemetrexed	Nonsquamous; second line	Pemetrexed vs. docetaxel	PFS 2.9 months in both arms; OS 8.3 vs. 7.9 (NS)	Docetaxel increased risk of febrile neutropenia, alopecia	Hanna et al. (2004)
Docetaxel	Any histology; second line	Docetaxel (75 mg/m^2 every 3 weeks) vs. vinorelbine or ifosfamide	OS at 1 year (21% vs. 19%, $p = 0.025$)	Higher grade 4 neutropenia with docetaxel	TAX320 (Fossella et al. 2000)
Docetaxel + Ramucirumab	Any histology; second line	Docetaxel + Ramucirumab versus docetaxel	PFS: 4.5 vs. 3.0 (HR 0.76, $p < 0.0001$); OS: 10.5 vs. 9.1 (HR 0.86, $p = 0.024$)	Neutropenia, fatigue, stomatitis	Garon et al. (2014)
Gemcitabine	Any histology; third line	Best supportive care (BSC)	No difference in OS (5.7 vs. 5.9) Tumor response: 19% (13–27) in gemcitabine arm. Quality of life: SS14 score improvement at 4 weeks: 22% with gemcitabine vs. 9% with BSC ($p = 0.0014$)	Neutropenia, nausea, pulmonary toxicity, alopecia	Anderson et al. (2000)

PFS progression-free survival, *OS* overall survival, *SS14* commonly reported symptoms from the EORTC quality of life questionnaire-C30 and LC13 scales

7 Antibody-Drug Conjugates

Antibody-drug conjugates (ADCs) are monoclonal antibodies targeting tumor-specific cell-surface proteins, that are conjugated to cytotoxic agents. This enables targeted delivery of cytotoxic chemotherapy to cancer cells. A number of ADCs recently have shown significant promise in different contexts and are under vigorous development for multiple indications. The HER2-targeted ADCs, trastuzumab emtansine (T-DM1) and trastuzumab deruxtecan (T-DXd), have shown promising activity in patients with previously treated advanced HER2-overexpressing or HER2-mutant NSCLC (Peters et al. 2019; Li et al. 2020; Tsurutani et al. 2020). A phase II trial of ado-trastuzumab emtansine in heavily pretreated advanced HER2-mutant NSCLC patients showed a partial response rate of 44% (95% CI, 22–69%) and a median PFS of 5 months (95% CI, 3–9 months) (Li et al. 2018). A phase I trial of trastuzumab deruxtecan demonstrated an ORR of 72.7% (8/11) and median PFS of 11.3 months (95% CI, 8.1–14.3) in HER2-mutant NSCLC (Tsurutani et al. 2020). Interim analysis of a subsequent phase II trial (DESTINY-Lung01) showed an ORR of 61.9% (95% CI, 45.6–76.4%) in 42 patients with an estimated PFS of 14 months (95% CI, 6.4–14.0 months) (Smit et al. 2020). Additional studies assessing the benefit of T-DXd have been initiated in HER2-overexpressing NSCLC in the frontline setting (NCT04686305). Initial results from a phase I trial examining U3-1402, an ADC targeting the HER3 receptor attached to a novel topoisomerase I inhibitor, showed a response rate of 31% in TKI-resistant, EGFR-mutant NSCLC (Janne et al. 2019).

Several other promising ADCs are under investigation. A phase I study of datopotamab deruxtecan, a trophoblast cell-surface antigen 2 (TROP2)-targeting ADC, showed an ORR of up to 25% and a disease control rate of up to 80% in heavily pretreated patients with advanced NSCLC (Spira et al. 2021; Sands et al. 2019) and a phase 3 study comparing its activity to standard docetaxel chemotherapy is ongoing in the second-line setting (NCT04656652). A DM4-conjugated ADC against carcinoembryonic antigen-related cell-adhesion molecule 5 anti-(CEACAM5) demonstrated an ORR of 20.3% and median PFS of 5.6 months in the high expressor subgroup of patients with advanced NSCLC (Gazzah et al. 2020). A phase II study of telisotuzumab vedotin, an MMAE drug conjugate targeting c-MET, has also shown promising activity in patients with c-MET-positive advanced NSCLC with an ORR of 18.8% ($n = 16$) (Strickler et al. 2018).

8 Small Cell Lung Cancer

Small cell lung cancers make up 10–15% of all lung cancer diagnoses and are most closely associated with heavy smoking as well as endocrine and immunological paraneoplastic syndromes (Saltos et al. 2020). Staging remains based on the original VA staging system classifying small cell lung cancers as limited- and extensive-stage disease with patients with limited-stage defined by the ability to fit all known disease into a radiation portal (generally matching TNM stages of stage I–IIIC) and such patients are treated with curative intent. Small cell lung cancer is a highly aggressive neoplasm characterized by fast doubling time and rapid proliferation of tumor cells leading to explosive disease progression and metastatic disease spread limiting the utility of localized therapies, such as surgery. Small cell lung cancer was recognized early as highly sensitive to platinum or anthracycline-based chemotherapy regimens and indeed combination chemotherapy with a platinum/etoposide-based doublet chemotherapy regimen remains the mainstay of therapy (Remon et al. 2021). In limited-stage small cell lung cancer, patients receive combination chemotherapy (usually with cisplatin-based doublet) with concurrent radiation (Turrisi et al. 1999) followed by prophylactic cranial irradiation for appropriate patients (Aupérin et al. 1999). The use of cisplatin is the standard of care, but for patients who are not CDDP candidates, carboplatin is appropriate to use, however carries more substantial myelotoxicity. Current research focuses mainly on proper integration of checkpoint inhibitor therapy to extend the benefit of combined modality therapy in patients with LS-SCLC.

In extensive-stage small cell lung cancer, platinum plus etoposide has been the standard of care for decades and their superiority has been confirmed via multiple studies including meta-analyses (Pujol et al. 2000; Mascaux et al. 2000). Generally, carboplatin is preferred over CDDP due to its more favorable side effect profile (Rossi et al. 2012). Other combinations, for example, cisplatin/irinotecan, have demonstrated initial promise in Asian studies but their benefit could not be confirmed in other populations (Lima et al. 2010). More recently, major progress has been achieved by the integration of anti-PD-L1 antibodies (atezolizumab or durvalumab) based on the results of the pivotal IMPOWER133 (Liu et al. 2021) and CASPIAN studies (Goldman et al. 2021) demonstrating significant benefits with the addition of checkpoint inhibitor therapy. The IMPOWER133 study compared Carboplatin/Etoposide with atezolizumab/placebo for 4 cycles followed by atezolizumab versus placebo maintenance and showed a significant OS benefit for the experimental arm (12.3 vs. 10.3 months, HR 0.76). Similarly, the CASPIAN study also showed a similar OS benefit (13 vs. 10.3 months, HR 0.73) with the addition of durvalumab to platinum-based doublet chemotherapy (both CDDP and Carboplatin allowed). In the CASPIAN study, up to 6 cycles of doublet chemotherapy were permitted in the control arm while 4 cycles were given in the experimental arm. Similar to the IMPOWER133 study, induction therapy was followed by maintenance durvalumab versus placebo. In addition to the notable OS benefits, both studies also highlight a small but real fraction of long-term responders with the use of checkpoint inhibitor therapy with an approximately 10% improvement in 2-year OS. Neither PD-L1 testing nor TMB assessment could be validated as clinically useful biomarkers in this context. Combination chemo/immunotherapy carries expected chemotherapy and immunotherapy toxicities without novel toxicity signals noted. These studies have established a new standard of care for patients with ES-SCLC with chemo/immunotherapy followed by maintenance immunotherapy and future studies will need to build upon this new foundation. Studies with the anti-PD-1 checkpoint inhibitors nivolumab (Leal et al. 2020) (NCT03382561) and pembrolizumab (Rudin et al. 2020) also demonstrated benefits concurrent with platinum-based combination chemotherapy in the first-line setting but have not been approved by the FDA for frontline indications and their prior approvals in the second- and beyond-line settings recently had been withdrawn.

Unfortunately, despite early chemotherapy sensitivity, resistance and progression commonly develop in limited-stage and essentially uniformly in extensive-stage disease. Upon progression, second-line chemotherapy has modest activity in platinum-sensitive (usually defined as progression >90 days since last platinum-based chemotherapy) and very limited activity in platinum-refractory disease (Lara et al. 2015). Up until recently the only FDA-approved therapy for second-line use has been topotecan (von Pawel et al. 1999) originally approved based upon studies demonstrating similar activity and better tolerability over the traditional CAV triplet chemotherapy regimen. Topotecan while originally developed as a 5-day intravenous regimen can also be administered using an oral formulation (Eckardt et al. 2007). While not FDA approved for this indication, irinotecan also has significant activity (Noronha et al. 2020b; Pillai and Owonikoko 2014). A novel liposomal formulation of irinotecan with enhanced drug delivery to tumors (Leonard et al. 2017) is now being developed with promising early results demonstrating a response rate of 33% and recently received FDA breakthrough designation (Paz-Ares et al. 2019). Other agents with documented single-agent activity are taxanes (Smit et al. 1998) as well as temozolomide which has notable CNS activity (Pietanza et al. 2012) as well as the third-generation anthracycline, amrubicin (Onoda et al. 2006). Recently, a novel marine agent lurbinectedin (Trigo et al. 2020) received accelerated approval by the FDA based on the results of a phase 2 study of 105 patients demonstrating a response rate of 35% in patients with pretreated small cell lung cancer, and notable activity

(ORR of 22.2%) was observed in the platinum-refractory subset as well. This novel agent has multiple mechanisms of action (Leal et al. 2010) including DNA damage and transcriptional modulation, and its key toxicity is bone marrow suppression. The phase 3 ATLANTIS study (Farago et al. 2019) (NCT02566993) of a lower dose of lurbinectedin in combination with doxorubicin failed to reach its prespecified endpoint of OS benefit over the control arm (investigator's choice—topotecan or CAV) in the second-line management of ES-SCLC. Retreatment with a frontline platinum/etoposide regimen can have significant activity and might be used preferentially in patients with late recurrence (more than 6 months from last platinum-based therapy) (Baize et al. 2020).

The atypical Notch ligand DLL-3 has been identified as a neuroendocrine marker that is frequently expressed in small cell lung cancer and has been assessed as a potential target. Despite initial promise (Rudin et al. 2017), phase 3 studies with the antibody-drug conjugate Rovalpituzumab tesirine (Rova-T) have been disappointing principally due to poor tolerance (Blackhall et al. 2021). Further studies are ongoing with less toxic targeting strategies, including, for example, the bispecific T-cell engager AMG757 with a possibly better therapeutic window (Serzan et al. 2020). Further advances in the management of SCLC are expected based on emerging molecularly defined subtypes of SCLC with specific treatment vulnerabilities (Rudin et al. 2019; Stewart et al. 2020).

9 Conclusion

While major advances allow a growing proportion of patients with NSCLC to derive very significant benefits from biomarker-informed targeted and immunotherapeutic options, systemic chemotherapy remains a key component of lung cancer management with notable synergies with targeted and immunotherapeutic agents and now forming the backbone of a novel class of promising antibody-drug conjugates. Continued investment in the development and optimization of chemotherapeutic options will yield further benefits to permit optimal treatment outcomes for the large majority of patients diagnosed with lung cancer.

References

Adrianzen Herrera D, Ashai N, Perez-Soler R, Cheng H (2019) Nanoparticle albumin bound-paclitaxel for treatment of advanced non-small cell lung cancer: an evaluation of the clinical evidence. Expert Opin Pharmacother 20(1):95–102

Aggarwal C, Thompson JC, Chien AL, Quinn KJ, Hwang WT, Black TA et al (2020) Baseline plasma tumor mutation burden predicts response to pembrolizumab-based therapy in patients with metastatic non-small cell lung cancer. Clin Cancer Res 26(10):2354–2361

Aggarwal C, Rolfo CD, Oxnard GR, Gray JE, Sholl LM, Gandara DR (2021) Strategies for the successful implementation of plasma-based NSCLC genotyping in clinical practice. Nat Rev Clin Oncol 18(1):56–62

Albain KS, Swann RS, Rusch VW, Turrisi AT 3rd, Shepherd FA, Smith C et al (2009) Radiotherapy plus chemotherapy with or without surgical resection for stage III non-small-cell lung cancer: a phase III randomised controlled trial. Lancet (London, England) 374(9687):379–386

Alexander M, Ko B, Lambert R, Gadgeel S, Halmos B (2020) The evolving use of pembrolizumab in combination treatment approaches for non-small cell lung cancer. Expert Rev Respir Med 14(2):137–147

American Cancer Society. Cancer Statistics Center. http://cancerstatisticscenter.cancer.org. Accessed 24 May 2020

Anderson H, Hopwood P, Stephens RJ, Thatcher N, Cottier B, Nicholson M et al (2000) Gemcitabine plus best supportive care (BSC) vs BSC in inoperable non-small cell lung cancer—a randomized trial with quality of life as the primary outcome. UK NSCLC Gemcitabine Group. Non-Small Cell Lung Cancer. Br J Cancer 83(4):447–453

Antonia SJ, Villegas A, Daniel D, Vicente D, Murakami S, Hui R et al (2017) Durvalumab after chemoradiotherapy in stage III non-small-cell lung cancer. N Engl J Med 377(20):1919–1929

Antonia SJ, Villegas A, Daniel D, Vicente D, Murakami S, Hui R et al (2018) Overall survival with durvalumab after chemoradiotherapy in stage III NSCLC. N Engl J Med 379(24):2342–2350

Arriagada R, Bergman B, Dunant A, Le Chevalier T, Pignon JP, Vansteenkiste J (2004) Cisplatin-based adjuvant chemotherapy in patients with completely resected non-small-cell lung cancer. N Engl J Med 350(4):351–360

Atagi S, Kawahara M, Yokoyama A, Okamoto H, Yamamoto N, Ohe Y et al (2012) Thoracic radiotherapy with or without daily low-dose carboplatin in elderly patients with non-small-cell lung cancer: a randomised, controlled, phase 3 trial by the Japan Clinical Oncology Group (JCOG0301). Lancet Oncol 13(7):671–678

Aupérin A, Arriagada R, Pignon JP, Le Péchoux C, Gregor A, Stephens RJ et al (1999) Prophylactic cranial irradiation for patients with small-cell lung cancer in complete remission. Prophylactic Cranial Irradiation Overview Collaborative Group. N Engl J Med 341(7):476–484

Aupérin A, Le Péchoux C, Rolland E, Curran WJ, Furuse K, Fournel P et al (2010) Meta-analysis of concomitant versus sequential radiochemotherapy in locally advanced non-small-cell lung cancer. J Clin Oncol 28(13):2181–2190

Baize N, Monnet I, Greillier L, Geier M, Lena H, Janicot H et al (2020) Carboplatin plus etoposide versus topotecan as second-line treatment for patients with sensitive relapsed small-cell lung cancer: an open-label, multicentre, randomised, phase 3 trial. Lancet Oncol 21(9):1224–1233

Belani CP, Choy H, Bonomi P, Scott C, Travis P, Haluschak J et al (2005) Combined chemoradiotherapy regimens of paclitaxel and carboplatin for locally advanced non-small-cell lung cancer: a randomized phase II locally advanced multi-modality protocol. J Clin Oncol 23(25):5883–5891

Blackhall F, Jao K, Greillier L, Cho BC, Penkov K, Reguart N et al (2021) Efficacy and safety of rovalpituzumab tesirine compared with topotecan as second-line therapy in DLL3-high SCLC: results from the phase 3 TAHOE study. J Thorac Oncol 16:1547–1558

Borghaei H, Langer CJ, Paz-Ares L, Rodríguez-Abreu D, Halmos B, Garassino MC et al (2020) Pembrolizumab plus chemotherapy versus chemotherapy alone in patients with advanced non-small cell lung cancer without tumor PD-L1 expression: a pooled analysis of 3 randomized controlled trials. Cancer 126(22):4867–4877

Carbone DP, Reck M, Paz-Ares L, Creelan B, Horn L, Steins M et al (2017) First-line nivolumab in stage IV or recurrent non-small-cell lung cancer. N Engl J Med 376(25):2415–2426

Cascone T, William WN Jr, Weissferdt A, Leung CH, Lin HY, Pataer A et al (2021) Neoadjuvant nivolumab or nivolumab plus ipilimumab in operable non-small cell lung cancer: the phase 2 randomized NEOSTAR trial. Nat Med 27(3):504–514

Ciuleanu T, Brodowicz T, Zielinski C, Kim JH, Krzakowski M, Laack E et al (2009) Maintenance pemetrexed plus best supportive care versus placebo plus best supportive care for non-small-cell lung cancer: a randomised, double-blind, phase 3 study. Lancet (London, England) 374(9699):1432–1440

Cortot AB, Audigier-Valette C, Molinier O, Le Moulec S, Barlesi F, Zalcman G et al (2020) Weekly paclitaxel plus bevacizumab versus docetaxel as second- or third-line treatment in advanced non-squamous non-small-cell lung cancer: results of the IFCT-1103 ULTIMATE study. Eur J Cancer (Oxford, England: 1990) 131:27–36

Curran WJ Jr, Paulus R, Langer CJ, Komaki R, Lee JS, Hauser S et al (2011) Sequential vs. concurrent chemoradiation for stage III non-small cell lung cancer: randomized phase III trial RTOG 9410. J Natl Cancer Inst 103(19):1452–1460

D'Addario G, Pintilie M, Leighl NB, Feld R, Cerny T, Shepherd FA (2005) Platinum-based versus non-platinum-based chemotherapy in advanced non-small-cell lung cancer: a meta-analysis of the published literature. J Clin Oncol 23(13):2926–2936

Dillman RO, Seagren SL, Propert KJ, Guerra J, Eaton WL, Perry MC et al (1990) A randomized trial of induction chemotherapy plus high-dose radiation versus radiation alone in stage III non-small-cell lung cancer. N Engl J Med 323(14):940–945

Douillard JY, Rosell R, De Lena M, Carpagnano F, Ramlau R, Gonzáles-Larriba JL et al (2006) Adjuvant vinorelbine plus cisplatin versus observation in patients with completely resected stage IB-IIIA non-small-cell lung cancer (Adjuvant Navelbine International Trialist Association [ANITA]): a randomised controlled trial. Lancet Oncol 7(9):719–727

Eckardt JR, von Pawel J, Pujol JL, Papai Z, Quoix E, Ardizzoni A et al (2007) Phase III study of oral compared with intravenous topotecan as second-line therapy in small-cell lung cancer. J Clin Oncol 25(15):2086–2092

Emens LA, Middleton G (2015) The interplay of immunotherapy and chemotherapy: harnessing potential synergies. Cancer Immunol Res 3(5):436–443

Farago AF, Drapkin BJ, Lopez-Vilarino de Ramos JA, Galmarini CM, Núñez R, Kahatt C et al (2019) ATLANTIS: a phase III study of lurbinectedin/doxorubicin versus topotecan or cyclophosphamide/doxorubicin/vincristine in patients with small-cell lung cancer who have failed one prior platinum-containing line. Future Oncol (London, England) 15(3): 231–239

Felip E, Altorki N, Zhou C, Csőszi T, Vynnychenko I, Goloborodko O, et al (2021) Adjuvant atezolizumab after adjuvant chemotherapy in resected stage IB-IIIA non-small-cell lung cancer (IMpower010): a randomised, multicentre, open-label, phase 3 trial. Lancet (London, England) 398(10308):1344–1357

Forde PM, Chaft JE, Pardoll DM (2018) Neoadjuvant PD-1 blockade in resectable lung cancer. N Engl J Med 379(9):e14

Forde PM, Spicer J, Lu S, et al (2021) Nivolumab (NIVO) + platinum-doublet chemotherapy (chemo) vs chemo as neoadjuvant treatment (tx) for resectable (IB-IIIA) non-small cell lung cancer (NSCLC) in the phase 3 CheckMate 816 trial. In: AACR annual meeting, 10–15 Apr 2021, Virtual. Abstract CT003

Forde PM, Spicer J, Lu S, Provencio M, Mitsudomi T, Awad MM, et al. Neoadjuvant Nivolumab plus Chemotherapy in Resectable Lung Cancer. The New England journal of medicine. 2022.

Fossella FV, DeVore R, Kerr RN, Crawford J, Natale RR, Dunphy F et al (2000) Randomized phase III trial of docetaxel versus vinorelbine or ifosfamide in patients with advanced non-small-cell lung cancer previously treated with platinum-containing chemotherapy regimens. The TAX 320 Non-Small Cell Lung Cancer Study Group. J Clin Oncol 18(12):2354–2362

Furuse K, Fukuoka M, Kawahara M, Nishikawa H, Takada Y, Kudoh S et al (1999) Phase III study of concurrent versus sequential thoracic radiotherapy in combination with mitomycin, vindesine, and cisplatin in unresectable stage III non-small-cell lung cancer. J Clin Oncol 17(9):2692–2699

Gadgeel S, Rodríguez-Abreu D, Speranza G, Esteban E, Felip E, Dómine M et al (2020) Updated analysis from KEYNOTE-189: pembrolizumab or placebo plus pemetrexed and platinum for previously untreated metastatic nonsquamous non-small-cell lung cancer. J Clin Oncol 38(14):1505–1517

Gandhi L, Rodriguez-Abreu D, Gadgeel S, Esteban E, Felip E, De Angelis F et al (2018) Pembrolizumab plus chemotherapy in metastatic non-small-cell lung cancer. N Engl J Med 378(22):2078–2092

Garon EB, Ciuleanu TE, Arrieta O, Prabhash K, Syrigos KN, Goksel T et al (2014) Ramucirumab plus docetaxel versus placebo plus docetaxel for second-line treatment of stage IV non-small-cell lung cancer after disease progression on platinum-based therapy (REVEL): a multicentre, double-blind, randomised phase 3 trial. Lancet (London, England) 384(9944):665–673

Garon EB, Kim JS, Govindan R (2021) Pemetrexed maintenance with or without pembrolizumab in nonsquamous non-small cell lung cancer: a cross-trial comparison of KEYNOTE-189 versus PARAMOUNT, PRONOUNCE, and JVBL. Lung Cancer (Amsterdam, Netherlands) 151:25–29

Gatzemeier U, Pluzanska A, Szczesna A, Kaukel E, Roubec J, De Rosa F et al (2007) Phase III study of erlotinib in combination with cisplatin and gemcitabine in advanced non-small-cell lung cancer: the Tarceva Lung Cancer Investigation Trial. J Clin Oncol 25(12):1545–1552

Gazzah A, Ricordel C, Cousin S, Cho BC, Calvo E, Kim TM et al (2020) Efficacy and safety of the antibody-drug conjugate (ADC) SAR408701 in patients (pts) with non-squamous non-small cell lung cancer (NSQ NSCLC) expressing carcinoembryonic antigen-related cell adhesion molecule 5 (CEACAM5). J Clin Oncol 38(15_Suppl):9505

Giaccone G, Herbst RS, Manegold C, Scagliotti G, Rosell R, Miller V et al (2004) Gefitinib in combination with gemcitabine and cisplatin in advanced non-small-cell lung cancer: a phase III trial—INTACT 1. J Clin Oncol 22(5):777–784

Goldman JW, Dvorkin M, Chen Y, Reinmuth N, Hotta K, Trukhin D et al (2021) Durvalumab, with or without tremelimumab, plus platinum-etoposide versus platinum-etoposide alone in first-line treatment of extensive-stage small-cell lung cancer (CASPIAN): updated results from a randomised, controlled, open-label, phase 3 trial. Lancet Oncol 22(1):51–65

Gray JE, Villegas A, Daniel D, Vicente D, Murakami S, Hui R et al (2020) Three-year overall survival with durvalumab after chemoradiotherapy in stage III NSCLC-update from PACIFIC. J Thorac Oncol 15(2):288–293

Gridelli C, Gallo C, Di Maio M, Barletta E, Illiano A, Maione P et al (2004) A randomised clinical trial of two docetaxel regimens (weekly vs 3 week) in the second-line treatment of non-small-cell lung cancer. The DISTAL 01 study. Br J Cancer 91(12): 1996–2004

Hanna N, Shepherd FA, Fossella FV, Pereira JR, De Marinis F, von Pawel J et al (2004) Randomized phase III trial of pemetrexed versus docetaxel in patients with non-small-cell lung cancer previously treated with chemotherapy. J Clin Oncol 22(9):1589–1597

Hanna NH, Schneider BJ, Temin S, Baker S Jr, Brahmer J, Ellis PM et al (2020) Therapy for stage IV non-small-cell lung cancer without driver alterations: ASCO and OH (CCO) joint guideline update. J Clin Oncol 38(14):1608–1632

Hellmann MD, Ciuleanu TE, Pluzanski A, Lee JS, Otterson GA, Audigier-Valette C et al (2018) Nivolumab plus Ipilimumab in lung cancer with a high tumor mutational burden. N Engl J Med 378(22):2093–2104

Herbst RS, Prager D, Hermann R, Fehrenbacher L, Johnson BE, Sandler A et al (2005) TRIBUTE: a phase III trial of erlotinib hydrochloride (OSI-774) combined with carboplatin and paclitaxel chemotherapy in advanced non-small-cell lung cancer. J Clin Oncol 23(25):5892–5899

Herbst RS, Baas P, Kim DW, Felip E, Pérez-Gracia JL, Han JY et al (2016) Pembrolizumab versus docetaxel for previously treated, PD-L1-positive, advanced non-small-cell lung cancer (KEYNOTE-010): a randomised controlled trial. Lancet (London, England) 387(10027):1540–1550

Herbst RS, Giaccone G, de Marinis F, Reinmuth N, Vergnenegre A, Barrios CH et al (2020) Atezolizumab for first-line treatment of PD-L1-selected patients with NSCLC. N Engl J Med 383(14):1328–1339

Hong DS, Fakih MG, Strickler JH, Desai J, Durm GA, Shapiro GI et al (2020) KRAS(G12C) inhibition with sotorasib in advanced solid tumors. N Engl J Med 383(13):1207–1217

Hosomi Y, Morita S, Sugawara S, Kato T, Fukuhara T, Gemma A et al (2020) Gefitinib alone versus gefitinib plus chemotherapy for non-small-cell lung cancer with mutated epidermal growth factor receptor: NEJ009 study. J Clin Oncol 38(2):115–123

Janne PA, Yu HA, Johnson ML, Steuer CE, Vigliotti M, Iacobucci C et al (2019) Safety and preliminary antitumor activity of U3-1402: a HER3-targeted antibody drug conjugate in EGFR TKI-resistant, EGFRm NSCLC. J Clin Oncol 37(15_Suppl):9010

Jotte R, Cappuzzo F, Vynnychenko I, Stroyakovskiy D, Rodríguez-Abreu D, Hussein M et al (2020) Atezolizumab in combination with carboplatin and nab-paclitaxel in advanced squamous NSCLC

(IMpower131): results from a randomized phase III trial. J Thorac Oncol 15(8):1351–1360

Karnofsky DA (1948) Chemotherapy of neoplastic disease; agents of clinical value. N Engl J Med 239(8):299–305

Kim SY, Halmos B (2020) Choosing the best first-line therapy: NSCLC with no actionable oncogenic driver. Lung Cancer Manag 9(3):Lmt36

Kreuter M, Vansteenkiste J, Fischer JR, Eberhardt W, Zabeck H, Kollmeier J et al (2013) Randomized phase 2 trial on refinement of early-stage NSCLC adjuvant chemotherapy with cisplatin and pemetrexed versus cisplatin and vinorelbine: the TREAT study. Ann Oncol 24(4):986–992

Langer CJ, Gadgeel SM, Borghaei H, Papadimitrakopoulou VA, Patnaik A, Powell SF et al (2016) Carboplatin and pemetrexed with or without pembrolizumab for advanced, non-squamous non-small-cell lung cancer: a randomised, phase 2 cohort of the open-label KEYNOTE-021 study. Lancet Oncol 17(11):1497–1508

Lara PN Jr, Moon J, Redman MW, Semrad TJ, Kelly K, Allen JW et al (2015) Relevance of platinum-sensitivity status in relapsed/refractory extensive-stage small-cell lung cancer in the modern era: a patient-level analysis of southwest oncology group trials. J Thorac Oncol 10(1):110–115

Le Chevalier T, Arriagada R, Quoix E, Ruffie P, Martin M, Tarayre M et al (1991) Radiotherapy alone versus combined chemotherapy and radiotherapy in nonresectable non-small-cell lung cancer: first analysis of a randomized trial in 353 patients. J Natl Cancer Inst 83(6):417–423

Leal JF, Martínez-Díez M, García-Hernández V, Moneo V, Domingo A, Bueren-Calabuig JA et al (2010) PM01183, a new DNA minor groove covalent binder with potent in vitro and in vivo anti-tumour activity. Br J Pharmacol 161(5):1099–1110

Leal T, Wang Y, Dowlati A, Lewis DA, Chen Y, Mohindra AR et al (2020) Randomized phase II clinical trial of cisplatin/carboplatin and etoposide (CE) alone or in combination with nivolumab as frontline therapy for extensive-stage small cell lung cancer (ES-SCLC): ECOG-ACRIN EA5161. J Clin Oncol 38(15_Suppl):9000

Leonard SC, Lee H, Gaddy DF, Klinz SG, Paz N, Kalra AV et al (2017) Extended topoisomerase 1 inhibition through liposomal irinotecan results in improved efficacy over topotecan and irinotecan in models of small-cell lung cancer. Anticancer Drugs 28(10):1086–1096

Li BT, Shen R, Buonocore D, Olah ZT, Ni A, Ginsberg MS et al (2018) Ado-trastuzumab emtansine for patients with HER2-mutant lung cancers: results from a phase II basket trial. J Clin Oncol 36(24):2532–2537

Li BT, Michelini F, Misale S, Cocco E, Baldino L, Cai Y et al (2020) HER2-mediated internalization of cytotoxic agents in ERBB2 amplified or mutant lung cancers. Cancer Discov 10(5):674–687

Liang J, Bi N, Wu S, Chen M, Lv C, Zhao L et al (2017) Etoposide and cisplatin versus paclitaxel and carboplatin with concurrent thoracic radiotherapy in unresectable stage III non-small cell lung cancer: a multicenter randomized phase III trial. Ann Oncol 28(4):777–783

Lim E, Harris G, Patel A, Adachi I, Edmonds L, Song F (2009) Preoperative versus postoperative chemotherapy in patients with resectable non-small cell lung cancer: systematic review and indirect comparison meta-analysis of randomized trials. J Thorac Oncol 4(11):1380–1388

Lima JP, dos Santos LV, Sasse EC, Lima CS, Sasse AD (2010) Camptothecins compared with etoposide in combination with platinum analog in extensive stage small cell lung cancer: systematic review with meta-analysis. J Thorac Oncol 5(12):1986–1993

Liu SV, Reck M, Mansfield AS, Mok T, Scherpereel A, Reinmuth N et al (2021) Updated overall survival and PD-L1 subgroup analysis of patients with extensive-stage small-cell lung cancer treated with atezolizumab, carboplatin, and etoposide (IMpower133). J Clin Oncol 39(6):619–630

Marrone KA, Naidoo J, Brahmer JR (2016) Immunotherapy for lung cancer: no longer an abstract concept. Semin Respir Crit Care Med 37(5):771–782

Mascaux C, Paesmans M, Berghmans T, Branle F, Lafitte JJ, Lemaitre F et al (2000) A systematic review of the role of etoposide and cisplatin in the chemotherapy of small cell lung cancer with methodology assessment and meta-analysis. Lung Cancer (Amsterdam, Netherlands) 30(1):23–36

Minami S, Kijima T (2015) Pemetrexed in maintenance treatment of advanced non-squamous non-small-cell lung cancer. Lung Cancer (Auckland, NZ) 6:13–25

Mino-Kenudson M, Le Stang N, Daigneault JB, Nicholson AG, Cooper WA, Roden AC et al (2021) The International Association for the Study of Lung Cancer global survey on programmed death-ligand 1 testing for NSCLC. J Thorac Oncol 16(4):686–696

Mok TSK, Wu YL, Kudaba I, Kowalski DM, Cho BC, Turna HZ et al (2019) Pembrolizumab versus chemotherapy for previously untreated, PD-L1-expressing, locally advanced or metastatic non-small-cell lung cancer (KEYNOTE-042): a randomised, open-label, controlled, phase 3 trial. Lancet (London, England) 393(10183):1819–1830

Mok T, Camidge DR, Gadgeel SM, Rosell R, Dziadziuszko R, Kim DW et al (2020) Updated overall survival and final progression-free survival data for patients with treatment-naive advanced ALK-positive non-small-cell lung cancer in the ALEX study. Ann Oncol 31(8):1056–1064

Morita R, Asahina H, Tanaka K, Saito R, Sugawara S, Ko R, Azuma K, Morita S, Saijo Y, Maemondo M, Seike M, Isamu O, Sugio K, Kobayashi K (2020) 382MO—The preliminary safety result of a phase II study of osimertinib in combination with platinum + pemetrexed in patients with previously untreated EGFR-mutated advanced NSCLC (NEJ032C/LOGIK1801: OPAL). Ann Oncol 31(Suppl_6):S1386–S1406. https://doi.org/10.1016/annonc/annonc367

Nagano T, Kim YH, Goto K, Kubota K, Ohmatsu H, Niho S et al (2010) Re-challenge chemotherapy for relapsed non-small-cell lung cancer. Lung Cancer (Amsterdam, Netherlands) 69(3):315–318

Non-small Cell Lung Cancer Collaborative Group (1995) Chemotherapy in non-small cell lung cancer: a meta-analysis using updated data on individual patients from 52 randomised clinical trials. BMJ (Clin Res Ed) 311(7010):899–909

Noronha V, Patil VM, Joshi A, Menon N, Chougule A, Mahajan A et al (2020a) Gefitinib versus gefitinib plus pemetrexed and carboplatin chemotherapy in EGFR-mutated lung cancer. J Clin Oncol 38(2):124–136

Noronha V, Sekhar A, Patil VM, Menon N, Joshi A, Kapoor A et al (2020b) Systemic therapy for limited stage small cell lung carcinoma. J Thorac Dis 12(10):6275–6290

Onoda S, Masuda N, Seto T, Eguchi K, Takiguchi Y, Isobe H et al (2006) Phase II trial of amrubicin for treatment of refractory or relapsed small-cell lung cancer: Thoracic Oncology Research Group Study 0301. J Clin Oncol 24(34):5448–5453

Pakkala S, Ramalingam SS (2018) Personalized therapy for lung cancer: striking a moving target. JCI Insight 3(15):e120858

Paz-Ares L, Luft A, Vicente D, Tafreshi A, Gümüş M, Mazières J et al (2018) Pembrolizumab plus chemotherapy for squamous non-small-cell lung cancer. N Engl J Med 379(21):2040–2051

Paz-Ares L, Spigel D, Chen Y, et al (2019) Initial efficacy and safety results of irinotecan liposome injection (NAL-IRI) in patients with small cell lung cancer. In: IASLC 20th world conference on lung cancer, 7–10 Sept 2019, Barcelona, Spain. Abstract OA03.03

Paz-Ares L, Vicente D, Tafreshi A, Robinson A, Soto Parra H, Mazières J et al (2020) A randomized, placebo-controlled trial of pembrolizumab plus chemotherapy in patients with metastatic squamous NSCLC: protocol-specified final analysis of KEYNOTE-407. J Thorac Oncol 15(10):1657–1669

Paz-Ares L, Ciuleanu T-E, Cobo M, Schenker M, Zurawski B, Menezes J, Richardet E, Bennouna J, Felip E, Juan-Vidal O, Alexandru A, Sakai H, Lingua v, Salman P, Souquet P-J, De Marchi P, Martin C, Pérol M, Scherpereel, Lu S, John T, Carbone DP, Meadows-Shropshire S, Agrawal S, Oukessou A, Yan J, Reck M. First-line nivolumab plus ipilimumab combined with two cycles of chemotherapy in patients with non-small-cell lung cancer (CheckMate 9LA): an international, randomised, open-label, phase 3 trial. Lancet Oncol 2021;22(2):198-211. doi: https://doi.org/10.1016/S1470-2045(20)30641-0.

Paz-Ares L, O'Brien M, Mauer M, Dafni U, Oselin K, Havel L, et al (2022) VP3-2022: Pembrolizumab (pembro) versus placebo for early-stage non-small cell lung cancer (NSCLC) following complete resection and adjuvant chemotherapy (chemo) when indicated: Randomized, triple-blind, phase III EORTC-1416-LCG/ETOP 8-15 – PEARLS/KEYNOTE-091 study. Annals of Oncology 33(4):451–453

Peters S, Stahel R, Bubendorf L, Bonomi P, Villegas A, Kowalski DM et al (2019) Trastuzumab emtansine (T-DM1) in patients with previously treated HER2-overexpressing metastatic non-small cell lung cancer: efficacy, safety, and biomarkers. Clin Cancer Res 25(1):64–72

Pietanza MC, Kadota K, Huberman K, Sima CS, Fiore JJ, Sumner DK et al (2012) Phase II trial of temozolomide in patients with relapsed sensitive or refractory small cell lung cancer, with assessment of methylguanine-DNA methyltransferase as a potential biomarker. Clin Cancer Res 18(4):1138–1145

Pignon JP, Tribodet H, Scagliotti GV, Douillard JY, Shepherd FA, Stephens RJ et al (2008) Lung adjuvant cisplatin evaluation: a pooled analysis by the LACE Collaborative Group. J Clin Oncol 26(21): 3552–3559

Pillai RN, Owonikoko TK (2014) Small cell lung cancer: therapies and targets. Semin Oncol 41(1):133–142

Provencio M, Nadal E, Insa A, García-Campelo MR, Casal-Rubio J, Dómine M et al (2020) Neoadjuvant chemotherapy and nivolumab in resectable non-small-cell lung cancer (NADIM): an open-label, multicentre, single-arm, phase 2 trial. Lancet Oncol 21(11):1413–1422

Pujol JL, Carestia L, Daurès JP (2000) Is there a case for cisplatin in the treatment of small-cell lung cancer? A meta-analysis of randomized trials of a cisplatin-containing regimen versus a regimen without this alkylating agent. Br J Cancer 83(1):8–15

Pujol JL, Paul S, Chouaki N, Peterson P, Moore P, Berry DA et al (2007) Survival without common toxicity criteria grade 3/4 toxicity for pemetrexed compared with docetaxel in previously treated patients with advanced non-small cell lung cancer (NSCLC): a risk-benefit analysis. J Thorac Oncol 2(5):397–401

Puri S, Saltos A, Perez B, Le X, Gray JE (2020) Locally advanced, unresectable non-small cell lung cancer. Curr Oncol Rep 22(4):31

Ramakrishnan R, Gabrilovich DI (2013) Novel mechanism of synergistic effects of conventional chemotherapy and immune therapy of cancer. Cancer Immunol Immunother 62(3):405–410

Ramalingam SS, Dahlberg SE, Belani CP, Saltzman JN, Pennell NA, Nambudiri GS et al (2019) Pemetrexed, bevacizumab, or the combination as maintenance therapy for advanced nonsquamous non-small-cell lung cancer: ECOG-ACRIN 5508. J Clin Oncol 37(26):2360–2367

Ramalingam SS, Vansteenkiste J, Planchard D, Cho BC, Gray JE, Ohe Y et al (2020) Overall survival with osimertinib in untreated, EGFR-mutated advanced NSCLC. N Engl J Med 382(1):41–50

Reck M, Rodríguez-Abreu D, Robinson AG, Hui R, Csőszi T, Fülöp A et al (2016) Pembrolizumab versus chemotherapy for PD-L1-positive non-small-cell lung cancer. N Engl J Med 375(19):1823–1833

Reck M, Garassino MC, Imbimbo M, Shepherd FA, Socinski MA, Shih JY et al (2018) Antiangiogenic therapy for patients with aggressive or refractory advanced non-small cell lung cancer in the second-line setting. Lung Cancer (Amsterdam, Netherlands) 120:62–69

Reck M, Rodríguez-Abreu D, Robinson AG, Hui R, Csőszi T, Fülöp A et al (2019) Updated analysis of KEYNOTE-024: pembrolizumab versus platinum-based chemotherapy for advanced non-small-cell lung cancer with PD-L1 tumor proportion score of 50% or greater. J Clin Oncol 37(7):537–546

Reck M, Ciuleanu T-E, Dols MC, Schenker M, Zurawski B, Menezes J et al (2020) Nivolumab (NIVO) + ipilimumab (IPI) + 2 cycles of platinum-doublet chemotherapy (chemo) vs 4 cycles chemo as first-line (1L) treatment (tx) for stage IV/recurrent non-small cell lung cancer (NSCLC): CheckMate 9LA. Presented at: ASCO20 virtual scientific program. J Clin Oncol 38(Suppl):Abstr 9501

Remon J, Aldea M, Besse B, Planchard D, Reck M, Giaccone G et al (2021) Small cell lung cancer: a slightly less orphan disease after immunotherapy. Ann Oncol 32:698–709

Robert C (2020) A decade of immune-checkpoint inhibitors in cancer therapy. Nat Commun 11(1):3801

Roche (2021) Pivotal phase III study shows Roche's Tecentriq helped people with early lung cancer live longer without their disease returning. News release. Roche. 22 Mar 2021. https://www.roche.com/media/releases/med-cor-2021-03-22.htm. Accessed 22 Mar 2021

Rockswold GL, Ramsey HE, Buker GD (1970) The results of treatment of lung cancer by surgery, radiation and chemotherapy at a USPHS hospital. Mil Med 135(5):362–368

Rosell R, Gómez-Codina J, Camps C, Maestre J, Padille J, Cantó A et al (1994) A randomized trial comparing preoperative chemotherapy plus surgery with surgery alone in patients with non-small-cell lung cancer. N Engl J Med 330(3):153–158

Rossi A, Di Maio M, Chiodini P, Rudd RM, Okamoto H, Skarlos DV et al (2012) Carboplatin- or cisplatin-based chemotherapy in first-line treatment of small-cell lung cancer: the COCIS meta-analysis of individual patient data. J Clin Oncol 30(14):1692–1698

Rossi G, Alama A, Genova C, Rijavec E, Tagliamento M, Biello F et al (2018) The evolving role of pemetrexed disodium for the treatment of non-small cell lung cancer. Expert Opin Pharmacother 19(17):1969–1976

Rudin CM, Pietanza MC, Bauer TM, Ready N, Morgensztern D, Glisson BS et al (2017) Rovalpituzumab tesirine, a DLL3-targeted antibody-drug conjugate, in recurrent small-cell lung cancer: a first-in-human, first-in-class, open-label, phase 1 study. Lancet Oncol 18(1):42–51

Rudin CM, Poirier JT, Byers LA, Dive C, Dowlati A, George J et al (2019) Molecular subtypes of small cell lung cancer: a synthesis of human and mouse model data. Nat Rev Cancer 19(5):289–297

Rudin CM, Awad MM, Navarro A, Gottfried M, Peters S, Csőszi T et al (2020) Pembrolizumab or placebo plus etoposide and platinum as first-line therapy for extensive-stage small-cell lung cancer: randomized, double-blind, phase III KEYNOTE-604 study. J Clin Oncol 38(21):2369–2379

Saltos A, Shafique M, Chiappori A (2020) Update on the biology, management, and treatment of small cell lung cancer (SCLC). Front Oncol 10:1074

Sands JM, Shimizu T, Garon EB, Greenberg J, Guevara FM, Heist RS et al (2019) First-in-human phase 1 study of DS-1062a in patients with advanced solid tumors. J Clin Oncol 37(15_Suppl):9051

Scagliotti GV, Parikh P, von Pawel J, Biesma B, Vansteenkiste J, Manegold C et al (2008) Phase III study comparing cisplatin plus gemcitabine with cisplatin plus pemetrexed in chemotherapy-naive patients with advanced-stage non-small-cell lung cancer. J Clin Oncol 26(21):3543–3551

Scagliotti GV, Pastorino U, Vansteenkiste JF, Spaggiari L, Facciolo F, Orlowski TM et al (2012) Randomized phase III study of surgery alone or surgery plus preoperative cisplatin and gemcitabine in stages IB to IIIA non-small-cell lung cancer. J Clin Oncol 30(2):172–178

Schiller JH, Harrington D, Belani CP, Langer C, Sandler A, Krook J et al (2002) Comparison of four chemotherapy regimens for advanced non-small-cell lung cancer. N Engl J Med 346(2):92–98

Senan S, Brade A, Wang LH, Vansteenkiste J, Dakhil S, Biesma B et al (2016) PROCLAIM: randomized phase III trial of pemetrexed-cisplatin or etoposide-cisplatin plus thoracic radiation therapy followed by consolidation chemotherapy in locally advanced non-squamous non-small-cell lung cancer. J Clin Oncol 34(9):953–962

Serzan MT, Farid S, Liu SV (2020) Drugs in development for small cell lung cancer. J Thorac Dis 12(10):6298–6307

Seto T, Azuma K, Yamanaka T, Sugawara S, Yoshioka H, Wakuda K et al (2020) Randomized phase III study of continuation maintenance bevacizumab with or without pemetrexed in advanced nonsquamous non-small-cell lung cancer: COMPASS (WJOG5610L). J Clin Oncol 38(8):793–803

Sharma J, Shum E, Chau V, Paucar D, Cheng H, Halmos B (2017) The evolving role of biomarkers in personalized lung cancer therapy. Respiration 93(1):1–14

Shu CA, Gainor JF, Awad MM, Chiuzan C, Grigg CM, Pabani A et al (2020) Neoadjuvant atezolizumab and chemotherapy in patients with resectable non-small-cell lung cancer: an open-label, multicentre, single-arm, phase 2 trial. Lancet Oncol 21(6):786–795. https://doi.org/10.1016/S1470-2045(20)30140-6

Sirotnak FM, Zakowski MF, Miller VA, Scher HI, Kris MG (2000) Efficacy of cytotoxic agents against human tumor xenografts is markedly enhanced by coadministration of ZD1839 (Iressa), an inhibitor of EGFR tyrosine kinase. Clin Cancer Res 6(12):4885–4892

Smit EF, Fokkema E, Biesma B, Groen HJ, Snoek W, Postmus PE (1998) A phase II study of paclitaxel in heavily pretreated patients with small-cell lung cancer. Br J Cancer 77(2):347–351

Smit EF, Nakagawa K, Nagasaka M, Felip E, Goto Y, Li BT et al (2020) Trastuzumab deruxtecan (T-DXd; DS-8201) in patients with HER2-mutated metastatic non-small cell lung cancer (NSCLC): interim results of DESTINY-Lung01. J Clin Oncol 38(15_Suppl):9504

Socinski MA, Jotte RM, Cappuzzo F, Orlandi F, Stroyakovskiy D, Nogami N et al (2018a) Atezolizumab for first-line treatment of metastatic nonsquamous NSCLC. N Engl J Med 378(24):2288–2301

Socinski MA, Jotte RM, Cappuzzo F, Orlandi FJ, Stroyakovskiy D, Nogami N et al (2018b) Overall survival (OS) analysis of IMpower150, a randomized Ph 3 study of atezolizumab (atezo) + chemotherapy (chemo) ± bevacizumab (bev) vs chemo + bev in 1L nonsquamous (NSQ) NSCLC. J Clin Oncol 36(15_Suppl):9002

Socinski MA, Jotte RM, Cappuzzo F, Mok TSK, West H, Nishio M et al (2019) IMpower150: analysis of efficacy in patients (pts) with liver metastases (mets). J Clin Oncol 37(15_Suppl):9012

Song WA, Zhou NK, Wang W, Chu XY, Liang CY, Tian XD et al (2010) Survival benefit of neoadjuvant chemotherapy in non-small cell lung cancer: an updated meta-analysis of 13 randomized control trials. J Thorac Oncol 5(4):510–516

Soria JC, Mauguen A, Reck M, Sandler AB, Saijo N, Johnson DH et al (2013) Systematic review and meta-analysis of randomised, phase II/III trials adding bevacizumab to platinum-based chemotherapy as first-line treatment in patients with advanced non-small-cell lung cancer. Ann Oncol 24(1):20–30

Spira A, Lisberg AE, Sands JM (2021) Datopotamab deruxtecan (Dato-DXd; DS-1062), a TROP2 ADC, in patients with advanced NSCLC: updated results of TROPION-PanTumor01 phase 1 study. In: 2020 World conference on lung cancer. Abstract OA0303. Presented 29 Jan 2021

Stewart CA, Gay CM, Xi Y, Sivajothi S, Sivakamasundari V, Fujimoto J et al (2020) Single-cell analyses reveal increased intratumoral heterogeneity after the onset of therapy resistance in small-cell lung cancer. Nat Cancer 1:423–436

Strauss GM, Herndon JE 2nd, Maddaus MA, Johnstone DW, Johnson EA, Harpole DH et al (2008) Adjuvant paclitaxel plus carboplatin compared with observation in stage IB non-small-cell lung cancer: CALGB 9633 with the Cancer and Leukemia Group B, Radiation Therapy Oncology Group, and North Central Cancer Treatment Group Study Groups. J Clin Oncol 26(31):5043–5051

Strickler JH, Weekes CD, Nemunaitis J, Ramanathan RK, Heist RS, Morgensztern D et al (2018) First-in-human phase I, dose-escalation and -expansion study of telisotuzumab vedotin, an antibody-drug conjugate targeting c-met, in patients with advanced solid tumors. J Clin Oncol 36(33):3298–3306

Trigo J, Subbiah V, Besse B, Moreno V, López R, Sala MA et al (2020) Lurbinectedin as second-line treatment for patients with small-cell lung cancer: a single-arm, open-label, phase 2 basket trial. Lancet Oncol 21(5):645–654

Tsurutani J, Iwata H, Krop I, Jänne PA, Doi T, Takahashi S et al (2020) Targeting HER2 with trastuzumab deruxtecan: a dose-expansion, phase I study in multiple advanced solid tumors. Cancer Discov 10(5):688–701

Turrisi AT 3rd, Kim K, Blum R, Sause WT, Livingston RB, Komaki R et al (1999) Twice-daily compared with once-daily thoracic radiotherapy in limited small-cell lung cancer treated concurrently with cisplatin and etoposide. N Engl J Med 340(4):265–271

von Pawel J, Schiller JH, Shepherd FA, Fields SZ, Kleisbauer JP, Chrysson NG et al (1999) Topotecan versus cyclophosphamide, doxorubicin, and vincristine for the treatment of recurrent small-cell lung cancer. J Clin Oncol 17(2):658–667

Wakelee HA, Dahlberg SE, Keller SM, Tester WJ, Gandara DR, Graziano SL et al (2016) E1505: adjuvant chemotherapy +/− bevacizumab for early stage NSCLC—outcomes based on chemotherapy subsets. J Clin Oncol 34(15_Suppl):8507

Wang J, Chen J, Guo Y, Wang B, Chu H (2017) Strategies targeting angiogenesis in advanced non-small cell lung cancer. Oncotarget 8(32):53854–53872

Weiss GJ, Langer C, Rosell R, Hanna N, Shepherd F, Einhorn LH et al (2006) Elderly patients benefit from second-line cytotoxic chemotherapy: a subset analysis of a randomized phase III trial of pemetrexed compared with docetaxel in patients with previously treated advanced non-small-cell lung cancer. J Clin Oncol 24(27):4405–4411

West H, McCleod M, Hussein M, Morabito A, Rittmeyer A, Conter HJ et al (2019) Atezolizumab in combination with carboplatin plus nab-paclitaxel chemotherapy compared with chemotherapy alone as first-line treatment for metastatic non-squamous non-small-cell lung cancer (IMpower130): a multicentre, randomised, open-label, phase 3 trial. Lancet Oncol 20(7):924–937

Winton T, Livingston R, Johnson D, Rigas J, Johnston M, Butts C et al (2005) Vinorelbine plus cisplatin vs. observation in resected non-small-cell lung cancer. N Engl J Med 352(25):2589–2597

Wu YL, Lee JS, Thongprasert S, Yu CJ, Zhang L, Ladrera G et al (2013) Intercalated combination of chemotherapy and erlotinib for patients with advanced stage non-small-cell lung cancer (FASTACT-2): a randomised, double-blind trial. Lancet Oncol 14(8):777–786

Wu YL, Tsuboi M, He J, John T, Grohe C, Majem M et al (2020) Osimertinib in resected EGFR-mutated non-small-cell lung cancer. N Engl J Med 383(18):1711–1723

Yu HA, Schoenfeld AJ, Makhnin A, Kim R, Rizvi H, Tsui D et al (2020) Effect of osimertinib and bevacizumab on progression-free survival for patients with metastatic EGFR-mutant lung cancers: a phase 1/2 single-group open-label trial. JAMA Oncol 6(7):1048–1054

Zhou Y, Lin Z, Zhang X, Chen C, Zhao H, Hong S et al (2019) First-line treatment for patients with advanced non-small cell lung carcinoma and high PD-L1 expression: pembrolizumab or pembrolizumab plus chemotherapy. J Immunother Cancer 7(1):120

Targeted Therapies in Non-small Cell Lung Cancer

Jessica R. Bauman and Martin J. Edelman

Contents

1	Introduction	347
2	**Driver Mutations: Discovery and Biology**	348
3	**Epidemiology and Treatment by Mutation**	351
3.1	EGFR	351
3.2	EGFR Exon 20 Insertion	354
3.3	ALK	354
3.4	ROS1	357
3.5	RET	357
3.6	NTRK	359
3.7	BRAF	359
3.8	MET	360
3.9	KRAS	361
3.10	HER2	362
3.11	Other Mutations on the Horizon	363
4	**Immunotherapy and the Targetable Mutations**	363
5	**Brain Metastases**	364
6	**Co-mutations and Outcomes**	364
7	**Squamous Cell NSCLC and Small Cell Lung Cancer and Targeted Therapies**	364
8	**Future Directions**	364
	References	364

J. R. Bauman · M. J. Edelman (✉)
Department of Hematology/Oncology, Fox Chase Cancer Center, Philadelphia, PA, USA
e-mail: martin.edelman@fccc.edu

1 Introduction

Historically, platinum-doublet chemotherapy was the mainstay of treatment for all patients with advanced non-small cell lung cancer (NSCLC). With platinum-doublet treatment, patients had a median overall survival of approximately 8 months and a 1-year survival of 33% (Schiller et al. 2002). In the last 20 years, however, there have been remarkable advances in the understanding of the pathophysiology, immunology, genetics, and heterogeneity of NSCLC, which has led to a myriad of new drug approvals based upon improvements in survival and quality of life (Ramalingam et al. 2020; Peters et al. 2017, 2020; Hirsch et al. 2017; Chen et al. 2013). Previously, we approached all patients with NSCLC as a homogenous population. We now base treatment on each patient's histology, molecular sequencing, and biomarkers of immune response. In this chapter, we will provide an overview of the discovery and biology of driver mutations and discuss the seven mutational targets for which treatment is currently fully approved (EGFR, ALK, ROS, RET, TRK, MET, BRAF, KRAS) and others for which investigational agents are likely to be approved in the near future (Her2). In addition, we will discuss some particular areas of interest with targeted therapies including brain metastases, issues of immunotherapy, and the influence of co-mutations and potential combinations with other agents.

2 Driver Mutations: Discovery and Biology

Molecular sequencing of the DNA and more recently RNA of NSCLC, particularly adenocarcinoma, has transformed our approach to selecting treatment for patients with advanced NSCLC. Once we considered lung cancer signaling and pathobiology to be too complex to target a single pathway. This paradigm shifted with the discovery of epidermal growth factor receptor (EGFR) mutations in NSCLC as the predictor of responsiveness to EGFR tyrosine kinase inhibitors (TKIs) (Lynch et al. 2004). EGFR TKIs were initially developed as a general approach to treatment of NSCLC because downstream signaling through EGFR dimerization was known to lead to cell proliferation and survival. However, multiple trials of EGFR inhibitors in nonbiomarker selected NSCLC showed only a 10–18% overall response rate (ORR) in pretreated patients with advanced NSCLC (Fukuoka et al. 2003; Kris et al. 2003; Sequist and Lynch 2008). Astute investigators observed that there appeared to be a subpopulation with dramatic responses to EGFR TKIs—patients who were younger, with adenocarcinoma histology, women, of East Asian descent, those who developed a rash with treatment, and/or those who were never smokers (Sequist and Lynch 2008). In light of these observations and the growing understanding of the molecular underpinnings of cancer in general, three groups sequenced the DNA of the tumors from patients with NSCLC with exceptional responses to EGFR TKIs vs. nonresponders and discovered activating mutations in the EGFR tyrosine kinase domain in those patients with exceptional responses (Lynch et al. 2004; Paez et al. 2004; Pao et al. 2004). The EGFR mutations discovered led to constitutive activation of the receptor with increased growth factor signaling, resulting in an oncogene-addicted tumor that was exquisitely sensitive to EGFR inhibition. This remarkable discovery began the era of understanding oncogene-addicted biology and treatment in NSCLC, depicted in Fig. 1 (Zhu et al. 2017).

It is now recognized that over half of patients with the adenocarcinoma subtype of NSCLC (approximately 40–50%) have specific molecular alterations, which has led to an explosion of oncogene-selected clinical trials as well as FDA approvals of over 20 targeted agents for 7 different driver mutations by the beginning of 2021 (Table 1). Consequently, next-generation sequencing (NGS) is now recommended for all patients with a new diagnosis of advanced NSCLC (Fig. 2) (Hirsch et al. 2017; Sholl et al. 2015). The specific incidences of the various mutations are quite variable from study to study for several reasons. The technology to assess for mutations has evolved considerably in the past few years and previously undetected mutations are now reported. Additionally, there is a clear variability in the occurrence of some mutations, with a very high incidence of EGFR mutations reported in China and other Asian countries (30–50%) vs. a much lower incidence in the United States and Western Europe (10–15%) (Zhang et al. 2020). Additionally, there is probably an element of referral bias in terms of the patients for whom analysis is obtained (likely more frequent in never smokers and high-income individuals) as well as the institutions performing the studies.

Although these targeted drugs are clear success stories in NSCLC therapeutics with significant reduction in symptoms and prolongation of survival for the majority of patients, disease progression is almost universal. This development of acquired resistance is the Achille's heel of targeted therapies and at the center of ongoing research in molecularly driven NSCLC. While details vary, the primary processes for most mutations and the consequences are very similar. A mutation resulting in a component of a pathway leading to cell growth and proliferation occurs (Fig. 1). The mutation is usually in the exon coding for a kinase domain, i.e., part of the molecule that transfers a phosphate group to a downstream part of the pathway that results in continued activity despite the lack of an upstream stimulus. In some instances (e.g., MET exon 14 skipping), the mutation occurs in the regulatory domain responsible for the

Targeted Therapies in Non-small Cell Lung Cancer

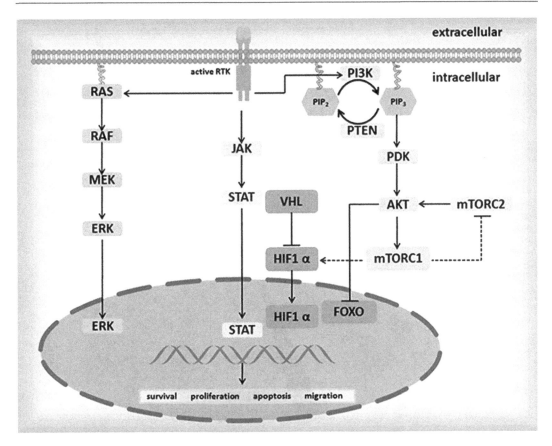

Fig. 1 Oncogene-addicted NSCLC

Table 1 Molecular targets and agents for NSCLC

Target[a]	FDA approved agents	FDA-approved agents (off label use)	Investigational
EGFR	Gefitinib, erlotinib, afatinib, dacomitinib, osimertinib		
ALK	Crizotinib, ceritinib, alectinib, brigatinib, lorlatinib		Entrectinib, ensartinib
BRAF	Dabrafenib + trametinib	Vemurafenib	
KRAS	None	Sotorasib	Adagrasib
EGFR exon 20	Mobocertinib, amivantamab		Osimertinib (high dose), poziotinib
HER2	None	Afatinib, ado-trastuzumab emtansine, neratinib, dacomitinib	Trastuzumab deruxtecan
MET	Tepotinib, capmatinib	Crizotinib, cabozantinib	Savolitinib, ficlatuzumab, onartuzumab, tivantinib
RET	Selpercatinib, pralsetinib	Cabozantinib, vandetanib, sunitinib	
NTRK	Larotrectinib, entrectinib		Ropotrectinib; taletrectinib
NRG1		Afatinib	Anti-HER3 therapy (GSK2849330)
ROS1	Crizotinib, entrectinib	Ceritinib, lorlatinib, cabozantinib	Ropotrectinib; taletrectinib

[a] Consolidated from Hirsch et al. (2017), Chu (2020), Halliday et al. (2019), Guo et al. (2019), Genova et al. (2020), Drilon et al. (2018b)

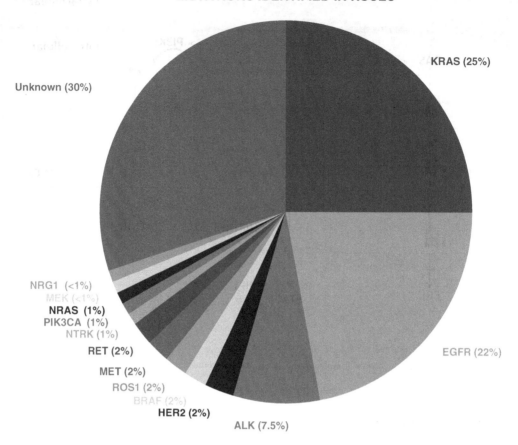

Fig. 2 Frequency of driver mutations identified in NSCLC. Frequencies are a combination of data from those in Tsao et al. (2016) and in Sholl et al. (2015)

termination or attenuation of signaling (Salgia 2017). Resistance to targeted agents can occur through several mechanisms: the emergence of clones that have abnormalities (including mutations, gene amplification, overexpression) that bypass the initial driver, mutations within the same pathway, mutations that have a higher affinity for the native substrate and therefore outcompete the TKI or that physically obstruct the kinase domain (gatekeeper) or those that alter the charge characteristics at the entrance to the kinase domain and consequently prevent the approach of the TKI (solvent front mutations). In this chapter, for each genetic mutation, we will summarize the epidemiology, pathologic features, prognosis, treatment options, and current strategies for acquired resistance. We will also touch upon other issues with targeted therapy including immunotherapy, brain metastases, co-mutations, and targeted therapy in squamous cell carcinoma and small cell.

3 Epidemiology and Treatment by Mutation

3.1 EGFR

Activating EGFR mutations occur in up to 20% of patients with lung adenocarcinoma and in approximately 50% of never smokers (Sholl et al. 2015; Shigematsu et al. 2005). They are most commonly found in patients who are younger, female, East-Asian, never smokers, and/or with adenocarcinoma histology. However, EGFR mutations have been noted across all ages, sex, ethnicity, smoking status, and histologies, and therefore it is necessary to evaluate all nonsquamous carcinoma patients for this mutation. The most common activating EGFR mutations, seen in 90% of patients, are deletion mutations in exon 19 or point mutations in exon 21 (L858R). The other 10% ("uncommon mutations") include exon 18 point mutations and exon 20 point or insertion mutations (Hirsch et al. 2017; Sequist and Lynch 2008; Shigematsu et al. 2005; O'Kane et al. 2017).

There are five EGFR TKIs that have been approved by the U.S. Food and Drug Administration (FDA) and European Medicines Agency (EMA) for advanced EGFR-mutated NSCLC: two first-generation TKIs, gefitinib and erlotinib, two second-generation TKIs, afatinib and dacomitinib, and one third-generation TKI, osimertinib. A sixth agent, icotinib, is approved for use in China. Eleven major randomized controlled trials have demonstrated superiority of EGFR TKIs initially to chemotherapy and now to earlier generations of EGFR inhibitors (Table 2) (Mok et al. 2009, 2017a; Mitsudomi et al. 2010; Maemondo et al. 2010; Zhou et al. 2011; Rosell et al. 2012; Sequist et al. 2013; Wu et al. 2014, 2015, 2017; Soria et al. 2018). Collectively, these trials demonstrated clear benefits in regard to progression-free survival, ORR, and quality of life in comparison to chemotherapy, with ORR between 60–80% and PFS from 9 to 17 months. An overall survival benefit was not initially observed in the early trials, which was thought to be related to small samples sizes and significant crossover. However, the frontline osimertinib trial, FLAURA, did show an improvement in OS compared to first-generation TKIs with a median OS of 38.6 months compared to 31.8 months when compared to gefitinib or erlotinib (Ramalingam et al. 2020). There was also superiority in intracranial activity with osimertinib, which was a key factor for the improved outcomes. The intracranial response rate was 91% compared with 68%, and the CNS PFS was not reached in the osimertinib arm, compared with 13.9 months with standard TKI. Osimertinib was also substantially less toxic, with a lower incidence of rash and diarrhea compared with prior agents. As a result, osimertinib has become the de facto standard of care for frontline treatment of advanced EGFR-mutated NSCLC.

Despite remarkable responses to frontline EGFR TKIs, patients inevitably develop disease progression with acquired resistance. Mechanisms of resistance differ based on which generation of EGFR-TKI is used in the frontline setting, and both EGFR-dependent and EGFR-independent mechanisms are observed (Fig. 3) (Lim et al. 2018; Lovly et al. 2017). For first- and second-generation TKIs, the most common mechanism of resistance is the development of a T790M mutation, which occurs in up to 50% of patients (Lim et al. 2018; Zhang and Yuan 2016). The T790M mutation is a gatekeeper mutation in the EGFR kinase domain which leads to both interference of drug binding and increased affinity of the active site for ATP vs. drug. Osimertinib targets both EGFR-sensitizing mutations and the T790M mutation. The drug was first evaluated in patients who developed resistance to first-generation TKIs. In the AURA clinical trial, patients with T790M-positive NSCLC who progressed on frontline EGFR TKIs were randomized to osimertinib or platinum-doublet chemotherapy. Patients treated with osimertinib showed improvement in ORR and PFS, though no benefit was noted in OS, again likely due to crossover (Mok et al. 2017a; Papadimitrakopoulou et al. 2020). For patients treated with osimertinib in the frontline setting, T790M mutations are not commonly seen but development of C797S mutations can occur in up to 7% of patients (Ramalingam et al. 2018). EGFR-independent

Table 2 Trial summary for patients with EGFR mutations

Trial and year	N	Comparator arms	Response rate (%)	Median PFS (mo)	HR (95% CI)	OS (months)	HR (95% CI)
IPASS; 2009 (Mok et al. 2009)	261	Gefitinib / Carbo/paclitaxel	71 / 47	9.6 / 6.3	0.48 (0.36–0.64)	18.8 / 17.4	0.90 (0.79–1.02)
WJTOG 3405; 2010 (Mitsudomi et al. 2010)	228	Gefitinib / Cisplatin/docetaxel	62 / 31	9.2 / 6.3	0.49 (0.35–0.71)	27.7 / 26.6	0.89 (0.483)
NEJ002; 2009 (Maemondo et al. 2010)	194	Gefitinib / Carbo/paclitaxel	74 / 31	10.4 / 5.5	0.36 (0.25–0.51)	30.5 / 23.6	$P = 0.31$
OPTIMAL; 2011 (Zhou et al. 2011, 2015)	154	Erlotinib / Carbo/gemcitabine	83 / 36	13.1 / 4.6	0.16 (0.10–0.26)	22.8 / 27.2	1.19 (0.83–1.71)
EURTAC; 2012 (Rosell et al. 2012)	174	Erlotinib / Platinum doublet	58 / 15	9.7 / 5.2	0.37 (0.25–0.54)	19.3 / 19.5	1.04 (0.65–1.68)
LUX-Lung 3; 2013 (Sequist et al. 2013; Yang et al. 2015)	345	Afatinib / Cisplatin/pem	56 / 23	11.1 / 6.9	0.58 (0.43–0.78)	25.8 / 24.5	0.75–1.11
LUX-Lung 6; 2014 (Wu et al. 2014; Yang et al. 2015)	364	Afatinib / Cisplatin/gemcitabine	67 / 23	11.0 / 5.6	0.20–0.39		
ENSURE; 2015 (Wu et al. 2015)	217	Erlotinib / Cisplatin/gemcitabine	63 / 34	11.0 / 5.5	0.34 (0.22–0.51)	26.3 / 25.5	0.91 (0.63–1.31)
AURA3; 2017 (Mok et al. 2017a; Papadimitrakopoulou et al. 2020)	419	Osimertinib / Cis/carbo + pem	71 / 31	10.1 / 4.4	0.30 (0.23–0.41)	27 / 23	0.87 (0.67–1.12)
FLAURA; 2018 (Ramalingam et al. 2020; Soria et al. 2018)	556	Osimertinib / Erlotinib or gefitinib	80 / 76	17.2 / 8.5	0.46 (0.37–0.57)	38.6 / 31.8	0.80 (0.64–0.997)
ARCHER 1050; 2017 (Wu et al. 2017; Mok et al. 2018)	452	Dacomitinib / Gefitinib	75 / 72	14.7 / 9.2	0.59 (0.47–0.74)	34 / 27	0.76 (0.58–0.99)
NEJ009; 2020 (Hosomi et al. 2020)	345	Gefitinib + carbo/pem / Gefitinib	84 / 67	20.9 / 11.9	0.49 (0.39–0.62)	50.9 / 38.8	0.72 (0.55–0.95)
Tata; 2020 (Noronha et al. 2020)	350	Gefitinib + carbo/pem / Gefitinib	75 / 63	16 / 8	0.51 (0.39–0.66)	NR / 17	0.45 (0.31–0.65)
NEJ026; 2019 (Saito et al. 2019)	228	Erlotinib + bevacizumab / Erlotinib	72 / 66	16.9 / 13.3	0.61 (0.42–0.88)	51 / 46	1.00 (0.68–1.48)
RELAY; 2019 (Nakagawa et al. 2019)	449	Erlotinib + ramucirumab / Erlotinib	76 / 75	19.4 / 12.4	0.59 (0.46–0.76)	NR / NR	0.83 (0.53–1.30)
ADAURA; 2020 (Wu et al. 2020a)	682	Osimertinib in resected EGFR NSCLC vs. placebo	n/a	2 year DFS: 90% vs. 44%	CI: 37–51	Not mature	

Abbreviations: *NR* not reached, *carbo* carboplatin, *cis* cisplatin, *pem* pemetrexed, *PFS* progression-free survival, *OS* overall survival, *HR* hazard ratio

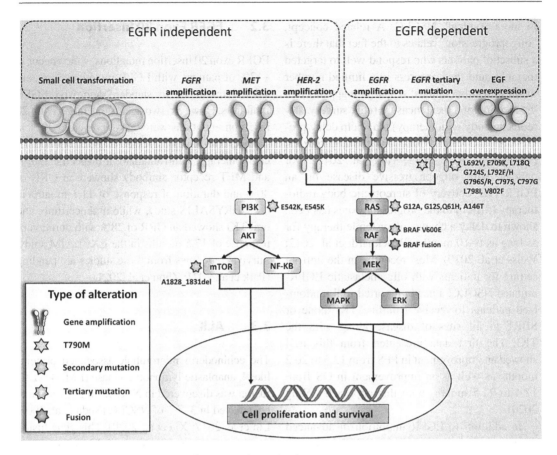

Fig. 3 EGFR-independent and -dependent mechanisms of resistance

mechanisms of acquired resistance that are most common include MET, HER2, or FGFR amplification, as well as mutations in KRAS, PIK3Ca, or BRAF V600E (Lim et al. 2018). Additionally, transformation to small cell carcinoma has been noted. Multiple trials targeting these various mechanisms of acquired resistance are underway, though the most standard treatment at progression after EGFR TKIs is chemotherapy.

In addition to targeting resistance mechanisms, alternative approaches to improve outcomes for patients with EGFR-mutated NSCLC include combining TKIs with chemotherapy or VEGF-targeting treatment. Two frontline trials done in Japan (Hosomi et al. 2020) and India (Noronha et al. 2020) added platinum-doublet chemotherapy to gefitinib compared to gefitinib alone (Table 2). Both of these showed improvements in PFS and OS, albeit with an increase in toxicity in the combination arm. Impressively, the median OS of the NEJ009 trial was 51 months, which is the longest OS ever seen in this population (Hosomi et al. 2020). Trials combining EGFR TKIs with VEGF inhibition with either bevacizumab or ramucirumab have also shown promise, with improvements in PFS, though no impact on OS (Table 2) (Saito et al. 2019; Nakagawa et al. 2019).

The addition of radiation in unique circumstances for patients with EGFR-mutated NSCLC is also being studied, both upfront and at progression. The concept of oligometastatic disease, i.e., that some patients with metastatic disease may have a limited number of sites of disease amenable to local management as opposed to a systemic disease, was first proposed by Hellman and Weichselbaum in 1995 (Hellman and Weichselbaum 1995). The incidence of this syndrome appears to be more frequent in patients with driver mutation related disease as opposed to more "typical" NSCLC. A related concept, "oligoprogression" relates to the fact that there is a subset of patients who respond well to targeted therapies and then progress in a limited number of sites. In either clinical scenario, it appears that the addition of a local measure (e.g., surgery, stereotactic body radiotherapy) may help delay progression and extend time on frontline therapy (Weickhardt et al. 2012; Yu et al. 2013). For patients with oligoprogressive disease on an EGFR TKI, delivery of stereotactic body radiotherapy (SBRT) to the progressing sites has been shown to delay a change of systemic therapy for as long as 6–10 months (Weickhardt et al. 2012; Weiss et al. 2019). Most recently, in the upfront setting for patients with oligometastatic EGFR-mutated NSCLC, a newly reported trial randomized patients to receive frontline TKI alone or SBRT to all sites of disease along with the TKI. The first data presented from this trial showed an improvement in PFS from 12.5 to 20.2 months as well as an improvement in OS from 17.4 to 22.5 months with this approach (Wang 2020).

In addition to EGFR inhibition in advanced disease, there is a new role for EGFR inhibition in the adjuvant setting post-surgery for patients with EGFR-mutated NSCLC. In the phase III study, ADAURA, 682 patients with completely resected, stage IB–IIIA EGFR-positive lung cancer, were randomized between osimertinib or placebo for 3 years. Disease-free survival was significantly longer in the patients treated with osimertinib; at 24 months, 89% of the osimertinib group and 52% of those in the placebo were alive and disease free (HR 0.2 (0.14–0.30)) (Wu et al. 2020a). Although survival data is immature, the FDA has approved osimertinib based on these results. Despite the impressive nature of the PFS, these data must be viewed with some caution as a similarly designed trial employing gefitinib failed to demonstrate an improved OS versus chemotherapy (Zhong et al. 2021).

Overall, patients with EGFR-mutated NSCLC have benefited from significant improvements in ORR, duration of response, quality of life, and survival with EGFR TKI therapy. Acquired resistance remains a clinical conundrum and an area of active research.

3.2 EGFR Exon 20 Insertion

EGFR exon 20 insertion mutations, which occur in ~12% of patients with EGFR mutations, are considered resistance to standard approved EGFR inhibitors. However, two agents that target exon 20 insertion mutations were just approved in 2021 in patients who have progressed on platinum doublet chemotherapy. Amivantamab, a bispecific EGFR and MET receptor antibody showed an ORR of 40% and duration of response of 11.1 months in the CHRYSALIS study, while mobocertinib, and oral TKI showed an ORR of 28% with duration of response of 17.5 months in the EXCLAIM study. Survival outcomes from these studies are pending (Park et al. 2021; Zhou et al. 2021).

3.3 ALK

The echinoderm microtubule-associated protein-like 4, anaplastic lymphoma kinase (EML4-ALK) fusion was discovered in NSCLC in 2007 and can be detected in 3–7% of NSCLC (Soda et al. 2007; Lin et al. 2017; Xia et al. 2020). This gene fusion develops from an inversion on the short arm of chromosome 2 that joins the 5′ end of the EML4 gene with the 3′ end of the ALK gene, creating the EML4-ALK chimeric protein (Xia et al. 2020). The ALK protein is a receptor tyrosine kinase in the insulin receptor superfamily and more than 20 different ALK fusion partners have been detected in rearrangements (Lin et al. 2017). The rearrangements lead to constitutive activation of ALK, triggering downstream pathways to signal unchecked through JAK/STAT, PI3K/AKT, and MEK/ERK to drive cell growth and survival. ALK rearrangements can be detected with fluorescence in situ hybridization (FISH), immunohistochemistry (IHC), or next-generation sequencing (NGS). As with EGFR, patients with ALK fusions are usually younger, have adenocarcinoma histology, and are scant or never smokers.

Since its discovery in NSCLC in 2007, five ALK inhibitors are now approved for the treatment of ALK-rearranged NSCLC with numerous clinical trials showing exquisite sensitivity to ALK inhibition: crizotinib, ceritinib, alectinib, brigatinib, and lorlatinib (Table 3) (Peters et al.

Table 3 Trial summary for ALK and ROS1 clinical trials

Trial and year	N	Arms	Response rate (%)	Median PFS (months)	HR (95% CI)	OS (months)	HR (95% CI)
ALK							
PROFILE 1001; 2010 (Kwak et al. 2010)	82	Crizotinib	57	Estimated 6 months, 72%	n/a	n/a	n/a
PROFILE 1007; 2013 (Shaw et al. 2013)	347	Crizotinib vs. second-line chemotherapy	65 20	7.7 3.0	0.49 (0.37–0.64)	20.3 22.8	1.02 (0.68–1.54)
PROFILE 1014; 2014 (Solomon et al. 2014, 2018a)	343	Crizotinib vs. first-line carbo/cis + pemetrexed	74 45	10.9 7.0	0.45 (0.35–0.6)	NR 47.5	0.346 (0.08–0.72)
ASCEND-4; 2017 (Soria et al. 2017)	376	Ceritinib vs. first-line carbo/cis + pemetrexed	73 27	16.6 8.1	0.55 (0.42–0.73)	NR 26.2	0.73 (0.5–1.08)
ALEX; 2017 (Peters et al. 2017; Mok et al. 2020)	303	Alectinib vs. crizotinib	83 76	35 11	0.47 (0.34–0.65)	NR 57.4	67 (0.46–0.98)
ALTA 1L; 2018 (Camidge et al. 2018, 2020)	275	Brigatinib vs. crizotinib	74 62	24 11	0.49 (0.35–0.68)	NR NR	0.92 (0.57–1.47)
2018 (Solomon et al. 2018b)	276	Lorlatinib	90 (TKI naïve) 47 (1 prior TKI) 39 (2+ prior TKIs)	NR (11.4 months-NR)	n/a	n/a	n/a
CROWN III (Shaw et al. 2020)	296	Lorlatinib vs. crizotinib	81 62	NR 9.1	0.21 (0.14–0.31)	NR NR	0.72 (0.41–1.25)
ROS1							
PROFILE 1001; 2014 (Shaw et al. 2014, 2019b)	50	Crizotinib	72	19.3	n/a	51	n/a
2017 (Lim et al. 2017)	32	Ceritinib	62	9.3	n/a	24	n/a
STARTRK; 2020 (Drilon et al. 2020a)	53	Entrectinib	77	19.0	n/a	Not reported	n/a
2019 (Shaw et al. 2019a)	69	Lorlatinib	62 (TKI naïve) 35 (prior TKI)	21 (TKI naïve) 8.5 (prior TKI)	n/a	Not reported	n/a

NR not reached, *carbo* carboplatin, *cis* cisplatin, *TKI* tyrosine kinase inhibitor, *PFS* progression-free survival, *OS* overall survival, *HR* hazard ratio

2017; Xia et al. 2020; Kwak et al. 2010; Soria et al. 2017; Camidge et al. 2018; Shaw et al. 2019a). Crizotinib was the first ALK inhibitor to demonstrate activity and earn FDA approval based on a phase I/II study of crizotinib in patients with ALK-positive NSCLC by FISH, which showed an ORR of 57% (Kwak et al. 2010). Crizotinib's efficacy was then confirmed in two trials comparing crizotinib to cytotoxic chemotherapy in the second- and then first-line setting for patients with ALK-positive NSCLC, which showed ORR of 65–75% compared to 20–45% and PFS of 7–11 months compared to 2–7 months, respectively (Shaw et al. 2013; Solomon et al. 2014). Survival favored the crizotinib arm, though there was high crossover between arms likely blunting the effect (Solomon et al. 2018a).

After crizotinib, three second-generation ALK inhibitors, ceritinib, alectinib, and brigatinib, were developed with improved potency against ALK and with better CNS penetrance (Peters et al. 2017; Soria et al. 2017; Camidge et al. 2018). All three were initially studied in the crizotinib resistant setting, showing ORR of 50–60% post crizotinib but subsequently were moved into the first-line setting (Lin et al. 2017). Ceritinib was studied in the phase III ASCEND-4, which compared first-line ceritinib to chemotherapy with platinum and pemetrexed, showing an improved PFS of 16.6 vs. 8.1 months and ORR of 73% vs. 27% (Soria et al. 2017). Alectinib was studied in the global phase III ALEX trial, which compared first-line alectinib to crizotinib, showing an improved PFS of 35 vs. 11 months and ORR of 83% vs. 75% with an improvement of OS of not reached vs. 57 months with crizotinib (Peters et al. 2017; Mok et al. 2020). Brigatinib was studied in the phase III ALTA-1L trial, which compared first-line brigatinib to crizotinib, showing an improved PFS of 24 vs. 11 months and ORR of 74% vs. 62% (Camidge et al. 2018, 2020). Overall survival remains immature. Additionally, intracranial efficacy was improved for all three second-generation ALK inhibitors. Based on this improved efficacy, the second-generation inhibitors have become standard of care in the frontline setting, with alectinib being the drug of choice due to length of follow-up, CNS activity, and improved toxicity profile.

Lorlatinib is the fifth ALK drug to receive FDA approval initially in the setting of resistance, but more recently as frontline therapy. Lorlatinib is a third-generation ALK inhibitor that was developed to overcome resistance to earlier ALK inhibitors, in particular the resistance mutation G1202R and to better penetrate the blood brain barrier. The phase II study of lorlatinib showed an ORR of 70% in patients previously treated with crizotinib and of 39% in patients previously treated with two or more ALK TKIs with a median duration of response (DOR) of 12.5 months (Solomon et al. 2018b). In the frontline setting, the CROWN III trial compared lorlatinib to crizotinib, which demonstrated an improved ORR of 76% vs. 58% and an improved median PFS of not reached vs. 9.3 months with a 12 month PFS of 80% vs. 35% as well as improved intracranial efficacy (66% vs. 20%) (Shaw et al. 2020).

Despite these remarkable responses and drug approvals for ALK-mutated NSCLC, development of resistance to ALK inhibition remains a formidable problem (Lin et al. 2017). ALK-dependent and ALK-independent mechanisms of resistance have been identified. ALK-dependent mechanisms involve mutations in the ALK kinase domain that reactivate the kinase by impacting the drug binding to the kinase, altering the confirmation, or modifying the ATP-binding affinity of the kinase as well as amplification of ALK (Sharma et al. 2018). These mutations can differ based on the ALK inhibitor employed. The most common mutations arising in the presence of crizotinib are L1196M, C1156Y, S1206Y, G1202R, 1151Tins, and G1269A. After ceritinib, R1275Q, L1152P, D1203, G1202R, F1174C, L1198F, and C1156Y have been described. After alectinib, I1171T, V1180L, and G1202R have been described, and G1202R, S1206C, and the co-mutation F1174V + L1198F are seen after brigatinib. An L1198F mutation has been seen after lorlatinib. Some of these mutations confer sensitivity to a different ALK inhibitor, while others are pan-resistant.

ALK-independent mechanisms of resistance have also been noted, which activate bypass signaling pathways (Lin et al. 2017; Sharma et al. 2018; McCoach et al. 2018). These include EGFR activation, KRAS mutation, PIK3CA, MET, and SRC activation. Transformation to small cell has also rarely been described. Strategies to target these resistance mutations are being developed. Additionally, strategies that combine ALK inhibition with a second drug to delay the development of resistance are also being studied, such as an ALK inhibitor with an inhibitor of MEK, VEGF, CDK 4/6, mTOR, or MET, among others (Sharma et al. 2018; Bayliss et al. 2016).

3.4 ROS1

Approximately 1–2% of NSCLC harbor ROS1 chromosomal rearrangements (Bergethon et al. 2012; Morris et al. 2019; Davies and Doebele 2013). ROS1 is a receptor tyrosine kinase in the insulin receptor family and rearrangements result in fusion genes that constitutively activate ROS1 kinase activity, leading to upregulation of MAPK/ERK, PI3K/AKT, and JAK signaling pathways that in turn drives proliferation, survival, and oncogenesis (Morris et al. 2019). In addition to NSCLC, ROS1 rearrangements have been noted in several tumors including glioblastoma, cholangiocarcinoma, ovarian cancer, and gastric cancer and are diagnosed using a FISH break-part assay or with an NGS panel (Davies and Doebele 2013). There are numerous fusion partners, but cluster of differentiation 74 (CD74) is most common in NSCLC. Generally, alterations in EGFR, ALK, and ROS1 are mutually exclusive, though there have been cases of additional mutations with ROS1 reported (Morris et al. 2019). Like EGFR and ALK, these rearrangements are also more common in patients who are light or never smokers, younger, and with adenocarcinoma histology.

Several TKIs have demonstrated clinical activity in patients with ROS1 rearrangements—crizotinib, entrectinib, ceritinib, and lorlatinib, while others are in development. Crizotinib was the first drug approved based on a single-arm study of crizotinib in patients with NSCLC with ROS1 rearrangements (Shaw et al. 2014). Crizotinib is a multikinase TKI that has affinity for ROS1, ALK, and MET (Morris et al. 2019). The ORR in this population was 72% and PFS was 19.2 months. OS was a remarkable 51 months (Shaw et al. 2019b). Entrectinib showed similar outcomes and also had activity in the brain, though is not effective in patients resistant to crizotinib (Drilon et al. 2020a; Roys et al. 2019). Ceritinib and lorlatinib have also demonstrated activity in ROS1 NSCLC, but only lorlatinib has shown activity in both crizotinib-naïve and -resistant patients, though neither are approved by the FDA for ROS1-NSCLC (Table 3) (Shaw et al. 2019a; Lim et al. 2017). The investigational agent, repotrectinib, also has shown powerful ROS1 activity (Mok et al. 2017b). It is also important to note that although there is some overlap between ALK and ROS1 inhibitors, not all ALK inhibitors have ROS1 activity.

Similar to other targeted populations, acquired resistance inevitably develops for patients with ROS1 rearrangements. The most common mechanisms of resistance include gatekeeper mutations (L2026M) or solvent front mutations (G2032R; D2033N) in the kinase domain as well as off-target alterations in bypass signaling pathways such as KIT or EGFR activation (Morris et al. 2019; Roys et al. 2019). Lorlatinib and repotrectinib in particular appear to have activity in several of these ROS1-dependent resistance mechanisms. Additionally, due to difference in blood brain penetrance of different TKIs, brain metastases may factor into decision-making of which TKI to consider both upfront and at the development of resistance.

3.5 RET

As with ROS1 NSCLC, REarranged during Transfection (RET) rearrangements occur in 1–2% of NSCLC and are more common in younger, never-smoking patients with adenocarcinoma histology (Ackermann et al. 2019; Li et al. 2019). Although RET rearrangements are seen in NSCLC, oncogenic RET mutations or rearrangements have been seen in several tumor types, most commonly in medullary thyroid cancer (mutations) and papillary thyroid cancer (rearrangements) (Li et al. 2019). Normal RET signaling involves ligands belonging to the glial-derived neurotrophic factor (GDNF) family, but like in other targeted populations, mutations and fusions result in ligand-independent, constitutive kinase activation resulting in enhanced cell proliferation, survival, and oncogenesis (Ackermann et al. 2019). In NSCLC, KIF5B-RET is the most common (70–90%) fusion partner, but other partners include CCDC6, NCOA4, and TRIM33.

The initial iteration of treatment for patients with RET-rearranged NSCLC involved multitarget TKIs, with activity seen with vandetanib, cabozantinib, and lenvatinib. Vandetanib inhibits VEGF, EGFR, and RET, and a clinical trial with 17 pretreated patients with RET-NSCLC showed an ORR of 53%, PFS of 4.7 months, and OS of 11.1 months (Lee et al. 2017). Cabozantinib, which inhibits VEGF, MET, and RET, and lenvatinib, which inhibits VEGF, FGFR, KIT, and RET, showed only modest activity with ORR ~20% and PFS of 4.7 and 7.3 months, respectively (Drilon et al. 2016; Hida et al. 2019). Overall, while these initial studies with multitarget TKIs were intriguing, the treatments were toxic and PFS only modest.

More recently, two TKIs with more selective RET inhibition, selpercatinib and pralsetinib, have been developed and were both approved by the FDA in 2020 (Table 4). Selpercatinib was approved based on the LIBRETTO-001 phase 1–2 trial of selpercatinib in patients ($n = 105$) with previously treated RET-NSCLC. Selpercatinib had an ORR of 64% and a duration of response of 17.5 months (Drilon et al. 2020b). Pralsetinib was approved based on the ARROW study ($n = 114$) that showed a 57% ORR and duration of response of 9.0 months (Markham 2020). Both showed intracranial activity and a low-grade toxicity profile in comparison to the multitarget TKIs.

Although these drugs have just been approved, resistance mechanisms are being elucidated that appear similar to other targetable populations

Table 4 Trial summary for MET, BRAF, NTRK, KRAS, Her2 clinical trials

Oncogene/agent (study)	n	Response rate (%)	Median PFS (months)	OS (months)
MET				
Capmatinib (GEOMETRY-1) (Wolf et al. 2020)	97	68 (tx naïve) 41 (prior tx)	5.4 (tx naïve) 12.4 (prior tx)	NS
Tepotinib (VISION) (Paik et al. 2020)	152	46	8.5	17.5
BRAF				
Dabrafenib (Planchard et al. 2016)	84	33	5.5	12.7
Vemurafenib (Hyman et al. 2015)	20	42	7.3	NR
Dabrafenib + trametinib (Planchard et al. 2017)	36	64	14.6	24.6
NTRK				
Larotrectinib[a] (Drilon et al. 2018a)	55	75	NR	NS
Entrectinib[a] (STARTRK) (Doebele et al. 2020)	54	57	11.2	21 (estimated)
KRAS				
Sotorasib (CODEBREAK 100) (Hong et al. 2020b)	59	32.2	6.3	NS
Adagrasib (KRYSTAL-1) (Janne et al. 2020)	51	45	NS	NS
Her2				
Ado-trastuzumab emtansine (Li et al. 2018)	18	44	5	NS
Trastuzumab deruxtecan (DESTINY LUNG-01) (Smit et al. 2020)	42	62	14	NS

NR not reached, NS not stated
[a] Multiple tumor types

with RET-dependent resistance seen with the development of solvent front (G810R, G810S, and G810C) mutations impacting the binding of drug to receptor (Solomon et al. 2020). Additionally, RET-independent mechanisms have also been noted with MET and KRAS amplification (Lin et al. 2020). Future strategies will include next-generation RET drugs with activity against these resistance mutations as well as other combination approaches.

3.6 NTRK

Neurotrophic tropomyosin-related kinase (NTRK) 1, 2, and 3 rearrangements are very rare in NSCLC, as less than 1% of patients harbor this mutation and have similar characteristics to the populations above being younger, never smokers, and have adenocarcinoma histology (Farago et al. 2018). These rearrangements can be identified using DNA- or RNA-based next-generation sequencing and immunohistochemistry (IHC), as well as by FISH (Hong et al. 2020a; Drilon et al. 2018a). In addition to NSCLC, NTRK rearrangements are seen in multiple adult and pediatric tumors including mammary analog secretory carcinoma, sarcoma, thyroid, breast and gastrointestinal carcinoma, and melanoma (Hong et al. 2020a). The fusion genes lead to the constitutive expression of a chimeric oncoprotein that leads to kinase-independent downstream signaling and oncogenesis.

Two drugs are currently FDA-approved for patients with NTRK-positive NSCLC, larotrectinib and entrectinib, which are both well tolerated (Table 4). Larotrectinib was approved based on a multitumor study of NTRK fusion-positive tumors with dramatic, durable responses seen across ages, tumor types, and TRK fusion partners, including NSCLC. Of 55 patients enrolled, the ORR was 75%, PFS of 28.3 months, and OS of 44.4 months (Drilon et al. 2018a; Haratake and Seto 2021). Entrectinib was approved based on the combined data from the STARTRK studies in multiple solid tumor types that demonstrated a 57% ORR and a median PFS of 11.2 months, though the ORR of NSCLC on the study was 70%.

Like in ROS1 and RET tumors, mechanisms of acquired resistance include solvent front mutations as well as other mutations in the kinase domain including at the gatekeeper position (NTRK1 F589L) (Drilon et al. 2018a). Next-generation inhibitors such as repotrectinib that target these mutations are already underway (Haratake and Seto 2021).

3.7 BRAF

BRAF kinase is part of the signaling cascade that begins with activation of the EGFR receptor and terminates in the nucleus with the result of cell grown and proliferation (O'Leary et al. 2019). There are three major classes of BRAF mutations: Class 1 and 2 which are activating mutations and Class 3 which is "kinase dead." At this time, only the Class 1 BRAF V600E (Val 600 Glu) can be effectively targeted. The V600E mutation occurs in 1–2% of NSCLC adenocarcinomas (O'Leary et al. 2019). Unlike other activating mutations, BRAF V600E mutations can occur in current or former smokers as well as in never or scant smokers and is associated with the adenocarcinoma histology (Leonetti et al. 2018).

BRAF V600E was identified as a target in melanoma some years ago and experience with that malignancy demonstrated that BRAF inhibition by itself resulted in compensatory MEK signaling and led to the occurrence of new skin cancers. Consequently, studies of BRAF inhibitors in NSCLC are usually combined with MEK inhibitors. Studies in BRAF V600E-mutated NSCLC demonstrate that in addition to preventing secondary cancers, inhibition of MEK results in enhanced antitumor activity in the form of increased response rate and progression-free survival.

Single agent BRAF inhibition with dabrafenib or vemurafenib demonstrated a 33–42% response rate with median OS >12 months (Table 4) (Planchard et al. 2016; Hyman et al. 2015). First-line therapy of NSCLC patients with BRAF V600E mutations with dual BRAF and MEK inhibition appears to demonstrate improved activity. The combination of dabrafenib with trametinib ($n = 57$) shows a 64% response rate and median overall survival of 24.6 months with primarily grade 1/2 side effects that were gastrointestinal in nature, leading to the FDA approval of this combination (Planchard et al. 2017).

As with other targets, resistance develops with secondary resistance mechanisms due to reactivation of ERK signaling through the MAPK pathway as well as bypass of the MAPK pathway (Leonetti et al. 2018). Third-generation RAF inhibitors are currently in early-phase trials.

3.8 MET

Mesenchymal-to-epithelial transition (MET) is a receptor tyrosine kinase that is activated by the ligand hepatocyte growth factor (HGF) (Salgia 2017; Guo et al. 2019). MET activation leads to downstream signaling through the RAS/RAF/MAPK and PI3K/ALT/mTOR pathways to promote oncogenesis, similar to other driver mutations in NSCLC, and when targeted can lead to cancer regression. As seen with HER2 alterations (see below), there are three types of MET alterations that have been identified in NSCLC: MET or its ligand, HGF, protein overexpression of MET of its ligand HGF, MET gene amplification, and MET gene mutations (Salgia 2017). Although 35–72% of NSCLC shows MET or HGF protein overexpression, no studies have shown that protein overexpression serves as an oncogenic driver. Of the alterations, MET mutations and gene amplification have been most successfully targeted. The most common mutations are those known as exon 14 skip mutations, which are found in the splice site of MET that result in skipping exon 14. These occur in 3–4% of adenocarcinomas, 2% of squamous cell carcinomas, and in 22% of the rare sarcomatoid NSCLC histology (Salgia 2017; Liu et al. 2016). The skip mutation results in the loss of the binding site for c-CBL which prevents degradation of MET and consequently results in overexpression.

MET inhibitors in development for exon 14 skip mutations are categorized into type I and type II TKIs, with type I binding to MET in its catalytically active confirmation and type II binding to MET in its inactive confirmation. Crizotinib, capmatinib, and tepotinib are all type I MET TKIs. Crizotinib was the initial TKI shown to have activity in patients with MET-exon-14 skip mutations as it is a MET inhibitor in addition to ALK and ROS1, and a small single-arm study showed an ORR of 33% and a median PFS of 7.3 months (Drilon et al. 2020c). However, since this initial experience, two more selective MET inhibitors are now approved by the FDA for MET-exon-14 skip mutations: capmatinib and tepotinib (Table 4) (Wolf et al. 2020; Paik et al. 2020). The phase 2 GEOMETRY-1 study enrolled patients with MET-exon 14 NSCLC and all patients received capmatinib (Wolf et al. 2020). Patients who had received 1–2 lines of therapy had an ORR of 41%, DOR of 9.7 months, and PFS of 5.4 months, whereas those who were treatment naïve had an ORR of 68%, DOR of 12.6 months, and PFS of 12.4 months; capmatinib also showed intracranial activity (intracranial RR of 54%). The phase 2 VISION study was a single-arm study of tepotinib in MET-exon 14 NSCLC, which showed an ORR of 46% and DOR of 10–15 months depending on which type of biopsy group they were in. Tepotinib also demonstrated intracranial activity. Both of these drugs were well tolerated with edema as the most common side effect. Type II MET TKIs include cabozantinib, merestinib, and glesatinib, which have limited data available.

In contrast to MET mutations, MET gene amplification is seen in treatment naïve NSCLC (2–5%) as well as in EGFR-NSCLC as a mechanism of acquired resistance (5–22%), though there is no clear consensus of how to measure and define MET amplification, which makes interpretation of clinical trial data challenging (Salgia 2017; Lim et al. 2018). Despite this, there is accumulating data that MET amplification may serve as an oncogenic driver. The GEOMETRY-1 study of capmatinib included cohorts of patients with NSCLC with MET gene amplification by gene copy number (GCN) (Wolf et al. 2020). In the cohort with low GCN, patients had an ORR of approximately 10% with PFS of 3 months and the cohort were closed for futility. However, those with a GCN of >10 had an ORR of 29% in those previously treated and of 40% in treatment naïve patients with a DOR of 8.3 and 7.5 months, and PFS of 4.1 and 4.2 months, respectively. Additionally, there are several ongoing studies in MET amplification-positive, EGFR-mutated NSCLC that show early signs of clinical benefit (Guo et al. 2019; Sequist et al. 2020; Wu et al. 2020b). One example is a phase 2 trial of tepotinib in combination with gefitinib in patients with MET-amplified, EGFR-mutant NSCLC who had progressed on frontline therapy (Wu et al. 2020b). In this phase 2 study, patients with MET-amplified, EGFR-mutant NSCLC were randomized between chemotherapy tepotinib in combination with gefitinib vs. chemotherapy. Patients who received tepotinib + gefitinib had a PFS of 16.6 months compared to 4.2 months with an OS of 37.3 vs. 13.1 months. Confirmatory studies are ongoing.

Sequencing resistant tumors has identified both on-target and off-target resistance mutations (Recondo et al. 2020). In a small retrospective study of patients who had been treated with a type I or type II MET inhibitor, 35% of patients developed on-target mechanisms of resistance including MET kinase domain mutations (H1094, G1163, L1195, D1228, and Y1230) or focal amplification of the MET exon-14 allele. Off-target mechanisms were identified in 45% of patients, including acquired KRAS mutations, or amplification of EGFR, KRAS, HER3, and/or BRAF. In this small study, in two of the six patients with on-target mutations, switching between a type I and II MET TKI led to a partial response with the new MET inhibitor. In a second small study of resistance mutations in patients with MET exon-14 mutations, alterations were found in the PIK3CA pathway including mutations in PIK3CA and loss of PTEN (Jamme et al. 2020). In a cancer cell model of these combination mutations, inhibiting both MET and PIK3Ca reduced cell growth significantly. Both of these studies suggest that targeting the mechanisms of resistance in patients with MET alterations will be an important area of future research and trial development.

3.9 KRAS

The Kirsten rat sarcoma viral oncogene homolog (K-ras) was first described almost 40 years ago. It is one of the most common abnormalities in epithelial cancers, specifically adenocarcinomas. In NSCLC, activating KRAS mutations are seen in approximately 20–40% of adenocarcinomas but are very infrequent in squamous histology (Moore et al. 2020). KRAS is a GTPase that is an intracellular intermediate messenger. Until recently, KRAS was considered to be "undruggable" for several reasons. First, unlike EGFR, ALK, and others, the phosphorylation aspects took place in the context of a cycling from an inactive GDP-bound state to an active GTP-bound state and back again catalyzed by GTP-activating proteins (GAPS). This is very different than the typical tyrosine kinase that transfers a phosphate group from ATP to a downstream messenger. Second, the enzymatic part of the protein is very shallow and lacks a defined binding pocket for which a drug can be designed to directly bind to the site. Third, there is an extraordinarily high affinity (nanomolar) of the GTP substrate for KRAS, making it difficult for a drug to outcompete.

There are a number of different KRAS protein mutations, mostly occurring at codons 12 and 13, including G12C, G12D, G12S, G12A, G13D, and others. Recent work indicates that specific mutations may have distinct characteristics in terms of cancer etiology and behavior. While most KRAS mutations are associated with tobacco use, KRAS mutations (specifically G12D) may occur in never smokers as well (Ferrer et al. 2018).

Over the years, a number of approaches have been taken to target KRAS. These have included efforts to disrupt the binding of KRAS to the cell surface membrane with farnesyl transferase inhibitors, blockade of upstream activating factors and downstream signaling amongst others. Some of these efforts continue. However, a major breakthrough has been the development of specific KRAS inhibitors.

Ostrem and colleagues overcame the issue of direct targeting of KRAS by developing an allosteric inhibitor that specifically bound to the cysteine in the mutated protein (Ostrem et al. 2013). Binding the cysteine results in a conformational change in the KRAS protein that keeps it in the inactive GDP-bound state. This has led to the development of a series of KRAS G12C inhibitors that are highly active and remarkably nontoxic.

Sotorasib (AMG 510), the first KRASG12C inhibitor to be reported and FDA approved, has demonstrated considerable activity with remarkably little toxicity (Table 4). In the phase I trial, 59 NSCLC patients had received at least first-line platinum-based therapy and most (89.8%) had received anti-PD-1/L1 immunotherapy (Hong et al. 2020b). Across a range of doses, 88.1% had disease control and 32.2% had a confirmed response. The median duration of stable disease was 4.0 months and median PFS for all NSCLC patients was 6.3 months. This benefit was achieved with only mild to moderate toxicity, primarily nausea, diarrhea, and fatigue. Based on this data, sotorasib was FDA approved in May 2021.

Adagrasib (MRTX849) is another selective KRAS G12C inhibitor that has entered clinical trials. The KRYSTAL-1 trial was a phase 1/2 that entered patients with multiple solid tumors, including NSCLC, and evaluated the single agent as well as combinations with pembrolizumab, afatanib, and cetuximab (in colorectal cancer). The recommended single agent dose, 600 mg bid, exceeded the dose demonstrated to inhibit KRAS G12C in the least sensitive animal models. Similar to sotorasib, most of the toxicity was gastrointestinal in nature and grade 1 and 2 in severity. Of 51 NSCLC patients treated at the 600 mg bid dose level, 49 had disease control and the objective response rate was 45%. Many of the responses were durable, with most patients still on therapy at the time of the initial report, some for >12 months (Janne et al. 2020).

3.10 HER2

Three types of human epithelial growth factor 2 (HER2) alterations have been identified in NSCLC: protein overexpression, gene amplification, and gene mutations (Jebbink et al. 2020). Gene mutations, however, are the only alterations that have been associated with a consistent and durable response to targeted therapies. Approximately 3% of lung adenocarcinomas harbor HER2 mutations, most commonly seen as an in-frame exon 20 insertion mutation (Y772_A775) in the tyrosine kinase domain, which leads to increased HER2 kinase activity and increased cell survival and tumorgenicity (Jebbink et al. 2020). HER2 mutations like many above are more frequently found in those who are younger, female, and/or never smokers (Pillai et al. 2017).

Two therapeutic approaches have been studied to target HER2 mutations—tyrosine kinase inhibitors or monoclonal antibodies/antibody drug conjugates (ADC). Approaches using afatinib (a pan-HER tyrosine kinase inhibitor) or trastuzumab (a monoclonal antibody against HER2) have been studied retrospectively and appear to have moderate activity (Mazieres et al. 2016). The European EUHER2 cohort showed that patients with HER2-mutant NSCLC treated with trastuzumab-based combination therapy had an ORR of 50%, disease control rate (DCR) of 75%, and PFS of 5.1 months. Those treated with afatinib had an ORR of 18.2%, DCR of 64%, and PFS of 4.8 months (Mazieres et al. 2016). Multiple other TKIs are currently under study (Jebbink et al. 2020; Wang et al. 2019). HER2 ADCs also show promising activity, which deliver a cytotoxic payload to HER2-positive tumor cells. Ado-trastuzumab emtansine (T-DM1) was studied in a phase II basket study with 18 lung cancer patients where the ORR was 44% HER2, the PFS was 5 months, and IHC did not predict response (Table 4) (Li et al. 2018). A new HER2 ADC, trastuzumab deruxtecan, is being studied in the DESTINY-Lung01 study, which has shown an ORR of 62% and estimated PFS of 14 months (Smit et al. 2020).

As HER2 targeting drugs for HER-mutant specific NSCLC are in their infancy, so is understanding the mechanisms of acquired resistance. One in vitro study of a novel HER2 inhibitor, poziotinib, identified a secondary point mutation in C805S as a potential mechanism of acquired resistance that interferes in the binding of poziotinib (Koga et al. 2018). In this study, HSP90 inhibition was able to overcome this resistance and thus opens up a novel therapeutic pathway to consider in clinical trials if documentation of this mutation is confirmed in patients.

3.11 Other Mutations on the Horizon

Several other mutations in both squamous and nonsquamous NSCLC are categorized as likely oncogenic driver mutations and have drugs in clinical development, including neuregulin 1 gene (NRG1) fusions, Phosphatidylinositol-3 kinase, catalytic (PI3KCA) mutations, fibroblast growth factor receptor (FGFR) alterations, and discoidin domain receptor 2 gene (DDR2) mutations. NRG1 fusions have been reported in 0.2–0.8% of NSCLC as well as multiple other solid tumors including cholangiocarcinoma, thyroid, ovarian, pancreas, and breast cancers (Guo et al. 2019; Chu 2020). NRG1 is a ligand of HER3, which has led to the exploration of pan-HER inhibitors for patients with some evidence of early activity. PIK3CA amplification is more common in squamous NSCLC (33–37%) than in adenocarcinoma (5–6%), while PIK3CA mutations occur in 2–5% of NSCLC (Guo et al. 2019). Both pan-PI3K and selective PI3K inhibitors have been studied, but thus far clinical development has been disappointing (Tan 2020; Bade and Dela Cruz 2020; Langer et al. 2019). FGFR alterations are more common in squamous cell carcinoma and can include point mutations (2–3%), amplification (25%), and translocations (1–3%) (Chu 2020). Early trials with selective FGFR inhibitors and multitarget inhibitors have been disappointing, but research is ongoing to better define the population (Guo et al. 2019). Finally, DDR2 mutations have been seen in 4% of squamous NSCLC and trials of dasatinib in this population are ongoing (Hammerman et al. 2011).

4 Immunotherapy and the Targetable Mutations

Immunotherapy with PD-1 inhibition has also transformed treatment of lung cancer; however, benefit from immunotherapy as monotherapy in most patients with targetable mutations has been lacking (Borghaei et al. 2015). Tumors with oncogenic driver mutations such as EGFR and ALK generally have a lower tumor mutational burden and low PD-L1 expression, with responses in the single digits (Offin et al. 2019; Gainor et al. 2016). Additionally, early attempts to combine these new and remarkably active approaches in NSCLC therapeutics have also met with disappointing results, both due to toxicity and due to relative lack of efficacy. An unexpectedly high incidence of pneumonitis led to the early discontinuation of osimertinib/immunotherapy combinations in EGFR-mutated disease (Oxnard et al. 2020). Similarly, in a small study of nivolumab in combination with crizotinib, the study was stopped due to significant rates of hepatotoxicity and lower than expected responses in patients with ALK-mutated disease (Spigel et al. 2018).

Two notable exceptions are patients with KRAS or BRAF mutations. Patients with either of these mutations are more likely to benefit from immunotherapy with improved response and survival (Liu et al. 2020; Dudnik et al. 2018). Both of these mutations are more commonly found in patients who are current or former smokers, which supports this finding as the benefits of immunotherapy have been more pronounced in those patients with exposure to smoking. Likely, this difference can be accounted for by the more inflamed tumor microenvironment and higher levels of PD-L1 expression in these tumors.

5 Brain Metastases

The presence of CNS disease has been classically viewed with dread and considered to be a major adverse prognostic factor, frequently excluding patients from clinical trials. Part of this approach is a historical artifact of imaging technology and part from the actual physiological issues (e.g., blood brain barrier) associated with brain metastases. As discussed above, many of the new targeted therapies in NSCLC, particularly those targeting EGFR, ALK, ROS1, and RET, have demonstrated unequivocal activity in CNS disease and can frequently allow for delay or elimination of radiotherapy or surgery (Peters et al. 2017; Soria et al. 2018; Drilon et al. 2020a,b).

6 Co-mutations and Outcomes

The advent of routine NGS as well as increasing data from whole exome and genome sequencing (WES, WGS) has demonstrated the complexity of even driver mutation NSCLC. It is relatively common to find both additional mutations within clones as well as other clones characterized by different mutations. Co-mutations may greatly influence the activity of targeted therapies, including initial response, duration of response, and mechanism of resistance (Skoulidis and Heymach 2019). For example, a patient with EGFR-mutated disease may have subclones of disease with p53 and RB mutations. Such patients frequently develop SCLC as a mechanism of resistance to EGFR TKIs (Gini et al. 2020). It is likely that further research will result in the development of multiple targeted therapies to address these issues.

7 Squamous Cell NSCLC and Small Cell Lung Cancer and Targeted Therapies

To date, almost all targetable mutations and approaches have occurred in nonsquamous NSCLC. Finding agents for specific targetable mutations the squamous histology was the initial focus of the Lung Master Protocol (LUNG-MAP) launched by the U.S. National Cancer Institute and led by the Southwest Oncology Group with the support of the U.S. FDA and other interested parties. Though several trials have been completed, none have been successful in developing a targeted agent in this entity (Redman et al. 2020).

Small cell lung cancer has also been the focus of a number of efforts to develop specific agents targeted against known mutations or expression patterns. Recent studies have targeted DLL-3 and GD-2 and others have not demonstrated activity sufficient for approval (Morgensztern et al. 2019; Edelman et al. 2020).

8 Future Directions

The discovery of the biology and pathogenesis of oncogenic driver NSCLC has transformed the treatment options we have to offer patients and their overall prognosis, with over 20 approved treatments for 8 types of mutations and more approvals imminent. Acquired resistance is the common theme across all drivers, and continued understanding of these mechanisms and how to counteract them remains the mainstay of ongoing research.

References

Ackermann CJ, Stock G, Tay R, Dawod M, Gomes F, Califano R (2019) Targeted therapy for RET-rearranged non-small cell lung cancer: clinical development and future directions. Onco Targets Ther 12:7857–7864

Bade BC, Dela Cruz CS (2020) Lung cancer 2020: epidemiology, etiology, and prevention. Clin Chest Med 41:1–24

Bayliss R, Choi J, Fennell DA, Fry AM, Richards MW (2016) Molecular mechanisms that underpin EML4-ALK driven cancers and their response to targeted drugs. Cell Mol Life Sci 73:1209–1224

Bergethon K, Shaw AT, Ou SH et al (2012) ROS1 rearrangements define a unique molecular class of lung cancers. J Clin Oncol 30:863–870

Borghaei H, Paz-Ares L, Horn L et al (2015) Nivolumab versus docetaxel in advanced nonsquamous non-small-cell lung cancer. N Engl J Med 373:1627–1639

Camidge DR, Kim HR, Ahn MJ et al (2018) Brigatinib versus crizotinib in ALK-positive non-small-cell lung cancer. N Engl J Med 379:2027–2039

Camidge DR, Kim HR, Ahn MJ et al (2020) Brigatinib versus crizotinib in advanced ALK inhibitor-naive ALK-positive non-small cell lung cancer: second interim analysis of the phase III ALTA-1L trial. J Clin Oncol 38:3592–3603

Chen G, Feng J, Zhou C et al (2013) Quality of life (QoL) analyses from OPTIMAL (CTONG-0802), a phase III, randomised, open-label study of first-line erlotinib versus chemotherapy in patients with advanced EGFR mutation-positive non-small-cell lung cancer (NSCLC). Ann Oncol 24:1615–1622

Chu QS (2020) Targeting non-small cell lung cancer: driver mutation beyond epidermal growth factor mutation and anaplastic lymphoma kinase fusion. Ther Adv Med Oncol 12:1758835919895756

Davies KD, Doebele RC (2013) Molecular pathways: ROS1 fusion proteins in cancer. Clin Cancer Res 19:4040–4045

Doebele RC, Drilon A, Paz-Ares L et al (2020) Entrectinib in patients with advanced or metastatic NTRK fusion-positive solid tumours: integrated analysis of three phase 1-2 trials. Lancet Oncol 21:271–282

Drilon A, Rekhtman N, Arcila M et al (2016) Cabozantinib in patients with advanced RET-rearranged non-small-cell lung cancer: an open-label, single-centre, phase 2, single-arm trial. Lancet Oncol 17:1653–1660

Drilon A, Laetsch TW, Kummar S et al (2018a) Efficacy of larotrectinib in TRK fusion-positive cancers in adults and children. N Engl J Med 378: 731–739

Drilon A, Somwar R, Mangatt BP et al (2018b) Response to ERBB3-directed targeted therapy in NRG1-rearranged cancers. Cancer Discov 8: 686–695

Drilon A, Siena S, Dziadziuszko R et al (2020a) Entrectinib in ROS1 fusion-positive non-small-cell lung cancer: integrated analysis of three phase 1-2 trials. Lancet Oncol 21:261–270

Drilon A, Oxnard GR, Tan DSW et al (2020b) Efficacy of selpercatinib in RET fusion-positive non-small-cell lung cancer. N Engl J Med 383:813–824

Drilon A, Clark JW, Weiss J et al (2020c) Antitumor activity of crizotinib in lung cancers harboring a MET exon 14 alteration. Nat Med 26:47–51

Dudnik E, Peled N, Nechushtan H et al (2018) BRAF mutant lung cancer: programmed death ligand 1 expression, tumor mutational burden, microsatellite instability status, and response to immune check-point inhibitors. J Thorac Oncol 13:1128–1137

Edelman MJ, Dvorkin M, Laktionov K, Navarro A, Juan-Vidal O, Kozlov V, Golden G, Jordan O, Deng CQ (2020) The anti-disialoganglioside (GD2) antibody dinutuximab (D) for second-line treatment (2LT) of patients (pts) with relapsed/refractory small cell lung cancer (RR SCLC): results from part 2 of the open-label, randomized, phase 2/3 distinct study. J Clin Oncol 38:9017

Farago AF, Taylor MS, Doebele RC et al (2018) Clinicopathologic features of non-small-cell lung cancer harboring an NTRK gene fusion. JCO Precis Oncol 2018. https://doi.org/10.1200/PO.18.00037

Ferrer I, Zugazagoitia J, Herbertz S, John W, Paz-Ares L, Schmid-Bindert G (2018) KRAS-mutant non-small cell lung cancer: from biology to therapy. Lung Cancer 124:53–64

Fukuoka M, Yano S, Giaccone G et al (2003) Multi-institutional randomized phase II trial of gefitinib for previously treated patients with advanced non-small-cell lung cancer (the IDEAL 1 trial) [corrected]. J Clin Oncol 21:2237–2246

Gainor JF, Shaw AT, Sequist LV et al (2016) EGFR mutations and ALK rearrangements are associated with low response rates to PD-1 pathway blockade in non-small cell lung cancer: a retrospective analysis. Clin Cancer Res 22:4585–4593

Genova C, Rossi G, Tagliamento M et al (2020) Targeted therapy of oncogenic-driven advanced non-small cell lung cancer: recent advances and new perspectives. Expert Rev Respir Med 14:367–383

Gini B, Thomas N, Blakely CM (2020) Impact of concurrent genomic alterations in epidermal growth factor receptor (EGFR)-mutated lung cancer. J Thorac Dis 12:2883–2895

Guo Y, Cao R, Zhang X et al (2019) Recent progress in rare oncogenic drivers and targeted therapy for non-small cell lung cancer. Onco Targets Ther 12:10343–10360

Halliday PR, Blakely CM, Bivona TG (2019) Emerging targeted therapies for the treatment of non-small cell lung cancer. Curr Oncol Rep 21:21

Hammerman PS, Sos ML, Ramos AH et al (2011) Mutations in the DDR2 kinase gene identify a novel therapeutic target in squamous cell lung cancer. Cancer Discov 1:78–89

Haratake N, Seto T (2021) NTRK fusion-positive non-small-cell lung cancer: the diagnosis and targeted therapy. Clin Lung Cancer 22:1–5

Hellman S, Weichselbaum RR (1995) Oligometastases. J Clin Oncol 13:8–10

Hida T, Velcheti V, Reckamp KL et al (2019) A phase 2 study of lenvatinib in patients with RET fusion-positive lung adenocarcinoma. Lung Cancer 138:124–130

Hirsch FR, Scagliotti GV, Mulshine JL et al (2017) Lung cancer: current therapies and new targeted treatments. Lancet 389:299–311

Hong DS, DuBois SG, Kummar S et al (2020a) Larotrectinib in patients with TRK fusion-positive solid tumours: a pooled analysis of three phase 1/2 clinical trials. Lancet Oncol 21:531–540

Hong DS, Fakih MG, Strickler JH et al (2020b) KRAS(G12C) inhibition with sotorasib in advanced solid tumors. N Engl J Med 383:1207–1217

Hosomi Y, Morita S, Sugawara S et al (2020) Gefitinib alone versus gefitinib plus chemotherapy for non-small-cell lung cancer with mutated epidermal growth factor receptor: NEJ009 study. J Clin Oncol 38:115–123

Hyman DM, Puzanov I, Subbiah V et al (2015) Vemurafenib in multiple nonmelanoma cancers with BRAF V600 mutations. N Engl J Med 373:726–736

Jamme P, Fernandes M, Copin MC et al (2020) Alterations in the PI3K pathway drive resistance to MET inhibitors in NSCLC harboring MET exon 14 skipping mutations. J Thorac Oncol 15:741–751

Janne PA, Rybkin II, Spira AI, Riely GJ, Papadopoulos KP, Sabari JK, Johnson ML, Heist RS, Bazhenova L, Marce M, Pacheco JM, Leal TA, Velastegui K, Cornelius C, Olson P, Christensen JG, Kheoh T, Chao RC, Ou SHI (2020) KRYSTAL-1: activity and safety of adagrasib (MRTX849) in advanced/metastatic non-small-cell lung cancer (NSCLC) harboring KRAS G12C mutation. Eur J Cancer 138:Plenary Session

Jebbink M, de Langen AJ, Boelens MC, Monkhorst K, Smit EF (2020) The force of HER2—a druggable target in NSCLC? Cancer Treat Rev 86:101996

Koga T, Kobayashi Y, Tomizawa K et al (2018) Activity of a novel HER2 inhibitor, poziotinib, for HER2 exon 20 mutations in lung cancer and mechanism of acquired resistance: an in vitro study. Lung Cancer 126:72–79

Kris MG, Natale RB, Herbst RS et al (2003) Efficacy of gefitinib, an inhibitor of the epidermal growth factor receptor tyrosine kinase, in symptomatic patients with non-small cell lung cancer: a randomized trial. JAMA 290:2149–2158

Kwak EL, Bang YJ, Camidge DR et al (2010) Anaplastic lymphoma kinase inhibition in non-small-cell lung cancer. N Engl J Med 363:1693–1703

Langer CJ, Redman MW, Wade JL 3rd et al (2019) SWOG S1400B (NCT02785913), a phase II study of GDC-0032 (Taselisib) for previously treated PI3K-positive patients with stage IV squamous cell lung cancer (lung-MAP sub-study). J Thorac Oncol 14:1839–1846

Lee SH, Lee JK, Ahn MJ et al (2017) Vandetanib in pretreated patients with advanced non-small cell lung cancer-harboring RET rearrangement: a phase II clinical trial. Ann Oncol 28:292–297

Leonetti A, Facchinetti F, Rossi G et al (2018) BRAF in non-small cell lung cancer (NSCLC): pickaxing another brick in the wall. Cancer Treat Rev 66:82–94

Li BT, Shen R, Buonocore D et al (2018) Ado-trastuzumab emtansine for patients with HER2-mutant lung cancers: results from a phase II basket trial. J Clin Oncol 36:2532–2537

Li AY, McCusker MG, Russo A et al (2019) RET fusions in solid tumors. Cancer Treat Rev 81:101911

Lim SM, Kim HR, Lee JS et al (2017) Open-label, multicenter, phase II study of ceritinib in patients with non-small-cell lung cancer harboring ROS1 rearrangement. J Clin Oncol 35:2613–2618

Lim SM, Syn NL, Cho BC, Soo RA (2018) Acquired resistance to EGFR targeted therapy in non-small cell lung cancer: mechanisms and therapeutic strategies. Cancer Treat Rev 65:1–10

Lin JJ, Riely GJ, Shaw AT (2017) Targeting ALK: precision medicine takes on drug resistance. Cancer Discov 7:137–155

Lin JJ, Liu SV, McCoach CE et al (2020) Mechanisms of resistance to selective RET tyrosine kinase inhibitors in RET fusion-positive non-small-cell lung cancer. Ann Oncol 31:1725–1733

Liu X, Jia Y, Stoopler MB et al (2016) Next-generation sequencing of pulmonary Sarcomatoid carcinoma reveals high frequency of actionable MET gene mutations. J Clin Oncol 34:794–802

Liu C, Zheng S, Jin R et al (2020) The superior efficacy of anti-PD-1/PD-L1 immunotherapy in KRAS-mutant non-small cell lung cancer that correlates with an inflammatory phenotype and increased immunogenicity. Cancer Lett 470:95–105

Lovly CM, Iyengar P, Gainor JF (2017) Managing resistance to EFGR- and ALK-targeted therapies. Am Soc Clin Oncol Educ Book 37:607–618

Lynch TJ, Bell DW, Sordella R et al (2004) Activating mutations in the epidermal growth factor receptor underlying responsiveness of non-small-cell lung cancer to gefitinib. N Engl J Med 350:2129–2139

Maemondo M, Inoue A, Kobayashi K et al (2010) Gefitinib or chemotherapy for non-small-cell lung cancer with mutated EGFR. N Engl J Med 362:2380–2388

Markham A (2020) Pralsetinib: first approval. Drugs 80:1865–1870

Mazieres J, Barlesi F, Filleron T et al (2016) Lung cancer patients with HER2 mutations treated with chemotherapy and HER2-targeted drugs: results from the European EUHER2 cohort. Ann Oncol 27:281–286

McCoach CE, Le AT, Gowan K et al (2018) Resistance mechanisms to targeted therapies in ROS1(+) and ALK(+) non-small cell lung cancer. Clin Cancer Res 24:3334–3347

Mitsudomi T, Morita S, Yatabe Y et al (2010) Gefitinib versus cisplatin plus docetaxel in patients with non-small-cell lung cancer harbouring mutations of the epidermal growth factor receptor (WJTOG3405): an open label, randomised phase 3 trial. Lancet Oncol 11:121–128

Mok TS, Wu YL, Thongprasert S et al (2009) Gefitinib or carboplatin-paclitaxel in pulmonary adenocarcinoma. N Engl J Med 361:947–957

Mok TS, Wu YL, Ahn MJ et al (2017a) Osimertinib or platinum-pemetrexed in EGFR T790M-positive lung cancer. N Engl J Med 376:629–640

Mok TSK, Kim SW, Wu YL et al (2017b) Gefitinib plus chemotherapy versus chemotherapy in epidermal growth factor receptor mutation-positive non-small-cell lung cancer resistant to first-line gefitinib (IMPRESS): overall survival and biomarker analyses. J Clin Oncol 35:4027–4034

Mok TS, Cheng Y, Zhou X, Lee KH, Nakagawa K, Niho S, Lee M, Linke R, Rosell R, Corral J, Migliorino MR, Pluzanski A, Sbar EI, Wang T, White JL, Wu YL (2018) Improvement in overall survival in a randomized study that compared dacomitinib with gefitinib in patients with advanced non-small-cell lung cancer and EGFR-activating mutations. In: ASCO abstract 2018

Mok TCD, Gadgeel SM, Rosell R, Dziadziuszko R, Kim DW, Pérol M, Ou SI, Ahn JS, Shaw AT, Bordogna W, Smoljanović V, Hilton M, Ruf T, Noé J, Peters S (2020) Updated overall survival and final progression-free survival data for patients with treatment-naive advanced ALK-positive non-small-cell lung cancer in the ALEX study. Ann Oncol 31(8):1056

Moore AR, Rosenberg SC, McCormick F, Malek S (2020) RAS-targeted therapies: is the undruggable drugged? Nat Rev Drug Discov 19:533–552

Morgensztern D, Besse B, Greillier L et al (2019) Efficacy and safety of rovalpituzumab tesirine in third-line and beyond patients with DLL3-expressing, relapsed/refractory small-cell lung cancer: results from the phase II TRINITY study. Clin Cancer Res 25:6958–6966

Morris TA, Khoo C, Solomon BJ (2019) Targeting ROS1 rearrangements in non-small cell lung cancer: crizotinib and newer generation tyrosine kinase inhibitors. Drugs 79:1277–1286

Nakagawa K, Garon EB, Seto T et al (2019) Ramucirumab plus erlotinib in patients with untreated, EGFR-mutated, advanced non-small-cell lung cancer (RELAY): a randomised, double-blind, placebo-controlled, phase 3 trial. Lancet Oncol 20:1655–1669

Noronha V, Patil VM, Joshi A et al (2020) Gefitinib versus Gefitinib plus pemetrexed and carboplatin chemotherapy in EGFR-mutated lung cancer. J Clin Oncol 38:124–136

O'Kane GM, Bradbury PA, Feld R et al (2017) Uncommon EGFR mutations in advanced non small cell lung cancer. Lung Cancer 109:137–144

O'Leary CG, Andelkovic V, Ladwa R et al (2019) Targeting BRAF mutations in non-small cell lung cancer. Transl Lung Cancer Res 8:1119–1124

Offin M, Rizvi H, Tenet M et al (2019) Tumor mutation burden and efficacy of EGFR-tyrosine kinase inhibitors in patients with EGFR-mutant lung cancers. Clin Cancer Res 25:1063–1069

Ostrem JM, Peters U, Sos ML, Wells JA, Shokat KM (2013) K-Ras(G12C) inhibitors allosterically control GTP affinity and effector interactions. Nature 503:548–551

Oxnard GR, Yang JC, Yu H et al (2020) TATTON: a multi-arm, phase Ib trial of osimertinib combined with selumetinib, savolitinib, or durvalumab in EGFR-mutant lung cancer. Ann Oncol 31:507–516

Paez JG, Janne PA, Lee JC et al (2004) EGFR mutations in lung cancer: correlation with clinical response to gefitinib therapy. Science 304:1497–1500

Paik PK, Felip E, Veillon R et al (2020) Tepotinib in non-small-cell lung cancer with MET exon 14 skipping mutations. N Engl J Med 383:931–943

Pao W, Miller V, Zakowski M et al (2004) EGF receptor gene mutations are common in lung cancers from "never smokers" and are associated with sensitivity of tumors to gefitinib and erlotinib. Proc Natl Acad Sci U S A 101:13306–13311

Papadimitrakopoulou VA, Mok TS, Han JY et al (2020) Osimertinib versus platinum-pemetrexed for patients with EGFR T790M advanced NSCLC and progression on a prior EGFR-tyrosine kinase inhibitor: AURA3 overall survival analysis. Ann Oncol 31:1536–1544

Park K, Haura EB, Leighl NB et al (2021) Amivantamab in EGFR exon 20 insertion-mutated non-small-cell lung cancer progressing on platinum chemotherapy: initial results from the CHRYSALIS phase I study. J Clin Oncol 39(30):3391–3402. https://doi.org/10.1200/JCO.21.00662. Epub 2021 Aug 2

Peters S, Camidge DR, Shaw AT et al (2017) Alectinib versus crizotinib in untreated ALK-positive non-small-cell lung cancer. N Engl J Med 377:829–838

Peters S, Shaw AT, Besse B et al (2020) Impact of lorlatinib on patient-reported outcomes in patients with advanced ALK-positive or ROS1-positive non-small cell lung cancer. Lung Cancer 144:10–19

Pillai RN, Behera M, Berry LD et al (2017) HER2 mutations in lung adenocarcinomas: a report from the lung cancer mutation consortium. Cancer 123:4099–4105

Planchard D, Kim TM, Mazieres J et al (2016) Dabrafenib in patients with BRAF(V600E)-positive advanced non-small-cell lung cancer: a single-arm, multicentre, open-label, phase 2 trial. Lancet Oncol 17:642–650

Planchard D, Smit EF, Groen HJM et al (2017) Dabrafenib plus trametinib in patients with previously untreated BRAF(V600E)-mutant metastatic non-small-cell lung cancer: an open-label, phase 2 trial. Lancet Oncol 18:1307–1316

Ramalingam SS, Cheng Y, Zhou C, Ohe Y, Imamura F, Cho BC, Lin MC, Majem M, Shah R, Rukazenkov Y, Todd A, Markovets A, Barrett JC, Chmielecki J, Gray J (2018) Mechanisms of acquired resistance to first-line osimertinib: preliminary data from the phase III FLAURA study. Ann Oncol 29. https://doi.org/10.1093/annonc/mdy424.063

Ramalingam SS, Vansteenkiste J, Planchard D et al (2020) Overall survival with osimertinib in untreated, EGFR-mutated advanced NSCLC. N Engl J Med 382:41–50

Recondo G, Bahcall M, Spurr LF et al (2020) Molecular mechanisms of acquired resistance to MET tyrosine kinase inhibitors in patients with MET exon 14-mutant NSCLC. Clin Cancer Res 26:2615–2625

Redman MW, Papadimitrakopoulou VA, Minichiello K et al (2020) Biomarker-driven therapies for previously treated squamous non-small-cell lung cancer (Lung-MAP SWOG S1400): a biomarker-driven master protocol. Lancet Oncol 21:1589–1601

Rosell R, Carcereny E, Gervais R et al (2012) Erlotinib versus standard chemotherapy as first-line treatment for European patients with advanced EGFR mutation-positive non-small-cell lung cancer (EURTAC): a multicentre, open-label, randomised phase 3 trial. Lancet Oncol 13:239–246

Roys A, Chang X, Liu Y, Xu X, Wu Y, Zuo D (2019) Resistance mechanisms and potent-targeted therapies of ROS1-positive lung cancer. Cancer Chemother Pharmacol 84:679–688

Saito H, Fukuhara T, Furuya N et al (2019) Erlotinib plus bevacizumab versus erlotinib alone in patients with EGFR-positive advanced non-squamous non-small-cell lung cancer (NEJ026): interim analysis of an open-label, randomised, multicentre, phase 3 trial. Lancet Oncol 20:625–635

Salgia R (2017) MET in lung cancer: biomarker selection based on scientific rationale. Mol Cancer Ther 16:555–565

Schiller JH, Harrington D, Belani CP et al (2002) Comparison of four chemotherapy regimens for advanced non-small-cell lung cancer. N Engl J Med 346:92–98

Sequist LV, Lynch TJ (2008) EGFR tyrosine kinase inhibitors in lung cancer: an evolving story. Annu Rev Med 59:429–442

Sequist LV, Yang JC, Yamamoto N et al (2013) Phase III study of afatinib or cisplatin plus pemetrexed in patients with metastatic lung adenocarcinoma with EGFR mutations. J Clin Oncol 31:3327–3334

Sequist LV, Han JY, Ahn MJ et al (2020) Osimertinib plus savolitinib in patients with EGFR mutation-positive, MET-amplified, non-small-cell lung cancer after progression on EGFR tyrosine kinase inhibitors: interim results from a multicentre, open-label, phase 1b study. Lancet Oncol 21:373–386

Sharma GG, Mota I, Mologni L, Patrucco E, Gambacorti-Passerini C, Chiarle R (2018) Tumor resistance against ALK targeted therapy-where it comes from and where it goes. Cancers (Basel) 10:62

Shaw AT, Kim DW, Nakagawa K et al (2013) Crizotinib versus chemotherapy in advanced ALK-positive lung cancer. N Engl J Med 368:2385–2394

Shaw AT, Ou SH, Bang YJ et al (2014) Crizotinib in ROS1-rearranged non-small-cell lung cancer. N Engl J Med 371:1963–1971

Shaw AT, Solomon BJ, Chiari R et al (2019a) Lorlatinib in advanced ROS1-positive non-small-cell lung cancer: a multicentre, open-label, single-arm, phase 1-2 trial. Lancet Oncol 20:1691–1701

Shaw AT, Riely GJ, Bang YJ et al (2019b) Crizotinib in ROS1-rearranged advanced non-small-cell lung cancer (NSCLC): updated results, including overall survival, from PROFILE 1001. Ann Oncol 30:1121–1126

Shaw AT, Bauer TM, de Marinis F et al (2020) First-line lorlatinib or crizotinib in advanced ALK-positive lung cancer. N Engl J Med 383:2018–2029

Shigematsu H, Lin L, Takahashi T et al (2005) Clinical and biological features associated with epidermal growth factor receptor gene mutations in lung cancers. J Natl Cancer Inst 97:339–346

Sholl LM, Aisner DL, Varella-Garcia M et al (2015) Multi-institutional oncogenic driver mutation analysis in lung adenocarcinoma: the lung cancer mutation consortium experience. J Thorac Oncol 10:768–777

Skoulidis F, Heymach JV (2019) Co-occurring genomic alterations in non-small-cell lung cancer biology and therapy. Nat Rev Cancer 19:495–509

Smit ENK, Nagasaka M, Felip E, Goto Y, Li BT, Pacheco JM, Murakami H, Barlesi F, Nicholas Saltos A, Perol M, Udagawa H, Saxena K, Shiga R, Guevara FM, Acharyya S, Shahidi J, Planchard D, Janne PA (2020) Trastuzumab deruxtecan (T-DXd; DS-8201) in patients with HER2-mutated metastatic non-small cell lung cancer (NSCLC): interim results of DESTINY-Lung01. J Clin Oncol 38(15_Suppl):9504

Soda M, Choi YL, Enomoto M et al (2007) Identification of the transforming EML4-ALK fusion gene in non-small-cell lung cancer. Nature 448:561–566

Solomon BJ, Mok T, Kim DW et al (2014) First-line crizotinib versus chemotherapy in ALK-positive lung cancer. N Engl J Med 371:2167–2177

Solomon BJ, Kim DW, Wu YL et al (2018a) Final overall survival analysis from a study comparing first-line crizotinib versus chemotherapy in ALK-mutation-positive non-small-cell lung cancer. J Clin Oncol 36:2251–2258

Solomon BJ, Besse B, Bauer TM et al (2018b) Lorlatinib in patients with ALK-positive non-small-cell lung cancer: results from a global phase 2 study. Lancet Oncol 19:1654–1667

Solomon BJ, Tan L, Lin JJ et al (2020) RET solvent front mutations mediate acquired resistance to selective RET inhibition in RET-driven malignancies. J Thorac Oncol 15:541–549

Soria JC, Tan DSW, Chiari R et al (2017) First-line ceritinib versus platinum-based chemotherapy in advanced ALK-rearranged non-small-cell lung cancer (ASCEND-4): a randomised, open-label, phase 3 study. Lancet 389:917–929

Soria JC, Ohe Y, Vansteenkiste J et al (2018) Osimertinib in untreated EGFR-mutated advanced non-small-cell lung cancer. N Engl J Med 378:113–125

Spigel DR, Reynolds C, Waterhouse D et al (2018) Phase 1/2 study of the safety and tolerability of nivolumab plus crizotinib for the first-line treatment of anaplastic lymphoma kinase translocation—positive advanced non-small cell lung cancer (CheckMate 370). J Thorac Oncol 13:682–688

Tan AC (2020) Targeting the PI3K/Akt/mTOR pathway in non-small cell lung cancer (NSCLC). Thorac Cancer 11:511–518

Tsao AS, Scagliotti GV, Bunn PA Jr et al (2016) Scientific advances in lung cancer 2015. J Thorac Oncol 11:613–638

Wang XZM (2020) First-line tyrosine kinase inhibitor with or without aggressive upfront local radiation therapy in patients with EGFRm oligometastatic non-small cell lung cancer: interim results of a randomized phase III, open-label clinical trial. J Clin Oncol 38(Suppl 15):9508

Wang Y, Jiang T, Qin Z et al (2019) HER2 exon 20 insertions in non-small-cell lung cancer are sensitive to the irreversible pan-HER receptor tyrosine kinase inhibitor pyrotinib. Ann Oncol 30:447–455

Weickhardt AJ, Scheier B, Burke JM et al (2012) Local ablative therapy of oligoprogressive disease prolongs disease control by tyrosine kinase inhibitors in oncogene-addicted non-small-cell lung cancer. J Thorac Oncol 7:1807–1814

Weiss J, Kavanagh B, Deal A et al (2019) Phase II study of stereotactic radiosurgery for the treatment of patients with oligoprogression on erlotinib. Cancer Treat Res Commun 19:100126

Wolf J, Seto T, Han JY et al (2020) Capmatinib in MET exon 14-mutated or MET-amplified non-small-cell lung cancer. N Engl J Med 383:944–957

Wu YL, Zhou C, Hu CP et al (2014) Afatinib versus cisplatin plus gemcitabine for first-line treatment of Asian patients with advanced non-small-cell lung cancer harbouring EGFR mutations (LUX-Lung 6): an open-label, randomised phase 3 trial. Lancet Oncol 15:213–222

Wu YL, Zhou C, Liam CK et al (2015) First-line erlotinib versus gemcitabine/cisplatin in patients with advanced EGFR mutation-positive non-small-cell lung cancer: analyses from the phase III, randomized, open-label, ENSURE study. Ann Oncol 26:1883–1889

Wu YL, Cheng Y, Zhou X et al (2017) Dacomitinib versus gefitinib as first-line treatment for patients with EGFR-mutation-positive non-small-cell lung cancer (ARCHER 1050): a randomised, open-label, phase 3 trial. Lancet Oncol 18:1454–1466

Wu YL, Tsuboi M, He J et al (2020a) Osimertinib in resected EGFR-mutated non-small-cell lung cancer. N Engl J Med 383:1711–1723

Wu YL, Cheng Y, Zhou J et al (2020b) Tepotinib plus gefitinib in patients with EGFR-mutant non-small-cell lung cancer with MET overexpression or MET amplification and acquired resistance to previous EGFR inhibitor (INSIGHT study): an open-label, phase 1b/2, multicentre, randomised trial. Lancet Respir Med 8:1132–1143

Xia B, Nagasaka M, Zhu VW, Ou SI, Soo RA (2020) How to select the best upfront therapy for metastatic disease? Focus on ALK-rearranged non-small cell lung cancer (NSCLC). Transl Lung Cancer Res 9:2521–2534

Yang JC, Wu YL, Schuler M et al (2015) Afatinib versus cisplatin-based chemotherapy for EGFR mutation-positive lung adenocarcinoma (LUX-Lung 3 and LUX-Lung 6): analysis of overall survival data from two randomised, phase 3 trials. Lancet Oncol 16:141–151

Yu HA, Sima CS, Huang J et al (2013) Local therapy with continued EGFR tyrosine kinase inhibitor therapy as a treatment strategy in EGFR-mutant advanced lung cancers that have developed acquired resistance to EGFR tyrosine kinase inhibitors. J Thorac Oncol 8:346–351

Zhang K, Yuan Q (2016) Current mechanism of acquired resistance to epidermal growth factor receptor-tyrosine kinase inhibitors and updated therapy strategies in human nonsmall cell lung cancer. J Cancer Res Ther 12:C131–C1C7

Zhang B, Zhang L, Yue D et al (2020) Genomic characteristics in Chinese non-small cell lung cancer patients and its value in prediction of postoperative prognosis. Transl Lung Cancer Res 9:1187–1201

Zhong WZ, Wang Q, Mao WM et al (2021) Gefitinib versus vinorelbine plus cisplatin as adjuvant treatment for stage II-IIIA (N1-N2) EGFR-mutant NSCLC: final overall survival analysis of CTONG1104 phase III trial. J Clin Oncol 39:713–722

Zhou C, Wu YL, Chen G et al (2011) Erlotinib versus chemotherapy as first-line treatment for patients with advanced EGFR mutation-positive non-small-cell lung cancer (OPTIMAL, CTONG-0802): a multicentre, open-label, randomised, phase 3 study. Lancet Oncol 12:735–742

Zhou C, Wu YL, Chen G et al (2015) Final overall survival results from a randomised, phase III study of erlotinib versus chemotherapy as first-line treatment of EGFR mutation-positive advanced non-small-cell lung cancer (OPTIMAL, CTONG-0802). Ann Oncol 26:1877–1883

Zhu QG, Zhang SM, Ding XX, He B, Zhang HQ (2017) Driver genes in non-small cell lung cancer: characteristics, detection methods, and targeted therapies. Oncotarget 8:57680–57692

Zhou C, Ramalingam SS, Kim TM et al (2021) Treatment outcomes and safety of mobocertinib in platinum-pretreated patients with egfr exon 20 insertion–positive metastatic non–small cell lung cancer: a phase 1/2 open-label nonrandomized clinical trial. JAMA Oncol 7(12):e214761

Immunotherapy of Lung Cancer

Igor Rybkin and Shirish M. Gadgeel

Contents

1 Introduction.. 371
2 Second-Line Therapy for Non-small Cell Lung Cancer.. 372
3 Single-Agent Anti-PD-1/PD-L1 as First-Line Therapy in NSCLC...................... 372
4 Combination of Chemotherapy and Immune Checkpoint Inhibitors............. 373
5 Combination of Immune Checkpoint Inhibitors.. 374
6 Immunotherapy in Small Cell Lung Cancer.. 375
7 Immunotherapy in Stage III NSCLC............ 375
8 Rationale for Immunotherapy in the Management of Stage III NSCLC... 376
9 PACIFIC Trial and Beyond............................ 376
10 Perioperative Immunotherapy....................... 378
11 Immune-Related Toxicities with Immune Checkpoint Inhibitors..................................... 379
12 Future of Cancer Immunotherapy................ 380
References... 382

I. Rybkin · S. M. Gadgeel (✉)
Henry Ford Cancer Institute/Henry Ford Health System, Detroit, MI, USA
e-mail: irybkin1@hfhs.org; sgadgee1@hfhs.org

1 Introduction

The major therapeutic advance in the management of lung cancer patients is the introduction and use of drugs that inhibit immune checkpoint pathways. Several previous strategies failed to stimulate immune response against lung cancer and failed to demonstrate any meaningful benefit, making the clinical benefit observed with immune checkpoint inhibitors even more remarkable.

Immune checkpoints are present on the surface of T cells and other immune cells in the tumor microenvironment as well as in the regional lymph nodes and in the circulation. These checkpoints serve an important regulatory function in normal physiology by restricting the immune response and thus limiting damage to normal tissue at sites of inflammation. These checkpoints are "hijacked" by cancers to limit antitumor immune response. Immune checkpoint inhibitors release the inhibitory signals of immune checkpoints and result in the activation of T-cell response. Two classes of checkpoint inhibitors, one against CTLA-4 and the other against PD-1/PD-L1, have been evaluated in several cancers including NSCLC. The clinical benefits observed with these immune checkpoint inhibitors have not only led to the incorporation of these agents in the management of lung cancer patients but also prompted the evaluation of other approaches to enhance the antitumor immune response.

2 Second-Line Therapy for Non-small Cell Lung Cancer

Drugs targeting the PD-1/PD-L1 axis were first evaluated in patients with progressive NSCLC following therapy with a platinum-based combination therapy. Several agents in randomized phase III trial demonstrated significant survival advantage compared to docetaxel chemotherapy. The median survival with these agents ranged from 9.2 to 12.2 months. The most striking feature of these trials was the sustained benefit observed in approximately 10% of the patients. The survival advantage was observed despite no or minimal advantage in terms of progression-free survival. Benefit was observed irrespective of tumor PD-L1 expression. However, probability of benefit was greater in patients with tumors that expressed PD-L1 and more so in patients with higher tumor PD-L1 expression.

3 Single-Agent Anti-PD-1/PD-L1 as First-Line Therapy in NSCLC

The clinical benefits observed with drugs targeting the PD-1/PD-L1 axis in the second-line setting prompted clinical trials evaluating these drugs in the first-line setting.

KEYNOTE-024 was a pivotal trial paving the way for use of immune checkpoint inhibitors in the frontline therapy setting (Reck et al. 2016). In this phase III, open-label trial, patients with advanced-stage NSCLC without EGFR or ALK sensitizing mutations and with PD-L1 22C3 PharmDx TPS ≥50% were randomized to receive in frontline therapy either pembrolizumab alone or investigator choice, histology-based platinum doublet chemotherapy. The primary endpoint, median PFS, was 10.3 months (95% CI, 6.7 to not reached) in pembrolizumab group versus 6.0 months (95% CI, 4.2–6.2; HR 0.5; 95% CI, 0.37–0.68; $p < 0.001$). Updated analysis of the secondary endpoint, median OS, showed 26.3 months (95% CI, 18.3–40.4) with pembrolizumab and 13.4 months (95% CI, 9.4–18.3 months; HR 0.62; 95% CI, 0.48–0.81) (Reck et al. 2019). Superiority of pembrolizumab was upheld even though 82 patients randomized to chemotherapy crossed over to pembrolizumab arm. This trial established pembrolizumab monotherapy as a standard of care for NSCLC patients with PD-L1 TPS ≥50%.

KEYNOTE-042, a randomized phase III trial, tested further role of immune checkpoint inhibitors in frontline settings in EGFR/ALK-negative, PD-L1 TPS ≥1% NSCLC patients, stratifying them based on the level of PD-L1 expression (Mok et al. 2019). Out of the total 902 patients with TPS ≥1%, 818 patients had TPS ≥20% and 599 patients TPS ≥50%. Median OS according to TPS population was 16.7 months (13.9–19.7) for pembrolizumab versus 12.1 months (11.3–13.3; HR 0.81, 0.71–0.93, $p = 0.0018$) for chemotherapy arm in TPS ≥1% group, 17.7 months (15.3–22.1) versus 13.0 months (11.6–15.3; HR 0.77, 95% CI, 0.64–0.92, $p = 0.002$) in TPS ≥20% group, and 20.0 months (95% CI, 15.4–24.9) versus 12.2 months (10.4–14.2; HR 0.69, 95% CI, 0.56–0.85, $p = 0.0003$) in TPS ≥50% group, respectively. This trial was the basis for FDA approval of pembrolizumab as a frontline therapy for NSCLC with PD-L1 TPS ≥1%. Despite this approval, the consensus is that the use of single agent pembrolizumab as the first-line therapy is restricted to patients with tumor PD-L1 TPS score of ≥50%.

Atezolizumab, an anti-PD-L1 inhibitory antibody, was also tested as a single-agent immune checkpoint inhibitor option in IMpower110 study, a randomized, open-label, phase III trial in EGFR/ALK-negative NSCLC with PD-L1 TPS ≥1% or more than 1% of PD-L1 expression in tumor-infiltrating immune cells (Herbst et al. 2020). The median OS, the primary endpoint, in the high PD-L1 expression population (TPS ≥50% or ≥10% expression in tumor-infiltrating immune cells) was 20.2 months in atezolizumab group versus 13.1 months in chemotherapy group (HR 0.59; $p = 0.01$). The drug now has FDA approval in patients with high tumor PD-L1.

4 Combination of Chemotherapy and Immune Checkpoint Inhibitors

Considering that PD-L1 low expressors have relatively limited benefit to the single-agent immune checkpoint inhibitors in the frontline settings, these agents were tested in combination with at the time standard of care, platinum doublet therapy.

KEYNOTE-189 and KEYNOTE-407 compared and established a role of pembrolizumab/histology-specific platinum doublet combination as a frontline option for nonsquamous and squamous cell lung carcinoma, respectively.

KEYNOTE-189, a double-blind, phase III trial, randomized (in a 2:1 ratio) 616 patients with metastatic, treatment-naïve, EGFR/ALK-negative nonsquamous NSCLC to either pembrolizumab plus platinum/pemetrexed ($n = 410$) or placebo plus platinum/pemetrexed ($n = 206$) for four cycles, followed by maintenance pemetrexed plus pembrolizumab/placebo accordingly (Gandhi et al. 2018). The estimated rate of OS at 12 months was 69.2% (95% CI, 64.1–73.8) in the pembrolizumab/chemotherapy group versus 49.4% (42.1–56.2) in the placebo/chemotherapy group (HR 0.49; 95% CI, 0.38–0.64). The updated analysis at median follow-up of 23.1 months demonstrated that the estimated rates of OS at 24 months were 45.5% and 29.9%, respectively (Gadgeel et al. 2020). The updated median OS was twice as long in pembrolizumab/chemotherapy group, 22.0 months (95% CI, 19.5–25.2) versus 10.7 months (8.7–13.6) in the placebo/chemotherapy group (HR 0.56; 95% CI, 0.45–0.70). Superior outcomes of pembrolizumab/chemotherapy arms persisted in the updated analysis even though 54% (111/206) of patients in the chemotherapy arm crossed over to the pembrolizumab monotherapy or other PD-1/PD-L1 inhibitors. OS and PFS data from this trial suggest that there is a particular benefit in combining pembrolizumab with chemotherapy. Importantly, addition of pembrolizumab resulted in PFS and OS benefits regardless of the PD-L1 expression level, including patients with PD-L1 TPS ≤1%, although the magnitude of benefit was less dramatic than in patients with PD-L1 TPS ≥50%, but statistically significant.

KEYNOTE-407 had a similar design but enrolled metastatic squamous cell NSCLC patients, randomizing 559 patients (1:1 ratio) to carboplatin with paclitaxel (or nab-paclitaxel) combined with either pembrolizumab or placebo for the first 4 cycles, followed by pembrolizumab/placebo maintenance for up to 35 cycles (Paz-Ares et al. 2018). In the protocol-specified final analysis, at a median follow-up of 14.3 months, the median OS was 17.1 months (95% CI, 14.4–19.9) in the pembrolizumab/chemotherapy group and 11.6 months (10.1–13.7) in the chemotherapy group (HR 0.71; 95% CI, 0.58–0.88) (Paz-Ares et al. 2020). Like KEYNOTE-189 trial, the benefit of adding pembrolizumab was seen in both PD-L1-expressing patients (TPS ≥1%) and PD-L1-negative patients (TPS ≤1%).

Based on the results of the KEYNOTE-189 and KEYNOTE-407 trials, the FDA approved pembrolizumab in combination with platinum doublet chemotherapy in the frontline settings in NSCLC, regardless of the level of PD-L1 expression and in the absence of EGFR or ALK activation genetic mutations.

The efficacy of PD-L1 inhibitory antibody, atezolizumab, in combination with carboplatin and nab-paclitaxel in the frontline therapy of metastatic nonsquamous NSCLC was tested in IMpower130 trial, an open-label, phase III study. IMpower130 allowed inclusion of EGFR- and ALK-positive NSCLC patients who progressed or were intolerant to at least one line of TKI-specific therapy. Median OS in atezolizumab/chemotherapy group was 18.6 months (95% CI, 16.0–21.2) versus 13.9 months (12.0–18.7) in the chemotherapy group (West et al. 2019).

Atezolizumab was also evaluated in combination with platinum doublet chemotherapy with bevacizumab, an inhibitor of vascular growth factor receptor (VGFR). IMpower150 randomly assigned patients to one of the three groups, where carboplatin with paclitaxel was combined with either bevacizumab (BCP, control group), atezolizumab (ACP), or atezolizumab plus bevacizumab (ABCP) (Socinski et al. 2018). The median PFS, a primary endpoint of the study, was longer in the ABCP group than in the BCP group (8.3 months versus 6.8 months; HR 0.62, 95% CI, 0.52–0.74). The median OS, a secondary endpoint, in these groups was 19.2 months and 14.7 months, respectively (HR 0.78, 95% CI, 0.64–0.96; $p = 0.02$).

Based on the results of IMpower130 and IMpower150 studies, the FDA approved atezolizumab in combination with carboplatin and nab-paclitaxel or in combination with carboplatin with paclitaxel and bevacizumab. Nonetheless, due to the lack of the high-quality direct comparison of ACP group versus ABCP and ACP group versus BCP group, the exact degree of benefit from the atezolizumab/bevacizumab combination remains unclear and use of platinum doublet/atezolizumab/bevacizumab in real-life practice remains limited.

5 Combination of Immune Checkpoint Inhibitors

CheckMate-227 was an open-label, multipart, phase III study randomizing EGFR/ALK-negative NSCLC patients based on their level of PD-L1 expression. Patients with PD-L1 TPS ≥1% were randomized to nivolumab plus ipilimumab versus nivolumab monotherapy versus platinum doublet chemotherapy. Cohort of patients with PD-L1 TPS ≤1% were randomized to nivolumab plus ipilimumab versus nivolumab with platinum doublet chemotherapy versus chemotherapy. The primary endpoint was OS in nivolumab plus ipilimumab versus chemotherapy arms in PD-L1 TPS ≥1% population. The median OS was 17.1 months (95% CI, 15.0–20.1) in nivolumab plus ipilimumab and 14.9 (95% CI, 12.7–16.7; $p = 0.007$) in chemotherapy group (Hellmann et al. 2019). The 3-year OS rates were 33% for nivolumab plus ipilimumab and 22% for chemotherapy. Nivolumab monotherapy group had a median OS of 15.7 months and 3-year OS rate of 29%, although the study was not designed for direct comparison of this group to nivolumab plus ipilimumab group. It is worth to mention that in PD-L1 TPS ≤1% population, nivolumab plus ipilimumab showed median OS and 3-year OS rate to be almost identical to the PD-L1 TPS ≥1% population, 17.2 months and 34%, respectively. Based on this trial, the FDA granted approval for nivolumab plus ipilimumab as the frontline therapy in EGFR/ALK-negative NSCLC PD-L1 TPS ≥1% patients. The combination was not approved for PD-L1 TPS ≤1% NSCLC as this dataset was not a part of primary endpoint analysis, although the results were intriguing and hypothesis generating.

An interesting and promising study design was implemented in CheckMate-9LA study, where the pair of nivolumab every 3 weeks and ipilimumab every 6 weeks was combined with platinum-based chemotherapy for the first two cycles, followed by maintenance nivolumab/ipilimumab combination for up to 2 years, as compared to the control arm receiving four cycles of histology-specific platinum-based chemotherapy followed by maintenance pemetrexed in nonsquamous NSCLC. In this randomized, open-label, international, phase III study, 719 patients were randomly assigned to the experimental arm and 358 patients to the standard-of-care control arm. Immunotherapy group demonstrated superior median OS, with 15.6 months (95% CI, 13.9–20.0) versus 10.9 months (9.5–12.6; HR 0.66, 95% CI, 0.55–0.80) for experimental and control arms, respectively (Paz-Ares et al. 2021). It is worth to notice that serious treatment-related adverse events were more frequent (30%) in the experimental group compared to the control group (18%), although the frequency of treatment-related deaths was equal between the groups (2%). The FDA approved the use of nivolumab/ipilimumab/chemotherapy combination for two cycles followed by nivolumab/ipilimumab maintenance as a frontline therapy of NSCLC regardless of the histology or PD-L1 level of expression.

6 Immunotherapy in Small Cell Lung Cancer

Effectiveness of immune checkpoint inhibitors in the small cell lung cancer was initially tested in the third line and above, but quickly moved to the frontline settings.

IMpower133 is a phase III, double-blind study that randomly assigned patients with extensive-stage (ES) SCLC to four cycles of carboplatin plus etoposide at the standard doses with atezolizumab (201 patients) or placebo (202 patients), followed by the maintenance of atezolizumab or placebo, according to the initial assignment (Horn et al. 2018). The median OS in the atezolizumab group was 12.3 months (95% CI, 10.8–15.9) and 10.3 months (9.3–11.3) in the placebo group (HR 0.70; 95% CI, 054–0.91; $p = 0.007$), with the rate of OS at 12 months 51.7% (95% CI, 44.4–59.0) and 38.2% (31.2–45.3). It is worthwhile to mention that during the maintenance phase, prophylactic cranial irradiation (PCI) was permitted, but not mandatory. Consolidative thoracic radiation was not allowed. No excessive toxicity related to the PCI concomitantly with durvalumab was reported, although atezolizumab arm had one case of Guillain-Barre syndrome, a rare and severe complication of immunotherapy. The FDA approved atezolizumab in combination with carboplatin and etoposide, for the first-line treatment of adult patients with extensive-stage small cell lung cancer.

CASPIAN, a controlled, open-label, Phase III trial, randomly assigned patients (in 1:1:1 ratio) to either durvalumab plus platinum/etoposide, durvalumab plus tremelimumab (anti-CTLA-4 inhibitory antibodies) plus platinum/etoposide, or platinum/etoposide alone. The trial allowed cisplatin (75–80 mg/m^2) or carboplatin (AUC 5–6), and etoposide (80–100 mg/m^2) at investigator choice. In the investigational arms, up to four cycles of immunochemotherapy were given followed by maintenance durvalumab alone. In the control group, patients could be given up to six cycles of platinum/etoposide followed by PCI (investigator's discretion). In-study crossover from the control arm to investigational arms was not allowed (Paz-Ares et al. 2019). In the planned interim analysis, median OS in the durvalumab plus platinum/etoposide group was 13.0 (95% CI, 11.5–14.8) versus 10.3 months (9.3–11.2) in the platinum/etoposide group (HR 0.73; 95% CI, 0.59–0.91; $p = 0.0047$), and the rates of OS at 18 months were 34% (26.9–41.0) and 25% (18.4–31.6), respectively. An updated analysis at a median follow-up of 25.1 months showed no statistically significant benefit of durvalumab/tremelimumab combination compared to the platinum/etoposide group (HR 0.82; 95% CI, 0.68–1.00), with median OS of 10.4 months (9.6–12.0) versus 10.5 months (9.3–11.2) (Goldman et al. 2021). However, durvalumab plus platinum/etoposide continued to demonstrate clinical benefit, with median OS of 12.9 months (95% CI, 11.3–14.7) versus 10.5 months (9.3–11.2) in the platinum/etoposide group (HR 0.75; 95% CI, 0.62–0.91). The FDA approved durvalumab in combination with etoposide and either carboplatin or cisplatin as a first-line treatment of adult patients with extensive-stage small cell lung cancer.

Pembrolizumab in combination with chemotherapy was also evaluated in randomized phase III trial KEYNOTE-604. The study showed improved PFS but failed to show survival advantage. Therefore, this drug has not received approval by the US FDA for the treatment of SCLC.

7 Immunotherapy in Stage III NSCLC

Stage III or locally advanced NSCLC is characterized by invasion of the mediastinum by the primary tumor or metastases to the mediastinal lymph nodes. Approximately 25–30% of NSCLC patients at diagnosis have locally advanced disease. Locally advanced NSCLC is characterized by local disease in the chest with the presence of systemic micrometastatic disease. Management of these patients therefore requires both local and systemic therapy. Most of these patients are considered inoperable due to both surgical and medical reasons. The standard therapy for unresectable stage III NSCLC is concurrent chemotherapy and radiation therapy. Though such therapy does improve survival, only 20% of the patients are alive for 5 years or longer. Over the years, several strategies have been evaluated to improve outcomes, including intensification of the radiation dose, induction/consolidation chemotherapy, and use of targeted agents without any significant improvement in survival, and in some instances these strategies resulted in increased toxicities and worse outcomes.

8 Rationale for Immunotherapy in the Management of Stage III NSCLC

Immune checkpoint inhibitors have an established role in the management of stage IV NSCLC. Initially, these agents were evaluated following disease progression on platinum-based chemotherapy and subsequently as first-line therapy either by themselves or in combination with platinum-based chemotherapy. In both these clinical settings, immune checkpoint inhibitors have improved survival. In addition, a small proportion of patients can achieve long-term disease control. These results have prompted the evaluation of these agents in earlier stages of NSCLC.

Preclinical studies suggest that radiation therapy through its cytotoxic effects may result in the release of tumor antigens, which could prime the immune system and enhance the effects of immune checkpoint inhibitors. These studies have prompted the evaluation of immune checkpoint inhibitors both during concurrent chemotherapy and radiation therapy and following concurrent chemotherapy and radiation therapy.

9 PACIFIC Trial and Beyond

The phase III PACIFIC trial evaluated the role of durvalumab in patients who had completed concurrent chemotherapy and radiation therapy for unresectable stage III NSCLC. Patients enrolled had received definitive radiation therapy between 54 and 66 Gy and had received at least two cycles of platinum-based chemotherapy administered concurrently with radiation therapy. Approximately 25% of the patients had received induction chemotherapy prior to concurrent chemotherapy and radiation therapy. The most common chemotherapy regimens utilized were carboplatin and paclitaxel (33.9%) and cisplatin and etoposide (21.7%) (Antonia et al. 2017).

Of the 713 patients randomized 2:1 to durvalumab or placebo, 709 received at least one dose of the study drug. The co-primary endpoints of the trial were progression-free survival (PFS) and overall survival (OS). Durvalumab was administered at a dose of 10 mg/kg every 2 weeks for 1 year. At a median follow-up of 25 months, the median PFS with durvalumab was 17.2 months as compared to 5.6 months with placebo (HR 0.51, 95% CI, 0.41–0.63), and the median OS was not reached with durvalumab and was 28.7 months with placebo (HR 0.68, 95% CI, 0.469–0.997) (Antonia et al. 2018). Recently, the investigators published updated results of the PACIFIC trial. The median survival of patients randomized to durvalumab was 47.5 months (29.1 months with placebo), and the 4-year PFS was 35.3% (19.3% with placebo) (Faivre-Finn et al. 2021). The median number of durvalumab infusions was 20 (1–27). In addition, the median time to death or distant metastases was longer with durvalumab (28.2 months) as compared to placebo (16.2 months), with less brain metastases detected in durvalumab patients.

The rates of adverse events and severe adverse events were very similar between patients who received durvalumab and patients who received placebo. However, the rate of discontinuation of therapy due to adverse events occurred in 15.4% of durvalumab patients and 9.8% of placebo patients. The most common cause of discontinuation of durvalumab was pneumonitis. The rate of all-grade pneumonitis was 33.9% in durvalumab patients versus 24.8% among patients who received placebo. Immune-related adverse events were reported in 24% of durvalumab patients and in 8% of placebo patients.

Similar results were reported by Hoosier Oncology Group with pembrolizumab in a phase II trial. In this trial, patients who had received concurrent chemotherapy and radiation and did not have progression of disease were treated with consolidation pembrolizumab. The primary endpoint of the study was the median time to metastatic disease or death (TMDD). Ninety-three patients were enrolled on the trial. With a median follow-up of 32.2 months, the median TMDD was 30.7 months (95% CI, 18.7 months–NR). The median PFS was 18.7 months (95% CI, 12.4–33.8), and the median OS was 35.8 months (95% CI, 24.2 months–NR). Grade ≥3 pneumonitis was observed in 6.5% of the patients, with one patient experiencing grade 5 pneumonitis (Durm et al. 2020).

The results from the PACIFIC trial have established consolidation durvalumab as the standard of care following treatment of stage III NSCLC patients with concurrent chemotherapy and radiation therapy.

PACIFIC results have spurred interest in evaluating the use of checkpoint inhibitors to further improve the outcomes in stage III NSCLC patients beyond consolidation durvalumab. A number of trials are evaluating the addition of checkpoint inhibitors to concurrent chemotherapy and radiation (Table 1). Several phase II studies have evaluated the feasibility of combining checkpoint inhibitors with concurrent chemotherapy and radiation. These studies have shown that it is feasible to administer checkpoint inhibitors without increased toxicities, specifically pneumonitis (Jabbour et al. 2021). PACIFIC 2 trial is comparing durvalumab with chemotherapy and radiation followed by consolidation durvalumab versus concurrent chemotherapy and radiation followed by consolidation with placebo. The results of this trial if positive will fail to identify the utility of adding durvalumab to concurrent chemotherapy and radiation. ECOG EA5181 is evaluating the addition of durvalumab with concurrent chemotherapy and radiation followed by durvalumab versus concurrent chemotherapy and radiation followed by consolidation durvalumab, which potentially will answer this question.

Table 1 Ongoing immunotherapy trials in stage III NSCLC

Trial	Phase	Experimental intervention	Primary endpoint
PACIFIC 2	III	Durvalumab concurrent with chemotherapy and radiation followed by durvalumab compared to placebo with concurrent chemotherapy and radiation followed by placebo	Progression-free survival
EA5181	III	Durvalumab with concurrent chemotherapy and radiation followed by durvalumab compared to concurrent chemotherapy and radiation followed by durvalumab	Overall survival
BTCRC-LUN16-081	II	Consolidation nivolumab versus nivolumab plus ipilimumab following concurrent chemotherapy and radiation	Progression-free survival
CheckMate-73L	III	Nivolumab with concurrent chemotherapy and radiation followed by nivolumab and ipilimumab (arm A) or nivolumab (arm B) or concurrent chemotherapy and radiation followed by durvalumab (arm C)	Progression-free survival and overall survival

10 Perioperative Immunotherapy

Immune checkpoint inhibitors are also being evaluated as part of neoadjuvant and adjuvant therapy in patients with resectable lung cancer (Table 2). Several feasibility studies evaluated neoadjuvant immunotherapy as single agents. In these trials, neoadjuvant therapy was feasible and did not impact the ability to perform surgery, and there was not an increased incidence of postoperative complications from such therapy. The complete pathologic response rate in these trials ranged from 5% to 18% (Forde et al. 2018). In the neoadjuvant NADIM phase II trial, 46 stage IIIA patients were treated with neoadjuvant nivolumab and carboplatin and paclitaxel. Of the 41 patients who underwent surgery, complete pathologic response was observed in 26 patients (56%) (Provencio et al. 2020). The primary endpoint of this study was the progression-free survival at 24 months and it was 77%.

Recently, Forde et al. presented the results of CheckMate-816, a trial evaluating the addition of nivolumab to neoadjuvant platinum-based chemotherapy compared to neoadjuvant platinum-based chemotherapy alone in patients with stage IB–IIIA NSCLC (per TNM 7th edition). The study had dual endpoints of pathologic complete response rate and clinical event-free survival rate. The investigators presented the results of the pathologic complete response. Among patients who received neoadjuvant nivolumab and chemotherapy, the pathologic complete response rate was 24% as compared to 2.2% among patients who received chemotherapy alone [AACR 2021, Forde]. There was no increased postoperative complications, and neoadjuvant chemotherapy and nivolumab did not impact the ability to perform surgery. Data on event-free survival rate was not presented.

The correlation of complete pathologic response rate to survival is not well established in prospective trials. However, in a meta-analysis of neoadjuvant trials, there was a strong correlation between pathologic response rate and survival. It is unclear if regulatory authorities will accept the pathologic response rate as an endpoint (Waser et al. 2020).

Immune checkpoint inhibitors are also being evaluated in the adjuvant setting (Table 3). Recently, it was announced in a press release that in the IMpower010 trial, adjuvant atezolizumab following surgery and adjuvant chemotherapy improved disease-free survival in all randomized stage II–IIIA patients. The magnitude of benefit was more pronounced in patients with PD-L1-positive tumors. Several trials are evaluating adjuvant checkpoint inhibitors administered with or following adjuvant chemotherapy.

Based on all the above data, it is expected that immune checkpoint inhibitors will become an integral part of management of stage II and stage IIIA NSCLC patients who have resectable or unresectable tumors.

Table 2 Ongoing neoadjuvant trials

Trial	Phase	Stage	Experimental intervention	Primary endpoint
IMpower030	III	II–IIIA–T3N2	Atezolizumab plus chemotherapy compared to placebo plus chemotherapy. Following surgery, patients who received neoadjuvant atezolizumab will receive 16 cycles of atezolizumab	Event-free survival
KEYNOTE-671	III	II–IIIA–IIIB (N2 only)	Pembrolizumab plus chemotherapy compared to placebo plus chemotherapy. Following surgery, patients will receive adjuvant pembrolizumab or placebo for 13 cycles	Event-free survival/overall survival
AEGEAN	III	II–IIIB (N2)	Durvalumab plus chemotherapy compared to placebo plus chemotherapy	Major pathologic response/ event-free survival

Table 3 Ongoing adjuvant trials

Trial	Phase	Stage	Experimental intervention	Primary endpoint
ANVIL	III	IB–IIIA	Nivolumab versus observation. Patients may or may not have received adjuvant chemotherapy and/or radiation therapy	Disease-free survival/overall survival
KEYNOTE-091	III	T ≥4 cm, II–IIIA 7th edition	Pembrolizumab versus placebo. Patients may or may not have received adjuvant chemotherapy	Disease-free survival
IMpower010	III	T ≥4 cm, II–IIIA 7th edition	Atezolizumab versus observation. Patients must be eligible to receive platinum-based chemotherapy and should have received prior to randomization to atezolizumab or observation	Disease-free survival

11 Immune-Related Toxicities with Immune Checkpoint Inhibitors

Immune checkpoint inhibitors are associated with unique adverse events that result from the activation of immune response and resemble autoimmune disorders (Marin-Acevedo et al. 2019). Though certain organs and tissues are more commonly affected, adverse events from immune checkpoint inhibitors can impact any organ in the body (Table 4).

Immune-related adverse events can occur at any time following initiation of immune checkpoint inhibitor therapy. Most immune-related adverse events occur within 6 months, but delayed onset of adverse events including after discontinuation of immune checkpoint inhibitors has been observed. Therefore, there is a need for both detailed baseline assessment and frequent clinical evaluations and laboratory assessments during therapy with checkpoint inhibitors to prevent, diagnose, and manage these adverse events. Baseline assessments should include the history of any autoimmune disorders and laboratory tests for thyroid and adrenal function and hepatitis serologies. Patients with a history of autoimmune disorders requiring immunosuppressive therapy are generally not treated with immune checkpoint inhibitors. Similarly, patients with a history of organ transplants are excluded from such therapy (Table 5).

Development of any symptoms, laboratory abnormalities, or signs of immune-mediated adverse events requires immediate initiation of immune-suppressive therapy, primarily steroids. Adverse events refractory to steroids are treated with infliximab, a tumor necrosis factor (TNF)-blocking agent, or mycophenolate mofetil, an inhibitor of inosine monophosphate dehydrogenase, an enzyme involved in the synthesis of guanosine nucleotides. Infliximab is avoided in patients with hepatitis due to concerns of hepatotoxicity with this agent. Therapy with immune checkpoint inhibitors is put on hold with the development of immune-mediated adverse events, particularly if the adverse event requires therapy. Notable exceptions are endocrine abnormalities, which could be managed with hormone replacement therapy. Immune checkpoint inhibitors could be restarted once immune-related adverse events recover to ≤grade 1 toxicity without requiring steroids or requiring very low doses of steroids. Certain immune-mediated adverse events such as pneumonitis or neurologic adverse events may require permanent discontinuation of immune checkpoint inhibitors even after the patient recovers from these adverse events.

The rate of ≥grade 3 adverse events with PD-1 signaling pathway-directed agents is about 10%. Immune-mediated adverse events are more common with anti-CTLA-4-containing regimens with notable exception of type I diabetes that is more common with PD-1 signaling pathway

Table 4 Efficacy of FDA-approved immune checkpoint inhibitors as a monotherapy in the frontline therapy (control arm for all trials—platinum doublet chemotherapy)

Drug(s)	Indication(s)	ORR (%)	mPFS (months)	mOS (months)	Study
Pembrolizumab	PD-L1 TPS ≥50%	45 vs. 28	10.6 vs. 6.0	26.3 vs. 13.4	K-024
	PD-L1 TPS ≥1%	27 vs. 27	5.4 vs. 6.5	16.7 vs. 12.1	K-042
Atezolizumab	PD-L1 ≥50%, or ≥10% immune cells	38 vs. 29	6.8 vs. 5.0	20.2 vs. 13.1	IMp110
Cemiplimab[a]	PD-L1 TPS ≥50%	39 vs. 20	8.2 vs. 5.7	NR vs. 14.2	E-L1

[a]EMPOWER-Lung 1 is an open-label, randomized, phase III study conducted globally, outside of the United States, randomly assigning advanced-stage NSCLC to cemiplimab, anti-PD-1 antibodies, or histology-specific platinum doublet chemotherapy (Sezer et al. 2021)

inhibitors. The rate of immune-mediated adverse events is no more when immune checkpoint inhibitors are combined with chemotherapy. Retrospective data suggests that the development of immune-mediated adverse events may predict for better outcomes. In addition, use of steroids to manage immune-mediated adverse events may not lead to inferior outcomes. It is imperative that the therapy with steroids or other immune-suppressive therapy to manage immune-mediated adverse events not be withheld due to concerns about tumor progression.

Immune-mediated adverse events
Common adverse events
Cutaneous—rash, pruritus without rash
Gastrointestinal—diarrhea, colitis, hepatitis
Endocrine—thyroid abnormalities (hypothyroidism more common than hyperthyroidism), adrenal insufficiency, hypophysitis
Pulmonary—pneumonitis
Musculoskeletal—myositis, arthritis
Uncommon adverse events
Cardiovascular—myocarditis, pericarditis
Renal—interstitial nephritis, granulomatous nephritis
Endocrine—type I diabetes
Ophthalmic—episcleritis, conjunctivitis, uveitis
Hematologic—hemolytic anemia, neutropenia, thrombocytopenia
Neurologic—myasthenia gravis, Guillain-Barre syndrome, peripheral neuropathies

12 Future of Cancer Immunotherapy

Despite the successes observed with immune checkpoint inhibitors, only a minority of patients achieve long-term benefit. Many patients either derive no benefit or derive limited benefit. Therefore, there remains a need to investigate novel approaches to activate the immune system to treat cancers and identify biomarkers that can define cancer patients most likely to derive benefit from a specific immunotherapeutic agent. There is also a need to understand the mechanisms of resistance to immunotherapy agents. Finally, investigations to define biomarkers that can predict for immune therapy-related toxicities are crucial (Murciano-Goroff et al. 2020).

Currently, the only biomarker utilized to define the use of immunotherapy in lung cancer patients is PD-L1. It is well recognized that it is an imperfect biomarker since all patients with high PD-L1 lung cancers do not benefit from PD-1 signaling pathway agents though the probability of benefit is higher and patients with low or no PD-L1 lung cancers may derive clinical benefit. Tumor mutation burden (TMB) has also been assessed as a biomarker, and this marker also has limitations. As with PD-L1, TMB is also an imperfect marker. Currently, in the United States, pembrolizumab is approved for patients with advanced cancers who have high tumor mutational burden. Combination of these markers may provide greater differentiation of patients most likely to derive benefit from checkpoint inhibitors. However, prospective data is lacking for analyzing the combination of biomarkers to define patient populations for treatment with immune checkpoint inhibitors.

Beyond CTLA-4 and PD-1, several other immune checkpoints can be targets for therapeutic intervention. These include LAG3, TIGIT, and TIM3, and currently drugs targeting these immune checkpoints are being evaluated in combination with PD-1/PD-L1 inhibitors for a vari-

Table 5 Efficacy of FDA-approved immune checkpoint inhibitor-based frontline therapies (control arm for all trials—platinum doublet chemotherapy)

Drug(s)	Indication(s)	ORR (%)	mPFS (months)	mOS (months)	Study
Nivolumab + ipilimumab	PD-L1 ≥1%	36 vs. 30	5.1 vs. 5.6	17.1 vs. 14.9	CM-227
Nivolumab + ipilimumab + platinum doublet	NSCLC	38 vs. 25	6.7 vs. 5.0	15.6 vs. 10.9	CM-9LA
Pembrolizumab + platinum + pemetrexed	NSCLC, nonsquamous	48 vs. 19	9.0 vs. 4.9	22.0 vs. 10.7	K-189
Pembrolizumab + carboplatin + paclitaxel/nab-paclitaxel	NSCLC, squamous	62 vs. 38	8.0 vs. 5.1	17.1 vs. 11.6	K-407
Atezolizumab + carboplatin + nab-paclitaxel	NSCLC, nonsquamous	49 vs. 32	7.0 vs. 5.5	18.6 vs. 13.9	IMp130
Atezolizumab + carboplatin + paclitaxel + bevacizumab	NSCLC, nonsquamous	63 vs. 48	8.3 vs. 6.8	19.2 vs. 14.7	IMp150[a]

[a]In this phase III study, control arm was treated with bevacizumab + platinum doublet chemotherapy

ety of cancers. Several bispecific antibodies are currently in development. Blinatumomab is a bispecific antibody with two variable segments, one that targets CD19 on B lymphocytes and the other that targets CD3 on T cells. The drug is approved for the treatment of B-cell acute lymphoblastic leukemia in the first or second remission. Similar drugs are in development for several cancers including lung cancer. Dual-affinity antibodies that block two separate immune checkpoints simultaneously such as PD-1 and CTLA-4 or PD-1 and LAG3 are also in clinical development. Finally, drugs that could activate and modify innate immune system such as oncolytic viruses and STING pathway activators are also being evaluated in clinical trials. Appropriate selection of patients for such novel agents to maximize benefit and minimize toxicity will be crucial in these ongoing trials.

References

Antonia SJ, Villegas A, Daniel D, Vicente D, Murakami S, Hui R, Yokoi T, Chiappori A, Lee KH, de Wit M, Cho BC, Bourhaba M, Quantin X, Tokito T, Mekhail T, Planchard D, Kim YC, Karapetis CS, Hiret S, Ostoros G, Kubota K, Gray JE, Paz-Ares L, de Castro Carpeno J, Wadsworth C, Melillo G, Jiang H, Huang Y, Dennis PA, Ozguroglu M, Investigators P (2017) Durvalumab after chemoradiotherapy in stage III non-small-cell lung cancer. N Engl J Med 377(20):1919–1929. https://doi.org/10.1056/NEJMoa1709937

Antonia SJ, Villegas A, Daniel D, Vicente D, Murakami S, Hui R, Kurata T, Chiappori A, Lee KH, de Wit M, Cho BC, Bourhaba M, Quantin X, Tokito T, Mekhail T, Planchard D, Kim YC, Karapetis CS, Hiret S, Ostoros G, Kubota K, Gray JE, Paz-Ares L, de Castro Carpeno J, Faivre-Finn C, Reck M, Vansteenkiste J, Spigel DR, Wadsworth C, Melillo G, Taboada M, Dennis PA, Ozguroglu M, Investigators P (2018) Overall survival with durvalumab after chemoradiotherapy in stage III NSCLC. N Engl J Med 379(24):2342–2350. https://doi.org/10.1056/NEJMoa1809697

Durm GA, Jabbour SK, Althouse SK, Liu Z, Sadiq AA, Zon RT, Jalal SI, Kloecker GH, Williamson MJ, Reckamp KL, Langdon RM, Kio EA, Gentzler RD, Adesunloye BA, Harb WA, Walling RV, Titzer ML, Hanna NH (2020) A phase 2 trial of consolidation pembrolizumab following concurrent chemoradiation for patients with unresectable stage III non-small cell lung cancer: Hoosier Cancer Research Network LUN 14-179. Cancer 126(19):4353–4361. https://doi.org/10.1002/cncr.33083

Faivre-Finn C, Vicente D, Kurata T, Planchard D, Paz-Ares L, Vansteenkiste JF, Spigel DR, Garassino MC, Reck M, Senan S, Naidoo J, Rimner A, Wu YL, Gray JE, Ozguroglu M, Lee KH, Cho BC, Kato T, de Wit M, Newton M, Wang L, Thiyagarajah P, Antonia SJ (2021) Four-year survival with durvalumab after chemoradiotherapy in stage III NSCLC—an update from the PACIFIC trial. J Thorac Oncol 16(5):860–867. https://doi.org/10.1016/j.jtho.2020.12.015

Forde PM, Chaft JE, Smith KN, Anagnostou V, Cottrell TR, Hellmann MD, Zahurak M, Yang SC, Jones DR, Broderick S, Battafarano RJ, Velez MJ, Rekhtman N, Olah Z, Naidoo J, Marrone KA, Verde F, Guo H, Zhang J, Caushi JX, Chan HY, Sidhom JW, Scharpf RB, White J, Gabrielson E, Wang H, Rosner GL, Rusch V, Wolchok JD, Merghoub T, Taube JM, Velculescu VE, Topalian SL, Brahmer JR, Pardoll DM (2018) Neoadjuvant PD-1 blockade in resectable lung cancer. N Engl J Med 378(21):1976–1986. https://doi.org/10.1056/NEJMoa1716078

Gadgeel S, Rodriguez-Abreu D, Speranza G, Esteban E, Felip E, Domine M, Hui R, Hochmair MJ, Clingan P, Powell SF, Cheng SY, Bischoff HG, Peled N, Grossi F, Jennens RR, Reck M, Garon EB, Novello S, Rubio-Viqueira B, Boyer M, Kurata T, Gray JE, Yang J, Bas T, Pietanza MC, Garassino MC (2020) Updated analysis from KEYNOTE-189: pembrolizumab or placebo plus pemetrexed and platinum for previously untreated metastatic nonsquamous non-small-cell lung cancer. J Clin Oncol 38(14):1505–1517. https://doi.org/10.1200/JCO.19.03136

Gandhi L, Rodriguez-Abreu D, Gadgeel S, Esteban E, Felip E, De Angelis F, Domine M, Clingan P, Hochmair MJ, Powell SF, Cheng SY, Bischoff HG, Peled N, Grossi F, Jennens RR, Reck M, Hui R, Garon EB, Boyer M, Rubio-Viqueira B, Novello S, Kurata T, Gray JE, Vida J, Wei Z, Yang J, Raftopoulos H, Pietanza MC, Garassino MC, KEYNOTE-189 Investigators (2018) Pembrolizumab plus chemotherapy in metastatic non-small-cell lung cancer. N Engl J Med 378(22):2078–2092. https://doi.org/10.1056/NEJMoa1801005

Goldman JW, Dvorkin M, Chen Y, Reinmuth N, Hotta K, Trukhin D, Statsenko G, Hochmair MJ, Ozguroglu M, Ji JH, Garassino MC, Voitko O, Poltoratskiy A, Ponce S, Verderame F, Havel L, Bondarenko I, Kazarnowicz A, Losonczy G, Conev NV, Armstrong J, Byrne N, Thiyagarajah P, Jiang H, Paz-Ares L, CASPIAN Investigators (2021) Durvalumab, with or without tremelimumab, plus platinum-etoposide versus platinum-etoposide alone in first-line treatment of extensive-stage small-cell lung cancer (CASPIAN): updated results from a randomised, controlled, open-label, phase 3 trial. Lancet Oncol 22(1):51–65. https://doi.org/10.1016/S1470-2045(20)30539-8

Hellmann MD, Paz-Ares L, Bernabe Caro R, Zurawski B, Kim SW, Carcereny Costa E, Park K, Alexandru A, Lupinacci L, de la Mora Jimenez E, Sakai H, Albert I, Vergnenegre A, Peters S, Syrigos K, Barlesi F, Reck M, Borghaei H, Brahmer JR, O'Byrne KJ, Geese WJ,

Bhagavatheeswaran P, Rabindran SK, Kasinathan RS, Nathan FE, Ramalingam SS (2019) Nivolumab plus ipilimumab in advanced non-small-cell lung cancer. N Engl J Med 381(21):2020–2031. https://doi.org/10.1056/NEJMoa1910231

Herbst RS, Giaccone G, de Marinis F, Reinmuth N, Vergnenegre A, Barrios CH, Morise M, Felip E, Andric Z, Geater S, Ozguroglu M, Zou W, Sandler A, Enquist I, Komatsubara K, Deng Y, Kuriki H, Wen X, McCleland M, Mocci S, Jassem J, Spigel DR (2020) Atezolizumab for first-line treatment of PD-L1-selected patients with NSCLC. N Engl J Med 383(14):1328–1339. https://doi.org/10.1056/NEJMoa1917346

Horn L, Mansfield AS, Szczesna A, Havel L, Krzakowski M, Hochmair MJ, Huemer F, Losonczy G, Johnson ML, Nishio M, Reck M, Mok T, Lam S, Shames DS, Liu J, Ding B, Lopez-Chavez A, Kabbinavar F, Lin W, Sandler A, Liu SV, IMpower133 Study Group (2018) First-line atezolizumab plus chemotherapy in extensive-stage small-cell lung cancer. N Engl J Med 379(23):2220–2229. https://doi.org/10.1056/NEJMoa1809064

Jabbour SK, Lee KH, Frost N, Breder V, Kowalski DM, Pollock T, Levchenko E, Reguart N, Martinez-Marti A, Houghton B, Paoli JB, Safina S, Park K, Komiya T, Sanford A, Boolell V, Liu H, Samkari A, Keller SM, Reck M (2021) Pembrolizumab plus concurrent chemoradiation therapy in patients with unresectable, locally advanced, stage III non-small cell lung cancer: the phase 2 KEYNOTE-799 nonrandomized trial. JAMA Oncol. https://doi.org/10.1001/jamaoncol.2021.2301

Marin-Acevedo JA, Chirila RM, Dronca RS (2019) Immune checkpoint inhibitor toxicities. Mayo Clin Proc 94(7):1321–1329. https://doi.org/10.1016/j.mayocp.2019.03.012

Mok TSK, Wu YL, Kudaba I, Kowalski DM, Cho BC, Turna HZ, Castro G Jr, Srimuninnimit V, Laktionov KK, Bondarenko I, Kubota K, Lubiniecki GM, Zhang J, Kush D, Lopes G, KEYNOTE-042 Investigators (2019) Pembrolizumab versus chemotherapy for previously untreated, PD-L1-expressing, locally advanced or metastatic non-small-cell lung cancer (KEYNOTE-042): a randomised, open-label, controlled, phase 3 trial. Lancet 393(10183):1819–1830. https://doi.org/10.1016/S0140-6736(18)32409-7

Murciano-Goroff YR, Warner AB, Wolchok JD (2020) The future of cancer immunotherapy: microenvironment-targeting combinations. Cell Res 30(6):507–519. https://doi.org/10.1038/s41422-020-0337-2

Paz-Ares L, Luft A, Vicente D, Tafreshi A, Gumus M, Mazieres J, Hermes B, Cay Senler F, Csoszi T, Fulop A, Rodriguez-Cid J, Wilson J, Sugawara S, Kato T, Lee KH, Cheng Y, Novello S, Halmos B, Li X, Lubiniecki GM, Piperdi B, Kowalski DM, KEYNOTE-407 Investigators (2018) Pembrolizumab plus chemotherapy for squamous non-small-cell lung cancer. N Engl J Med 379(21):2040–2051. https://doi.org/10.1056/NEJMoa1810865

Paz-Ares L, Dvorkin M, Chen Y, Reinmuth N, Hotta K, Trukhin D, Statsenko G, Hochmair MJ, Ozguroglu M, Ji JH, Voitko O, Poltoratskiy A, Ponce S, Verderame F, Havel L, Bondarenko I, Kazarnowicz A, Losonczy G, Conev NV, Armstrong J, Byrne N, Shire N, Jiang H, Goldman JW, CASPIAN Investigators (2019) Durvalumab plus platinum-etoposide versus platinum-etoposide in first-line treatment of extensive-stage small-cell lung cancer (CASPIAN): a randomised, controlled, open-label, phase 3 trial. Lancet 394(10212):1929–1939. https://doi.org/10.1016/S0140-6736(19)32222-6

Paz-Ares L, Vicente D, Tafreshi A, Robinson A, Soto Parra H, Mazieres J, Hermes B, Cicin I, Medgyasszay B, Rodriguez-Cid J, Okamoto I, Lee S, Ramlau R, Vladimirov V, Cheng Y, Deng X, Zhang Y, Bas T, Piperdi B, Halmos B (2020) A randomized, placebo-controlled trial of pembrolizumab plus chemotherapy in patients with metastatic squamous NSCLC: protocol-specified final analysis of KEYNOTE-407. J Thorac Oncol 15(10):1657–1669. https://doi.org/10.1016/j.jtho.2020.06.015

Paz-Ares L, Ciuleanu TE, Cobo M, Schenker M, Zurawski B, Menezes J, Richardet E, Bennouna J, Felip E, Juan-Vidal O, Alexandru A, Sakai H, Lingua A, Salman P, Souquet PJ, De Marchi P, Martin C, Perol M, Scherpereel A, Lu S, John T, Carbone DP, Meadows-Shropshire S, Agrawal S, Oukessou A, Yan J, Reck M (2021) First-line nivolumab plus ipilimumab combined with two cycles of chemotherapy in patients with non-small-cell lung cancer (CheckMate 9LA): an international, randomised, open-label, phase 3 trial. Lancet Oncol 22(2):198–211. https://doi.org/10.1016/S1470-2045(20)30641-0

Provencio M, Nadal E, Insa A, Garcia-Campelo MR, Casal-Rubio J, Domine M, Majem M, Rodriguez-Abreu D, Martinez-Marti A, De Castro Carpeno J, Cobo M, Lopez Vivanco G, Del Barco E, Bernabe Caro R, Vinolas N, Barneto Aranda I, Viteri S, Pereira E, Royuela A, Casarrubios M, Salas Anton C, Parra ER, Wistuba I, Calvo V, Laza-Briviesca R, Romero A, Massuti B, Cruz-Bermudez A (2020) Neoadjuvant chemotherapy and nivolumab in resectable non-small-cell lung cancer (NADIM): an open-label, multicentre, single-arm, phase 2 trial. Lancet Oncol 21(11):1413–1422. https://doi.org/10.1016/S1470-2045(20)30453-8

Reck M, Rodriguez-Abreu D, Robinson AG, Hui R, Csoszi T, Fulop A, Gottfried M, Peled N, Tafreshi A, Cuffe S, O'Brien M, Rao S, Hotta K, Leiby MA, Lubiniecki GM, Shentu Y, Rangwala R, Brahmer JR, Investigators, K.-. (2016) Pembrolizumab versus chemotherapy for PD-L1-positive non-small-cell lung cancer. N Engl J Med 375(19):1823–1833. https://doi.org/10.1056/NEJMoa1606774

Reck M, Rodriguez-Abreu D, Robinson AG, Hui R, Csoszi T, Fulop A, Gottfried M, Peled N, Tafreshi A, Cuffe S, O'Brien M, Rao S, Hotta K, Vandormael K, Riccio A, Yang J, Pietanza MC, Brahmer JR (2019) Updated analysis of KEYNOTE-024: pembrolizumab versus platinum-based chemotherapy for advanced non-small-cell lung cancer with PD-L1 tumor proportion score of 50% or greater. J Clin Oncol 37(7):537–546. https://doi.org/10.1200/JCO.18.00149

Sezer A, Kilickap S, Gumus M, Bondarenko I, Ozguroglu M, Gogishvili M, Turk HM, Cicin I, Bentsion D, Gladkov O, Clingan P, Sriuranpong V, Rizvi N, Gao B, Li S, Lee S, McGuire K, Chen CI, Makharadze T, Paydas S, Nechaeva M, Seebach F, Weinreich DM, Yancopoulos GD, Gullo G, Lowy I, Rietschel P (2021) Cemiplimab monotherapy for first-line treatment of advanced non-small-cell lung cancer with PD-L1 of at least 50%: a multicentre, open-label, global, phase 3, randomised, controlled trial. Lancet 397(10274):592–604. https://doi.org/10.1016/S0140-6736(21)00228-2

Socinski MA, Jotte RM, Cappuzzo F, Orlandi F, Stroyakovskiy D, Nogami N, Rodriguez-Abreu D, Moro-Sibilot D, Thomas CA, Barlesi F, Finley G, Kelsch C, Lee A, Coleman S, Deng Y, Shen Y, Kowanetz M, Lopez-Chavez A, Sandler A, Reck M, IMpower150 Study Group (2018) Atezolizumab for first-line treatment of metastatic nonsquamous NSCLC. N Engl J Med 378(24):2288–2301. https://doi.org/10.1056/NEJMoa1716948

Waser NA, Adam A, Schweikert B, Vo L, McKenna M, Breckenridge M, Penrod JR, Goring S (2020) 1243P Pathologic response as early endpoint for survival following neoadjuvant therapy (NEO-AT) in resectable non-small cell lung cancer (rNSCLC): systematic literature review and meta-analysis. Ann Oncol 31:S806. https://doi.org/10.1016/j.annonc.2020.08.116

West H, McCleod M, Hussein M, Morabito A, Rittmeyer A, Conter HJ, Kopp HG, Daniel D, McCune S, Mekhail T, Zer A, Reinmuth N, Sadiq A, Sandler A, Lin W, Ochi Lohmann T, Archer V, Wang L, Kowanetz M, Cappuzzo F (2019) Atezolizumab in combination with carboplatin plus nab-paclitaxel chemotherapy compared with chemotherapy alone as first-line treatment for metastatic non-squamous non-small-cell lung cancer (IMpower130): a multicentre, randomised, open-label, phase 3 trial. Lancet Oncol 20(7):924–937. https://doi.org/10.1016/S1470-2045(19)30167-6

Combined Radiotherapy and Chemotherapy: Theoretical Considerations and Biological Premises

Michael K. Farris, Cole Steber, Corbin Helis, and William Blackstock

Contents

1 Introduction 385
2 Exploitable Mechanisms 386
3 Clinical Implications 387
4 Future Considerations 392
References 394

Abstract

Understanding the general radiobiological principles at play in the setting of combined radiation and chemotherapy is essential to appreciate how this approach has evolved over time into the standard of care for locally advanced non-small cell lung cancer (NSCLC).

The basic biological pathways through which these modalities interact with each other as well as cancerous and noncancerous cells have been described over the last several decades. Key mechanisms reviewed below include spatial cooperation, independent cell kill, protection of normal tissues, and finally enhancement of tumor response (i.e., radio-sensitization or radio-enhancement). Translation of these principles into clinical trials has slowly enhanced our understanding of each, and revealed potential exploits that can guide us toward further improving the therapeutic ratio in lung cancer treatment.

Modern radiation therapy techniques as well as newly identified targeted drugs and immunotherapies will continue to evolve our understanding in this setting.

1 Introduction

Over the last 60 years, the combination of chemotherapy and radiation therapy (RT) has become a standard of care in many cancer types. Locally advanced non-small cell lung cancer (LA-NSCLC) and limited-stage small cell lung cancer (LS-SCLC) in particular have been extensively studied in the prospective setting with a wide variety of regimens. Over time, the dramatically different treatment approaches that have been used have helped us form a better understanding of how to exploit the underlying cancer

Michael K. Farris and Cole Steber share co-first author credit and contributed equally to this chapter.

M. K. Farris (✉) · C. Steber
C. Helis · W. Blackstock
Wake Forest School of Medicine, Comprehensive Cancer Center, Winston-Salem, NC, USA
e-mail: mfarris@wakehealth.edu

biology, and enhance the therapeutic ratio. The potential benefits of a concurrent approach have been demonstrated when compared against clearly inferior outcomes of RT alone, and lackluster outcomes of induction or sequential approaches.

To unlock the full potential of concurrent chemoradiation, it is helpful to first understand the basic principles and mechanisms behind each modality. These insights will help guide future avenues of study that incorporate newer systemic agents with more precise methods of RT delivery.

2 Exploitable Mechanisms

The four basic mechanisms through which RT and chemotherapy interact were established by Steel and Peckham in the 1970s (Steel and Peckham 1979). These include spatial cooperation, toxicity independence, protection of normal tissues, and enhancement of tumor response.

The first mechanism, *spatial cooperation*, arises when disease that exists in different anatomical locations might be missed by one agent, but dealt with by another. In the case of lung cancer, an example would be targeted RT to obvious intrathoracic gross disease, while systemic chemotherapy helps to address potential microscopic subclinical disease outside the RT portals.

The nature of spatial differences in agents operating under this mechanism does not require direct interaction between the two treating agents. In other words, there is no required modification assumed. If individual agents are addressing the disease in different sites independently and not overlapping in their effect, then one would want to give the best of either agent. In clinical practice, exploitation is best illustrated when RT and chemotherapy are delivered sequentially. This would enable both the radiation and chemo to be given at their full (most effective) dose without fear of overlapping toxicities and allows targeting of different anatomical sites of disease. The choice of sequencing would be dependent on the site which is at the highest risk of acute failure (locoregional or distant).

The next mechanism, *toxicity independence*, occurs when two agents can be given simultaneously without having to reduce their dose levels. If these two agents do not interact negatively with one another to diminish tumoricidal effectiveness, even the addition of one agent at less than full dose should overall improve the therapeutic ratio to some degree when both are used together. When applied to the treatment of lung cancer, exploitation of nonoverlapping toxicities between RT and certain chemotherapies can act on intrathoracic disease and occult systemic disease simultaneously leading to a higher immediate cell kill than would be obtained by either treatment alone. This scenario does not require interaction between RT and chemotherapy.

Another mechanism termed *protection of normal tissues* can allow for higher doses of RT or chemotherapy than would ordinarily be tolerated. Hopefully, this would improve cancer control while maintaining or decreasing expected toxicity and thereby improve the therapeutic ratio. Generally, this mechanism is illustrated through the addition of a third agent, which does not interfere with the ability of either chemotherapy or RT to kill tumor cells, but does limit the impact of either treatment on nearby normal cells. Such a mechanism can only apply if tumor cells are not protected to the same degree as normal tissue.

Although it is not commonly exploited in the clinic, the injection of amifostine prior to head and neck RT to protect against RT-induced xerostomia is a classic example of this in practice. Amifostine is a thiol prodrug that once activated can scavenge free radicals. Since radiation does much of its damage through free radical creation, the scavenging of free radicals may limit toxicity if the unwanted free radicals that are produced in normal tissues can be selectively eliminated. In theory, tumor cells which may have hypovascularity and lower pH are slower to take up amifostine, and therefore it should be preferentially absorbed more often in normal tissues than in tumors (Koukourakis 2002). While studies have demonstrated some suggestion of efficacy, it has not caught on for routine use in clinic (Brizel et al. 2000). Difficult logistics of administration just prior to RT, as well as other issues including nausea and blood pressure effects, have limited widespread routine use. Even so, it serves as an excellent example of the potential ways that this mechanism could be exploited to enhance the therapeutic ratio. There are other novel radioprotectors currently being investigated, such as avasopasem, a novel superoxide dismutase mimetic (see Sect. 4).

The last mechanism, *enhancement of tumor response*, occurs when a combination of agents produces a greater effect together than that expected from either individual agent. It could be argued that induction systemic therapy, when utilized to reduce tumor bulk and allow for smaller fields or dose escalation, is a type of exploitation of this approach. Adaptive chemoradiation techniques looking at decreasing treatment volumes mid treatment with subsequent dose escalation operate on the same principle. Another example of exploitation of enhanced tumor response can be found in the use of radiosensitizers. Oxygen is the most efficient radiosensitizer of hypoxic tumor cells and when present can "latch on to" damaged DNA forming peroxides. This essentially fixates the damage that has been initiated by RT through the creation of free radicals and hydrogen abstraction. While not routinely used in clinic, techniques have been investigated that capitalize on the enhancement of tumor response by increasing oxygenation and blood flow with carbogen and nicotinamide. Similarly, oxygen mimetics have been studied as well including nitroimidazoles (nimorazole, misonidazole, etanidazole). In the clinical setting, these drugs often required high doses and were associated with peripheral neuropathy (Rojas et al. 1996; Wardman 2019).

Some drugs, such as tirapazamine, can operate through exploitation of normal tissue protection and enhanced tumor response. Tirapazamine is a prodrug that is selectively converted into its toxic form in the hypoxic environment of tumor cells (Evans et al. 1998).

Other specific molecular mechanisms that are already being exploited in certain cancers include enhanced DNA damage and repair, cell cycle synchronization, enhanced apoptosis, angiogenesis pathway disruption, and inhibition of cell proliferation. Many of these pathways are differentially expressed in tumors and normal tissues, which may help in achieving an improved therapeutic ratio.

Any of these mechanisms above could be exploited to provide an improved therapeutic strategy compared with RT or chemotherapy alone. Importantly, more than one mechanism may be simultaneously exploited. For example, if one attempts to achieve enhancement of tumor response using chemotherapy agents that have no overlapping toxicity with radiation therapy, there may also be (1) a benefit from the simple addition of antitumor effects (independent cell kill), while (2) chemotherapy may also deal with the disease outside the radiation therapy treatment field (spatial cooperation). When assessing tumor cell kill after delivery of a combination of agents, the overall effect may be additive, infra-additive, or supra-additive (synergistic).

As our understanding of cancer molecular biology continues to evolve, new opportunities for exploitation will arise. This is especially true with improvements in radiation delivery and the advent of new targeted therapies and immunotherapies.

3 Clinical Implications

For patients with LA-NSCLC, definitive conventional RT alone has led to unsatisfactory outcomes. RTOG 73-01 demonstrated high rates of intrathoracic failure at 33% for patients treated with 60 Gy on RTOG 73-01 (Perez et al. 1980). Multiple approaches have since been attempted to improve local control in these patients using altered RT fractionation as well as the addition of chemotherapy to RT concurrently or in various combinations (induction, consolidation, or both).

In the 1970s, there was increased interest in the use of radiosensitizers such as misonidazole. This was of particular interest in helping to improve local control and increasing hypoxic cell kill. An RTOG study investigated the concurrent use of misonidazole in a phase I/II study with a hypofractionated regimen with 6 Gy delivered twice weekly in 3 weeks for

36 Gy total (Simpson et al. 1987). This hypofractionated versus conventional fractionated regimen was phased out for practical reasons as delivery of misonidazole required precisely timed injection prior to each dose of radiation. Furthermore, the high doses of misonidazole utilized were associated with significant neuropathy. The results were not favorable. No benefit was found in the misonidazole group compared to a placebo group receiving the same course of radiation or a conventional arm receiving 60 Gy in 6 weeks receiving no drug. Investigation into the use of misonidazole in LA-NSCLC fell out of favor as a result, and likewise the use of hypofractionated RT alone for LA-NSCLC was less common until more recent investigations.

After encouraging results from several clinical trials investigating the combination of chemotherapy and radiation therapy, further investigation was warranted. Induction therapy was felt a promising approach that might allow exploitation of the spatial cooperation mechanism. This was of particular interest for LA-NSCLC, where distant failure due to occult extrathoracic disease was the predominant mode of failure following definitive treatment. This prompted a phase II study designed by the RTOG to evaluate induction vinblastine and cisplatin followed by irradiation at day 50 with 63 Gy delivered in 7 weeks concurrent with another cycle of the chemotherapy (Sause et al. 1992). After demonstration of tolerance for the regimen and a 2-year survival of 34%, the phase III RTOG 88-08 compared patients treated with 60 Gy of conventional RT vs. induction cisplatin/vinblastine followed by standard RT or hyperfractionated RT to 69.6 Gy delivered at 1.2 Gy delivered BID. Results showed a superior 1-year survival at 60% with the induction chemo and standard RT regimen to both of the other two arms ($p = 0.03$). Another study (CALGB 8433) investigating induction chemotherapy with the same induction regimen followed by conventional RT to 60 Gy versus RT alone to the same dose was completed prior to this and found a similar finding of improved survival in the combination therapy group (Dillman et al. 1990).

Other studies examining induction therapy prior to radiation included the study by Le Chevalier et al., which compared radiotherapy alone with those receiving a four-drug chemotherapy regimen including vindesine, cyclophosphamide, cisplatin, and lomustine given in three monthly cycles before and after radiation therapy (Le Chevalier et al. 1991). With the knowledge that preoperative chemotherapy had been shown to increase the 5-year survival rates of LA-NSCLC that undergo surgical resection, the EORTC 08941 study was designed to compare patients with IIIA-N2 disease randomized to surgery or radiation therapy, both after induction therapy with a platinum-based chemotherapy (van Meerbeeck et al. 2007). Induction chemotherapy obtained a response rate of 61%. Patients treated with surgery required post-op RT 40% of the time, and the median overall survival (OS) for patients assigned to resection was 16.4 versus 17.5 months with radiotherapy.

Despite confirming an improvement in the sequential use of induction chemotherapy followed by RT, one question that remained about induction chemotherapy was this: Did it matter when given prior to chemoradiation? This question was investigated by CALGB 39801, which randomized patients to immediate concurrent chemoradiation with weekly carboplatin/paclitaxel or the experimental arm giving two cycles of carboplatin/paclitaxel followed by the same course of chemoradiation (Vokes et al. 2007). Survival differences were not found to be significantly different, but patients experienced grade 4 toxicity more often at 40% when induction chemotherapy was included versus 26% without. This study highlights that unfortunately independent cell kill may be minimal when considering the induction chemotherapy regimens that are followed by chemoradiation. The reported induction response in this study showed partial response in 31%, stable disease in 39%, and progression in 6% of patients.

While induction chemotherapy may enable exploitation of the spatial cooperation between the modalities, it does not enable exploitation on the other mechanisms including enhancement of tumor response or radiosensitization. Due to the nonoverlapping portions of the two treatment modalities, there is no enhancement of tumor response that can be reasonably expected.

Early examples of combining chemotherapy and RT concurrently included the phase II and III studies by Sause et al. as well as the study by Schaake-Koning et al. (Sause et al. 1992, 1995; Schaake-Koning et al. 1992). In the latter study, cisplatin was investigated as a potential therapy to enhance or potentiate radiation damage in tumors. Much of this was derived from in vitro and animal studies as well as the early clinical trials using cisplatin in head and neck chemoradiation regimens. The study by Schaake-Koning et al. was designed to randomize patients with NSCLC to a split-course radiation therapy alone with a total dose of 55 Gy and two other arms with either weekly (30 mg/m^2) or daily (5 mg/m^2) cisplatin utilizing the same radiotherapy (Schaake-Koning et al. 1992). This study found a survival and local control benefit to the arm receiving daily cisplatin over the radiation therapy-alone group, but those patients receiving daily cisplatin had worse rates of nausea and vomiting at around 80% compared to 25%, respectively.

After experiences with dose escalation using conventional radiation therapy at 2 Gy/fx in RTOG 73-01, investigators turned to dose escalation using hyperfractionated (>2 Gy/fx) regimens such as in RTOG 83-11, which established that 69.6 Gy delivered in 1.2 Gy BID was a preferred hyperfractionated dose fractionation (Cox et al. 1990). Hyperfractionation was strongly considered as a method of increasing tumor cell kill while sparing normal tissues by taking advantage of the differences in the α/β ratios between tumors and normal tissues. Multiple studies examined the possible combination approach of concurrent chemotherapy and hyperfractionation (Jeremic et al. 1995, 1996; Sause et al. 1995).

One concern with the implementation of these regimens was for worsened acute toxicity that may occur when delivering chemotherapy during a course of hyperfractionated radiotherapy. In the studies by Jeremic et al., hyperfractionated radiation therapy was given with a total dose of either 64.8 or 69.6 Gy and concurrent carboplatin/etoposide given either every other week (Jeremic et al. 1995) or daily (Jeremic et al. 1996). These studies did show a benefit in survival, and this was likely due to the improved local control seen in the arms that included concurrent chemotherapy along with the hyperfractionated radiation therapy and a lack of significant improvement in the rate of distant metastases. Acute and late grade 4 toxicity was significantly worse in patients receiving 200 mg of carboplatin/etoposide and hyperfractionated radiation therapy to 64.8 Gy (Jeremic et al. 1995). However, when carboplatin/etoposide was given at 100 or 50 mg, there were no differences in acute and late high-grade toxicities.

Further investigation into concurrent chemotherapy and hyperfractionated RT began after confirmation that giving induction chemotherapy followed by concurrent chemoradiation could be tolerated in trials such as the CALGB 8433 and RTOG 88-08 (Dillman et al. 1990; Sause et al. 1995). Several RTOG trials including RTOG 90-15, RTOG 91-06, and RTOG 92-04 were designed to assess the combination of concurrent chemotherapy and hyperfractionated RT (Byhardt et al. 1995; Komaki et al. 2002; Lee et al. 1996). These studies found that this combined approach resulted in increased, but acceptable, acute toxicity and found significant prolongation of time to in-field progression in the hyperfractionated arms that also included concurrent chemotherapy. In RTOG 92-04, there was increased chronic esophagitis seen in the patients that had hyperfractionated RT concurrent with chemotherapy as opposed to conventional RT concurrent with chemotherapy. There was evidence of improved tumor control with improved time to in-field progression favoring the chemotherapy/hyperfractionated RT arm, but in the end this arm was not able to demonstrate improved OS over chemo/conventional RT arm (Komaki et al. 2002).

The rationale for the concurrent chemoradiation is to improve locoregional (intrathoracic) tumor control. Although concurrent chemotherapy may potentially have acted on the disease outside the radiation therapy treatment field, due to its delivery with lower systemic doses it was assumed from the onset that this type of administration would not have a major effect on systemic disease outside the radiotherapy treatment field and exploitation of the mechanism of spatial cooperation would be minimal. Likewise, since the dose of chemotherapy was often lower (in several of the studies low-dose chemo was given daily) this likely decreases the ability for the given chemotherapy agent to exploit the mechanism of independent cell kill. The lack of independent cell kill pertains to the disease within the thorax as well as any microscopic distant disease. In contrast, the mechanisms exploited by induction chemotherapy include spatial cooperation and independent cell kill.

Since concurrent chemotherapy has minimal exploitation of spatial cooperation and independent cell kill, its role in LA-NSCLC is to act primarily as a radiosensitizer and exploit the mechanism of enhancement of tumor response. In order to provide radiosensitization in the concurrent setting, the agent is ideally present at the time of irradiation. This was reflected in early trials such as the drug being given prior to the daily radiation therapy fraction (Schaake-Koning et al. 1992) or in between the two daily fractions (Jeremic et al. 1995, 1996). With the drug present at the time of irradiation, it allows both modification of the initial radiation damage and decrease/inhibition of the repair of radiation damage. Concurrent chemotherapy may affect cell cycle progression, and modification of cell synchrony was investigated by Chen et al. (2003) in a phase I/II study of concurrent pulsed low-dose paclitaxel and provided high levels of local control. Other processes of concurrent chemotherapy to be considered are improved drug access to tumor after radiation therapy as well as reduction in tumor bulk leading to increased tumor cell proliferation and thereby increased chemosensitivity of surviving tumor cells. With these processes at play, one may expect consolidation chemotherapy as a good way to exploit these processes. Early studies investigating consolidation chemotherapy after chemoradiation appeared promising in several prospective phase II studies (Gandara et al. 2006; Lau et al. 2001; Sekine et al. 2006). Randomized phase III studies such as Hanna et al. (2008) or Ahn et al. (2015) showed no difference in treatment outcome between concurrent chemoradiation alone and the same concurrent chemoradiation followed by consolidation chemotherapy. Results such as this confirmed that concurrent chemoradiation without any consolidation chemotherapy offers the best treatment outcome.

Trials such as the RTOG 9410 sought to answer the question on induction versus concurrent sequencing. RTOG 9410 randomized patients with LA-NSCLC to three arms: arm 1 with chemotherapy with vinblastine/cisplatin induction followed by conventional RT, arm 2 with concurrent chemotherapy with vinblastine/cisplatin chemotherapy with conventional RT, and arm 3 with cisplatin/etoposide with hyperfractionated RT (Curran et al. 2011). This study found that concurrent chemotherapy provided long-term survival compared to sequential chemotherapy with higher acute but similar late toxicities. Additionally, this trial did not show a clear benefit in a hyperfractionated course of radiation over a conventional one when given with concurrent chemotherapy, as similarly shown in head and neck cancer on RTOG 0129 (Nguyen-Tan et al. 2014). Explanations for this include worse acute nonhematologic toxicity in the hyperfractionated arm, which may have offset any benefit that this more aggressive concurrent regimen may have provided in terms of in-field disease control.

Despite the success in exploiting the mechanism of enhanced tumor response with concurrent chemoradiation, it is not without its trade-offs. There is evidence of overlapping toxicities and thus not entirely exploiting the mechanism of independent toxicity. The enhancement in cell kill that is found within tumor cells when giving concurrent chemotherapy also appears to enhance normal tissue response to radiation therapy. This has led to increased toxicity of normal tissues such as the esophagus and lung parenchyma, which occur more often in the concurrent arms of trials. Concurrent studies showed that the type and magnitude of toxicity largely depend on the dose and sequence of chemotherapy administered. In multiple concurrent chemotherapy RTOG studies (90-15, 91-06, 92-04) (Byhardt et al. 1995; Komaki et al. 2002; Lee et al. 1996), platinum-based doublets were used and the incidence of grade 3+ nonhematological toxicity ranged from 24% to 53%, being 34% when pooled together (Byhardt et al. 1998). In more contemporary studies, using paclitaxel and carboplatin such as RTOG 0617, the standard-dose RT arm had overall 76% grade 3+ events, 20% grade 3+ pulmonary events, and 7% grade 3+ esophagitis (Bradley et al. 2015). Secondary analysis of RTOG 0617 demonstrates how improvement in radiation therapy treatment techniques such as intensity-modulated radiotherapy (IMRT) and volumetric modulated arc therapy (VMAT) and improved dose delivery have allowed for increased normal tissue sparing, which has decreased rates of higher grade toxicity in patients undergoing concurrent chemoradiation (Chun et al. 2017).

Hypofractionation (generally defined as doses of radiation therapy >2 Gy per fraction) and accelerated radiation have been investigated in multiple studies and have been shown to improve OS for patients with NSCLC (Mauguen et al. 2012). A major potential advantage of hypofractionation is the ability to overcome accelerated repopulation of tumor cells, which may begin after 3–4 weeks of radiation therapy, improving the therapeutic ratio (Fowler and Chappell 2000). However, historically there has been concern over excess late toxicity with hypofractionated radiation due to the relatively higher biologically effective doses of radiation delivered to normal tissues compared with tumor with increasing fraction size.

The advent of new technologies such as intensity-modulated radiation therapy (IMRT) and image-guided radiation therapy (IGRT), as well as improved anatomic imaging, has allowed for increasingly precise delivery of radiation therapy while minimizing the radiation dose delivered to normal structures. This has had the greatest impact on early-stage NSCLC, where SBRT using very hypofractionated regimens is now the standard of care for medically inoperable patients. More recent investigations have included the use of these advanced radiation therapy techniques to attempt to further escalate the dose of radiotherapy without excessive toxicity.

RTOG 0617 was a 2 × 2 armed phase III trial investigating the use of standard fractionated dose-escalated radiation therapy with concurrent chemotherapy as well as the use of concurrent and adjuvant cetuximab (Bradley et al. 2015). The initial report and long-term follow-up confirm that cetuximab was not found to improve treatment outcomes and that radiation dose escalation to 74 Gy was found to have a detrimental effect on survival than standard-dose radiation therapy (Bradley et al. 2020). The reasons for this finding have been unclear, but are generally thought to be due to late normal tissue complications that outweighed any benefit from dose escalation.

A recent study reported that only a small number of patients derived benefit from dose escalation to 74 Gy, while in a much larger proportion (approximately 40% of all patients), 74 Gy was still not an adequate dose to achieve tumor control (Scott et al. 2021). This is consistent with both local relapse rates of approximately 40% seen in NSCLC treated with combined chemoradiotherapy, and data suggesting a BED_{10} of >100–105 Gy is needed to achieve optimal tumor control in the setting of SBRT for early-stage NSCLC (Grills et al. 2012; Onishi et al. 2004). Further attempts at hypofractionated dose escalation in locally advanced NSCLC have also been made. The Alliance CALGB 31102 protocol was a phase I study of concurrent chemotherapy with accelerated hypofractionated RT, escalating dose by progressive hypofractionation (60 Gy delivered in 27, 24, 22, and 20 fractions, respectively) (Urbanic et al. 2018). Hypofractionated radiation therapy was given with standard-dose concurrent carboplatin/paclitaxel. Twenty-six percent of patients had grade 3 or greater toxicity and three cases of grade 5 toxicity were observed. As a result, the maximum tolerated dose was set at 60 Gy in 24 fractions (BED_{10} = 75 Gy). Local progression occurred in only 24% of patients using this treatment paradigm suggesting an improvement in tumor control, but to date this dose fractionation scheme has not been tested in a randomized trial (Urbanic et al. 2018).

A phase I dose escalation trial of hypofractionated radiation therapy alone reported a maximum tolerated dose in a similar range, and as with Alliance CALGB 31102, much of the high-grade toxicity was related to damage to the proximal tracheobronchial tree (Cannon et al. 2013; Urbanic et al. 2018). As similar dose-limiting toxicities were seen when ablative doses of radiation were delivered to central lesions on early SBRT protocols, the proximal tracheobronchial tree is likely to be a major dose-limiting organ in node-positive lung cancer (Tekatli et al. 2016; Timmerman et al. 2010). With these limitations and the typical distribution of disease in lung malignancies with involved lymph nodes, it is unlikely that even with modern radiation techniques it would be possible to escalate the doses of radiation therapy sufficiently to control gross disease without concurrent systemic therapy.

A major recent advance in the treatment of NSCLC has been the advent of immunotherapy agents such as pembrolizumab, nivolumab, and durvalumab. The recently published PACIFIC trial reported significant improvements in progression-free survival (median progression-free survival of 17.2 vs. 5.6 months) and OS (3-year OS of 57% vs. 43.5%) with the addition of consolidation durvalumab to concurrent chemoradiotherapy (Antonia et al. 2018; Gray et al. 2020). This combined approach that takes advantage of both the enhancement of tumor response seen with concurrent chemoradiotherapy and the spatial cooperation of sequential chemotherapy and radiation has showed significantly improved outcomes over prior treatment strategies for locally advanced NSCLC and represents the current standard of care.

4 Future Considerations

There are multiple ongoing investigations into combined chemotherapy and hypofractionated radiation therapy for lung cancer. One promising avenue is the use of a simultaneous integrated boost technique to deliver higher doses of radiation therapy to areas of gross disease while limiting doses to normal tissues. An interim analysis of a randomized phase II trial using this technique to deliver up to 72 Gy in 30 fractions has shown promising toxicity results (Moningi et al. 2019).

An additional promising modality currently under investigation is the use of PET-adapted radiation therapy to deliver higher doses to areas of metabolically active disease after initial therapy. A single-arm phase II study showed promising local control, and the randomized RTOG 1106 evaluating this technique has completed accrual (NCT01507428) (Kong et al. 2017).

In addition to advanced radiation techniques, novel radioprotector agents are also under investigation. Avasopasem (GC4419) is a novel superoxide dismutase mimetic that has shown very promising results in the reduction of severe oral mucositis in patients undergoing chemoradiotherapy for oral cavity and oropharyngeal carcinoma. This and similar agents are currently being investigated for both concurrent chemoradiotherapy and SBRT for lung cancers (NCT04225026 and NCT04476797).

Induction and concurrent chemotherapy/radiation therapy trials in locally advanced lung cancer

Induction chemotherapy (IC) trials	Treatment arms	Chemo dose	RT dose	Outcome	Severe toxicity
CALGB 8433 (Dillman et al. 1990)	Arm 1: IC followed by RT; Arm 2: RT alone	Cisplatin 100 mg/m^2 on days 1, 29; vinblastine 5 mg/m^2 on days 1, 8, 15, 22, 29	40 Gy in 20 fractions with a boost of 20 Gy in 10 fractions	Median OS arm 1 vs. 2: 13.8 vs. 9.7 months	Arm 1 vs. 2 G3+ infections: 7% vs. 3%, severe weight loss 14% vs. 6%, G3+ esophagitis 1% vs. 1%
(Le Chevalier et al. 1991)	Arm 1: RT alone; Arm 2: IC for ×3 monthly cycles followed by RT	Vindesine 1.5 mg/m^2 on days 1, 2; lomustine 50 mg/m^2 days 2, 25 and 25 mg/m^2 on day 3; cisplatin 100 mg/m^2 on day 2; cyclophosphamide 200 mg/m^2 on days 2–4	65 Gy in 26 fractions	Median OS arm 1 vs. 2: 10 vs. 12 months	Arm 1 vs. 2 G3+ pulmonary toxicity: 4.5% vs. 2.8%
RTOG 8808/ ECOG 4588 (Sause et al. 1995)	Arm 1: RT alone; Arm 2: IC followed by RT; Arm 3: hyperfractionated RT	Cisplatin 100 mg/m^2 on days 1, 29; vinblastine 5 mg/m^2 weekly ×5	60 Gy in 30 fractions; 69.6 Gy delivered 1.2 BID	Median OS arm 1, 2, 3: 11.4 vs. 13.8 vs. 12.3 months	G3+ nonheme toxicity in arms 1, 2, 3: 22%, 26%, 19%
Concurrent chemoradiation (cCRT) trials (Schaake-Koning et al. 1992)	Arm 1: split-course RT alone; Arm 2: cCRT as split-course RT (weekly chemo); Arm 3: cCRT as split-course RT (daily chemo)	Cisplatin 30 mg/m^2 weekly; cisplatin 6 mg/m^2 daily	30 Gy in 10 fractions, 3-week rest, 25 Gy in 10 fractions	1-year OS arm 1, 2, 3: 46%, 44%, 54%	Arms 1, 2, 3 G3+ esophagitis: 0%, 1%, 5%; G3+ heme: 0%, 1%, 3%
RTOG 9015 (Byhardt et al. 1995)	Phase 2: concurrent HFRT	Cisplatin 75 mg/m^2 days 1, 29, 50; vinblastine 5 mg/m^2 weekly ×5	69.6 Gy in 1.2 Gy BID fractions	Median OS: 12.2 months	G3+ esophagitis: 24%, G4+ heme: 45%
(Jeremic et al. 1996)	Arm 1: HFRT alone; Arm 2: concurrent HFRT	Daily carboplatin 50 mg/m^2 and etoposide 50 mg	69.6 Gy in 1.2 Gy BID fractions	Median OS arm 1 vs. 2: 14 vs. 22 months	Arms 1 vs. 2 G3+ esophagitis: 6% vs. 8%; G3+ heme: 0% vs. 3%
RTOG 9106 (Lee et al. 1996)	Phase 2: concurrent HFRT	Two cycles of oral etoposide 100 mg daily for 2 weeks and cisplatin 50 mg/m^2 on days 1, 8	69.6 Gy in 1.2 Gy BID fractions	Median OS: 18.9 months	G3+ esophagitis: 53%; G3+ pulmonary: 25%; G4 heme: 57%
CALGB 39801 (Vokes et al. 2007)	Arm 1: cCRT; Arm 2: IC followed by cCRT	IC: ×2 cycles of carboplatin AUC 6; paclitaxel 200 mg/m^2; concurrent weekly carboplatin AUC 2; paclitaxel 50 mg/m^2	66 Gy in 33 fractions	Median OS arm 1 vs. 2: 12 vs. 14 months	IC G3+ neutropenia: 38%; Arm 1 vs. 2 G3+ esophagitis: 32% vs. 36%, G3+ dyspnea: 14% vs. 19%

(Continued)

(Continued)

Induction chemotherapy (IC) trials	Treatment arms	Chemo dose	RT dose	Outcome	Severe toxicity
RTOG 9410 (Curran et al. 2011)	Arm 1: IC followed by RT; Arm 2: cCRT; Arm 3: concurrent HFRT	IC: cisplatin 100 mg/m^2 on days 1, 29; vinblastine 5 mg/m^2 weekly ×5; Arm 2: same chemo given with RT; Arm 3: concurrent cisplatin 50 mg/m^2 days 1, 8, 29, 36 and oral etoposide 50 mg BID for 5 days starting with cisplatin cycle	Arms 1 and 2: 60 Gy in 30 fractions; Arm 3: 69.6 Gy in 1.2 Gy BID fractions	Median OS arms 1, 2, 3: 14.6 vs. 17 vs. 15.6 months	Arms 1, 2, 3 G3+ esophagitis: 4%, 23%, 45%; G3+ pulmonary: 9%, 4%, 3%, worst heme: 80%, 87%, 71%, worst nonheme: 35%, 53%, 67%
RTOG 0617 (Bradley et al. 2015)	Arm 1: standard-dose RT cCRT; Arm 2: high-dose RT cCRT; Arm 3: standard-dose RT cCRT + cetux; Arm 4: high-dose RT cCRT + cetux	Concurrent weekly carboplatin AUC 2 and paclitaxel 45 mg/m^2 followed by ×2 cycles of consolidation carboplatin AUC 6 and paclitaxel 200 mg/m^2; cetuximab 400 mg/m^2 loading dose with weekly 250 mg/m^2	Standard-dose RT: 60 Gy in 30 fractions; high-dose RT: 74 Gy in 37 fractions	Median OS arm 1, 2, 3, 4: 28.7 vs. 20.3 vs. 25 vs. 24 months	Arms 1, 2, 3, 4 G3+ esophagitis: 7%, 15%, 7%, 19%; G3+ pulmonary: 15%, 9%, 18%, 17%
PACIFIC trial (Gray et al. 2020)	Arm 1: cCRT followed by consolidation durvalumab; Arm 2: cCRT alone	Concurrent platinum-based chemotherapy for at least 2 cycles; consolidation durvalumab 10 mg/kg every 2 weeks for up to 12 months	54–66 Gy	3-year OS arm 1 vs. 2: 57% vs. 43.5%; median OS arm 1 vs. 2: not reached vs. 29.1 months	Arm 1 vs. 2: G3/4 pneumonitis: 1.9% vs. 1.7%; max G3/4 adverse event any cause: 30.5% vs. 26.1%

References

Ahn JS, Ahn YC, Kim JH, Lee CG, Cho EK, Lee KC et al (2015) Multinational randomized phase III trial with or without consolidation chemotherapy using docetaxel and cisplatin after concurrent chemoradiation in inoperable stage III non-small-cell lung cancer: KCSG-LU05-04. J Clin Oncol 33(24):2660–2666. https://doi.org/10.1200/jco.2014.60.0130

Antonia SJ, Villegas A, Daniel D, Vicente D, Murakami S, Hui R et al (2018) Overall survival with durvalumab after chemoradiotherapy in stage III NSCLC. N Engl J Med 379(24):2342–2350. https://doi.org/10.1056/NEJMoa1809697

Bradley JD, Paulus R, Komaki R, Masters G, Blumenschein G, Schild S et al (2015) Standard-dose versus high-dose conformal radiotherapy with concurrent and consolidation carboplatin plus paclitaxel with or without cetuximab for patients with stage IIIA or IIIB non-small-cell lung cancer (RTOG 0617): a randomised, two-by-two factorial phase 3 study. Lancet Oncol 16(2):187–199. https://doi.org/10.1016/S1470-2045(14)71207-0

Bradley JD, Hu C, Komaki RR, Masters GA, Blumenschein GR, Schild SE et al (2020) Long-term results of NRG oncology RTOG 0617: standard- versus high-dose chemoradiotherapy with or without cetuximab for unresectable stage III non-small-cell lung cancer. J Clin Oncol 38(7):706–714. https://doi.org/10.1200/jco.19.01162

Brizel DM, Wasserman TH, Henke M, Strnad V, Rudat V, Monnier A et al (2000) Phase III randomized trial of amifostine as a radioprotector in head and neck cancer. J Clin Oncol 18(19):3339–3345. https://doi.org/10.1200/jco.2000.18.19.3339

Byhardt RW, Scott CB, Ettinger DS, Curran WJ, Doggett RL, Coughlin C et al (1995) Concurrent hyperfractionated irradiation and chemotherapy for unresectable nonsmall cell lung cancer. Results of Radiation Therapy Oncology Group 90-15. Cancer 75(9):2337–2344. https://doi.org/10.1002/1097-0142(19950501)75:9<2337::aid-cncr2820750924>3.0.co;2-k

Byhardt RW, Scott C, Sause WT, Emami B, Komaki R, Fisher B et al (1998) Response, toxicity, failure patterns, and survival in five Radiation Therapy Oncology Group (RTOG) trials of sequential and/or concurrent chemotherapy and radiotherapy for locally advanced non-small-cell carcinoma of the lung. Int J Radiat Oncol Biol Phys 42(3):469–478. https://doi.org/10.1016/s0360-3016(98)00251-x

Cannon DM, Mehta MP, Adkison JB, Khuntia D, Traynor AM, Tomé WA et al (2013) Dose-limiting toxicity after hypofractionated dose-escalated radiotherapy in non-small-cell lung cancer. J Clin Oncol 31(34):4343–4348. https://doi.org/10.1200/jco.2013.51.5353

Chen Y, Pandya K, Keng PC, Johnstone D, Li J, Lee YJ et al (2003) Phase I/II clinical study of pulsed paclitaxel radiosensitization for thoracic malignancy: a therapeutic approach on the basis of preclinical research of human cancer cell lines. Clin Cancer Res 9(3):969–975

Chun SG, Hu C, Choy H, Komaki RU, Timmerman RD, Schild SE et al (2017) Impact of intensity-modulated radiation therapy technique for locally advanced non-small-cell lung cancer: a secondary analysis of the NRG oncology RTOG 0617 randomized clinical trial. J Clin Oncol 35(1):56–62. https://doi.org/10.1200/jco.2016.69.1378

Cox JD, Azarnia N, Byhardt RW, Shin KH, Emami B, Pajak TF (1990) A randomized phase I/II trial of hyperfractionated radiation therapy with total doses of 60.0 Gy to 79.2 Gy: possible survival benefit with greater than or equal to 69.6 Gy in favorable patients with Radiation Therapy Oncology Group stage III non-small-cell lung carcinoma: report of Radiation Therapy Oncology Group 83-11. J Clin Oncol 8(9):1543–1555. https://doi.org/10.1200/jco.1990.8.9.1543

Curran WJ Jr, Paulus R, Langer CJ, Komaki R, Lee JS, Hauser S et al (2011) Sequential vs. concurrent chemoradiation for stage III non-small cell lung cancer: randomized phase III trial RTOG 9410. J Natl Cancer Inst 103(19):1452–1460. https://doi.org/10.1093/jnci/djr325

Dillman RO, Seagren SL, Propert KJ, Guerra J, Eaton WL, Perry MC et al (1990) A randomized trial of induction chemotherapy plus high-dose radiation versus radiation alone in stage III non-small-cell lung cancer. N Engl J Med 323(14):940–945. https://doi.org/10.1056/nejm199010043231403

Evans JW, Yudoh K, Delahoussaye YM, Brown JM (1998) Tirapazamine is metabolized to its DNA-damaging radical by intranuclear enzymes. Cancer Res 58(10):2098–2101

Fowler JF, Chappell R (2000) Non-small cell lung tumors repopulate rapidly during radiation therapy. Int J Radiat Oncol Biol Phys 46(2):516–517. https://doi.org/10.1016/s0360-3016(99)00364-8

Gandara DR, Chansky K, Albain KS, Gaspar LE, Lara PN Jr, Kelly K et al (2006) Long-term survival with concurrent chemoradiation therapy followed by consolidation docetaxel in stage IIIB non-small-cell lung cancer: a phase II Southwest Oncology Group Study (S9504). Clin Lung Cancer 8(2):116–121. https://doi.org/10.3816/CLC.2006.n.039

Gray JE, Villegas A, Daniel D, Vicente D, Murakami S, Hui R et al (2020) Three-year overall survival with durvalumab after chemoradiotherapy in stage III NSCLC-update from PACIFIC. J Thorac Oncol 15(2):288–293. https://doi.org/10.1016/j.jtho.2019.10.002

Grills IS, Hope AJ, Guckenberger M, Kestin LL, Werner-Wasik M, Yan D et al (2012) A collaborative analysis of stereotactic lung radiotherapy outcomes for early-stage non-small-cell lung cancer using daily online cone-beam computed tomography image-guided radiotherapy. J Thorac Oncol 7(9):1382–1393. https://doi.org/10.1097/JTO.0b013e318260e00d

Hanna N, Neubauer M, Yiannoutsos C, McGarry R, Arseneau J, Ansari R et al (2008) Phase III study of cisplatin, etoposide, and concurrent chest radiation with or without consolidation docetaxel in patients with inoperable stage III non-small-cell lung cancer: the Hoosier Oncology Group and U.S. Oncology. J Clin Oncol 26(35):5755–5760. https://doi.org/10.1200/jco.2008.17.7840

Jeremic B, Shibamoto Y, Acimovic L, Djuric L (1995) Randomized trial of hyperfractionated radiation therapy with or without concurrent chemotherapy for stage III non-small-cell lung cancer. J Clin Oncol 13(2):452–458. https://doi.org/10.1200/jco.1995.13.2.452

Jeremic B, Shibamoto Y, Acimovic L, Milisavljevic S (1996) Hyperfractionated radiation therapy with or without concurrent low-dose daily carboplatin/etoposide for stage III non-small-cell lung cancer: a randomized study. J Clin Oncol 14(4):1065–1070. https://doi.org/10.1200/jco.1996.14.4.1065

Komaki R, Seiferheld W, Ettinger D, Lee JS, Movsas B, Sause W (2002) Randomized phase II chemotherapy and radiotherapy trial for patients with locally advanced inoperable non-small-cell lung cancer: long-term follow-up of RTOG 92-04. Int J Radiat Oncol Biol Phys 53(3):548–557. https://doi.org/10.1016/s0360-3016(02)02793-1

Kong FM, Ten Haken RK, Schipper M, Frey KA, Hayman J, Gross M et al (2017) Effect of midtreatment PET/CT-adapted radiation therapy with concurrent chemotherapy in patients with locally advanced non-small-cell lung cancer: a phase 2 clinical trial. JAMA Oncol 3(10):1358–1365. https://doi.org/10.1001/jamaoncol.2017.0982

Koukourakis MI (2002) Amifostine in clinical oncology: current use and future applications. Anticancer Drugs 13(3):181–209. https://doi.org/10.1097/00001813-200203000-00001

Lau D, Leigh B, Gandara D, Edelman M, Morgan R, Israel V et al (2001) Twice-weekly paclitaxel and weekly carboplatin with concurrent thoracic radiation followed by carboplatin/paclitaxel consolidation for stage III non-small-cell lung cancer: a California Cancer Consortium phase II trial. J Clin Oncol 19(2):442–447. https://doi.org/10.1200/jco.2001.19.2.442

Le Chevalier T, Arriagada R, Quoix E, Ruffie P, Martin M, Tarayre M et al (1991) Radiotherapy alone versus combined chemotherapy and radiotherapy in nonresectable non-small-cell lung cancer: first analysis of a randomized trial in 353 patients. J Natl Cancer Inst 83(6):417–423. https://doi.org/10.1093/jnci/83.6.417

Lee JS, Scott C, Komaki R, Fossella FV, Dundas GS, McDonald S et al (1996) Concurrent chemoradiation therapy with oral etoposide and cisplatin for locally advanced inoperable non-small-cell lung cancer: radiation therapy oncology group protocol 91-06. J Clin Oncol 14(4):1055–1064. https://doi.org/10.1200/jco.1996.14.4.1055

Mauguen A, Le Péchoux C, Saunders MI, Schild SE, Turrisi AT, Baumann M et al (2012) Hyperfractionated or accelerated radiotherapy in lung cancer: an individual patient data meta-analysis. J Clin Oncol 30(22):2788–2797. https://doi.org/10.1200/jco.2012.41.6677

Moningi S, Nguyen QN, Lin SH, Jeter MD, O'Reilly MS, Chang JY et al (2019) Phase II trial of intensity-modulated photon or scanning beam proton therapy both with simultaneous integrated boost dose escalation to the gross tumor volume with concurrent chemotherapy for stage II/III non-small cell lung cancer—interim analysis. Int J Radiat Oncol Biol Phys 105(1, Supplement):E522. https://doi.org/10.1016/j.ijrobp.2019.06.2416

Nguyen-Tan PF, Zhang Q, Ang KK, Weber RS, Rosenthal DI, Soulieres D et al (2014) Randomized phase III trial to test accelerated versus standard fractionation in combination with concurrent cisplatin for head and neck carcinomas in the Radiation Therapy Oncology Group 0129 trial: long-term report of efficacy and toxicity. J Clin Oncol 32(34):3858–3866. https://doi.org/10.1200/jco.2014.55.3925

Onishi H, Araki T, Shirato H, Nagata Y, Hiraoka M, Gomi K et al (2004) Stereotactic hypofractionated high-dose irradiation for stage I nonsmall cell lung carcinoma: clinical outcomes in 245 subjects in a Japanese multi-institutional study. Cancer 101(7):1623–1631. https://doi.org/10.1002/cncr.20539

Perez CA, Stanley K, Rubin P, Kramer S, Brady L, Perez-Tamayo R et al (1980) A prospective randomized study of various irradiation doses and fractionation schedules in the treatment of inoperable non-oat-cell carcinoma of the lung. Preliminary report by the Radiation Therapy Oncology Group. Cancer 45(11):2744–2753. https://doi.org/10.1002/1097-0142(19800601)45:11<2744::aid-cncr2820451108>3.0.co;2-u

Rojas A, Hirst VK, Calvert AS, Johns H (1996) Carbogen and nicotinamide as radiosensitizers in a murine mammary carcinoma using conventional and accelerated radiotherapy. Int J Radiat Oncol Biol Phys 34(2):357–365. https://doi.org/10.1016/0360-3016(95)02087-x

Sause WT, Scott C, Taylor S, Byhardt RW, Banker FL, Thomson JW et al (1992) Phase II trial of combination chemotherapy and irradiation in non-small-cell lung cancer, Radiation Therapy Oncology Group 88-04. Am J Clin Oncol 15(2):163–167. https://doi.org/10.1097/00000421-199204000-00014

Sause WT, Scott C, Taylor S, Johnson D, Livingston R, Komaki R et al (1995) Radiation Therapy Oncology Group (RTOG) 88-08 and Eastern Cooperative Oncology Group (ECOG) 4588: preliminary results of a phase III trial in regionally advanced, unresectable non-small-cell lung cancer. J Natl Cancer Inst 87(3):198–205. https://doi.org/10.1093/jnci/87.3.198

Schaake-Koning C, van den Bogaert W, Dalesio O, Festen J, Hoogenhout J, van Houtte P et al (1992) Effects of concomitant cisplatin and radiotherapy on inoperable non-small-cell lung cancer. N Engl J Med 326(8):524–530. https://doi.org/10.1056/nejm199202203260805

Scott JG, Sedor G, Scarborough JA, Kattan MW, Peacock J, Grass GD et al (2021) Personalizing radiotherapy prescription dose using genomic markers of radiosensitivity and normal tissue toxicity in NSCLC. J Thorac Oncol 16(3):428–438. https://doi.org/10.1016/j.jtho.2020.11.008

Sekine I, Nokihara H, Sumi M, Saijo N, Nishiwaki Y, Ishikura S et al (2006) Docetaxel consolidation therapy following cisplatin, vinorelbine, and concurrent thoracic radiotherapy in patients with unresectable stage III non-small cell lung cancer. J Thorac Oncol 1(8):810–815

Simpson JR, Bauer M, Wasserman TH, Perez CA, Emami B, Wiegensberg I et al (1987) Large fraction irradiation with or without misonidazole in advanced non-oat cell carcinoma of the lung: a phase III randomized trial of the RTOG. Radiation Therapy Oncology Group. Int J Radiat Oncol Biol Phys 13(6):861–867. https://doi.org/10.1016/0360-3016(87)90100-3

Steel GG, Peckham MJ (1979) Exploitable mechanisms in combined radiotherapy-chemotherapy: the concept of additivity. Int J Radiat Oncol Biol Phys 5(1):85–91. https://doi.org/10.1016/0360-3016(79)90044-0

Tekatli H, Haasbeek N, Dahele M, De Haan P, Verbakel W, Bongers E et al (2016) Outcomes of hypofractionated high-dose radiotherapy in poor-risk patients with "ultracentral" non-small cell lung cancer. J Thorac Oncol 11(7):1081–1089. https://doi.org/10.1016/j.jtho.2016.03.008

Timmerman R, Paulus R, Galvin J, Michalski J, Straube W, Bradley J et al (2010) Stereotactic body radiation therapy for inoperable early stage lung cancer. JAMA 303(11):1070–1076. https://doi.org/10.1001/jama.2010.261

Urbanic JJ, Wang X, Bogart JA, Stinchcombe TE, Hodgson L, Schild SE et al (2018) Phase 1 study of accelerated hypofractionated radiation therapy with concurrent chemotherapy for stage III non-small cell lung cancer: CALGB 31102 (Alliance). Int J Radiat Oncol Biol Phys 101(1):177–185. https://doi.org/10.1016/j.ijrobp.2018.01.046

van Meerbeeck JP, Kramer GW, Van Schil PE, Legrand C, Smit EF, Schramel F et al (2007) Randomized controlled trial of resection versus radiotherapy after induction chemotherapy in stage IIIA-N2 non-small-cell lung cancer. J Natl Cancer Inst 99(6):442–450. https://doi.org/10.1093/jnci/djk093

Vokes EE, Herndon JE 2nd, Kelley MJ, Cicchetti MG, Ramnath N, Neill H et al (2007) Induction chemotherapy followed by chemoradiotherapy compared with chemoradiotherapy alone for regionally advanced unresectable stage III non-small-cell lung cancer: Cancer and Leukemia Group B. J Clin Oncol 25(13):1698–1704. https://doi.org/10.1200/jco.2006.07.3569

Wardman P (2019) Nitroimidazoles as hypoxic cell radiosensitizers and hypoxia probes: misonidazole, myths and mistakes. Br J Radiol 92(1093):20170915. https://doi.org/10.1259/bjr.20170915

Mechanisms of Action of Radiotherapy and Immunotherapy in Lung Cancer: Implications for Clinical Practice

Kewen He, Ugur Selek, Hampartsoum B. Barsoumian, Duygu Sezen, Matthew S. Ning, Nahum Puebla-Osorio, Jonathan E. Schoenhals, Dawei Chen, Carola Leuschner, Maria Angelica Cortez, and James W. Welsh

Contents

1	Introduction	400
2	**Interactions Between Radiation and Immunotherapy in Lung Cancer**	401
2.1	Radiation Dose and Fractionation	401
2.2	Photon (X-Ray) Therapy Versus Proton Therapy	402
2.3	FLASH-RT	402
3	**Effects of Radiation Therapy with Immunotherapy on Immune Cells**	402
3.1	CD4 and CD8 T Cells	402
3.2	Regulatory T Cells	404
3.3	Macrophages	405
3.4	B Cells and NK Cells	405
3.5	Dendritic Cells	406
4	**Strategies to Enhance the Effectiveness of Radio-Immunotherapy Combinations**	408
4.1	RadScopal™: Combining High-Dose RT with Low-Dose RT	408
4.2	Pulsed RT with CTLA-4 Inhibitors	409
References		409

K. He
Department of Radiation Oncology, Unit 97, The University of Texas MD Anderson Cancer Center, Houston, TX, USA

Department of Radiation Oncology, Shandong Cancer Hospital Affiliated to Shandong University, Jinan, China

U. Selek
Department of Radiation Oncology, Koç University School of Medicine, Istanbul, Turkey

Abstract

Radiotherapy (RT) remains an essential component of treatment for localized or advanced lung cancer that is not amenable to surgery. Immunotherapies such as checkpoint inhibitors have attracted much attention in recent years and offer promise for the treatment of several types of cancer; however, response

H. B. Barsoumian · M. S. Ning · N. Puebla-Osorio · C. Leuschner · M. A. Cortez · J. W. Welsh (✉)
Department of Radiation Oncology, Unit 97, The University of Texas MD Anderson Cancer Center, Houston, TX, USA
e-mail: jwelsh@mdanderson.org

D. Sezen
Department of Radiation Oncology, Unit 97, The University of Texas MD Anderson Cancer Center, Houston, TX, USA

Department of Radiation Oncology, Koç University School of Medicine, Istanbul, Turkey

J. E. Schoenhals
Department of Radiation Oncology, Unit 97, The University of Texas MD Anderson Cancer Center, Houston, TX, USA

University of Texas Southwestern Medical Center, UT Southwestern, Dallas, TX, USA

D. Chen
Department of Radiation Oncology, Shandong Cancer Hospital Affiliated to Shandong University, Jinan, China

rates and overall survival in patients with lung cancer remain low. Combining RT with immunotherapy is actively being explored as a way of boosting the effectiveness of both types of therapy. Here, we discuss various aspects and types of RT and their activity in combination with immunotherapy, including radiation dose and fractionation, modality (photons versus protons), and ultrahigh dose rate (FLASH) radiation. We then review the basic mechanisms of how RT interacts with immunotherapy in lung cancer in terms of the type of immune cell, e.g., CD8/CD4 T cells, Tregs, macrophages, natural killer (NK) cells, B cells, and dendritic cells. We also introduce promising new RT methods that involve "pulsed" dosing or high-dose plus low-dose RT, and their role in treating multiple isocenters of disease. We hope to provide some implications for better clinical practice.

1 Introduction

Radiotherapy (RT) remains the primary treatment regimen for localized and advanced lung cancer that is not amenable to surgery. Despite local and systemic therapies, long-term control without systemic relapse presents a major challenge in the treatment of NSCLC patients. Immune checkpoint inhibitors (ICIs) targeting programmed death 1 (PD-1), programmed death ligand 1 (PD-L1), or cytotoxic T lymphocyte antigen-4 (CTLA-4) have significantly improved survival of lung cancer patients during the past 6 years. ICIs target negative immune regulators on T cells (PD-1 or CTLA-4), resulting in their activation, or inhibitory pathways on tumors (PD-L1) that facilitate escape of immune surveillance, thus enhancing antitumor immune response and host-mediated eradication of malignant cells (Fitzgerald and Simone II 2020). Although 26–45% of lung cancer patients respond to ICI, some patients progress and acquire resistance. Resistance to immunotherapy is driven by tumor immunity and presence of an immune-suppressive tumor microenvironment (TME). High density of the stroma hinders immune cell infiltration into the TME and facilitates deactivation of immune cells. Mounting evidence showed improvement of responses for the combination of RT and immunotherapy (J. W. Welsh et al. 2019; Theelen et al. 2019; Antonia et al. 2018; Verma et al. 2018a; D. Chen et al. 2020a; Verma et al. 2018b). The analysis of the mechanisms of action for the combination of RT and immunotherapy is crucial for the rational design of a treatment regimen that improves clinical outcomes for ICI-resistant patients.

The cytotoxic effect of RT-induced DNA damage has been recognized as the primary antitumor function of radiation, but RT can also induce immunogenic death in tumor, i.e., cell death that effectively exposes tumor-associated antigens (TAAs) (Ko and Formenti 2019). TAAs released from dying tumor cells are captured by dendritic cells (DCs) and antigen-presenting cells (APCs). APCs present neoantigens to T cells, stimulating the adaptive immune system that triggers the immune response cascade against tumors cells including T-cell priming, clonal expansion, and release of effector T cells that home to tumors, and reprogramming of the TME into an inflamed environment (D. S. Chen and Mellman 2013). Tumor cells damaged by RT activate APCs by releasing "danger" molecules such as calreticulin, high-mobility group box 1 protein (HMGB1), and adenosine triphosphate (ATP), which are part of the damage-associated molecule patterns (DAMPs) (Di Virgilio et al. 2017). These processes trigger a potent inflammatory cytokine response that promotes DC maturation, upregulation of co-stimulatory signals that facilitate cross-priming of cytotoxic CD8$^+$ T lymphocytes, and upregulation of chemokine receptors that promote DC migration to the draining lymph nodes (Herrera et al. 2017). The potential of RT to trigger antigen-specific, adaptive immunity is referred to as the "in situ" vaccination.

In addition to priming antitumor immunity, RT can convert the TME from an immune-suppressive state to tumor-lysing state by generating inflammatory responses through the induction of inflammatory mediators such as interferons (IFNs) and chemokines that attract T cells (Lugade et al. 2008). Low-dose RT (i.e., doses of <2 Gy) repolarized tumor-associated macrophages from pro-tumorigenic M2 phenotype to antitumor M1 phenotype. M1 macrophages express inducible nitric oxide synthase (iNOS), which increases the infiltration of effector cells into the TME through the expression of the adhesion molecule VCAM1 in the tumor endothelium. RT also induced chemokines such as CXCL9, CXCL10, CXCL11, and CXCL16 that facilitate homing of T cells to tumors (Klug et al. 2013; Matsumura et al. 2008; S. S. Kim et al. 2020c). Recent studies also showed that low-dose RT reversed immune suppression in the TME and maximized systemic outcomes in lung adenocarcinoma mouse model (Barsoumian et al. 2020).

In this chapter, we first discuss how various forms of RT act in combination with immunotherapy, including the influence of radiation dose and fractionation, radiation modality (photons versus protons), and use of ultralow dose rate (FLASH) RT. We then review the basic mechanisms of the action of RT with immunotherapy in lung cancer in terms of the type of immune cell, such as CD8/CD4 T cells, T regulatory cells (Tregs), macrophages, natural killer (NK) cells, B cells, and DCs.

2 Interactions Between Radiation and Immunotherapy in Lung Cancer

2.1 Radiation Dose and Fractionation

Standard of care for non-small cell lung cancer (NSCLC) includes RT as monotherapy or in combination with surgery and chemotherapy. RT delivered in multiple repetitive fractions killed tumor cells while preserving normal tissue repair during the time interval between fractions. In NSCLC patients with node-positive or locally advanced operable disease, conventional fractionated RT can be used in various treatment time points. In resectable locally advanced disease (stage IIIA), platinum-based chemotherapy is preferred before or after primary surgery, while adjuvant RT is indicated in cases with N2 lymph node involvement. Preoperative chemoradiotherapy is another option in the treatment of resectable N2 disease. Definitive concurrent or sequential chemoradiation is the primary treatment in unresectable locally advanced NSCLC (Duma et al. 2019). Large-field irradiation is highly toxic to peripheral lymphocytes and circulating blood pool, because peripheral lymphocytes are highly radiosensitive and radiation doses as low as 0.2 Gy can cause lymphopenia (Heylmann et al. 2018). Although RT induces immune stimulation and chemokine secretion that attract cytotoxic T lymphocytes (CTL), conventional fractionation RT may be contraindicated (Lee Jr. et al. 2018) as low absolute lymphocyte count (ALC) is associated with poor prognosis (D. Chen et al. 2020b; Huemer et al. 2019).

Technical improvements provide a safe administration of high radiation doses in single or in hypofractionated schemes. Stereotactic ablative radiation therapy (SABR) has emerged as a viable treatment option in patients with early-stage and node-negative disease (Timmerman et al. 2018) while preserving surrounding tissues and reducing lymphopenia. Results from preclinical studies evaluating the effects from hypofractionated and ablative treatment regimens are limited and contradictory. In two preclinical carcinoma models, fractionated (8 Gy × 3 and 6 Gy × 5) but not single-dose radiotherapy (20 Gy × 1) induced an abscopal effect when combined with anti-CTLA-4 antibody (Dewan et al. 2009). On the other hand, a single high dose in the range of 12 and 18 Gy was associated with the induction of the DNA exonuclease, Trex1, thus removing cytosolic DNA (Vanpouille-Box et al. 2017a). The accumulation of cytosolic DNA in irradiated cancer cells is crucial for the activation of the cGAS-STING (cyclic GMP-AMP synthase/stimulator of interferon genes) pathway and production of type I interferons to elicit anticancer immune responses (Deng et al. 2014).

2.2 Photon (X-Ray) Therapy Versus Proton Therapy

Although modern photon radiation techniques are administered safely to most patients, they cause toxicity to vital organs. While photon radiation traverses the entire body causing an exit dose, proton beam therapy (PBT) has a sharp dose buildup and drop-off part, eliminating any exit dose (Lee Jr. et al. 2018). Normal tissues, lymphocytes, and immune cells were preserved with particle therapies while providing a similar tumor dose level reached by photons (Baumann et al. 2020). Photon-based radiation plans often include low-dose baths due to the exit dose and overlapping treatment fields (J. Welsh et al. 2011). In this context, particle therapy is superior in reducing the low-dose regions and preventing ALC decrease (Tang et al. 2014; N. Kim et al. 2020b).

Protons and other charged particles have unique biological characteristics compared to photons. They are biologically stratified as high-linear energy transfer (LET) radiation and generate complex DNA damage, including two or more lesions in one or two helical turns of DNA (Asaithamby et al. 2011). Consequently, different DNA repair pathways induced with high LET radiation may have different effects on immune response. Additionally, PD-L1 expression on cancer cells was upregulated in response to DNA double-strand breaks, although its translation to practice needs additional clinical research (Asaithamby et al. 2011; Durante and Formenti 2020).

Numerous studies showed dosimetric superiority of PBT in NSCLC, particularly in the nearby critical structures (Zou et al. 2020; Teoh et al. 2020). Proton therapy may be advantageous in treating central, previously irradiated, and locally advanced tumors. Considering the high cost of the PBT, this treatment may be limited to patients that have inaccessible tumors (Mesko and Gomez 2018).

Due to their unique radiobiological and dosimetric properties, protons and other charged particles may be less toxic to immune cells. Effects of protons or carbon on the immune response remain to be demonstrated.

2.3 FLASH-RT

Ultrahigh dose rate RT, known as FLASH-RT, is a promising technique in which radiation is delivered at very high dose rates, i.e., more than 100 Gy/s, compared with conventional dose rate RT (Tubin et al. 2020). Normal tissues remained unharmed even after high-dose exposure in a single fraction known as FLASH effect. A comparison of thorax-radiated mice using single-fraction FLASH-RT or conventional RT showed that a higher dose of 30 Gy was required to cause similar pulmonary fibrosis levels as seen following 17 Gy at conventional dose rates (Favaudon et al. 2014). The same pattern was observed for eliciting TGF-β signaling. FLASH-RT also reduced any effects of organ or tumor motion. The tissue protection during FLASH-RT is due to the induction of a massive oxygen consumption and a transient protective hypoxia in normal tissues (Bourhis et al. 2019). Radiation-induced hypoxia triggers instantly a series of radiochemical reactions. The interactions between FLASH-RT and immune cells remain under investigation. However, considering the short irradiation time, fewer circulating lymphocytes were affected by FLASH-RT compared to conventional radiation. By minimizing the irradiated amount of blood chromosomal damage can be reduced (Wilson et al. 2019). In a mouse model for NSCLC, pulsed-FLASH and FLASH radiation-induced recruitment of $CD3^+$ T lymphocytes compared to conventional proton radiation and both $CD4^+$ and $CD8^+$ cells were enhanced in the tumor core (Rama et al. 2019).

3 Effects of Radiation Therapy with Immunotherapy on Immune Cells

3.1 CD4 and CD8 T Cells

In addition to the effects described in the preceding sections, RT increased the repertoire of tumor-infiltrating T cells, such as activated memory $CD4^+$ and $CD8^+$ T cells (McGee et al. 2018), induced transformation of peripheral $CD8^+$ T cells (Zhang et al. 2017), optimized the CD8:CD4 ratio, and increased the polyfunctionality of CD4⁺ T cells (Doescher et al. 2018). All these effects were further enhanced when utilized in combination with ICI (Rudqvist et al. 2018). Kinetic studies of intra-tumoral immune cell activation during RT confirmed active changes of CD4⁺ and proliferating CD8⁺ T cells as well as MHC class I upregulation. The release of TAAs following RT resulted in enhanced uptake and cross-presentation. RT-induced danger signals, chemokines, and inflammatory cytokines modified the TME by recruiting immune cells to both local and distant (abscopal) nonirradiated areas (Jesenko et al. 2020). Notably, cGAS/STING signaling has been identified as a major pathway involved in RT-mediated antitumor effects (Jesenko et al. 2020). RT-induced cytosolic DNA release triggers release of type I interferon through the cGAS/STING pathway, and priming of cytotoxic CD8⁺ T cells that facilitate systemic anticancer effects (Yamazaki and Galluzzi 2020).

These processes culminate in a multilayered stimulation of the immune system and modification of the TME (Gong et al. 2017) and provide a strong rationale for combinations of RT and ICIs. In mouse models of NSCLC, RT stimulated neoantigen expression, tumor PD-L1 expression (via IFN-γ/STAT3 signaling) (K. J. Kim et al. 2017), and MHC class I expression; reversed exhaustion of CD8 T cells; and increased tumor-infiltrating CD8⁺ T cells within the TME (Gong et al. 2017). Increase in peripheral CD8⁺ T cells and CD8⁺/CD4⁺ T-cell ratio has been associated with clinical benefit in a phase I trial of stereotactic ablative RT with ipilimumab (Tang et al. 2017).

In clinical studies the combination of pembrolizumab (PD-1 checkpoint inhibitor) and hypofractionated RT increased immune response and showed evidence of abscopal effects (tumor regression in distant nonirradiated metastases). A pooled analysis of randomized phase I/II trials of pembrolizumab ± RT significantly increased responses and improved outcomes among patients with metastatic NSCLC. Notably, the best abscopal response rate and best abscopal disease control rate of 42% and 65% were noted with combination therapy, compared to 20% and 43%, respectively, for pembrolizumab alone (Theelen et al. 2020), along with increased median PFS (4–9 months) and OS (9–19 months). Adaptive immune resistance was reversed with a combination of PD-1 blockade and hypofractionated RT, resulting in enhancement of CD8⁺ T cell-dependent local and distant tumor control (Morisada et al. 2018). Interestingly, an exploratory analysis of the phase I/II trial for lung and liver lesions found significantly increased PFS with combination therapy even among patients with low PD-L1 expression: median 21 months versus 5 months without RT (J. Welsh et al. 2020). These studies suggest the ability of RT to reinvigorate host anticancer immunity in combination with immune checkpoint inhibition (J. Welsh et al. 2020).

While RT synergized with ICI, alternative approaches are still needed for non-responding patients. Combinations of RT with IL-2 have demonstrated potential (Jing et al. 2019) in further enhancing the activation of highly cytolytic effector phenotype CD8⁺ T cells (Monjazeb et al. 2014) and cytokine-driven clonal expansion of antigen-specific CD4 T cells (Fujimura et al. 2013). In an osteosarcoma model, the efficacy of RT with an immunocomplex of IL-2 and its monoclonal antibody (IL-2/S4B6) was investigated. The combination treatment significantly reduced tumor volume along with irradiated as well as untreated sites by 99% and 58%, respectively, induced CD8⁺ T cells, and prolonged survival (Takahashi et al. 2017).

cGAS/STING agonists are tested to further enhance immunostimulatory effects (Le Naour et al. 2020), with promising therapeutic candidates in development for combination with RT (Storozynsky and Hitt 2020). Many of these developments apply nanotechnology: engineering antigen-capturing nanoparticles to deliver tumor-specific peptides to antigen-presenting cells, supported by mechanistic studies on expansion of CD8⁺ cytotoxic T cells within a melanoma model (Min et al. 2017). In colorectal cancer xenograft models, RT-activated hafnium oxide nanoparticles (NBTXR3) resulted in enhanced cell destruction, double-stranded DNA breaks, and micronuclei formation, and further increased the stimulation of the cGAS/STING pathway (Marill et al. 2019). A novel formulation of an inhalable nanoparticulate cGAS/STING agonist synergized with RT, resulting in long-term control of bilateral lung metastases (in both the treated and untreated lung), was associated with long-term survival in mouse models (Liu et al. 2019).

Novel therapies targeting DNA damage response inhibitors induced similar inflammatory type I interferon responses by a different mechanism. DNA damage-induced PD-L1 expression is also upregulated by ATM/ATR/Chk1 kinase activities, and inhibition of DNA repair (via siRNA silencing of ATM or pharmacologic blockade) resulted in type I IFN release, further enhanced by RT to increase PD-L1 expression and $CD8^+$ T-cell proliferation (associated with superior tumor response in pancreatic cancer mouse models) (Gutiontov and Weichselbaum 2019).

In murine xenograft models of hepatocellular carcinoma, the ATR kinase inhibitor, AZD6738, enhanced RT-stimulated $CD8^+$ T-cell infiltration, activation, and proliferation, as well as IFN-γ production (even more so than RT plus anti-PD-L1 alone). The triple combination (RT + anti-PD-L1 + AZD6738) furthermore led to more robust and persistent anticancer immunity than RT plus anti-PD-L1 alone, as demonstrated by decreased recurrence among these mouse models (Sheng et al. 2020). Further support for AZD6738 has been independently demonstrated in mouse models of Kras-mutant cancer, with attenuation of RT-induced $CD8^+$ T-cell exhaustion via inhibition of RT-induced PD-L1 upregulation on cancer cells—thereby enhancing RT cytotoxic effects while potentiating RT immune response (Vendetti et al. 2018).

3.2 Regulatory T Cells

Regulatory T cells (Tregs), which express high levels of CD25 and Foxp3, are essential for normal homeostasis. They play a crucial role in cancer-mediated immunosuppression as tumors recruit and induce Tregs to downregulate T-cell responses and promote tolerance. Multiple mechanisms of immunosuppression are associated with Tregs, including IL-2 sequestration; conversion of extracellular ATP to adenosine through CD39 and CD73; direct interactions with APCs through Fas-FasL, granzyme B, and perforin; driving IDO expression in APCs; and various checkpoint pathways, including LAG3, TIM3, PD-1, TIGIT, and CTLA-4 (reviewed in J. H. Kim et al. (2020a), and Lucca and Dominguez-Villar (2020)). Tregs can also secrete inhibitory cytokines including TGF-β and IL-10, which suppress cytotoxic immune cells in the TME (Jarnicki et al. 2006).

As noted earlier in this chapter, radiation has both immunostimulatory and immunosuppressive effects. Increase of Tregs during RT has been associated to the relative radioresistance of Tregs compared to cytotoxic T cells (reviewed in Persa et al. 2015). Balogh and colleagues demonstrated reduced levels on apoptosis in $CD4^+$ Foxp3+ Tregs compared to $CD4^+$ Foxp3− T cells, as well as increased repopulation following 2 Gy (Balogh et al. 2013). However, results are conflicting regarding the immune-suppressive function of Tregs after radiation. While an in vitro study showed reduction in Treg suppression after 30 Gy (Cao et al. 2009), in mice, whole-body radiation doses of 2 Gy (Qu et al. 2010b) or 5 Gy (Qu et al. 2010a) retained Treg immune suppression.

Tregs in cancer can be targeted in several ways. First, antibodies targeting one or more of the numerous molecules expressed by Tregs (e.g., CTLA-4) may result in preferential depletion of this cell type. In one study, selective depletion of CTLA-4 with an antibody had antitumor effects in the mouse colorectal adenocarcinoma models CT26 and MC38, and this effect was linked to preferential Treg depletion at the tumor site (Selby et al. 2013). In melanoma patients CTLA-4 inhibition caused only partial Treg reduction (Simpson et al. 2013). Other checkpoint inhibitors such as TIGIT, LAG3, and TIM3 may target subsets of Tregs (Fourcade et al.

2018). Tregs express high levels of co-stimulatory molecules including GITR, ICOS, CD27, and OX40. We have shown that a GITR-depleting antibody reduced Tregs in a NSCLC murine model (Schoenhals et al. 2018). Targeting Treg trafficking through CCR4 or low-dose chemotherapy (i.e., cyclophosphamide) may further reduce Tregs in tumors (Maeda et al. 2019; Scurr et al. 2017).

There are multiple clinical trials aimed at targeting Tregs in cancer in combination with RT. One study is looking to use low-dose cyclophosphamide in combination with RT and anti-PD-L1 in patients with head and neck cancer (NCT03844763). Another study is using a DC vaccine and an anti-CD27 antibody in combination with RT and temozolomide for glioblastoma (NCT03688178). We are currently running a phase I/II trial using anti-GITR, anti-PD-1, and anti-CTLA-4 with or without SBRT for solid tumors (NCT04021043).

3.3 Macrophages

In the TME, monocytes represent precursor cells that differentiate into antitumor M1 macrophage (CD11b$^+$ Ly6C$^+$ F4/80$^+$ CD38^{hi}) or pro-tumorigenic M2 macrophage (CD11b$^+$ Ly6C$^+$ F4/80$^+$ CD206$^+$ or CD163$^+$), while immature monocytes become monocytic myeloid-derived suppressor cell (M-MDSC) (murine CD11b$^+$ Ly6C$^+$ F4/80$^-$, human CD11b$^+$ CD14$^+$ CD33$^+$ HLA-DR$^{low/-}$). The ratio of M1/M2 macrophage predicts the response to immunotherapy (Macciò et al. 2020) that is driven by Tregs, TGF-β-suppressive cytokine, and presence of cancer-associated fibroblasts (CAFs) in the stroma. Altogether, the tumor forms a physical and cellular barrier that inhibits infiltration and function of effector T cells and NK cells, and ultimately evades detection. M1/M2 macrophages are associated with Th1/Th2 immune responses in the TME (Jayasingam et al. 2019; Almatroodi et al. 2016) such as secretion of IL-4 by M2 macrophages promoting Th2 T cell-based responses leading to secretion of anti-inflammatory cytokines (IL-4, IL-5, IL-10, and IL-13). In contrast, M1 macrophages produce IL-12 cytokine and promote Th1 T cells, which in turn produce IL-2, IFN-γ, TNF-α, and pro-inflammatory/effector cytokines.

High doses of RT may tip the balance toward M2 macrophage polarization and increased MDSC recruitment, partially by inducing IL-6 cytokine and CXCL12 chemokine production (Wu et al. 2013). Low doses of radiation (≤2 Gy) favor M1 macrophage polarization and reduced TGF-β levels (Klug et al. 2013; Barsoumian et al. 2020). Immuno-oncology (IO) agents targeting macrophages or TME are currently tested in preclinical and clinical studies for efficacy and reversal of M2 macrophages to M1. Macrophage-targeting drugs include Toll-like receptor agonists such as monophosphoryl lipid A (MPLA) working on TLR4 (Fensterheim et al. 2018); CpG-based vaccines activating TLR9 (Krieg 2007); RNA-based vaccines activating TLR3 and initiating RIG-I pathway, culminating in the production of type I interferons (Vidyarthi et al. 2018); cGAS/STING pathway agonists (Pan et al. 2020); CD40 agonists (Yasmin-Karim et al. 2018); and MerTK inhibitors that turn immunologically "cold" tumors into "hot" (Caetano et al. 2019). Tregs can be targeted through CTLA-4, TGF-β, TGF-βR, GITR, TIGIT, or CCR8 blockade that promotes and maintains the M1 macrophage phenotype (Bose et al. 2019; Schoenhals et al. 2018; Fourcade et al. 2018).

3.4 B Cells and NK Cells

Tumor-infiltrating B cells are heterogeneous cell populations with tumor-promoting or tumor-suppressor properties (Helmink et al. 2020). B cells associated with tertiary lymphoid structures (TLSs) consist of a T-cell zone containing CD4$^+$ T cells, CD8$^+$ T cells, mature DCs, and Tregs providing antigen recognition, processing, and presentation (Dieu-Nosjean et al. 2014; Tsou et al. 2016), and secretion of inflammatory cytokines.

TLSs correlated with favorable clinical outcomes (Sautes-Fridman et al. 2019; Dieu-Nosjean et al. 2014; Helmink et al. 2020) through generating an adaptive immune response (Dieu-Nosjean et al. 2014; Sautes-Fridman et al. 2019; Tsou et al. 2016). B cells can cross-present TAAs to CD8$^+$ T cells and facilitate antitumor immune response by production of tumor-specific antibodies with ADCC and phagocytosis capacities, supporting tumor-associated macrophages, and DCs (S. S. Wang et al. 2019a).

High levels of tumor-infiltrating T cells and B cells with increased B-cell receptor diversity can predict improved OS in breast, lung, melanoma, and lung adenocarcinoma (Iglesia et al. 2016); the latter showed six B cell-specific genes positively associated as independent factors of overall survival. Patients with lower risk scores had better responses to RT and immunotherapy indicating that tumor-infiltrating B cells are a favorable prognostic and response factor (Han et al. 2020). RT-induced antitumor immune responses were attributed to MHC-I-restricted CD8$^+$ cytotoxic T cells, but MHC-II-restricted B cells and NK cells are also important drivers of antitumor immunity. Infiltration of B cells into tumors also facilitates robust interactions with CD8$^+$ T cells, as B cells recruit CD8$^+$ T cells via the chemokine CXCL9 (Hladikova et al. 2019). RT may strengthen this interaction, by enhancing clonality and somatic hypermutation of tumor-infiltrating B cells. RT combined with anti-PD-1 therapy promoted antigen-specific and memory B cells in squamous cell carcinomas (S. S. Kim et al. 2020c). RT increased the numbers of intra-tumoral cytotoxic CD8$^+$ T cells in both primary (irradiated) tumors and secondary (unirradiated) tumors in a mouse model (Niknam et al. 2018) and enhanced chemokine production including CXCL9, CXCL10, CXCL11, and CXCL16 (Meng et al. 2010; Matsumura et al. 2008; S. S. Kim et al. 2020c). B cells are engaging NK cells via the interaction of CD48 (on the B cells) and CD244 (on the NK cells), and ADCC (Gao et al. 2005), and production of IFN-γ (Michael et al. 1989), thereby promoting differentiation of B cells (Gao et al. 2001). This interaction also promotes B-cell class switch recombination (Gao et al. 2005). B cells promote a Th2-type response by inducing the expression of IL-13 in NK cells (Gao et al. 2006). NK cells have strong antitumor activity (Morvan and Lanier 2016) by mediating ADCC through FcγRs (i.e., FcγR IIIa/CD16a and FcγR IIc/CD32c) and the Fc region of tumor-specific antibodies (Tsou et al. 2016), which may also affect the function of Fc receptor-expressing granulocytes, DCs, and MDSCs (Tsou et al. 2016). Activation of NK cells via the NKG2D receptor was demonstrated in irradiated tumor cell lines that expressed NKG2D ligands (J. Y. Kim et al. 2006). In a mouse model for solid tumors, adoptive transfer of ex vivo-activated NK cells combined with RT prolonged survival (Ames et al. 2015). In sum, RT seems to enhance the cross talk between B cells and NK cells and reprogram the tumor microenvironment in favor of antitumor outcomes.

3.5 Dendritic Cells

High-dose stereotactic RT triggers release of TAAs, as well as danger signals (ATP, HMGB1, heat-shock proteins, and RNA/DNA fragments) that activate professional APCs such as DCs. Immature DCs capture antigens at infection or tumor sites and traffic into draining lymph nodes (dLN) and spleen to present these antigens to T cells. Mature DCs usually express higher levels of MHC-I, MHC-II, and co-stimulatory molecules CD80, CD86, OX40L, 4-1BBL, and Flt3 receptor. DCs can also be activated through the stimulation of Toll-like receptors such as TLR2, TLR4, TLR3, TLR7, TLR8, and TLR9 to produce pro-inflammatory cytokines that drive Th1/Th2/Th17 T-cell responses. DCs are generally divided into two major categories: conventional dendritic cells (cDCs) of myeloid lineage, phenotypically characterized as CD11c$^+$CD11b$^+$, and plasmacytoid dendritic cells (pDCs), phenotypically characterized in mice as CD11c⁺PDCA1⁺ and in humans as CD11c⁺CD303⁺. Subcategories also include CD11c⁺CD11b⁻ DCs, further divided into CD11c⁺CD8α⁺ lymphoid DCs and CD11c⁺CD103⁺ nonlymphoid migratory DCs, although both subtypes may share similar molecular factors, such as BATF3 and IRF8 (Mildner and Jung 2014). Few reports also observed the presence of CD11c⁺CD8α⁺CD103⁺ population that can be either stimulatory or tolerogenic. For example, CD11c⁺CD8⁺ DCs are tolerogenic in the gastrointestinal tract and tumors with high expression of IDO1 or arginase enzymes (Mellor et al. 2003; Bhatt et al. 2014), but also stimulatory against lung infections (Dunne et al. 2009).

We recently showed that high-dose RT (36 Gy total given in three 12 Gy fractions) increased the levels of pDCs in the TME 3–5 days postradiation, which in turn express high levels of TLR9 and can be further stimulated to promote local and abscopal responses (Younes et al. 2021). Similarly, high-dose RT increased the levels of CD11c⁺CD103⁺ DCs in the spleens of treated mice associated with systemic antitumor response (Niknam et al. 2018). RT can activate DCs through the release of nuclear DNA fragments from irradiated tumor cells and the initiation of the cGAS/STING pathway and produce type I interferons. IFN-β for example increased MHC-I expression, restored sensitivity to anti-PD-1 treatment, and enhanced T-cell priming (X. Wang et al. 2017b). Higher RT doses (>15 Gy per fraction) may induce the expression of TREX1 exonuclease which degrades cytoplasmic DNA and inhibits interferon production through the cGAS/STING pathway (Vanpouille-Box et al. 2017b).

In another approach, depleting DCs by using CD11c-targeting antibodies in a mouse model of lymphoma was shown to reduce both CD8⁺ T-cell activation and antitumor activity of 10 Gy local RT given with either a CD40 agonist or a TLR7 agonist (Dovedi et al. 2016). In a mammary carcinoma model, DCs were critical for RT-mediated abscopal effects, and subsequent administration of the growth factor Fms-like tyrosine kinase receptor 3 ligand (Flt3L) further enhanced the generation and maturation of DCs, and slowed secondary tumor growth (Demaria et al. 2004). The TLR3 agonist poly(I:C) boosted the function of cDCs and improved the immunogenicity of cold tumors, like pancreatic and oral squamous cell carcinomas, especially with RT (single dose of 12 Gy) (Blair et al. 2020). In a phase I trial of 15 cancer patients, DCs were pulsed with autologous tumor lysates and injected back intradermally along with poly-ICLC (Hiltonol) at specified time points (Rodríguez-Ruiz et al. 2018). Six of the patients also received stereotactic RT (8 Gy × 3 fractions or 6 Gy × 5 fractions) to lesions injected with Hiltonol, out of which 5 patients reached stable disease (SD) after 7 weeks. One patient with metastatic prostate cancer also presented with an abscopal response in thoracic lesions upon 3-month follow-up (Rodríguez-Ruiz et al. 2018). DCs were loaded with antigens released from apoptotic heat-shocked tumor cells and given to 28 esophageal cancer patients (once per week for a total of four injections) who also received conventional adjuvant radiotherapy (60 Gy total, 2 Gy/fraction over 6 weeks). Patients in the vaccination group showed higher levels of IL-12 and IFN-γ Th1 cytokines and elevated percentages of IFN-γ⁺ CD8⁺ T cells (C. Wang et al. 2017a). Finally, the future efficacy of RT + dendritic cell-based vaccines can be improved by the addition of checkpoint inhibitors such as anti-CTLA-4 and anti-PD-1 to overcome T-cell exhaustion and further promote abscopal responses in metastatic solid tumors (Y. Wang et al. 2019b).

A schematic overview of the effects of RT and immunotherapy on immune cell populations and functional interactions between lymphocytes in antitumor adaptive immune responses triggered by RT is provided in Fig. 1.

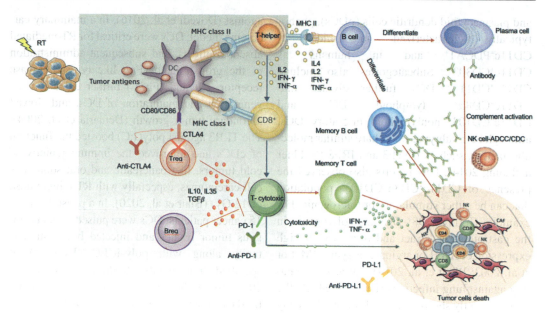

Fig. 1 Schematic overview of the effects of radiotherapy and immunotherapy on immune cells. Radiation therapy (RT) induces immunogenic cell death in cancer cells, releasing tumor neoantigens and activating antigen-presenting dendritic cells (DCs), which in turn migrate to local lymph nodes. In the lymph node, activated DCs present antigens to CD8+ T cells through MHC-I molecules and CD4+ T cells through MHC-II molecules. Clones of activated helper T cells produce cytokines that initiate B cells and CD8+ T cells, which become cytotoxic T cells. The latter ultimately leave the lymph node and travel to sites where cells bearing the target antigen reside, initiating a cytotoxic antitumor response. Conversely, at the time of the initial response to antigen, CTLA-4 expressed on regulatory T cells (Tregs) binds to CD80/CD86 on antigen-presenting cells (APCs) and inhibits T-cell activation. Anti-CTLA-4 antibody is thought to regulate T-cell proliferation early in an immune response, primarily in lymph nodes, whereas anti-PD-1/PD-L1 antibody suppresses T cells later in an immune response, primarily in peripheral tissues. In addition, the initiated B cells mature into effector B cells and can further differentiate into plasma cells, which can produce antibodies against tumor-specific antigens. These antibodies in turn act directly against their target proteins, triggering NK cell-directed antibody-dependent cellular cytotoxicity (ADCC) or complement-dependent cytotoxicity (CDC) reactions. Effector B cells can also enhance T-cell responses by producing stimulatory cytokines. As T cells and B cells mature into effector cells, a subset of each differentiates into memory cells and can immediately become effector cells upon re-exposure to the same tumor-specific antigen. Conversely, regulatory B cell (Bregs) can act in concert with Tregs to suppress antitumor immune responses. *IFN* interferon, *IL* interleukin, *TGF* tumor growth factor, *TNF* tumor necrosis factor

4 Strategies to Enhance the Effectiveness of Radio-Immunotherapy Combinations

4.1 RadScopal™: Combining High-Dose RT with Low-Dose RT

As discussed elsewhere throughout this chapter, TME and stroma are critical components that suppress host immune responses that can be targeted through RT (Jarosz-Biej et al. 2019). While high-dose RT may prime the immune system, it may also have immune-suppressive effects in the TME by recruiting Tregs, MDSCs, and tumor-infiltrating macrophages (Darragh et al. 2018). Although low-dose radiation did not directly kill tumor cells, it modulates the immune-suppressive TME (Klug et al. 2013; De Palma et al. 2013) by promoting the M1 macrophage subtype and reducing inhibitory TGF-β levels (Barsoumian et al. 2020; Patel et al. 2021).

Increasing evidence emerged that cancer immunotherapy is more effective for patients with limited disease burden (Arina et al. 2020; Brooks and Chang 2019). Therefore, RT plays a critical role in debulking of tumors and modulating of the stroma to enhance immunotherapy efficacy. Often irradiation of multiple sites might not be possible; partial irradiation of all lesions is another efficient option (Luke et al. 2018). Welsh et al. have developed a novel technique introduced as "RadScopal™," using high-dose RT (>20 Gy in ≥2 Gy fractions) to "prime" T cells followed by low-dose RT (≤20 Gy in <2 Gy fractions) to "pull" in the T cells, supporting that specific RT techniques can enhance the abscopal effect (Patel et al. 2021; Barsoumian et al. 2020).

4.2 Pulsed RT with CTLA-4 Inhibitors

The addition of CTLA-4 inhibitors to traditionally fractionated RT boosts the activation of T-cell clones with high-affinity T-cell receptors, expanding the repertoire of those cells peripherally and leading to robust activation of tumor-reactive T cells and formation of memory T cells. However, this combination typically does not reach the threshold needed to induce abscopal effects, which may explain at least in part why abscopal effects are rarely observed in clinical practice. On the other hand, when CTLA-4 inhibitors are given with RT delivered in "pulses" (i.e., when 2–4 lesions are treated at a time in three irradiation cycles given 3 months apart), the repeated exposure of the host immune system to the same tumor antigens would presumably lead to faster deployment of memory T cells to carry out effector functions. Similarly, the differentiation of memory B cells into plasma cells could produce 10–100 times the number of antibodies than those that are secreted during the primary immune response. One might thus assume that the adaptive immune response triggered by pulsed RT could reach the abscopal threshold and have a greater chance of producing a systemic response, which presumably could be further improved by the concurrent use of anti-CTLA-4.

These suppositions are the subject of active investigation in our lab, with the corresponding ongoing preclinical and clinical studies.

References

Almatroodi SA, McDonald CF, Darby IA, Pouniotis DS (2016) Characterization of M1/M2 tumour-associated macrophages (TAMs) and Th1/Th2 cytokine profiles in patients with NSCLC. Cancer Microenviron 9(1):1–11. https://doi.org/10.1007/s12307-015-0174-x

Ames E, Canter RJ, Grossenbacher SK, Mac S, Smith RC, Monjazeb AM et al (2015) Enhanced targeting of stem-like solid tumor cells with radiation and natural killer cells. Oncoimmunology 4(9):e1036212. https://doi.org/10.1080/2162402X.2015.1036212

Antonia SJ, Villegas A, Daniel D, Vicente D, Murakami S, Hui R et al (2018) Overall survival with durvalumab after chemoradiotherapy in stage III NSCLC. N Engl J Med 379(24):2342–2350. https://doi.org/10.1056/NEJMoa1809697

Arina A, Gutiontov SI, Weichselbaum RR (2020) Radiotherapy and immunotherapy for cancer: from "systemic" to "multisite". Clin Cancer Res 26(12):2777–2782. https://doi.org/10.1158/1078-0432.CCR-19-2034

Asaithamby A, Hu B, Chen DJ (2011) Unrepaired clustered DNA lesions induce chromosome breakage in human cells. Proc Natl Acad Sci U S A 108(20):8293–8298. https://doi.org/10.1073/pnas.1016045108

Balogh A, Persa E, Bogdándi EN, Benedek A, Hegyesi H, Sáfrány G et al (2013) The effect of ionizing radiation on the homeostasis and functional integrity of murine splenic regulatory T cells. Inflamm Res 62(2):201–212. https://doi.org/10.1007/s00011-012-0567-y

Barsoumian HB, Ramapriyan R, Younes AI, Caetano MS, Menon H, Comeaux NI et al (2020) Low-dose radiation treatment enhances systemic antitumor immune responses by overcoming the inhibitory stroma. J Immunother Cancer 8(2):e000537. https://doi.org/10.1136/jitc-2020-000537

Baumann BC, Mitra N, Harton JG, Xiao Y, Wojcieszynski AP, Gabriel PE et al (2020) Comparative effectiveness of proton vs photon therapy as part of concurrent chemoradiotherapy for locally advanced cancer. JAMA Oncol 6(2):237–246. https://doi.org/10.1001/jamaoncol.2019.4889

Bhatt S, Qin J, Bennett C, Qian S, Fung JJ, Hamilton TA et al (2014) All-trans retinoic acid induces arginase-1 and inducible nitric oxide synthase-producing dendritic cells with T cell inhibitory function. J Immunol 192(11):5098–5108. https://doi.org/10.4049/jimmunol.1303073

Blair TC, Bambina S, Alice AF, Kramer GF, Medler TR, Baird JR et al (2020) Dendritic cell maturation defines immunological responsiveness of tumors to radiation therapy. J Immunol 204(12):3416–3424. https://doi.org/10.4049/jimmunol.2000194

Bose D, Banerjee S, Chatterjee N, Das S, Saha M, Saha KD (2019) Inhibition of TGF-β induced lipid droplets switches M2 macrophages to M1 phenotype. Toxicol In Vitro 58:207–214. https://doi.org/10.1016/j.tiv.2019.03.037

Bourhis J, Sozzi WJ, Jorge PG, Gaide O, Bailat C, Duclos F et al (2019) Treatment of a first patient with FLASH-radiotherapy. Radiother Oncol 139:18–22. https://doi.org/10.1016/j.radonc.2019.06.019

Brooks ED, Chang JY (2019) Time to abandon single-site irradiation for inducing abscopal effects. Nat Rev Clin Oncol 16(2):123–135. https://doi.org/10.1038/s41571-018-0119-7

Caetano MS, Younes AI, Barsoumian HB, Quigley M, Menon H, Gao C et al (2019) Triple therapy with MerTK and PD1 inhibition plus radiotherapy promotes abscopal antitumor immune responses. Clin Cancer Res 25(24):7576–7584. https://doi.org/10.1158/1078-0432.CCR-19-0795

Cao M, Cabrera R, Xu Y, Liu C, Nelson D (2009) Gamma irradiation alters the phenotype and function of CD4+CD25+ regulatory T cells. Cell Biol Int 33(5):565–571. https://doi.org/10.1016/j.cellbi.2009.02.007

Chen DS, Mellman I (2013) Oncology meets immunology: the cancer-immunity cycle. Immunity 39(1):1–10. https://doi.org/10.1016/j.immuni.2013.07.012

Chen D, Patel RR, Verma V, Ramapriyan R, Barsoumian HB, Cortez MA et al (2020a) Interaction between lymphopenia, radiotherapy technique, dosimetry, and survival outcomes in lung cancer patients receiving combined immunotherapy and radiotherapy. Radiother Oncol 150:114–120. https://doi.org/10.1016/j.radonc.2020.05.051

Chen D, Verma V, Patel RR, Barsoumian HB, Cortez MA, Welsh JW (2020b) Absolute lymphocyte count predicts abscopal responses and outcomes in patients receiving combined immunotherapy and radiation therapy: analysis of 3 phase 1/2 trials. Int J Radiat Oncol Biol Phys 108(1):196–203. https://doi.org/10.1016/j.ijrobp.2020.01.032

Darragh LB, Oweida AJ, Karam SD (2018) Overcoming resistance to combination radiation-immunotherapy: a focus on contributing pathways within the tumor microenvironment. Front Immunol 9:3154. https://doi.org/10.3389/fimmu.2018.03154

De Palma M, Coukos G, Hanahan D (2013) A new twist on radiation oncology: low-dose irradiation elicits immunostimulatory macrophages that unlock barriers to tumor immunotherapy. Cancer Cell 24(5):559–561. https://doi.org/10.1016/j.ccr.2013.10.019

Demaria S, Ng B, Devitt ML, Babb JS, Kawashima N, Liebes L et al (2004) Ionizing radiation inhibition of distant untreated tumors (abscopal effect) is immune mediated. Int J Radiat Oncol Biol Phys 58(3):862–870. https://doi.org/10.1016/j.ijrobp.2003.09.012

Deng L, Liang H, Xu M, Yang X, Burnette B, Arina A et al (2014) STING-dependent cytosolic DNA sensing promotes radiation-induced type I interferon-dependent antitumor immunity in immunogenic tumors. Immunity 41(5):843–852. https://doi.org/10.1016/j.immuni.2014.10.019

Dewan MZ, Galloway AE, Kawashima N, Dewyngaert JK, Babb JS, Formenti SC et al (2009) Fractionated but not single-dose radiotherapy induces an immune-mediated abscopal effect when combined with anti-CTLA-4 antibody. Clin Cancer Res 15(17):5379–5388. https://doi.org/10.1158/1078-0432.CCR-09-0265

Di Virgilio F, Dal Ben D, Sarti AC, Giuliani AL, Falzoni S (2017) The P2X7 receptor in infection and inflammation. Immunity 47(1):15–31. https://doi.org/10.1016/j.immuni.2017.06.020

Dieu-Nosjean MC, Goc J, Giraldo NA, Sautes-Fridman C, Fridman WH (2014) Tertiary lymphoid structures in cancer and beyond. Trends Immunol 35(11):571–580. https://doi.org/10.1016/j.it.2014.09.006

Doescher J, Jeske S, Weissinger SE, Brunner C, Laban S, Bölke E et al (2018) Polyfunctionality of CD4. Strahlenther Onkol 194(5):392–402. https://doi.org/10.1007/s00066-018-1289-z

Dovedi SJ, Lipowska-Bhalla G, Beers SA, Cheadle EJ, Mu L, Glennie MJ et al (2016) Antitumor efficacy of radiation plus immunotherapy depends upon dendritic cell activation of effector CD8+ T cells. Cancer Immunol Res 4(7):621–630. https://doi.org/10.1158/2326-6066.CIR-15-0253

Duma N, Santana-Davila R, Molina JR (2019) Non-small cell lung cancer: epidemiology, screening, diagnosis, and treatment. Mayo Clin Proc 94(8):1623–1640. https://doi.org/10.1016/j.mayocp.2019.01.013

Dunne PJ, Moran B, Cummins RC, Mills KH (2009) CD11c+CD8alpha+ dendritic cells promote protective immunity to respiratory infection with Bordetella pertussis. J Immunol 183(1):400–410. https://doi.org/10.4049/jimmunol.0900169

Durante M, Formenti S (2020) Harnessing radiation to improve immunotherapy: better with particles? Br J Radiol 93(1107):20190224. https://doi.org/10.1259/bjr.20190224

Favaudon V, Caplier L, Monceau V, Pouzoulet F, Sayarath M, Fouillade C et al (2014) Ultrahigh dose-rate FLASH irradiation increases the differential response between normal and tumor tissue in mice. Sci Transl Med 6(245):245ra93. https://doi.org/10.1126/scitranslmed.3008973

Fensterheim BA, Young JD, Luan L, Kleinbard RR, Stothers CL, Patil NK et al (2018) The TLR4 agonist monophosphoryl lipid A drives broad resistance to infection via dynamic reprogramming of macrophage metabolism. J Immunol 200(11):3777–3789. https://doi.org/10.4049/jimmunol.1800085

Fitzgerald K, Simone CB II (2020) Combining immunotherapy with radiation therapy in non-small cell lung cancer. Thorac Surg Clin 30(2):221–239. https://doi.org/10.1016/j.thorsurg.2020.01.002

Fourcade J, Sun Z, Chauvin JM, Ka M, Davar D, Pagliano O et al (2018) CD226 opposes TIGIT to disrupt Tregs in melanoma. JCI Insight 3(14):e121157. https://doi.org/10.1172/jci.insight.121157

Fujimura K, Oyamada A, Iwamoto Y, Yoshikai Y, Yamada H (2013) CD4 T cell-intrinsic IL-2 signaling differentially affects Th1 and Th17 development. J Leukoc Biol 94(2):271–279. https://doi.org/10.1189/jlb.1112581

Gao N, Dang T, Yuan D (2001) IFN-gamma-dependent and -independent initiation of switch recombination by NK cells. J Immunol 167(4):2011–2018. https://doi.org/10.4049/jimmunol.167.4.2011

Gao N, Dang T, Dunnick WA, Collins JT, Blazar BR, Yuan D (2005) Receptors and counterreceptors involved in NK-B cell interactions. J Immunol 174(7):4113–4119. https://doi.org/10.4049/jimmunol.174.7.4113

Gao N, Schwartzberg P, Wilder JA, Blazar BR, Yuan D (2006) B cell induction of IL-13 expression in NK cells: role of CD244 and SLAM-associated protein. J Immunol 176(5):2758–2764. https://doi.org/10.4049/jimmunol.176.5.2758

Gong X, Li X, Jiang T, Xie H, Zhu Z, Zhou F et al (2017) Combined radiotherapy and anti-PD-L1 antibody synergistically enhances antitumor effect in non-small cell lung cancer. J Thorac Oncol 12(7):1085–1097. https://doi.org/10.1016/j.jtho.2017.04.014

Gutiontov SI, Weichselbaum RR (2019) STING (or SRC) like an ICB: priming the immune response in pancreatic cancer. Cancer Res 79(15):3815–3817. https://doi.org/10.1158/0008-5472.CAN-19-1700

Han L, Shi H, Luo Y, Sun W, Li S, Zhang N et al (2020) Gene signature based on B cell predicts clinical outcome of radiotherapy and immunotherapy for patients with lung adenocarcinoma. Cancer Med 9(24):9581–9594. https://doi.org/10.1002/cam4.3561

Helmink BA, Reddy SM, Gao J, Zhang S, Basar R, Thakur R et al (2020) B cells and tertiary lymphoid structures promote immunotherapy response. Nature 577(7791):549–555. https://doi.org/10.1038/s41586-019-1922-8

Herrera FG, Bourhis J, Coukos G (2017) Radiotherapy combination opportunities leveraging immunity for the next oncology practice. CA Cancer J Clin 67(1):65–85. https://doi.org/10.3322/caac.21358

Heylmann D, Badura J, Becker H, Fahrer J, Kaina B (2018) Sensitivity of CD3/CD28-stimulated versus non-stimulated lymphocytes to ionizing radiation and genotoxic anticancer drugs: key role of ATM in the differential radiation response. Cell Death Dis 9(11):1053. https://doi.org/10.1038/s41419-018-1095-7

Hladikova K, Koucky V, Boucek J, Laco J, Grega M, Hodek M et al (2019) Tumor-infiltrating B cells affect the progression of oropharyngeal squamous cell carcinoma via cell-to-cell interactions with CD8(+) T cells. J Immunother Cancer 7(1):261. https://doi.org/10.1186/s40425-019-0726-6

Huemer F, Lang D, Westphal T, Gampenrieder SP, Hutarew G, Weiss L et al (2019) Baseline absolute lymphocyte count and ECOG performance score are associated with survival in advanced non-small cell lung cancer undergoing PD-1/PD-L1 blockade. J Clin Med 8(7):1014. https://doi.org/10.3390/jcm8071014

Iglesia MD, Parker JS, Hoadley KA, Serody JS, Perou CM, Vincent BG (2016) Genomic analysis of immune cell infiltrates across 11 tumor types. J Natl Cancer Inst 108(11):djw144. https://doi.org/10.1093/jnci/djw144

Jarnicki AG, Lysaght J, Todryk S, Mills KH (2006) Suppression of antitumor immunity by IL-10 and TGF-beta-producing T cells infiltrating the growing tumor: influence of tumor environment on the induction of CD4+ and CD8+ regulatory T cells. J Immunol 177(2):896–904. https://doi.org/10.4049/jimmunol.177.2.896

Jarosz-Biej M, Smolarczyk R, Cichon T, Kulach N (2019) Tumor microenvironment as a "game changer" in cancer radiotherapy. Int J Mol Sci 20(13). https://doi.org/10.3390/ijms20133212

Jayasingam SD, Citartan M, Thang TH, Mat Zin AA, Ang KC, Ch'ng ES (2019) Evaluating the polarization of tumor-associated macrophages into M1 and M2 phenotypes in human cancer tissue: technicalities and challenges in routine clinical practice. Front Oncol 9:1512. https://doi.org/10.3389/fonc.2019.01512

Jesenko T, Bosnjak M, Markelc B, Sersa G, Znidar K, Heller L et al (2020) Radiation induced upregulation of DNA sensing pathways is cell-type dependent and can mediate the off-target effects. Cancers (Basel) 12(11):3365. https://doi.org/10.3390/cancers12113365

Jing H, Hettich M, Gaedicke S, Firat E, Bartholomä M, Niedermann G (2019) Combination treatment with hypofractionated radiotherapy plus IL-2/anti-IL-2 complexes and its theranostic evaluation. J Immunother Cancer 7(1):55. https://doi.org/10.1186/s40425-019-0537-9

Kim JY, Son YO, Park SW, Bae JH, Chung JS, Kim HH et al (2006) Increase of NKG2D ligands and sensitivity to NK cell-mediated cytotoxicity of tumor cells by heat shock and ionizing radiation. Exp Mol Med 38(5):474–484. https://doi.org/10.1038/emm.2006.56

Kim KJ, Kim JH, Lee SJ, Lee EJ, Shin EC, Seong J (2017) Radiation improves antitumor effect of immune checkpoint inhibitor in murine hepatocellular carcinoma model. Oncotarget 8(25):41242–41255. https://doi.org/10.18632/oncotarget.17168

Kim JH, Kim BS, Lee SK (2020a) Regulatory T cells in tumor microenvironment and approach for anticancer immunotherapy. Immune Netw 20(1):e4. https://doi.org/10.4110/in.2020.20.e4

Kim N, Myoung Noh J, Lee W, Park B, Park H, Young Park J et al (2020b) Proton beam therapy reduces the risk of severe radiation-induced lymphopenia during chemoradiotherapy for locally advanced non-small cell lung cancer: a comparative analysis of proton versus photon therapy. Radiother Oncol 156:166–173. https://doi.org/10.1016/j.radonc.2020.12.019

Kim SS, Shen S, Miyauchi S, Sanders PD, Franiak-Pietryga I, Mell L et al (2020c) B cells improve overall survival in HPV-associated squamous cell carcinomas and are activated by radiation and PD-1 blockade. Clin Cancer Res 26(13):3345–3359. https://doi.org/10.1158/1078-0432.CCR-19-3211

Klug F, Prakash H, Huber PE, Seibel T, Bender N, Halama N et al (2013) Low-dose irradiation programs macrophage differentiation to an iNOS(+)/M1 phenotype that orchestrates effective T cell immunotherapy. Cancer Cell 24(5):589–602. https://doi.org/10.1016/j.ccr.2013.09.014

Ko EC, Formenti SC (2019) Radiation therapy to enhance tumor immunotherapy: a novel application for an established modality. Int J Radiat Biol 95(7):936–939. https://doi.org/10.1080/09553002.2019.1623429

Krieg AM (2007) Development of TLR9 agonists for cancer therapy. J Clin Invest 117(5):1184–1194. https://doi.org/10.1172/JCI31414

Le Naour J, Zitvogel L, Galluzzi L, Vacchelli E, Kroemer G (2020) Trial watch: STING agonists in cancer therapy. Oncoimmunology 9(1):1777624. https://doi.org/10.1080/2162402X.2020.1777624

Lee HJ Jr, Zeng J, Rengan R (2018) Proton beam therapy and immunotherapy: an emerging partnership for immune activation in non-small cell lung cancer. Transl Lung Cancer Res 7(2):180–188. https://doi.org/10.21037/tlcr.2018.03.28

Liu Y, Crowe WN, Wang L, Lu Y, Petty WJ, Habib AA et al (2019) An inhalable nanoparticulate STING agonist synergizes with radiotherapy to confer long-term control of lung metastases. Nat Commun 10(1):5108. https://doi.org/10.1038/s41467-019-13094-5

Lucca LE, Dominguez-Villar M (2020) Modulation of regulatory T cell function and stability by co-inhibitory receptors. Nat Rev Immunol 20(11):680–693. https://doi.org/10.1038/s41577-020-0296-3

Lugade AA, Sorensen EW, Gerber SA, Moran JP, Frelinger JG, Lord EM (2008) Radiation-induced IFN-gamma production within the tumor microenvironment influences antitumor immunity. J Immunol 180(5):3132–3139. https://doi.org/10.4049/jimmunol.180.5.3132

Luke JJ, Lemons JM, Karrison TG, Pitroda SP, Melotek JM, Zha Y et al (2018) Safety and clinical activity of pembrolizumab and multisite stereotactic body radiotherapy in patients with advanced solid tumors. J Clin Oncol 36(16):1611–1618. https://doi.org/10.1200/JCO.2017.76.2229

Macciò A, Gramignano G, Cherchi MC, Tanca L, Melis L, Madeddu C (2020) Role of M1-polarized tumor-associated macrophages in the prognosis of advanced ovarian cancer patients. Sci Rep 10(1):6096. https://doi.org/10.1038/s41598-020-63276-1

Maeda S, Murakami K, Inoue A, Yonezawa T, Matsuki N (2019) CCR4 blockade depletes regulatory T cells and prolongs survival in a canine model of bladder cancer. Cancer Immunol Res 7(7):1175–1187. https://doi.org/10.1158/2326-6066.CIR-18-0751

Marill J, Mohamed Anesary N, Paris S (2019) DNA damage enhancement by radiotherapy-activated hafnium oxide nanoparticles improves cGAS-STING pathway activation in human colorectal cancer cells. Radiother Oncol 141:262–266. https://doi.org/10.1016/j.radonc.2019.07.029

Matsumura S, Wang B, Kawashima N, Braunstein S, Badura M, Cameron TO et al (2008) Radiation-induced CXCL16 release by breast cancer cells attracts effector T cells. J Immunol 181(5):3099–3107. https://doi.org/10.4049/jimmunol.181.5.3099

McGee HM, Daly ME, Azghadi S, Stewart SL, Oesterich L, Schlom J et al (2018) Stereotactic ablative radiation therapy induces systemic differences in peripheral blood immunophenotype dependent on irradiated site. Int J Radiat Oncol Biol Phys 101(5):1259–1270. https://doi.org/10.1016/j.ijrobp.2018.04.038

Mellor AL, Baban B, Chandler P, Marshall B, Jhaver K, Hansen A et al (2003) Cutting edge: induced indoleamine 2,3 dioxygenase expression in dendritic cell subsets suppresses T cell clonal expansion. J Immunol 171(4):1652–1655. https://doi.org/10.4049/jimmunol.171.4.1652

Meng Y, Mauceri HJ, Khodarev NN, Darga TE, Pitroda SP, Beckett MA et al (2010) Ad.Egr-TNF and local ionizing radiation suppress metastases by interferon-beta-dependent activation of antigen-specific CD8+ T cells. Mol Ther 18(5):912–920. https://doi.org/10.1038/mt.2010.18

Mesko S, Gomez D (2018) Proton therapy in non-small cell lung cancer. Curr Treat Options Oncol 19(12):76. https://doi.org/10.1007/s11864-018-0588-z

Michael A, Hackett JJ, Bennett M, Kumar V, Yuan D (1989) Regulation of B lymphocytes by natural killer cells. Role of IFN-gamma. J Immunol 142(4):1095–1101

Mildner A, Jung S (2014) Development and function of dendritic cell subsets. Immunity 40(5):642–656. https://doi.org/10.1016/j.immuni.2014.04.016

Min Y, Roche KC, Tian S, Eblan MJ, McKinnon KP, Caster JM et al (2017) Antigen-capturing nanoparticles improve the abscopal effect and cancer immunotherapy. Nat Nanotechnol 12(9):877–882. https://doi.org/10.1038/nnano.2017.113

Monjazeb AM, Tietze JK, Grossenbacher SK, Hsiao HH, Zamora AE, Mirsoian A et al (2014) Bystander activation and anti-tumor effects of CD8+ T cells following Interleukin-2 based immunotherapy is independent of CD4+ T cell help. PLoS One 9(8):e102709. https://doi.org/10.1371/journal.pone.0102709

Morisada M, Clavijo PE, Moore E, Sun L, Chamberlin M, Van Waes C et al (2018) PD-1 blockade reverses adaptive immune resistance induced by high-dose hypofractionated but not low-dose daily fractionated radiation. Oncoimmunology 7(3):e1395996. https://doi.org/10.1080/2162402X.2017.1395996

Morvan MG, Lanier LL (2016) NK cells and cancer: you can teach innate cells new tricks. Nat Rev Cancer 16(1):7–19. https://doi.org/10.1038/nrc.2015.5

Niknam S, Barsoumian HB, Schoenhals JE, Jackson HL, Yanamandra N, Caetano MS et al (2018) Radiation followed by OX40 stimulation drives local and abscopal antitumor effects in an anti-PD1-resistant lung tumor model. Clin Cancer Res 24(22):5735–5743. https://doi.org/10.1158/1078-0432.Ccr-17-3279

Pan BS, Perera SA, Piesvaux JA, Presland JP, Schroeder GK, Cumming JN et al (2020) An orally available non-nucleotide STING agonist with antitumor activity. Science 369(6506):eaba6098. https://doi.org/10.1126/science.aba6098

Patel RR, Verma V, Barsoumian HB, Ning MS, Chun SG, Tang C et al (2021) Use of multi-site radiation therapy for systemic disease control. Int J Radiat Oncol Biol Phys 109(2):352–364. https://doi.org/10.1016/j.ijrobp.2020.08.025

Persa E, Balogh A, Sáfrány G, Lumniczky K (2015) The effect of ionizing radiation on regulatory T cells in health and disease. Cancer Lett 368(2):252–261. https://doi.org/10.1016/j.canlet.2015.03.003

Qu Y, Jin S, Zhang A, Zhang B, Shi X, Wang J et al (2010a) Gamma-ray resistance of regulatory CD4+CD25+Foxp3+ T cells in mice. Radiat Res 173(2):148–157. https://doi.org/10.1667/RR0978.1

Qu Y, Zhang B, Liu S, Zhang A, Wu T, Zhao Y (2010b) 2-Gy whole-body irradiation significantly alters the balance of CD4+ CD25− T effector cells and CD4+ CD25+ Foxp3+ T regulatory cells in mice. Cell Mol Immunol 7(6):419–427. https://doi.org/10.1038/cmi.2010.45

Rama N, Saha T, Shukla S, Goda C, Milewski D, Mascia A et al (2019) Improved tumor control through T-cell infiltration modulated by ultra-high dose rate proton FLASH using a clinical pencil beam scanning proton system. Int J Radiat Oncol Biol Phys 105:S164–S165

Rodríguez-Ruiz ME, Perez-Gracia JL, Rodríguez I, Alfaro C, Oñate C, Pérez G et al (2018) Combined immunotherapy encompassing intratumoral poly-ICLC, dendritic-cell vaccination and radiotherapy in advanced cancer patients. Ann Oncol 29(5):1312–1319. https://doi.org/10.1093/annonc/mdy089

Rudqvist NP, Pilones KA, Lhuillier C, Wennerberg E, Sidhom JW, Emerson RO et al (2018) Radiotherapy and CTLA-4 blockade shape the TCR repertoire of tumor-infiltrating T cells. Cancer Immunol Res 6(2):139–150. https://doi.org/10.1158/2326-6066.CIR-17-0134

Sautes-Fridman C, Petitprez F, Calderaro J, Fridman WH (2019) Tertiary lymphoid structures in the era of cancer immunotherapy. Nat Rev Cancer 19(6):307–325. https://doi.org/10.1038/s41568-019-0144-6

Schoenhals JE, Cushman TR, Barsoumian HB, Li A, Cadena AP, Niknam S et al (2018) Anti-glucocorticoid-induced tumor necrosis factor-related protein (GITR) therapy overcomes radiation-induced Treg immunosuppression and drives abscopal effects. Front Immunol 9:2170. https://doi.org/10.3389/fimmu.2018.02170

Scurr M, Pembroke T, Bloom A, Roberts D, Thomson A, Smart K et al (2017) Low-dose cyclophosphamide induces antitumor T-cell responses, which associate with survival in metastatic colorectal cancer. Clin Cancer Res 23(22):6771–6780. https://doi.org/10.1158/1078-0432.CCR-17-0895

Selby MJ, Engelhardt JJ, Quigley M, Henning KA, Chen T, Srinivasan M et al (2013) Anti-CTLA-4 antibodies of IgG2a isotype enhance antitumor activity through reduction of intratumoral regulatory T cells. Cancer Immunol Res 1(1):32–42. https://doi.org/10.1158/2326-6066.CIR-13-0013

Sheng H, Huang Y, Xiao Y, Zhu Z, Shen M, Zhou P et al (2020) ATR inhibitor AZD6738 enhances the antitumor activity of radiotherapy and immune checkpoint inhibitors by potentiating the tumor immune microenvironment in hepatocellular carcinoma. J Immunother Cancer 8(1):e000340. https://doi.org/10.1136/jitc-2019-000340

Simpson TR, Li F, Montalvo-Ortiz W, Sepulveda MA, Bergerhoff K, Arce F et al (2013) Fc-dependent depletion of tumor-infiltrating regulatory T cells co-defines the efficacy of anti-CTLA-4 therapy against melanoma. J Exp Med 210(9):1695–1710. https://doi.org/10.1084/jem.20130579

Storozynsky Q, Hitt MM (2020) The impact of radiation-induced DNA damage on cGAS-STING-mediated immune responses to cancer. Int J Mol Sci 21(22):8877. https://doi.org/10.3390/ijms21228877

Takahashi Y, Yasui T, Minami K, Tamari K, Otani K, Seo Y et al (2017) Radiation enhances the efficacy of antitumor immunotherapy with an immunocomplex of interleukin-2 and its monoclonal antibody. Anticancer Res 37(12):6799–6806. https://doi.org/10.21873/anticanres.12140

Tang C, Liao Z, Gomez D, Levy L, Zhuang Y, Gebremichael RA et al (2014) Lymphopenia association with gross tumor volume and lung V5 and its effects on non-small cell lung cancer patient outcomes. Int J Radiat Oncol Biol Phys 89(5):1084–1091. https://doi.org/10.1016/j.ijrobp.2014.04.025

Tang C, Welsh JW, de Groot P, Massarelli E, Chang JY, Hess KR et al (2017) Ipilimumab with stereotactic ablative radiation therapy: phase I results and immunologic correlates from peripheral T cells. Clin Cancer Res 23(6):1388–1396. https://doi.org/10.1158/1078-0432.CCR-16-1432

Teoh S, Fiorini F, George B, Vallis KA, Van den Heuvel F (2020) Proton vs photon: a model-based approach to patient selection for reduction of cardiac toxicity in locally advanced lung cancer. Radiother Oncol 152:151–162. https://doi.org/10.1016/j.radonc.2019.06.032

Theelen WSME, Peulen HMU, Lalezari F, van der Noort V, de Vries JF, Aerts JGJV et al (2019) Effect of pembrolizumab after stereotactic body radiotherapy vs pembrolizumab alone on tumor response in patients with advanced non-small cell lung cancer: results of the PEMBRO-RT phase 2 randomized clinical trial. JAMA Oncol. https://doi.org/10.1001/jamaoncol.2019.1478

Theelen WSME, Chen D, Verma V, Hobbs BP, Peulen HMU, Aerts JGJV et al (2020) Pembrolizumab with or without radiotherapy for metastatic non-small-cell lung cancer: a pooled analysis of two randomised trials. Lancet Respir Med. https://doi.org/10.1016/S2213-2600(20)30391-X

Timmerman RD, Paulus R, Pass HI, Gore EM, Edelman MJ, Galvin J et al (2018) Stereotactic body radiation therapy for operable early-stage lung cancer: findings from the NRG Oncology RTOG 0618 Trial. JAMA Oncol 4(9):1263–1266. https://doi.org/10.1001/jamaoncol.2018.1251

Tsou P, Katayama H, Ostrin EJ, Hanash SM (2016) The emerging role of B cells in tumor immunity. Cancer Res 76(19):5597–5601. https://doi.org/10.1158/0008-5472.CAN-16-0431

Tubin S, Yan W, Mourad WF, Fossati P, Khan MK (2020) The future of radiation-induced abscopal response: beyond conventional radiotherapy approaches. Future Oncol 16(16):1137–1151. https://doi.org/10.2217/fon-2020-0063

Vanpouille-Box C, Alard A, Aryankalayil MJ, Sarfraz Y, Diamond JM, Schneider RJ et al (2017a) DNA exonuclease Trex1 regulates radiotherapy-induced tumour immunogenicity. Nat Commun 8:15618. https://doi.org/10.1038/ncomms15618

Vanpouille-Box C, Formenti SC, Demaria S (2017b) TREX1 dictates the immune fate of irradiated cancer cells. Oncoimmunology 6(9):e1339857. https://doi.org/10.1080/2162402X.2017.1339857

Vendetti FP, Karukonda P, Clump DA, Teo T, Lalonde R, Nugent K et al (2018) ATR kinase inhibitor AZD6738 potentiates CD8+ T cell-dependent antitumor activity following radiation. J Clin Invest 128(9):3926–3940. https://doi.org/10.1172/JCI96519

Verma V, Cushman TR, Selek U, Tang C, Welsh JW (2018a) Safety of combined immunotherapy and thoracic radiation therapy: analysis of 3 single-institutional phase I/II trials. Int J Radiat Oncol Biol Phys 101(5):1141–1148. https://doi.org/10.1016/j.ijrobp.2018.04.054

Verma V, Cushman TR, Tang C, Welsh JW (2018b) Toxicity of radiation and immunotherapy combinations. Adv Radiat Oncol 3(4):506–511. https://doi.org/10.1016/j.adro.2018.08.003

Vidyarthi A, Khan N, Agnihotri T, Negi S, Das DK, Aqdas M et al (2018) TLR-3 stimulation skews M2 macrophages to M1 through IFN-αβ signaling and restricts tumor progression. Front Immunol 9:1650. https://doi.org/10.3389/fimmu.2018.01650

Wang C, Pu J, Yu H, Liu Y, Yan H, He Z et al (2017a) A dendritic cell vaccine combined with radiotherapy activates the specific immune response in patients with esophageal cancer. J Immunother 40(2):71–76. https://doi.org/10.1097/CJI.0000000000000155

Wang X, Schoenhals JE, Li A, Valdecanas DR, Ye H, Zang F et al (2017b) Suppression of type I IFN signaling in tumors mediates resistance to anti-PD-1 treatment that can be overcome by radiotherapy. Cancer Res 77(4):839–850. https://doi.org/10.1158/0008-5472.CAN-15-3142

Wang SS, Liu W, Ly D, Xu H, Qu L, Zhang L (2019a) Tumor-infiltrating B cells: their role and application in anti-tumor immunity in lung cancer. Cell Mol Immunol 16(1):6–18. https://doi.org/10.1038/s41423-018-0027-x

Wang Y, Zenkoh J, Gerelchuluun A, Sun L, Cai S, Li X et al (2019b) Administration of dendritic cells and anti-PD-1 antibody converts X-ray irradiated tumors into effective in situ vaccines. Int J Radiat Oncol Biol Phys 103(4):958–969. https://doi.org/10.1016/j.ijrobp.2018.11.019

Welsh J, Gomez D, Palmer MB, Riley BA, Mayankkumar AV, Komaki R et al (2011) Intensity-modulated proton therapy further reduces normal tissue exposure during definitive therapy for locally advanced distal esophageal tumors: a dosimetric study. Int J Radiat Oncol Biol Phys 81(5):1336–1342. https://doi.org/10.1016/j.ijrobp.2010.07.2001

Welsh JW, Tang C, de Groot P, Naing A, Hess KR, Heymach JV et al (2019) Phase II trial of ipilimumab with stereotactic radiation therapy for metastatic disease: outcomes, toxicities, and low-dose radiation-related abscopal responses. Cancer Immunol Res 7(12):1903–1909. https://doi.org/10.1158/2326-6066.CIR-18-0793

Welsh J, Menon H, Chen D, Verma V, Tang C, Altan M et al (2020) Pembrolizumab with or without radiation therapy for metastatic non-small cell lung cancer: a randomized phase I/II trial. J Immunother Cancer 8(2):e001001. https://doi.org/10.1136/jitc-2020-001001

Wilson JD, Hammond EM, Higgins GS, Petersson K (2019) Ultra-high dose rate (FLASH) radiotherapy: silver bullet or fool's gold? Front Oncol 9:1563. https://doi.org/10.3389/fonc.2019.01563

Wu CT, Chen MF, Chen WC, Hsieh CC (2013) The role of IL-6 in the radiation response of prostate cancer. Radiat Oncol 8:159. https://doi.org/10.1186/1748-717X-8-159

Yamazaki T, Galluzzi L (2020) Mitochondrial control of innate immune signaling by irradiated cancer cells. Oncoimmunology 9(1):1797292. https://doi.org/10.1080/2162402X.2020.1797292

Yasmin-Karim S, Bruck PT, Moreau M, Kunjachan S, Chen GZ, Kumar R et al (2018) Radiation and local anti-CD40 generate an effective. Front Immunol 9:2030. https://doi.org/10.3389/fimmu.2018.02030

Younes AI, Barsoumian HB, Sezen D, Verma V, Patel R, Wasley M et al (2021) Addition of TLR9 agonist immunotherapy to radiation improves systemic antitumor activity. Transl Oncol 14(2):100983. https://doi.org/10.1016/j.tranon.2020.100983

Zhang T, Yu H, Ni C, Liu L, Lv Q, Zhang Z et al (2017) Hypofractionated stereotactic radiation therapy activates the peripheral immune response in operable stage I non-small-cell lung cancer. Sci Rep 7(1):4866. https://doi.org/10.1038/s41598-017-04978-x

Zou Z, Bowen SR, Thomas HMT, Sasidharan BK, Rengan R, Zeng J (2020) Scanning beam proton therapy versus photon IMRT for stage III lung cancer: comparison of dosimetry, toxicity, and outcomes. Adv Radiat Oncol 5(3):434–443. https://doi.org/10.1016/j.adro.2020.03.001

Part IV

Current Treatment Strategies in Early-Stage Non-small Cell Lung Cancer

Early Non-small Cell Lung Cancer: The Place of Radical Non-SABR Radiation Therapy

Tathagata Das and Matthew Hatton

Contents

1 **Introduction** 418
2 **Curative Radiotherapy** 418
2.1 Patient Selection 418
2.2 Principles Underlying Radiotherapy Treatment 419
2.3 Initial Radical Radiotherapy Experience 419
3 **Current Radiation Practice** 420
4 **Fractionation** 423
4.1 Split Course 423
4.2 Hypofractionation 423
4.3 Hyperfractionation 424
4.4 Accelerated Radiotherapy 425
4.5 Continuous Hyperfractionated Accelerated Radiotherapy (CHART) 425
5 **Dose Escalation** 426
5.1 Isotoxic Radiotherapy 427
6 **Summary** 427
References 428

T. Das · M. Hatton (✉)
Weston Park Hospital, Sheffield, UK
e-mail: matthewhatton@nhs.net

Abstract

The evidence for radiotherapy as a potentially curative treatment for early lung cancer has gradually accumulated over the past 50 years with our conventional gold standard of 60 Gy in 30 fractions over 6 weeks established in the 1980s. A multimodality approach is now standard for the management of most presentations of lung cancer with concurrent chemoradiotherapy/immunotherapy combinations being standard of care for stage III disease. In parallel, technological developments enabled us to establish stereotactic ablative body radiotherapy (SABR) as the standard of care for inoperable stage I disease.

Unfortunately, a significant proportion of patients presenting to our day-to-day practice will not be best served by the gold standard treatments of SABR or the concurrent chemoradiotherapy/immunotherapy combinations. For these patients, it is the use of non-SABR radiation schedules that offers potentially curative treatment as a single modality or combined with chemotherapy. Awareness and interest in an accelerated approach have been increased by the COVID-19 pandemic. This chapter reviews the evidence for non-SABR radiation schedules as they continue to have an important role in the management of early-stage NSCLC in combination with all other aspects of care in the control of symptoms and maintenance of quality of life.

1 Introduction

Lung cancer accounts for 13% of cancer diagnosed in the United Kingdom with approximately 47,000 new cases per annum (https://www.nhs.uk/conditions/lung-cancer/). With "emergency presentation" being the commonest route to diagnosis, around three-quarters of patients have a late stage of disease at presentation (Suhail et al. 2019; Knight et al. 2017). It is estimated that around 60% of patients require radiotherapy during the course of their disease (Tyldesley et al. 2001) and when used some survival improvement is reported for all stages (Cheng et al. 2019). However, the technological advances seen in radiation planning and delivery since the turn of the century mean that the largest gains are seen for patients with the earlier stage I–III disease (Goldstraw et al. 2016).

It is hoped that we are in the advent of population screening for lung cancer following studies that confirm that low-dose CT screening is associated with reduced lung cancer mortality (de Koning et al. 2020). The UK lung cancer pilot screening trial has confirmed the feasibility of this approach noting that 86% of the identified cases had early-stage (stage I and II) lung cancer (Field et al. 2016). Unfortunately, the UK lung cancer screening program has been deferred by the COVID-19 pandemic, but it is still reasonable to expect that as screening programs are rolled out the proportion of patients diagnosed with an earlier stage of disease will increase over the coming years.

Radiotherapy is not the only therapeutic area to see significant advances over the recent years, and the standards of care for both surgery and systemic anticancer therapy are well documented in other chapters. This means that the management of early-stage lung NSCLC is increasing in complexity and the importance of multidisciplinary team assessment of patient-specific factors like respiratory function and comorbidity should not be underestimated. Noting that concurrent chemoradiotherapy (cCRT) is covered by Jeremić et al. (2021), we will review the evidence for radical, non-SABR radiotherapy outside that setting as single- or multimodality treatment.

2 Curative Radiotherapy

Surgery remains the cornerstone of curative treatment in NSCLC but only 20–30% of patients have resectable disease after careful staging procedures and one-third of these patients are considered unsuitable for surgery. In this context, radiotherapy has been developed as an alternative locoregional treatment and is indicated for early stage I–II NSCLC when the patient declines surgery or is medically inoperable. Radiotherapy is also delivered with curative intent as part of the multimodality approach that is the standard of care for patients presenting with stage III disease.

2.1 Patient Selection

A number of factors have been shown to predict for an increased chance of long-term survival following radical radiotherapy, and accurate staging is required when selecting patients for treatment. Tumor stage/size is of prime importance with smaller lesions having a higher probability of local control, good performance status (PS (WHO 0 or 1)), and minimal weight loss (<10%) being also predictive of long-term survival, and these are factors that should play a role in patient selection. Clinical trials reporting outcomes for cCRT include only 2% of patients with a PS of 2 (Aupérin et al. 2010). Even if reversible components of a poor PS are addressed, this is one group of patients who could struggle to complete the treatment course.

The elderly patient is another cohort underrepresented in cCRT studies; for example, only 13% of patients were 70 years or older in the concurrent treatment arms in the meta-analysis reported by Auperin et al. (2010). In a pooled analysis of individual patient data on cCRT for stage III NSCLC in patients aged over 70 years who participated in the US National Cancer Institute Cooperative Group studies, older patients experienced worse survival outcomes, increased toxicity, and a higher rate of treatment-related death than younger patients (Stinchcombe et al. 2017). This suggests that a more comprehensive geriatric assessment may have value in elderly patients to ensure that the most appropriate strategy to deliver "curative" radiotherapy is selected. For example, Antonio et al. (2018) studied patients over 75 with stage III NSCLC, with a combination of activities of daily living, instrumental activities of daily living [IADL] scales, and comorbidity scores, and showed that higher scores were associated with shorter survival and a higher risk of grade 3–4 toxicity.

The other factor in patient selection is coexisting morbidities, which can be associated with toxicity in patients receiving both concurrent and sequential CRT (Driessen et al. 2016). In particular, it needs to be remembered that pneumonitis/fibrosis from radiotherapy may result in an unacceptable level of pulmonary restriction. There are no published guidelines to indicate the lower limit of pulmonary function needed for radical radiotherapy treatment, but it is widely accepted that caution is needed when FEV1 or DLCO is <40% predicted value (Charloux 2011; Brunelli et al. 2009).

It is within these groups of patients with higher risks of significant toxicity where consideration of alternative treatment strategies that employ radical non-SABR regimens using sequential CRT or radiotherapy alone will enable a "curative" dose of radiotherapy to be given.

2.2 Principles Underlying Radiotherapy Treatment

In the early development of radiation treatment, it was found that one large dose might have profound effects on tumors, but the equally profound effects on normal tissues limited clinical usefulness. The response to this limitation was the application of the basis radiobiological principles of repair, redistribution, resistance, repopulation, and reoxygenation. Cells are more sensitive to radiation during the mitotic phase of the cell cycle, and the use of multiple small doses favors the cells that are quiescent and able to repair the sublethal damage before the next cell division. This means that radiation will have more effect on rapidly dividing (tumor) cells in comparison to the more slowly dividing normal tissues which underpins the development of fractionated treatment. In addition, fractionation increases tumor cell kill by allowing the redistribution of tumor cells into more sensitive phases of the cell cycle and gives time to improve the oxygenation of tumor cells and reduce the effects of hypoxia which is an important radio-resistance mechanism for cancer cells.

The outcome of treatment will depend on the total dose delivered and both normal and malignant tissues have sigmoid dose-response relationships. A certain radiation dose must be given before a response is seen, tissues (normal and malignant) respond soon after treatment is begun, and a maximal reaction can be expected between 3 and 4 weeks after initiating therapy. These factors have led to the classical radiation schedule delivering one fraction per day (usually 1.8–2 Gy), 5 days per week over 5–7 weeks. In 1982, the RTOG 73-01 trial reported 3-year survival rates of 6%, 10%, and 15% after doses of 40 Gy, 50 Gy, and 60 Gy, respectively (Perez et al. 1982), that set the conventional standard of 60 Gy in 30 fractions over 6 weeks.

The most important aim of radical radiotherapy treatment in NSCLC is to gain local control of the disease within the thorax. The RTOG study was one of the first to document that failure of local control impacted survival with 3-year survival falling from 22% in those who had the disease controlled within the thorax to 10% in those who relapsed locally (Perez et al. 1982), and it is clear that poor outcomes relate to both distant metastases and a failure to eradicate the local disease.

2.3 Initial Radical Radiotherapy Experience

2.3.1 Stage I/II NSCLC

There were no randomized trials addressing the benefit of radical radiotherapy in stage I/II disease with results from series published in the 1980s and 1990s reporting 5-year survivals ranging from 6% to 50% (Table 1). Supporting evidence from patients treated between 1998 and 2001 (4357 patients) comes from the SEER data, which confirmed a significantly better survival from patients with stage I/II disease who received radiotherapy when compared with untreated patients (stage 1 median survival of 21 vs.

Table 1 Reported survival in selected studies (1980–2020) for stage I–II NSCLC treated with radiotherapy alone

First author	Year	Stage	No. of patients/ (treatment)	Median survival (months)	5-year survival (%)
Cooper (Cooper et al. 1985)	1985	T1–3	72		6
Haffty (Haffty et al. 1988)	1988	I	43	28	21
Noordijk (Noordijk et al. 1988)	1988		50	27	16
Zhang (Zhang et al. 1989)	1989	I, II	44	>36	32
Burt (Burt et al. 1989)	1990	T1–3 N0 T1 N0	133 29		27 50
Sandler (Sandler et al. 1990)	1990	I	77	20	10
Talton (Talton et al. 1990)	1990	T1–3 N0	77	16	17
Dosoretz (Dosoretz et al. 1992)	1992	T1–2	152	17	10
Kasowitz (Kaskowitz et al. 1993)	1993	T1–2	53	21	6
Slotman (Slotman et al. 1994)	1994	I	47	20	15
Gauden (Gauden et al. 1995)	1995	I	347	28	27
Graham (Graham et al. 1995)	1995	T1 N0 T1 N0 no wt loss	35 25	~16	29 40
Krol (Krol et al. 1996)	1996	I I (<4 cm)	108 89	~24	15
Morita (Morita et al. 1997)	1997	T1–2	149	27	22
Wisnivesky (Wisnivesky et al. 2005)	2005	I, II	3588	21	11
Nyman (Nyman et al. 2016)	2016	T1–T2 N0 T1–T2 N0	53 (conformal) 49 (SABR)	–	59 (3 years) 54 (3 years)
Ball (Ball et al. 2019)	2019	T1–T2a N0 T1–T2a N0	35 (conformal) 66 (SABR)	36 60	59 (2 years) 77 (2 years)

14 months). Though survival rates at 5 years were not significantly different (11 vs. 10%), the study concluded that there was an observed improvement in the median survival of 5–7 months when radiotherapy had been given (Wisnivesky et al. 2005).

2.3.2 Stage III NSCLC

Some historical results for radical radiotherapy in stage III disease are documented in Table 2. There was a small survival advantage shown in a randomized trial compared to no treatment. This was performed in 1968 with doses and techniques that now would be considered suboptimal (Roswit et al. 1968). There have been no trials comparing palliative and radical dose of radiotherapy, and most series report a 2-year survival of around 15% and document a tail of long-term survivors. A review of 26 series containing 4796 patients treated to a dose greater than 40 Gy demonstrated an exponential survival curve with 7% alive at 5 years (Katz and Alberts 1983), and the RTOG 7301 study (Perez et al. 1982) established an international standard radical radiotherapy schedule of 60 Gy in 30 fractions in the 1980s.

3 Current Radiation Practice

The radiotherapy results achieved in the 1980s and 1990s were inferior to surgery and clearly unsatisfactory. Since then, the technical delivery of radiotherapy treatment of lung cancer has changed considerably, and target volume delineation has improved with the use of staging PET/CT scanning (Konert et al. 2015) and information

Table 2 Survival in selected trials for locally advanced lung cancer treated with radiotherapy, 1980–2020

First author	Year	Patient numbers	Treatment Gy/week/fractions	2/3/5-year survival (%)	Median OS (months)
Perez (Perez et al. 1982)	1982	378	60/6/30	19/–/5	
Arriagada (Arriagada et al. 1991)	1991	177	65/6.5/32	14/–/–	
Schaake-Koning (Schaake-Koning et al. 1992) (Split course)	1992	114	55/7/20	13/2/–	
		110	RT	19/13/–	
		107	cCRT (weekly cisplatin)	26/16/–	
			cCRT (daily cisplatin)		
Wurschmidt (Wurschmidt et al. 1994)	1994	206	>60/>6/>25	36/–/5	
Sause (Sause et al. 1995)	1995	452	69.6/6/58	–/–/6	
			60.0/6/30	–/–/5	
			sCRT 60.0/6/30	–/–/8	
Saunders (Saunders et al. 1999)	1999	224	60/6/30	21/–/–	
Ball (Ball et al. 1999)	1999	51	60/6/30	26/–/–	
De Ruysscher (Du Ruysscher et al. 2007)	2007	48	61.2–68.4/3.5/34–38	36/–/–	
Hanna (Hanna et al. 2008)	2008	243	59.4/6.5/33		
			cCRT vs.	–/26/–	
			cCRT + docetaxel	–/27/–	
Auperin (Aupérin et al. 2010)	2010	1205	sCRT	–/–/11	
			cCRT	–/–/15	
Baumann (Baumann et al. 2011) (CHARTWEL)	2011	406	60/2.5/40	31/22/11	14
			66/6.5/33	32/18/7	14
Din OS (Din et al. 2013)	2013	609	55/20/4	50/36/20	24
Bradley (Bradley et al. 2020) (RTOG 0617)	2015	544	cCRT 60/6/30	60/–/32	28
			cCRT 74/7.5/37	45/–/18	20
Hatton (Hatton et al. 2016) (CHARTED)	2015	18	57.6–64.8/2.5/38–42	49/–/–	24
Iyengar (Iyengar et al. 2016)	2016	60	60–66/6–6.5/30–33		12
			60/–/15		
Cho (Cho et al. 2016)	2016	124	60/3–4/15–20	59/–/–	
Antonia (Antonia et al. 2018) (PACIFIC)	2017	236	cCRT	55/44/36	29
			vs.		
		473	cCRT + immunotherapy	66/57/50	47
Fenwick (Fenwick et al. 2020) (IDEAL)	2020	120	cCRT 63–71/5/30	68/–/–	22
			cCRT 63–73/6/30	50/–/–	41
Haslet (Haslett et al. 2020) ISO-IMRT	2020	37	61.2–79.2/3.5–4.5/34–44	34/–/–	18

RT radiotherapy alone, *sCRT* sequential chemoradiotherapy, *cCRT* concurrent chemoradiotherapy

from diagnostic procedures such as endoscopic bronchial ultrasound (EBUS) (Peeters et al. 2016). The technical delivery of radiotherapy has evolved through three-dimensional planning techniques to using intensity-modulated radiotherapy treatment (IMRT) reducing radiotherapy dose to critical normal structures. Four-dimensional CT scanning to visualize tumor motion and computerized planning systems give us increasingly more accurate estimates of tumor and organ-at-risk doses. The use of arc therapy and image guidance methods (IGRT, e.g., cone beam CT (CBCT)) prior to each treatment dramatically improves the accuracy of patient positioning and tumor localization (Bissonnette et al. 2009). These advances give the ability to deliver radical treatment to larger tumors and patients with poorer fitness levels. As the technology

Table 3 Schematic to illustrate fractionation schedules used in the treatment of NSCLC

	Fractions	* Size Gy	*/day	week
Conventional	***** ***** ***** ***** ***** ***** **	2	1	6+
Split course	***** ***** ***** *****	>2	1	>5
Hypofractionated	***** ***** ***** *****	>2	1	<5
Hyperfractionated	***** ***** ***** ***** ***** ***** ***** ***** ***** ***** ***** *****	1–1.3	2	6
CHART	************ ************ ************	1.5	3	2
CHARTWEL/HART	***** ***** *** ***** ***** *** ***** ***** ***	1.6	3	2.5
SABR	* * * * *	>7	Alt days	1–2

* Radiotherapy fraction

advance continues, there is reasonable expectation that this ability will increase as approaches like MRI-linacs and proton treatment are developed. However, these novel approaches do need rigorous testing before being adopted into our routine practice. Boosting radiotherapy (Cooke et al. 2021; Kong et al. 2021) doses to subvolumes based on the variation in tracer update seen on PET is an example of an approach that is yet to show sufficient improvement in survival outcome for widespread adoption.

Taken alongside the development of a number of alternative fractionation radiotherapy schedules (Table 3) that exploit the radiobiological differences between normal tissue and tumor responses, the radical non-SABR schedules will retain an important place in the treatment of early-stage NSCLC.

Although surgery remains the treatment of choice for patients with early-stage disease, its position is increasingly challenged by SABR which for those patients with small localized tumors and inoperable disease is now the standard of care. For these patients, there is evidence from randomized studies of better outcomes for SABR when compared to more conventionally fractionated radiotherapy (Nyman et al. 2016; Ball et al. 2019). However, treatment volume constraints and proximity to central organs at risk (OARs) can limit the use of SABR. Guideline recommendations focus on T1–2 tumors (or T3 tumors by virtue of invading chest wall) with a maximum size of 5 cm, 2 cm away from critical central structures (UK SABR Consortium 2019). It is for patients with more advanced disease or who fall outside these SABR selection criteria for which a more conventionally fractionated treatment is still needed.

Patients with stage II/III disease should be assessed for multimodality treatment which often combines radical radiotherapy with systemic treatment. The NSCLC Collaborative Group meta-analysis established the benefits (treatment of micrometastasis) and toxicities of adding chemotherapy to conventionally fractionated radiotherapy with a 4% improvement in 2-year survival (NSCLC Collaborative Group 1995). Many chemotherapy agents have a radiation-sensitizing effect, and the additional improvement in local control offered by concurrent chemoradiotherapy was established by a meta-analysis of 14 trials that have compared concurrent treatment with radiotherapy alone. This confirmed the benefit of concomitant chemoradiotherapy on the overall survival (hazard ratio [HR], 0.84; 95% CI: 0.74–0.95; $p = 0.004$), with an absolute benefit of 4.5% at 5 years (Aupérin et al. 2010). This data established concurrent chemoradiotherapy as the standard of care. Further studies looking at the addition of adjuvant or consolidation chemotherapy to the concurrent treatment proved disappointing. A phase III study of concurrent chemoradiotherapy with or without consolidation docetaxel in stage III NSCLC was terminated early as the group receiving docetaxel showed excessive grade 3–5 toxicity (28.8% vs.

8.1%) compared to the observation arm, and the median survival was 21.2 months in the group receiving docetaxel and 23.2 months in the observation group (Hanna et al. 2008). The addition of immunotherapy following concurrent treatment has significantly improved outcomes for selected patients. The PACIFIC trial demonstrated that durvalumab significantly improved progression-free survival as compared to placebo among patients with stage III, unresectable non-small cell lung cancer (NSCLC) who did not have disease progression after concurrent chemoradiotherapy. The 5-year survival rate was 42.9% in the durvalumab group, as compared with 33.4% in the placebo group, HR 0.72 (95% CI: 0.59–0.89) (Spigel et al. 2022).

It needs to be remembered that the potential toxicity from these approaches can be significant and a fair proportion of patients seen in day-to-day practice would not have met the inclusion criteria for these multimodality studies. Hence, performance status, age, and comorbidities will continue to exclude a high number of patients from the concurrent form of treatment. For these patients, sequential chemoradiotherapy or single-modality radiotherapy may be the most appropriate treatment, and strategies that can improve outcomes are reviewed below.

4 Fractionation

Fractionation is aimed at taking advantage of the five radiobiological principles: (reoxygenation, repair, redistribution, resistance, and repopulation). Several fractionation schedules have been developed to take advantage of different radiobiological properties of tumor and normal tissues (Table 3) aiming to improve the local control rates to feed through to a reduction in distant metastasis and an improvement in survival.

4.1 Split Course

A split-course schedule uses daily fractions for 1–2 weeks with a rest period of 2–4 weeks to allow recovery of the normal tissues, and then treatment was restarted usually following the same schedule. The major drawback of this approach is tumor repopulation in the rest period, and it requires the addition of chemotherapy radiosensitizers to produce outcomes comparable with other fractionation approaches (Schaake-Koning et al. 1992).

4.2 Hypofractionation

Hypofractionated schedules aim to complete treatment in around 4 weeks, which is primarily done by increasing the fraction size. These approaches were initially adopted for convenience of departments lacking treatment capacity or for patients who were living long distances from the radiation treatment units. However, it is now recognized that accelerated repopulation of tumor cells can occur 28 days after the start of a course of radiation treatment (Withers et al. 1988; Maciejewski et al. 1989), which gives a strong scientific rationale for this approach. The regimen of 55 Gy in 20 daily fractions over 4 weeks is one of the most commonly used fractionations in the United Kingdom (Din et al. 2013) with a biological effective dose equivalent to 65 Gy delivered using conventional fractionation. Review of its use as a standard treatment for 563 patients with stage 1–III NSCLC in our center showed a 2-year overall survival rate of 48% with outcomes matching those treated with the CHART fractionation (Robinson et al. 2019).

Using the National Cancer Database, Iocolano et al. (2020) compared the outcomes for hypofractionated and conventional radiotherapy for stage III NSCLC patients treated with radiotherapy alone between 2004 and 2014. A total of 6490 patients were evaluated (conventional—5378, hypofractionated—1112) reporting that the use of hypofractionated treatment was associated with older age, lower biological effective dose (BED10), academic facility type, higher T stage, and lower N stage. The initial analysis showed an inferior OS (median 9.9 vs. 11.1 months, $p < 0.001$) for the hypofractionated schedules, but once the imbalance in covariates was adjusted for, the difference in survival was no longer significant ($p = 0.1$).

Concerns persist with the hypofractionated approach and are dominated by late radiation toxicity involving central and perihilar structures (Cannon et al. 2013). Despite this, a wide variety of hypofractionated schedules have been tested. Thirion et al. (2004) have reported on giving 72 Gy in 24 fractions over 5 weeks to patients with stage I–IIIB NSCLC and demonstrated that treatment was well tolerated with no reported late grade 3/4 toxicities. In a further phase I/II trial in 55 patients to determine the maximum tolerated dose delivered within 6 weeks (Belderbos et al. 2006), fraction size was fixed at 2.25 Gy and if more than 30 fractions were prescribed, twice-daily fractionation was used. The relative mean lung dose was used to divide patients into five risk groups, and safe dose escalation was achieved to 74.25 Gy and 94.5 Gy in the highest and lowest risk groups, respectively. Dieleman et al. (2018) retrospectively reviewed their experience using 74 Gy in 24 fractions with low-dose daily cisplatin as a radiation sensitizer reporting a grade III+ toxicity rate of 20% and a 40% survival rate at 5 years.

A prospective phase I dose escalation trial for patients of poor performance status with stage ≥II NSCLC not suitable for surgery, SABR, or chemoradiation increased doses (50 Gy, 55 Gy, or 60 Gy) validated OAR constraints for a 15-fraction schedule in the IMRT/IGRT era (Westover et al. 2015). The subsequent randomized phase III study that compared 60 Gy in 15 or 30 fractions in patients with PS ≥2 stage II–III NSCLC has published interim results (Iyengar et al. 2016) reporting less toxicity in the 15-fraction arm. Cho et al. (2016) retrospectively reviewed hypofractionated RT for medically inoperable T1–T3 N0 NSCLC using a risk-adaptive dose schedule (60 Gy in 4, 15, or 20 fractions depending on the location, size, and geometry of the tumor in relation to the esophagus). The 15 and 20 fraction schedules were used on the more central tumors with 4% grade 3 pneumonitis and no grade 4–5 pneumonitis or grade 2–5 esophagitis reported. A higher dose hypofractionated regime of 60 Gy/15 fractions (BED_{10} 90 Gy) has been reported by Sunnybrook in patients with stage I–III NSCLC. Forty-seven patients (52.8%) had stage II–III disease, and the 2-year survival rate was 68% for this group (Zeng et al. 2018).

4.3 Hyperfractionation

It is early verses late adverse effects of radiotherapy that underpin this approach. Early effects are observed in rapidly proliferating tissues such as the skin, mucosa, and bone marrow and are influenced by the daily dose rather than the fraction size. However, late effects are directly due to the damage induced to slowly proliferating tissues such as muscle, bone, and lung where fraction size is the key factor, with larger fractions increasing the risk of late damage. It is this late damage that can have profound effects on the quality of life and hence limit the total radiation dose. Most tumors act like rapidly proliferating tissue, so by giving several small fractions per day, the effect on the tumor may be increased while the risk of late normal tissue effects is decreased. Hyperfractionation may also allow an increase in the total dose if the time interval between the different fractions allows the more efficient repair in the normal rapidly proliferating tissues (when compared to the tumor) to take place.

The classical hyperfractionated schedule uses 2 fractions a day of 1–1.2 Gy separated by a 6-h interval while keeping the same total dose as the classical once-daily fraction regimens. This approach was investigated by the RTOG in a three-arm trial phase III study comparing the classical schedule of 60 Gy and 69.6 Gy with two daily fractions of 1.2 Gy, and induction chemotherapy with cisplatin and vinblastine followed by 60 Gy in 6 weeks (Sause et al. 1995; Cox et al. 1990). The 1-, 2-, and 3-year survival rates were 46%, 19%, and 6%, respectively, after 60 Gy and 51%, 24%, and 13% after the hyperfractionated schedule. With an 8% increase in biological total radiation dose, the study was underpowered for the comparison between the radiotherapy arms showing no statistical significance difference; however, both arms reported inferior outcomes in comparison to the sequential CRT. Single-center experience of the hyperfractionated schedule confirmed that treatment was well tolerated when given alone or with concurrent low-dose paclitaxel/carboplatin reporting median and 5-year survivals of 29 months/29% and 39 months/36% for the two groups, respectively (Jeremic and Milicic 2008).

4.4 Accelerated Radiotherapy

An increase in total dose using a conventional radiation schedule will also prolong treatment. Repopulation is an important issue, and the increase in treatment time will reduce the efficacy of the extra dose delivered and may be a contributory factor to the results reported in the RTOG 0617 study where worse outcomes were seen in the experimental (74 Gy) dose-escalated group compared to those receiving the standard 60 Gy (Bradley et al. 2020). Accelerated fractionation aims to reduce the duration of treatment with the goal of avoiding tumor repopulation with evidence suggesting that repopulation starts at 28 days after the beginning of radiotherapy (Withers et al. 1988; Maciejewski et al. 1989).

Ball et al. (1999) accelerated treatment into a 3-week schedule that gave 60 Gy in twice-daily fractions that maintained the fraction size at 2 Gy. They showed that the acute and late tolerance of the esophagus had become the limiting factor for accelerated radiotherapy schedules with the rates of grade 3 and 4 esophagitis which were 9% and 0%, respectively, for the conventional fractionated arm and 31% and 4% for the accelerated schedule and six patients requiring dilatation of an esophageal stricture. Using this twice-daily fractionation and reducing the fraction size to 1.6 Gy, Sibley et al. (1999) showed that dose escalation was feasible using conformal techniques and a dose of 80 Gy in 5 weeks was reached. A further phase I/II dose study escalated dose according to the risk of radiation pneumonitis with three risk groups defined on the basis of V20 values. Twice-daily fractions of 1.8 Gy were given, and a dose of 68.4 Gy over 25 days was reached (Du Ruyssscher et al. 2007). These two studies confirm that dose escalation for accelerated treatment is possible with response rates and 2-year survivals offering some encouragement.

4.5 Continuous Hyperfractionated Accelerated Radiotherapy (CHART)

The first large published randomized trial that directly compared an accelerated schedule with a conventional fractionation in the radical treatment of NSCLC used CHART (Saunders et al. 1999). This schedule further accelerated treatment by continuing the radiotherapy through the weekend so that treatment was completed in 12 days (54 Gy in 1.5 Gy fractions given three times/day with a minimum interfraction interval of 6 h). The study randomized 563 patients comparing CHART to a classical radiation schedule of 60 Gy in daily fractions in 6 weeks. The 2-, 3-, and 5-year survival rates were 21%, 13%, and 7%, respectively, after conventional radiation and 30%, 18%, and 12% after CHART. The differences were highly significant due to an improvement in local control and a 9% reduction of distant metastasis. The acute morbidity, mainly dysphagia, was higher in the CHART group with moderate or severe dysphagia reported in 49% vs. 19% for CHART and conventional radiotherapy, respectively. Importantly, no difference was seen between the two arms in late morbidity.

The 10% improvement in 2-year survival documented in the CHART trial is comparable to the improvement seen by the addition of chemotherapy to more conventionally fractionated radiotherapy regimes. A nine-center observational study reported the results for 849 patients treated with CHART in routine practice (Sanganalmath et al. 2018). It confirmed that CHART was deliverable with 99% of patients completing the treatment and less than 5% suffering grade 3 or greater toxicity. This series reported a median survival of 22 months and 2- and 3-year survival rates of 47% and 32%, respectively, which suggest that the survivals reported in the original CHART study can be reproduced in day-to-day practice. Within this cohort of patients, 26% had sequential chemotherapy/CHART supporting the evidence gained from the INCH (Induction Chemotherapy and CHART) trial that this combined chemoradiotherapy schedule can be delivered with acceptable levels of toxicity (Hatton et al. 2011).

Despite this evidence base, CHART has not been widely adopted as a standard schedule largely due to the difficulty of weekend working. This led to the development of accelerated, hyperfractionated radiotherapy schedules that avoid treatment over the weekend. CHARTWEL (CHART Week-End-Less) was developed at Mount Vernon Hospital and delivered a dose escalation of 60 Gy over an 18-day period maintaining the three-times daily treatment with 1.5 Gy fractions which are delivered 5 days per week. Encouraging results from the phase II trial (Saunders et al. 2002) which report a 2-year survival rate in the region of 45% meant that the regime was taken into a phase III randomized study recruiting 406 patients (Baumann et al. 2011). The 2-year survival rate reported for the CHARTWEL arm was only 31%, and no significant differences in outcome were seen when compared to the standard conventionally fractionated schedule.

A similar result was seen in the ECOG 2597 trial where two cycles of induction chemotherapy were given as standard and then randomized between hyperfractionated accelerated radiotherapy (HART—57.6 Gy in 1.5 Gy tds for 2½ weeks) and conventional radiotherapy (64 Gy in 32 daily fractions). The trial was closed early due to slow accrual, although a 15% improvement in favor of HART in 2- and 3-year survival was reported that did not reach statistical significance (Belani et al. 2005). As these trials seem to yield conflicting results, a meta-analysis of modified radiotherapy fractionation was performed in 2012 (Mauguen et al. 2012). It identified ten studies that had recruited 2000 patients with non-small cell lung cancer and concluded that modified fractionation improved overall survival when compared with conventional schedules (HR = 0.88, 95% CI: 0.80–0.97; $p = 0.009$) giving an absolute benefit of 2.5% (8.3–10.8%) at 5 years. However, this was at the expense of an increased risk of acute esophageal toxicity (odds ratio [OR] = 2.44 in NSCLC and OR = 2.41 in SCLC; $p < 0.001$).

Results suggest that modified radiotherapy schedules have a place in the treatment of NSCLC particularly for the elderly and other patients who may not have the reserve to cope with combined chemoradiotherapy treatment (Zehentmayr et al. 2020). The benefits and toxicities for the combination of chemotherapy and conventionally fractionated radiotherapy are well established, and a similar evidence base needs to be developed for the accelerated radiotherapy schedules over the next few years.

5 Dose Escalation

A second approach to improving local control rates is to escalate the radiotherapy dose to the tumor, and the technical radiotherapy developments like IMRT and IGRT have made this feasible. Initial dose escalation studies concentrated on the delivery of extra fractions, and these studies confirm that a significantly higher dose could be delivered with long-term toxicity follow-up confirming that such an approach is safe with acceptable levels of pulmonary toxicity (Saunders et al. 2002; Kong et al. 2005; Arriagada et al. 2004). These studies increased the numbers of daily fractions and extended the duration of treatment. However, the RTOG 0617 study (Bradley et al. 2020) where the dose was escalated to 74 Gy over 7.5 weeks in the concurrent chemoradiotherapy setting provided a reality check showing that both local control and survival were worse in the dose-escalated arm when compared to the standard 60 Gy over 6 weeks.

Radiobiological modeling suggests that dose escalation to improve the tumor control probability (TCP) is likely to be more effective if the overall treatment time is fixed rather than fixing the dose per fraction, and dose escalation typically adds 1–2% local control for each 1% increase in dose (Fenwick et al. 2009). It is also increasingly recognized that there is an accelerated tumor clonogen proliferation, which becomes clinically relevant for NSCLC approximately 3–4 weeks after initiation of radiotherapy (Withers et al. 1988; Maciejewski et al. 1989; Fowler and Chappell 2000). Therefore, fractionation techniques that can avoid prolongation of treatment time are attractive, and dose escalations using modified fractionation are discussed below.

5.1 Isotoxic Radiotherapy

A number of these dose escalation strategies employ the isotoxic approach pioneered by the MAASTRO group allowing individualized dose escalation using hyperfractionated accelerated RT based on predefined mean lung dose (MLD) in stage I–III patients. They demonstrated, with 3D CRT delivered two times a day over 4 weeks, that increasing the radiation dose to prespecified normal tissue dose constraints could lead to increased tumor control probability with the same normal tissue complication probability (van Baardwijk et al. 2010). However, it should be noted that fewer than 10% of patients received the maximum dose of 79.2 Gy in 44 fractions twice daily (van Baardwijk et al. 2012). Since this study has been reported, IMRT techniques have become part of routine practice giving the potential to use the isotoxic approach to escalate the dose delivered to the target increasing tumor control probability with the same normal tissue complication probability (Chan et al. 2014).

To explore this approach, Cancer Research UK funded four parallel dose escalation studies to intensify accelerated schedules used in the United Kingdom. The first, CHART-ED (Hatton et al. 2016), reported no dose-limiting toxicities with a straight dose escalation (using additional twice-daily fractions of 1.8 Gy) to 64.8 Gy in 17 days, a dose increase with the potential to increase local tumor control by 30%. The IDEAL-CRT trial escalated to 73 Gy in 30 fractions over 6-week schedule with dose escalation calculated on an individual patient basis according to lung or esophageal radiation dose. Both reported encouraging 2-year survival figures: 52% and 65%, respectively.

Following the confirmation of low toxicity with the original IDEAL-CRT trial (Fenwick et al. 2020), a further accelerated schedule was investigated where the overall treatment time was shortened from 6 weeks to 5 weeks by treating with RT twice a day on 1 day each week (but not on the day of chemotherapy). This portion of the study recruited 36 patients with a minimum follow-up of 6 months, and no excess toxicity has been seen (ref as above for ideal). The I-START trial (Lester et al. 2018) individualized the RT dose in a similar way to IDEAL-CRT using a 20# schedule to deliver 52–65 Gy over 4 weeks following sequential chemotherapy. It recruited 80 patients and concluded that escalation of the prescription dose to 65 Gy is safe and feasible if the predefined organs-at-risk dose volume constraints are met with very low rates of esophagitis pneumonitis seen. Isotoxic IMRT (Haslett et al. 2020) treated patients twice daily over 4 weeks to a maximum of 79.2 Gy using prespecified normal tissue doses. Thirty-seven patients were recruited with a median prescribed tumor dose of 77.4 Gy (61.2–79.2 Gy). The maximum dose of 79.2 Gy was achieved in 14 (37.8%) patients. Grade 3 esophagitis was reported in two patients, and no patients developed grade 3–4 pneumonitis. There were three grade 5 events.

A systematic review of sequential chemoradiotherapy using modified dose escalation regimens suggests that this approach could yield similar outcomes to concomitant treatment (Zehentmayr et al. 2020). Two-year local control rates were documented as 56% vs. 59%, and overall survival was reported as 18.3 vs. 16.7 months, respectively. It was noted that the risk of acute esophagitis was higher in the modified regimes and that overall survival was better for those where the diagnostic workup included PET/CT.

6 Summary

A multimodality approach is now the standard for the management of most presentations of lung cancer. The evidence for radiotherapy as a potentially curative treatment for early lung cancer has gradually accumulated over the past 50 years. The median survival for patients treated in the studies that established our conventional gold standard of 60 Gy in 30 fractions over 6 weeks was less than 10 months. The addition of sequential chemotherapy increased the reported median survival to 14–15 months in the 1990s for patients with stage III disease. In the following decade, concurrent chemoradiotherapy gave a further improvement to 16–17 months and established that approach as our standard of care. The first decade of this century was characterized by real advances in the technical delivery of radiotherapy, which have led to SABR becoming our standard-of-care treatment for stage I disease. That decade also saw improvements in imaging that gave more accurate staging of disease improving median survival for stage III disease to 24 months in PET/CT staged patients. The addition of immunotherapy to our treatment algorithms has been the step change that has taken place over the last decade improving median survivals for the concurrently treated stage III patient to around 36 months, with many open studies looking to give us an evidence base for use of these combinations in the earlier stages of the disease.

Unfortunately, a significant proportion of patients presenting to us in our day-to-day practice will not be best served by the gold standard treatments of SABR or the concurrent chemoradiotherapy/immunotherapy combinations. For these patients, it is the use of non-SBRT radiation schedules that offers potentially curative treatment either as a single modality or combined with chemotherapy. In these settings, there is good evidence that accelerated treatment schedules improve outcomes; for example, CHART (Saunders et al. 1999; Sanganalmath et al. 2018) was shown to produce a better 2-year survival rate than conventional fractionation with a median and 2-year survival that matched those reported for sequential chemoradiotherapy. The case for dose escalation is not as clear-cut with the RTOG 0617 (Bradley et al. 2020) study clearly demonstrating that extending a conventionally fractionated treatment is not the approach to forward. However, as reported by Zehentmayr et al. (2020), dose escalation of accelerated fractionations has the potential of broadening treatment options, an approach support by the UK studies piloting four such regimes which were delivered with acceptable toxicity and 2-year survivals between 34% and 65% (Hatton et al. 2016; Fenwick et al. 2020; Lester et al. 2018; Haslett et al. 2020).

The use of non-SBRT radiation schedules will maintain an important role in the management of early-stage NSCLC, which can be offered as potential curative treatment or in combination with all other aspects of care in the control of symptoms and maintenance of quality of life. Awareness and interest in an accelerated approach have been increased by the COVID-19 pandemic with centers adopting schedules that can reduce the risk of COVID exposure in a vulnerable population and ease pressures on busy radiotherapy departments (Faivre-Finn et al. 2020). It must be remembered that a number of these schedules that have a modest evidence base and prospective data collection of the toxicity and outcomes of those being adopted into routine practice will greatly enhance our understanding. This is in addition to research efforts directed toward establishing the role of modified schedules with novel systemic treatments like immunotherapy and application of new technologies.

Acknowledgments The review and comments on the manuscript by Dr. Patricia Fisher are greatly appreciated.

References

Antonia SJ, Villegas A, Daniel D, Vicente D, Murakami S, Hui R et al (2018) Overall survival with durvalumab after chemoradiotherapy in stage III NSCLC. N Engl J Med 379:2342–2350. https://doi.org/10.1056/NEJMoa1809697

Antonio M, Saldana J, Linares J, Ruffinelli JC, Palmero R, Navarro A et al (2018) Geriatric assessment may help decision-making in elderly patients with inoperable, locally advanced non-small-cell lung cancer. Br J Cancer 118:639–647. https://doi.org/10.1038/bjc.2017.455

Arriagada R, Le Chevalier T, Quoix E, Ruffie P, de Cremoux H, Douillard JY et al (1991) Effect of chemotherapy on locally advanced non-small lung carcinoma: a randomized study of 353 patients. Int J Radiat Oncol Biol Phys 20:1183–1190. https://doi.org/10.1016/0360-3016(91)90226-t

Arriagada R, Komaki R, Cox JD (2004) Radiation dose escalation in non-small cell carcinoma of the lung. Semin Radiat Oncol 14:287–291

Aupérin A, Le Pechoux C, Rolland E, Curran WJ, Furuse K, Fournel P et al (2010) Meta-analysis of concomitant versus sequential radiochemotherapy in locally advanced non-small-cell lung cancer. J Clin Oncol 28:2181–2190

Ball D, Bishop J, Smith J, O'Brien P, Davis S, Ryan G et al (1999) A randomised phase III study of accelerated or standard fraction radiotherapy with or without concurrent carboplatin in inoperable non-small cell lung cancer: final report of an Australian multicentre trial. Radiother Oncol 52:129–136. https://doi.org/10.1016/s0167-8140(99)00093-6

Ball D, Mai GT, Vinod D et al (2019) Stereotactic ablative body radiotherapy versus standard radiotherapy in inoperable stage 1 non-small-cell lung cancer (TROG 09.02 CHISEL): a multicentre, phase 3, open-label, randomised, controlled trial. Lancet Oncol 20:494–503

Baumann M, Herrmann T, Koch R, Matthiessen W, Appold S, Wahlers B, et al, On behalf of the CHARTWEL-Bronchus Group (2011) Final results of the randomized phase III CHARTWEL-trial (ARO 97-1) comparing hyperfractionated-accelerated vs conventionally fractionated radiotherapy in non-small cell lung cancer (NSCLC). Radiother Oncol 100:76–85. https://doi.org/10.1016/j.radonc.2011.06.031

Belani CP, Wang W, Johnson DH, Wagner H, Schiller J, Veeder M et al (2005) Phase III study of the Eastern Cooperative Oncology Group (ECOG 2597): induction chemotherapy followed by either standard thoracic radiotherapy or hyperfractionated accelerated radiotherapy for patients with unresectable stage IIIA and B non-small-cell lung cancer. J Clin Oncol 23(16):3760–3767. https://doi.org/10.1200/JCO.2005.09.108

Belderbos JSA, De Jaeger K, Heemsbergen WD, Seppenwoolde Y, Bass P, Boersma LJ et al (2006) Final results of a phase I/II dose escalation trial in non-small-cell lung cancer using three-dimensional conformal radiotherapy. Int J Radiat Oncol Biol Phys 66:126–134. https://doi.org/10.1016/j.ijrobp.2006.04.034

Bissonnette JP, Purdie TG, Higgins JA, Li W, Bezjak A (2009) Cone-beam computed tomographic image guidance for lung cancer radiation therapy. Int J Radiat Oncol Biol Phys 73:927–934

Bradley JD, Hu C, Komaki RR, Masters GA, Blumenschein GR, Schild SE et al (2020) Long-term results of NRG Oncology RTOG 0617: standard- versus high-dose chemoradiotherapy with or without cetuximab for unresectable stage III non-small-cell lung cancer. J Clin Oncol 38(7):706–714. https://doi.org/10.1200/JCO.19.01162

Brunelli A, Charloux A, Bolliger CT, Rocco G, Sculier J-P, Varela G et al (2009) ERS/ESTS clinical guidelines on fitness for radical therapy in lung cancer patients (surgery and chemo-radiotherapy). Eur Respir J 34:17–41

Burt PA, Hancock BM, Stout R (1989) Radical radiotherapy for carcinoma of the bronchus: an equal alternative to radical surgery? Clin Oncol 1:86–90. https://doi.org/10.1016/s0936-6555(89)80041-x

Cannon DM, Mehta MP, Adkison JB, Khuntia D, Traynor AM, Tomé WA et al (2013) Dose-limiting toxicity after hypofractionated dose-escalated radiotherapy in non-small-cell lung cancer. J Clin Oncol 31(34):4343–4348

Chan C, Lang S, Rowbottom C, Guckenberger M, Faivre-Finn C, IASLC Advanced Radiation Technology Committee (2014) Intensity-modulated radiotherapy for lung cancer: current status and future developments. J Thorac Oncol 9(11):1598–1608. https://doi.org/10.1097/JTO.0000000000000346

Charloux A (2011) Fitness for radical treatment of lung cancer patients. Breathe 7:221–228

Cheng M, Jolly S, Quarshie WO, Kapadia N, Vigneau FD, Kong FS (2019) Modern radiation further improves survival in non-small cell lung cancer: an analysis of 288,670 patients. J Cancer 10(1):168–177

Cho WK, Noh JM, Ahn YC, Oh D, Pyo H (2016) Radiation therapy alone in cT1-3N0 non-small cell lung cancer patients who are unfit for surgical resection or stereotactic radiation therapy: comparison of risk-adaptive dose schedules. Cancer Res Treat 48:1187–1195. https://doi.org/10.4143/crt.2015.391

Cooke S, De Ruysscher D, Reymen B, Lambrecht M, Fredberg PG, Faivre-Finn C et al (2021) Local, regional and pulmonary failures in the randomised PET-boost trial for NSCLC. J Thorac Oncol 16(3 Suppl):113, Abstract OA02.05

Cooper JD, Pearson FD, Todd TR, Patterson GA, Ginsberg RJ, Basiuk J et al (1985) Radiotherapy alone for patients with operable carcinoma of the lung. Chest 87:289–292. https://doi.org/10.1378/chest.87.3.289

Cox JD, Azarnia N, Byhardt RW, Shin KH, Emami B, Pajak TF et al (1990) A randomized phase II/III trial of hyper-fractionated radiation therapy with total doses of 60.0 Gy to 79.2 Gy possible survival benefit with greater than or equal to 69.6 Gy in favorable patients with Radiation Therapy Oncology Group Stage III non-small cell lung carcinoma: report of Radiation Therapy Oncology Group 83–11. J Clin Oncol 8:1543–1555. https://doi.org/10.1200/JCO.1990.8.9.1543

de Koning HJ, van der Aalst CM, de Jong PA, Scholten E, Nackaerts K, Heuvelmans MA et al (2020) Reduced lung-cancer mortality with volume CT screening in a randomized trial. N Engl J Med 382:503–513. https://doi.org/10.1056/NEJMoa1911793

Dieleman EMT, Uitterhoeve ALJ, van Hoek MW, van Os RM, Wiersma J, Koolen MGJ et al (2018) Concurrent daily cisplatin and high-dose radiation therapy in patients with stage III non-small cell lung cancer. Int J Radiat Oncol Biol Phys 102(3):543–551. https://doi.org/10.1016/j.ijrobp.2018.07.188

Din OS, Harden SV, Hudson E, Mohammed N, Pemberton LS, Lester JF et al (2013) Accelerated hypo-fractionated radiotherapy for non-small cell lung cancer: results from 4 UK centres. Radiother Oncol 109(1):8–12

Dosoretz DE, Katin MJ, Blitzer PH, Rubenstein JH, Salenis S, Rashid M et al (1992) Radiation therapy in the management of medically inoperable carcinoma of the lung: results and implications for future treatment strategies. Int J Radiat Oncol Biol Phys 24:3–9. https://doi.org/10.1016/0360-3016(92)91013-D

Driessen EJM, Bootsma GP, Hendriks LEL, van den Berkmortel FM, Bogaarts BA, van Loon JGM et al (2016) Stage III non-small cell lung cancer in the elderly: patient characteristics predictive for tolerance and survival of chemoradiation in daily clinical practice. Radiother Oncol 121:26–31

Du Ruysscher D, Wanders R, Van Haren E, Minken A, Bentzen SM, Lambin P et al (2007) Hi-CHART: a phase I/II study on the feasibility of high-dose continuous hyper-fractionated accelerated radiotherapy in patients with in-operable non-small cell lung cancer. Int J Radiat Oncol Biol Phys 71:132–138. https://doi.org/10.1016/j.ijrobp.2007.09.048

Faivre-Finn C, Fenwick JD, Franks KN, Harrow S, Hatton MQF, Hiley C et al (2020) Reduced fractionation in lung cancer patients treated with curative-intent radiotherapy during the COVID-19 pandemic. Clin Oncol 32:481–489. https://doi.org/10.1016/j.clon.2020.05.001

Fenwick JD, Nahum AE, Malik ZI, Eswar CV, Hatton MQ, Laurence VM et al (2009) Escalation and intensification of radiotherapy for stage III non-small cell lung cancer: opportunities for treatment improvement. Clin Oncol 21:343–360. https://doi.org/10.1016/j.clon.2008.12.011

Fenwick JD, Landau DB, Baker AT, Bates AT, Eswar C, Garcia-Alonso A et al (2020) Long-term results from the IDEAL-CRT phase 1/2 trial of isotoxically dose-escalated radiation therapy and concurrent chemotherapy for stage II/III non-small cell lung cancer. Int J Radiat Oncol Biol Phys 106(4):733–742

Field JK, Duffy SW, Baldwin DR, Whynes DK, Devaraj A, Brain KE, Eisen T et al (2016) UK Lung Cancer RCT Pilot Screening Trial: baseline findings from the screening arm provide evidence for the potential implementation of lung cancer screening. Thorax 71:161–170

Fowler JF, Chappell R (2000) Non-small cell lung tumors repopulate rapidly during radiation therapy. Int J Radiat Oncol Biol Phys 46:516–517

Gauden S, Ramsay J, Tripciony L (1995) The curative treatment by radiotherapy alone of stage I non-small cell lung cancer. Chest 108:1278–1282. https://doi.org/10.1378/chest.108.5.1278

Goldstraw P, Chansky K, Crowley J et al (2016) The IASLC Lung Cancer Staging Project: proposals for revision of the TNM stage groupings in the forthcoming (eighth) edition of the TNM classification for lung cancer. J Thorac Oncol 11:39–51

Graham PH, Gebski VJ, Stat M, Langlands AO (1995) Radical radiotherapy for early non-small cell lung cancer. Int J Radiat Oncol Biol Phys 31:261–266. https://doi.org/10.1016/0360-3016(94)E0137-9

Haffty BG, Goldberg NB, Gerstley J, Fisher DB, Peschel RD (1988) Results of radical radiotherapy in clinical stage I technically operable non-small cell lung cancer. Int J Radiat Oncol Biol Phys 15:69–73. https://doi.org/10.1016/0360-3016(88)90348-3

Hanna NH, Neubauer M, Ansari R et al (2008) Phase III study of cisplatin, etoposide, and concurrent chest radiation with or without consolidation docetaxel in patients with inoperable stage III non-small-cell lung cancer: the Hoosier Oncology Group and U.S. Oncology. J Clin Oncol 26(35):5755–5760

Haslett K, Ashcroft L, Bayman N, Franks K, Groom N, Hanna G et al (2020) Isotoxic intensity modulated radiotherapy (IMRT) in stage III non-small cell lung cancer (NSCLC): a feasibility study. Int J Radiat Oncol Biol Phys. https://doi.org/10.1016/j.ijrobp.2020.11.040

Hatton M, Lyn E, Nankivell M, Stephens R, Pugh C, Navani N et al (2011) Induction chemotherapy and continuous hyperfractionated accelerated radiotherapy (CHART): the MRC INCH randomised trial. Int J Radiat Oncol Biol Phys 81:712–718

Hatton M, Hill R, Fenwick J, Morgan S, Wilson P, Atherton P et al (2016) Continuous hyperfractionated accelerated radiotherapy – escalated dose (CHART-ED): a phase I study. Radiother Oncol 118:471–477

Iocolano M, Wild AT, Hannum M, Zhang Z, Simone CB, Gelblum D et al (2020) Hypofractionated vs. conventional radiation therapy for stage III non-small cell lung cancer treated without chemotherapy. Acta Oncol 59(2):164–170. https://doi.org/10.1080/0284186X.2019.1675907

Iyengar P, Westover KD, Court LE, Patel MK, Shivnani AT, Saunders MW et al (2016) A phase III randomized study of image guided conventional (60 Gy/30 fx) versus accelerated, hypofractionated (60 Gy/15 fx) radiation for poor performance status stage II and III NSCLC patients—an interim analysis. Int J Radiat Oncol Biol Phys 96:E451. https://doi.org/10.1016/j.ijrobp.2016.06.1763

Jeremic B, Milicic B (2008) From conventionally fractionated radiation therapy to hyper-fractionated radiation therapy alone and with concurrent chemotherapy in patients with early stage non-small cell lung cancer. Cancer 112:876–884

Jeremić B, Dubinsky P, Milisavljević S, Kiladze I (2021) Combined radiation therapy and chemotherapy as an exclusive treatment option in locally advanced inoperable non-small cell lung cancer. Medical Radiology. https://doi.org/10.1007/174_2021_277

Kaskowitz L, Graham MV, Emami B, Halverson KJ, Rush C (1993) Radiation therapy alone for stage I non-small cell lung cancer. Int J Radiat Oncol Biol Phys 27:517–523. https://doi.org/10.1016/0360-3016(93)90374-5

Katz HR, Alberts RW (1983) A comparison of high dose continuous and split course irradiation in non-oat cell carcinoma of the lung. Am J Clin Oncol 6(4):445–457. https://doi.org/10.1097/00000421-198308000-00010

Knight SB, Crosbie PA, Balata H, Chudziak J, Hussell T, Dive C (2017) Progress and prospects of early detection in lung cancer. Open Biol 7(9):170070. https://doi.org/10.1098/rsob.170070

Konert T, Vogel W, MacManus MP, Nestle U, Belderbos J, Gregoire V et al (2015) PET/CT imaging for target volume delineation in curative intent radiotherapy of non-small cell lung cancer: IAEA consensus report 2014. Radiother Oncol 116:27–34

Kong FM, Ten Haken RK, Schipper MJ et al (2005) High-dose radiation improved local tumor control and overall survival in patients with inoperable/unresectable non-small-cell lung cancer: long-term results of a radiation dose escalation study. Int J Radiat Oncol Biol Phys 63:324–333

Kong F, Hu C, Machtay M, Matuszak M, Xiao Y, Ten Haken R et al (2021) Randomized phase II trial (RTOG1106) on mid treatment PET/CT guided adaptive radiotherapy in locally advanced non-small cell lung cancer. J Thorac Oncol 16(3 Suppl):112, Abstract OA02.04

Krol AD, Aussems P, Noordijk EM, Hermans J, Leer JW et al (1996) Local irradiation alone for peripheral stage I lung cancer: could we omit local nodal irradiation? Int J Radiat Oncol Biol Phys 34:297–302. https://doi.org/10.1016/0360-3016(95)00227-8

Lester JF, Courtier N, Eswar C, Mohammed N, Fenwick J, Griffiths G et al (2018) Initial results of the phase Ib/II, I-START trial - isotoxic accelerated radiotherapy for the treatment of stage II–IIIB NSCLC. J Clin Oncol. https://doi.org/10.1200/JCO.2018.36.15_suppl.e20551

Maciejewski B, Withers HR, Taylor JMG et al (1989) Dose fractionation and regeneration in radiotherapy for cancer of the oral cavity and oropharynx: tumor dose–response and repopulation. Int J Radiat Oncol Biol Phys 16:831–843

Mauguen A, Le Péchoux C, Saunders MI, Schild SE, Turrisi AT, Baumann M et al (2012) Hyperfractionated or accelerated radiotherapy in lung cancer: an individual patient data meta-analysis. J Clin Oncol 30(22):2788–2797. https://doi.org/10.1200/JCO.2012.41.6677

Morita K, Fuwa N, Suzuki Y, Nishio M, Sakai K, Tamaki Y et al (1997) Radical radiotherapy for medically inoperable non-small cell lung cancer in clinical stage I: a retrospective analysis of 149 patients. Radiother Oncol 42:31–36. https://doi.org/10.1016/S0167-8140(96)01828-2

Noordijk EM, Van Poest Clement E, Hermans J, Wever AMJ, Leer JWH (1988) Radiotherapy as an alternative to surgery in elderly patients with resectable lung cancer. Radiother Oncol 13:83–89. https://doi.org/10.1016/0167-8140(88)90029-1

NSCLC Collaborative Group (1995) Chemotherapy in non-small cell lung cancer: a meta-analysis using updated data on individual patients from 52 randomized clinical trials. Br Med J 311:899–909

Nyman J, Hallqvist A, Lund J, Brustugun O, Bergman B et al (2016) SPACE – a randomized study of SBRT vs conventional fractionated radiotherapy in medically inoperable stage I NSCLC. Radiother Oncol 121:1–8

Peeters ST, Dooms C, Van Baardwijk A, Dingemans AMC, Martinussen H, Vansteenkiste J et al (2016) Selective mediastinal node irradiation in non-small cell lung cancer in the IMRT/VMAT era: how to use E(B)US-NA information in addition to PET-CT for delineation? Radiother Oncol 120:273–278

Perez CA, Stanley K, Grundy G et al (1982) Impact of irradiation technique and tumour extent in tumour control and survival of patients with unresectable non-oat cell carcinoma of the lung: report by the Radiation Therapy Oncology Group. Cancer 50:1091–1099

Robinson SD, Tahir BA, Absalom KAR, Lankathilake A, Das T, Lee C et al (2019) Radical accelerated radiotherapy for non-small cell lung cancer (NSCLC): a 5-year retrospective review of two dose fractionation schedules. Radiother Oncol 143:37–43. https://doi.org/10.1016/j.radonc.2019.08.025

Roswit B, Patno ME, Rapp R (1968) The survival of patients with inoperable lung cancer: a large randomized study of radiation therapy verses placebo. Radiology 90:688–697

Sandler HM, Curran WJ, Turrisi AT (1990) The influence of tumour size and pre-treatment staging on outcome following radiation therapy alone for stage I non-small cell lung cancer. Int J Radiat Oncol Biol Phys 19:9–13. https://doi.org/10.1016/0360-3016(90)90127-6

Sanganalmath P, Lester JE, Bradshaw AG, Das T, Esler C, Roy AEF et al (2018) Continuous hyperfractionated accelerated radiotherapy (CHART) for non-small cell lung cancer (NSCLC): 7 years' experience from nine UK centres. Clin Oncol 30:144–150. https://doi.org/10.1016/j.clon.2017.12.019

Saunders M, Dische S, Barrett A, Harvey A, Griffiths G, Parmar M (1999) Continuous, hyper-fractionated, accelerated radiotherapy (CHART) versus conventional radiotherapy in non-small cell lung cancer: mature data from the randomised multicentre trial. Radiother Oncol 52:137–148. https://doi.org/10.1016/s0167-8140(99)00087-0

Saunders MI, Rojas A, Lyn BE, Wilson E, Phillips H (2002) Dose escalation with CHARTWEL (continuous hyper-fractionated accelerated radiotherapy week end less) combined with neo-adjuvant chemotherapy in the treatment of locally advanced non-small cell lung cancer. Clin Oncol 14:352–360. https://doi.org/10.1053/clon.2002.0121

Sause WT, Scott C, Taylor S, Johnson D, Livingston R, Komaki R et al (1995) Radiation Therapy Oncology Group (RTOG) 88-08 and Eastern Cooperative Oncology Group (ECOG) 4588: preliminary results of a phase III trial in regionally advanced unresectable non-small-cell lung cancer. J Natl Cancer Inst 87(3):198–205. https://doi.org/10.1093/jnci/87.3.198

Schaake-Koning C, van den Bogaert W, Dalesio O et al (1992) Effects of concomitant cisplatin and radiotherapy on inoperable non-small cell lung cancer. N Engl J Med 326:524–530

Sibley GS, Maguire PD, Anscher MA, Light K, Antoine P, Marks LB (1999) High-dose accelerated radiotherapy for non-small cell lung cancer: 7360 cGy and beyond. Int J Radiat Biol Phys 45:241

Slotman BJ, Njo H, Karim A (1994) Curative radiotherapy for technically operable stage 1 non-small cell lung cancer. Int J Radiat Oncol Biol Phys 29:33–37. https://doi.org/10.1016/0360-3016(94)90223-2

Spigel DR, Faivre-Finn C, Gray JE, Vicente D, Planchard D, Paz-Ares L et al (2022) Five-year survival outcomes from the PACIFIC Trial: durvalumab after chemoradiotherapy in stage III non-small-cell lung cancer. J Clin Oncol 40(12):1301–1311

Stinchcombe TE, Zhang Y, Vokes EE, Schiller JH, Bradley JD, Kelly K et al (2017) Pooled analysis of individual patient data on concurrent chemoradiotherapy for stage III non–small-cell lung cancer in elderly patients compared with younger patients who participated in US National Cancer Institute Cooperative Group Studies. J Clin Oncol 35:2885–2892

Suhail A, Crocker CE, Das B, Payne JI, Manos D (2019) Initial presentation of lung cancer in the emergency department: a descriptive analysis. CMAJ Open 7(1):E117–E123. https://doi.org/10.9778/cmajo.2018006

Talton BM, Constable WC, Kersh CR (1990) Curative radiotherapy in non-small cell carcinoma of the lung. Int J Radiat Oncol Biol Phys 19:15–21. https://doi.org/10.1016/0360-3016(90)90128-7

Thirion P, Holmberg O, Collins CD, O'Shea C, Moriarty M, Pomeroy M et al (2004) Escalated dose for non-small-cell lung cancer with accelerated hypofractionated three-dimensional conformal radiation therapy. Radiother Oncol 71:163–166. https://doi.org/10.1016/j.radonc.2003.09.006

Tyldesley S, Boyd C, Schulze K, Walker H, Mackillop WJ (2001) Estimating the need for radiotherapy for lung cancer: an evidence-based, epidemiologic approach. Int J Radiat Oncol Biol Phys 49:973–985

UK SABR Consortium (2019) Stereotactic ablative body radiation therapy (SABR): a resource. v6.1. https://www.sabr.org.uk/wp-content/uploads/2019/04/SABRconsortium-guidelines-2019-v6.1.0.pdf

van Baardwijk A, Wanders S, Boersma L, Borger J, Oellers M, Dingemans AMC et al (2010) Mature results of an individualized radiation dose prescription study based on normal tissue constraints in stages I to III non-small-cell lung cancer. J Clin Oncol 28(8):1380–1386

van Baardwijk A, Reymen B, Wanders S, Borger J, Ollers M, Dingemans AM et al (2012) Mature results of a phase II trial on individualised accelerated radiotherapy based on normal tissue constraints in concurrent chemo-radiation for stage III nonsmall cell lung cancer. Eur J Cancer 48(15):2339–2346

Westover KD, Loo BW Jr, Gerber DE, Iyengar P, Choy H, Diehn M et al (2015) Precision hypofractionated radiation therapy in poor performing patients with non-small cell lung cancer: phase 1 dose escalation trial. Int J Radiat Oncol Biol Phys 93:72–81. https://doi.org/10.1016/j.ijrobp.2015.05.004

Wisnivesky JP, Bonomi M, Henschke C (2005) Radiation therapy for the treatment of stage I–II non-small cell lung cancer. Chest 128:1461–1467

Withers HR, Taylor JMG, Maciejewski B (1988) The hazard of accelerated tumor clonogen repopulation during radiotherapy. Acta Oncol 27:131–146

Wurschmidt F, Bunemann H, Bunemann C, Beck-Bornholdt HP, Heilmann HP et al (1994) Inoperable non-small cell lung cancer: a retrospective analysis of 427 patients treated with high dose radiotherapy. Int J Radiat Oncol Biol Phys 28:583–588. https://doi.org/10.1016/0360-3016(94)90182-1

Zehentmayr F, Grambozov B, Kaiser J, Fastner G, Sedlmayer F (2020) Radiation dose escalation with modified fractionation schedules for locally advanced NSCLC: a systematic review. Thorac Cancer 11:1375–1385. https://doi.org/10.1111/1759-7714.13451

Zeng K, Poon I, Ung Y, Zhang L, Cheung P (2018) Accelerated hypofractionated radiation therapy for centrally located lung tumors not suitable for stereotactic body radiation therapy (SBRT) or concurrent chemoradiotherapy (CRT). Int J Radiat Oncol Biol Phys 102:e719–ee20

Zhang HX, Yin WB, Zhang LJ, Yang ZY, Zhang ZX, Wang M et al (1989) Curative radiotherapy of early operable non-small cell lung cancer. Radiother Oncol 14:89–94. https://doi.org/10.1016/0167-8140(89)90052-2

Never-Ending Story: Surgery Versus SBRT in Early-Stage NSCLC

James Taylor, Pamela Samson, William Stokes, and Drew Moghanaki

A reliable way to make people believe in falsehoods is frequent repetition, because familiarity is not easily distinguished from truth.

Daniel Kahneman, Thinking, Fast and Slow

Contents

1 Introduction 433
2 Defining the Standard of Care 434
3 How Did Surgery Become and Continue to Be the "Standard"? 434
3.1 Tradition and Dogma 434
3.2 Retrospective Comparisons 435
3.3 The Promise of Staging the Mediastinum More Comprehensively 436
4 Conundrum of Post-SBRT Radiographic Scars 437
5 Difficulty with Defining Medical Operability 438
6 The Future Landscape Is Evolving 439
6.1 Future of Pathologic Assessment 439
6.2 The Future of Local Control and Procedural Risk 439
6.3 Defining Synergistic Approaches 440
7 How to Think About Surgery Versus SBRT in the Modern Era 440
References 441

J. Taylor
Sidney Kimmel Cancer Center at Thomas Jefferson University, Philadelphia, PA, USA

P. Samson
Siteman Cancer Center at Washington University, St Louis, MO, USA

W. Stokes
Winship Cancer Institute of Emory University, Atlanta, GA, USA

D. Moghanaki (✉)
UCLA Health Jonsson Cancer Center, Los Angeles, CA, USA
e-mail: DMoghanaki@mednet.ucla.edu

1 Introduction

The purpose of this chapter is to examine the never-ending story and debates regarding the roles of surgery versus stereotactic body radiation therapy (SBRT) for medically operable patients with early-stage non-small cell lung cancer (NSCLC). Technical approaches to optimize the safety and efficacy of each of these treatments are described elsewhere in this textbook. We will use a historical framework to inform the current discussions with an evaluation of belief systems that may be anchored to the hope and promise of each treatment. We will also describe how the changing landscape of cancer treatment is already influencing future narratives about surgery or SBRT as the combination of systemic therapies is raising questions about the value of each treatment being given alone. By the end of this chapter, the authors hope that readers will better appreciate the nuances of this never-ending story and be able to engage in a more informed discussion if ever pulled into a debate about surgery vs. SBRT for early-stage NSCLC.

2 Defining the Standard of Care

Before discussing the premise behind surgery as the standard of care for early-stage NSCLC, the definition of the standard of care itself should first be evaluated. From a legal perspective, the concept of standard of care, like medicine itself, has evolved and is open to interpretation. According to Peter Moffett's *The Standard of Care: A Legal History and Definitions: The Bad and Good News*, there are three definitions of the standard of care that have occurred over time, which may vary by region (Moffett and Moore 2011):

- The initial definition was based on custom, "that which is typically done is what is considered standard."
- The twentieth-century definition included a clause, "that which is customarily done plus anything that seems reasonable even if not typically done."
- The more recent definition is even more broad, "that which a minimally competent physician in the same field would do under a similar circumstance."

Given the ambiguities of these definitions, it is not clear that surgery can be considered the "only" standard of care for early-stage NSCLC. Clearly, SBRT could also meet this definition, and thus all patients should be informed about both treatment options. The legal ramifications of restricting knowledge about SBRT can be epitomized by a unanimous ruling in the UK Supreme Court, which opined that physicians are legally negligent whenever they fail to disclose alternative treatments, particularly if a complication occurs following a treatment that was the only one offered (Dyer 2015).

The standard of care must also be considered from an ethical perspective that respects patient autonomy, justice, beneficence, and nonmaleficence. Patients must be given the freedom to choose and not be coerced. The treatment being offered must provide a benefit that outweighs the risks, and alternative options should be presented to preserve patient autonomy. For the majority of patients, surgical resection of early-stage lung cancer is straightforward and entails a limited convalescence period that lasts only several weeks. However, some may endure prolonged periods of postoperative suffering and premature death that today can be avoided with a recommendation for SBRT instead of surgery. A key ethical dilemma that this presents is that patients with stage I NSCLC are almost always asymptomatic and readily agree to surgery after an informed consent process that informs them that surgical resection will help them live a longer and better life. Yet, some may endure a catastrophic complication and death within 90 days even though they could have lived at least several years with no treatment at all.

3 How Did Surgery Become and Continue to Be the "Standard"?

To inform how surgery became and continues to be the standard of care, several points must be considered: first, a strong history of tradition and dogma in the field of thoracic surgery; second, the obfuscation in retrospective comparisons of surgery versus SBRT (Stokes and Rusthoven 2018); and third, the unconfirmed promise of intraoperative mediastinal staging in the era of PET staging.

3.1 Tradition and Dogma

The first successful pneumonectomy for lung cancer was performed by Dr. Evarts Graham in 1933, and the case report was published in the *Journal of the American Medical Association* (Graham et al. 1984). Following the success of that operation, his patient went on to live for 30 years to confirm that surgical removal of early-stage lung cancer could lead to long-term cures. The tumor was removed with a pneumonectomy given the centrally located tumor. Graham referred to the surgical procedure as "the only method that at present can offer any hope" for lung cancer and would go on to say that at present there had not been any "record in the literature of the successful treatment by radiotherapy of a single case." Like other brilliant surgeons of his era, Graham subscribed to Halsted's theory of centrifugal tumor spread where the only hopes of achieving cure relied on maximal resection with exceedingly large surgical margins that could only be achieved with a pneumonectomy (Halsted 1907). This preference for radical resections was not unique to lung cancer surgery and extended throughout surgical disciplines to include the radical neck dissection for squamous cell tumors of the head and neck and the pelvic exenteration for gynecological malignancies (Subramanian et al. 2006; Moghanaki and Chang 2016). While Graham continues to be heralded for introducing the utility of surgical resection of early-stage lung cancer, a lesser known fact is that all of his next 19 patients died from a postoperative complication to provide him with a 95% mortality rate with his first 20 cases (Horn et al. 2008). Nonetheless, the influence of survivor bias prevailed, and the pneumonectomy became the operative treatment of choice for the management of lung cancer for decades to come (Horn et al. 2008).

The postoperative mortality rate following radical pneumonectomies continued to be as high as 20% (Gutierrez and Pickren 1974). Yet, it would be many years later before the radical pneumonectomy would be challenged by limited resection. In fact, pneumonectomy was considered by many surgeons as the only reasonable option as evidenced by the opinion of famous surgeons Ochsner and DeBakey who stated, "The performance of a simple lobectomy in carcinoma of the lung is just as illogical as partial removal of the breast in mammary carcinoma" (Ochsner and Debakey 1999). However, the work of Dr. Shimkin using data collected from the Ochsner and Overholt clinics demonstrated that patients with localized lung cancer had improved survival compared with those with advanced disease in a surgical agnostic manner (Shimkin et al. 1962). Dr. Shimkin and colleagues suggested that more extensive resections increased mortality without improving total survival, and the use of lobectomy and sublobar resections eventually emerged (Shimkin et al. 1962).

Meanwhile, there continued to be a paucity of data comparing radiation therapy with surgery for lung cancer treatment until a landmark trial was published in 1963 by Morrison and colleagues from the Hammersmith Hospital in London (Morrison et al. 1963). This was the first and only completed randomized clinical trial of surgery vs. radiotherapy with a total of 58 patients enrolled. Treatment with radiotherapy used an 8-million-volt linear accelerator to a dose of 45 Gy that is considered palliative by today's standards. The study was conducted over a decade before the introduction of computed tomography imaging, and the radiation therapy treatment fields consisted of large overlapping anterior-posterior portals aimed at X-ray defined targets. Surgery was performed by either pneumonectomy or lobectomy, also using outdated techniques. The results demonstrated improved overall survival at 1 year with surgery, but by 4 years the benefit of surgery had lost its statistical significance (23% vs. 7%, "differences are almost significant at the 5% level"). The authors concluded that "radical surgery has been compared with supervoltage radiotherapy in the treatment of operable carcinoma and the results of surgical resection were significantly better" (Morrison et al. 1963). Following this study, no other head-to-head randomized trials of surgery versus any form of radiotherapy in medically operable patients with early-stage lung cancer would be completed. Thus, the data from this single randomized trial with 58 patients using outdated techniques provided the scientific evidence base that surgery must be the standard of care for early-stage lung cancer and supported a dogma that has been passed down through successive generations of trainees to this date.

3.2 Retrospective Comparisons

Since the publication of the Hammersmith randomized trial in 1963, technological advances led to the development of SBRT, and a series of phase I and II clinical trials demonstrated better-than-expected results with SBRT (Chang et al. 2015; Timmerman et al. 2018). These data, reported predominantly from cohorts of frail and elderly populations who were medically inoperable, led to a growth of interest in SBRT with increasing numbers of operable patients preferring a nonsurgical option (Haque et al. 2018). This would eventually inspire a series of flawed retrospective studies to compare the outcomes after SBRT versus surgery that provide a dominant fuel for the never-ending debates.

A key problem with retrospective studies of surgery versus SBRT is that they compare cohorts of patients who were deemed medically operable and a population that was either counseled to be a poor surgical candidate or who decided that they might not fare well after a trip to the operating room (Cornwell and Moghanaki 2018). This comparative conundrum has been well described by Rusthoven and colleagues who termed this type of bias as "confounding by operability" (Stokes and Rusthoven 2018). It is described by a scenario where patients who are selected for treatment according to guidelines have limited access to alternative options such as SBRT given the potential medical and legal ramifications of endorsing a nonstandard of care. Various statistical methods have been used to adjust for imbalances in patient cohorts to approximate a randomized scenario. However, datasets that perform such exercises are unable to account for confounding that may include weak grip strength, unstable gait, poor support systems at home, limited vision, hearing impairment, or cognitive deficits, all of which are routinely considered when evaluating a patient's fitness for surgery. Population-based observational studies that compare treatment outcomes without randomization are unavoidably clouded by bias and frequently incomplete or incorrect data (Harbeck et al. 2000; Rossouw et al. 2009; Soni et al. 2019; Park et al. 2012; Farjah et al. 2009).

In 2019, a publication by Soni et al. highlighted the limitations of comparative efficacy research by querying MEDLINE between 2000 and 2016 for observational studies that retrospectively compared two treatment regimens for any cancer diagnosis using SEER, SEER-Medicare, or the National Cancer Database (Soni et al. 2019). They selectively matched these studies to randomized trials that evaluated the same treatment regimens. Their results found no significant correlation between the hazard ratio estimates reported by observational studies versus randomized trials outcomes. Only 40% of the matched studies were in agreement regarding treatment effects (κ, 0.037; 95% CI, −0.027 to 0.1), and only 62% of the observational study HRs fell within the 95% CIs of the randomized trials. The authors concluded that "there was no agreement beyond what is expected by chance, regardless of reporting quality or statistical rigor of the observational study" (Soni et al. 2019).

Unfortunately, a lack of awareness about the limitations of retrospective comparisons of non-randomized treatments has contributed to the propagation of misinformation that at times has been used to deliberately interfere with the conduct of randomized clinical trials of surgery versus SBRT that would benefit the lung cancer community. A commonly cited example stems from a 2017 editorial commentary that opined as follows: "Until we have a trial that proves SBRT is better than observation, we are committing academic medical malpractice by embarking on another surgical RCT (Flores 2018). As doctors and investigators, we must not subject healthy curable individuals to an unproven therapy under the guise of an RCT. The only logical next step is to first prove whether or not SBRT is better than observation. Only then can we advance to the next step of comparing SBRT with surgery in healthy patients" (Flores 2018). While some may believe that these statements are appropriate arguments in an intellectual debate, it actually undermines progress and sheds light on heuristics and a lack of support for scientific progress.

3.3 The Promise of Staging the Mediastinum More Comprehensively

Another commonly discussed advantage of surgical resection over SBRT is the rigid concern about more comprehensive assessment of lymph nodes to inform patients and clinicians about adjuvant therapy decisions. However, the randomized Z0030 trial which randomized 1111 patients with clinically node-negative patients to mediastinal sampling versus dissection found no difference in the overall survival. Certainly, even with the best imaging and staging workup, surgery can detect occult nodal disease through a more comprehensive intraoperative mediastinal lymph node dissection in approximately 10–15% of patients (Pignon et al. 2008, 2020; Douillard et al. 2006). However, relying on earlier access to postoperative cisplatin-containing adjuvant chemotherapy options that have been shown to improve survival, the 5% overall survival benefit in the few patients who are upstaged and recover enough to receive it raises serious questions about a "surgery for all" recommendation. A closer look at the evidence base for adjuvant therapy that was updated by Pignon et al. in 2008 summarized the data on patients who enrolled in clinical trials between 1994 and 2001, well before the introduction of FDG PET/CT staging for routine clinical care (Pignon et al. 2020). In 2014, Louie et al. described that if 100 patients with clinical stage I NSCLC underwent up-front surgery with mediastinal staging, and if 15 were upstaged with nodal sampling, only 10 out of 100 would receive adjuvant therapy (Louie et al. 2015). This is based on evidence from multiple studies that demonstrate that only two out of three postoperative patients agree to adjuvant chemotherapy (Felip et al. 2020). Louie et al. extrapolated the 5% OS benefit at 5 years in the 10 out of 100 upstaged patients to ultimately translate it into only a 0.5% survival benefit at 5 years. Therefore, 200 patients would need to undergo invasive mediastinal staging to extend 1 person's life, a benefit that would disappear if the postoperative mortality of the 200 patients exceeded 0.5%. The 200 patients would also be at risk for postoperative complications, a prolonged convalescence period, and more limited treatment options if they developed a secondary lung cancer, which occurs in approximately 15–20% of lung cancer survivors (Louie et al. 2015; Pasini et al. 2003).

4 Conundrum of Post-SBRT Radiographic Scars

While the above concerns continue to perpetuate a false premise that surgery is the optimal management option for patients with early-stage NSCLC, a visible challenge exists for clinicians who manage patients with SBRT and often have to interpret posttreatment radiographic scars during surveillance imaging (pun intended). While posttreatment scars are frequently visible after lung cancer resection, they do not often evolve to create diagnostic dilemmas. Notwithstanding, posttreatment scars after SBRT can at times be notoriously difficult to interpret given their propensity to wax and wane for many in patients without local progression (Ronden et al. 2018a). Investigators have described a list of radiographic high-risk features that are associated with the likelihood of benign versus malignant radiographic progressions of post-SBRT scars (Ronden et al. 2018a; Huang et al. 2013). However, an attempted validation study that investigated these high-risk features was sobering (Ronden et al. 2018b). As reported in 2018 by Ronden et al., five clinicians with expertise in lung SBRT were presented 747 follow-up scans on 88 patients without tumor progression who had a median overall survival of 62 months after SBRT (range: 31–96 months). The clinicians were blinded to the outcome of these patients and reported at least one high-risk feature in 98% of patients. High-risk features were reported for 64% of patients in the first year of surveillance and 86% thereafter, demonstrating the increased frequency of abnormal radiographic findings over time. Serial growth on successive scans was identified in 14% of patients, and two or three previously defined high-risk features were scored in 53% and 23% of patients, respectively. The potential consequences of these false-positive findings were further characterized with 57%, 23%, and 14% of patients being recommended a shorter interval CT scan, a FDG PET/CT scan, or biopsy by at least one observer (Ronden et al. 2018b).

To move the field forward, a pictorial essay has been published that describes 15 distinct radiographic changes that can be used to distinguish post-SBRT scars with high-risk features (Ronden et al. 2018a). Primers have been written for radiologists and nonradiation oncologists to raise awareness that the evolution of scars after SBRT is infrequently associated with malignant progression (Huang et al. 2015). However, more research is needed to avoid the risk of invasive procedures for patients who develop concerning abnormal scars, particularly as there have been reports of post-SBRT salvage lobectomies in patients who were found to have no histopathological evidence of malignancy (Antonoff et al. 2016; Taira et al. 2014). This management challenge has emerged as a pivotal point of debate that presents a formidable challenge for those who espouse SBRT as a preferred alternative to surgery.

5 Difficulty with Defining Medical Operability

As the fields of thoracic surgery and radiation oncology move forward, and the criteria for matching patients with early-stage NSCLC to surgery or SBRT, an important consideration is that the definition of medically operable can be variable among studies, institutions, and surgeons alike. This creates difficult challenges for individual patient clinical decision-making, which has become increasingly difficult when knowing that SBRT is a reasonable alternative.

Classic determinants of operability have historically included comorbidity (and whether or not these are controlled), pulmonary function (FEV1 percent predicted, DLCO, and ventilation-perfusion ratio), as well as functional elements including in-office walk tests and stair climbing. Interestingly, there is data to suggest that surgeons can both under- and overestimate operability. For example, Puri and colleagues applied the definition of high-risk operable patients from the American College of Surgery Oncology Group (ACOSOG) trials z4032, z4033, and z4099 to their institutional series of over 1000 patients that received surgical resection (Puri et al. 2014). In these clinical trials, high-risk status included FEV1 ≤50% predicted, DLCO ≤50%, age ≥75 years old, poor ejection fraction, pulmonary hypertension, as well as cutoffs for P_{O2} and P_{CO2}. Of note, patients enrolled in these trials would have received sublobar resection. In the Puri et al. institutional series, almost 20% of patients met these risk criteria. When compared to "normal-risk" patients, it was found that the patients meeting the high-risk criteria were less likely to undergo lobectomy (60% versus 76%, $p < 0.001$), but it did not show any difference in postoperative complications (28% versus 26%) or 30-day mortality (1% versus 2%). The conclusion of this analysis was that even with a substantial proportion of high-risk patients receiving lobectomy, there was no difference in morbidity or mortality when compared to normal-risk patients.

Conversely, previous work has demonstrated how surgeons may overestimate operability. In an institutional series of all stage I NSCLC patients (who were treated with either surgery or SBRT), Samson and colleagues identified factors independently associated with the receipt of SBRT, which included age, FEV1 percent predicted, and a diagnosis of congestive heart failure (Samson et al. 2019). This was used to create a training/validation model to predict patient treatment allocation based on these variables associated with SBRT. When the model was applied to this decade-long series of approximately 1200 patients, it was found that the 3-year overall survival rate of surgical patients for whom the model allocated surgery was 88%, while the 3-year overall survival of surgical patients that the model allocated to SBRT was only 36%. When comparing patients that were allocated to SBRT and the treatment they actually received, it was found that there was no significant difference in the 3-year overall survival rate (32% for SBRT versus 36% for surgical patients).

6 The Future Landscape Is Evolving

6.1 Future of Pathologic Assessment

Despite current practice patterns within the oncology community that prioritize tissue diagnosis and local control, their importance is starting to be questioned given lung cancer is often a systemic disease. Important advances in imaging, targeted therapies, immunotherapy, and biomarker assays are now challenging surgeons and radiation oncologists to think about broader aspects of care for patients who present with presumed local-only disease. For example, the recently published ADAURA trial demonstrated a dramatic reduction of postoperative progression and death at 24 months in patients with resected NSCLC who harbored EGFR+ driver mutations with the adjuvant osimertinib (Wu et al. 2020). Although this trial has not yet demonstrated an overall survival benefit, this may follow with longer follow-up given that the hazard ratio for progression-free survival was 0.17 with a 99.06% confidence interval of 0.11–0.26 ($p < 0.001$) (Wu et al. 2020). Given this efficacy, advancements in targeted therapy and immunotherapy for relapsed or metastatic disease may likely soon abrogate the historically important role of earlier detection of occult nodal disease and mitigate the need for invasive mediastinal staging beyond that which endobronchial ultrasound sampling can achieve.

The introduction of blood-based biomarkers presents yet another challenge to the importance of invasive mediastinal staging. The NCCN guidelines already recommend liquid biopsies for patients with NSCLC when a biopsy of the primary tumor poses significant procedural risks or when the patient is too sick to undergo invasive procedures (Ettinger et al. 2018; Revelo et al. 2019). For colorectal cancers, DNA-based assays during posttreatment surveillance have already begun to complement traditional invasive assessments such as colonoscopy for annual screenings. Significant investments have been made to further develop blood-based assays for cancer care, and once validated they could serve a routine role for disease monitoring after up-front surgery or SBRT. Thus, the traditional pathologic assessment of lymph nodes may be destined to eventually become an antiquated procedure of the past.

6.2 The Future of Local Control and Procedural Risk

Beyond the questions about invasive nodal assessments, there is emerging uncertainty about the importance of surgical resection to ensure complete eradication of the primary tumor in patients who often harbor microscopic metastatic disease. As advancements in systemic therapies, immunotherapies, and potentially gene therapies take a more central role, new debates have emerged regarding whether a future with improved systemic therapy will justify the risks of surgical resection. Will any form of local control be sufficient or will debate remain over small differences in local control between operative and nonoperative strategies?

When considering the 3–7% primary tumor control advantage with surgery (100% with surgery versus 93–97% with SBRT), it is instructive to consider the benefits of video-assisted thoracoscopic surgery (VATS) that has reduced the morbidity of surgical intervention for lung cancer. Unfortunately, VATS is not broadly available, and resections via thoracotomy continue to be performed around the world (Verstegen et al. 2013; Allen et al. 2006; Ferguson et al. 2014). As such, postoperative complications are reported in approximately 38% of patients including a major cardiovascular event in every 1 out of 25 patients. Prolonged hospitalizations of >30 days occur in around 5% of patients and are associated with significant morbidity and an approximate 10% mortality rate (Ferguson et al. 2014). In an analysis of 3516 lung cancer patients, the National Veterans Affairs Surgical Quality Improvement Program (VASQIP) reported a 30-day mortality rate of 4% in patients undergoing surgery for early-stage lung cancer (Harpole et al. 1999). Historically,

30-day endpoints have been used as a standard metric for postoperative mortality data. However, it has been argued that this metric fails to capture all treatment-related deaths as many patients may die after this time during prolonged recoveries or at other facilities following a transfer from the surgical center. An analysis including more than 6000 patients who underwent resection for lung cancer at a single academic institution over a 12-year period revealed that >50% of all perioperative deaths occurred after transfer or discharge from the treating center (Senthi and Senan 2014; Kim et al. 2014). Updated reports that use a 90-day mortality metric have provided evidence that the surgical mortality rate at 90 days has been generally double the 30-day rate (Harpole et al. 1999; Senthi and Senan 2014).

Although less common, it must be noted that SBRT is not without significant risks and morbidity. There have been multiple reports that demonstrate full-dose SBRT to tumors that are in close proximity to or abut the proximal bronchial tree can lead to fatal complications via stenosis, hemoptysis, or severe radiation pneumonitis (Timmerman et al. 2003; McGarry et al. 2005; Lindberg et al. 2021). Refinements in SBRT planning techniques with strict constraints on the ipsilateral bronchi and use of three-dimensional daily image-guided techniques using cone beam computed tomography before each treatment delivery have reduced the incidence of severe or fatal complications to case reports with multiple prospective clinical trials reporting a 0% rate of treatment-related mortality at 5 years (Hof et al. 2007; Onishi et al. 2007; Chang et al. 2021). Nonetheless, tumors that abut the proximal bronchus are still considered high risk for SBRT and may be better treated with alternative strategies such as conventional fraction or even surgery whenever patients are operable.

6.3 Defining Synergistic Approaches

Finally, in the era of immunotherapy, additional questions have emerged regarding the potential of synergy with SBRT and immunotherapy to eradicate micrometastatic disease. As such, removal of the tumor might not be the best option as it would preclude the opportunity for SBRT to introduce neoantigens and stimulate the immune system further (Corso et al. 2011, 2017; Fields and Muraro 2017). This hypothesis is currently being tested in three phase III randomized clinical trials that are randomizing patients with operable and inoperable stage I NSCLC to SBRT with or without immune checkpoint inhibitors (SWOG 1914, PACIFIC-4, KEYNOTE-867) (National Cancer Institute 2021; AstraZeneca 2021; Merck Sharp and Dohme Corp. 2021). Patients with operable disease are also being studied with preoperative checkpoint inhibitors and SBRT as reported by Altorki et al., who recently published the results of a phase II trial ($n = 60$) that randomized patients with operable stage I–III NSCLC to preoperative durvalumab with or without attenuated doses of SBRT (8 Gy × 3). The results demonstrated a 53% vs. 7% rate of major pathological response, respectively, with a 27% rate of complete pathological response in patients who received the combination. Thus, a future state of NSCLC care may begin with biomarker analyses, combination SBRT + immunotherapy for local control, followed by targeted therapy, gene therapy, or immunotherapy with no more blood drawn than what would typically be needed for a comprehensive metabolic panel.

7 How to Think About Surgery Versus SBRT in the Modern Era

The answers are simple. It begins with recognizing that we have never truly known how a patient with early-stage NSCLC might fare after SBRT instead of surgery. Those who counsel patients with early-stage lung cancer about their treatment options, if honest, will admit that the literature has yet to inform us whether surgery or SBRT is more effective whenever early-stage tumors are small or large, are growing within a certain location within a lobe, have a certain radiographic characteristic, or are found to have a particular histopathological finding after biopsy. We believe that as some point in the future, genomic and radiomic biomarkers can help us classify patients who will have better outcomes with surgery or SBRT. For example, the recently demonstrated association of KEAP1/NFE2L2 mutations with radioresistance suggests that these tumors should be resected instead of treated with SBRT (Binkley et al. 2020). Yet, we are worried that many clinicians will be unable to follow the nuances of scientific discoveries, and opt to rely on their confirmation bias for surgery being the best option in all situations unless the risk is "too high". This is because many are insufficiently trained to understand the limitations of retrospective investigations or recognize comparisons that are flawed. The reported outcomes with SBRT are destined to improve over time to a point that it will very likely demonstrate equivalent or even longer survival rates than surgical series have been able to report. This will not necessarily be a result of additional technological advances in the delivery of SBRT, but instead because of an ongoing gradual shift in the health of patients who are being referred to or preferring SBRT instead of surgery. Survival rates after SBRT are now higher than ever before and are being reported with longer follow-up. For example, the MD Anderson clinical trial titled "Lung Cancer Stereotactic Ablative Radiotherapy in Stage I Non-small Cell Lung Cancer Patients Who Can Undergo Lobectomy (STARS)" recently reported a 5-year overall survival rate of 87% with a median follow-up of 61 months among 80 patients with operable stage I NSCLC who refused surgery.

To move everyone into the future of high-quality care for patients with early-stage NSCLC, we believe that all medical centers should by now have assembled multidisciplinary thoracic oncology teams who meet regularly to discuss each case, evaluate the nuances of radiographic and pathological findings, and work collaboratively to safeguard each patient's preferences, particularly as clinicians are generally conflicted since they were trained to deliver only one type of treatment modality. The multidisciplinary team should continuously review the literature to stay up to date as the current pace of new FDA approvals for NSCLC therapies does not appear to be slowing. Strategies to overcome unsubstantiated concerns about biopsy-related complications should be addressed to reduce the frequency of empiric surgery or SBRT in patients without histopathological confirmation of lung cancer. Consideration should be given for empiric SBRT instead of empiric lobectomy whenever tumors are located in the middle of a lobe and are not amenable to a sublobar resection. Multidisciplinary teams should also give thoughtful consideration to alternative treatments such as cryotherapy and microwave ablation in select situations.

Finally, we wish to emphasize that a successful thoracic oncology team includes not only a surgical and radiation oncologist, but also a medical oncologist, pulmonologist, diagnostic and interventional radiologist, and pathologist who each have a particular interest in lung cancer. Channels of communication must be wide open among the team members, and intimidation with dogma and heuristics must be addressed and discouraged until they stop. Each patient who seeks our care hopes that their clinicians have their best interest in mind, work well together, and are not blinded by personal bias. Finally, patients should have an opportunity to learn about each treatment directly from the clinician who delivers that care given that their expertise cannot be substituted by someone without formal training in another discipline. And, of course, each patient's preferences should be respected whenever they are presented with management options so that their values are honored given the probability of recurrence after up-front surgery or SBRT.

References

Allen MS, Darling GE, Pechet TTV et al (2006) Morbidity and mortality of major pulmonary resections in patients with early-stage lung cancer: initial results of the randomized, prospective ACOSOG Z0030 trial. Ann Thorac Surg 81(3):1013–1020. https://doi.org/10.1016/j.athoracsur.2005.06.066

Antonoff MB, Correa AM, Sepesi B et al (2016) Salvage pulmonary resection after stereotactic body radiotherapy: a feasible and safe option for local failure in selected patients. J Thorac Cardiovasc Surg 154(2):689–699. https://doi.org/10.1016/j.jtcvs.2017.03.142

AstraZeneca. Durvalumab vs placebo with stereotactic body radiation therapy in early stage unresected non-small cell lung cancer patients (PACIFIC-4). ClinicalTrials.gov. Identifier: NCT 03833154. https://clinicaltrials.gov/ct2/show/NCT03833154. Updated 19 Apr 2021. Accessed 31 May 2021

Binkley MS, Jeon YJ, Nesselbush M et al (2020) KEAP1/NFE2L2 mutations predict lung cancer radiation resistance that can be targeted by glutaminase inhibition. Cancer Discov 10(12):1826–1841. https://doi.org/10.1158/2159-8290.CD-20-0282

Chang JY, Senan S, Paul MA et al (2015) Stereotactic ablative radiotherapy versus lobectomy for operable stage I non-small-cell lung cancer: a pooled analysis of two randomised trials. Lancet Oncol 16(6):630–637. https://doi.org/10.1016/S1470-2045(15)70168-3

Chang JY, Mehran RJ, Feng L et al (2021) Stereotactic ablative radiotherapy in operable stage I NSCLC patients: long-term results of the expanded STARS clinical trial. J Clin Oncol 39:2–3

Cornwell LD, Moghanaki D (2018) Collaborating to assess the role of stereotactic body radiation therapy in medically operable stage I non-small cell lung cancer. J Thorac Dis 10(Suppl 26):S3311–S3313. https://doi.org/10.21037/jtd.2018.08.83

Corso CD, Ali AN, Diaz R (2011) Radiation-induced tumor neoantigens: imaging and therapeutic implications. Am J Cancer Res 1(3):390–412

Corso CD, Park HS, Moreno AC et al (2017) Stage I lung SBRT clinical practice patterns. Am J Clin Oncol Cancer Clin Trials 40(4):358–361. https://doi.org/10.1097/COC.0000000000000162

Douillard J, Rosell R, De Lena M et al (2006) Adjuvant vinorelbine plus cisplatin versus observation in patients with completely resected stage IB–IIIA non-small-cell lung cancer (Adjuvant Navelbine International Trialist Association [ANITA]): a randomised controlled trial. Lancet Oncol 7:719–727. https://doi.org/10.1016/S1470-2045(06)70804-X

Dyer C (2015) Doctors should not cherry pick what information to give patients, court rules. BMJ 350:h1414. https://doi.org/10.1136/bmj.h1414

Ettinger DS, Aisner DL, Wood DE et al (2018) NCCN guidelines® insights: non-small cell lung cancer, featured updates to the NCCN guidelines. J Natl Compr Canc Netw 16(7):807–821. https://www.nccn.org/login?ReturnURL=https://www.nccn.org/professionals/physician_gls/pdf/nscl.pdf

Farjah F, Flum DR, Varghese TK, Symons RG, Wood DE, J. Maxwell Chamberlain Memorial Paper for General Thoracic Surgery (2009) Surgeon specialty and long-term survival after pulmonary resection for lung cancer. Ann Thorac Surg 87(4):995–1006. https://doi.org/10.1016/j.athoracsur.2008.12.030

Felip E, Rosell R, Maestre A et al (2020) Preoperative chemotherapy plus surgery versus surgery plus adjuvant chemotherapy versus surgery alone in early-stage non-small-cell lung cancer. J Clin Oncol 28(19). https://doi.org/10.1200/JCO.2009.27.6204

Ferguson MK, Saha-Chaudhuri P, Mitchell JD, Varela G, Brunelli A (2014) Prediction of major cardiovascular events after lung resection using a modified scoring system. Ann Thorac Surg 97(4):1135–1140. https://doi.org/10.1016/j.athoracsur.2013.12.032

Fields RC, Muraro E (2017) Local high-dose radiotherapy induces systemic immunomodulating effects of potential therapeutic relevance in oligometastatic. Breast Cancer 8:1476. https://doi.org/10.3389/fimmu.2017.01476

Flores RM (2018) Lung cancer randomized controlled trials should compare stereotactic body radiation therapy with observation, NOT surgery. J Thorac Cardiovasc Surg 155(1):403–404. https://doi.org/10.1016/j.jtcvs.2017.08.058

Graham E A, Singer J J (1984) Landmark article Oct 28, 1933. Successful removal of an entire lung for carcinoma of the bronchus. By Evarts A. Graham and J. J. Singer. JAMA. 13;251(2):257–60. https://doi.org/10.1001/jama.251.2.257.

Gutierrez AC, Pickren JW (1974) Surgical therapy of lung cancer. Am Assoc Thorac Surg 71(4):581–591. https://doi.org/10.1016/S0022-5223(19)40182-7

Halsted WS (1907) The results of radical operations for the cure of carcinoma of the breast. Ann Surg 46(1):1–19. https://doi.org/10.1097/00000658-190707000-00001

Haque W, Szeja S, Tann A et al (2018) Changes in treatment patterns and overall survival in patients with early-stage non-small cell lung cancer in the United States after the incorporation of stereotactic ablative radiation therapy. Am J Clin Oncol 41(3):259–266. https://doi.org/10.1097/COC.0000000000000265

Harbeck N, Alt U, Berger U et al (2000) Long-term follow-up confirms prognostic impact of PAI-1 and cathepsin D and L in primary breast cancer. Int J Biol Markers 15(1):79–83. https://doi.org/10.1177/172460080001500115

Harpole J, De Camp J, Daley J et al (1999) Prognostic models of thirty-day mortality and morbidity after major pulmonary resection. J Thorac Cardiovasc Surg 117(5):969–979. https://doi.org/10.1016/S0022-5223(99)70378-8

Hof H, Muenter M, Oetzel D, Hoess A, Debus J, Herfarth K (2007) Stereotactic single-dose radiotherapy (radiosurgery) of early stage nonsmall-cell lung cancer (NSCLC). Cancer 110(1):148–155. https://doi.org/10.1002/cncr.22763

Horn L, Johnson DH, Evarts A (2008) Graham and the first pneumonectomy for lung cancer. J Clin Oncol 26(19):3268–3275. https://doi.org/10.1200/JCO.2008.16.8260

Huang K, Senthi S, Palma DA et al (2013) High-risk CT features for detection of local recurrence after stereotactic ablative radiotherapy for lung cancer. Radiother Oncol 109(1):51–57. https://doi.org/10.1016/j.radonc.2013.06.047

Huang K, Palma DA, IASLC Advanced Radiation Technology Committee (2015) Follow-up of patients after stereotactic radiation for lung cancer. J Thorac

Oncol 10(3):412–419. https://doi.org/10.1097/JTO.0000000000000435

Kim AW, McMillan RR, Towe CW et al (2014) Thirty-day mortality underestimates the risk of early death after major resections for thoracic malignancies. Ann Thorac Surg 98(5):1774–1775. https://doi.org/10.1016/j.athoracsur.2014.06.024

Lindberg K, Grozman V, Karlsson K, Kristiansen C, Jeppesen S (2021) The HILUS-trial—a prospective Nordic multicenter phase 2 study of ultracentral lung tumors treated with stereotactic body radiotherapy. J Thorac Oncol. https://doi.org/10.1016/j.jtho.2021.03.019

Louie AV, Palma DA, Dahele M, Rodrigues GB, Senan S (2015) Management of early-stage non-small cell lung cancer using stereotactic ablative radiotherapy: controversies, insights, and changing horizons. Radiother Oncol 114(2):138–147. https://doi.org/10.1016/j.radonc.2014.11.036

Wu Y-L, Goldman JW, Laktionov K et al (2020) Osimertinib in resected EGFR-mutated non-small-cell lung cancer. N Engl J Med 383:1711–1723. https://doi.org/10.1056/NEJMoa2027071

McGarry RC, Papiez L, Williams M, Whitford T, Timmerman RD (2005) Stereotactic body radiation therapy of early-stage non-small-cell lung carcinoma: phase I study. Int J Radiat Oncol Biol Phys 63(4):1010–1015. https://doi.org/10.1016/j.ijrobp.2005.03.073

Merck Sharp & Dohme Corp. Efficacy and safety study of stereotactic body radiotherapy (SBRT) with or without pembrolizumab (MK-3475) in adults with unresected stage I or IIA non-small cell lung cancer (NSCLC) (MK-3475-867/KEYNOTE-867). ClinicalTrials.gov. Identifier: NCT 03924869. https://clinicaltrials.gov/ct2/show/NCT03924869. Updated 24 May 2021. Accessed 31 May 2021

Moffett P, Moore G (2011) The standard of care: legal history and definitions: the bad and good news. West J Emerg Med 12(1):109–112

Moghanaki D, Chang JY (2016) Is surgery still the optimal treatment for stage I non-small cell lung cancer? Transl Lung Cancer Res 5(2):183–189. https://doi.org/10.21037/tlcr.2016.04.05

Morrison R, Deeley TJ, Cleland WP (1963) The treatment of carcinoma of the bronchus: a clinical trial to compare surgery and supervoltage radiotherapy. Lancet 2:683–684

National Cancer Institute. Testing the addition of the drug atezolizumab to the usual radiation treatment for patients with early non-small cell lung cancer. ClinicalTrials.gov. Identifier: NCT 04214262. https://clinicaltrials.gov/ct2/show/NCT04214262. Updated 28 May 2021. Accessed 31 May 2021

Ochsner A, Debakey M (1999) Primary pulmonary malignancy: treatment by total pneumonectomy; analysis of 79 collected cases and presentation of 7 personal cases. Ochsner J 1(3):109–10925

Onishi H, Shirato H, Nagata Y et al (2007) Hypofractionated stereotactic radiotherapy (HypoFXSRT) for stage I non-small cell lung cancer: updated results of 257 patients in a Japanese multi-institutional study. J Thorac Oncol 2(7 Suppl 3):S94–S100. https://doi.org/10.1097/JTO.0b013e318074de34

Park HS, Lloyd S, Decker RH, Wilson LD, Yu JB (2012) Limitations and biases of the surveillance, epidemiology, and end results database. Curr Probl Cancer 36(4):216–224. https://doi.org/10.1016/j.currproblcancer.2012.03.011

Pasini F, Verlato G, Durante E et al (2003) Persistent excess mortality from lung cancer in patients with stage I non-small-cell lung cancer, disease-free after 5 years. Br J Cancer 88:1666–1668. https://doi.org/10.1038/sj.bjc.6600991

Pignon JP, Scagliotti GV, Douillard J et al (2008) Lung adjuvant cisplatin evaluation: a pooled analysis by the LACE collaborative group. J Clin Oncol 26(21):3552–3559. https://doi.org/10.1200/JCO.2007.13.9030

Pignon J, Tribodet H, Scagliotti GV et al (2020) Lung adjuvant cisplatin evaluation: a pooled analysis by the LACE Collaborative Group. J Clin Oncol 26:21. https://doi.org/10.1200/JCO.2007.13.9030

Puri V, Crabtree TD, Bell JM et al (2014) National cooperative group trials of "high-risk" patients with lung cancer: are they truly. Ann Thorac Surg 97(5):1678–1685. https://doi.org/10.1016/j.athoracsur.2013.12.028

Revelo AE, Martin A, Velasquez R et al (2019) Liquid biopsy for lung cancers: an update on recent developments. Ann Transl Med 7(7):1–13. https://doi.org/10.21037/atm.2019.03.28

Ronden MI, Palma D, Slotman BJ (2018a) Brief report on radiological changes following stereotactic ablative radiotherapy (SABR) for early-stage lung tumors: a pictorial essay. J Thorac Oncol 13(6):855–862. https://doi.org/10.1016/j.jtho.2018.02.023

Ronden MI, van Sörnsen de Koste JR, Johnson C et al (2018b) Incidence of high-risk radiologic features in patients without local recurrence after stereotactic ablative radiation therapy for early-stage non-small cell lung cancer. Int J Radiat Oncol Biol Phys 100(1):115–121. https://doi.org/10.1016/j.ijrobp.2017.09.035

Rossouw JE, Anderson GL, Prentice RL et al (2009) Risks and benefits of estrogen plus progestin in healthy postmenopausal women. JAMA 288(3):321–333. http://www.ncbi.nlm.nih.gov/pubmed/12117397

Samson P, Roach MC Jr, Carpenter L et al (2019) Algorithm assignment to stereotactic body radiation therapy is associated with high risk of post-surgical serious adverse events in stage I non-small cell lung cancer patients. Radiat Oncol Biol 105(1):E530–E531. https://doi.org/10.1016/j.ijrobp.2019.06.2436

Senthi S, Senan S (2014) Surgery for early-stage lung cancer: post-operative 30-day versus 90-day mortality and patient-centred care. Eur J Cancer 50(3):675–677. https://doi.org/10.1016/j.ejca.2013.09.029

Shimkin MB, Connelly RR, Marcus SC, Cutler SJ (1962) Pneumonectomy and lobectomy in bronchogenic carcinoma. A comparison of end results of the Overholt and Ochsner clinics. J Thorac Cardiovasc Surg 44(4):503–519. https://doi.org/10.1016/s0022-5223(19)32943-5

Soni PD, Hartman HE, Dess RT et al (2019) Comparison of population-based observational studies with randomized trials in oncology. J Clin Oncol 37(14):1209–1216. https://doi.org/10.1200/JCO.18.01074

Stokes WA, Rusthoven CG (2018) Surgery vs. SBRT in retrospective analyses: confounding by operability is the elephant in the room. J Thorac Dis 10(Suppl 17):S2007–S2010. https://doi.org/10.21037/jtd.2018.05.40

Subramanian S, Chiesa F, Lyubaev V, Aidarbekova A (2006) The evolution of surgery in the management of neck metastases. Acta Otorhinolaryngol Ital 26(6):309–316

Taira N, Kawabata T, Ichi T et al (2014) Salvage operation for late recurrence after stereotactic body radiotherapy for lung cancer: two patients with no viable cancer cells. Ann Thorac Surg 97(6):2167–2171. https://doi.org/10.1016/j.athoracsur.2013.07.123

Timmerman R, Papiez L, McGarry R et al (2003) Extracranial stereotactic radioablation: results of a phase I study in medically inoperable stage I non-small cell lung cancer. Chest 124(5):1946–1955. https://doi.org/10.1378/chest.124.5.1946

Timmerman RD, Paulus R, Pass HI et al (2018) Stereotactic body radiation therapy for operable early-stage lung cancer findings from the NRG oncology RTOG 0618 trial. JAMA Oncol 4(9):1263–1266. https://doi.org/10.1001/jamaoncol.2018.1251

Verstegen NE, Oosterhuis JWA, Palma DA et al (2013) Stage I-II non-small-cell lung cancer treated using either stereotactic ablative radiotherapy (SABR) or lobectomy by video-assisted thoracoscopic surgery (VATS): outcomes of a propensity score-matched analysis. Ann Oncol 24(6):1543–1548. https://doi.org/10.1093/annonc/mdt026

Stereotactic Ablative Radiotherapy for Early-Stage Lung Cancer

Dat T. Vo, John H. Heinzerling, and Robert D. Timmerman

Contents

1 Introduction.. 445
2 **Techniques and Technological Advances in SAbR for Lung Tumors**............... 447
2.1 Patient Positioning and Immobilization.......... 447
2.2 Daily Imaging for Patient Repositioning Prior to Treatment............................. 448
2.3 Tumor Motion Assessment............................ 449
2.4 Tumor Motion Control................................. 450
2.5 Target Volume Delineation and Treatment Planning.. 451
3 **Radiobiological Aspects of SAbR**.................. 453
3.1 Tumor Biology... 453
3.2 Normal Tissue Radiobiology and Tolerance... 455
4 **Clinical Results in Primary Lung Cancer**.... 457
4.1 Medically Inoperable Patients with Early-Stage Lung Cancer.................... 457
4.2 Medically Operable Patients....................... 462
4.3 Surveillance After SAbR............................. 463
5 **Conclusions and Future Considerations**...... 463
References.. 464

D. T. Vo · R. D. Timmerman (✉)
Department of Radiation Oncology, UT Southwestern Medical Center, Dallas, TX, USA
e-mail: Robert.Timmerman@UTSouthwestern.edu

J. H. Heinzerling
Levine Cancer Institute, Atrium Health, Southeast Radiation Oncology Group, Charlotte, NC, USA

Abstract

Stereotactic ablative radiotherapy (SAbR), also known as stereotactic body radiation therapy (SBRT), utilizes advanced techniques of immobilization, image guidance, and unique field arrangements to deliver precise, oligofractionated radiotherapy to a variety of tumor types. SAbR has been established as a technologically innovative therapy for early-stage non-small cell lung cancer (NSCLC) and has emerged as the standard treatment option for medically inoperable patients through completion of prospective, multi-institutional trials. Recent trials continue to evaluate the role of SAbR in the medically operable and borderline operable population and will compare surgical resection and SAbR as treatment modalities in these patients. This chapter reviews the techniques utilized in SAbR, the evidence for use of SAbR in early-stage lung cancer, its extension of use to medically operable patients, and the toxicities associated with this technique.

1 Introduction

Stereotactic radiosurgery first emerged as a technique in the 1950s by such innovators as Lars Leksell to treat intracranial neoplasms using single large-dose treatments (Leksell 1951). These treatments were a fundamental change from the perception of conventionally fractionated radiotherapy (CFRT) classically used to exploit the radiobiological differences between normal and neoplastic tissues. Leksell established the principles of immobilization and precise targeting utilizing a frame with fiducial markers to define an intracranial coordinate system that allowed treatment guidance, patient immobilization, and facilitated accurate dose delivery with maximization of normal tissue sparing. Leksell constructed a treatment machine with multiple, noncoplanar cobalt-60 sources arranged in a hemisphere that allowed by the emitted γ-rays to converge on a target with high conformality and dose falloff to spare adjacent normal tissue.

Based on the success of intracranial radiosurgery, pioneers such as A.J. Hamilton, Henric Blomgren, Ingmar Lax, and Minoru Uematsu developed technologies that would allow similar treatment accuracy for targets within the body (Hamilton et al. 1995; Lax et al. 1994; Blomgren et al. 1995; Uematsu et al. 1998). The first stereotactic experience utilized a stereotactic radiosurgery frame, with a modified linear accelerator, to radiate the spine in patients with metastatic cancer (Hamilton et al. 1995). While tumors within the skull have no additional movement once the skull has been immobilized, body tumors are subject to forces within the body such as respiratory breathing, cardiac contraction, and gastrointestinal peristalsis. The Swedish researchers extended patient immobilization and fiducial targeting to the body through construction of a body frame and attempted to reduce internal motion of targets related to respiration in order to allow high doses of radiation to be administered extracranially. New dosimetric methods were created to use multiple, non-coplanar beams with compact aperture dimensions to mimic the convergence of beams seen in Gamma Knife® treatments. These methods to treat body tumors have collectively been termed stereotactic ablative radiotherapy (SAbR) (Loo et al. 2011), also known as stereotactic body radiation therapy (SBRT) (Timmerman et al. 2003a, b). SAbR is defined by the American College of Radiology (ACR) and the American Society of Radiation Oncology (ASTRO) as a treatment strategy used to deliver a radiation dose to a well-defined extracranial target in five fractions or less, utilizing higher doses per fraction than compared to CFRT (Chao et al. 2020).

SAbR is radiobiologically unique from CFRT. SAbR treatments cause dramatic effects within targeted tissues, disruption of both cell division and function, leading to the associated term "ablative" radiotherapy. An order of magnitude of higher fractional doses of 10–20 Gy compared to conventional fraction doses of 1.8–2 Gy leads to biologic ablation of cells, leaving them dysfunctional not only to divide but also to perform other cellular functions. In order to model the biological effects of SAbR on cancer cells, the universal survival curve was constructed by combining the linear quadratic (LQ) model, which approximates the effects of CFRT, with that of the multitarget model, which better approximates the effects of ablative doses of radiation (Park et al. 2008). In addition to the tumoricidal effects of SAbR on the tumor itself, there are effects of SAbR on the tumor microenvironment, particularly in regard to vascular damage and the immune system. It is thought that radiation doses of 10 Gy or higher per fraction cause significant vascular damage, likely through damage of endothelial cells, resulting in destruction of the tumor microenvironment and indirect tumor cell death (Park et al. 2012). There may also be an immunomodulatory role for SAbR as it can promote anticancer immunity from the induction of necrosis/necroptosis and senescence, modes of cell death that are considered pro-inflammatory (Haikerwal et al. 2015). Normal tissue toxicity is also affected by these ablative effects, and thus it is essential to avoid unnecessary treatment of normal tissue surrounding the target. Improvements in imaging, targeting, onboard image guidance, dosimetric methods, and radiation delivery devices collectively allow a geometric avoidance of surrounding normal tissues, making these high-dose-per-fraction treatments possible despite their profound potency.

It is estimated that there are approximately 228,820 new cases of lung cancer per year in the

United States, with approximately 90% being non-small cell lung cancer (Siegel et al. 2020). About 30% of these cases present with early-stage disease, with an approximate 5-year survival rate of 60–70% with surgical resection (Naruke et al. 1988; Nesbitt et al. 1995). While surgical resection is the standard therapy in these patients, many patients cannot tolerate surgery because of comorbidities related to lung and cardiac function. In the past, these patients were treated with conventional radiation typically given to a dose of approximately 45–66 Gy in fractions of 1.8–2.0 Gy over 6 weeks, resulting in a 5-year survival rate of approximately 10–30% (Kaskowitz et al. 1993; Wisnivesky et al. 2005). Exploration of high-dose-per-fraction treatments for primary lung cancer has now shown high rates of local control and survival more comparable to surgical series. The techniques utilized in SAbR treatments, the unique biologic effects, the associated toxicity, and its careful exploration through prospective clinical trials in patients with early-stage lung cancer will be discussed below.

2 Techniques and Technological Advances in SAbR for Lung Tumors

Safe and effective SAbR treatments require ensuring accuracy and precision achieved by reliable and reproducible patient immobilization; daily image guidance for precise repositioning prior to treatment; assessment and accounting for tumor and organ motion consistently between planning and treatment; and use of multiple, non-coplanar treatment fields to ensure adequate target coverage with rapid falloff of dose to surrounding normal tissues. These principles allow the reduction of normal tissue exposure to high and intermediate doses, minimizing the probability of normal tissue complications while ensuring accurate high-dose delivery to the target. Because of the proximity to several critical structures including normal lung tissue, bronchi, chest wall, esophagus, heart, brachial plexus, and spinal cord, realization of these SAbR principles is of greatest importance to ensure safe treatment with minimal toxicity while achieving adequate tumor control. For CFRT, emphasis on correlation of the static treatment plan to actual treatment is less critical than for SAbR because of the large margins placed around the target, the homogeneous dose distributions, and the more "forgiving" fractionation typically seen with limited-field CFRT. This, however, is not the case for SAbR treatments, and all effort should be made to ensure the accuracy of equipment used in simulation, planning, and treatment delivery. Recently, the American Association of Physicists in Medicine (AAPM) published their best practice guidelines for SAbR treatments including equipment and QA procedures (Benedict et al. 2010). Many of the technological advances within radiation therapy have been developed to allow increased safety of oligofractionated treatment and will be discussed here.

2.1 Patient Positioning and Immobilization

Because SAbR treatments are often longer than conventional radiotherapy treatment sessions, consistent, reproducible, and comfortable patient immobilization is essential for ensuring treatment accuracy (Yang and Timmerman 2018). Several available systems designed for stereotactic patient positioning and immobilization are currently commercially available and include body frames, vacuum cushions, and thermal plastic restraints. Some of these devices feature a fiducial system mimicking that of brain radiosurgery headframes that are rigidly attached and registered to the target. Fiducials are simply reliable "markers" whose position can be consistently and confidently correlated to both the target (tumor) and treatment device (frame) (Fig. 1).

"Frame" systems provide both immobilization and a fiducial system that can approximate initial target localization independently from other image guidance systems (e.g., room lasers and cone beam CT), which is then enhanced and adjusted by utilizing image guidance (Lax et al. 1994; Herfarth et al. 2001; Wang et al. 2006; Murray et al. 2007; Yoon et al. 2006). We find

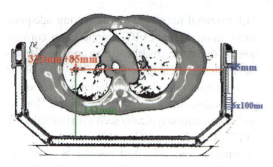

Fig. 1 Example of fiducial system in a stereotactic body frame with coordinates corresponding to target location

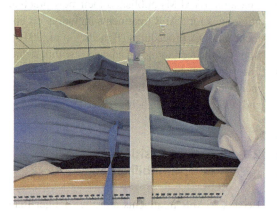

Fig. 2 Example of frame system, the Elekta stereotactic body frame showing external coordinate system, vacuum pillow, and integrated respiratory motion control with abdominal compression

that the use of a body frame is associated with suitable immobilization for SAbR for a variety of tumor sites, including that of lung (Foster et al. 2013). With a body frame, patients are moved to the coordinates of the tumor in the stereotactic frame followed by shifting the isocenter of the linear accelerator to the treatment isocenter, based on these coordinates. In addition, these systems often integrate motion control techniques such as abdominal compression used to coach the chest wall breathing approach (Fig. 2).

While many centers continue to utilize frame-based approaches for immobilization, some centers have relied on frameless-based immobilization strategies. "Frameless" systems rely on the combination of markers and imaging methods to effectively relocate a reference position within the patient. Many commercially based frameless immobilization devices exist, including vacuum-based system like the Elekta BodyFIX system or the full-body immobilization device like the CIVCO Body Pro-Lok ONE system. Frameless rigid immobilization with high-quality image guidance can potentially provide adequate immobilization for the accurate delivery of SAbR (Dahele et al. 2012; Josipovic et al. 2012). The use of flattening-filter free radiation delivery can significantly reduce the time required for immobilization and risk for translational and rotational error (Peguret et al. 2013). In addition, implanted fiducial seeds within the tumor can be accurately relocated on a daily basis using imaging techniques (Murphy 1997; Chang et al. 2003; Wulf et al. 2000; Fuss et al. 2004). Other technologies that can be used for SAbR treatments include electromagnetic transponders that can be tracked throughout treatment to ensure accurate positioning during the entire treatment course (Balter et al. 2005).

As with any system, assessment must be made by each institution on its ability to achieve accuracy in its primary objective: consistent patient immobilization and target localization. Staff training and quality assurance programs are essential for proper implication of any device, no matter its claimed accuracy. Since no one system has been shown to be superior, achieving patient comfort that avoids positions in which the patient fights gravity or requires cumbersome positions to support is of utmost importance when incorporating SAbR into any radiation oncology program.

2.2 Daily Imaging for Patient Repositioning Prior to Treatment

Image guidance provides target localization and validation of patient position prior to treatment. Typically, this is performed with computed tomography (CT) (CT-on-rails) or cone beam CT (CBCT) incorporated into the treatment unit (Jaffray et al. 2002) (Fig. 3). Because lung tumors are very distinct on CT scan, pretreatment reference volumes can be registered to the image and adjustments can be reliably made on the day of treatment. Appropriate adjustments are made

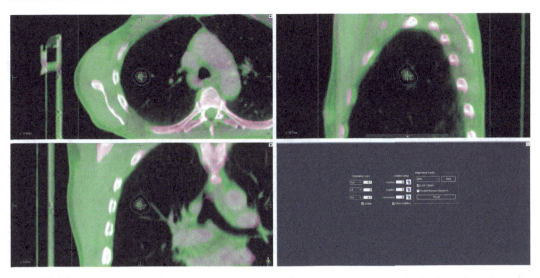

Fig. 3 Example of CBCT to validate target position prior to SBRT lung treatment. After realignment of CBCT to the planning CT, couch shifts are shown in the bottom right and are applied prior to treatment

typically with couch shifts to align pretreatment target position to the newly acquired CT data. CBCT offers improved tumor localization accuracy over bony matching using orthogonal kV imaging (Corradetti et al. 2013). CBCT scans are often slow in acquisition time and thus are more like slow CT to estimate respiratory-associated motion prior to treatment (Wang et al. 2007), but improvements are being made including respiratory-correlated CBCT or 4D CBCT to attempt to characterize motion on a daily basis immediately prior to treatment (Sonke et al. 2005; Nakagawa et al. 2013). Advanced image guidance, typically including mounted in-room kV imagers, has allowed monitoring of target or fiducial position during treatment as well (Verellen et al. 2003; Chang et al. 2003; Shirato et al. 1999). This has minimized uncertainty associated with external reference points and has allowed accurate internal tumor localization in near real time.

2.3 Tumor Motion Assessment

Because of their proximity to moving organs such as the diaphragm and heart, lung tumors have significant motion up to 5 cm (Mageras et al. 2004). This motion can vary quite significantly depending on tumor location as well as from patient to patient (Stevens et al. 2001; Liu et al. 2006; Heinzerling et al. 2008). Classic 3D imaging with fast spiral CT studies can misrepresent target position by obtaining images of the tumor in a specific phase of the respiratory cycle, leading to extreme errors in target position definition (Chen et al. 2004) (Fig. 4). Additionally, tumors also have rotational movement that must be considered for radiotherapy planning and treatment (Paganelli et al. 2015).

Thus, a personalized assessment for each patient is required to characterize tumor motion. This was typically achieved in the past with fluoroscopy and more recently with 4D computed tomography (4D CT) (Fig. 5), during which several CT images are obtained over multiple respiratory cycles and correlated with a surrogate for breathing motion. Images are then reconstructed into several respiratory phases (typically ten) to show anatomy through an entire respiratory cycle.

Other techniques to quantify target motion include slow CT (Lagerwaard et al. 2001), breath-hold techniques (Mageras et al. 2004; Scherman Rydhog et al. 2017), and respiratory-correlated PET/CT or MRI (Koch et al. 2004; Lee et al. 2016; Oliver et al. 2015). If tumor motion exceeds 5–10 mm, tumor motion control as described below is recommended so as to avoid excess toxicity.

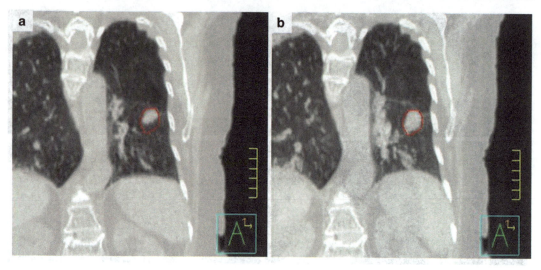

Fig. 4 Example of target definition on fast, spiral CT (**a**) compared to maximum-intensity projection (MIP) from 4D CT (**b**) showing underestimation of target excursion on fast CT

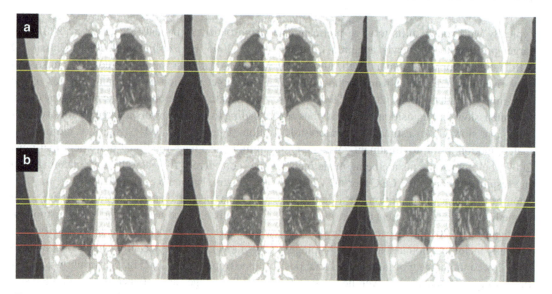

Fig. 5 (**a**) 4D CT in the coronal plane showing a T1 tumor in inhalation, exhalation, and maximum-intensity projection (MIP) with lines demarcating the tumor craniocaudal motion envelope (also known as the internal target volume, ITV), and (**b**) the poor correlation of tumor and diaphragm motion between inhalation and exhalation (i.e., the diaphragm moves considerably more than the tumor)

2.4 Tumor Motion Control

Several methods exist to control tumor motion and include techniques to reduce tumor motion (dampening), correlate treatment with tumor position (gating), or track the tumor position (chasing). Ways to dampen tumor motion include abdominal compression, which places a pressure device on the abdomen to dampen the motion of the diaphragm (Lax et al. 1994; Heinzerling et al. 2008; Negoro et al. 2001; Bouilhol et al. 2013). Other techniques such as deep inspiration breath hold or active breathing control (ABC) arrest or freeze the tumor in a reproducible position within the respiratory cycle (Yin et al. 2001; Murphy et al. 2002; Josipovic et al. 2019). Respiratory gating utilizes respiratory cycle monitoring combined with a surrogate to trigger the delivery of radiation during a specific segment of the respiratory cycle (expiration or inspiration) (Vedam et al. 2001; Kini et al. 2003; Jang et al. 2014; Saito et al. 2014). Finally, tumor tracking systems actually move the radiation beam path to follow the motion of the tumor (Kuriyama et al. 2003; Sharp et al. 2004; Shirato et al. 2000; Menten et al. 2016; Inoue et al. 2013; Bibault et al. 2012). Regardless of the method used, careful assurance of accuracy, reproducibility, as well as prudent implementation of motion data into treatment planning are essential for precise treatment delivery.

2.5 Target Volume Delineation and Treatment Planning

Target volumes are defined using mechanisms that quantify both tumor volume and tumor motion such as four-dimensional CT described above. The gross tumor volume (GTV) is typically defined on CT in lung windowing. In certain cases, when the tumor is hard to differentiate from surrounding normal structures, MRI or PET/CT can be useful to accurately determine tumor volume. A good example of this is in lung tumors adjacent to the chest wall or associated with lung atelectasis or consolidation (Fig. 6). In these situations, PET/CT can be helpful for delineating targets more precisely.

Typically in SAbR, like in brain radiosurgery, the GTV is equal to the clinical target volume (CTV), keeping the volume of normal tissues exposed to high doses to a minimum. An internal target volume or ITV can also be delineated based on the volume needed to encompass tumor motion. An additional margin is then added to the defined volume to account for daily setup error and machine tolerances, which constitutes the planning treatment volume (PTV).

SAbR requires conformal dose distributions that allow rapid dose falloff outside of the tumor

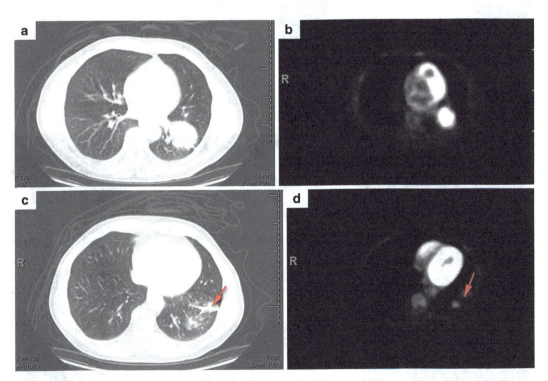

Fig. 6 PET/CT showing primary lung tumor with high SUV (**a**, **b**) with distal consolidation showing low SUV uptake (**c**, **d**). Use of PET/CT for tumor delineation in this case allows decreased target volume and better sparing of normal tissue dose

volume. This is accomplished by utilizing beams that are highly shaped to the target allowing sharp collimation of beam fluence outside of the target and using multiple beams (typically 10–15) or large-angle arc rotations (Liu et al. 2006; Cardinale et al. 1999; Papiez et al. 2003; Giglioli et al. 2017). Use of nonopposing beams is encouraged to ovoid overlap of dose at points of entrance and exit. In most circumstances, non-coplanar beams are also preferred to provide more isotropic dose falloff in all directions. Typical beam arrangements for lung SBRT are seen in Fig. 7.

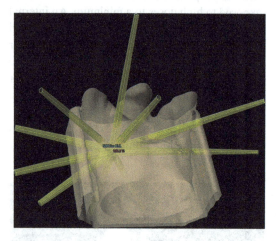

Fig. 7 Typical non-coplanar beam arrangement for SAbR treatment of lung tumors

The resulting dose distribution seen in Fig. 8 shows relatively isotropic dose falloff in all directions. Reducing high-dose spillage outside of the intended treatment volume is critical for preventing normal tissue toxicity of organs at risk. Ablation is likely to occur not only in the target itself, but also in the shell of normal tissue immediately outside of the PTV. Thus, the intermediate- and high-dose spillage outside of the target is directly related to the toxicity that can occur with SAbR. Tubular structures within the lung can be obliterated and cause subsequent downstream effects such as atelectasis or consolidation. Because of this, SAbR protocols commonly define criteria related to the conformality of target dose and the compactness of intermediate dose. Examples of this include evaluations of parameters such as "R50" defined as the ratio of the 50% prescription isodose volume to the PTV (assessing intermediate-dose compactness) and "D2cm" defined as the maximum dose 2 cm from the PTV in any direction (avoiding extreme polarization of dose).

These parameters, which change with PTV dimensions, allow evaluation of intermediate-dose spillage that can cause more global organ damage. Conformality index or the ratio of the prescription isodose volume to the PTV (assessing high-dose compactness) should be kept

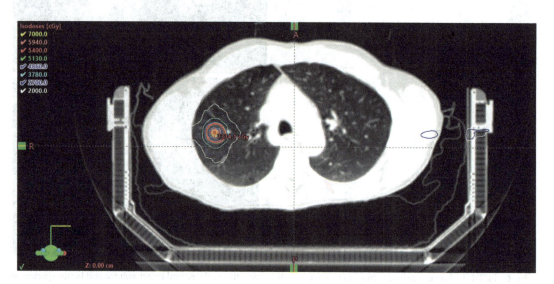

Fig. 8 Dose distribution of left-sided primary lung tumor showing isotropic dose falloff with non-coplanar beam arrangement

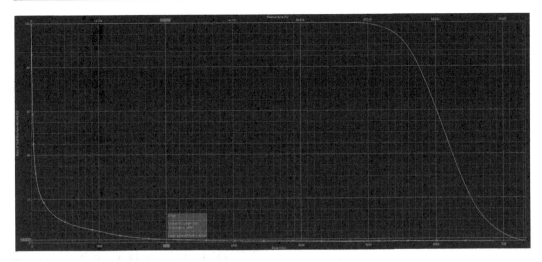

Fig. 9 Dose-volume histogram from SAbR primary lung treatment to 54 Gy in three fractions showing low V20 (<5%)

below 1.2, and typical PTV coverage should be 95–100% with 99% of the PTV covered by 90% of prescription dose. In addition, normal tissue dose constraints are being developed and modified based on the existing data from patients treated with SAbR to help predict toxicity based on dose-volume relationships (Kim et al. 2017). These constraints specifically relate to total dose, fractionation, and volume of specific normal tissues. Because dose-volume relationships in the setting of hypofractionation are not well understood, these constraints are frequently modified based on the patient outcome data in ongoing multicenter trials evaluating SAbR. Figure 9 shows an example of a typical dose-volume histogram for a stage I lung cancer treatment indicating good target coverage and lung sparing.

Notice that despite the high prescription dose (60 Gy in three fractions), the volume of lung getting 20 Gy (V20) is quite low (5%) compared to what is normally seen in CFRT (20–35%). Yet, because this dose is given in three fractions, using classic parameters such as V20 can be misleading and lead to excessive toxicity. A better parameter for evaluating pneumonitis for a three-fraction therapy would be V11.4, which should ideally be kept below 37% (Kim et al. 2017).

3 Radiobiological Aspects of SAbR

3.1 Tumor Biology

Conventional understanding of tumor radiobiology has been mostly obtained through experimentation of lower doses per fraction when compared to SAbR, which involves very high doses in few fractions. Because of these origins, traditional radiobiology has been challenged when applied to ablative, oligofractionated treatments. Typically, the cell survival curve for ionizing radiation has been used to describe the surviving fraction versus dose and classically has been illustrated by the linear-quadratic (LQ) formula (Hall et al. 1972; Rossi and Kellerer 1972) (Fig. 10).

With CFRT, daily doses ranging from 1.5 to 3.0 Gy are used which occur on the "shoulder" of the survival curve, allowing cells to be able to repair some of the radiation damage. Higher fractional doses (>3–5 Gy) occur on the linear portion of the curve predicting a constant proportion of cell kill. Several authors have challenged the LQ model for daily doses beyond the shoulder (6–8 Gy), claiming that it grossly overestimates cell kill in this range (Marks 1995; Guerrero and Li 2004; Park et al. 2008). Several modifications

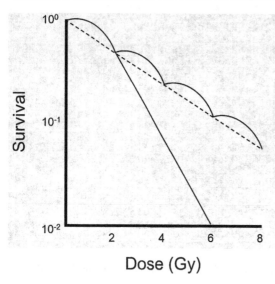

Fig. 10 A plot of the logarithm of cell survival with increasing single-fraction dose is initially curvilinear (known as the shoulder) followed by a linear relationship. Giving the same total dose of radiation by multiple smaller fractions (e.g., 2 Gy) repeats the shoulder with each fraction resulting in considerably more cell survival than for a single large dose. The linear-quadratic formalism appropriately models the curvilinear shoulder portion of the survival curve but overestimates cell loss in the linear portion

have been proposed to correctly model SAbR dose-response curves, including utilization of the older multitarget model to ascertain a "single-fraction equivalent dose" for oligofractionated treatments ranging from 7 to 10 Gy, thus eliminating any influence of the classic LQ model (Marks 1995; Park et al. 2008). Another proposal modifies the existing LQ model by incorporating aspects of the lethal-potentially lethal model, which accounts for ongoing radiation repair processes that occur during radiation exposure (Guerrero and Li 2004). Regardless of the proposal, the predicted tumor cell kill becomes significantly different when compared to the LQ model, preventing overestimation of cell kill for large fraction sizes used in SAbR.

These newly proposed models have created important implications when dose fractionation schemes are compared for SAbR. In addition, factors such as treatment delivery time and dose rate become significant considerations for predicting cell kill during SAbR. For example, evaluation of clonogenic survival in vitro when exposed to high doses of radiation from 12 to 18 Gy shows that in glioma cell lines, cell kill can be significantly affected by treatment duration changing from 1.5 to 2 h (Benedict et al. 1997). A review of this topic has concluded that for treatments lasting longer than 30 min, significant loss of cytotoxicity may be seen in high-dose-per-fraction treatments (Fowler et al. 2004). More research is needed both in vitro and in vivo to better model high-dose-fractional treatments (Timmerman and Story 2006), including different radiobiologic effects of SAbR such as vascular and stromal effects that are not seen with CFRT (Kirkpatrick and Dewhirst 2008; Fuks and Kolesnick 2005), normal tissue effects after SAbR, preservation of immune response (Lee et al. 2009; Curiel 2007), and combination of effective mechanisms with targeted drugs or immunotherapy.

Clinical studies of SAbR for early-stage lung cancer have conferred high tumor control probabilities (TCP). Early studies of clinical data suggest that biological effective doses (BED) greater than 100 Gy ($\alpha/\beta = 10$) are effective for optimal local control (Onishi et al. 2004; Wulf et al. 2005). For early-stage lung cancer treated with SAbR, clinical data suggests that there is a sigmoidal function between tumor control probability and BED with a TCP $\geq$90% for BED $\geq$159 $Gy_{8.6}$ (Mehta et al. 2012). Accounting for fractionation schedules, higher biological effective doses account for higher tumor control probabilities, perhaps not related to alternative biological pathways (Brown et al. 2013). In addition, shorter treatment durations have improved local control when patients completed SAbR in $\leq$10 days, compared to those with treatment durations $\geq$11 days, suggesting that SAbR may reduce the effects from accelerated tumor repopulation, especially from highly proliferative tumors such as lung cancer (Kestin et al. 2014). Reoxygenation of tumor cells may have an effect on the efficacy of SAbR as there may be heterogeneous areas of well-oxygenated cells and hypoxic cells, depending on the rate of cellular proliferation and location relative to tumor vasculature. Classically, hypoxic cells are radioresistant to CFRT, and the optimal fractionation schedule to take advantage of reoxygenation to impart radiosensitivity in subsequent fractions of radiation with SAbR is unknown (Shibamoto et al. 2016). Hypoxic cell radiosensitizers have been investigated as a strategy to augment the tumor cell killing effects of SAbR, although the high dose per fraction with SAbR can generate efficient cell kill, overcoming hypoxic radioresistance (Brown et al. 2010; Meyer and Timmerman 2011).

Further studies have been explored to explain the increased tumor control probability with suggestions that there may be additional or unrecognized biological processes beyond the canonical principles in radiobiology, that is, repair, repopulation, redistribution, reoxygenation, and radiosensitivity. Damage to the tumor vasculature and endothelial cells with subsequent damage to the tumor microenvironment may contribute to increased cytotoxicity from the effects of large radiation dose per fraction (Garcia-Barros et al. 2003; Park et al. 2012). Moreover, SAbR has a profound effect on the immune system. Radiation therapy is commonly thought to have an immunosuppressive effect on antitumor immunity. However, in certain circumstances, ionizing radiation may have an immunostimulatory effect, with novel mechanisms being elucidated such as immunogenic cell death (Golden et al. 2012; Song et al. 2019). SAbR may also promote anticancer immunity by inducing necrosis/necroptosis and senescence, which are modes of cell death that are considered pro-inflammatory (Haikerwal et al. 2015; Song et al. 2019). Current trends in research include studying novel strategies to enhance the immunostimulatory aspects of SAbR or overcome the immunosuppressive effects of radiation therapy.

3.2 Normal Tissue Radiobiology and Tolerance

With high-dose-per-fraction treatments given with SAbR, different types of normal tissue can possess unique radiation tolerance characteristics. Serial structures such as airways, nerves, vessels, and bowel are linear or branching structures where damage at any point along their path can cause downstream dysfunction. This is in contrast to parallel structures such as lung alveoli, kidney nephrons, and gland acini, where damage to one portion does not necessarily affect adjacent tissue. Within the thorax, both serial and parallel normal tissues exist in close proximity including serially functioning small and large airways, esophagus, and brachial plexus adjacent to parallel functioning alveoli/capillary complexes. In addition, the heart, pericardium, pleura, bones, and chest wall, which are difficult to assign as parallel versus serial, have unique mechanisms of injury and tolerance to high-dose-per-fraction treatment.

Direct damage to parallel functioning tissues such as the alveoli occurs at relatively low threshold dose; however, the overall volume of parallel tissue in a healthy organ is typically very large. Much of this parallel functioning tissue constitutes a reserve (i.e., functional capacity beyond what is actually needed for activities of daily life). So long as the reserve (extra volume of tissue) is preserved, patients will avoid symptomatic dysfunction. Unlike serially functioning tissues, delivering damaging dose above the threshold creates little additional dysfunction within parallel tissue; rather, the key to avoiding toxicity is to minimize exposing volumes of tissue at or above the threshold dose. As SAbR is inherently a volume-sparing technique, parallel tissue dysfunction can be dramatically minimized compared to conventional, large-volume irradiation techniques. For instance, rates of pneumonitis seen in SAbR for lung tumors are far less than those in CFRT (Timmerman et al. 2003a, b). Therefore, as discussed above, the dose falloff region or "gradient region" should be strategically reduced to ensure that damage to parallel structures is kept to a minimum.

Radiation-induced lung toxicities often manifest as radiation pneumonitis and lung fibrosis, and recent Radiation Therapy Oncology Group (RTOG) studies include a constraint on the lung-GTV structure where V20 is required to be less than 10%. Similar damage can be inflicted on blood vessels traveling along the routes of these airways. Loss of lung parenchymal function (either ventilation or perfusion) most often leads to effects on oxygenation parameters including arterial oxygen pressure on room air (PaO_2) and diffusing capacity MY for carbon monoxide (DLCO) after high-dose-per-fraction treatment (Timmerman et al. 2003a, b). In the medically inoperable population studied in RTOG 0236, SAbR resulted in minimal changes or decline in arterial blood gases or oxygen saturation (Stanic et al. 2014). Long-term studies of lung SAbR demonstrated no significant long-term changes in PFTs, including FEV1 and DLCO with an insignificant dependence on dose-effect relationship (Stephans et al. 2009; Guckenberger et al. 2013). Moreover, poor baseline pulmonary function did not predict for radiation pneumonitis or decreased overall survival in RTOG 0236 (Stanic et al. 2014). In addition, the increasing recognition of the importance of critical volume-dose constraints provides a safe and effective parameter in the protection of normal and functional tissue, such as the lung (Ritter et al. 2017).

In contrast to CFRT, which often causes minor, repairable irritation of serially functioning airways, SAbR dose schedules can cause significant damage to large and small airways within the lung leading to mucosal injury and downstream collapse. Because downstream effects are related to upstream damage, targets in close proximity to large airways such as those near the hilum and central chest are especially prone to high levels of downstream damage and should be treated with great care (see section on central tumors for more discussion). Injury to the proximal bronchial tree can result in impaired pulmonary toilet, post-obstructive pneumonia, airway stenosis, occlusion, fistula formation, or fatal complications (Joyner et al. 2006; Haseltine et al. 2016; Timmerman et al. 2006). For centrally located lesions, it may be advantageous from a safety perspective to offer a SAbR regimen of five fractions. In the RTOG 0813 clinical trial evaluating SAbR in medically inoperable patients with centrally located early-stage lung cancers, a maximum tolerated dose was not found up to 60 Gy in five fractions (Bezjak et al. 2019).

Other serial tissues can also show dramatic differences in toxicity between what is classically seen in CFRT versus SAbR. Esophagitis, while commonly seen with CFRT, is typically self-limiting and resolves 2–4 weeks after treatment completion. After SAbR, however, high dose to the serial esophageal tissue can cause deep esophageal ulcers, strictures, and tracheoesophageal fistula formation. One study of 56 patients treated with CyberKnife suggested a complication probability of 50% for grade 2 esophageal toxicity with a D_{max} of 43.4 Gy and D_{1cc} of 32.9 Gy (Nuyttens et al. 2016). This suggests that conservative measures must be taken to protect the esophagus with SAbR (Abelson et al. 2012; Wang et al. 2020). Pleural and pericardial effusions can also develop with SAbR dose schedules due to irritation of the pericardium or pleura, especially in tumors adjacent to the heart or chest wall (Horne et al. 2018). Typically, these fluid collections will reabsorb without any necessary intervention, but they are important to characterize because of their absence in CFRT. Other, more rare late effects with SAbR that have been described in serial tissues include aneurysms, fistulas, and neuropathies and should caution investigators to monitor doses to all serial functioning tissues including large blood vessels and large nerves such as brachial plexus and intercostal nerves (Shaikh and Turaka 2014; Manyam et al. 2019; Lindberg et al. 2019). Sadly, in 2021, it was difficult to identify the actual route of the phrenic nerve on available imaging so as to identify its dose tolerance.

The chest wall is also susceptible to toxicity, usually manifesting as severe pain from intercostal neuropathy or rib fracture. It has been suggested to keep the V30Gy less than 30 cm³ to reduce the risk of chest wall toxicity (Dunlap et al. 2010; Stephans et al. 2012; Voruganti et al. 2020). However, this strategy inherently spills more dose into the lung; hence, it is not used at our center. More follow-up is still needed from previously completed clinical trials to describe other late effects of SAbR that have not yet manifested themselves.

4 Clinical Results in Primary Lung Cancer

SAbR provides a local, ablative dose particularly effective at eradicating gross visible tumor, making it an ideal treatment for limited visible disease without regional or distant spread. In contrast, SAbR is not particularly appropriate for treating microscopic disease either adjuvantly or prophylactically because of its likelihood of causing collateral damage to normal tissues with high-dose-per-fraction treatment. A disease that is localized after ideal staging workup and has a low probability of regional or distant metastatic spread represents the ideal setting for which the principles of SAbR could be applied and provide benefit when compared to those of CFRT. Thus, typically advanced small cell lung cancer and advanced (node positive) non-small cell lung cancer (NSCLC) are conditions where SAbR is unlikely to be used effectively except possibly as a boost to gross disease (Feddock et al. 2013; Hepel et al. 2016; Higgins et al. 2017). Early-stage NSCLC and limited lung metastases in patients with controlled systemic disease are diseases where the principles of SAbR could be exploited to achieve higher rates of tumor control.

4.1 Medically Inoperable Patients with Early-Stage Lung Cancer

Surgical resection remains the standard therapy for patients with stage I non-small cell lung cancer (NSCLC), with 5-year survival rate of approximately 60–70% (Naruke et al. 1988; Nesbitt et al. 1995). Patients determined to be medically inoperable have been treated in the past with standard fractionated radiotherapy, typically given to a dose of approximately 45–66 Gy in fractions of 1.8–2 Gy over 6 weeks, with 5-year survival rate of approximately 10–30% (Kaskowitz et al. 1993; Wisnivesky et al. 2005). Based on data suggesting a dose-response relationship in these patients, use of oligofractionated SAbR was first explored in the inoperable patient population.

Early retrospective experience using SAbR for primary lung tumors showed effective responses for primary lung tumors with a wide variety of dose fractionation schemes (Blomgren et al. 1995; Uematsu et al. 1998, 2001; Nyman et al. 2006). Yet, many of the criteria for patients to be treated differed, and most of the experiences had small patient numbers treated with quite variable dose fractionation schemes. In addition, patients were typically treated at one center, and often the follow-up was short, making reporting of late toxicities seen with these treatments inadequate. Consequently, to truly study SAbR within an interpretable forum, investigation with clear, predefined selection criteria, consistent doses, strict quality assurance, and adequate follow-up is needed through the use of prospective trials.

Indiana University carried out a phase I dose escalation study in patients with stage I medically inoperable NSCLC to both evaluate toxicity for SAbR in primary lung cancer and determine the maximum tolerated dose (MTD) (Timmerman et al. 2003a, b; McGarry et al. 2005). Forty-seven patients with T1–2N0 NSCLC were treated with consistent SAbR techniques in three fractions. Independent escalation trials were performed for three different tumor cohorts: T1, T <5, and T2 5–7 cm. All intrathoracic tumor locations were treated including central tumors. Doses were escalated from 24 Gy over three fractions (8 Gy per fraction) up to 72 Gy in three fractions (24 Gy per fraction). The MTD was not reached for T1 or T2 tumors <5 cm despite reaching doses of 60–66 Gy in three fractions. For T2 tumors larger than 5 cm, the MTD was determined to be 66 Gy in three fractions after dose-limiting toxicity that included pneumonia, and pericardial effusion was seen at the 72 Gy dose level. Impressive tumor response was seen at all dose levels (Fig. 11), but on longer follow-up, 10 local failures were seen out of 47 patients at a median follow-up of 15.2 months. Nine of the ten failures were in patients who received ≤16 Gy per fraction. As patients continued to be followed up, radiologic changes surrounding the tumor were seen including fibrotic changes in the lung (Matsuo et al. 2007) but were not typically asso-

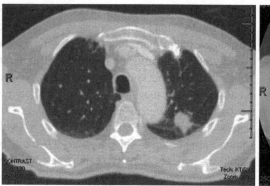
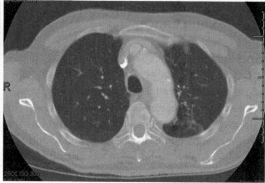

Fig. 11 Example of response seen after SAbR in early-stage primary lung cancer. Dramatic tumor response can be seen as early as 2–3 months with total radiologic disappearance often by 1 year

ciated with any symptoms. Often, these changes can be mistaken for tumor recurrence (Matsuo et al. 2007; Takeda et al. 2008). However, follow-up PET scans and biopsies showed no evidence of tumor recurrence in the majority of patients treated in the higher dose cohorts.

Because of the encouraging tumor response and tolerable toxicity seen in the phase I experience, the Indiana group further evaluated SAbR in this patient population with a 70-patient phase II trial (Timmerman et al. 2006; Fakiris et al. 2009). Small tumors were treated with 60 Gy in three fractions, while larger tumors received 66 Gy in three fractions, with 35 patients enrolled to each cohort. The study was powered for a target local control rate of 80%, which would represent a dramatic improvement over results seen with CFRT. Patients continued to be followed up for toxicity related to treatment. The initial results of the trial were published early because of new detection of treatment-related toxicity not seen in the phase I trial (Timmerman et al. 2006). Actuarial 2-year local control rate was 95% with a median follow-up of 17.5 months, and overall survival was 56% at 2 years. The majority of deaths were found to be related to comorbid illnesses seen in this frail patient population, rather than death associated with lung cancer. Again, toxicity was tolerable, with less than 20% of patients experiencing high-grade toxicity, but there were six treatment-related deaths. Severe toxicity (grades 3–5) was significantly more likely to occur in patients with "central" tumors, defined as tumors near the proximal bronchial tree (see Sect. 5). The trial was recently updated after a median follow-up of 50 months showing 3-year local control and survival rates of 88% and 42%, respectively (Fakiris et al. 2009).

Based on the encouraging results seen in the Indiana experience, the Radiation Therapy Oncology Group initiated a multi-institutional phase II study in 2002. RTOG 0236 completed accrual of 59 patients in October of 2006. Eligible patients were purely medically inoperable (not confounded by those refusing surgery) and included peripheral T1 or T2/3 tumors ≤5 cm. Patients with tumors within 2 cm of the "proximal bronchial tree" (Fig. 12) were excluded based on the toxicity seen in the phase II study from Indiana University.

Patients were treated to 60 Gy in three fractions based on planning without tissue heterogeneity correction (assuming that the body is solid water). Forty-four patients had T1 tumors, 11 had T2 tumors, and no patients enrolled had T3 tumors. Extensive central accreditation, conduct, and dosimetry constraints were developed prior to the opening of the trial by the RTOG Lung, Physics, and Image-Guided Therapy committees to ensure meaningful quality assurance of SAbR techniques and that patients received consistent treatment according to protocol guidelines at all of the participating centers. The first results of this trial were published in the 2010 theme issue on cancer for the Journal of the American Medical Association (Timmerman et al. 2010). Severe

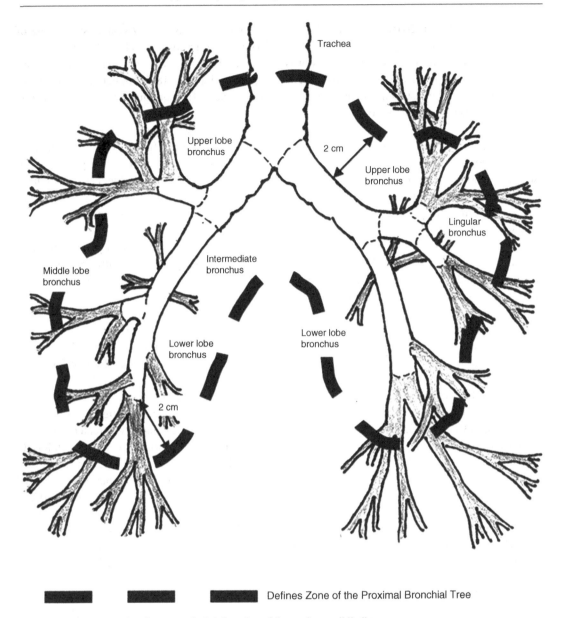

Fig. 12 Diagram showing the anatomical delineation of "central or perihilar" tumors

toxicity was limited in this trial, with only 12.7% of patients with grade 3 treatment-related toxicity and only 3.6% with grade 4 toxicity. Only one failure was seen at the primary tumor site, leading to a 3-year primary tumor control rate of 98%. The local control rate was determined to be 91% with three additional patients having failure within the involved lobe outside of the treated area. Regional failure within hilar or mediastinal lymph nodes was low despite nonsurgical staging, with a 3-year locoregional control rate of 87%. Eleven patients, however, failed in distant sites, the majority within 1 year of treatment. Despite these failures, disease-free and overall survivals were also encouraging in this trial with 3-year rates of 48% and 56%, respectively.

The long-term 5-year results of RTOG 0236 were more recently published (Timmerman et al. 2018a). The 5-year recurrence rates were as follows: primary tumor 7.3%, primary tumor and involved lobe (local) 20.0%, regional 10.9%, local-regional 25.5%, and disseminated 23.6%. The disease-free survival rate at 5 years was 25.5%, and overall survival rate was 40.0%. The further follow-up demonstrated that there are additional recurrences, stemming from the untreated areas of the lung, outside of the primary targeted tumor. Grade 3 toxicity occurred in 27.3% of patients, and 3.6% of patients had grade 4 toxicity, with the majority of the adverse effects related to the pulmonary or musculoskeletal categories.

Other multicenter prospective trials utilizing SAbR in the medically inoperable population have been performed. The Dutch Group has published prospective results of SAbR where treatment was based on patient characteristics related to tumor size and location (Lagerwaard et al. 2008). After treating 200-plus patients (80% were medically inoperable), local control rate was over 90% while severe late toxicity was under 5% with their "risk-adapted" approach. A Nordic study group similarly reported 65% 2-year overall survival rate in a group of 57 medically inoperable patients. Local control rate at 2 years was 93% using their three-fraction SAbR regimen (Baumann et al. 2009).

The Japanese Clinical Oncology Group conducted a study, JCOG0403, of SAbR in 169 patients with operable and inoperable T1 tumors using four fractions of 12 Gy, demonstrating local control rate of 87.3% in inoperable patients and 85.4% in operable patients, a study based on the data from their initial phase I–II study (Nagata et al. 2005, 2015). The Japanese Clinical Oncology Group is currently conducting a randomized phase III trial comparing 55 Gy in four fractions versus 42 Gy in four fractions (Kimura et al. 2017). The dose of 42 Gy in four fractions prescribed to the PTV was determined to be an equivalent dose to the previously utilized 48 Gy in four fractions prescribed to a central tumor point, using the superposition algorithm, density correction, and $D_{95\%}$ prescribing method for dose calculation (Kawahara et al. 2017).

Similarly, Sun et al. demonstrated that local disease recurrence was 8.1%, regional disease recurrence was 13.6%, and distant disease recurrence was 13.8% at 7 years, using a dose of 50 Gy in four fractions for clinical stage I NSCLC (Sun et al. 2017). Second lung primary carcinoma developed in 18.5% of patients, underscoring the need for continued surveillance in this group of patients.

A randomized, phase II study was recently reported evaluating SAbR versus stereotactic body proton therapy (SBPT) for patients with high-risk, medically inoperable, early-stage non-small cell lung cancer, with a dose of 50 Gy (relative biological effectiveness) in four fractions (Nantavithya et al. 2018). The trial closed early due to poor accrual with only 21 patients enrolled but did show a 3-year local control rate of 87.5% of patients who received SAbR versus 90.0% in the SBPT assignment.

The RTOG recently completed a randomized phase II study, RTOG 0915, comparing two different "gentler" radiotherapy schedules, 34 Gy delivered in one fraction and 48 Gy in four fractions (Videtic et al. 2015, 2019). The goal of the trial was to determine the regimen with the least toxicity while maintaining a high level of tumor control at 1 year of equal to or greater than 90%, as demonstrated by more potent dosing in RTOG 0236. The intended goal of the study was to eventually compare with the fractionation schedule of 54 Gy in three fractions, as used in RTOG 0236. A total of 84 out of 94 patients accrued were eligible for analysis, demonstrating that the primary tumor failure rates were similar in both arms, with a primary tumor failure rate of 10.6% in the 34 Gy arm and 6.8% in the 48 Gy arm. The rate of grade ≥3 protocol-specified adverse events at 1 year, the primary endpoint of the RTOG 0915, was 10.3% in the single-fraction arm and 13.3% in the four-fraction arm.

Recently, two publications have compared SAbR to conventionally fractionated radiation therapy for patients with early-stage non-small cell lung cancer. The SPACE trial is the first randomized phase II trial comparing SAbR versus conventionally fractionated radiation therapy (Nyman et al. 2016). One hundred and two patients with stage I medically inoperable NSCLC were randomized to 66 Gy delivered in 3 fractions, prescribed at the isocenter, versus 70 Gy delivered in 35 fractions. The SPACE trial did not show any statistically significant difference in progression-free survival or overall survival, but patients who received SAbR had improved toxicity and health-related quality of life over conventionally fractionated radiation therapy. The CHISEL trial recruited 101 patients with inoperable peripherally located stage I non-small cell lung cancer and evaluated SAbR (given as 54 Gy in 3 fractions or 48 Gy in 4 fractions) versus external beam radiation therapy given at 66 Gy in 33 fractions or 50 Gy in 20 fractions (Ball et al. 2019). Local control rate at 2 years with SAbR was significantly better at 89% than standard radiotherapy, which had a 2-year local control rate of 65%. This improvement in local control translated into an improved 2-year overall survival rate of 77% versus 59% in the standard radiotherapy group. While there are differences in the diagnostic workup and SAbR dosimetry and planning, these two studies suggest that SAbR is equally efficacious or even superior to conventionally fractionated radiation therapy. Similar to the CHISEL results, retrospective studies and one systematic review suggest that SAbR confers a survival benefit over standard radiotherapy (Hegi et al. 2018; von Reibnitz et al. 2018; Haque et al. 2018). The Ontario Clinical Oncology Group (OCOG)-LUSTRE Trial has been activated to evaluate SAbR, given at 48 Gy in 4 fractions, versus a hypofractionated course of radiotherapy at 60 Gy delivered in 15 fractions with a planned sample size of 324 patients (Swaminath et al. 2017).

From the initial experience from Indiana, severe toxicity was high in tumors within the central lung, leading to exclusion of these patients in the subsequent RTOG 0236 trial (Timmerman et al. 2006). In the 4-year Indiana phase II trial results, there was no significant difference in survival or toxicity between patients with peripheral and patients with central tumors, albeit "central" was defined differently for the 2009 report (Fakiris et al. 2009). To further investigate the optimal regimen for centrally located tumors, the RTOG conducted a seamless phase I–II trial, NRG Oncology/RTOG 0813, to address the question of escalating doses in five fractions for centrally located tumors. Patients started at a dose of 50 Gy in five fractions with escalation up to 12.0 Gy per fraction, in 0.5 Gy-per-fraction increments, to determine the maximally tolerated dose for central tumors in the inoperable patient population. The results were published in 2018, enrolling 120 patients with biopsy-proven T1–T2 (≤5 cm) centrally located NSCLC (Bezjak et al. 2019). The 12.0 Gy-per-fraction arm was associated with a dose-limiting toxicity probability of 7.2% and 2-year local control rate of 87.9%.

The first toxicity analysis of the Nordic HILUS-Trial was presented at the 2016 IASLC 17th World Conference on Lung Cancer, where patients with centrally located tumor (defined as ≤1 cm from the proximal bronchial tree) either from primary NSCLC or progressive metastasis from another tumor were treated with 56 Gy in eight fractions (Lindberg et al. 2017). The 74 enrolled patients were stratified to tumors located close to a main bronchus or tumors close to a lobar bronchus. In this initial presentation, 28% of patients experienced grade 3–5 toxicity with six patients experiencing lethal hemoptysis and one patient suffering from lethal pneumonitis. Grade 4–5 side effects occurred more often in patients with primary NSCLC (19%), compared to those with centrally located metastatic cancer (3%). The European Organisation for Research and Treatment of Cancer (EORTC) launched the LungTech phase II trial (EORTC 22113-08113-LungTech), where patients with early-stage, centrally located, inoperable NSCLC will receive 60.0 Gy in eight fractions (Adebahr et al. 2015; Lambrecht et al. 2016).

Because of these favorable local control and survival results from these SAbR prospective trials with results that are only modestly poorer than the results with definitive surgical resection despite the frail population in which the study was conducted (Naruke et al. 1988; Nesbitt et al. 1995; Ginsberg and Rubinstein 1995), exploration of utilizing SAbR techniques within the medically operable population was deemed feasible and is discussed below.

4.2 Medically Operable Patients

Because of the high tumor control and acceptable toxicity seen with SAbR for early-stage NSCLC in the inoperable population, the use of SAbR in patients able to undergo surgical resection is being explored in the United States, Europe, and Asia. A large retrospective experience from Japan included a significant number of operable patients and showed a 3-year survival rate of 88% (Onishi et al. 2004). In the JCOG0403 prospective trial of SAbR, the 64 enrolled, operable patients had a 3-year local control rate of 85.4% and 3-year overall survival rate of 76.5% (Nagata et al. 2015). There was no grade 4 or 5 toxicity detected in the study. The most common pattern of failure was distant metastases in 33% of patients followed by regional nodal failures in 25% of patients.

RTOG 0618 was a single-arm phase II study of 33 accrued patients, of which 26 were evaluable, with operable T1–T2, N0 NSCLC, with no tumor larger than 5 cm (Timmerman et al. 2018b). All patients have FEV1 and DLCO greater than 35% predicted arterial oxygen tension greater than 60 mmHg, arterial carbon dioxide tension less than 50 mmHg, and no severe underlying medical problems. SAbR was given at 54 Gy in three fractions, prescribed to the PTV. Only one patient had a primary tumor recurrence with an estimated 4-year primary tumor control and local control rate of 96%. The 4-year locoregional control rate was 88%, driven by regional failures in three patients, and disseminated recurrence occurred in five patients, giving a 4-year disseminated failure rate of 12%. The toxicity profile was acceptable with no patients experiencing a grade 4–5 treatment-related adverse event. Given these findings, SAbR for patients with operable early-stage NSCLC may be a suitable treatment alternative to surgery, and several randomized phase III trials have commenced evaluating SAbR against surgical resection.

Many retrospective and database studies have attempted to compare SAbR and surgery for early-stage lung cancer but have been subjected to selection biases and lack of control on confounding variables. Initially, three prospective, randomized trials were opened, comparing surgery and SAbR for stage I operable NSCLC, the STARS trial (NCT00840749), the ROSEL trial (NCT00687986), and the ACOSOG Z4099/RTOG 1021 trial (NCT01336894). Unfortunately, all three were closed early due to slow accrual. A pooled analysis was performed of the STARS and ROSEL trial for a total of 58 patients, showing a 3-year overall survival rate of 95% in patients who received SAbR, compared to 79% of patients in the surgery group (Chang et al. 2015). The 3-year recurrence-free survival was 86% in the SAbR group versus 80% in the surgery group. No patients in the SAbR arm had grade 4 events or treatment-related death, while 1 patient (4%) died of surgical complications and 12 (44%) patients had grade 3–4 treatment-related adverse events. The results of ACOSOG Z4099/RTOG 1021 trial have not been reported (Fernando and Timmerman 2012).

Three other randomized, phase III trials have recently been activated, the JoLT-Ca STABLEMATES trial (NCT02468024), VALOR trial (NCT02984761), and SABRTooth trial (NCT02629458). As of October 2020, a total of 169 patients have been enrolled on the STABLEMATES trial. The SABRTooth trial recently reported their results, demonstrating that only 24 patients were randomized in the study, out of a total of 106 patients deemed eligible, as 41% of patients preferred SAbR and 18% preferred surgery. Only 15 patients underwent their assigned treatment, citing a variety of different barriers to trial recruitment (Snee et al. 2016; Franks et al. 2020).

In a unique single-arm phase II study of a combined approach of neoadjuvant SAbR followed by surgery 10 weeks later, the rate of pCR, determined by the uptake of hematoxylin-eosin (H&E) staining and morphologic appearance of tumor cells, was 60% (95% confidence interval, 44–76%) (Palma et al. 2019). This result is discordant from the high rates of local control demonstrated by multiple prior studies, as described above. Many limitations likely existed in this study, including the optimal method for determining tumor viability, the short time between radiation therapy and surgery, and difficulties in assessing reproductive viability (Ozsahin et al.

2019; Connolly et al. 2019). Nonetheless, SAbR is an effective treatment for patients who are medically inoperable and those who refuse surgery.

4.3 Surveillance After SAbR

After the completion of SAbR, based on the international expert consensus, it is recommended that patients receive surveillance CT imaging 3, 6, and 12 months after completion of SAbR in the first year, every 6 months in the second year, and annually from years 3 to 5. PET/CT or CT imaging is suitable in patients where there is a suspicion for local recurrence (Nguyen et al. 2018). Findings that potentially suggest local recurrence include infiltration into adjacent organs/structures, sustained growth over serial scans, bulging margins, mass-like growth, predominantly spherical growth and craniocaudal growth, and airspace obliteration/loss of air bronchograms.

5 Conclusions and Future Considerations

Stereotactic ablative radiotherapy (SAbR) has utilized innovation within the engineering and physics of radiation therapy to increase treatment accuracy and to allow delivery of oligofractionated, ablative doses of radiation. This technological advancement has allowed the exploration of high-dose-per-fraction treatments, leading to observation of unique radiobiological outcomes that have challenged the principles of conventional fractionation. The technologic and biologic benefits of SAbR have been observed most dramatically in patients with early-stage lung cancer. Use of SAbR in these patients has now been established as the standard treatment option for medically inoperable patients through careful study in the prospective, multi-institutional clinical trials described above. In 2017, the ASTRO released the executive summary of evidence-based guidelines for the use of stereotactic ablative radiotherapy in early-stage non-small cell lung cancer, which offers guidance including patient selection, choice of fractionation, and use of surgery versus SAbR in medically operable patients (Videtic et al. 2017).

Toxicity of this treatment has been well characterized in the clinical trials, allowing for appropriate selection of candidates for SAbR. Because of the encouraging control rates seen in medically inoperable patients, study of SAbR has now been extended to medically operable patients and is being compared to surgical resection in ongoing randomized clinical trials.

As systemic therapy becomes more effective for solid tumors, it was thought that local treatments such as radiotherapy and surgical resection would be less utilized in cancer therapy. Interestingly, however, the opposite is occurring within oncologic therapy. As systemic therapy proves to be more effective, local failure is becoming an increasingly more common method of failure, making local control progressively more critical to patient outcome. Thus, the techniques and ablative doses utilized with SAbR will become more important not only in early-stage disease, but also in metastatic disease as a measure for consolidation or ablation of resistant cancer deposits after systemic therapy. In addition, customization of therapy to patient-specific tumor characteristics will become increasingly important in the future as biological, clinical, and technical research within oncology creates paradigms to facilitate adaptive therapy. Within adaptive therapy, pretreatment diagnostic information including imaging, staging, and tissue characteristics (proteomic, genomics, and predictive assays) will be integrated to design patient-specific therapy. Patients can be monitored during treatment with similar methods, and treatments can be adjusted including the need for adjuvant therapies and to avoid toxicity from treatment. This paradigm avoids the "one-size-fits-all" mantra in the current oncologic therapy and utilizes a tailored approach to constantly reevaluate and respond to queues in order to redirect therapy toward better patient outcome. As we continue toward this goal of adapting therapy, it will continue to be crucial to utilize well-designed prospective trials so that therapeutic tools such as SAbR can be refined to their optimal potential.

References

Abelson JA, Murphy JD, Loo BW Jr, Chang DT, Daly ME, Wiegner EA, Hancock S, Chang SD, Le QT, Soltys SG, Gibbs IC (2012) Esophageal tolerance to high-dose stereotactic ablative radiotherapy. Dis Esophagus 25:623–629

Adebahr S, Collette S, Shash E, Lambrecht M, Le Pechoux C, Faivre-Finn C, De Ruysscher D, Peulen H, Belderbos J, Dziadziuszko R, Fink C, Guckenberger M, Hurkmans C, Nestle U (2015) LungTech, an EORTC phase II trial of stereotactic body radiotherapy for centrally located lung tumours: a clinical perspective. Br J Radiol 88:20150036

Ball D, Mai GT, Vinod S, Babington S, Ruben J, Kron T, Chesson B, Herschtal A, Vanevski M, Rezo A, Elder C, Skala M, Wirth A, Wheeler G, Lim A, Shaw M, Schofield P, Irving L, Solomon B, Trog Chisel Investigators (2019) Stereotactic ablative radiotherapy versus standard radiotherapy in stage 1 non-small-cell lung cancer (TROG 09.02 CHISEL): a phase 3, open-label, randomised controlled trial. Lancet Oncol 20:494–503

Balter JM, Wright JN, Newell LJ, Friemel B, Dimmer S, Cheng Y, Wong J, Vertatschitsch E, Mate TP (2005) Accuracy of a wireless localization system for radiotherapy. Int J Radiat Oncol Biol Phys 61:933–937

Baumann P, Nyman J, Hoyer M, Wennberg B, Gagliardi G, Lax I, Drugge N, Ekberg L, Friesland S, Johansson KA, Lund JA, Morhed E, Nilsson K, Levin N, Paludan M, Sederholm C, Traberg A, Wittgren L, Lewensohn R (2009) Outcome in a prospective phase II trial of medically inoperable stage I non-small-cell lung cancer patients treated with stereotactic body radiotherapy. J Clin Oncol 27:3290–3296

Benedict SH, Lin PS, Zwicker RD, Huang DT, Schmidt-Ullrich RK (1997) The biological effectiveness of intermittent irradiation as a function of overall treatment time: development of correction factors for linac-based stereotactic radiotherapy. Int J Radiat Oncol Biol Phys 37:765–769

Benedict SH, Yenice KM, Followill D, Galvin JM, Hinson W, Kavanagh B, Keall P, Lovelock M, Meeks S, Papiez L, Purdie T, Sadagopan R, Schell MC, Salter B, Schlesinger DJ, Shiu AS, Solberg T, Song DY, Stieber V, Timmerman R, Tome WA, Verellen D, Wang L, Yin FF (2010) Stereotactic body radiation therapy: the report of AAPM Task Group 101. Med Phys 37:4078–4101

Bezjak A, Paulus R, Gaspar LE, Timmerman RD, Straube WL, Ryan WF, Garces YI, Pu AT, Singh AK, Videtic GM, McGarry RC, Iyengar P, Pantarotto JR, Urbanic JJ, Sun AY, Daly ME, Grills IS, Sperduto P, Normolle DP, Bradley JD, Choy H (2019) Safety and efficacy of a five-fraction stereotactic body radiotherapy schedule for centrally located non-small-cell lung cancer: NRG oncology/RTOG 0813 trial. J Clin Oncol 37:1316–1325

Bibault JE, Prevost B, Dansin E, Mirabel X, Lacornerie T, Lartigau E (2012) Image-guided robotic stereotactic radiation therapy with fiducial-free tumor tracking for lung cancer. Radiat Oncol 7:102

Blomgren H, Lax I, Naslund I, Svanstrom R (1995) Stereotactic high dose fraction radiation therapy of extracranial tumors using an accelerator. Clinical experience of the first thirty-one patients. Acta Oncol 34:861–870

Bouilhol G, Ayadi M, Rit S, Thengumpallil S, Schaerer J, Vandemeulebroucke J, Claude L, Sarrut D (2013) Is abdominal compression useful in lung stereotactic body radiation therapy? A 4DCT and dosimetric lobe-dependent study. Phys Med 29:333–340

Brown JM, Diehn M, Loo BW Jr (2010) Stereotactic ablative radiotherapy should be combined with a hypoxic cell radiosensitizer. Int J Radiat Oncol Biol Phys 78:323–327

Brown JM, Brenner DJ, Carlson DJ (2013) Dose escalation, not "new biology," can account for the efficacy of stereotactic body radiation therapy with non-small cell lung cancer. Int J Radiat Oncol Biol Phys 85:1159–1160

Cardinale RM, Wu Q, Benedict SH, Kavanagh BD, Bump E, Mohan R (1999) Determining the optimal block margin on the planning target volume for extracranial stereotactic radiotherapy. Int J Radiat Oncol Biol Phys 45:515–520

Chang SD, Main W, Martin DP, Gibbs IC, Heilbrun MP (2003) An analysis of the accuracy of the CyberKnife: a robotic frameless stereotactic radiosurgical system. Neurosurgery 52:140–146; discussion 46–47

Chang JY, Senan S, Paul MA, Mehran RJ, Louie AV, Balter P, Groen HJ, McRae SE, Widder J, Feng L, van den Borne BE, Munsell MF, Hurkmans C, Berry DA, van Werkhoven E, Kresl JJ, Dingemans AM, Dawood O, Haasbeek CJ, Carpenter LS, De Jaeger K, Komaki R, Slotman BJ, Smit EF, Roth JA (2015) Stereotactic ablative radiotherapy versus lobectomy for operable stage I non-small-cell lung cancer: a pooled analysis of two randomised trials. Lancet Oncol 16:630–637

Chao ST, Dad LK, Dawson LA, Desai NB, Pacella M, Rengan R, Xiao Y, Yenice KM, Rosenthal SA, Hartford A (2020) ACR-ASTRO practice parameter for the performance of stereotactic body radiation therapy. Am J Clin Oncol 43:545–552

Chen GT, Kung JH, Beaudette KP (2004) Artifacts in computed tomography scanning of moving objects. Semin Radiat Oncol 14:19–26

Connolly JG, Jones GD, Caso R, Jones DR (2019) Stereotactic ablative radiotherapy for operable stage I non-small cell lung cancer: not ready for prime time. Ann Transl Med 7:S234

Corradetti MN, Mitra N, Bonner Millar LP, Byun J, Wan F, Apisarnthanarax S, Christodouleas J, Anderson N, Simone CB 2nd, Teo BK, Rengan R (2013) A moving target: image guidance for stereotactic body radiation therapy for early-stage non-small cell lung cancer. Pract Radiat Oncol 3:307–315

Curiel TJ (2007) Tregs and rethinking cancer immunotherapy. J Clin Invest 117:1167–1174

Dahele M, Verbakel W, Cuijpers J, Slotman B, Senan S (2012) An analysis of patient positioning during stereotactic lung radiotherapy performed without rigid external immobilization. Radiother Oncol 104:28–32

Dunlap NE, Cai J, Biedermann GB, Yang W, Benedict SH, Sheng K, Schefter TE, Kavanagh BD, Larner JM (2010) Chest wall volume receiving >30 Gy predicts risk of severe pain and/or rib fracture after lung stereotactic body radiotherapy. Int J Radiat Oncol Biol Phys 76:796–801

Fakiris AJ, McGarry RC, Yiannoutsos CT, Papiez L, Williams M, Henderson MA, Timmerman R (2009) Stereotactic body radiation therapy for early-stage non-small-cell lung carcinoma: four-year results of a prospective phase II study. Int J Radiat Oncol Biol Phys 75:677–682

Feddock J, Arnold SM, Shelton BJ, Sinha P, Conrad G, Chen L, Rinehart J, McGarry RC (2013) Stereotactic body radiation therapy can be used safely to boost residual disease in locally advanced non-small cell lung cancer: a prospective study. Int J Radiat Oncol Biol Phys 85:1325–1331

Fernando HC, Timmerman R (2012) American College of Surgeons oncology group Z4099/radiation therapy oncology group 1021: a randomized study of sublobar resection compared with stereotactic body radiotherapy for high-risk stage I non-small cell lung cancer. J Thorac Cardiovasc Surg 144:S35–S38

Foster R, Meyer J, Iyengar P, Pistenmaa D, Timmerman R, Choy H, Solberg T (2013) Localization accuracy and immobilization effectiveness of a stereotactic body frame for a variety of treatment sites. Int J Radiat Oncol Biol Phys 87:911–916

Fowler JF, Welsh JS, Howard SP (2004) Loss of biological effect in prolonged fraction delivery. Int J Radiat Oncol Biol Phys 59:242–249

Franks KN, McParland L, Webster J, Baldwin DR, Sebag-Montefiore D, Evison M, Booton R, Faivre-Finn C, Naidu B, Ferguson J, Peedell C, Callister MEJ, Kennedy M, Hewison J, Bestall J, Gregory WM, Hall P, Collinson F, Olivier C, Naylor R, Bell S, Allen P, Sloss A, Snee M (2020) SABRTOOTH: a randomised controlled feasibility study of stereotactic ablative radiotherapy (SABR) with surgery in patients with peripheral stage I non-small cell lung cancer (NSCLC) considered to be at higher risk of complications from surgical resection. Eur Respir J 56:2000118

Fuks Z, Kolesnick R (2005) Engaging the vascular component of the tumor response. Cancer Cell 8:89–91

Fuss M, Salter BJ, Cheek D, Sadeghi A, Hevezi JM, Herman TS (2004) Repositioning accuracy of a commercially available thermoplastic mask system. Radiother Oncol 71:339–345

Garcia-Barros M, Paris F, Cordon-Cardo C, Lyden D, Rafii S, Haimovitz-Friedman A, Fuks Z, Kolesnick R (2003) Tumor response to radiotherapy regulated by endothelial cell apoptosis. Science 300:1155–1159

Giglioli FR, Clemente S, Esposito M, Fiandra C, Marino C, Russo S, Strigari L, Villaggi E, Stasi M, Mancosu P (2017) Frontiers in planning optimization for lung SBRT. Phys Med 44:163–170

Ginsberg RJ, Rubinstein LV (1995) Randomized trial of lobectomy versus limited resection for T1 N0 non-small cell lung cancer. Lung cancer study group. Ann Thorac Surg 60:615–622; discussion 22–23

Golden EB, Pellicciotta I, Demaria S, Barcellos-Hoff MH, Formenti SC (2012) The convergence of radiation and immunogenic cell death signaling pathways. Front Oncol 2:88

Guckenberger M, Klement RJ, Kestin LL, Hope AJ, Belderbos J, Werner-Wasik M, Yan D, Sonke JJ, Bissonnette JP, Xiao Y, Grills IS (2013) Lack of a dose-effect relationship for pulmonary function changes after stereotactic body radiation therapy for early-stage non-small cell lung cancer. Int J Radiat Oncol Biol Phys 85:1074–1081

Guerrero M, Li XA (2004) Extending the linear-quadratic model for large fraction doses pertinent to stereotactic radiotherapy. Phys Med Biol 49:4825–4835

Haikerwal SJ, Hagekyriakou J, MacManus M, Martin OA, Haynes NM (2015) Building immunity to cancer with radiation therapy. Cancer Lett 368:198–208

Hall EJ, Gross W, Dvorak RF, Kellerer AM, Rossi HH (1972) Survival curves and age response functions for Chinese hamster cells exposed to x-rays or high LET alpha-particles. Radiat Res 52:88–98

Hamilton AJ, Lulu BA, Fosmire H, Stea B, Cassady JR (1995) Preliminary clinical experience with linear accelerator-based spinal stereotactic radiosurgery. Neurosurgery 36:311–319

Haque W, Verma V, Polamraju P, Farach A, Butler EB, Teh BS (2018) Stereotactic body radiation therapy versus conventionally fractionated radiation therapy for early stage non-small cell lung cancer. Radiother Oncol 129:264–269

Haseltine JM, Rimner A, Gelblum DY, Modh A, Rosenzweig KE, Jackson A, Yorke ED, Wu AJ (2016) Fatal complications after stereotactic body radiation therapy for central lung tumors abutting the proximal bronchial tree. Pract Radiat Oncol 6:e27–e33

Hegi F, D'Souza M, Azzi M, De Ruysscher D (2018) Comparing the outcomes of stereotactic ablative radiotherapy and non-stereotactic ablative radiotherapy definitive radiotherapy approaches to thoracic malignancy: a systematic review and meta-analysis. Clin Lung Cancer 19:199–212

Heinzerling JH, Anderson JF, Papiez L, Boike T, Chien S, Zhang G, Abdulrahman R, Timmerman R (2008) Four-dimensional computed tomography scan analysis of tumor and organ motion at varying levels of abdominal compression during stereotactic treatment of lung and liver. Int J Radiat Oncol Biol Phys 70:1571–1578

Hepel JT, Leonard KL, Safran H, Ng T, Taber A, Khurshid H, Birnbaum A, Group Brown University Oncology Research, Wazer DE, DiPetrillo T (2016) Stereotactic body radiation therapy boost after concurrent chemoradiation for locally advanced non-small cell lung cancer: a phase 1 dose escalation study. Int J Radiat Oncol Biol Phys 96:1021–1027

Herfarth KK, Debus J, Lohr F, Bahner ML, Rhein B, Fritz P, Hoss A, Schlegel W, Wannenmacher MF (2001) Stereotactic single-dose radiation therapy of liver tumors: results of a phase I/II trial. J Clin Oncol 19:164–170

Higgins KA, Pillai RN, Chen Z, Tian S, Zhang C, Patel P, Pakkala S, Shelton J, Force SD, Fernandez FG, Steuer CE, Owonikoko TK, Ramalingam SS, Bradley JD, Curran WJ (2017) Concomitant chemotherapy and radiotherapy with SBRT boost for unresectable stage III non-small cell lung cancer: a phase I study. J Thorac Oncol 12:1687–1695

Horne ZD, Richman AH, Dohopolski MJ, Clump DA, Burton SA, Heron DE (2018) Stereotactic body radiation therapy for isolated hilar and mediastinal non-small cell lung cancers. Lung Cancer 115:1–4

Inoue T, Katoh N, Onimaru R, Shimizu S, Tsuchiya K, Suzuki R, Sakakibara-Konishi J, Shinagawa N, Oizumi S, Shirato H (2013) Stereotactic body radiotherapy using gated radiotherapy with real-time tumor-tracking for stage I non-small cell lung cancer. Radiat Oncol 8:69

Jaffray DA, Siewerdsen JH, Wong JW, Martinez AA (2002) Flat-panel cone-beam computed tomography for image-guided radiation therapy. Int J Radiat Oncol Biol Phys 53:1337–1349

Jang SS, Huh GJ, Park SY, Yang PS, Cho EY (2014) The impact of respiratory gating on lung dosimetry in stereotactic body radiotherapy for lung cancer. Phys Med 30:682–689

Josipovic M, Persson GF, Logadottir A, Smulders B, Westmann G, Bangsgaard JP (2012) Translational and rotational intra- and inter-fractional errors in patient and target position during a short course of frameless stereotactic body radiotherapy. Acta Oncol 51:610–617

Josipovic M, Aznar MC, Thomsen JB, Scherman J, Damkjaer SM, Nygard L, Specht L, Pohl M, Persson GF (2019) Deep inspiration breath hold in locally advanced lung cancer radiotherapy: validation of intrafractional geometric uncertainties in the INHALE trial. Br J Radiol 92:20190569

Joyner M, Salter BJ, Papanikolaou N, Fuss M (2006) Stereotactic body radiation therapy for centrally located lung lesions. Acta Oncol 45:802–807

Kaskowitz L, Graham MV, Emami B, Halverson KJ, Rush C (1993) Radiation therapy alone for stage I non-small cell lung cancer. Int J Radiat Oncol Biol Phys 27:517–523

Kawahara D, Ozawa S, Kimura T, Saito A, Nishio T, Nakashima T, Ohno Y, Murakami Y, Nagata Y (2017) Marginal prescription equivalent to the isocenter prescription in lung stereotactic body radiotherapy: preliminary study for Japan clinical oncology group trial (JCOG1408). J Radiat Res 58:149–154

Kestin L, Grills I, Guckenberger M, Belderbos J, Hope AJ, Werner-Wasik M, Sonke JJ, Bissonnette JP, Xiao Y, Yan D, Group Elekta Lung Research (2014) Dose-response relationship with clinical outcome for lung stereotactic body radiotherapy (SBRT) delivered via online image guidance. Radiother Oncol 110:499–504

Kim DWN, Medin PM, Timmerman RD (2017) Emphasis on repair, not just avoidance of injury, facilitates prudent stereotactic ablative radiotherapy. Semin Radiat Oncol 27:378–392

Kimura T, Nagata Y, Eba J, Ozawa S, Ishikura S, Shibata T, Ito Y, Hiraoka M, Nishimura Y, Group Radiation Oncology Study Group of the Japan Clinical Oncology (2017) A randomized phase III trial of comparing two dose-fractionations stereotactic body radiotherapy (SBRT) for medically inoperable stage IA non-small cell lung cancer or small lung lesions clinically diagnosed as primary lung cancer: Japan Clinical Oncology Group Study JCOG1408 (J-SBRT trial). Jpn J Clin Oncol 47:277–281

Kini VR, Vedam SS, Keall PJ, Patil S, Chen C, Mohan R (2003) Patient training in respiratory-gated radiotherapy. Med Dosim 28:7–11

Kirkpatrick JP, Dewhirst MW (2008) Analytic solution to steady-state radial diffusion of a substrate with first-order reaction kinetics in the tissue of a Krogh's cylinder. Radiat Res 169:350–354

Koch N, Liu HH, Starkschall G, Jacobson M, Forster K, Liao Z, Komaki R, Stevens CW (2004) Evaluation of internal lung motion for respiratory-gated radiotherapy using MRI: part I—correlating internal lung motion with skin fiducial motion. Int J Radiat Oncol Biol Phys 60:1459–1472

Kuriyama K, Onishi H, Sano N, Komiyama T, Aikawa Y, Tateda Y, Araki T, Uematsu M (2003) A new irradiation unit constructed of self-moving gantry-CT and linac. Int J Radiat Oncol Biol Phys 55:428–435

Lagerwaard FJ, Van Sornsen de Koste JR, Nijssen-Visser MR, Schuchhard-Schipper RH, Oei SS, Munne A, Senan S (2001) Multiple "slow" CT scans for incorporating lung tumor mobility in radiotherapy planning. Int J Radiat Oncol Biol Phys 51:932–937

Lagerwaard FJ, Haasbeek CJ, Smit EF, Slotman BJ, Senan S (2008) Outcomes of risk-adapted fractionated stereotactic radiotherapy for stage I non-small-cell lung cancer. Int J Radiat Oncol Biol Phys 70:685–692

Lambrecht M, Melidis C, Sonke JJ, Adebahr S, Boellaard R, Verheij M, Guckenberger M, Nestle U, Hurkmans C (2016) Lungtech, a phase II EORTC trial of SBRT for centrally located lung tumours—a clinical physics perspective. Radiat Oncol 11:7

Lax I, Blomgren H, Naslund I, Svanstrom R (1994) Stereotactic radiotherapy of malignancies in the abdomen. Methodological aspects. Acta Oncol 33:677–683

Lee Y, Auh SL, Wang Y, Burnette B, Wang Y, Meng Y, Beckett M, Sharma R, Chin R, Tu T, Weichselbaum RR, Fu YX (2009) Therapeutic effects of ablative radiation on local tumor require CD8+ T cells: changing strategies for cancer treatment. Blood 114:589–595

Lee D, Greer PB, Ludbrook J, Arm J, Hunter P, Pollock S, Makhija K, O'Brien RT, Kim T, Keall P (2016) Audiovisual biofeedback improves cine-magnetic resonance imaging measured lung tumor motion consistency. Int J Radiat Oncol Biol Phys 94:628–636

Leksell L (1951) The stereotaxic method and radiosurgery of the brain. Acta Chir Scand 102:316–319

Lindberg K, Bergstrom P, Brustugun OT, Engelholm S, Grozman V, Hoyer M, Karlsson K, Khalil A, Kristiansen C, Lax I, Loden B, Nyman J, Persson G, Rogg L, Wersall P, Lewensohn R (2017) The Nordic HILUS-trial—first report of a phase II trial of SBRT of centrally located lung tumors. J Thorac Oncol 12: S340

Lindberg K, Grozman V, Lindberg S, Onjukka E, Lax I, Lewensohn R, Wersall P (2019) Radiation-induced brachial plexus toxicity after SBRT of apically located lung lesions. Acta Oncol 58:1178–1186

Liu R, Buatti JM, Howes TL, Dill J, Modrick JM, Meeks SL (2006) Optimal number of beams for stereotactic body radiotherapy of lung and liver lesions. Int J Radiat Oncol Biol Phys 66:906–912

Loo BW Jr, Chang JY, Dawson LA, Kavanagh BD, Koong AC, Senan S, Timmerman RD (2011) Stereotactic ablative radiotherapy: what's in a name? Pract Radiat Oncol 1:38–39

Mageras GS, Pevsner A, Yorke ED, Rosenzweig KE, Ford EC, Hertanto A, Larson SM, Lovelock DM, Erdi YE, Nehmeh SA, Humm JL, Ling CC (2004) Measurement of lung tumor motion using respiration-correlated CT. Int J Radiat Oncol Biol Phys 60:933–941

Manyam BV, Verdecchia K, Rogacki K, Reddy CA, Zhuang T, Videtic GMM, Azok JT, Stephans KL (2019) Investigation of brachial plexus dose that exceeds RTOG constraints for apical lung tumors treated with four- or five-fraction stereotactic body radiation therapy. J Radiosurg SBRT 6:189–197

Marks LB (1995) Extrapolating hypofractionated radiation schemes from radiosurgery data: regarding Hall et al., IJROBP 21:819–824; 1991 and Hall and Brenner, IJROBP 25:381–385; 1993. Int J Radiat Oncol Biol Phys 32:274–276

Matsuo Y, Nagata Y, Mizowaki T, Takayama K, Sakamoto T, Sakamoto M, Norihisa Y, Hiraoka M (2007) Evaluation of mass-like consolidation after stereotactic body radiation therapy for lung tumors. Int J Clin Oncol 12:356–362

McGarry RC, Papiez L, Williams M, Whitford T, Timmerman RD (2005) Stereotactic body radiation therapy of early-stage non-small-cell lung carcinoma: phase I study. Int J Radiat Oncol Biol Phys 63:1010–1015

Mehta N, King CR, Agazaryan N, Steinberg M, Hua A, Lee P (2012) Stereotactic body radiation therapy and 3-dimensional conformal radiotherapy for stage I non-small cell lung cancer: a pooled analysis of biological equivalent dose and local control. Pract Radiat Oncol 2:288–295

Menten MJ, Fast MF, Nill S, Kamerling CP, McDonald F, Oelfke U (2016) Lung stereotactic body radiotherapy with an MR-linac—quantifying the impact of the magnetic field and real-time tumor tracking. Radiother Oncol 119:461–466

Meyer J, Timmerman R (2011) Stereotactic ablative radiotherapy in the framework of classical radiobiology: response to Drs. Brown, Diehn, and Loo. Int J Radiat Oncol Biol Phys 79:1599–1600; author reply 600

Murphy MJ (1997) An automatic six-degree-of-freedom image registration algorithm for image-guided frameless stereotaxic radiosurgery. Med Phys 24:857–866

Murphy MJ, Martin D, Whyte R, Hai J, Ozhasoglu C, Le QT (2002) The effectiveness of breath-holding to stabilize lung and pancreas tumors during radiosurgery. Int J Radiat Oncol Biol Phys 53:475–482

Murray B, Forster K, Timmerman R (2007) Frame-based immobilization and targeting for stereotactic body radiation therapy. Med Dosim 32:86–91

Nagata Y, Takayama K, Matsuo Y, Norihisa Y, Mizowaki T, Sakamoto T, Sakamoto M, Mitsumori M, Shibuya K, Araki N, Yano S, Hiraoka M (2005) Clinical outcomes of a phase I/II study of 48 Gy of stereotactic body radiotherapy in 4 fractions for primary lung cancer using a stereotactic body frame. Int J Radiat Oncol Biol Phys 63:1427–1431

Nagata Y, Hiraoka M, Shibata T, Onishi H, Kokubo M, Karasawa K, Shioyama Y, Onimaru R, Kozuka T, Kunieda E, Saito T, Nakagawa K, Hareyama M, Takai Y, Hayakawa K, Mitsuhashi N, Ishikura S (2015) Prospective trial of stereotactic body radiation therapy for both operable and inoperable T1N0M0 non-small cell lung cancer: Japan clinical oncology group study JCOG0403. Int J Radiat Oncol Biol Phys 93:989–996

Nakagawa K, Haga A, Kida S, Masutani Y, Yamashita H, Takahashi W, Sakumi A, Saotome N, Shiraki T, Ohtomo K, Iwai Y, Yoda K (2013) 4D registration and 4D verification of lung tumor position for stereotactic volumetric modulated arc therapy using respiratory-correlated cone-beam CT. J Radiat Res 54:152–156

Nantavithya C, Gomez DR, Wei X, Komaki R, Liao Z, Lin SH, Jeter M, Nguyen QN, Li H, Zhang X, Poenisch F, Zhu XR, Balter PA, Feng L, Choi NC, Mohan R, Chang JY (2018) Phase 2 study of stereotactic body radiation therapy and stereotactic body proton therapy for high-risk, medically inoperable, early-stage non-small cell lung cancer. Int J Radiat Oncol Biol Phys 101:558–563

Naruke T, Goya T, Tsuchiya R, Suemasu K (1988) Prognosis and survival in resected lung carcinoma based on the new international staging system. J Thorac Cardiovasc Surg 96:440–447

Negoro Y, Nagata Y, Aoki T, Mizowaki T, Araki N, Takayama K, Kokubo M, Yano S, Koga S, Sasai K, Shibamoto Y, Hiraoka M (2001) The effectiveness of an immobilization device in conformal radiotherapy for lung tumor: reduction of respiratory tumor movement and evaluation of the daily setup accuracy. Int J Radiat Oncol Biol Phys 50:889–898

Nesbitt JC, Putnam JB Jr, Walsh GL, Roth JA, Mountain CF (1995) Survival in early-stage non-small cell lung cancer. Ann Thorac Surg 60:466–472

Nguyen TK, Senan S, Bradley JD, Franks K, Giuliani M, Guckenberger M, Landis M, Loo BW Jr, Louie AV,

Onishi H, Schmidt H, Timmerman R, Videtic GMM, Palma DA (2018) Optimal imaging surveillance after stereotactic ablative radiation therapy for early-stage non-small cell lung cancer: findings of an international Delphi consensus study. Pract Radiat Oncol 8:e71–e78

Nuyttens JJ, Moiseenko V, McLaughlin M, Jain S, Herbert S, Grimm J (2016) Esophageal dose tolerance in patients treated with stereotactic body radiation therapy. Semin Radiat Oncol 26:120–128

Nyman J, Johansson KA, Hulten U (2006) Stereotactic hypofractionated radiotherapy for stage I non-small cell lung cancer—mature results for medically inoperable patients. Lung Cancer 51:97–103

Nyman J, Hallqvist A, Lund JA, Brustugun OT, Bergman B, Bergstrom P, Friesland S, Lewensohn R, Holmberg E, Lax I (2016) SPACE—a randomized study of SBRT vs conventional fractionated radiotherapy in medically inoperable stage I NSCLC. Radiother Oncol 121:1–8

Oliver JA, Budzevich M, Zhang GG, Dilling TJ, Latifi K, Moros EG (2015) Variability of image features computed from conventional and respiratory-gated PET/CT images of lung cancer. Transl Oncol 8: 524–534

Onishi H, Araki T, Shirato H, Nagata Y, Hiraoka M, Gomi K, Yamashita T, Niibe Y, Karasawa K, Hayakawa K, Takai Y, Kimura T, Hirokawa Y, Takeda A, Ouchi A, Hareyama M, Kokubo M, Hara R, Itami J, Yamada K (2004) Stereotactic hypofractionated high-dose irradiation for stage I nonsmall cell lung carcinoma: clinical outcomes in 245 subjects in a Japanese multiinstitutional study. Cancer 101:1623–1631

Ozsahin M, Slotman BJ, Bourhis J (2019) Reproductive viability of cells following preoperative stereotactic ablative radiotherapy. Int J Radiat Oncol Biol Phys 105:233–234

Paganelli C, Lee D, Greer PB, Baroni G, Riboldi M, Keall P (2015) Quantification of lung tumor rotation with automated landmark extraction using orthogonal cine MRI images. Phys Med Biol 60:7165–7178

Palma DA, Nguyen TK, Louie AV, Malthaner R, Fortin D, Rodrigues GB, Yaremko B, Laba J, Kwan K, Gaede S, Lee T, Ward A, Warner A, Inculet R (2019) Measuring the integration of stereotactic ablative radiotherapy plus surgery for early-stage non-small cell lung cancer: a phase 2 clinical trial. JAMA Oncol 5:681–688

Papiez L, Timmerman R, DesRosiers C, Randall M (2003) Extracranial stereotactic radioablation: physical principles. Acta Oncol 42:882–894

Park C, Papiez L, Zhang S, Story M, Timmerman RD (2008) Universal survival curve and single fraction equivalent dose: useful tools in understanding potency of ablative radiotherapy. Int J Radiat Oncol Biol Phys 70:847–852

Park HJ, Griffin RJ, Hui S, Levitt SH, Song CW (2012) Radiation-induced vascular damage in tumors: implications of vascular damage in ablative hypofractionated radiotherapy (SBRT and SRS). Radiat Res 177:311–327

Peguret N, Dahele M, Cuijpers JP, Slotman BJ, Verbakel WF (2013) Frameless high dose rate stereotactic lung radiotherapy: intrafraction tumor position and delivery time. Radiother Oncol 107:419–422

Ritter TA, Matuszak M, Chetty IJ, Mayo CS, Wu J, Iyengar P, Weldon M, Robinson C, Xiao Y, Timmerman RD (2017) Application of critical volume-dose constraints for stereotactic body radiation therapy in NRG radiation therapy trials. Int J Radiat Oncol Biol Phys 98:34–36

Rossi HH, Kellerer AM (1972) Radiation carcinogenesis at low doses. Science 175:200–202

Saito T, Matsuyama T, Toya R, Fukugawa Y, Toyofuku T, Semba A, Oya N (2014) Respiratory gating during stereotactic body radiotherapy for lung cancer reduces tumor position variability. PLoS One 9:e112824

Scherman Rydhog J, Riisgaard de Blanck S, Josipovic M, Irming Jolck R, Larsen KR, Clementsen P, Lars Andersen T, Poulsen PR, Fredberg Persson G, Munck Af Rosenschold P (2017) Target position uncertainty during visually guided deep-inspiration breath-hold radiotherapy in locally advanced lung cancer. Radiother Oncol 123:78–84

Shaikh T, Turaka A (2014) Predictors and management of chest wall toxicity after lung stereotactic body radiotherapy. Cancer Treat Rev 40:1215–1220

Sharp GC, Jiang SB, Shimizu S, Shirato H (2004) Prediction of respiratory tumour motion for real-time image-guided radiotherapy. Phys Med Biol 49:425–440

Shibamoto Y, Miyakawa A, Otsuka S, Iwata H (2016) Radiobiology of hypofractionated stereotactic radiotherapy: what are the optimal fractionation schedules? J Radiat Res 57(Suppl 1):i76–i82

Shirato H, Shimizu S, Shimizu T, Nishioka T, Miyasaka K (1999) Real-time tumour-tracking radiotherapy. Lancet 353:1331–1332

Shirato H, Shimizu S, Kunieda T, Kitamura K, van Herk M, Kagei K, Nishioka T, Hashimoto S, Fujita K, Aoyama H, Tsuchiya K, Kudo K, Miyasaka K (2000) Physical aspects of a real-time tumor-tracking system for gated radiotherapy. Int J Radiat Oncol Biol Phys 48:1187–1195

Siegel RL, Miller KD, Jemal A (2020) Cancer statistics, 2020. CA Cancer J Clin 70:7–30

Snee MP, McParland L, Collinson F, Lowe CM, Striha A, Baldwin DR, Naidu B, Sebag-Montefiore D, Gregory WM, Bestall J, Hewison J, Hinsley S, Franks K (2016) The SABRTooth feasibility trial protocol: a study to determine the feasibility and acceptability of conducting a phase III randomised controlled trial comparing stereotactic ablative radiotherapy (SABR) with surgery in patients with peripheral stage I non-small cell lung cancer (NSCLC) considered to be at higher risk of complications from surgical resection. Pilot Feasibility Stud 2:5

Song CW, Glatstein E, Marks LB, Emami B, Grimm J, Sperduto PW, Kim MS, Hui S, Dusenbery KE, Cho LC (2019) Biological principles of stereotactic body radiation therapy (SBRT) and stereotactic radiation surgery (SRS): indirect cell death. Int J Radiat Oncol Biol Phys. https://doi.org/10.1016/j.ijrobp.2019.02.047

Sonke JJ, Zijp L, Remeijer P, van Herk M (2005) Respiratory correlated cone beam CT. Med Phys 32:1176–1186

Stanic S, Paulus R, Timmerman RD, Michalski JM, Barriger RB, Bezjak A, Videtic GM, Bradley J (2014) No clinically significant changes in pulmonary function following stereotactic body radiation therapy for early- stage peripheral non-small cell lung cancer: an analysis of RTOG 0236. Int J Radiat Oncol Biol Phys 88:1092–1099

Stephans KL, Djemil T, Reddy CA, Gajdos SM, Kolar M, Machuzak M, Mazzone P, Videtic GM (2009) Comprehensive analysis of pulmonary function test (PFT) changes after stereotactic body radiotherapy (SBRT) for stage I lung cancer in medically inoperable patients. J Thorac Oncol 4:838–844

Stephans KL, Djemil T, Tendulkar RD, Robinson CG, Reddy CA, Videtic GM (2012) Prediction of chest wall toxicity from lung stereotactic body radiotherapy (SBRT). Int J Radiat Oncol Biol Phys 82:974–980

Stevens CW, Munden RF, Forster KM, Kelly JF, Liao Z, Starkschall G, Tucker S, Komaki R (2001) Respiratory-driven lung tumor motion is independent of tumor size, tumor location, and pulmonary function. Int J Radiat Oncol Biol Phys 51:62–68

Sun B, Brooks ED, Komaki RU, Liao Z, Jeter MD, McAleer MF, Allen PK, Balter PA, Welsh JD, O'Reilly MS, Gomez D, Hahn SM, Roth JA, Mehran RJ, Heymach JV, Chang JY (2017) 7-year follow-up after stereotactic ablative radiotherapy for patients with stage I non-small cell lung cancer: results of a phase 2 clinical trial. Cancer 123:3031–3039

Swaminath A, Wierzbicki M, Parpia S, Wright JR, Tsakiridis TK, Okawara GS, Kundapur V, Bujold A, Ahmed N, Hirmiz K, Kurien E, Filion E, Gabos Z, Faria S, Louie AV, Owen T, Wai E, Ramchandar K, Chan EK, Julian J, Cline K, Whelan TJ (2017) Canadian phase III randomized trial of stereotactic body radiotherapy versus conventionally hypofractionated radiotherapy for stage I, medically inoperable non-small-cell lung cancer—rationale and protocol design for the Ontario Clinical Oncology Group (OCOG)-LUSTRE trial. Clin Lung Cancer 18:250–254

Takeda A, Kunieda E, Takeda T, Tanaka M, Sanuki N, Fujii H, Shigematsu N, Kubo A (2008) Possible misinterpretation of demarcated solid patterns of radiation fibrosis on CT scans as tumor recurrence in patients receiving hypofractionated stereotactic radiotherapy for lung cancer. Int J Radiat Oncol Biol Phys 70:1057–1065

Timmerman RD, Story M (2006) Stereotactic body radiation therapy: a treatment in need of basic biological research. Cancer J 12:19–20

Timmerman R, Papiez L, McGarry R, Likes L, DesRosiers C, Frost S, Williams M (2003a) Extracranial stereotactic radioablation: results of a phase I study in medically inoperable stage I non-small cell lung cancer. Chest 124:1946–1955

Timmerman R, Papiez L, Suntharalingam M (2003b) Extracranial stereotactic radiation delivery: expansion of technology beyond the brain. Technol Cancer Res Treat 2:153–160

Timmerman R, McGarry R, Yiannoutsos C, Papiez L, Tudor K, DeLuca J, Ewing M, Abdulrahman R, DesRosiers C, Williams M, Fletcher J (2006) Excessive toxicity when treating central tumors in a phase II study of stereotactic body radiation therapy for medically inoperable early-stage lung cancer. J Clin Oncol 24:4833–4839

Timmerman R, Paulus R, Galvin J, Michalski J, Straube W, Bradley J, Fakiris A, Bezjak A, Videtic G, Johnstone D, Fowler J, Gore E, Choy H (2010) Stereotactic body radiation therapy for inoperable early stage lung cancer. JAMA 303:1070–1076

Timmerman RD, Hu C, Michalski JM, Bradley JC, Galvin J, Johnstone DW, Choy H (2018a) Long-term results of stereotactic body radiation therapy in medically inoperable stage I non-small cell lung cancer. JAMA Oncol 4:1287–1288

Timmerman RD, Paulus R, Pass HI, Gore EM, Edelman MJ, Galvin J, Straube WL, Nedzi LA, McGarry RC, Robinson CG, Schiff PB, Chang G, Loo BW Jr, Bradley JD, Choy H (2018b) Stereotactic body radiation therapy for operable early-stage lung cancer: findings from the NRG oncology RTOG 0618 trial. JAMA Oncol 4:1263–1266

Uematsu M, Shioda A, Tahara K, Fukui T, Yamamoto F, Tsumatori G, Ozeki Y, Aoki T, Watanabe M, Kusano S (1998) Focal, high dose, and fractionated modified stereotactic radiation therapy for lung carcinoma patients: a preliminary experience. Cancer 82: 1062–1070

Uematsu M, Shioda A, Suda A, Fukui T, Ozeki Y, Hama Y, Wong JR, Kusano S (2001) Computed tomography-guided frameless stereotactic radiotherapy for stage I non-small cell lung cancer: a 5-year experience. Int J Radiat Oncol Biol Phys 51:666–670

Vedam SS, Keall PJ, Kini VR, Mohan R (2001) Determining parameters for respiration-gated radiotherapy. Med Phys 28:2139–2146

Verellen D, Soete G, Linthout N, Van Acker S, De Roover P, Vinh-Hung V, Van de Steene J, Storme G (2003) Quality assurance of a system for improved target localization and patient set-up that combines real-time infrared tracking and stereoscopic X-ray imaging. Radiother Oncol 67:129–141

Videtic GM, Hu C, Singh AK, Chang JY, Parker W, Olivier KR, Schild SE, Komaki R, Urbanic JJ, Timmerman RD, Choy H (2015) A randomized phase 2 study comparing 2 stereotactic body radiation therapy schedules for medically inoperable patients with stage I peripheral non-small cell lung cancer: NRG oncology RTOG 0915 (NCCTG N0927). Int J Radiat Oncol Biol Phys 93:757–764

Videtic GMM, Donington J, Giuliani M, Heinzerling J, Karas TZ, Kelsey CR, Lally BE, Latzka K, Lo SS, Moghanaki D, Movsas B, Rimner A, Roach M, Rodrigues G, Shirvani SM, Simone CB 2nd, Timmerman R, Daly ME (2017) Stereotactic body radiation therapy for early-stage non-small cell lung cancer: executive summary of an ASTRO evidence-based guideline. Pract Radiat Oncol 7:295–301

Videtic GM, Paulus R, Singh AK, Chang JY, Parker W, Olivier KR, Timmerman RD, Komaki RR, Urbanic JJ, Stephans KL, Yom SS, Robinson CG, Belani CP, Iyengar P, Ajlouni MI, Gopaul DD, Gomez Suescun JB, McGarry RC, Choy H, Bradley JD (2019) Long-term follow-up on NRG oncology RTOG 0915 (NCCTG N0927): a randomized phase 2 study comparing 2 stereotactic body radiation therapy schedules for medically inoperable patients with stage I peripheral non-small cell lung cancer. Int J Radiat Oncol Biol Phys 103:1077–1084

von Reibnitz D, Shaikh F, Wu AJ, Treharne GC, Dick-Godfrey R, Foster A, Woo KM, Shi W, Zhang Z, Din SU, Gelblum DY, Yorke ED, Rosenzweig KE, Rimner A (2018) Stereotactic body radiation therapy (SBRT) improves local control and overall survival compared to conventionally fractionated radiation for stage I non-small cell lung cancer (NSCLC). Acta Oncol 57:1567–1573

Voruganti IS, Donovan E, Walker-Dilks C, Swaminath A (2020) Chest wall toxicity after stereotactic radiation in early lung cancer: a systematic review. Curr Oncol 27:179–189

Wang L, Feigenberg S, Chen L, Pasklev K, Ma CC (2006) Benefit of three-dimensional image-guided stereotactic localization in the hypofractionated treatment of lung cancer. Int J Radiat Oncol Biol Phys 66:738–747

Wang Z, Wu QJ, Marks LB, Larrier N, Yin FF (2007) Cone-beam CT localization of internal target volumes for stereotactic body radiotherapy of lung lesions. Int J Radiat Oncol Biol Phys 69:1618–1624

Wang C, Rimner A, Gelblum DY, Dick-Godfrey R, McKnight D, Torres D, Flynn J, Zhang Z, Sidiqi B, Jackson A, Yorke E, Wu AJ (2020) Analysis of pneumonitis and esophageal injury after stereotactic body radiation therapy for ultra-central lung tumors. Lung Cancer 147:45–48

Wisnivesky JP, Bonomi M, Henschke C, Iannuzzi M, McGinn T (2005) Radiation therapy for the treatment of unresected stage I-II non-small cell lung cancer. Chest 128:1461–1467

Wulf J, Hadinger U, Oppitz U, Olshausen B, Flentje M (2000) Stereotactic radiotherapy of extracranial targets: CT-simulation and accuracy of treatment in the stereotactic body frame. Radiother Oncol 57:225–236

Wulf J, Baier K, Mueller G, Flentje MP (2005) Dose-response in stereotactic irradiation of lung tumors. Radiother Oncol 77:83–87

Yang M, Timmerman R (2018) Stereotactic ablative radiotherapy uncertainties: delineation, setup and motion. Semin Radiat Oncol 28:207–217

Yin F, Kim JG, Haughton C, Brown SL, Ajlouni M, Stronati M, Pamukov N, Kim JH (2001) Extracranial radiosurgery: immobilizing liver motion in dogs using high-frequency jet ventilation and total intravenous anesthesia. Int J Radiat Oncol Biol Phys 49:211–216

Yoon SM, Choi EK, Lee SW, Yi BY, Ahn SD, Shin SS, Park HJ, Kim SS, Park JH, Song SY, Park CI, Kim JH (2006) Clinical results of stereotactic body frame based fractionated radiation therapy for primary or metastatic thoracic tumors. Acta Oncol 45:1108–1114

Role of Postoperative Radiation Therapy in Non-Small Cell Lung Cancer

Alexander K. Diaz and Chris R. Kelsey

Contents

1 Introduction 471
2 **Patterns and Rates of Local/Regional Progression** 472
2.1 Patterns of Progression 472
2.2 Rates of Local/Regional Progression 472
3 **Postoperative RT—Randomized Trials and the PORT Meta-Analysis** 473
4 **Postoperative RT—Stage I/II NSCLC** 474
5 **Postoperative RT—Stage III NSCLC** 475
6 **Indications for PORT** 476
7 **Toxicity/Mortality** 477
8 **PORT and Adjuvant Chemotherapy** 477
9 **Radiation Doses and Techniques** 478
10 **Conclusions and Future Directions** 478
References 480

Abstract

Patients who undergo surgery for non-small cell lung cancer are at relatively high risk of local/regional recurrence, especially those with involved mediastinal lymph nodes. Postoperative radiation therapy (PORT) has been shown to decrease the risk of local/regional recurrence but its effect on overall survival remains unclear due to the competing risks of distant metastases and treatment-related morbidity and mortality. The randomized LungART study sought to examine the benefit of PORT, using modern techniques and doses, in patients with mediastinal lymph node involvement (N2) receiving adjuvant chemotherapy. Preliminary results show an improvement in local/regional control but no improvement in overall survival. While many guidelines continue to recommend PORT in the setting of positive margins or mediastinal lymph node involvement, these recommendations may change based on the final results of the LungART trial.

A. K. Diaz · C. R. Kelsey (✉)
Duke University Medical Center, Durham, NC, USA
e-mail: christopher.kelsey@duke.edu

1 Introduction

Lung cancer is the leading cause of cancer mortality in the USA with ~135,000 estimated deaths in 2020 (Siegel et al. 2020). Non-small cell lung cancer (NSCLC) accounts for ~85% of new cases. Surgery is generally pursued for medically operable patients with early-stage NSCLC. Adjuvant therapy is not routinely recommended for smaller primary tumors without regional lymph node involvement. Chemotherapy, typically a cisplatin-based doublet, improves survival when hilar or mediastinal lymph nodes are involved and is occasionally advised for patients with larger primary tumors even in the setting of negative lymph nodes (NSCLC Meta-analyses Collaborative Group et al. 2010). A recent randomized study demonstrated that adjuvant osimertinib also improves outcomes in resected EGFR+ disease (Wu et al. 2020).

The role of postoperative radiotherapy (PORT) in resected lung cancer remains uncertain. The risk of local/regional recurrence is relatively high after surgery, particularly for patients with involved mediastinal lymph nodes. PORT has been shown in multiple randomized studies to reduce this risk. However, PORT also causes acute side effects and has long-term risks, particularly in a vulnerable population of patients who have recently undergone thoracic surgery. Whether PORT improves overall survival in resected NSCLC remains unclear. Indeed, a prior meta-analysis, admittedly evaluating prospective studies that utilized antiquated radiation techniques, suggested that PORT may actually *decrease* survival (Anon 1998). This chapter will comprehensively review the rational and role of PORT and provide general recommendations and guidelines.

2 Patterns and Rates of Local/Regional Progression

2.1 Patterns of Progression

An understanding of lobe-specific lymphatic spread can guide rational PORT volumes. There are three scenarios in which patterns of lung cancer progression have been studied—anatomical investigations (Riquet et al. 1989; Hata 1990), surgical series evaluating lobe-specific patterns of lymphatic spread after mediastinoscopy (Nohl-Oser 1972) or mediastinal lymph node dissection (Libshitz et al. 1986; Ishida et al. 1990; Asamura et al. 1999), and imaging studies evaluating patterns of regional progression after surgery (Kelsey et al. 2006; Billiet et al. 2016). The mediastinal lymph nodes are a complex system and malignant progression does not always follow predictable patterns, but relatively consistent patterns of lymphatic drainage can be concluded from these studies. To summarize:

1. Direct spread to the mediastinum, bypassing the hilum, is common.
2. Right lung tumors drain predominantly into the ipsilateral mediastinum with infrequent contralateral involvement.
3. Left upper lobe tumors commonly involve the anterior mediastinal lymph node stations (levels 5 and 6).
4. Left lower lobe tumors commonly involve the contralateral mediastinum by first spreading to level 7 and then to 4R and 2R.
5. Subcarinal lymph nodes are frequently involved by both upper and lower lobe tumors.
6. Supraclavicular lymph node involvement typically arises from high paratracheal disease (2R and 2 L), not simply from tumors in the upper lobes.

2.2 Rates of Local/Regional Progression

Before reviewing rates of local and/or regional progression after surgery for NSCLC (hereafter simplified as "local/regional"), it would be prudent to recognize that significant differences in the definition of "local" or "local/regional" failure have been used in various studies. This introduces some challenges in understanding patterns of failure after surgery. From a radiation oncology standpoint, an ideal definition would include sites of progression that would be included in a typical postoperative RT field, and therefore potentially prevented with treatment. This would include the surgical margin (e.g., bronchial stump after lobectomy), ipsilateral hilum, and mediastinum. The contralateral hilum and supraclavicular fossa are not generally included in standard PORT fields, so excluding these from the definition of local/regional failure would be ideal. Some studies have included failure in the ipsilateral lung as a "local" failure. This too is problematic from a practical standpoint since PORT volumes obviously do not include the entire ipsilateral lung and such failures are more likely distant metastases or secondary primary tumors. Finally, some studies have scored local/regional failures only when there was no evidence of distant failure at the time of progression (Ginsberg and Rubinstein 1995). Since a distant failure occurs concomitantly with ~50% of local/regional failures, this will significantly underreport the true rate of malignant progression in local/regional sites after surgery.

For early-stage NSCLC (stage I-II), using an ideal definition of local/regional failure as noted above, a large series from Duke University Medical Center reported a 23% 5-year actuarial risk of local failure after surgery (Kelsey et al. 2009). A follow-up multi-institutional study using the same definition reported a similar rate of local recurrence in early-stage NSCLC (Kelsey et al. 2013). Studies have identified several potential risk factors for local/regional recurrence including more limited surgical procedures (wedge or segmentectomy) (Ginsberg and Rubinstein 1995; Kelsey et al. 2009; Harpole Jr et al. 1996; Warren and Faber 1994; Lee et al. 1999; Martini et al. 1995; Varlotto et al. 2010; Guerra et al. 2013), positive surgical margins (Lee et al. 1999; Hsu et al. 2004; Sawyer et al. 1997a; Sawyer et al. 1997b), lack of or limited mediastinal sampling (Martini et al. 1995; Lardinois et al. 2005; Hung et al. 2012), stage (Kelsey et al. 2009; Lee et al. 1999; Sawyer et al. 1997b), extent of regional lymph node involvement (Hsu et al. 2004; Fujimoto et al. 2006), size of the primary tumor (Lee et al. 1999; Guerra et al. 2013; Saynak et al. 2011), squamous histology (Kelsey et al. 2009; Sawyer et al. 1999), visceral pleural invasion (Guerra et al. 2013; Fujimoto et al. 2006), and lymphovascular space invasion (Kelsey et al. 2009; Varlotto et al. 2010; Saynak et al. 2011), among others. However, risk factors for local/regional recurrence have not been consistent across studies. Currently, only positive margins, which are relatively rare after lobectomy, are deemed sufficiently worrisome to warrant postoperative RT in early-stage NSCLC.

The risk of local/regional recurrence is higher for N2 disease. In the LungART trial the risk of mediastinal recurrence was 46% without PORT (Pechoux et al. 2020). Prospective and retrospective studies have consistently reported rates of local failure ~50–60% (Sawyer et al. 1997b; Taylor et al. 2003; Pass et al. 1992; Betticher et al. 2006). Such high rates of local/regional failure are not surprising. Microscopic deposits of tumor likely infiltrate throughout the mediastinal lymphatic network, making a curative en bloc "cancer resection" impractical.

3 Postoperative RT— Randomized Trials and the PORT Meta-Analysis

The publication of the PORT meta-analysis in 1998 had a dramatic effect on the recommendations for, and subsequent utilization of, radiation therapy in the management of resected NSCLC. Comprising nine prospective randomized trials with over 2,100 patients treated between 1965 and 1995, the PORT meta-analysis evaluated the role of PORT in N0, N1, and N2 disease (Anon 1986, 1998; Van Houtte et al. 1980; Lafitte et al. 1996; Stephens et al. 1996; Dautzenberg et al. 1999; Debevec et al. 1996; Feng et al. 2000) (Table 1). Collectively, PORT was associated with an absolute survival *reduction* of 7% at 2 years with survival curves continuing to separate over time. This was despite a decreased risk of local/regional failure (PORT improved local/regional control by 24%). The detriment in survival was stage dependent. PORT was most detrimental in patients with N0 disease, a bit less detrimental in the N1 cohort, and rather equivocal without clear benefit or harm in those with N2 disease. Notably, all patients, regardless of stage, were treated with similar radiation fields and doses.

There have been many critiques of the PORT meta-analysis citing the antiquated radiation

Table 1 Randomized trials of postoperative RT in NSCLC

Trial	n	Stage	Local control (crude[a]) S vs S + RT	Overall survival (5 years[a]) S vs S + RT
Studies in the 1998 PORT meta-analysis				
Van Houtte (Van Houtte et al. 1980) (1966–1975)	224	I	81% vs 96%	43% vs 24%
LCSG (Anon 1986) (1978–1985)	230	II-III	81% vs 99%	41% vs 41%[b,c]
Lafitte (Lafitte et al. 1996) (1985–1991)	132	IB	81% vs 85%	52% vs 35%
Stephens (Stephens et al. 1996) (1986–1993)	308	II-III	32% vs 43%[c]	20% vs 21%[c]
Dautzenberg (Dautzenberg et al. 1999) (1986–1994)	728	I-III	66% vs 72%[d]	43% vs 30%
Debevec (Debevec et al. 1996) (1988–1992)	74	I-III	72% vs 84%	28% vs 33%[c]
Feng (Feng et al. 2000) (1982–1995)	366	II-III	67% vs 87%	41% vs 43%
Studies not in the 1998 PORT meta-analysis				
Mayer (Mayer et al. 1997) (not stated)	155	I-III	76% vs 94%	20% vs 30%
Trodella (Trodella et al. 2002) (1989–1997)	104	I	77% vs 98%	58% vs 67%
LungART (Pechoux et al. 2020) (2007–2018)	504	III	54% vs 75%	69% vs 67%[e]

[a] Unless otherwise noted
[b] 4 year data
[c] Estimated from graphs provided
[d] 5-year actuarial
[e] 3-year overall survival

techniques, excessive doses, and large fields (among other factors) that might have contributed to the observed findings. What is incontrovertible is that PORT can do harm. If the reduction in survival due to treatment-related mortality was similar across stages, which is a reasonable hypothesis given similar treatment approaches despite stage, then one might postulate that the marked reduction in survival in stage I disease was due to significant treatment-related mortality that far exceeded the increase in cause-specific survival due to improved local control. As patients with stage I NSCLC are at relatively low risk for local/regional failure, and expected to gain little from PORT, this explanation seems congruent. However, as PORT neither improved, nor reduced, overall survival in N2 disease, then one might postulate that radiation therapy had a significant positive effect on cause-specific survival in this cohort but it was completely nullified by treatment-related mortality. Thus, if radiation techniques could be improved, with a concomitant decrease in treatment-related mortality, then PORT may prove beneficial in resected NSCLC, particularly N2 disease.

4 Postoperative RT—Stage I/II NSCLC

In an early randomized trial included in the PORT meta-analysis, PORT was associated with a significant *reduction* in 5-year overall survival in the subset of patients with stage I NSCLC (24% vs 43%) (Van Houtte et al. 1980). This finding was supported when all the studies were combined in the meta-analysis.

On the other hand, in a small Italian phase III study that was published after the PORT meta-analysis, 104 patients with completely resected stage I NSCLC were randomized to observation or PORT. PORT consisted of three-dimensional treatment planning targeting only the bronchial stump and ipsilateral hilum to a dose of 50.4 Gy in 1.8 Gy daily fractions. Only one local recurrence was observed in the PORT arm compared to 12 such events in controls ($P = 0.0019$), translating to improved 5-year overall survival (67% vs 58%, $P = 0.048$) (Trodella et al. 2002). Although the radiation approach and results of this study are intriguing, they had no effect on the general sentiment that PORT should not be administered to patients with resected stage I disease. Further, when these data were incorporated into an update of the PORT meta-analysis, the deleterious effect of adjuvant radiotherapy in stage I disease persisted (Burdett and Stewart 2005).

Similar to stage I (N0) disease, adjuvant radiation therapy was associated with inferior survival in patients with N1 disease in the PORT meta-analysis, though to a lesser degree (Anon 1998). In the Adjuvant Navelbine International Trialist Association (ANITA) trial, where PORT was not a randomized variable, the effect of PORT on survival varied as a function of systemic therapy. For patients with N1 disease receiving chemotherapy, PORT was associated with shorter survival, whereas those in the observation arm appeared to benefit from radiotherapy. These data must be interpreted with caution, however, as radiotherapy was not controlled for and was ultimately left to institutional discretion (Douillard et al. 2008). Taken altogether, except in the case of positive surgical margins, PORT is not recommended in early-stage NSCLC.

5 Postoperative RT—Stage III NSCLC

National guidelines for many years have recommended PORT in patients with resected N2 (IIIA) NSCLC (National Comprehensive Cancer Network 2020), in part due to findings from the ANITA randomized trial (Douillard et al. 2006). In this study, 840 patients with completely resected stage IB-IIIA NSCLC were randomized to either postoperative cisplatin and vinorelbine ($n = 407$) or observation ($n = 433$). The administration of PORT was left to institutional discretion. Slightly more than one-third of patients with N1 disease (36.6%) received PORT compared to half of those with N2. Subset analysis revealed longer 5-year survival in those with N2 disease receiving both PORT and chemotherapy (47% vs 34% chemotherapy alone), whereas a detrimental effect of PORT was seen in the study's N1 cohort receiving chemotherapy (40% vs 56%) (Douillard et al. 2008).

Since its publication, the ANITA study has been the only phase III trial cited as justification for PORT in patients with N2 disease. Two population-based studies have also lended credence to this recommendation. Utilizing data from the National Cancer Institute's Surveillance, Epidemiology, and End Results (SEER) Program between 1998 and 2002, PORT was associated with improved survival in patients with resected N2 disease (hazard ratio = 0.855; 95% CI, 0.762 to 0.959; $P = 0.0077$) (Lally et al. 2006), which was also observed more recently upon query of the National Cancer Database (resected N2 NSCLC treated between 2004 and 2006) (median survival 42 months vs 38 months, $p = 0.048$) (Mikell et al. 2015). However, given these studies were not randomized trials, many felt the issue remained unresolved.

With this in mind, a European collaborative study, led by investigators in France, embarked upon the Lung Adjuvant Radiotherapy Trial (LungART) (Pechoux et al. 2020). In this phase III study, 501 surgically resected patients with either pathologically or cytologically documented N2 mediastinal disease were randomized between 2007 and 2018 to PORT ($n = 252$) or no further therapy ($n = 249$). All patients were intended to receive either neoadjuvant or adjuvant chemotherapy. PORT (54 Gy) was supposed to be initiated within 4–8 weeks after surgery or 2–6 weeks after completion of adjuvant chemotherapy. Participants were stratified based on treatment center, administration of chemotherapy, squamous cell histology versus non-squamous histology, extent of mediastinal lymph node involvement (0 vs 1 vs 2+ stations), and whether or not pre-treatment PET-CT was acquired. Disease-free survival was the primary endpoint, with overall survival and toxicity evaluated as secondary endpoints.

Baseline characteristics were balanced between groups with most patients being male, undergoing lobectomy, having multilevel N2 involvement, diagnosed with adenocarcinoma, and receiving postoperative chemotherapy. Most patients received 3-dimensional conformal radiotherapy (89%). Various dosimetric parameters were collected including lung V20 Gy (median 23%), mean heart dose (median 13.4 Gy), and heart V35 Gy (median 15%). Preliminary data failed to demonstrate a benefit of PORT with regard to 3-year disease-free survival (47% vs 44%) or overall survival (67% vs 69%) (Pechoux et al. 2020). PORT was associated with a lower risk of local/regional recurrence in the mediastinum (46% vs 25%) but also a higher risk of cardiopulmonary complications (2% vs 16%). The study has yet to be published in the peer-reviewed literature.

6 Indications for PORT

National Comprehensive Cancer Network (NCCN) guidelines currently recommend PORT for patients with positive surgical margins and N2 mediastinal lymph node involvement (National Comprehensive Cancer Network 2020). European guidelines, on the other hand, advocate for PORT only in the setting of positive margins (Postmus et al. 2017). In the setting of a complete resection, even with N2 disease, the "addition of PORT is not routinely recommended, but may be an option following individual risk assessment."

Assessing risk, both of disease recurrence and toxicity, is necessary in the decision-making process. Radiation therapy can decrease the risk of local/regional recurrence but we would be remiss to minimize or forget that the treatment comes at a cost. Therefore, making an appropriate recommendation not only relies upon recognizing a high-risk population that stands to gain from PORT but also ensuring any detriment incurred from radiotherapy does not negate or exceed the benefit. We currently recommend that PORT be considered in the following circumstances:

1. N2 lymph node involvement. Several factors should be considered in a patient with pathologic N2 involvement. These include response to preoperative chemotherapy (Früh et al. 2019), completeness of lymph node dissection at the time of surgery, microscopic versus macroscopic N2 involvement, presence of extracapsular extension, whether additional adjuvant therapy will be administered (e.g., osimertinib), and so forth. Final results from the LungART trial will undoubtedly affect national and international guidelines respecting this indication.

2. Positive margins. Though lacking randomized data, basic oncologic principles would suggest that a compromised surgical margin should be addressed with PORT. This is supported by a number of well-established guidelines due to the high-risk for recurrence (National Comprehensive Cancer Network 2020; Rodrigues et al. 2015).

3. Inadequate lymph node sampling/dissection in high-risk settings. This is less frequently encountered in the modern era given robust guidelines on extent of lymph node sampling/dissection that should accompany lung cancer resection. PORT could be considered in select patients at high-risk of harboring microscopic disease who undergo insufficient mediastinal lymph node sampling (e.g., a large central right upper lobe tumor without 4R and 7 sampling). Just as lobectomy has long been regarded as the standard approach for lung cancer resection, mediastinal lymph node dissection too was thought to provide an oncologic benefit over less comprehensive lymphadenectomy (Martini 1995). Yet, the matter is far from settled as only 1 of 3 small-scale prospective trials demonstrated a survival advantage (Sugi et al. 1998; Wu et al. 2002; Izbicki et al. 1998). The American College of Surgery Oncology Group Z0030 Trial compared mediastinal lymph node dissection ($n = 525$) to sampling ($n = 498$) in

patients with early-stage NSCLC (T1–2, N0-nonhilar N1) and found no differences in median survival or local, regional, and distant recurrence (Darling et al. 2011). However, it must be noted patients underwent extensive lymph node sampling (levels 2R/4R/7/10R for right lung tumors and 5/6/7/10 L on the left) prior to intra-operative randomization.

7 Toxicity/Mortality

Lung resection, regardless of extent, places increased demand on the remaining parenchyma for ventilation and oxygenation. Thoracic radiation, even when highly conformal, augments this burden by further damaging some viable tissue. Of course, this is occurring in a patient population with varying degrees of diminished functional lung capacity given the role of smoking in tumorigenesis. Additionally, data has emerged demonstrating a linear relationship between ischemic cardiac events and radiation dose to the heart (Darby et al. 2013). Patients with lung cancer often have underlying cardiac disease. The PORT meta-analysis and LungART study confirmed that radiation therapy carries a cost. Balancing the risks of PORT with the potential benefits has proved to be challenging.

Two randomized studies in the 1980s and 1990s, included in the PORT meta-analysis, reported higher rates of cardiopulmonary death in patients receiving PORT (Anon 1986; Dautzenberg et al. 1999). In the PORT meta-analysis, separation of the survival curves was clearly evident by 6 months raising the possibility that at least some of these events were related to acute treatment-related toxicities (Anon 1998), likely cardiopulmonary in origin.

There is reason to suspect that at least part of the potential toxicity of PORT observed in prior studies may be offset by the use of newer radiation techniques. Indeed, the studies outlined above and many others documenting the morbidity/mortality associated with PORT used less conformal techniques than what is routinely employed today. Utilizing data from the National Cancer Institute's Surveillance, Epidemiology, and End Results (SEER) Program, investigators observed an association between PORT and an increased risk of heart disease mortality in patients diagnosed between 1983 and 1988 (HR, 1.49; 95% CI, 1.11–2.01 [$P = 0.0090$]), that was not maintained over the ensuing 5 years (HR, 1.08; 95% CI, 0.79–1.48 [$P = 0.6394$]) (Lally et al. 2007). More recent data found no differences in quality of life, pulmonary function tests, or cardiopulmonary symptoms between patients who underwent PORT compared to those who did not (Kepka et al. 2011).

Preliminary data from the LungART trial does suggest, however, that cardiopulmonary complications may persist after PORT despite modern techniques. Of the 99 deaths assessed in those receiving PORT, 16 (16%) were attributable to cardiopulmonary complications compared to only 2 (2%) of patients who died without receiving PORT ($n = 102$) (Pechoux et al. 2020). These data suggest that if PORT is pursued, rigorous minimization of dose to the heart and lungs is critical. Most patients treated in the LungART study were treated with 3-dimensional techniques. Intensity-modulated radiation therapy (IMRT) may be prudent in some cases.

8 PORT and Adjuvant Chemotherapy

A number of large randomized studies have established the role of adjuvant platinum-based chemotherapy for resected NSCLC. In the International Adjuvant Lung Cancer Trial (IALT), chemotherapy (consisting of cisplatin with an additional vinca alkaloid) led to significantly improved disease-free and overall survival. The use of PORT was left to the discretion of treating institutions but was to be administered following chemotherapy. Nearly one-third of study participants received radiation, the majority of those with N2 disease. However, there was no significant interaction between the effect of chemotherapy and PORT ($p = 0.66$) (Anon 2004).

Another investigation establishing adjuvant cisplatin as standard of care is the National Cancer Institute of Canada Clinical Trials Group

JBR.10 trial. This phase 3 study conducted from 1994–2001 demonstrated improved disease-free and overall survival in patients with completely resected stage IB or II NSCLC receiving vinorelbine and cisplatin (Winton et al. 2005). PORT was not allowed.

More recently, osimertinib has shown promise in resected locally advanced NSCLC. This third generation tyrosine kinase inhibitor exhibits a 200-fold selectivity for the T790M/L858R protein over wild-type EGFR. Although initially fast-tracked by the United States Food and Drug Administration for metastatic disease, its use in *EGFR*-mutant resected stage IB-IIIA disease yielded significantly improved disease-free survival compared with surgery alone (Wu et al. 2020). Long-term results to assess overall survival are awaited.

In patients who undergo surgery for NSCLC and are found to have pN2 disease, it is recommended that adjuvant chemotherapy be pursued first as long as surgical margins are negative. If PORT is recommended, it should be given after recovery from chemotherapy. This sequencing reflects the known benefit of adjuvant chemotherapy and the uncertain benefit of PORT. In the setting of positive margins, many guidelines recommend concurrent chemotherapy and PORT (National Comprehensive Cancer Network 2020; Rodrigues et al. 2015). If the patient received neoadjuvant chemotherapy, then PORT can proceed after recovery from surgery, generally 4–6 weeks later.

9 Radiation Doses and Techniques

There are no prospective studies evaluating the optimal dose of PORT in resected NSCLC. It would therefore seem prudent to utilize doses that are used in other settings when microscopic disease is being addressed. Therefore, we recommend 45–50 Gy in 1.8–2 Gy fractions in the setting of a margin negative resection, which is consistent with national guidelines. Higher doses, potentially with concurrent chemotherapy, would be appropriate in settings of microscopically, and especially macroscopic, residual disease. In such settings 54–60 Gy is recommended. Doses higher than 60 Gy should not be utilized. Either 3D or IMRT is reasonable, as long as lung and heart constraints can be met. Restricting lung V20 to 15–20% and mean heart dose <10 Gy would be ideal.

PORT volumes vary considerably in both prospective studies and clinical practice. At one extreme, the entire mediastinum, ipsilateral hilum, and bronchial stump are included in the clinical target volume. At the other, only involved mediastinal and hilar lymph node stations are encompassed. Given the known toxicity of PORT, and concern for treatment-related mortality given the PORT meta-analysis, we would generally advocate for smaller, rather than larger, radiation fields. Treatment of the bronchial stump/ipsilateral hilum should be considered if either the bronchial or vascular margin is close or there were involved hilar lymph nodes. With widely negative margins (peripheral tumor) and a thorough hilar lymph node dissection which shows no evidence of malignancy, it would seem reasonable to exclude the hilum. All involved mediastinal lymph node stations should be included in the CTV, even if those stations are found to be negative after preoperative chemotherapy. Finally, additional select mediastinal stations may also be included depending upon imaging, surgical, and pathological findings. For example, if level 7 was not sampled/dissected during a right lower lobectomy, and disease was detected in 4R, it may be reasonable to also include level 7. Such decisions require clinical judgment and depend upon a number of factors. A representative case is shown in Fig. 1.

10 Conclusions and Future Directions

A 1995 meta-analysis showed that adjuvant chemotherapy, using long-term alkylating agents, was associated with inferior survival in NSCLC, on the same order as what was found in the 1998 PORT meta-analysis (Group N-SCLCC, Non-small Cell Lung Cancer Collaborative Group

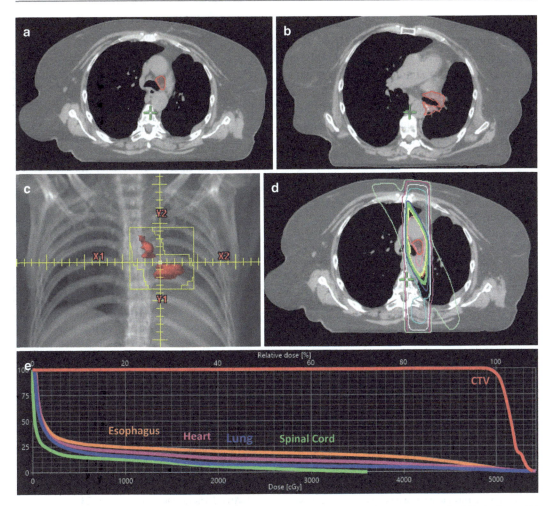

Fig. 1 A 55 y/o female is found to have an incidental 3.8 cm left lower lobe mass on CT scan. On PET-CT the mass was hypermetabolic as well as left hilar and a 4 L lymph node. Biopsies of both the mass and the 4 L lymph node during bronchoscopy using endobronchial ultrasound showed adenocarcinoma without any driver mutations. Biopsies of 4R and 7 were negative She underwent 3 cycles of neoadjuvant carboplatin and paclitaxel with CT imaging showing a partial response. She then underwent left lower lobectomy and left hilar and mediastinal lymph node dissection. Due to surgical limitations, 4 L could not be re-sampled. Disease was noted in a 10 L lymph node but 4R and 7 were again negative. She then received PORT to the 4 L (**panel a**) and left hilar (**panel b**) lymph node stations using 3D conformal techniques (50 Gy in 2 Gy fractions) (**panel c** and **d**). Dosimetric values were as follows: Lung V20 8%, mean esophageal dose 10 Gy, mean heart dose 7.6 Gy, spinal cord Dmax 36 Gy (**panel e**)

1995). A non-statistically significant advantage was observed for cisplatin-based chemotherapy. Knowing that the development of distant metastases was a significant obstacle to cure in resected lung cancer, our colleagues in medical oncology persisted in evaluating new drug combinations and administrative schedules. Eventually, individual randomized studies (Douillard et al. 2006; Anon 2004) and subsequent meta-analyses have confirmed that adjuvant chemotherapy improves survival in resected NSCLC (NSCLC Meta-analyses Collaborative Group et al. 2010).

Local/regional failure remains a significant hindrance and PORT clearly reduces this risk. In the LungART study, the risk of local/regional recurrence was 25% and 46% with and without PORT, respectively. However, the risks of PORT remain problematic, even using more moderate doses with conventional fractionation and modern treatment planning. Although local recurrence was reduced, the LungART study did not show a statistically significant improvement in survival with PORT and at the time of this writing has only been reported in abstract form. A careful review of toxicity, dosimetric data, and patterns of failure may help better guide PORT in the modern era.

References

Annon (1998) Postoperative radiotherapy in non-small-cell lung cancer: systematic review and meta-analysis of individual patient data from nine randomised controlled trials. PORT Meta-analysis Trialists Group. Lancet 352(9124):257–263

Anon (1986) Effects of postoperative mediastinal radiation on completely resected stage II and stage III epidermoid cancer of the lung. N Engl J Med 315(22):1377–1381

Anon (2004) Cisplatin-based adjuvant chemotherapy in patients with completely resected non–small-cell lung cancer. N Engl J Med 350(4):351–360

Asamura H, Nakayama H, Kondo H, Tsuchiya R, Naruke T (1999) Lobe-specific extent of systematic lymph node dissection for non–small cell lung carcinomas according to a retrospective study of metastasis and prognosis. J Thorac Cardiovasc Surg 117(6):1102–1111

Betticher DC, Hsu Schmitz S-F, Tötsch M, Hansen E, Joss C, von Briel C et al (2006) Prognostic factors affecting long-term outcomes in patients with resected stage IIIA pN2 non-small-cell lung cancer: 5-year follow-up of a phase II study. Br J Cancer 94(8):1099–1106

Billiet C, De Ruysscher D, Peeters S, Decaluwé H, Vansteenkiste J, Dooms C et al (2016) Patterns of locoregional relapses in patients with contemporarily staged stage III-N2 NSCLC treated with induction chemotherapy and resection: implications for postoperative radiotherapy target volumes. J Thorac Oncol 11(9):1538–1549

Burdett S, Stewart L (2005) PORT meta-analysis group. Postoperative radiotherapy in non-small-cell lung cancer: update of an individual patient data meta-analysis. Lung Cancer 47(1):81–83

Darby SC, Ewertz M, McGale P, Bennet AM, Blom-Goldman U, Brønnum D et al (2013) Risk of ischemic heart disease in women after radiotherapy for breast cancer. N Engl J Med 368(11):987–998

Darling GE, Allen MS, Decker PA, Ballman K, Malthaner RA, Inculet RI et al (2011) Randomized trial of mediastinal lymph node sampling versus complete lymphadenectomy during pulmonary resection in the patient with N0 or N1 (less than hilar) non–small cell carcinoma: results of the American College of Surgery Oncology Group Z0030 Trial [Internet]. J Thorac Cardiovasc Surg 141:662–670. https://doi.org/10.1016/j.jtcvs.2010.11.008

Dautzenberg B, Arriagada R, Boyer Chammard A, Jarema A, Mezzetti M, Mattson K et al (1999) A controlled study of postoperative radiotherapy for patients with completely resected nonsmall cell lung carcinoma. Cancer 86(2):265–273

Debevec M, Bitenc M, Vidmar S, Rott T, Orel J, Strojan P et al (1996) Postoperative radiotherapy for radically resected N2 non-small-cell lung cancer (NSCLC): randomised clinical study 1988–1992. Lung Cancer 14(1):99–107

Douillard J-Y, Rosell R, De Lena M, Carpagnano F, Ramlau R, Gonzáles-Larriba JL et al (2006) Adjuvant vinorelbine plus cisplatin versus observation in patients with completely resected stage IB--IIIA non-small-cell lung cancer (Adjuvant Navelbine International Trialist Association [ANITA]): a randomised controlled trial. Lancet Oncol 7(9):719–727

Douillard J-Y, Rosell R, De Lena M, Riggi M, Hurteloup P, Mahe M-A et al (2008) Impact of postoperative radiation therapy on survival in patients with complete resection and stage I, II, or IIIA non-small-cell lung cancer treated with adjuvant chemotherapy: the adjuvant Navelbine International Trialist Association (ANITA) Randomized Trial. Int J Radiat Oncol Biol Phys 72(3):695–701

Feng QF, Wang M, Wang LJ, Yang ZY, Zhang YG, Zhang DW et al (2000) A study of postoperative radiotherapy in patients with non–small-cell lung cancer: a randomized trial. Int J Radiat Oncol Biol Phys 47(4):925–929

Früh M, Betticher DC, Stupp R, Xyrafas A, Peters S, Ris HB et al (2019) Multimodal treatment in operable stage III NSCLC: a pooled analysis on long-term results of three SAKK trials (SAKK 16/96, 16/00, and 16/01). J Thorac Oncol 14(1):115–123

Fujimoto T, Cassivi SD, Yang P, Barnes SA, Nichols FC, Deschamps C et al (2006) Completely resected N1 non-small cell lung cancer: factors affecting recurrence and long-term survival. J Thorac Cardiovasc Surg 132(3):499–506

Ginsberg RJ, Rubinstein LV (1995) Randomized trial of lobectomy versus limited resection for T1 N0 non-small cell lung cancer. Ann Thorac Surg 60(3):615–623

Group N-SCLCC, Non-small Cell Lung Cancer Collaborative Group (1995) Chemotherapy in non-small cell lung cancer: a meta-analysis using updated data on individual patients from 52 randomised clinical trials [Internet]. BMJ 311:899–909. https://doi.org/10.1136/bmj.311.7010.899

Guerra JLL, Lopez Guerra JL, Gomez DR, Lin SH, Levy LB, Zhuang Y et al (2013) Risk factors for local and regional recurrence in patients with resected N0–N1 non-small-cell lung cancer, with implications for patient selection for adjuvant radiation therapy [Internet]. Ann Oncol 24:67–74. https://doi.org/10.1093/annonc/mds274

Harpole DH Jr, Hemdon JE II, Young WG Jr, Wolfe WG, Sabiston DC Jr (1996) Stage I nonsmall cell lung cancer: A multivariate analysis of treatment methods and patterns of recurrencee. Division of Thoracic Surgery, Brigham and Women's Hospital, 75 Francis Street, Boston, MA 02115. Cancer 1995;76:787–796. Lung Cancer 14(1):165

Hata E (1990) Rationale for extended lymphadenectomy for lung cancer. Theor Surg 5:19–25

Hsu H-C, Wang C-J, Huang E-Y, Sun L-M (2004) Postoperative adjuvant thoracic radiotherapy for patients with completely resected non-small cell lung cancer with nodal involvement: outcome and prognostic factors. Br J Radiol 77(913):43–48

Hung J-J, Jeng W-J, Hsu W-H, Chou T-Y, Huang B-S, Wu Y-C (2012) Predictors of death, local recurrence, and distant metastasis in completely resected pathological stage-I non–small-cell lung cancer. J Thorac Oncol 7(7):1115–1123

Ishida T, Yano T, Maeda K, Kaneko S, Tateishi M, Sugimachi K (1990) Strategy for lymphadenectomy in lung cancer three centimeters or less in diameter. Ann Thorac Surg 50(5):708–713

Izbicki JR, Passlick B, Pantel K, Pichlmeier U, Hosch SB, Karg O et al (1998) Effectiveness of radical systematic mediastinal lymphadenectomy in patients with resectable non-small cell lung cancer: results of a prospective randomized trial. Ann Surg 227(1):138–144

Kelsey CR, Light KL, Marks LB (2006) Patterns of failure after resection of non–small-cell lung cancer: Implications for postoperative radiation therapy volumes. Int J Radiat Oncol Biol Phys 65(4):1097–1105

Kelsey CR, Marks LB, Hollis D, Hubbs JL, Ready NE, D'Amico TA et al (2009) Local recurrence after surgery for early stage lung cancer: an 11-year experience with 975 patients. Cancer 115(22):5218–5227

Kelsey CR, Higgins KA, Peterson BL, Chino JP, Marks LB, D'Amico TA et al (2013) Local recurrence after surgery for non–small-cell lung cancer: a recursive partitioning analysis of multi-institutional data. J Thorac Cardiovasc Surg 146(4):768–73.e1

Kepka L, Bujko K, Orlowski TM, Jagiello R, Salata A, Matecka-Nowak M et al (2011) Cardiopulmonary morbidity and quality of life in non-small cell lung cancer patients treated with or without postoperative radiotherapy. Radiother Oncol 98(2):238–243

Lafitte JJ, Ribet ME, Prévost BM, Gosselin BH, Copin M-C, Brichet AH (1996) Postresection irradiation for T2 N0 M0 non–small cell carcinoma: a prospective, randomized study. Ann Thorac Surg 62(3):830–834

Lally BE, Zelterman D, Colasanto JM, Haffty BG, Detterbeck FC, Wilson LD (2006) Postoperative radiotherapy for stage II or III non-small-cell lung cancer using the surveillance, epidemiology, and end results database. J Clin Oncol 24(19):2998–3006

Lally BE, Detterbeck FC, Geiger AM, Thomas CR Jr, Machtay M, Miller AA et al (2007) The risk of death from heart disease in patients with nonsmall cell lung cancer who receive postoperative radiotherapy: analysis of the surveillance, epidemiology, and end results database. Cancer 110(4):911–917

Lardinois D, Suter H, Hakki H, Rousson V, Betticher D, Ris H-B (2005) Morbidity, survival, and site of recurrence after mediastinal lymph-node dissection versus systematic sampling after complete resection for non-small cell lung cancer. Ann Thorac Surg 80(1):268–275

Lee JH, Machtay M, Kaiser LR, Friedberg JS, Hahn SM, McKenna MG et al (1999) Non-small cell lung cancer: prognostic factors in patients treated with surgery and postoperative radiation therapy. Radiology 213(3):845–852

Libshitz HI, McKenna RJ Jr, Mountain CF (1986) Patterns of mediastinal metastases in bronchogenic carcinoma. Chest 90(2):229–232

Martini N (1995) Mediastinal lymph node dissection for lung cancer. The memorial experience. Chest Surg Clin N Am 5(2):189–203

Martini N, Bains MS, Burt ME, Zakowski MF, McCormack P, Rusch VW et al (1995) Incidence of local recurrence and second primary tumors in resected stage I lung cancer. J Thorac Cardiovasc Surg 109(1):120–129

Mayer R, Smolle-Juettner FM, Szolar D, Stuecklschweiger GF, Quehenberger F, Friehs G et al (1997) Postoperative radiotherapy in radically resected non-small cell lung cancer. Chest 112(4):954–959

Mikell JL, Gillespie TW, Hall WA, Nickleach DC, Liu Y, Lipscomb J et al (2015) Postoperative radiotherapy is associated with better survival in non–small cell lung cancer with involved N2 lymph nodes: results of an analysis of the National Cancer Data Base. J Thorac Oncol 10(3):462–471

National Comprehensive Cancer Network (2020) NCCN Clinical Practice Guidelines in Oncology: Non-Small Cell Lung Cancer. Report No.: Version 2.2021

Nohl-Oser HC (1972) An investigation of the anatomy of the lymphatic drainage of the lungs as shown by the lymphatic spread of bronchial carcinoma. Ann R Coll Surg Engl 51(3):157–176

NSCLC Meta-analyses Collaborative Group, Arriagada R, Auperin A, Burdett S, Higgins JP, Johnson DH et al (2010) Adjuvant chemotherapy, with or without postoperative radiotherapy, in operable non-small-cell lung cancer: two meta-analyses of individual patient data. Lancet 375(9722):1267–1277

Pass HI, Pogrebniak HW, Steinberg SM, Mulshine J, Minna J (1992) Randomized trial of neoadjuvant therapy for lung cancer: interim analysis. Ann Thorac Surg 53(6):992–998

Pechoux CL, Le Pechoux C, Pourel N, Barlesi F, Faivre-Finn C, Lerouge D et al (2020) LBA3_PR An international randomized trial, comparing post-operative conformal radiotherapy (PORT) to no PORT, in patients with completely resected non-small cell lung cancer (NSCLC) and mediastinal N2 involvement: primary end-point analysis of LungART (IFCT-0503, UK NCRI, SAKK) NCT00410683 [Internet]. Ann Oncol 31:S1178. https://doi.org/10.1016/j.annonc.2020.08.2280

Postmus PE, Kerr KM, Oudkerk M, Senan S, Waller DA, Vansteenkiste J et al (2017) Early and locally advanced non-small-cell lung cancer (NSCLC): ESMO clinical practice guidelines for diagnosis, treatment and follow-up. Ann Oncol 28(suppl_4):iv1–i21

Riquet M, Hidden G, Debesse B (1989) Direct lymphatic drainage of lung segments to the mediastinal nodes. An anatomic study on 260 adults. J Thorac Cardiovasc Surg 97(4):623–632

Rodrigues G, Choy H, Bradley J, Rosenzweig KE, Bogart J, Curran WJ et al (2015) Adjuvant radiation therapy in locally advanced non-small cell lung cancer: Executive summary of an American Society for Radiation Oncology (ASTRO) evidence-based clinical practice guideline [Internet]. Pract Radiat Oncol 5:149–155. https://doi.org/10.1016/j.prro.2015.02.013

Sawyer TE, Bonner JA, Gould PM, Foote RL, Deschamps C, Trastek VF et al (1997a) Effectiveness of postoperative irradiation in stage IIIA non–small cell lung cancer according to regression tree analyses of recurrence risks. Ann Thorac Surg 64(5):1402–1407

Sawyer TE, Bonner JA, Gould PM, Foote RL, Deschamps C, Trastek VF et al (1997b) The impact of surgical adjuvant thoracic radiation therapy for patients with nonsmall cell lung carcinoma with ipsilateral mediastinal lymph node involvement. Cancer 80(8):1399–1408

Sawyer TE, Bonner JA, Gould PM, Foote RL, Deschamps C, Lange CM et al (1999) Factors predicting patterns of recurrence after resection of N1 non-small cell lung carcinoma. Ann Thorac Surg 68(4):1171–1176

Saynak M, Veeramachaneni NK, Hubbs JL, Nam J, Qaqish BF, Bailey JE et al (2011) Local failure after complete resection of N0–1 non-small cell lung cancer. Lung Cancer 71(2):156–165

Siegel RL, Miller KD, Jemal A (2020 Jan) Cancer statistics, 2020. CA Cancer J Clin 70(1):7–30

Stephens RJ, Girling DJ, Bleehen NM, Moghissi K, Yosef HM, Machin D (1996) The role of post-operative radiotherapy in non-small-cell lung cancer: a multicentre randomised trial in patients with pathologically staged T1-2, N1-2, M0 disease. Medical Research Council lung cancer working party. Br J Cancer 74(4):632–639

Sugi K, Nawata K, Fujita N, Ueda K, Tanaka T, Matsuoka T et al (1998) Systematic lymph node dissection for clinically diagnosed peripheral non-small-cell lung cancer less than 2 cm in diameter. World J Surg 22(3):290–294. discussion 294–5

Taylor NA, Liao ZX, Stevens C, Walsh G, Roth J, Putnam J et al (2003) Postoperative radiotherapy increases locoregional control of patients with stage IIIA non–small-cell lung cancer treated with induction chemotherapy followed by surgery [Internet]. Int J Radiat Oncol Biol Phys 56:616–625. https://doi.org/10.1016/s0360-3016(03)00063-4

Trodella L, Granone P, Valente S, Valentini V, Balducci M, Mantini G et al (2002) Adjuvant radiotherapy in non-small cell lung cancer with pathological stage I: definitive results of a phase III randomized trial. Radiother Oncol 62(1):11–19

Van Houtte P, Rocmans P, Smets P, Goffin J-C, Lustmanmaréchal J, Vanderhoeft P et al (1980) Postoperative radiation therapy in lung cancer: a controlled trial after resection of curative design. Int J Radiat Oncol Biol Phys 6(8):983–986

Varlotto JM, Recht A, Flickinger JC, Medford-Davis LN, Dyer A-M, DeCamp MM (2010) Varying recurrence rates and risk factors associated with different definitions of local recurrence in patients with surgically resected, stage I nonsmall cell lung cancer [Internet]. Cancer 116(10):2390–2400. https://doi.org/10.1002/cncr.25047

Warren WH, Faber LP (1994) Segmentectomy versus lobectomy in patients with stage I pulmonary carcinoma. Five-year survival and patterns of intrathoracic recurrence. J Thorac Cardiovasc Surg 107(4):1087–1093. discussion 1093–4

Winton T, Livingston R, Johnson D, Rigas J, Johnston M, Butts C et al (2005) Vinorelbine plus cisplatin vs. observation in resected non–small-cell lung cancer. N Engl J Med 352(25):2589–2597

Wu YL, Huang Z-F, Wang S-Y, Yang X-N, Ou W (2002) A randomized trial of systematic nodal dissection in resectable non-small cell lung cancer. Lung Cancer 36(1):1–6

Wu Y-L, Tsuboi M, He J, John T, Grohe C, Majem M et al (2020 Oct 29) Osimertinib in resected EGFR-mutated non-small-cell lung cancer. N Engl J Med 383(18):1711–1723

The Role of Thermal Ablation in the Treatment of Stage I Non-small Cell Lung Cancer

Roberto B. Kutcher-Diaz, Aaron Harman, and John Varlotto

Contents

1 Introduction 484
2 Patient Selection and Evaluation 484
3 Technique 486
4 Results 489
5 Follow-Up 496
6 Summary 499
References 499

R. B. Kutcher-Diaz · A. Harman
Department of Radiology, UMass Memorial Medical Center, Worcester, MA, USA
e-mail: roberto.kutcher-diaz@umassmemorial.org;
Aaron.Harman@umassmemorial.org

J. Varlotto (✉)
Department of Oncology, Joan C. Edwards School of Medicine, Marshall University, Huntington, WV, USA
e-mail: varlotto@marshall.edu

Abstract

Currently, the standard of care for Stage I non-small cell lung cancer (NSCLC) is surgical resection. Although this treatment modality has been demonstrated to have 5-year survival rates approaching 80%, patients who are medically inoperable account for around 18–22% of this population (Raz et al. 2007). Interest has thus turned toward nonsurgical treatments, such as Stereotactic Body Radiation Therapy (SBRT) and ablation, that might improve the otherwise dismal 13–14-month median survival of untreated Stage I disease. Over the past 10 years, data on the safety and efficacy of the three types of ablation which includes radiofrequency ablation (RFA), microwave ablation (MWA), and cryoablation (CA) have bolstered their place in the armamentarium of minimally invasive therapies. Recent advancements in thermal ablation therapies have overcome some of the anatomic limitations that were initially encountered with RFA (e.g., treatment of only small peripheral lesions located distal to vasculature, large airways, and the mediastinum). The most common complications associated with thermal ablation include pneumothorax, pulmonary hemorrhage, and pleural effusion.

Irrespective of thermal ablative technique, tumor size <3 cm has been found to be the most important factor in predicting local control. Local progression rates in recent literature range from 15% to 44% with mean overall survivals of 34–57 months. Although the safety and efficacy of percutaneous thermal ablation have been documented over the past 20 years, randomized trials are needed to determine the relative benefit of these procedures when compared to alternatives such as SBRT and sublobar resection.

1 Introduction

In the setting of NSCLC, thermal ablation was introduced as a tool of endoscopic and open surgical techniques. Sanderson et al. first reported the cryoablation of lung cancer in 1975 with the bronchoscopic treatment of an endobronchial squamous cell carcinoma. Interstitial hyperthermia via the radiofrequency ablation of a primary lung cancer was first described during an open thoracotomy by Lilly et al. in 1983. However, despite several decades since the initial applications, it was Dupuy's 2000 report of the delivery of ablation via a percutaneous approach, enabled by computerized tomography's visualization of lung, which transformed thermal ablation's role in NSCLC. Since then, thanks to its widespread availability and experience compared to other modalities, RFA has become the most studied of the ablative therapies for lung cancer.

Radiofrequency and microwave ablation are both hyperthermic techniques. However, whereas, RFA deposits energy via an electric current, MWA creates an electromagnetic field which rotates polar molecules at a high frequency. The heat created by these techniques induces cell membrane alteration, protein denaturation, and coagulative necrosis around the probes resulting in tumor cell death. In contrast, cryoablation induces cell death by creating an ice ball around a probe containing pressurized argon gas. A series of freeze-thaw cycles create intracellular and extracellular ice crystals and induce osmotic shifts that result in tissue necrosis and apoptosis. All three modalities of ablation can indirectly stimulate the immune system with the release of large amounts of tumor antigen and tissue debris into the systemic circu-

lation (Fietta et al. 2009; Widenmeyer et al. 2011; Kim and Erinjeri 2019).

The purpose of this chapter is to describe the technique, results, complications, and follow-up evaluation of Stage I non-small cell lung cancer patients treated with RFA, MWA, and CA. The results from multicenter studies of RFA will also be compared to similar studies of stereotactic body radiation therapy (SBRT) and sublobar resection that are also mostly performed in patients who are unable to undergo the standard of care resection (lobectomy).

2 Patient Selection and Evaluation

The treatment approach for effective management of early-stage NSCLC is evolving to mirror complex disease presentations and patient situations, as well as to accommodate the many different therapeutic options. For early-stage lung cancer, surgery offers survival rates as high as 79.5% at 5 years (Koike et al. 1998). However, approximately 25% of patients with Stage I disease are medically inoperable due to cardiac and pulmonary comorbidities (Donington et al. 2012). The NCCN, ACCP, and ESMO guidelines contemplate thermal ablation as an option (in selected clinical scenarios) for these high-risk patients. According to the NCCN guidelines, image-guided thermal ablation may be an option for patients with inoperable Stage IA disease not undergoing definitive RT or SBRT (see Table 1

Table 1 High operative risk patients who may benefit from thermal ablation for lung cancer (Dupuy et al. 2015)

Major criteria (one of the following)
• FEV1 or DCLO ≤50%
Minor criteria (two or more)
• FEV1 or DLCO between 51% and 60%
• Advanced age ≥75 years
• Pulmonary hypertension
• LVEF ≤40%
• Resting or exercise PaO_2 <55 mmHg
• pCO_2 >45 mmHg
• Modified Medical Research Council (MMRC) Dyspnea Scale ≥3

for high risk for lobectomy criteria), multiple lung cancers, or symptomatic locoregional recurrence after definitive treatment (NCCN NSCLC v1.2021 2021).

The decision to offer these methods of treatment is best considered in a multi-disciplinary group setting (Detterbeck et al. 2013). Thoracic surgeons, radiation oncologists, interventional radiologists, and medical oncologists should be involved in determining the most appropriate treatment strategy. This plan should include evaluation of surgical technique (lobectomy versus limited resection), conventional radiotherapy versus SBRT, and percutaneous thermal ablation or combined modality treatment. Thermal ablation can be considered as a sole treatment option or with other local modalities (external beam radiotherapy, SBRT, brachytherapy) to achieve local tumor obliteration with the goal of cure or palliation.

As with selection of patient for other curative treatments, a thorough diagnosis and staging should be performed. At our institution, FDG-PET as well as percutaneous biopsy (PNB) of extrathoracic lesions as necessary is part of the standard pretreatment staging. Nodal staging is preferred. If patients can tolerate general anesthesia, a mediastinoscopy is performed. Otherwise, a bronchoscopy with nodal sampling via endobronchial ultrasound (EBUS) is considered. As per past guidelines, if the staging work-up with FDG CT/PET is negative, patients with clinical T1 tumors in the outer 2/3 of the hemi-thorax can forego invasive nodal sampling (Detterbeck et al. 2007). Additionally, lung biopsy can also be performed in the same setting as lung ablation in patients without evidence of nodal or distant metastases.

Given the minimally invasive nature of image-guided ablation, few absolute contraindications exist, such as severe coagulopathy (Aufranc et al. 2019). Most patients who are able to tolerate a CT-guided needle biopsy of the lung are generally candidates for thermal ablation (McTaggart and Dupuy 2007). However, certain comorbidities and lesion characteristics are associated with poor outcomes. A Charlson Comorbidity Index score ≥ 5 portends significantly higher mortality following thermal ablation and could be used to identify patients who might not benefit from therapy (Simon et al. 2012). Although low FEV or DLCO do not necessarily preclude treatment, patients with severe emphysema and bullae are at increased risk for bronchopleural fistula (Palussière et al. 2017; Sidoff and Dupuy 2017). The need for placement of multiple probes as well as prior local treatment has been associated with an increased incidence of complications (McDevitt et al. 2016). Irregular tumor shape may result in incomplete treatment or suggest local spread beyond lesion margins on CT (Vogl et al. 2013). Studies across the thermal ablative modalities have consistently demonstrated that lesions >3 cm in diameter are associated higher rates of local recurrence (Simon et al. 2007; Healey et al. 2017; McDevitt et al. 2016).

Technical aspects of each therapy also make some lesions more suitable for treatment with one ablative modality versus another. Due to potential interference, patients with implanted cardiac devices may require device interrogation prior and after RFA (Skonieczki et al. 2011). Tumor proximity to mediastinal structures (<1 cm) which cannot be mitigated with displacement techniques is a contraindication to RFA and MWA (Palussière et al. 2018; Wolf et al. 2008). Cryoablation, unique in its preservation collagenous structures, enables the treatment of peripheral (subpleural) (Zhang et al. 2012) or central lesions abutting the main airways, pericardium, or large vessels (Colak et al. 2014). Cryoablation is debatably the ablation procedure of choice for subpleural lesions because it allows preservation of somatically innervated nerves of the parietal pleura which are more likely to be damaged by the RFA and MWA techniques resulting in great difficulties with post-procedural pain. Furthermore, CA is less likely to result in bronchopleural fistulas (Quirk et al. 2020). Additionally, CA's analgesic effect allows patients with contraindications to general anesthesia to undergo procedures with local anesthesia and sedation (Zhang et al. 2012). Lesions adjacent to vessels (<3 mm) are at higher risk of recurrence when treated by RFA (Gillams and Lees 2008) and cryoablation (Yashiro et al. 2013). Microwaves deliver more uniform energy and higher power to lung tissue (Brace et al. 2009) making MWA less susceptible to this heat sink effect (Vogl et al. 2013; Sidoff and Dupuy 2017). For this reason, the authors prefer to use microwave ablation for most lung tumors.

3 Technique

The authors' experience is with the Emprint (Medtronic, Dublin, Ireland) and Neuwave (Ethicon/Johnson & Johnson, Somerville, NJ) microwave ablation systems. The former allows for the use of one antenna at a time, and the latter allows for up to three antennae to be used simultaneously.

Prior to the procedure, the CT or PET/CT is reviewed to plan positioning of the patient and choice of antenna. Most antennae are either 15 or 17 gauge. Each manufacturer provides tables of ablation zone dimensions based on wattage and ablation time, which they have determined experimentally.

The procedure can be performed under conscious sedation or general anesthesia. General anesthesia is useful for patients who are unable to cooperate and for tumors at the lung bases which could be temporarily immobilized with apnea. If bleeding is a significant risk, double-lumen endotracheal tubes are recommended.

The antenna is placed into the tumor using CT-fluoroscopic guidance, which allows real-time needle guidance for speed and accuracy. Once the antenna is in place, a CT scan through the entire tumor and antenna is performed and positioning is carefully evaluated. We measure the distances from the probe outward based on our planned wattage and ablation time to ensure there will be a 1 cm margin around the tumor. Most often we use the highest of both wattage and time to create the largest ablation zone possible as long as there is not an adjacent critical structure. If a tumor is too large for a single antenna to provide adequate coverage, it is ideal to use a system which allows multiple antennae to be used simultaneously. A single antenna system can also be used with repositioning of the antenna between ablations as many times as needed. If a tumor is small enough that a single antenna can provide adequate coverage with a single session of ablation, the antenna is placed into the center of the tumor (Fig. 1). If the tumor requires two or more antennae for ade-

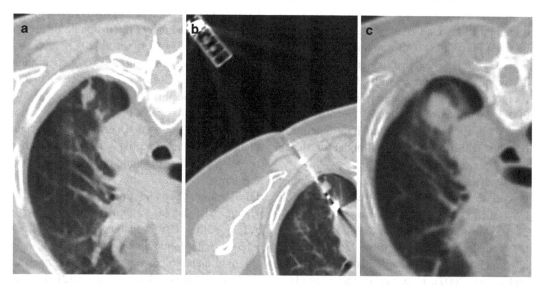

Fig. 1 An 80-year-old female with a history of left lung adenocarcinoma treated with SBRT a year prior. A 1 cm recurrent lesion was identified on surveillance (**a**) amenable to treatment by a single, centrally placed microwave antenna (**b**). The ablation zone is seen as an area of consolidation encompassing the nodule with wide margins (**c**)

quate coverage, the tumor is bracketed. The antennae are placed so that their ablation zones overlap, with no two antennae further than 2 cm apart. We often create coronal, sagittal, and oblique reconstructions of the scan to make measurements in as many planes as necessary. Once we are satisfied with the position of the antenna/antennae, we begin the ablation.

Assessment of adequate thermal ablation of the tumor requires demonstrating a minimal core tumor temperature of 60 °C and evaluating the thermal injury occurring to the normal lung surrounding the tumor. The latter has been shown using porcine lung models in which the ground-glass attenuation (GGA) CT scan changes taking place in the lung correspond to hemorrhage that occurs beyond the volume of tissue necrosis produced by thermal ablation (Yamamoto et al. 2005). Knowledge of pre-ablation lesion size is important so that thermal injury can be demonstrated beyond the margin of the lesion. This assessment can be made complex due to procedure-related enlargement of the solid portion of the tumor and the synchronous development of the peripheral zone of GGA. As a guideline, 0.5–1 cm of circumferential GGA surrounding the lesion indicates a satisfactory treatment endpoint (Fig. 1). Additional ablation with repositioning of the electrode needle should be considered to treat areas where GGA is absent. One group of investigators, however, cautioned that the extent of the GGA may not be indicative of the exact extent of coagulation necrosis (Hiraki et al. 2007).

Although the authors usually reserve cryoablation for lung tumors invading the chest wall given its proven efficacy with pain management (Fig. 2), many practitioners prefer it for early-stage NSCLC. The authors' experience is with the Cryocare (Healthtronics, Austin, TX) and Galil Medical (Boston Scientific, Marlborough, MA) cryoablation systems. Prior to the procedure, the CT or PET/CT is reviewed to plan positioning of the patient and choice of probe. Most cryoablation probes range from 13 to 17 gauge.

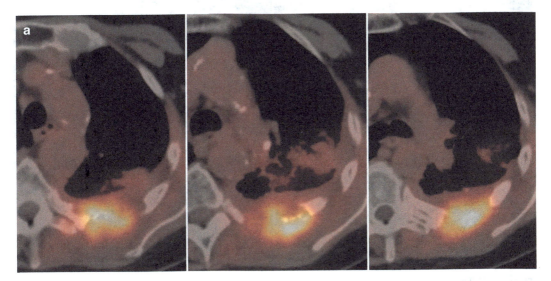

Fig. 2 A 78-year-old female with a history of Stage IIIA NSCLC of the left lower lobe treated by chemoradiation 8 months prior. Surveillance imaging showed recurrent disease with posterior chest wall and rib involvement (**a**), correlating with worsening pain affecting activities of daily living. Cryoablation was performed with eight probes spanning the lesion (**b**). Decreased pain following treatment allowed tapering and eventual discontinuation of opioids

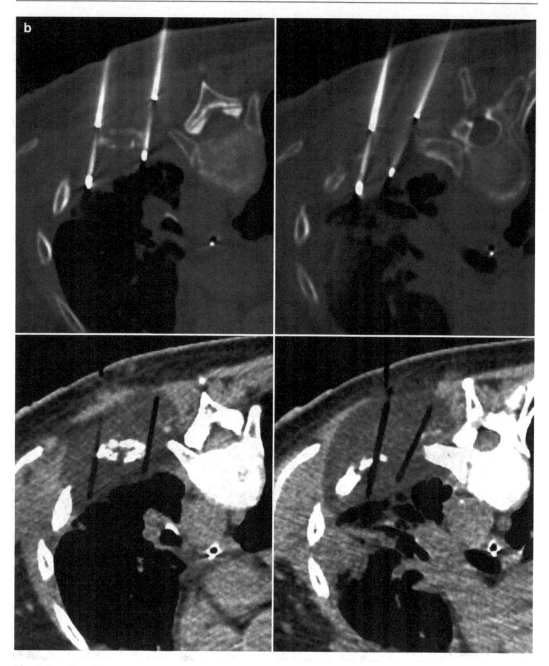

Fig. 2 (continued)

The probes are advanced into the tumor in the same way as microwave ablation antennae. Most practitioners perform three freeze-thaw cycles in lung tumors, as compared to soft tissue cryoablation in which 2 cycles are most commonly performed. The protocol at our institution is a 3-min freeze, 3-min passive thaw, 7-min freeze, 3-min passive thaw, 10-min freeze, and finally an active thaw until the antennae can be removed. The ice ball is typically less well visualized in lung as it is in soft tissue. However, the three freeze-thaw cycles produce hemorrhage within and around the tumor which more efficiently freezes the surrounding lung parenchyma.

Post-procedure recovery follows conscious sedation or post anesthesia recovery standards. We perform a chest radiograph in inspiration and expiration at 2 h following the procedure to exclude pneumothorax or occult pulmonary hemorrhage. Patients may be discharged 6–8 h after the procedure the same day or observed overnight as indicated. A mild fever due to the body's inflammatory response to ablation is common for the initial 2 days following the procedure (Yamamoto et al. 2005), and we recommend patients take ibuprofen around the clock for the first 2 days.

4 Results

Over the past decade, seven new prospective clinical trials have improved our understanding of the outcomes of thermal ablation in pulmonary tumors. Three of these studies (Ambrogi et al. 2011; Dupuy et al. 2015; Palussière et al. 2018) focus exclusively on patients with Stage I NSCLC. Table 2 summarizes the results of these trials including tumor type and size as well as the rates of local control, definition of local recurrence, and overall survival rates.

In general, the patients selected for ablation were mostly medically inoperable secondary to multiple medical comorbidities. Patients had good performance status (ECOG ≤2) and were not excluded on the basis of pulmonary function tests. Central tumors were avoided due if contiguous or in <1 cm proximity to vital structures. Patient follow-up in all series was generally only limited secondary to patient longevity.

Given the limits on assessing overall survival (OS) imposed by the cohort heterogeneity of retrospective studies, determining and improving local control rates (LCR) have been one of the principal outcomes.[1] Among other factors, such as proximity to large vessels and central location, tumor size has been identified as the strongest predictor of local recurrence (Gillams and Lees 2008; Hiraki et al. 2006; Vogl et al. 2013). Across ablative modalities, studies have identified a dichotomous response between tumors larger and smaller than 3 cm in diameter (Lee 2004; Simon et al. 2007; Healey et al. 2017; McDevitt et al. 2016). A recent meta-analysis of RFA and MWA for lung cancer and pulmonary metastases (Yuan et al. 2019) found aggregate 2-year local control rates of 62.1% (38.4–85.8, 95% CI) with RFA and 68.5% (51.8–85.1, 95% CI) with MWA.[2] Rates of 34–69% (McDevitt et al. 2016; Yashiro et al. 2013) have been reported on comparable cryoablation studies. In the setting of lung cancer, recent reports suggest improved control at 2 years with earlier disease (Stage IA, <3 cm): 64–88% (Simon et al. 2007; Huang et al. 2018) with RFA and 52–100% (McDevitt et al. 2016; Yamauchi et al. 2012; Zhang et al. 2012) with CA. In 2018, Palussière et al. reported a prospective, multicenter trial designed to assess local control with RFA of NSCLC Stage IA lesions. For a total of 3 years, they followed all participants by chest CT every 3 months for a year and whole-body CT every 6 months, and PET-CT at 3 months and 1 year. Their study showed a LCR of 84.38% (95% CI, [67.21–95.72]) at 1 year and 81.25% (95% CI, [54.35–95.95]) at 3 years. To date, the only prospective trials on cryoablation of lung tumors have been performed on metastatic disease with primary LCR of 80–94.2% at 1 year and 77.2–80% at 2 years (Kawamura et al. 2006; de Baere et al. 2015; Callstrom et al. 2020).

While most comparisons between MWA and RFA have shown no difference in LCR (Shi et al. 2017; Aufranc et al. 2019; Jiang et al. 2018; Yuan et al. 2019), Vogl et al. (2016) showed significantly improved control with MWA at 18 months (89.3% vs. 70.8%). On a meta-analysis comparing RFA, MWA, and CA which included studies of metastatic and primary lung cancers, Jiang et al. (2018) found a significantly higher rate of

---

[1] Local control most commonly refers to tumor at the ablated site with response defined in terms of RECIST or mRECIST criteria. Studies cited in this paragraph use this definition. However, some authors, for example Dupuy et al. (2015), define local control as encompassing any new tumor in the treated lobe.

[2] With regard to local control, no significant difference has been demonstrated between treatment of primary lung cancer and metastatic lung lesions (Lencioni et al. 2008; Healey et al. 2017).

Table 2 Thermal ablation trials

Author/patient population	Modality	Cohort size and tumor types	Lesion size	Local control	Survival	Complications
Kawamura et al. (2006) NSCLC and lung metastases Prospective	Cryo	35 Tumors • NSCLC: 8 (23%)	Mean: 1.33 cm (range, 0.06–3 cm)	Local control (all tumors): • 80% at 1 year • 80% at 28 months	*Not reported for NSCLC*	Pneumothorax[a]: 18% • Requiring chest tube: 1 • Requiring needle aspiration: 3 Phrenic nerve palsy: 4.5% (1)
Ambrogi et al. (2011) NSCLC Prospective	RFA	59 Tumors • NSCLC IA: 44 (75%) • NSCLC IB: 15 (25%)	Mean: 2.6 cm (range, 1.1–5 cm)	Complete response at 47 months: • NSCLC Stage I: 59% • NSCLC IA: 66% • NSCLC IB: 40%	Overall survival: • 83% at 1 year • 40% at 3 years • 25% at 5 years Cancer-related survival for Stage IA: • 95% at 1 year • 71% at 3 years • 52% at 5 years	Complications: • Grade 3: 5% PFTs: • No change in FEV, FVC at 3 or 6 months
Yang et al. (2014) NSCLC Retrospective	MWA	47 Tumors (NSCLC Stages IA and IB)	2.4–3.5 cm: 51% 3.6–5 cm: 49%	Local control (assessed by absence of enhancement): • 96% at 1 year • 64% at 3 years • 48% at 5 years	Overall survival: • 83% at 1 year • 40% at 3 years • 25% at 5 years OS for Stage IA: • 95% at 1 year • 71% at 3 years • 52% at 5 years OS significantly better in Stage IA than IB, $p = 0.016$	Major complications: 19% • Pneumothorax[a]: 5 • Pleural effusion: 3 • Bronchopleural fistula: 1
Moore et al. (2015) NSCLC Retrospective	Cryo	47 Tumors (NSCLC Stage IA) • 14 T1a • 33 T1b	Mean: 1.90 cm ± 0.5 (range: 0.5–3 cm)	85.1% at 5 years	Overall survival rates: • 89.4% at 1 year • 78.1% at 3 years • 67.8% at 5 years	Pneumothorax[a]: 15% • Requiring pigtail drain: 6 • Requiring surgical chest tube: 1 Pulmonary hemorrhage[b]: 4%
Gobara et al. (2016) NSCLC and Lung Metastases Prospective	RFA	33 Tumors • NSCLC Stage I: 7 (21%)	Mean: 1.5 cm (range, 1.0–2.4 cm)	Disease-free survival (NSCLC Stage I): • 71% at 1 year • 38% at 2 years	Overall survival (NSCLC Stage I): • 83% at 1 year • 63% at 2 year	Complications: • Grade 3: 12% (CTCAE v3.0) • Pneumothorax[a]: 6% • Pleural effusion[a]: 6%

Macchi/LUMIRA (Macchi et al. 2017) NSCLC Prospective	RFA vs. MWA	52 Tumors (NSCLC Stage IV) • RFA: 28 (54%) • MWA: 24 (46%)	Mean: 1.90 cm ± 0.89	Local control (assessed by absence of enhancement): • RFA: 75% at 1 year • MWA: 93.5% at 1 year No significant difference, $p = 0.098$	Overall survival: • RFA: 71.4% at 1 year • MWA: 66.7% at 1 year No significant difference, $p = 0.883$	Complications (pre- and post-procedure; grade not specified): • RFA: 57% • MWA: 33% No significant difference, $p = 0.051$ Intraprocedural pain (VAS: 0–10): • RFA: 3.25% • MWA: 1.79% Significant difference, $p = 0.0043$
Huang et al. (2018) NSCLC Retrospective	RFA	73 Tumors (NSCLC Stage IA)	Mean: 2.2 cm (range: 1–3 cm)	All (<3 cm) • 96% at 1 years • 88% at 2 years • 74% at 5 years <2 cm • 94.7% at 1 years • 94.7% at 2 years • 78.9% at 5 years	Overall survival: • 96% at 1 year • 86.5% at 2 years • 67.1% at 3 years • 36.3% at 5 years • 1% at 10 years	Pneumothorax[a]: 4% Moderate post-procedural pain (CTCAE v4.0): 6%

[a] Requiring chest tube placement
[b] Pulmonary hemorrhage requiring bronchoscopy

local progression with CA (23.7%) than with RFA (19.8%) and MWA (10.9%).

However, local control provides an incomplete picture of thermal ablation's overall effectiveness. A meta-analysis by Bi et al. (2016) comparing RFA with SBRT in patients with NSCLC Stage I found that despite the latter's better local control (55–88% at 3 years), there was no significant difference ($p = 0.77$) in OS (53–56% at 3 years, respectively). Likewise, despite a significantly higher rate of local progression with CA, Jiang et al. (2018) found no difference in OS in comparison to thermal ablative therapies. The uncoupling of these two outcomes is at least partly due to the ability to re-treat recurrent disease by repeat ablation without an increased complication rate (Hiraki et al. 2008; Lanuti et al. 2012; Yang et al. 2017). In a prospective clinical trial of RFA with overall survival as primary endpoint, Dupuy et al. (2015) found no significant relation between OS rates of 86.3% at 1 year and 69.8% at 2 years and the local control rates in the first-year posttreatment ($p = 0.49$). The authors hypothesized that this may be due to the "secondary assist rate" of repeat local therapy with thermal ablation or radiation therapy. In a recent multicenter prospective trial study of 32 patients with Stage IA NSCLC, Palussière et al. (2018) reported OS rates of 91.67% and 58.33% at 1 and 3 years, respectively. In this study, RFA treatment was repeated in two out of the five cases with local progression.

Survival data for MWA and cryoablation is limited to single-center, retrospective studies. In a study of MWA, Zheng et al. (2016) reported survival outcomes in 52 patients with T1–4, N0, M0 NSCLC: OS of 94.1% at 1 years and 76.9% at 3 years and a cancer-specific survival of 80% at 3 years. In a cohort of 47 Stage IA and IB NSCLC patients, Yang et al. (2014) found a size threshold of 3.5 cm to have significant effect on survival after MWA. In tumors smaller and larger than 3.5 cm, 3-year survival rates were 59% and 27%, respectively ($p = 0.016$). A prospective, randomized trial (LUMIRA) by Macchi et al. (2017) compared RFA and MWA in the setting of Stage IV NSCLC and found no differences in overall survival. Their findings echoed those of mixed metastasis/primary tumor studies comparing the MWA and RFA (Shi et al. 2017; Chi et al. 2018; Aufranc et al. 2019). In studies of Stage IA tumors (≤ 3 cm) treated with cryoablation, the 3-year and 5-year survival rates have been noted to be fairly impressive at 78.1%/88% (Moore et al. 2015/Yamauchi et al. 2012) and 67.8% (Moore et al. 2015), respectively.

Comparison of overall survival outcomes between thermal ablation and SBRT or surgery is challenging due to the frailty which preclude those treatments (Crabtree et al. 2013). However, comparative studies which take into account the comorbidity differences between these patients have found no significant differences in survival between thermal ablation, SBRT, and sublobar resection (Kwan et al. 2014; Bi et al. 2016; Iguchi et al. 2020).

However, to better assess the different modalities to treat Stage I NSCLC, large multicenter studies randomizing patients to the different treatment techniques are needed. The multicenter studies are needed to demonstrate that the promising results in individual centers can be successfully obtained in larger populations across multiple treatment centers. Unfortunately, two such efforts to compare stereotactic body radiation to lobectomy accrued only 58 patients between them (Chang et al. 2016). Until the performance of comparative randomized studies, we will have to rely on multi-institutional phase I/II studies. Table 3 displays the three multicenter studies of RFA in the treatment of Stage I NSCLC (Dupuy et al. 2015; Lencioni et al. 2008; Palussière et al. 2018) and includes median survival (if obtained) as well as the definition of local control and how local control was determined. Unfortunately, to the best of our knowledge, there are no such studies of MWA and CA in Stage I NSCLC. All patients in these three studies had biopsy-proven Stage I NSCLC. Because the ACOSOG trial's definition of local recurrence included the ipsilateral hilum as well as the treated lesion, while the Rapture study and the multicenter French study only assessed the treated lesion, the lower local control (59.8%) in ACOSOG Z4033/RFA as compared to the other two studies (87.5% crude,

Table 3 Multicenter studies of radiofrequency ablation

Study/modality	Patient #/ lesion size	Median F/U	Local control area and definition	Local control	PFTs	Survival	Complications
ACOSOG Z4033/ RFA (Dupuy et al. 2015)	54 ≤3 cm	24 months (all patients)	Same lobe or ipsil hilum Recurrence 1.25× any dimension compared to 3-month baseline or mass lesion >9 mm that enhanced 15HU	68.9%—1 year 59.8%—2 years	No change in FEV1 or DLCO FVC improved at 3, 24 months	86.3%—1 year 69.8%—2 year	11.8% Gr3 No Gr4–5 due to treatment
Rapture/RFA (Lencioni et al. 2008)	33 ≤3.5 cm	15 months	Treated lesion RECIST response, failure if <30% decrease in longest diameter compared to 1-month or contrast enhancement	87.5%[a]	No change in FEV, FVC At 1, 3, 6, 12 months	70%—1 year 48%—2 year	No change in SF-12 physical[b] or FACT-L[c]
Multicenter French (Palussière et al. 2018)	32 ≤3 cm	36 months (all patients)	Treated lesion Recurrence >20% longest diameter on 2 consecutive CT scans and/or PET + > mediastinum	84.4%—1 year 81.3%—2 years	No change in FEV1, FVC at 3 months	91.7%—1 year 58.3%—3 years	Global health status, physical function, pain, and dyspnea by QLQ C30[d]

[a] Defined as complete ablation lasting at least 1 year
[b] Short-form-12
[c] Functional assessment of cancer therapy—lung
[d] Quality of life questionnaire, core questionnaire

81.3% at 2 years) may have been partially explained by definition. As can be seen, all studies differed in how local recurrences were determined which may have affected recurrence rates and makes cross trial comparisons difficult. Unfortunately, all follow-up times were too short to assess long-term outcomes at 4–5 years or more. Pulmonary function tests appear to be unchanged in all three studies.

Table 4 displays the multi-institutional Phase I/II studies of SBRT performed by the RTOG/NRG Oncology Group (Timmerman et al. 2018a, b; Stanic et al. 2014; Videtic et al. 2018; Bezjak et al. 2019) and the one multi-institutional surgical study of sublobar resection (Fernando et al. 2014) that was completed during this century. Of note, all of the studies of SBRT were performed on medically inoperable patients except for RTOG 0618 which only contained 26 patients. The median follow-ups in these investigations are fairly long at 48 months except RTOG 0813 which, unlike the other studies, has a shorter follow-up and deals with central-based lesions and will be discussed separately below. Except RTOG 0813, all other studies treated peripheral lesions, 2 cm or greater from the proximal bronchial tree (Timmerman et al. 2006). Local failure for all studies was defined as local enlargement defined of at least a 20% increase in the longest diameter of the gross tumor volume per CT scan and evidence of tumor viability (uptake of a similar intensity as the pretreatment staging PET or by repeat biopsy-confirming carcinoma). Despite differences in dosing strategies (34 Gy/1 fraction, 48 Gy/4 fractions, 54 Gy/3fractions), primary control rates have remained high between 89.4% and 96%. Although the primary tumor control rates remain high, OS rates in the medically inoperable patients at 5 years remained relatively poor ranging between 29.6% and 41.1% suggesting that the patients in these studies had multiple medical comorbidities. It should be noted that RTOG 0236 had the highest rate of grade 3 or greater toxicity which may be explained by the lack of experience with SBRT during this early accrual period (2004–2006) or due to the higher biologically effective dose of the 54 Gy in 3 fraction regimen as compared to other dosing strategies which are shown to be just as effective and less aggressive, i.e., 48 Gy in 4 fractions.

RTOG 0813 (Bezjak et al. 2019) treated central-based lesions which were defined as being within or touching the zone 2 cm around the proximal bronchial tree (PBT) or immediately adjacent to the mediastinal or pericardial pleura. The 5-fraction dosing strategy started at 50 Gy in 5 fractions and escalated dose at 0.5 Gy/fraction until toxicity or the pre-defined maximum dose of 60 Gy was reached. A dose-limiting toxicity (DLT) was defined as any grade 3 or worse toxicity that occurred within 1 year from the start of SBRT and was thought to be due to treatment. The maximum tolerated dose was defined as the dose at which the DLT did not exceed 20%. The authors concluded that the maximum tolerated dose was 12 Gy/fraction which had a DLT of 7.2%. As expected, the local control rates at 2 years in the 11.5 and the 12.5 Gy arms were high at 89.4%. However, there were major flaws with the reporting/execution of this trial as follows:

1. Was this patient population truly at high risk for complications? Only 17% of patients had ultracentral tumors. The term ultracentral was not defined in this manuscript nor in the protocol, but although the definition varies, one reasonable definition of these very high-risk lesions is a tumor whose planning tumor volume overlaps the central bronchial tree, esophagus, or pulmonary artery (Giuliani et al. 2018). Unfortunately, this radiation strategy for these very high-risk tumors remains unknown despite the publication of this trial.
2. There was a high dropout rate. 120 patients were entered and only 100 were able to be analyzed.
3. Of the 100 patients that were able to be analyzed, 11 died within the first year and could not be evaluated for the DLT.
4. Toxicity from high dose radiation regimens is not limited to one year, but was only reported to 1 year in the abstract and result sections. Interestingly, in the discussion section of this manuscript, the authors noted that 4 patients

Table 4 Multicenter studies of techniques (stereotactic body radiation therapy and sublobar resection) that are also mostly used in patients who are not candidates for lobectomy

Study/modality	Patient #/tumors/dose	Median F/U	Local control definition	Local control	PFTs	Survival	Complications
RTOG 0236 (Timmerman et al. 2018a, b; Stanic et al. 2014) Medically inoperable	55 Biopsy + <5 cm 54 Gy in 3 Fr	48 months	Primary Tumor Control (PTC)-treated lesion Local-lesion and involved lobe	PTC—92.7% Local control—80.0% Regional—10.9% All 5 year rates	FEV1 and DLCO decline of 5.8, 6.3% at 2 years No change arterial or O₂ saturation	55.8%—3 years 40.0%—5 years	27.3% Gr 3 3.6% Gr 4
RTOG 0915 (Videtic et al. 2018) Medically inoperable	39 Biopsy + <5 cm 34 Gy in 1 Fr	48 months	Same as RTOG 0236	PTC—89.4% Local control—81.2% 5 year rates		61.3%—2 years 29.6%—5 years	2.6% Gr 3–5 1 grade 5
RTOG 0915 (Videtic et al. 2018) Medically inoperable	45 Biopsy + <5 cm 48 Gy in 4 Fr	48 months	Same as RTOG 0236	PTC—93.2% Local control—88.2% 5 year rates		77.7%—2 years 41.1%—5 years	11.1% Gr 3–5 1 grade 5
RTOG 0618 (Timmerman et al. 2018b) Medically operable	26 Biopsy + <5 cm 54 Gy in 3 Fr	48.1 months	Same as RTOG 0236	PTC—4 years 96% Local control—4 years 96%		56%—4 years	Grade 3–8% No Gr 4/5
RTOG 0813 (Bezjak et al. 2019) Medically inoperable	120 (71 evaluable in 11.5 and 12 Gy cohorts) Biopsy + <5 cm, centrally located 50–60 Gy in 5 Fr	37.9 months	Same as RTOG 0236	Local control—2 years 89.4% (11.5 Gy) 87.% (12 Gy)		67.9% (11.5 Gy)—2 years 72.7% (12.5 Gy)—2 years	Gr3–5 12.1% within first year in 11.5/12 Gy arms

had grade 5 events after 1 year (3 bronchopulmonary hemorrhages and 1 esophageal ulcer), 3 of which were in the 11.5 Gy arm and 1 was in the 12.0 Gy arm. Because the study was designed to report toxicity at 1 year, these four fatal events were not included in the primary calculations of the DLT.

As can be seen by the high rates of local control and long-term follow-up in the RTOG/NRG Group Lung SBRT trials (89.4–96% at 5 years) and sublobar resection results (86.0% at 5 years) noted from ACOSOG Z4032 (Fernando et al. 2014), we agree with the NCCN, ACCP, and ESMO guidelines as noted earlier in this chapter which limits ablation techniques to medically inoperable patients who cannot receive radiation. Because of the evolving efficacy of cryoablation in treating central lesion and because of potential toxicity of SBRT in treating ultracentral lesions in retrospective studies (Grade 3 or higher toxicity rates of 20–38% (Tekatli et al. 2016; Timmerman et al. 2006; Song et al. 2009) with fatal pulmonary hemorrhages as high as 13% (Tekatli et al. 2016)), we think that some of the lesions may be more safely treated with cryoablation as a sole modality and/or combined with a lower, safer radiation dose strategy.

Most adverse events associated with thermal ablation are usually encountered in the immediate intra- and post-procedural period. Pulmonary function, as measured by FEV1 and VC, is generally not significantly affected (Lencioni et al. 2008; Dupuy et al. 2015). A meta-analysis of RFA, MWA, and CA estimated major complications (defined as those requiring medical intervention) at 11.5% (Jiang et al. 2018). Post-procedure pneumothoraxes and pleural effusions, the most common complications, are associated with a 34% and 5–10% of hyperthermic ablations, respectively. However, pneumothoraxes and effusions requiring drainage occur in approximately 6–12% and 1–6% of interventions, respectively (Gobara et al. 2016; Yuan et al. 2019). The most commonly reported complications following cryoablation are pneumothorax (28–51%) and pulmonary hemorrhage (1–40%), requiring intervention after (4–26%) and 0–4% of cases, respectively (Yamauchi et al. 2012; Moore et al. 2015; Callstrom et al. 2020). Other rare, but serious complications listed included hemorrhage, ARDS, pleuritis, and bronchopleural fistula. Alexander et al. (2012) described the placement of endobronchial valves for RFA-related bronchopleural fistulas as a minimally invasive alternative to surgery.

5 Follow-Up

The appearances of treated lung cancer after thermal ablation are well documented (Bojarski et al. 2005; Wolf et al. 2008; Ito et al. 2012; Chheang et al. 2013). Changes in the treated zone after hyperthermic ablation (i.e., RFA or MWA) follow similar patterns. Following a baseline study within 6 weeks post-procedure, changes to tumor/ablation zone size and contrast-enhancement patterns may be followed with CT or PET/CT every 3–4 months (Ahmed et al. 2014). Immediate CT following RFA/MWA demonstrates GGA surrounding the tumor in 84% of cases and represents pulmonary bleeding and/or increased blood flow. The ablation zone usually remains larger during the first 3 months following the RFA/MWA procedure. During this time period, transient and reversible locoregional nodal enlargement can sometimes be appreciated (Sharma et al. 2007).

During cryoablation, perilesional hemorrhage usually develops after the first thaw cycle enabling visualization of the ice ball. The latter may be identified as decreased attenuation within soft tissue lesions surrounded by perilesional GGA. Within 1 week, the GGA changes to dense opacity (Yasui et al. 2004; Ito et al. 2012). Successful treatment is associated with a larger ablation zone than the original tumor size (Yamamoto et al. 2005), with the lethal zone in cryoablation being several millimeters central to the GGA margins (Chheang et al. 2013).

With both hyperthermic ablation techniques and CA, successful treatment is associated with progressive contraction of the lesion and resolution of any pleural changes distal to the immediate ablation zone (Fig. 3), as well as loss of

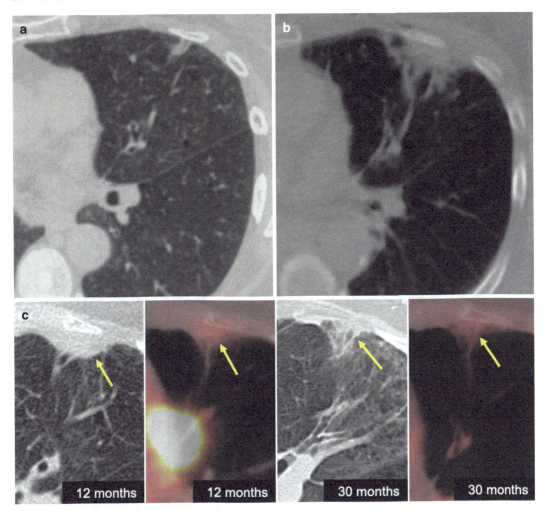

Fig. 3 A 67-year-old female with history of left breast cancer 12 years prior and large cell neuroendocrine carcinoma of the lung, recently treated with chemoradiation. The patient was referred for biopsy and possible microwave ablation of 1 cm left upper lobe nodule (**a**). Post-ablation CT demonstrates a 1 cm margin around the lesion (**b**). Surveillance imaging shows early consolidation followed by involution of the ablation zone without focal FDG avidity to suggest recurrence (**c**). The arrow shows continued evolution of the successfully-treated lesion over 30 months. Because of the relatively large size of the ablation zone, serial ct scan follow-up is recommended to assess treatment outcome

contrast enhancement of the lesion. A thin (<5 mm) pattern of peripheral/rim enhancement, corresponding to reactive hyperemia, is also associated with successful treatment (Anderson et al. 2009). Cavities develop within the ablation zone in up to 20–58% of patients following RFA/MWA and up to 80% following cryoablation. Most patients with cavities have no specific symptoms, and the cavities usually spontaneously contract with time (Okuma et al. 2007; Steinke et al. 2005; Wang et al. 2005). Other reactive CT findings that are considered to be benign include bubble lucencies and pleural thickening within or near the ablation zone (Pennathur et al. 2007). When pleural effusions occur, they are usually self-limiting, but can show FDG avidity (Higaki et al. 2008).

After 3 months, continued growth of the ablation zone should be viewed as suspicious for incomplete tumor destruction and recurrent tumor (Bojarski et al. 2005; Wang et al. 2005) (Fig. 4). Progressive, persistent, or minimally

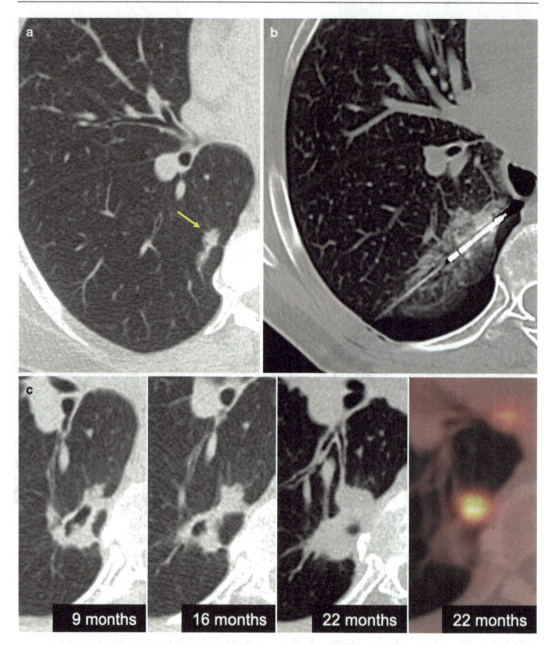

Fig. 4 A 57-year-old female with slow-growing right lower lobe nodule (**a**) who declined surgical resection. The arrow demonstrates the lung cancer prior to ablation. Ablation image shows antenna protruding into the pleural space leading to incomplete ablation of anterolateral aspect of lesion (**b**). Follow-up images show residual, growing mass at the anterior margin of the ablation zone with associated FDG avidity indicative of recurrence (**c**)

decreased FDG avidity at 3 months on PET/CT has been shown to predict local recurrence tumor. The use of FDG-PET may prove to be a predictive test for treatment failure or success. Immediate post-ablation inflammation may obscure residual/recurrent disease. Later assessment (usually after 1–2 months) can demonstrate three basic patterns as follows:

1. A diffuse increase followed by continued decreasing activity (Fig. 3).
2. Little change with subpleural lesions and rim activity followed by a collapse of the lesion with decreasing focal activity over time.
3. Immediate residual activity or eccentric residual activity invariably showing progression over time.

6 Summary

Since the first published report of modern percutaneous RFA for the treatment of lung neoplasms in 2000, a number of largely retrospective studies have demonstrated local control rates of 58–80%, with median follow-ups of 15–31 months. More recent studies with microwave ablation and cryoablation have shown similar outcomes. The primary complications of thermal ablation are pneumothorax and pleural effusion, occurring in 13–63% and 10–21%, respectively. RFA is most effective with non-subpleural, peripheral lesions due to less concern for the heat sink effect and due to the lower likelihood of complications. Prospective trials with careful long-term follow-up assessing a standard radiologic definition of local control and using a known toxicity scale (i.e., common terminology criteria for adverse events (CTCAE v5.0)) are greatly needed.

Due to the ability of SBRT to control greater than 90% of primary tumors at 5 years (Timmerman et al. 2018a, b; Stanic et al. 2014; Videtic et al. 2018; Bezjak et al. 2019) and because this technique does not require hospitalization, most medically inoperable Stage I NSCLC patient are treated with SBRT at the University of Massachusetts, especially for tumors that are not considered to be ultracentral (i.e., tumors whose planning target volume touches or overlaps the central bronchial tree, esophagus, or pulmonary artery). It is felt that due to the potential of SBRT-regimens to result in serious toxicity in ultracentral lesions, prospective trials of alternative safer radiation regimens with or without cryoablation or trials of cryoablation alone are needed. Thermal ablation is considered for small (<3 cm) peripheral tumors in medically inoperable patients who are not eligible for radiation. Thermal ablation is also considered for the rare patients experiencing primary tumor failure after SBRT.

References

Ahmed M, Solbiati L, Brace CL, Breen DJ, Callstrom MR, William Charboneau J, Chen M-H et al (2014) Image-guided tumor ablation: standardization of terminology and reporting criteria—a 10-year update. J Vasc Interv Radiol 25(11):1691–1705.e4. https://doi.org/10.1016/j.jvir.2014.08.027

Alexander ES, Healey TT, Martin DW, Dupuy DE (2012) Use of endobronchial valves for the treatment of bronchopleural fistulas after thermal ablation of lung neoplasms. J Vasc Interv Radiol 23(9):1236–1240

Ambrogi MC, Fanucchi O, Cioni R, Dini P, De Liperi A, Cappelli C, Davini F, Bartolozzi C, Mussi A (2011) Long-term results of radiofrequency ablation treatment of stage I non-small cell lung cancer: a prospective intention-to-treat study. J Thorac Oncol 6(12):2044–2051. https://doi.org/10.1097/JTO.0b013e31822d538d

Anderson EM, Lees WR, Gillams AR (2009) Early indicators of treatment success after percutaneous radiofrequency of pulmonary tumors. Cardiovasc Intervent Radiol 32(3):478–483. https://doi.org/10.1007/s00270-008-9482-6

Aufranc V, Farouil G, Abdel-Rehim M, Smadja P, Tardieu M, Aptel S, Guibal A (2019) Percutaneous thermal ablation of primary and secondary lung tumors: comparison between microwave and radiofrequency ablation. Diagn Interv Imaging 100(12):781–791. https://doi.org/10.1016/j.diii.2019.07.008

Bezjak A, Paulus R, Gaspar LE, Timmerman RD, Straube WL, Ryan WF, Garces Y et al (2019) Safety and efficacy of a five-fraction stereotactic body radiotherapy schedule for centrally located non-small-cell lung cancer: NRG Oncology/RTOG 0813 Trial. J Clin Oncol 37(15):1316–1325. https://doi.org/10.1200/JCO.18.00622

Bi N, Shedden K, Zheng X, Kong F-MS (2016) Comparison of the effectiveness of radiofrequency ablation with stereotactic body radiation therapy in inoperable stage I non-small cell lung cancer: a systemic review and pooled analysis. Int J Radiat Oncol Biol Phys 95(5):1378–1390. https://doi.org/10.1016/j.ijrobp.2016.04.016

Bojarski JD, Dupuy DE, Mayo-Smith WW (2005) CT imaging findings of pulmonary neoplasms after treatment with radiofrequency ablation: results in 32 tumors. Am J Roentgenol 185(2):466–471. https://doi.org/10.2214/ajr.185.2.01850466

Brace CL, Louis Hinshaw J, Laeseke PF, Sampson LA, Lee FT (2009) Pulmonary thermal ablation: comparison of radiofrequency and microwave devices by using gross pathologic and CT findings in a Swine model. Radiology 251(3):705–711. https://doi.org/10.1148/radiol.2513081564

Callstrom MR, Woodrum DA, Nichols FC, Palussiere J, Buy X, Suh RD, Abtin FG et al (2020) Multicenter study of metastatic lung tumors targeted by interventional cryoablation evaluation (SOLSTICE). J Thorac Oncol 15(7):1200–1209. https://doi.org/10.1016/j.jtho.2020.02.022

Chang JY, Senan S, Paul MA, Mehran RJ, Louie AV, Balter P, Greon HJM et al (2016) Stereotactic ablation radiotherapy versus lobectomy for operable stage I non-small cell lung cancer: a pooled analysis of two randomized trials. Lancet Oncol 16(6):630–637. https://doi.org/10.1016/S1470-2045(15)70168-3

Chheang S, Abtin F, Guteirrez A, Genshaft S, Suh R (2013) Imaging features following thermal ablation of lung malignancies. Semin Interv Radiol 30(02):157–168. https://doi.org/10.1055/s-0033-1342957

Chi J, Ding M, Shi Y, Wang T, Cui D, Tang X, Li P, Zhai B (2018) Comparison study of computed tomography-guided radiofrequency and microwave ablation for pulmonary tumors: a retrospective, case-controlled observational study. Thorac Cancer 9(10):1241–1248. https://doi.org/10.1111/1759-7714.12822

Colak E, Tatli S, Shyn PB, Tuncali K, Silverman SG (2014) CT-guided percutaneous cryoablation of central lung tumors. Diagn Interv Radiol 20(4):316–322. https://doi.org/10.5152/dir.2014.13440

Crabtree T, Puri V, Timmerman R, Fernando H, Bradley J, Decker PA, Paulus R, Putnam JB, Dupuy DE, Meyers B (2013) Treatment of stage I lung cancer in high-risk and inoperable patients: comparison of prospective clinical trials using stereotactic body radiotherapy (RTOG 0236), sublobar resection (ACOSOG Z4032), and radiofrequency ablation (ACOSOG Z4033). J Thorac Cardiovasc Surg 145(3):692–699. https://doi.org/10.1016/j.jtcvs.2012.10.038

de Baere T, Tselikas L, Woodrum D, Abtin F, Littrup P, Deschamps F, Suh R, Aoun HD, Callstrom M (2015) Evaluating cryoablation of metastatic lung tumors in patients—safety and efficacy: the ECLIPSE Trial—interim analysis at 1 year. J Thorac Oncol 10(10):1468–1474. https://doi.org/10.1097/JTO.0000000000000632

Detterbeck FC, Jantz MA, Wallace M, Vansteenkiste J, Silvestri GA, American College of Chest Physicians (2007) Invasive mediastinal staging of lung cancer: ACCP evidence-based clinical practice guidelines (2nd Edition). Chest 132(3 Suppl):202S–220S. https://doi.org/10.1378/chest.07-1362

Detterbeck FC, Lewis SZ, Diekemper R et al (2013) Executive Summary: diagnosis and management of lung cancer 3rd ed: American College of Chest Physicians evidence-based clinical practice guidelines. Chest 143(5 Suppl):7S–37S. https://doi.org/10.1378/chest.12-2377

Donington J, Ferguson M, Mazzone P, Handy J, Schuchert M, Fernando H, Loo B et al (2012) American College of Chest Physicians and Society of Thoracic Surgeons Consensus Statement for evaluation and management for high-risk patients with stage I non-small cell lung cancer. Chest 142(6):1620–1635. https://doi.org/10.1378/chest.12-0790

Dupuy DE, Fernando HC, Hillman S, Ng T, Tan AD, Sharma A, Rilling WS, Hong K, Putnam JB (2015) Radiofrequency ablation of stage IA non-small cell lung cancer in medically inoperable patients: results from the American College of Surgeons Oncology Group Z4033 (Alliance) Trial. Cancer 121(19):3491–3498. https://doi.org/10.1002/cncr.29507

Fernando HC, Landreneau RJ, Mandrekar SJ, Nichols FC, Hillman SL, Heron DE, Meyers BF et al (2014) Impact of brachytherapy on local recurrence rates after sublobar resection: results from ACOSOG Z4032 (Alliance), a phase III randomized trial for high-risk operable non-small-cell lung cancer. J Clin Oncol 32(23):2456–2462. https://doi.org/10.1200/JCO.2013.53.4115

Fietta AM, Morosini M, Passadore I, Cascina A, Draghi P, Dore R, Rossi S, Pozzi E, Meloni F (2009) Systemic inflammatory response and downmodulation of peripheral CD25+Foxp3+ T-regulatory cells in patients undergoing radiofrequency thermal ablation for lung cancer. Hum Immunol 70(7):477–486. https://doi.org/10.1016/j.humimm.2009.03.012

Gillams AR, Lees WR (2008) Radiofrequency ablation of lung metastases: factors influencing success. Eur Radiol 18(4):672–677. https://doi.org/10.1007/s00330-007-0811-y

Giuliani M, Mathew AS, Bahig H, Bratman SV, Filion E, Glick D, Louie AV et al (2018) SUNSET: stereotactic radiation for ultracentral non-small cell lung cancer - a safety and efficacy trial. Clin Lung Cancer 19(4):529–532

Gobara H, Arai Y, Kobayashi T, Yamakado K, Inaba Y, Kodama Y, Yamagami T et al (2016) Percutaneous radiofrequency ablation for patients with malignant lung tumors: a phase II prospective multicenter study (JIVROSG-0702). Jpn J Radiol 34(8):556–563. https://doi.org/10.1007/s11604-016-0557-z

Healey TT, March BT, Baird G, Dupuy DE (2017) Microwave ablation for lung neoplasms: a retrospective analysis of long-term results. J Vasc Interv Radiol 28(2):206–211. https://doi.org/10.1016/j.jvir.2016.10.030

Higaki F, Okumura Y, Sato S, Hiraki T, Gobara H, Mimura H, Akaki S, Tsuda T, Kanazawa S (2008) Preliminary retrospective investigation of FDG-PET/CT timing in follow-up of ablated lung tumor. Ann Nucl Med 22(3):157–163. https://doi.org/10.1007/s12149-007-0113-0

Hiraki T, Sakurai J, Tsuda T, Gobara H, Sano Y, Mukai T, Hase S et al (2006) Risk factors for local progression after percutaneous radiofrequency ablation of lung tumors: evaluation based on a preliminary review of 342 tumors. Cancer 107(12):2873–2880. https://doi.org/10.1002/cncr.22333

Hiraki T, Gobara H, Iishi T, Sano Y, Iguchi T, Fujiwara H, Tajiri N et al (2007) Percutaneous radiofrequency ablation for clinical stage I non-small cell lung cancer: results in 20 nonsurgical candidates. J Thorac Cardiovasc Surg 134(5):1306–1312. https://doi.org/10.1016/j.jtcvs.2007.07.013

Hiraki T, Mimura H, Gobara H, Sano Y, Fujiwara H, Date H, Kanazawa S (2008) Repeat radiofrequency ablation for local progression of lung tumors: does it have a role in local tumor control? J Vasc Interv Radiol 19(5):706–711. https://doi.org/10.1016/j.jvir.2007.12.441

Huang B-Y, Li X-M, Song X-Y, Zhou J-J, Shao Z, Yu Z-Q, Lin Y, Guo X-Y, Liu D-J, Li L (2018) Long-term results of CT-guided percutaneous radiofrequency ablation of inoperable patients with stage Ia non-small cell lung cancer: a retrospective cohort study. Int J Surg 53:143–150. https://doi.org/10.1016/j.ijsu.2018.03.034

Iguchi T, Hiraki T, Matsui Y, Mitsuhashi T, Katayama N, Katsui K, Soh J et al (2020) Survival outcomes of treatment with radiofrequency ablation, stereotactic body radiotherapy, or sublobar resection for patients with clinical stage I non-small-cell lung cancer: a single-center evaluation. J Vasc Interv Radiol 31(7):1044–1051. https://doi.org/10.1016/j.jvir.2019.11.035

Ito N, Nakatsuka S, Inoue M, Yashiro H, Oguro S, Izumi Y, Kawamura M, Nomori H, Kuribayashi S (2012) Computed tomographic appearance of lung tumors treated with percutaneous cryoablation. J Vasc Interv Radiol 23(8):1043–1052. https://doi.org/10.1016/j.jvir.2012.04.033

Jiang B, Mcclure MA, Chen T, Chen S (2018) Efficacy and safety of thermal ablation of lung malignancies: a network meta-analysis. Ann Thorac Med 13(4):243–250. https://doi.org/10.4103/atm.ATM_392_17

Kawamura M, Izumi Y, Tsukada N, Asakura K, Sugiura H, Yashiro H, Nakano K, Nakatsuka S, Kuribayashi S, Kobayashi K (2006) Percutaneous cryoablation of small pulmonary malignant tumors under computed tomographic guidance with local anesthesia for nonsurgical candidates. J Thorac Cardiovasc Surg 131(5):1007–1013. https://doi.org/10.1016/j.jtcvs.2005.12.051

Kim DH, Erinjeri JP (2019) Postablation immune microenvironment: synergy between interventional oncology and immuno-oncology. Semin Interv Radiol 36(04):334–342. https://doi.org/10.1055/s-0039-1696704

Koike T, Terashima M, Takizawa T, Watanabe T, Kurita Y, Yokoyama A (1998) Clinical analysis of small-sized peripheral lung cancer. J Thorac Cardiovasc Surg 115(5):1015–1020. https://doi.org/10.1016/S0022-5223(98)70399-X

Kwan SW, Mortell KE, Talenfeld AD, Brunner MC (2014) Thermal ablation matches sublobar resection outcomes in older patients with early-stage non-small cell lung cancer. J Vasc Interv Radiol 25(1):1–9.e1. https://doi.org/10.1016/j.jvir.2013.10.018

Lanuti M, Sharma A, Willers H, Digumarthy SR, Mathisen DJ, Shepard J-AO (2012) Radiofrequency ablation for stage I non-small cell lung cancer: management of locoregional recurrence. Ann Thorac Surg 93(3):921–27; discussion 927–988. https://doi.org/10.1016/j.athoracsur.2011.11.043

Lee JM, Jin GY, Nahum Goldberg S, Lee YC, Chung GH, Han YM, Lee SY, Kim CS (2004) Percutaneous radiofrequency ablation for inoperable non-small cell lung cancer and metastases: preliminary report. Radiology 230(1):125–134. https://doi.org/10.1148/radiol.2301020934

Lencioni R, Crocetti L, Cioni R, Suh R, Glenn D, Regge D, Helmberger T et al (2008) Response to radiofrequency ablation of pulmonary tumours: a prospective, intention-to-treat, multicentre clinical trial (the RAPTURE Study). Lancet 9(7):621–628. https://doi.org/10.1016/S1470-2045(08)70155-4

Lilly MB, Brezovich IA, Atkinson W, Chakraborty D, Durant JR, Ingram J, Mcelvein RB (1983) Hyperthermia with implanted electrodes: in vitro and in vivo correlations. Int J Radiat Oncol Biol Phys 9(3):373–382. https://doi.org/10.1016/0360-3016(83)90299-7

Macchi M, Belfiore MP, Floridi C, Serra N, Belfiore G, Carmignani L, Grasso RF et al (2017) Radiofrequency versus microwave ablation for treatment of the lung tumours: LUMIRA (Lung Microwave Radiofrequency) randomized trial. Med Oncol 34(5):96. https://doi.org/10.1007/s12032-017-0946-x

McDevitt JL, Mouli SK, Nemcek AA, Lewandowski RJ, Salem R, Sato KT (2016) Percutaneous cryoablation for the treatment of primary and metastatic lung tumors: identification of risk factors for recurrence and major complications. J Vasc Interv Radiol 27(9):1371–1379. https://doi.org/10.1016/j.jvir.2016.04.005

McTaggart RA, Dupuy DE (2007) Thermal ablation of lung tumors. Tech Vasc Interv Radiol 10(2):102–113. https://doi.org/10.1053/j.tvir.2007.09.004

Moore W, Talati R, Bhattacharji P, Bilfinger T (2015) Five-year survival after cryoablation of stage I non-small cell lung cancer in medically inoperable patients. J Vasc Interv Radiol 26(3):312–319. https://doi.org/10.1016/j.jvir.2014.12.006

National Comprehensive Cancer Network (2021) Non-small cell lung cancer (Version 1.2021). https://www.nccn.org/professionals/physician_gls/pdf/nscl.pdf. Accessed 1 Dec 2020

Okuma T, Matsuoka T, Yamamoto A, Oyama Y, Inoue K, Nakamura K, Inoue Y (2007) Factors contributing to cavitation after CT-guided percutaneous radiofrequency ablation for lung tumors. J Vasc Interv Radiol 18(3):399–404. https://doi.org/10.1016/j.jvir.2007.01.004

Palussière J, Catena V, Buy X (2017) Percutaneous thermal ablation of lung tumors – radiofrequency, microwave and cryotherapy: where are we going? Diagn Interv Imaging 98(9):619–625. https://doi.org/10.1016/j.diii.2017.07.003

Palussière J, Chomy F, Savina M, Deschamps F, Gaubert JY, Renault A, Bonnefoy O et al (2018) Radiofrequency ablation of stage IA non-small cell lung cancer in patients ineligible for surgery: results of a prospective multicenter phase II trial. J Cardiothorac Surg 13(1):91. https://doi.org/10.1186/s13019-018-0773-y

Pennathur A, Luketich JD, Abbas G, Chen M, Fernando HC, Gooding WE, Schuchert MJ, Gilbert S, Christie NA, Landreneau RJ (2007) Radiofrequency ablation for the treatment of stage I non-small cell lung cancer in high-risk patients. J Thorac Cardiovasc Surg 134(4):857–864. https://doi.org/10.1016/j.jtcvs.2007.04.060

Quirk MT, Lee S, Murali N, Genshaft S, Abtin F, Suh R (2020) Alternatives to surgery for early-stage lung cancer: thermal ablation. Clin Chest Med 41(2):197–200. https://doi.org/10.1016/j.ccm.2020.02.002

Raz DJ, Zell JA, Ignatius Ou S-H, Gandara DR, Anton-Culver H, Jablons DM (2007) Natural history of stage I non-small cell lung cancer. Chest 132(1):193–199. https://doi.org/10.1378/chest.06-3096

Sanderson DR, Neel HB, Payne WS, Woolner LB (1975) Cryotherapy for bronchogenic carcinoma: report of a case. Mayo Clin Proc 50(8):435–437

Sharma A et al (2007) PET findings following successful radiofrequency ablation of lung. RSNA

Shi F, Li G, Zhou Z, Rongde X, Li W, Zhuang W, Chen Z, Chen X (2017) Microwave ablation versus radiofrequency ablation for the treatment of pulmonary tumors. Oncotarget 8(65):109791–109798. https://doi.org/10.18632/oncotarget.22308

Sidoff L, Dupuy DE (2017) Clinical experiences with microwave thermal ablation of lung malignancies. Int J Hyperthermia 33(1):25–33. https://doi.org/10.1080/02656736.2016.1204630

Simon CJ, Dupuy DE, DiPetrillo TA, Safran HP, Alexander Grieco C, Ng T, Mayo-Smith WW (2007) Pulmonary radiofrequency ablation: long-term safety and efficacy in 153 patients. Radiology 243(1):268–275. https://doi.org/10.1148/radiol.2431060088

Simon TG, Beland MD, Machan JT, Dipetrillo T, Dupuy DE (2012) Charlson Comorbidity Index predicts patient outcome, in cases of inoperable non-small cell lung cancer treated with radiofrequency ablation. Eur J Radiol 81(12):4167–4172. https://doi.org/10.1016/j.ejrad.2012.06.007

Skonieczki BD, Wells C, Wasser EJ, Dupuy DE (2011) Radiofrequency and microwave tumor ablation in patients with implanted cardiac devices: is it safe? Eur J Radiol 79(3):343–346. https://doi.org/10.1016/j.ejrad.2010.04.004

Song SY, Choi W, Shin SS, Lee S-w, Ahn SD, Kim JH, Je HU et al (2009) Fractionated stereotactic body radiation therapy for medically inoperable stage I lung cancer adjacent to central large bronchus. Lung Cancer 66(1):89–93. https://doi.org/10.1016/j.lungcan.2008.12.016

Stanic S, Paulus R, Timmerman RD, Michalski JM, Barriger RB, Bezjak A, Videtic GMM, Bradley J (2014) No clinically significant changes in pulmonary function following stereotactic body radiation therapy for early-stage peripheral non-small cell lung cancer: an analysis of RTOG 0236. Int J Radiat Oncol Biol Phys 88(5):1092–1099. https://doi.org/10.1016/j.ijrobp.2013.12.050

Steinke K, Haghighi KS, Wulf S, Morris DL (2005) Effect of vessel diameter on the creation of ovine lung radiofrequency lesions in vivo: preliminary results. J Surg Res 124(1):85–91. https://doi.org/10.1016/j.jss.2004.09.008

Tekatli H, Haasbeek N, Dahele M, De Haan P, Verbakel W, Bongers E, Hashemi S et al (2016) Outcomes of hypofractionated high-dose radiotherapy in poor-risk patients with "ultracentral" non-small cell lung cancer. J Thorac Oncol 11(7):1081–1089. https://doi.org/10.1016/j.jtho.2016.03.008

Timmerman R, McGarry R, Yiannoutsos C, Papiez L, Tudor K, DeLuca J, Ewing M et al (2006) Excessive toxicity when treating central tumors in a phase II study of stereotactic body radiation therapy for medically inoperable early-stage lung cancer. J Clin Oncol 24(30):4833–4839. https://doi.org/10.1200/JCO.2006.07.5937

Timmerman RD, Chen H, Michalski JM, Bradley JC, Galvin J, Johnstone DW, Choy H (2018a) Long-term results of "stereotactic body radiation therapy in medically inoperable stage I non-small cell lung cancer". JAMA Oncol 4(9):1287–1288. https://doi.org/10.1001/jamaoncol.2018.1258

Timmerman R, Paulus R, Pass HI, Gore EM, Edelman MJ, Galvin J, Straube WL et al (2018b) Stereotactic body radiation therapy for operable early-stage lung cancer: findings from the NRG Oncology RTOG 0618 Trial. JAMA Oncol 4(9):1263–1266. https://doi.org/10.1001/jamaoncol.2018.1251

Videtic G, Paulus R, Singh AK, Chang JY, Parke W, Olivier K, Timmerman RD et al (2018) Long-term follow-up on NRG Oncology RTOG 0915 (NCCTG N0927): a randomized phase 2 study comparing 2 stereotactic body radiation therapy schedules for medically inoperable patients with stage I peripheral non-small cell lung cancer. Int J Radiat Oncol Biol Phys 103(5):1077–1084. https://doi.org/10.1016/j.ijrobp.2018.11.051

Vogl TJ, Worst TS, Naguib NNN, Ackermann H, Gruber-Rouh T, Nour-Eldin N-EA (2013) Factors influencing local tumor control in patients with neoplastic pulmonary nodules treated with microwave ablation: a risk-factor analysis. AJR Am J Roentgenol 200(3):665–672. https://doi.org/10.2214/AJR.12.8721

Vogl TJ, Eckert R, Naguib NNN, Beeres M, Gruber-Rouh T, Nour-Eldin N-EA (2016) Thermal ablation of colorectal lung metastases: retrospective comparison among laser-induced thermotherapy, radiofrequency ablation, and microwave ablation. AJR Am J Roentgenol 207(6):1340–1349. https://doi.org/10.2214/AJR.15.14401

Wang H, Littrup PJ, Duan Y, Zhang Y, Feng H, Nie Z (2005) Thoracic masses treated with percutaneous cryotherapy: initial experience with more than 200 procedures. Radiology 235(1):289–298. https://doi.org/10.1148/radiol.2351030747

Widenmeyer M, Shebzukhov Y, Haen SP, Schmidt D, Clasen S, Boss A, Kuprash DV et al (2011) Analysis of tumor antigen-specific T cells and antibodies in cancer patients treated with radiofrequency ablation. Int J Cancer 128(11):2653–2662. https://doi.org/10.1002/ijc.25601

Wolf FJ, Grand DJ, Machan JT, Dipetrillo TA, Mayo-Smith WW, Dupuy DE (2008) Microwave ablation of lung malignancies: effectiveness, CT findings, and safety in 50 patients. Radiology 247(3):871–879. https://doi.org/10.1148/radiol.2473070996

Yamamoto A, Nakamura K, Matsuoka T, Toyoshima M, Okuma T, Oyama Y, Ikura Y, Ueda M, Inoue Y (2005) Radiofrequency ablation in a porcine lung model: correlation between CT and histopathologic findings. AJR Am J Roentgenol 185(5):1299–1306. https://doi.org/10.2214/AJR.04.0968

Yamauchi Y, Izumi Y, Hashimoto K, Yashiro H, Inoue M, Nakatsuka S, Goto T et al (2012) Percutaneous cryoablation for the treatment of medically inoperable stage I non-small cell lung cancer. PloS One 7(3):e33223. https://doi.org/10.1371/journal.pone.0033223

Yang X, Ye X, Zheng A, Huang G, Ni X, Wang J, Han X, Li W, Wei Z (2014) Percutaneous microwave ablation of stage I medically inoperable non-small cell lung cancer: clinical evaluation of 47 cases. J Surg Oncol 110(6):758–763. https://doi.org/10.1002/jso.23701

Yang X, Ye X, Huang G, Han X, Wang J, Li W, Wei Z, Meng M (2017) Repeated percutaneous microwave ablation for local recurrence of inoperable stage I nonsmall cell lung cancer. J Cancer Res Ther 13(4):683–688. https://doi.org/10.4103/jcrt.JCRT_458_17

Yashiro H, Nakatsuka S, Inoue M, Kawamura M, Tsukada N, Asakura K, Yamauchi Y, Hashimoto K, Kuribayashi S (2013) Factors affecting local progression after percutaneous cryoablation of lung tumors. J Vasc Intervent Radiol 24(6):813–821. https://doi.org/10.1016/j.jvir.2012.12.026

Yasui K, Kanazawa S, Sano Y, Fujiwara T, Kagawa S, Mimura H, Dendo S et al (2004) Thoracic tumors treated with CT-guided radiofrequency ablation: initial experience. Radiology 231(3):850–857. https://doi.org/10.1148/radiol.2313030347

Yuan Z, Wang Y, Zhang J, Zheng J, Li W (2019) A meta-analysis of clinical outcomes after radiofrequency ablation and microwave ablation for lung cancer and pulmonary metastases. J Am Coll Radiol 16(3):302–314. https://doi.org/10.1016/j.jacr.2018.10.012

Zhang X, Tian J, Zhao L, Wu B, Kacher DS, Ma X, Liu S, Ren C, Xiao Y-Y (2012) CT-guided conformal cryoablation for peripheral NSCLC: initial experience. Eur J Radiol 81(11):3354–3362. https://doi.org/10.1016/j.ejrad.2012.04.035

Zheng A, Ye X, Yang X, Huang G, Gai Y (2016) Local efficacy and survival after microwave ablation of lung tumors: a retrospective study in 183 patients. J Vasc Interv Radiol 27(12):1806–1814. https://doi.org/10.1016/j.jvir.2016.08.013

Part V

Current Treatment Strategies in Locally Advanced and Metastatic Non-small Cell Lung Cancer

Lung Dose Escalation

Kenneth E. Rosenzweig

Contents

1. Introduction ... 508
2. Reducing Target Volumes ... 508
3. Reducing Normal Tissue Irradiation ... 509
4. Early Studies ... 510
5. Trials of Radiation Dose Intensification Without Concurrent Chemotherapy ... 510
6. Dose Escalation with Concurrent Chemotherapy ... 512
7. Randomized Trial of Dose Escalation ... 512
8. Adaptive Radiation ... 513
9. Immunotherapy ... 513
10. Conclusions ... 514
References ... 514

Abstract

RTOG 7301 established standard doses of radiation for the treatment of patients with stage III non-small cell lung cancer at 60 Gy in 2 Gy per fraction. However, overall survival was still poor and local failures were a continuing problem. Over the next 30 years, a number of single-institution and multi-institution studies have been performed, attempting to improve overall survival by reducing local failures through radiation dose escalation either alone or in combination with chemotherapy with promising results. NRG Oncology RTOG 0617 was a randomized trial that evaluated 60 versus 74 Gy with concurrent chemotherapy. Although the higher dose of radiation did not result in improved survival, there was a favorable rate of overall survival. The PACIFIC trial has established that the addition of immunotherapy after chemoradiation improved survival. New technology in radiation oncology has been developed that can improve tumor imaging, deliver more conformal RT with less dose to normal structures, and decrease the setup uncertainties, which has increased the therapeutic ratio and allows for safe dose escalation or reduced toxicity at standard doses. This chapter reviews these studies and discusses the current status of radiation dose escalation for patients with stage III NSCLC.

K. E. Rosenzweig (✉)
Icahn School of Medicine at Mount Sinai,
New York, NY, USA
e-mail: ken.rosenzweig@mountsinai.org

Abbreviations

3D	Three-dimensional
3D-CRT	Three-dimensional conformal radiotherapy
4D	Four-dimensional
BID	Twice daily
CALGB	Cancer and Leukemia Group B
CT	Computed tomography
CTV	Clinical tumor volume
DVH	Dose volume histogram
ENI	Elective nodal irradiation
FDG PET	Fluorodeoxyglucose positron emission tomography
GTV	Gross tumor volume
Gy	Gray
IMRT	Intensity-modulated radiation therapy
kV	Kilovoltage
MSKCC	Memorial Sloan Kettering Cancer Center
MTD	Maximum tolerated dose
NCCTG	North Central Cancer Treatment Group
NKI	Netherlands Cancer Institute
NSCLC	Non-small cell lung cancer
NTCP	Normal tissue complication probability
PT	Proton therapy
PTV	Planning target volume
rMLD	Relative mean lung dose
RT	Radiation therapy
RTOG	Radiation Therapy Oncology Group
SEER	Surveillance, Epidemiology, and End Results
UM	University of Michigan
UNC	University of North Carolina
V_{eff}	V effective

1 Introduction

Poor outcomes in patients with unresectable non-small cell lung cancer (NSCLC) have been attributed, in part, to low rates of local control with traditional doses of definitive radiotherapy (RT). Overall survival rates in NSCLC are expected to improve with better local control rates, which is possible with higher radiation dose levels. Unfortunately, the therapeutic ratio for treating lung cancer with radiation has traditionally been small, due to the sensitivity of the lung and resulting pneumonitis and esophagitis with higher radiation doses. Thus, dose escalation in patients with NSCLC has historically been a double-edged sword with improved local control rates with higher doses, but correspondingly higher treatment-related morbidity and mortality.

Over the last 30 years, the therapeutic ratio of RT for NSCLC has widened due to reduced normal lung tissue treated with high doses of radiation through a reduction in the target volume, more sophisticated radiation delivery systems, and a better understanding of the relationship between radiation dose volume histograms of critical organs and treatment-related morbidity. As a result, safe dose escalation over 60 Gy became feasible.

2 Reducing Target Volumes

Target volumes have reduced over the last 30 years due to reductions in (1) gross tumor volume (GTV), because of improved imaging; (2) clinical target volume (CTV), because of the elimination of elective nodal irradiation (ENI); and (3) planning target volume (PTV), because of reduced setup uncertainty from new imaging and immobilization techniques.

Although computed tomography (CT) scanners have been in use since 1973, it took close to 20 years for them to become integrated into RT treatment planning. CT scans provide three-dimensional (3D) information regarding tumor volume as well as demonstrate enlarged and pathologic lymph nodes. An analysis based on Surveillance, Epidemiology, and End Results (SEER) data showed that between 1994 and 2005, the use of CT-based simulation for the treatment of thoracic malignancies increased from 2.4% to 77.6%. Patients who had CT-based simulation also had an improved survival as compared to patients who received conventional simulation (Chen et al. 2011).

Over the last decade, fluorodeoxyglucose positron emission tomography (FDG PET) imaging has also been used in conjunction with CT to aid in identifying malignant lymph nodes that were not enlarged (negative on CT scan) and aid in separating the actual tumor from atelectasis due to obstruction from the tumor. Thus, GTVs have become easier to identify, and areas of uncertainties that were previously included in the GTV can now be more safely eliminated.

Historically, elective nodal regions have been irradiated to doses of 45–50 Gy as part of the target volume in patients with NSCLC. However, following various series identifying distant and local relapses as the primary sites of relapse, researchers began to selectively eliminate the traditional elective nodal sites (Bradley et al. 2005; Rosenzweig et al. 2007; Hayman et al. 2001). Elimination of these elective nodal sites considerably reduces irradiation to normal tissue, which can significantly impact treatment morbidity and mortality. In a phase III study from China (Yuan et al. 2007), patients were randomized to concurrent chemoradiation and either elective nodal irradiation (ENI) with 60–64 Gy of RT or no ENI and higher doses of RT (68–74 Gy). The group that received ENI demonstrated higher rates of pneumonitis (29% vs. 17%; $p = 0.044$), while better 2-year overall survival rates were found in the group treated with higher doses and no ENI (39.4% vs. 25.6%; $p = 0.048$). As a result, most thoracic radiation oncologists eliminated ENI from their treatment plan.

CTV and PTV margins in lung cancer treatment have been reduced due to several innovations. Margins for daily setup errors have been minimized through patient-specific immobilization devices, which, compared to no immobilization, are able to more accurately reproduce patient positioning at the time of simulation. Additionally, daily cone beam CT scans or orthogonal KV imaging allows for the repositioning of patients according to the internal anatomy or the actual tumor, thereby significantly reducing the margins allotted for setup errors compared with skin marks alone (Yeung et al. 2009). Lastly, with the use of respiratory gating systems and 4D CT scans, tumor motion can be objectively measured and accounted for, which can lead to smaller margins.

3 Reducing Normal Tissue Irradiation

Three-dimensional treatment planning became possible when CT scans were integrated into radiation treatment planning, allowing for more complex plans that better spared normal tissue and improved target coverage. Further improvements in target coverage and reductions in irradiated normal tissue have been achieved with the implementation of more conformal radiation delivery systems, including intensity-modulated radiotherapy (IMRT), image guidance, and proton therapy (Sura et al. 2008; Bral et al. 2010; Sejpal et al. 2011; Lazarev et al. 2021).

Protons, unlike photons, are charged particles that have physical characteristics that allow them to traverse a finite distance in the tissue, deposit a prescribed dose in the tumor, and then come to an abrupt halt, leaving negligible dose in normal structures beyond the tumor (Fig. 1). Because of this, protons can have a role in dose escalation for lung cancer. A phase I–II clinical trial from MDACC (Sejpal et al. 2011) compared toxicity outcomes in 62 patients with LA-NSCLC treated with concurrent proton beam therapy with patients receiving 3D CRT or IMRT. The investigators showed that rates of grade ≥ 3 pneumonitis and esophagitis were significantly lower with protons (2% and 5%, respectively) than 3D CRT (30% vs. 18%) or IMRT (9% vs. 44%), $p < 0.001$ for both. Additionally, median total prescription doses for proton-based and photon-based treatments were 74 and 63 Gy, respectively, further highlighting the potential of protons to deliver higher irradiation doses with fewer treatment-related sequelae.

NRG Oncology RTOG 1308 is a phase III randomized controlled trial comparing concurrent chemoradiation to 70 Gy with either photon or proton radiation followed by immunotherapy. Enrollment is currently ongoing and will help to determine whether proton therapy improves survival in LA-NSCLC.

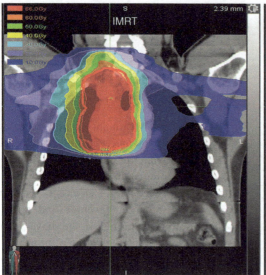 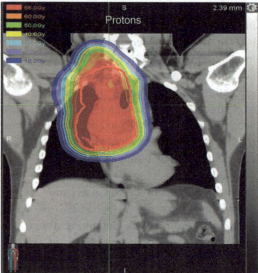

Fig. 1 Coronal CT images comparing a photon IMRT plan (left) with a proton plan (right). Normal tissue dose is represented by the colored isodose curves (blue, light blue, yellow, green). Less normal tissue dose is delivered with protons, allowing for dose escalation to 66.6 Gy. V_{20} in the photon and proton plans was 31% and 26%, respectively. (Figure courtesy of James Urbanic, MD, University of California San Diego)

The advent of image-guided radiation therapy (IGRT) has also improved the therapeutic ratio. IGRT typically consists of cone beam computed tomography (CBCT) within the treatment room to verify patient position. Adjustments can then be made when comparing that day's CBCT with imaging that was performed at the time of radiation planning prior to initiating treatment. A retrospective study at Wake Forest School of Medicine suggested a survival benefit in patients with locally advanced lung cancer who underwent daily CBCT (Kilburn et al. 2016).

4 Early Studies

Radiation Therapy Oncology Group (RTOG) trial 73-01 (Perez et al. 1980) was one of the first dose escalation studies. It established 60 Gy at 2 Gy per once-daily fraction as the standard of care for unresectable NSCLC. The study randomized 376 patients with T1–3 N0–2 NSCLC to either 40 Gy (either once daily at 2 Gy or split course at 4 Gy), 50 Gy, or 60 Gy. Radiation techniques were two-dimensional (2D), and treatment fields included full elective nodal irradiation. Intrathoracic relapses for 40 Gy split, 40 Gy, 50 Gy, and 60 Gy were 44%, 52%, 42%, and 33%, respectively. Overall survival rates also improved with increasing radiation dose levels at 24 and 30 months. However, severe or life-threatening toxicity developed more frequently in the 60 Gy arm. The study determined that 60 Gy should be the standard radiation treatment dose with which to compare future studies. Although higher doses were found to be associated with better outcomes, patients in both groups had high rates of extrathoracic and unirradiated lung relapses. Thus, treatment intensification was needed to improve outcomes.

5 Trials of Radiation Dose Intensification Without Concurrent Chemotherapy

RTOG 83-11 (Cox et al. 1990) was a phase I–II hyperfractionation dose escalation study that randomized 884 patients with inoperable NSCLC to doses of 60–79.2 Gy, in 1.2 Gy per twice-daily (BID) fraction. The overall survival rates for the entire cohort were not significantly affected by radiation dose. In a subgroup of good-performance-status patients, however, a survival advantage was seen at 12 and 24 months with radiation doses of 69.6 Gy or higher ($p = 0.07$). Based on the results of RTOG 83-11 and those from the Cancer and Leukemia Group B (CALGB) trial 84-33, which demonstrated a survival advantage to induction chemotherapy prior to standard 60 Gy at 2 Gy per once-daily fraction (Dillman et al. 1996), the RTOG developed protocol 88-08. RTOG 88-08 randomized 498 patients with stage II–IIIB NSCLC to 60 Gy at 2 Gy per once-daily fraction, 69.6 Gy at 1.2 Gy per BID fraction, or induction chemotherapy of cisplatin and vinblastine followed by 60 Gy at 2 Gy per once-daily fraction (Sause et al. 1995). The results showed a median survival of 11.4 months with 60 Gy of radiation alone and 12 months with hyperfractionated radiation to 69.6 Gy. Importantly, induction chemotherapy followed by 60 Gy had a median survival of 13.2 months, thus confirming what became the standard of care for stage III NSCLC.

Following this study, RTOG 93-11 evaluated dose escalation using once-daily doses of 2.15 Gy per fraction (without inhomogeneity corrections) to find the maximum tolerated dose (MTD) (Bradley et al. 2005). Patients were placed into dose escalation groups based on the volume of lung receiving 20 Gy (V_{20}). The results from the study demonstrated that doses for patients with a V_{20} <25% (small tumors) could be safely escalated to 83.8 Gy. In patients with a V_{20} between 25% and 36% (intermediate-sized tumors), the dose could be escalated to 77.4 Gy. Local-regional control still remained a problem despite these higher doses of radiation: the overall rate of relapse was 38%, and 18% of patients experienced only a local failure.

Memorial Sloan Kettering Cancer Center (MSKCC, New York, NY), University of Michigan (UM, Ann Arbor), and the Netherlands Cancer Institute (NKI, Amsterdam) performed their own single-institution dose escalation studies. From 1991 to 2003, MSKCC enrolled 104 patients, including 28% with stage I–II NSCLC and 68% with stage III NSCLC, in a three-dimensional conformal radiotherapy (3D CRT) study (Rosenzweig et al. 2005). The protocol incorporated lung DVH data to ensure that the normal tissue complication probability (NTCP) was limited to <25%. Eighty-four Gy was determined to be the MTD. Although this was a phase I study, the investigators found that with doses of >80 Gy, overall survival was improved in patients with stage I–II disease ($p = 0.05$) and in patients with stage III disease ($p = 0.02$). Furthermore, local control was improved with doses >80 Gy (88%) compared with doses <80 Gy (14%).

UM's phase I dose escalation study utilized lung DVH data to stratify patients into dose escalation groups (Hayman et al. 2001; Narayan et al. 2004). The study enrolled 104 patients, including 25 who received induction chemotherapy (allowed after 1997). The study results determined an MTD ranging from 65.1 Gy in patients with very large tumors to 102.9 Gy for early-stage tumors. Stage III patients were able to be treated to a dose of 75.6 Gy.

From 1998 through 2003, 88 patients were enrolled in a 3D CRT study by the NKI in a phase I–II dose escalation trial (Belderbos et al. 2006). Similar to the UM study, patients were separated into five risk groups based on their relative mean lung dose (rMLD). Typical stage III tumors were able to be treated safely with doses of 74–81 Gy.

Even though the use of concurrent chemotherapy (with adjuvant immunotherapy) is now considered the standard of care for stage III NSCLC, there are still some patients who are not able to tolerate concurrent treatment. A retrospective review of 338 patients who had definitive RT without concurrent chemotherapy revealed that doses of 66 Gy or greater were superior to less than 60 Gy in improving overall survival and local control (Sonnick et al. 2018). This suggests that it is reasonable to consider higher dose of RT when it is not being delivered with chemotherapy, assuming that normal tissue dose constraints are acceptable.

6 Dose Escalation with Concurrent Chemotherapy

A number of studies have evaluated concurrent chemoradiation for locally advanced NSCLC. After establishing the feasibility of concurrent chemoradiation to either 60 Gy in daily treatment or 69.6 Gy in BID treatment, a large phase III randomized controlled trial was performed.

RTOG 94-10 randomized 595 patients with stage II–III NSCLC to the gold standard of the time: induction chemotherapy followed by 60 Gy at 2 Gy per fraction (arm 1, similar to CALGB 84-33 and RTOG 88-08), to concurrent chemotherapy and 60 Gy at 2 Gy per fraction (arm 2), and to concurrent chemotherapy with RT dose escalation to 69.6 Gy at 1.2 Gy per BID fraction (arm 3). The primary objective of the trial was to evaluate whether concurrent chemotherapy and RT had a better overall survival than induction chemotherapy followed by RT. The trial demonstrated median survivals of 14.6, 17, and 15.6 months for arms 1, 2, and 3, respectively, thusly establishing concurrent chemoradiation to 60 Gy as the new standard of care (Curran et al. 2011). These results have been confirmed, and meta-analyses have shown improvement in overall survival with also an increase in side effects, including esophagitis (Xiao and Hong 2021).

As a follow-up study, RTOG 0117 was developed to evaluate dose escalation with concurrent chemotherapy utilizing modern RT techniques. In the phase I portion of the study, 17 patients with stage I–IIIB NSCLC were treated with escalating doses of RT. All patients received 3D CRT and were required to have a lung V_{20} <30%, mean esophagus dose <34 Gy, and an esophageal V_{55} of <30%. The maximal tolerated dose was 74 Gy, at which acceptable toxicity occurred with only one grade 4 event in seven patients (Bradley et al. 2010). The phase II portion of RTOG 0117 used the 74 Gy arm at 2 Gy per fraction from the phase I portion ($n = 9$) and enrolled another 46 patients. The results demonstrated a median survival of 21.6 months for patients with stage III NSCLC and with acceptable toxicity.

The North Central Cancer Treatment Group (NCCTG) and the University of North Carolina (UNC, Chapel Hill) conducted their own protocols investigating dose escalation with concurrent chemotherapy (Rosenman et al. 2002). The NCCTG 0028 was a phase I study where 15 patients with unresectable NSCLC underwent dose escalation from 70 to 78 Gy in 4 Gy increments. RT was delivered using 3D CRT, limiting the lung V_{20} <40%, and no ENI was delivered. The results found the MTD to be 74 Gy in combination with weekly carboplatin and paclitaxel, which were consistent with the findings of RTOG 0117. A UNC phase I–II protocol demonstrated a median survival of 24 months with only eight patients (13%) developing local-regional relapse as the only site of failure, although 35% of patients had a local failure as a component of their relapse. RTOG grade 3–4 esophagitis developed in only five patients (8%), and no grade 3–4 pneumonitis developed.

7 Randomized Trial of Dose Escalation

Due to the successes with RTOG 0117, and other dose escalation studies, RTOG began a randomized controlled trial, RTOG 0617, to confirm the benefits of radiation dose escalation with concurrent chemotherapy. The study was a 2 × 2 study on which patients with stage III NSCLC were randomized to either 60 or 74 Gy of radiation with concurrent weekly paclitaxel and carboplatin with or without cetuximab. The trial enrolled 544 patients with almost 500 available for analysis, making it one of the most successful phase III NSCLC trials done with radiation therapy.

The trial was stopped early when an interim analysis showed that there was a minimal likelihood that the experimental arm (74 Gy) would be superior to the standard dose of 60 Gy. With over 5 years of follow-up, the standard-dose arm had a rate of survival at 5 years of 32% versus 23% for the high-dose arm (Bradley et al. 2020). The rates of progression-free survival at 5 years were 18% and 13%, respectively. Additionally, the use of cetuximab did not improve survival either, with almost identical outcomes in both arms.

As might be expected, the failure of the high-dose arm to yield improved outcomes was surprising and concerning, especially when considering that phase I and II trials leading up to RTOG 0617 had been so promising. Extensive secondary analyses have been done to help elucidate the results. The long-term results showed that there were more fatal toxicity and fatal complications in the high-dose arm than in the standard-dose arm. Dysphagia and esophagitis were significantly higher with the higher dose as well. Grade 3 or worse pulmonary toxicity was essentially the same in both arms, 20.6% and 19.3%, respectively. The dose to the heart was also a significant predictor of poor outcome, with the percent of heart receiving either 5 or 30 Gy (V_5 or V_{30}) being a significant predictor in multivariable analysis for survival.

Cardiac dose is now emerging as a significant cause of dose-limiting toxicity in patients receiving thoracic radiation. Classic radiation-related heart toxicity includes pericardial effusion, acute coronary events (such as myocardial infarction), pericarditis, arrhythmia, and heart failure. A retrospective review of 127 patients who received high-dose radiation for stage III NSCLC revealed that increasing heart dose was associated with the likelihood of these side effects (Wang et al. 2017). Additionally, dose specific to the left anterior descending coronary vessel in the heart may also be predictive of cardiac toxicity (Atkins et al. 2021).

8 Adaptive Radiation

Adaptive radiation therapy (ART) is a technique to adjust the radiation treatment plan to changes observed during the course of treatment. Some examples of how ART could be incorporated into practice include redefining the tumor volume after it has decreased in size, accounting for re-expansion of the lung during treatment, or adapting to changes in pleural effusions or lung atelectasis. This is typically accomplished through the use of imaging such as cone beam computed tomography (CBCT). Newer radiation treatment machines incorporate magnetic resonance (MR) imaging into the linear accelerator. The goal of ART is to ensure that the delineated tumor volume is receiving the intended dose. But ART could also be a tool to allow for safe dose escalation if tumors shrink and increase their distance from organs at risk or in the specific case of lung cancer, if the lung increases in size.

A group from Aarhus University examined the use of ART in 233 patients and found that the mean lung dose decreased approximately 2 Gy, a meaningful change. Although it was not a goal of this report to assess for the ability to dose escalate, it would stand to reason that if the lung dose is increasing, a higher prescription dose would be achievable (Møller et al. 2016).

A phase II trial in 42 patients from UM obtained a mid-treatment PET and escalated dose to 83 Gy in 30 fractions to the smaller tumor volume. The treatment was well tolerated, and local control and overall survival were favorable (Kong et al. 2017).

RTOG 1106 was a randomized phase II trial where patients were treated with either a standard dose of 60 Gy or adaptive RT that was used to escalate doses up to 80.4 Gy to a smaller tumor volume. This was accomplished by reimaging midway through the treatment with PET/CT and creating a smaller tumor volume if possible, similar to the UM study. A report of this trial was presented at the 2020 World Conference of Lung Cancer and revealed that adaptive therapy could be safely delivered, but local-regional progression-free survival was unchanged.

9 Immunotherapy

The PACIFIC trial was a phase III randomized control trial that demonstrated that patients who were given the immune checkpoint inhibitor durvalumab at the conclusion of concurrent chemoradiation for locally advanced NSCLC had a significant improvement in survival (Antonia et al. 2017). The median time to death or distant metastasis improved from 16.2 to 28.3 months, an astounding improvement. Adjuvant durvalumab has rapidly become the standard of care in patients who have a response to chemoradiation.

The results of PACIFIC trial potentially call into the role that dose escalation plays in lung cancer. Using higher doses of radiation that may be associated with the significant toxicity seen in RTOG 0617 may be discouraged since it may prevent future treatment with immunotherapy. The PACIFIC trial used thoracic radiation doses that mostly ranged from 56 to 66 Gy. Further work will need to be done to assess whether higher doses have any interaction with the immune response.

10 Conclusions

Safer dose escalation with RT beyond standard doses of radiation established by RTOG 7301 has been possible with advances in imaging and radiation technology. Higher doses of radiation, even with the omission of ENI, appear to improve local-regional control; however, overall survival and distant metastases remain a huge problem. Dose escalation with concurrent chemotherapy has been possible, but the results of RTOG 0617 were disappointing since it demonstrated worse survival with high-dose radiation. The advent of immunotherapy in the treatment of all malignancies will likely revolutionize cancer therapy and have a lasting impact of the treatment on all patients with lung cancer. Future work in dose escalation will need to account for the immune response and other biologic determinants of tumor behavior.

References

Antonia SJ, Villegas A, Daniel D, Vicente D, Murakami S, Hui R, Yokoi T, Chiappori A, Lee KH, de Wit M, Cho BC, Bourhaba M, Quantin X, Tokito T, Mekhail T, Planchard D, Kim YC, Karapetis CS, Hiret S, Ostoros G, Kubota K, Gray JE, Paz-Ares L, de Castro Carpeño J, Wadsworth C, Melillo G, Jiang H, Huang Y, Dennis PA, Özgüroğlu M, PACIFIC Investigators (2017) Durvalumab after chemoradiotherapy in stage III non-small cell lung cancer. N Engl J Med 377:1919–1929

Atkins KM, Chaunzwa TL, Lamba N, Bitterman DS, Rawal B, Bredfeldt J, Williams CL, Kozono DE, Baldini EH, Nohria A, Hoffmann U, Aerts HJWL, Mak RH (2021) Association of left anterior descending coronary artery radiation dose with major adverse cardiac events and mortality in patients with non-small cell lung cancer. JAMA Oncol 7:206–219

Belderbos JS, Heemsbergen WD, de Jaeger K, Baas P, Lebesque JV (2006) Final results of a phase I/II dose escalation trial in non-small-cell lung cancer using three-dimensional conformal radiotherapy. Int J Radiat Oncol Biol Phys 66:126–134

Bradley J, Graham MV, Winter K, Purdy JA, Komaki R, Roa WH, Ryu JK, Bosch W, Emami B (2005) Toxicity and outcome results of RTOG 9311: a phase I-II dose-escalation study using three-dimensional conformal radiotherapy in patients with inoperable non-small-cell lung carcinoma. Int J Radiat Oncol Biol Phys 61:318–328

Bradley JD, Moughan J, Graham MV, Byhardt R, Govindan R, Fowler J, Purdy JA, Michalski JM, Gore E, Choy H (2010) A phase I/II radiation dose escalation study with concurrent chemotherapy for patients with inoperable stages I to III non-small-cell lung cancer: phase I results of RTOG 0117. Int J Radiat Oncol Biol Phys 77:367–372

Bradley JD, Paulus R, Komaki R, Masters G, Blumenschein G, Schild S, Bogart J, Hu C, Forster K, Magliocco A, Kavadi V, Garces YI, Narayan S, Iyengar P, Robinson C, Wynn RB, Koprowski C, Meng J, Beitler J, Gaur R, Curran W Jr, Choy H (2020) Long-term results of NRG Oncology RTOG 0617: standard versus high dose chemoradiotherapy w with or without cetuximab for unresectable stage III non-small cell lung cancer. J Clin Oncol 38:706–714

Bral S, Duchateau M, Versmessen H, Verdries D, Engels B, De Ridder M, Tournel K, Collen C, Everaert H, Schallier D, De Greve J, Storme G (2010) Toxicity report of a phase 1/2 dose-escalation study in patients with inoperable, locally advanced nonsmall cell lung cancer with helical tomotherapy and concurrent chemotherapy. Cancer 116:241–250

Chen AB et al (2011) Survival outcomes after radiation therapy for stage III non-small-cell lung cancer after adoption of computed tomography-based simulation. J Clin Oncol 17:2305–2311

Cox JD, Azarnia N, Byhardt RW, Shin KH, Emami B, Pajak TF (1990) A randomized phase I/II trial of hyperfractionated radiation therapy with total doses of 60.0 Gy to 79.2 Gy: possible survival benefit with greater than or equal to 69.6 Gy in favorable patients with Radiation Therapy Oncology Group stage III non-small-cell lung carcinoma: report of Radiation Therapy Oncology Group 83-11. J Clin Oncol 8:1543–1555

Curran WJ Jr, Paulus R, Langer CJ, Komaki R, Lee JS, Hauser S, Movsas B, Wasserman T, Rosenthal SA, Gore E, Machtay M, Sause W, Cox JD (2011) Sequential vs. concurrent chemoradiation for stage III non-small cell lung cancer: randomized phase III trial RTOG 9410. J Natl Cancer Inst 103: 1452–1460

Dillman RO, Herndon J, Seagren SL, Eaton WL Jr, Green MR (1996) Improved survival in stage III non-small-cell lung cancer: seven-year follow-up of cancer and leukemia group B (CALGB) 8433 trial. J Natl Cancer Inst 88:1210–1215

Hayman JA, Martel MK, Ten Haken RK, Normolle DP, Todd RF 3rd, Littles JF, Sullivan MA, Possert PW, Turrisi AT, Lichter AS (2001) Dose escalation in non-small-cell lung cancer using three-dimensional conformal radiation therapy: update of a phase I trial. J Clin Oncol 19:127–136

Kilburn JM, Soike MH, Lucas JT, Ayala-Peacock D, Blackstock W, Isom S, Kearns WT, Hinson WH, Miller AA, Petty WJ, Munley MT, Urbanic JJ (2016) Image guided radiation therapy may result in improved local control in locally advanced lung cancer patients. Pract Radiat Oncol 6:e73–e80

Kong FM, Ten Haken RK, Schipper M, Frey KA, Hayman J, Gross M, Ramnath N, Hassan KA, Matuszak M, Ritter T, Bi N, Wang W, Orringer M, Cease KB, Lawrence TS, Kalemkerian GP (2017) Effect of midtreatment PET/CT-adapted radiation therapy with concurrent chemotherapy in patients with locally advanced non-small-cell lung cancer: a phase 2 clinical trial. JAMA Oncol 3:1358–1365

Lazarev S, Rosenzweig K, Samstein R, Salgado LR, Hasan S, Press RH, Sharma S, Powell CA, Hirsch FR, Simone CB 2nd (2021) Where are we with proton beam therapy for thoracic malignancies? Current status and future perspectives. Lung Cancer 152:157–164

Møller DS, Holt MI, Alber M, Tvilum M, Khalil AA, Knap MM, Hoffmann L (2016) Adaptive radiotherapy for advanced lung cancer ensures target coverage and decreases lung dose. Radiother Oncol 121:32–38

Narayan S, Henning GT, Ten Haken RK, Sullivan MA, Martel MK, Hayman JA (2004) Results following treatment to doses of 92.4 or 102.9 Gy on a phase I dose escalation study for non-small cell lung cancer. Lung Cancer 44:79–88

Perez CA, Stanley K, Rubin P, Kramer S, Brady L, Perez-Tamayo R, Brown GS, Concannon J, Rotman M, Seydel HG (1980) A prospective randomized study of various irradiation doses and fractionation schedules in the treatment of inoperable non-oat-cell carcinoma of the lung: preliminary report by the Radiation Therapy Oncology Group. Cancer 45:2744–2753

Rosenman JG, Halle JS, Socinski MA, Deschesne K, Moore DT, Johnson H, Fraser R, Morris DE (2002) High-dose conformal radiotherapy for treatment of stage IIIA/IIIB non-small-cell lung cancer: technical issues and results of a phase I/II trial. Int J Radiat Oncol Biol Phys 54:348–356

Rosenzweig KE, Fox JL, Yorke E, Amols H, Jackson A, Rusch V, Kris MG, Ling CC, Leibel SA (2005) Results of a phase I dose-escalation study using three-dimensional conformal radiotherapy in the treatment of inoperable nonsmall cell lung carcinoma. Cancer 103:2118–2127

Rosenzweig KE, Sura S, Jackson A, Yorke E (2007) Involved-field radiation therapy for inoperable non-small-cell lung cancer. J Clin Oncol 25:5557–5561

Sause WT, Scott C, Taylor S, Johnson D, Livingston R, Komaki R, Emami B, Curran WJ, Byhardt RW, Turrisi AT et al (1995) Radiation Therapy Oncology Group (RTOG) 88-08 and Eastern Cooperative Oncology Group (ECOG) 4588: preliminary results of a phase III trial in regionally advanced, unresectable non-small-cell lung cancer. J Natl Cancer Inst 87:198–205

Sejpal S, Komaki R, Tsao A, Chang JY, Liao Z, Wei X, Allen PK, Lu C, Gillin M, Cox JD (2011) Early findings on toxicity of proton beam therapy with concurrent chemotherapy for nonsmall cell lung cancer. Cancer 117:3004–3013

Sonnick MA, Oro F, Yan B, Desai A, Wu AJ, Shi W, Zhang Z, Gelblum DY, Paik PK, Yorke ED, Rosenzweig KE, Chaft JE, Rimner A (2018) Identifying the optimal radiation dose in locally advanced non-small-cell lung cancer treated with definitive radiotherapy without concurrent chemotherapy. Clin Lung Cancer 19:e131–e140

Sura S, Gupta V, Yorke E, Jackson A, Amols H, Rosenzweig KE (2008) Intensity-modulated radiation therapy (IMRT) for inoperable non-small cell lung cancer: the Memorial Sloan-Kettering Cancer Center (MSKCC) experience. Radiother Oncol 87:17–23

Wang K, Eblan MJ, Deal AM, Lipner M, Zagar TM, Wang Y, Mavroidis P, Lee CB, Jensen BC, Rosenman JG, Socinski MA, Stinchcombe TE, Marks LB (2017) Cardiac toxicity after radiotherapy for stage III non-small-cell lung cancer: pooled analysis of dose-escalation trials delivering 70 to 90 Gy. J Clin Oncol 35:1387–1394

Xiao W, Hong M (2021) Concurrent vs sequential chemoradiotherapy for patients with advanced non-small-cell lung cancer. Medicine 100:e21455

Yeung AR, Li JG, Shi W, Newlin HE, Chvetsov A, Liu C, Palta JR, Olivier K (2009) Tumor localization using cone-beam CT reduces setup margins in conventionally fractionated radiotherapy for lung tumors. Int J Radiat Oncol Biol Phys 74:1100–1107

Yuan S, Sun X, Li M, Yu J, Ren R, Yu Y, Li J, Liu X, Wang R, Li B, Kong L, Yin Y (2007) A randomized study of involved-field irradiation versus elective nodal irradiation in combination with concurrent chemotherapy for inoperable stage III nonsmall cell lung cancer. Am J Clin Oncol 30:239–244

Multimodality Treatment of Stage IIIA/N2 NSCLC: Why Always NO to Surgery?

Branislav Jeremić, Ivane Kiladze, and Slobodan Milisavljevic

Contents

1 Introduction 518
2 Neoadjuvant Treatments Followed by Surgery Versus Exclusive Radiochemotherapy 519
3 Is There a Specific Stage IIIA/N2 Patient Subgroup Which Can Benefit from Surgical Multimodality Approach? 524
4 Specific Considerations of Radiochemotherapy 525
5 Conclusions and Future Endeavors 527

References 528

B. Jeremić (✉)
School of Medicine, University of Kragujevac, Kragujevac, Serbia
e-mail: nebareje@gmail.com

I. Kiladze
Caucasus Medical Center, Tbilisi, Georgia

S. Milisavljevic
University Clinical Center, School of Medicine, Kragujevac, Serbia

Abstract

The highest level of evidence from prospective randomized clinical trials (PRCTs) and meta-analyses (MAs) which have asked the question about optimal treatment approach in patients with Stage IIIA/pN2 non-small cell lung cancer (NSCLC) accumulated slowly in the past 25 years. They have mostly focused on the question of induction chemotherapy (CHT) or induction radiochemotherapy (RT-CHT) both followed by surgery and frequently compared it with exclusive RT-CHT. Seven PRCTs and five MAs which currently exist have investigated this issue. None of them showed any benefit for surgical multimodality approach over exclusive RT-CHT, except an unplanned, post-hoc analysis coming from a single PRCT, which concerned lobectomy-suitable candidates. While there are many retrospective studies which tried to identify patient subgroups favoring induction therapies followed by surgery, their results have never been reproduced even in retrospective setting. Importantly, no PRCT ever investigated potential pretreatment patient and/or tumor-related predictors favoring surgical multimodality and it remained unknown which, if any, patients may actually benefit from surgical multimodality approach. Exclusive RT-CHT achieves similar results to induction therapies followed by surgery but with less morbidity and mortality. Together with the lack of identified pretreatment predictors pointing towards surgery, they suggest that surgical bi- or trimodality approach should not be practiced outside well planned clinical trial.

1 Introduction

Stage III non-small cell lung cancer (NSCLC) is very heterogeneous disease, reflected in a number of T and N combinations currently existing (Rami-Porta et al. 2014; Goldstraw et al. 2016). It was usually divided between Stages IIIA and IIIB (now, IIIC as well) having different prognosis. While more advanced cases, those of Stage IIIB/C, are treated with concurrent radiochemotherapy (RT-CHT) (Aupérin et al. 2010; Liang et al. 2010; O'Rourke et al. 2010), in a more favorable setting of Stage IIIA, clinicians and researchers kept continuously observing poor results with surgery alone. It was shown that complete surgical resection for patients with Stage IIIA with N2-positive nodes is technically feasible; however, the 5-year survival for patients treated that way is about 10% (Shields 1990; Roth et al. 1994). Most patients who undergo primary resection of Stage IIIA tumors experience loco-regional and systemic relapses and die of the disease (Sugarbaker et al. 1995; Kumar et al. 1996; Livingston 1997). Different attempts to improve these results were undertaken employing intensified, mostly combined treatment approaches. Beside intensification of both RT (higher dose, altered fractionation) and CHT aspects (different drugs and dosing, targeted agents, and immunotherapy), attempts in the past 3 decades were made to include surgery as the part of the multimodality treatment approach. In particular, these efforts comprised surgery and adjuvant CHT and/or RT (Douillard et al. 2006; Yoshino et al. 2012), neoadjuvant CHT followed by surgery (Pass et al. 1992; Rosell et al. 1994; Roth et al. 1994; Shepherd et al. 1998; Johnstone et al. 2002; Nagai et al. 2003; Stephens et al. 2005; van Meerbeeck et al. 2007) and induction RT-CHT followed by surgery (Albain et al. 2009; Sorensen et al. 2013; Eberhardt et al. 2015). While Stage IIIA represents approximately 15% of all patients with NSCLC (van Meerbeeck et al. 2007; SEER 2010) and between 30% and 50% of those with Stage III (Goldstraw et al. 2007; Zeng et al. 2012; Shi et al. 2017), special emphasis in clinical research was made upon patients with N2 disease.

Attempts to properly stage and restage patients remain challenging and ever evolving effort, focusing naturally on tools used for N2 disease. In a systematic review (Candela and Detterbeck 2010) computerized tomography (CT) alone had significant false negative (FN) and false positive (FP) rate (approximately 30% each), and complete response (CR) on CT could not justify avoidance of surgery due to 50% FN rate. PET/CT (Positron emission tomography/CT) fared slightly better, but again, could not be suggested due to FN rate of 25% and FP rate of 33%. Achieving a complete response (CR) in mediastinum on PET was deemed not strong enough to justify avoidance of surgery due to the fact that up to one-third of patients had viable tumor cells in the resected specimen. Although remediastinoscopy had somewhat lower FN rate (25%) it, however, carried higher morbidity and mortality (1% vs 0.05%) when compared to first time mediastinoscopy (De Waele et al. 2008; Louie et al. 2011). Endobronchial ultrasound (EBUS) or Endoesophageal ultrasound (EEUS) followed by fine-needle biopsy (FN rate, 15%) (Candela and Detterbeck 2010) are becoming new standards, requesting, however, additional confirmation. Almost general consensus among pulmonologists and thoracic surgeons is that first time mediastinoscopy should be reserved for response evaluation and restaging post-induction therapy before surgery. This strategy seems conditional to meticulous planning at the time of initial staging of the mediastinum when EBUS/EEUS with fine-needle biopsy could be employed.

While evaluation of mediastinum, both before surgery and during the surgery, continues to be important and one may even say, a dominating aspect, in this setting many issues request additional efforts worldwide. While mediastinoscopy is considered by many gold standard, recent guidelines regarding its role in evaluation of N2 (De Leyn et al. 2007; Silvestri et al. 2013; De Leyn et al. 2014) as well the place and role of systematic LN dissection versus (selective) sampling of only LNs suspicious on imaging remain debated. Surgical evaluation of mediastinum, at least partially, also depends on both geography and the extent of surgery, but the degree of surgeon specialization and hospital volumes of patients undergoing lung cancer surgery as well (Ellis et al. 2011; Rocco et al. 2016).

For patients with Stage IIIA/N2 NSCLC, in spite of growing body of the data discussing how best to address diagnostic and treatment aspects of mediastinal lymph nodes (MLNs) owing to the data from prospective randomized clinical trials (PRCTs) and meta-analyses (MAs), these approaches remain largely unsolved. Frequently, they focused on clarifying important aspects of surgical multimodality (bimodality, trimodality) treatment approach in the setting of Stage IIIA/N2 NSCLC as opposed to non-surgical combined modality (RT-CHT). Another important question is, if one considers neadjuvant therapy followed by surgery as preferred treatment option in this setting, what is the optimal neoadjuvant part: neoadjuvant CHT alone or neoadjuvant RT-CHT or the intensified version of the latter, i.e., neoadjuvant CHT followed by concurrent RT-CHT? PRCTs have tried to enlighten this issue and existing five MAs (Shah et al. 2012; Xu et al. 2015; Guo et al. 2016; Chen et al. 2018; Tong et al. 2018) have added more substance to the highest level of evidence in this case (Table 1). These MAs have used different eligibility criteria which resulted in inclusion of different study types and the number of enrolled patients, but have reached quite similar conclusions. When investigated, neoadjuvant RT-CHT had a significant benefit in tumor response, pCR, N2 downstaging, pCR of N2 as well as higher number of patients achieving R0 resection. With some of the studies providing long term data, these benefits, no matter how important, never translated into a significant benefit in terms of either OS or PFS. They seem to have supported the view that adding RT to neoadjuvant CHT before surgery did not lead to benefit in these hard endpoints, which many use as justification to omit RT from pre-surgery part of the combined surgical modality approach in patients with Stage IIIA, mostly N2 disease.

2 Neoadjuvant Treatments Followed by Surgery Versus Exclusive Radiochemotherapy

Currently, there is not less than seven PRCTs (Shepherd et al. 1998; Johnstone et al. 2002; Stephens et al. 2005; van Meerbeeck et al. 2007; Albain et al. 2009; Sorensen et al. 2013; Eberhardt et al. 2015) (Table 2) and five MAs (Xu et al. 2015; Ren et al. 2015; McElnay et al. 2015; Xu et al. 2016; Pöttgen et al. 2017) (Table 3) focusing on the issue of optimal loco-regional treatment in Stage IIIA/N2 NSCLC. They have all investigated the issue of whether neoadjuvant CHT or neoadjuvant RT-CHT followed by surgery is superior to exclusive RT-CHT. Of PRCTs, two small trials (Shepherd et al. 1998; Stephens et al. 2005) compared RT alone with CHT followed by surgery with no difference being observed in terms of either MST or 2 years. OS between surgical and non-surgical arms, in spite of the significant difference in the results in surgical arms between the two studies. Treatment-related deaths also significantly differed in surgical arms in these two studies, being 8% in the study of Shepherd et al. (1998), vs 0% mortality in the study of Stephens et al. (2005). Both studies showed that RT, even if given alone, is not inferior to bimodal surgical approach, in spite of "modest" radical doses of 50–60 Gy in the study of Stephens et al. (2005). Two additional studies compared neoadjuvant CHT followed by surgery with CHT and RT given sequentially. Both the study of the Radiation Therapy Oncology Group (RTOG) (Johnstone et al. 2002) and the study from the European Organization for the Research and Treatment of Cancer (EORTC) (van Meerbeeck et al. 2007) also showed no advantage for bimodal surgical approach over sequential

Table 1 Meta-analyses characteristics and findings

Author (year)	Comparison	N	Type of studies	Summary of findings	Comment
Shah et al. (2012)	Induction CHT + surgery versus induction RT-CHT + surgery	7	RCT (one full) RCT (two abstracts) Phase II (one full) Retrospective (three full)	HR, 0.93; 95% CI, 0.54–1.62; $p = 0.81$ (2 RCTs; $n = 165$) HR, 0.77, 95% CI, 0.50–1.19; $p = 0.24$ (2 retrospective studies; $n = 183$)	• No benefit of adding RT to induction CHT in terms of OS • included retrospective studies and abstracts
Xu et al. (2015)	Induction CHT + surgery versus induction RT-CHT + surgery	3	RCT (three) (total $n = 229$)	OR, 3.61, 95% CI, 1.07–12.15; $p = 0.04$ (mediastinal LN pCR; 2 RCTs) HR, 0.79, 95% CI 0.57–1.09; $p = 0.15$ (OS, 3 RCTs) HR, 0.67; 95% CI 0.39–1.15; $p = 0.15$ (PFS, 2 RCTs)	• Benefit of adding RT in terms of mediastinal LN pCR • No benefit in terms of OS and PFS
Guo et al. (2016)	Induction CHT + surgery versus induction RT-CHT + surgery	12	Phase III RCT (three) Phase II (one) Retrospective (six) Abstracts (two) (total $n = 2,724$)	HR, 0.75, 95% CI, 0.63–0.89; $p = 0.001$ (tumor downstaging) ($n = 6$) HR, 0.72, 95% CI, 0.60–0.88; $p = 0.001$ (pCR) ($n = 6$) HR, 0.64, 95% CI, 0.48–0.85; $p = 0.002$ (local control) ($n = 5$) HR, 0.89, 95% CI, 0.68–1.19; $p = 0.44$ (5 years OS) ($n = 4$) HR, 0.74, 95% CI, 0.43–1.26; $p = 0.26$ (5 years PFS) ($n = 4$) HR, 0.77, 95% CI, 0.50–1.18, $p = 0.24$ (5 years OS) ($n = 2$) HR, 0.73, 95% CI, 0.51–1.07; $p = 0.20$ (5 years PFS) ($n = 2$)	• Difference favoring induction RT-CHT in tumor downstaging, pCR and local control, • No benefit in adding RT on OS or PFS • Different N studies used for different endpoints
Chen et al. (2018)	Induction CHT + surgery versus induction RT-CHT + surgery	3	Phase III RCT (three) (total $n = 334$)	OR, 0.51, 95% CI, 0.32–0.80; $p = 0.003$ (tumor response) OR, 0.32; 95% CI, 0.09–1.16, $p = 0.08$ (pathological CR) OR, 0.60, 95% CI, 0.35–1.00; $p = 0.05$ (mediastinal LN downstaging) OR, 0.50, 95% CI, 0.26–0.99; $p = 0.05$ (mediastinal LN pCR) OR, 0.46, 95% CI, 0.22–0.96; $p = 0.04$ (R0 resection) OR, 0.85, 95% CI, 0.53–1.36; $p = 0.49$ (PFS at 2 years) OR, 0.80, 95% CI, 0.44–1.47; $p = 0.47$ (PFS at 4 years) OR, 0.78, 95% CI, 0.34–1.78; $p = 0.55$ (PFS at 6 years) OR, 0.82, 95% CI, 0.53–1.82; $p = 0.39$ (OS at 2 years) OR, 0.98, 95% CI, 0.58–1.66; $p = 0.94$ (OS at 4 years) OR, 1.14, 95% CI, 0.59–2.20; $p = 0.71$ (OS at 6 years)	• Induction RT-CHT has a significant benefit in tumor response, pCR, N2 downstaging, pCR of N2 and higher number of patients with R0 resection • No more peri-intervention mortality in RT-CHT • No difference in OS and PFS after 2, 4, and 6 years
Tong et al. (2018)	Induction CHT + surgery versus induction RT-CHT + surgery	4	Phase III (three) (total $n = 461$)	OR, 1.97, 95% CI, 1.25–3.10; $p = 0.003$ (tumor response) OR, 1.97, 95% CI, 1.00–3.86; $p = 0.05$ (mediastinal LN pCR) OR, 0.91, 95% CI, 0.73–1.14; $p = 0.42$ (OS) OR, 1.01, 95% CI, 0.81–1.26; $p = 0.91$ (PFS)	• Induction RT-CHT improved ORR and pCR rate of N2 LNs • Induction RT-CHT did not significantly improve OS or PFS • Induction RT-CHT did not exacerbate the toxicity

RCT randomized controlled trial, *HR* hazard ratio, *CI* confidence intervals, *RT* radiation therapy, *CHT* chemotherapy, *OS* overall survival, *PFS* progression-free survival, *Tx* treatment, *MA* meta-analysis, *pCR* pathological complete response

Table 2 Prospective randomized trials (PRCTs) in patients with Stage IIIA NSCLC

Author (year)	Stage	N Pts	Treatment	MST (months)	OS (years)	Mortality (%)	Comment
Shepherd et al. (1998)	IIIA (pN2)	16	Induction CHT + S	18.7	40 (2 years)	0	No pCR; 8 pts. with POCHT
		15	RT alone	16.2	48 (2 years)	0	
Stephens et al. (2005)	T3, N1	24	Induction CHT + S	13.8	15 (2 years)	8	Only 4 (17%) pts. had complete resection; of these, 2 died after pneumonectomy
	T1–3, N2 (inoperable-unresectable)	24	RT alone	11.3	16 (2 years)	0	
Johnstone et al. (2002)	IIIA (T1–T3N2)	29	Induction CHT + S	19.4	70 (1 years)	7	Bulky N2 in 54% pts
		32	CHT + RT	17.4	66 (1 years)	3	
van Meerbeeck et al. (2007)	III/N2 (inoperable)	167	Induction CHT + S	16.4	16.4 (5 years)	9	PORT in 40% pts
		165	CHT + RT	17.5	17.5 (5 years)	<1	
Albain et al. (2009)	T1–3pN2	202	Induction RT-CHT + S	23.6	27.2 (5 years)	8	26% mortality in 54 pts. with pneumonectomy
		194	RT-CHT	22.2	20.3 (5 years)	2	
Eberhardt et al. (2015)	IIIA/pN2	81	Induction CHT + RT-CHT + S	n.r.	44 (5 years)	7.4	PET or PET/CT in 97% pts. 85 pts. not randomly assigned
	Selected IIIB	80	induction CHT + RT-CHT	n.r.	40 (5 years)	2.5	
Sorensen et al. (2013)	T1–3N2M0 (pN2)	170	Induction CHT + S + RT	17	20 (5 years)	n.r.	Still in an abstract form at the time of this publication
		171	CHT + RT	15	16 (5 years)		

MST median survival time, *OS* overall survival, *CHT* chemotherapy, *S* surgery, *pCR* pathological complete response, *POCHT* postoperative chemotherapy, *RT* radiotherapy, *PORT* postoperative radiotherapy, *PET* positron emission tomography, *CT* computed tomography, *n.r.* not reported

Table 3 Meta-analyses characteristics and findings based on included PRCTs

Author (year) (ref)	Comparison	N	Type of studies	Summary of findings	Comment
Xu et al. (2015)	Induction CHT ± RT + surgery versus concurrent or sequential RT-CHT	4	PRCT ($N = 820$)	OS (4 trials), HR, 0.95; 95% CI, 0.81–1.10; $p = 0.49$ PFS (2 trials), HR 0.90; 95% CI, 0.77–1.05; $p = 0.19$	• No superiority of either bimodality or trimodality surgical Tx over sequential or concurrent RT-CHT
Ren et al. (2015)	Induction CHT ± RT + surgery versus concurrent or sequential RT-CHT	3	PRCT ($N = 789$)	2-year OS: HR, 1.00; 95% CI, 0.85–1.17; $p = 0.98$ 4-year OS: HR,1.13; 95% CI, 0.85–1.51; $p = 0.39$ 3-year PFS (3 trials): HR, 1.05; 95% CI, 0.61–1.81; $p = 0.86$	• No superiority of either bimodality or trimodality surgical Tx over sequential or concurrent RT-CHT
McElnay et al. (2015)	Induction CHT + surgery versus Concurrent or sequential RT-CHT Induction RT-CHT + surgery versus Concurrent or sequential RT-CHT	4 2 6	PRCT ($N = 229$) (bimodality trials) PRCT ($N = 820$) (trimodality trials) PRCT ($N = 1,049$) (all trials combined)	HR, 1.01; 95% CI 0.82–1.23; $p = 0.954$ HR,0.87; 95% CI 0.75–1.01; $p = 0.068$ HR, 0.92; 95% CI, 0.81–1.03; $p = 0.157$	• No superiority of either bimodality or trimodality surgical Tx over sequential or concurrent RT-CHT
Xu et al. (2016)	Induction CHT ± RT + surgery versus concurrent or sequential RT-CHT	5	PRCT ($N = 851$)	HR, 0.94; 95% CI, 0.81–1.09; $p = 0.686$ PFS (2 PRCT and 1 retrospective study) HR 0.91; 95% CI 078–1.06; $p = 0.10$	• No superiority of either bimodality or trimodality surgical Tx over sequential or concurrent RT-CHT
Pöttgen et al. (2017)	Induction CHT ± RT + surgery versus concurrent or sequential RT-CHT	6 3	PRCT ($N = 1,322$) PRCT ($N = 889$)	OS, HR, 0.92, 95% CI, 0.82–0.04; $p = 0.78$ PFS, HR, 0.91, 95% CI, 0.73–1.13; $p = 0.91$	• No superiority of either bimodality or trimodality surgical Tx over sequential or concurrent RT-CHT

PRCT prospective randomized controlled trial, *HR* hazard ratio, *CI* confidence intervals, *RT* radiation therapy, *CHT* chemotherapy, *OS* overall survival, *PFS* progression-free survival, *Tx* treatment

CHT-RT approach. Similarly to studies from the above, they have observed significantly more toxic deaths in surgical arms (RTOG: 7% vs 3%; EORTC: 9% vs <1%). Finally, three most recent and, from the standpoint of combined RT-CHT, contemporary PRCTs (Albain et al. 2009; Sorensen et al. 2013; Eberhardt et al. 2015) compared either neoadjuvant RT-CHT followed by surgery or neoadjuvant CHT followed by concurrent RT-CHT followed by surgery or neoadjuvant CHT followed by surgery and RT with exclusive RT-CHT. All three studies reconfirmed that there is no advantage for any (bimodal, trimodal) surgical mutimodality approach over exclusive RT-CHT in this setting. What they have also reconfirmed was more toxic deaths in surgical arms: INT0139: 8% vs 2% (Albain et al. 2009) ESPATUE: 7.4% vs 2.5% (Eberhardt et al. 2015). Of serious concern was the finding of INT0139 (Albain et al. 2009) showing mortality of 26% when neoadjuvant RT-CHT was followed by right pneumonectomy. Postoperative mortality, as reported in these PRCTs were a 30-day mortality and not on a 90-day, the latter being mandatory as giving better insight into a hazardous surgical approach (Kim et al. 2012). As a summary of existing evidence from seven PRCTs, in spite of somewhat differing patients and study characteristics, currently there is not even a hint of advantage for any of the surgical multimodality approaches (neoadjuvant CHT followed by surgery or neoadjuvant RT-CHT followed by surgery or neoadjuvant CHT followed by RT-CHT followed by surgery) when compared to exclusive RT-CHT. Although formal HR QoL in this setting and costs of the treatment were not specifically addressed, it is very likely they would significantly favor RT-CHT. Finally, even if one argues that it is still plausible to offer surgical multimodality in this setting, why anyone would proceed with surgery if one can achieve the same results without it?

Five MAs (Xu et al. 2015; Ren et al. 2015; McElnay et al. 2015; Xu et al. 2015; Pöttgen et al. 2017) pooled the data from PRCTs which compared surgical bimodality or trimodality approach with exclusive RT-CHT (Table 3). These MAs have used somewhat different sources, but their findings were unequivocal: no MA found a significant difference between surgical multimodality approaches and exclusive RT-CHT. MAs, however, have not provided investigation of treatment-related morbidity and mortality, known from included PRCTs to be significantly higher in surgical arms.

Unfortunately, although both PRCTs and MAs represent the highest level of evidence nonbelievers in evidence based medicine neglected it, while critics offered various reasons to continue with surgical multimodality approaches. The reason most frequently cited as the "proof" for necessity to use surgery comes from a single, unplanned, post-hoc, subgroup analysis of INT0139 trial (Albain et al. 2009). Using a matched pair analysis this low level of evidence has shown that lobectomy-treated patients achieved better results than those treated with exclusive RT-CHT. What has rarely been emphasized was the fact that pathological response to neoadjuvant RT-CHT in this analysis could not be taken into account because the matching was done according to pretreatment factors and the type of surgery, questioning the validity of this finding for any serious consideration.

Additional aspects of RT-CHT should also be taken into account. In majority of PRCTs design of the non-surgical arms was far from being optimal. While in some PRCTs combined RT-CHT was administered as sequential approach (Table 2), it was proven to be significantly inferior to concurrent RT-CHT in a number of PRCTs and MAs (Aupérin et al. 2010; O'Rourke et al. 2010; Liang et al. 2010). Also, in PRCTs where concurrent RT-CHT was followed by surgery, the final 15Gy to 20Gy of the concurrent RT-CHT part was given after a gap (for assessment of response) of several weeks, introducing therefore, a treatment interruption and effectively becoming a split-course RT, known for decades as inferior to continuous course RT regimens.

Results of various retrospective studies have shown that exclusive RT-CHT, mostly a concurrent one, can achieve MST of 26–27 months and a 5-year OS of >30% (Taylor et al. 2004; MacManus et al. 2013). In a subset analysis of a pooled data from 5 prospective studies (3 PRTCs and 2 phase II trials), Jeremic et al. (2013) reported on 222 patients with Stage IIIA NSCLC which resembled surgical candidates due to good KPS (70–100) and weight loss <5%. In this favorable subset, exclusive concurrent RT-CHT produced the MST of 38 months with 5-year OS was 41%, all accompanied with low toxicity including zero mortality. Of special importance was that these results had been reached in patients clinically staged. They compare favorably to the best results achieved in various surgical combinations in this setting (Hancock et al. 2014; Boffa et al. 2017), ranging 35–38% at 5 years.

3 Is There a Specific Stage IIIA/N2 Patient Subgroup Which Can Benefit from Surgical Multimodality Approach?

Highest level of evidence showed that exclusive RT-CHT is not only as effective as surgical bi- or trimodality approaches, but less toxic and is likely offering superior QoL as well as definitely having better cost-benefit aspect, an important matter for both patients and hospital managers. However, one may perhaps argue that there could be a patient subgroup "hidden" within whole cohort of patients with Stage IIIA/N2 as having characteristics which could make it suitable for surgical multimodality approach. If so, which are those characteristics and how can one identify them? To be even more specific, which pretreatment patient-, and/or tumor-related factors could predict superior outcome of a surgical multimodality approach in a particular patient? Have potential predictors been investigated and, if they had, how it was done and which ones have been proven, so far?

Investigation of potential predicting factors is appropriately performed using an approach advocated more than 10 years ago (Clark et al. 2006; Clark 2008). It mandates using the setting of PRCTs where a potential predictor is separately investigated in all arms (e.g., surgical trimodality versus exclusive RT-CHT) used in a PRCT. In case there is a differential finding of the influence of one or more of these factors seen in the two treatment arms (e.g., females doing better in surgical multimodality approach but not in exclusive RT-CHT approach) this indicates female gender favors one treatment approach (in this case, surgical) over the other. Unfortunately, in the pioneering effort, and the most comprehensive review of the literature performed up to 2016, not a single PRCT was found using this approach to investigate whether any of the pretreatment patient- or tumor-related factors could predict favorable effect of surgical approaches over the non-surgical one (Jeremic et al. 2016). Furthermore, not a single Phase II study or a retrospective study ever investigated this issue. Importantly, however, almost 10 years ago, American College of Chest Physicians guidelines (Ramnath et al. 2013) clarified that there were no preoperative factors which can identify patients benefiting from surgery after neoadjuvant therapy. They recommended that the decision to pursue surgery be made before starting neoadjuvant therapy rather than after, considering upfront resection followed by adjuvant therapy as inappropriate in patients with N2 disease identified preoperatively.

It is, therefore, neither unexpected nor unjustified, that thoracic oncologists have turned to various, mostly single institutional, retrospective analysis to get better insight into particular characteristic which could identify patients benefiting from surgical multimodality approach. These attempts, however, were largely by-passing the T component of the disease, and almost uniquely focused on the issue of N2 disease. Various considerations of N2 disease appeared in the past 15 years. One of these (Detterbeck 2008) defined three different types of N2 disease having different postoperative prognosis: the "unsuspected N2," when it is found intraoperatively in such well-staged patients; the "ignored N2," patients with suspicious mediastinal nodes by image [computed tomography (CT) or/and positron emission tomography (PET)], who nevertheless undergo a resection without further staging investigations; and the "underappreciated N2," patients with subtle suspicion of N2 involvement such as those with central tumor, N1 node enlargement or big lung cancer (>3 cm), who do not undergo an invasive staging procedure (EBUS or mediastinoscopy), even though there is a well-documented 20% chance of N2 disease in this case despite normal CT and PET of the mediastinum. Obviously, while the first one is irrelevant before the surgical attack, still, however having prognostic implications, the second and third groups remain of major interest at the time of staging and likely restaging. In the most recent one discussion, the metastases of NSCLC to ipsilateral mediastinum (N2) were grouped into three categories: occult N2, resectable N2, and non-resectable N2 (Evison et al. 2017). It was shown (Andre et al. 2000) that proven pN2 carried better prognosis than cN2. Also, the number of lymph node (LN) stations involved was important, involvement of a single LN having better prognosis than when there was ≥ 2 LNs. The microscopic (p)N2 confined to a single LN carried better prognosis than microscopic (p)N2 in ≥ 2LNs. It was also better than cN2 disease in a single N2 and better than cN2 with respect to 5-year survival data (34%, 11%, 8%, and 3%, respectively). Another important finding from several retrospective studies (Obiols et al. 2014; Legras et al. 2014; Cho et al. 2014; Funakoshi et al. 2012) was that occurrence of unsuspected N2 was shown to be important prognostic factor in trimodality surgical approach. Multilevel positive LN compared to single level positive LN at initial mediastinoscopy was independent ominous prognostic factor (Misthos et al. 2008; Decaluwé et al. 2009; Funakoshi et al. 2012). To extend this, even in patients with persistent N2 disease, single level involvement carried better 5-year OS survival (37% vs 7%, $p < 0.005$). When various surgical variables were examined and entered into a multivariate analysis, complete resection and ypN category (ypN0-1 and ypN2-single level vs multilevel-ypN2 and ypN3) independently influenced OS. Matsunaga et al. (2014) retrospectively investigated various combinations of locations of primary tumors and mediastinal LNs in patients with cN2, c-IIIA, pN2. They have been grouped into either cN2α. [only involvement of upper mediastinal lymph nodes (UMLN) in upper lobe tumors (T) or only lower mediastinal lymph nodes (LMLN) in lower lobe T] or cN2β (involvement of LMLN in upper lobe T with or without UMLN or involvement of UMLN in lower lobe T with or without LMLN). cN2α achieved significantly better outcome (OS at 5 years: 29.5% vs 0%, $p = 0.0007$). Other (Farjah et al. 2009) developed and validated a prediction model for pN2 by using several risk factors (tumor location and size by CT, nodal disease by CT, maximum standardized uptake value (SUV) of the primary tumor, N1 by PET, and histology) and obtained significant performance characteristics in 93 patients with pN2 NSCLC. Some other (Ding et al. 2016) investigated the prognostic significances of the number of positive LNs (nN), the ratio of the number of positive to removed LNs [LN ratio (LNR)], combination of pN and nN (pN-nN), combination of pN and LNR (pN-LNR), and pN. In a high number of patients with pN2 ($n = 497$), pN-LNR was an independent prognostic factor as well as pN-nN, LNR, nN, or pN. In a series of 203 patients with induction therapy followed by surgery Kamel et al. (2017) identified patients with upper lobe tumors and less than 60% reduction in N2 SUVmax as more likely to have persistent N2 disease, a surrogate for a poor prognosis.

4 Specific Considerations of Radiochemotherapy

In the preceding sections, characteristics of RT as given in many neoadjuvant RT-CHT approaches (e.g., INT0139) have been emphasized as clearly suboptimal. Both the RT dose given with the neoadjuvant CHT (e.g., 45 Gy in 24 daily fractions), and the timing of the continuation till radical dose (e.g., 61 Gy) which always requested several weeks, had clearly questioned its effectiveness in this setting. This is even more so if one considers patients not undergoing surgery as less favorable ones. With more potent diagnostic and treatment capabilities occurring in the past decades, many researchers embarked on approach testing the question whether higher RT doses given in a neoadjuvant part with concurrent CHT would be beneficial. In one such attempt (Sonett et al. 2004), platinum-based CHT was given concurrently with higher RT doses (≥59 Gy) and achieved pathological downstaging in 85% patients, no residual LN was found in 82.5% patients, while pCR, 5-year OS, and 5-year PFS were 45%, 46.2%, and 56.4%, respectively. Lobectomy was successfully performed in 72.5% cases and pneumonectomy in 27.5% cases. These good results were accompanied with very low toxicity which dispersed the fear of higher RT dose initially considered as risky. In a retrospective study on 104 patients (Cerfolio et al. 2005), carboplatin-based CHT was given with RT doses which sometimes exceeded 60 Gy. Patients were divided between high dose RT (median, 60 Gy) and low dose RT (median, 45 Gy), the former achieving higher rate of pCR. No difference was found in major morbidity and mortality between the two groups although pneumonectomy carried a higher risk of complications. Additionally exploring impact of high dose RT (59.4 Gy) and concurrent 2 cycles of cisplatin/etoposide in cases when pneumonectomy followed it, researchers (Daly et al. 2006) observed that there is a high mortality risk (13.3%), but in that study mortality was only 5.6% in cases of right pneumonectomy. Past decade also brought similar results. Indeed, a recent RTOG 0229 study (Suntharalingam et al. 2012) proved in a phase II setting that 61Gy can efficiently be given with concurrent CHT before surgery. Further exploring this issue, Sher et al. (2015) used the National Cancer Data Base (NCDB) data in 1041 patients and explored the impact of possible dose escalation/response by dividing RT doses into a low (36–45 Gy), standard (45–54 Gy), and high (54–74 Gy) groups. On univariate analysis, patients treated with 45–54 Gy experienced prolonged OS (median 38.3 vs 31.8 vs 29.0 months for 45–54 Gy, 36–45 Gy and 54–74 Gy, respectively, $p = 0.0089$), which was confirmed on multivariate analysis. Residual nodal disease was seen less often after 54–74 Gy (25.5% vs 31.8% vs 37.5% for 54–74 Gy, 36–45 Gy and 45–54 Gy, respectively, $p = 0.0038$). There were no differences in positive surgical margin status or adverse surgical outcomes between the cohorts. The authors concluded that RT dose between 45 and 54 Gy was associated with superior survival in comparison with doses above and below this threshold, indicating that candidates for trimodality therapy did not seem to achieve additional benefit with dose escalation. These results likely biased by the lack of complete set of information not existing in the NCDB were effectively challenged by Allen et al. (2018) who reported on 48 patients treated with the median RT dose of 72 Gy (range, 60–72 Gy), vast majority of which received a concurrent cisplatin/etoposide. While 72% of patients eventually underwent lobectomy, 28% underwent pneumonectomy. The 30- and 90-day mortality rates were 0%. The nodal downstaging rate was 82% with pCR was 64%. The MST was 29.9 months, the median time to loco-regional progression was 35.1 months and the median time to distant progression was 39.3 months. Loco-regional failure was 8% and distant failure was 44%. They showed that high dose neoadjuvant RT-CHT was safe and effective. Most recently, short-term surgical results observed during two NRG oncology studies (Donington et al. 2020) after high dose concurrent RT-CHT was explored. Of a total of 126 patients, 74% had anatomic resection, of which 77 underwent lobectomy, and 16 underwent extended resection. R0 resections occurred in 91%. Grade 3 or 4 surgical adverse events were reported in 28%, 30-day mortality in 4%, and 90-day mortality in 5%. Patients undergoing extended resection experienced similar rates of grade 3 or 4 adverse events but higher 30-day (1.3% vs 18.8%) and 90-day mortality (2.6% vs 18.8%). This study showed that while lobectomy was safe following high dose concurrent RT-CHT, increased mortality was noted with extended resections.

While these results may indicate cautious optimism with high dose neoadjuvant concurrent RT-CHT, they also need to be placed into the context of both timing of surgery and efficacy of salvage surgery in cases when exclusive RT-CHT is given alone. Many studies published in the first decade of this millennium showed promising results, frequently however, including patients with earlier stages, likely biasing it towards better overall prognosis. Recent analysis of the NCDB data (Gao et al. 2017) included 1,623 patients treated with neoadjuvant RT-CHT where RT doses ranged 40–60 Gy. Patients were divided into 4 groups based on the interval between RT-CHT and surgery: 0 to ≤3, >3 to ≤6, >6 to ≤9, and > 9 to ≤12 weeks). Multivariate analysis demonstrated no significant difference in OS in those who underwent an operation within 6 weeks of neoadjuvant RT-CHT. However, significantly lower OS was observed in those having operation >6 and ≤9 weeks after neoadjuvant RT-CHT (HR, 1.33, 95% CI: 1.01–1.76, $p = 0.043$) and >9 and ≤12 weeks after NCRT (HR, 1.44, 95% CI: 1.04–2.01, $p = 0.030$). These results asked for keeping the time period between the end of RT-CHT and surgery short and avoiding unnecessary delays. Most recently, Rice et al. (2020) used the same source in 5946 patients, dividing surgical timing after neoadjuvant RT-CHT into short (<77 days), mid (77–114 days), and long (>114 days) delays. Mortality rates at 30-and 90-day were similar across all groups. Multivariate analysis demonstrated a significant difference in survival when patients underwent earlier operative intervention compared to late. Short, mid, and long delay groups 1-year OS was 82%, 83%, and 80% and 3-year OS was 59%, 58%, and 52%, respectively ($p = 0.0003$). The delay in surgical resection of Stage IIIA NSCLC was not associated increased early mortality, however it was associated with inferior 3-year OS.

Studies exploring impact of salvage surgery shed additional light into optimization of the treatment approaches in this setting, additionally influencing decision-making process in the past 2 decades. In a small single-institution study from Germany (Schreiner et al. 2018) salvage surgery after high dose definitive concurrent RT-CHT was shown to be effective and low toxic. RT dose ranged 59.4–72 Gy (median, 66 Gy). Median interval between definitive RT-CHT and salvage surgery was 6.7 months. Perioperative morbidity and 30-day mortality was 38% and 7.7%, respectively. Postoperative MST was 29.7 months and 5-year OS was 46%. Importantly, this cohort included patients with Stage IV and IIIB NSCLC, respectively. Italian study (Casiraghi et al. 2017) included 35 patients deemed eligible for lung cancer resection due to relapse after definitive RT-CHT (cisplatin-based RT; RT mean dose, 58 Gy). Complete resection was obtained in 77% patients. Median time from RT-CHT to resection was 7 months (range 1–39). Viable tumor was found in 89.6% patients. Major complications occurred in 25.7%. There were 5.7% perioperative deaths within 30 days. With a median follow-up of 13 months, postoperative 2- and 3-year OS after complete resection was 46% and 37%, respectively. Spanish study (Romero-Vielva et al. 2019) reported on 27 patients having salvage surgery after high dose RT and concurrent platinum-based CHT. Early postoperative deaths occurred in 4% of cases. The MST was 75.56 months, while 5-year OS was 53.3%. The median DFS was 14.97 months. Most recently, a study using NCDB data included more than 2000 patients and compared planned surgical trimodality therapy (RT doses >45 Gy followed by lobectomy or pneumonectomy ≤90 days from end of neoadjuvant RT-CHT) to exclusive RT-CHT (RT dose >59 Gy and lobectomy or pneumonectomy performed >90 days from exclusive RT-CHT completion) (Ye et al. 2020). Surgery occurred at a median of 41 days (range 1–90) after RT-CHT in the planned trimodality group and 114 days (91–440) in the salvage surgery group. There was no difference in 90-day mortality and no difference in 3–5-year OS. The authors concluded that salvage surgery remains a viable option for medically appropriate patients after exclusive RT-CHT.

5 Conclusions and Future Endeavors

The highest level of evidence (PRCTs and MAs) unequivocally documented lack of benefit of surgical multimodality approaches in patients with Stage IIIA/N2 NSCLC. Importantly, evidence points towards surgical approaches as having significantly higher morbidity and mortality and although not properly investigated, likely increased costs and decreased QoL. They all suggest RT-CHT as standard treatment option in this setting, in particular when modern RT-CHT is used, although and unfortunately, many individuals and medical commentators still advocate the use of bimodality or trimodality surgical approach.

Question, therefore, is not only what one should do in this setting, but how to secure that patients are offered appropriate treatment. Tumor board should be the place where all discussions are provided, enabling evidence to be used in the decision-making process, rather than pseudo expertise and wishful thinking. Because, as of the first half of 2021, not a single piece of the highest level of evidence supports the use of surgical multimodality approach. Or we will continue to accept a single, unplanned, post-hoc analysis from a single PRCT (Albain et al. 2009) as the evidence so strong that it outweighs 7 PRCTs and 5 MAs?

The story of surgery as potentially important part of multimodality approach does not, however, ends here. There is universal agreement on the necessity to produce more PRCTs although such endeavors, unfortunately too often, fail (poor accrual leading to prolonged recruitment times, consequential Will-Rogers phenomenon, but also poor implementation of the results of existing trials). Indeed, there are many current trials which test various generations of drugs (CHT, targeted agents, immunotherapy) in the neoadjuvant fashion. It is expected that they shed more lights into the matter of combined modality approaches in this setting.

While PRCTs remain the best available tool in clinical research in general, and one should be strongly encouraged to participate in one, could we use the time while we wait for results to come for something meaningful? What about using existing data from existing PRCTs to investigate possibly important pretreatment predictive (not prognostic!) factors which could help us in better study design in the future? Many interesting findings could easily be, retrospectively now, investigated. Importance of histology, for example, due to contrasting results of EORTC (van Meerbeeck et al. 2007) versus Scandinavian (Sorensen et al. 2013) study could be one such with significant impact in the pretreatment decision-making process. Emphasis on pretreatment patient- and tumor-related factors should help us identify patients where surgical multimodality approach may be preferred and do that before treatment starts. Perhaps, we start with this low cost and time efficient effort in our continuous quest towards optimized treatment approach in patients with Stage IIIA/N2 NSCLC.

References

Albain KS, Swann RS, Rusch VW et al (2009) Radiotherapy plus chemotherapy with or without surgical resection for stage III non-small-cell lung cancer: a phase III randomised controlled trial. Lancet 374:379–386

Allen AM, Shochat T, Flex D et al (2018) High-dose radiotherapy as neoadjuvant treatment in non-small-cell lung cancer. Oncology 95:13–19

Andre F, Grunenwald D, Pignon JP et al (2000) Survival of patients with resected N2 non-small-cell lung cancer: evidence for a subclassification and implications. J Clin Oncol 18:2981–2989

Aupérin A, Le Péchoux C, Rolland E et al (2010) Meta-analysis of concomitant versus sequential radiochemotherapy in locally advanced non-small-cell lung cancer. J Clin Oncol 28:2181–2190

Boffa D, Fernandez FG, Kim S et al (2017) Surgically managed clinical stage IIIA-clinical N2 lung cancer in the society of thoracic surgeons database. Ann Thorac Surg 104:395–403

Candela SC, Detterbeck FC (2010) A systematic review of restaging after induction therapy for stage IIIa lung cancer prediction of pathologic stage. J Thorac Oncol 5:389–398

Casiraghi M, Maisonneuve P et al (2017) Salvage surgery after definitive chemoradiotherapy for non-small cell lung cancer. Semin Thorac Cardiovasc Surg 29:233–241

Cerfolio RJ, Bryant AS, Spencer SA, Bartolucci AA (2005) Pulmonary resection after high-dose and low-dose chest irradiation. Ann Thorac Surg 80:1224–1230

Chen Y, Peng X, Zhou Y, Xia K, Zhuan W (2018) Comparing the benefits of chemoradiotherapy and chemotherapy for resectable stage III A/N2 non-small cell lung cancer: a meta-analysis. World J Surg Oncol 16:8

Cho HJ, Kim SR, Kim HR et al (2014) Modern outcome and risk analysis of surgically resected occult N2 non-small cell lung cancer. Ann Thorac Surg 97:1920–1925

Clark GM (2008) Prognostic factors versus predictive factors: examples from a clinical trial of erlotinib. Mol Oncol 1:406–412

Clark GM, Zborowski DM, Culbertson JL et al (2006) Clinical utility of epidermal growth factor receptor expression for selecting patients with advanced non-small cell lung cancer for treatment with erlotinib. J Thorac Oncol 1:837–846

Daly BDT, Fernando HC, Ketchedjian A et al (2006) Pneumonectomy after high-dose radiation and concurrent chemotherapy for nonsmall cell lung cancer. Ann Thorac Surg 82:227–231

De Leyn P, Lardinois D, Van Schil PE et al (2007) ESTS guidelines for preoperative lymph node staging for non-small cell lung cancer. Eur J Cardiothorac Surg 32:1–8

De Leyn P, Dooms C, Kuzdzal J et al (2014) Revised ESTS guidelines for preoperative mediastinal lymph node staging for non-small-cell lung cancer. Eur J Cardiothorac Surg 45:787–798

De Waele M, Serra-Mitjans M, Hendriks J et al (2008) Accuracy and survival of repeat mediastinoscopy after induction therapy for non-small cell lung cancer in a combined series of 104 patients. Eur J Cardiothorac Surg 33:824–828

Decaluwé H, De Leyn P, Vansteenkiste J et al (2009) Surgical multimodality treatment for baseline resectable stage IIIA-N2 non-small cell lung cancer. Degree of mediastinal lymph node involvement and impact on survival. Eur J Cardiothorac Surg 36:433–439

Detterbeck F (2008) What to do with 'surprise' N2?: intraoperative management of patients with non-small-cell lung cancer. J Thorac Oncol 3:289–302

Ding X, Hui Z, Dai H et al (2016) A proposal for combination of lymph node ratio and anatomic location of involved lymph nodes for nodal classification in non-small cell lung cancer. J Thorac Oncol 11:1565–1573

Donington JS, Paulus R, Edelman MJ, for the NRG Oncology Lung Group et al (2020) Resection following concurrent chemotherapy and high-dose radiation for stage IIIA non–small cell lung cancer. J Thorac Cardiovasc Surg 160:1331–1345.e1

Douillard JY, Rosell R, De Lena M et al (2006) Adjuvant vinorelbine plus cisplatin versus observation in patients with completely resected stage IB-IIIA non-small-cell lung cancer (Adjuvant Navelbine International Trialist Association [ANITA]): a randomised controlled trial. Lancet Oncol 7:719–727

Eberhardt WE, Pöttgen C, Gauler TC et al (2015) Phase III study of surgery versus definitive concurrent chemoradiotherapy boost in patients with resectable stage IIIA(N2) and selected IIIB non-small-cell lung cancer after induction chemotherapy and concurrent chemoradiotherapy (ESPATUE). J Clin Oncol 33:4194–4201

Ellis MC, Diggs BS, Vetto JT et al (2011) Intraoperative oncologic staging and outcomes for lung cancer resection vary by surgeon specialty. Ann Thorac Surg 92:1958–1963

Evison M, Clive A, Castle L et al (2017) Resectable clinical N2 non-small cell lung cancer; what is the optimal treatment strategy? An update by the British Thoracic Society Lung Cancer Specialist Advisory Group. J Thorac Oncol 12:1434–1341

Farjah F, Flum DR, Varghese TK Jr et al (2009) Surgeon specialty and long-term survival after pulmonary resection for lung cancer. Ann Thorac Surg 87:995–1004

Funakoshi Y, Takeuchi Y, Kusumoto H et al (2012) Which subgroup of patients with pathologic N2 non-small cell lung cancer benefit from surgery? J Cancer Res Clin Oncol 138:1027–1033

Gao SJ, Corso CD, Wang EH et al (2017) Timing of surgery after neoadjuvant chemoradiation in locally advanced non–small cell lung cancer. J Thorac Oncol 12:314–322

Goldstraw P, Crowley J, Chansky K et al (2007) The IASLC lung cancer staging project: proposals for the revision of the TNM stage groupings in the forthcoming (seventh) edition of the TNM classification of malignant tumours. J Thorac Oncol 2:706–714

Goldstraw P, Chansky K, Crowley J et al (2016) The IASLC lung cancer staging project: proposals for revision of the TNM stage groupings in the forthcoming (eighth) edition of the TNM classification for lung cancer. J Thorac Oncol 11:39–51

Guo SX, Jian Y, Chen YL et al (2016) Neoadjuvant chemoradiotherapy versus chemotherapy alone followed by surgery for resectable stage III non-small-cell lung cancer: a meta-analysis. Sci Rep 6:34388

Hancock J, Rosen J, Moreno A et al (2014) Management of clinical stage IIIA primary lung cancers in the National Cancer Database. Ann Thorac Surg 98:424–432

Jeremic B, Milicic B, Milisavljevic S (2013) Radiotherapy alone versus radiochemotherapy in patients with favorable prognosis clinical stage IIIa non small-cell lung cancer (NSCLC). Clin Lung Cancer 14:172–180

Jeremic B, Casas F, Dubinsky P et al (2016) Surgery in stage IIIA nonsmall cell lung cancer: lack of predictive and prognostic factors identifying any patient subgroup benefiting from it. Clin Lung Cancer 17:107–112

Johnstone DW, Byhardt RW, Ettinger D, Scott CB (2002) Phase III study comparing chemotherapy and radiotherapy with preoperative chemotherapy and surgical resection in patients with non-small-cell lung cancer with spread to mediastinal lymph nodes (N2); final report of RTOG 89-01. Radiation therapy oncology group. Int J Radiat Oncol Biol Phys 54:365–369

Kamel MK, Rahouma M, Ghaly G et al (2017) Clinical predictors of persistent mediastinal nodal disease after induction therapy for stage IIIA N2 non-small cell lung cancer. Ann Thorac Surg 103:281–286

Kim AW, Boffa DJ, Wang Z et al (2012) An analysis, systematic review, and meta-analysis of the perioperative mortality after neoadjuvant therapy and pneumonectomy for non-small cell lung cancer. J Thorac Cardiovasc Surg 143:55–63

Kumar P, Herndon J II, Langer M et al (1996) Patterns of disease failure after trimodality therapy of nonsmall cell lung carcinoma pathologic stage IIIA (N2): analysis of cancer and leukemia group B protocol 8935. Cancer 77:2393–2399

Legras A, Mordant P, Arame A et al (2014) Long-term survival of patients with pN2 lung cancer according to the pattern of lymphatic spread. Ann Thorac Surg 97:1156–1162

Liang H-Y, Zhou H, Li H-L et al (2010) Chemoradiotherapy for advanced non-small cell lung cancer: concurrent or sequential? It's no longer the question: a systematic review. Int J Cancer 127:718–728

Livingston RB (1997) Combined modality therapy of lung cancer. Clin Cancer Res 3:2638–2647

Louie BE, Kapur S, Farivar AS et al (2011) Safety and utility of mediastinoscopy in non-small cell lung cancer in a complex mediastinum. Ann Thorac Surg 92:278–283

MacManus MP, Everitt S, Bayne M et al (2013) The use of fused PET/CT images for patient selection and radical radiotherapy target volume definition in patients with non-small cell lung cancer: results of a prospective study with mature survival data. Radiother Oncol 106:292–298

Matsunaga T, Suzuki K, Takamochi K et al (2014) Time to refine N2 staging? cN2α and cN2β based on local regional involvement provide a more accurate prognosis in surgically treated IIIA non-small-cell lung cancer than N2 alone or the number of node stations involved. Eur J Cardiothorac Surg 46:86–91

McElnay PJ, Choong A, Jordan E et al (2015) Outcome of surgery versus radiotherapy after induction treatment in patients with N2 disease: systematic review and meta-analysis of randomised trials. Thorax 70:764–768

Misthos P, Sepsas E, Kokotsakis J, Skottis I, Lioulias A (2008) The significance of one-station N2 disease in the prognosis of patients with nonsmall-cell lung cancer. Ann Thorac Surg 86:1626–1630

Nagai K, Tsuchiya R, Mori T et al (2003) A randomized trial comparing induction chemotherapy followed by surgery with surgery alone for patients with stage IIIA N2 non-small cell lung cancer (JCOG 9209). J Thorac Cardiovasc Surg 125:254–260

O'Rourke N, Roqué I, Figuls M et al (2010) Concurrent chemoradiotherapy in non-small cell lung cancer. Cochrane Database Syst Rev 6:CD002140

Obiols C, Call S, Rami-Porta R et al (2014) Survival of patients with unsuspected pN2 non-small cell lung cancer after an accurate preoperative mediastinal staging. Ann Thorac Surg 97:957–964

Pass HI, Pogrebniak HW, Steinberg SM et al (1992) Randomized trial of neoadjuvant therapy for lung cancer: interim analysis. Ann Thorac Surg 53:992–998

Pöttgen C, Eberhardt W, Stamatis G, Stuschke M (2017) Definitive radiochemotherapy versus surgery with multimodality treatment in stage III non-small cell lung cancer (NSCLC) - a cumulative meta-analysis of the randomized evidence. Oncotarget 8 41670–41678.

Rami-Porta R, Bolejack V, Giroux DJ et al (2014) International association for the study of lung cancer Staging and Prognostic Factors Committee, Advisory Board Members and Participating Institutions The IASLC lung cancer staging project: the new database to inform the eighth edition of the TNM classification of lung cancer. J Thorac Oncol 9:1618–1624

Ramnath N, Dilling TJ, Harris LJ et al (2013) Treatment of stage III non-small cell lung cancer: diagnosis and management of lung cancer, 3rd ed: American College of Chest Physicians evidence-based clinical practice guidelines. Chest 143:e314S–e340S

Ren Z, Zhou S, Liu Z et al (2015) Randomized controlled trials of induction treatment and surgery versus combined chemotherapy and radiotherapy in stagesIIIA-N2 NSCLC: a systematic review and meta-analysis. J Thorac Dis 7:1414–1422

Rice JD, Heidel J, Trivedi JR, van Berkel VH (2020) Optimal surgical timing after neoadjuvant therapy for stage IIIa non-small cell lung cancer. Ann Thorac Surg 109:842–847

Rocco G, Nason K, Brunelli A et al (2016) Management of stage IIIA (N2) non-small cell lung cancer: a transatlantic perspective. Ann Thorac Surg 101: 1247–1250

Romero-Vielva L, Viteri S, Moya-Hornoc I et al (2019) Salvage surgery after definitive chemo-radiotherapy for patients with non-small cell lung cancer. Lung Cancer 133:117–122

Rosell R, Gomez-Codina J, Camps C et al (1994) A randomized trial comparing preoperative chemotherapy plus surgery with surgery alone in patients with non-small-cell lung cancer. N Engl J Med 330:153–158

Roth JA, Fossella F, Komaki R et al (1994) A randomized trial comparing perioperative chemotherapy and surgery with surgery alone in resectable stage IIIA non-small-cell lung cancer. J Natl Cancer Inst 86:673–680

Schreiner W, Dudek W, Lettmaier S, Fietkau R, Sirbu H (2018) Long-term survival after salvage surgery for local failure after definitive chemoradiation therapy for locally advanced non-small cell lung cancer. Thorac Cardiovasc Surg 66:135–141

Shah AA, Berry MF, Tzao C et al (2012) Induction chemoradiation is not superior to induction chemotherapy alone in stage IIIA lung cancer. Ann Thorac Surg 93:1807–1812

Shepherd FA, Johnston MR, Payne D et al (1998) Randomized study of chemotherapy and surgery versus radiotherapy for stage IIIA non-small-cell lung cancer: a National Cancer Institute of Canada Clinical Trials Group Study. Br J Cancer 78:683–685

Sher DJ, Fidler MJ, Seder CW, Liptay MJ, Koshy M (2015) Relationship between radiation therapy dose and outcome in patients treated with neoadjuvant chemoradiation therapy and surgery for stage IIIA non-small cell lung cancer: a population-based, comparative effectiveness analysis. Int J Radiat Oncol Biol Phys 92:307–316

Shi Y, Sun Y, Yu J et al (2017) China experts consensus on the diagnosis and treatment of advanced stage primary lung cancer. (2016 version). Asia Pac J Clin Oncol 13:87–103

Shields TW (1990) The significance of ipsilateral mediastinal lymph node metastasis (N2 disease) in non-small cell carcinoma of the lung: a commentary. J Thorac Cardiovasc Surg 99:48–53

Silvestri GA, Gonzalez AV, Jantz MA et al (2013) Methods for staging non-small cell lung cancer: diagnosis and management of lung cancer, 3rd ed: American College of Chest Physicians evidence-based clinical practice guidelines. Chest 143:e211S–e250S

Sonett JR, Suntharalingam M, Edelman MJ et al (2004) Pulmonary resection after curative intent radiotherapy (>59 Gy) and concurrent chemotherapy in non-small-cell lung cancer. Ann Thorac Surg 78:1200–1205

Sorensen JB, Riska H, Ravn J et al (2013) Scandinavian phase III trial of neoadjuvant chemotherapy in NSCLC stages IB-IIIA/T3. J Clin Oncol 31(Suppl):abstract 7504

Stephens RJ, Girling DJ, Hopwood P et al (2005) A randomised controlled trial of pre-operative chemotherapy followed, if feasible, by resection versus radiotherapy in patients with inoperable stage T3, N1, M0 or T1-3, N2, M0 non-small cell lung cancer. Lung Cancer 49:395–400

Sugarbaker DJ, Herndon J, Kohman LJ, Krasna MJ, Green MR, and the Cancer and Leukemia Group B Thoracic Surgery Group (1995) Results of cancer and leukemia group B protocol 8935: a multiinstitutional phase II trimodality trial for stage IIIA (N2) non-small-cell lung cancer. J Thorac Cardiovasc Surg 109:473–485

Suntharalingam M, Paulus R, Edelman MJ et al (2012) Radiation therapy oncology group protocol 02-29: a phase II trial of neoadjuvant therapy with concurrent chemotherapy and full-dose radiation therapy followed by surgical resection and consolidative therapy for locally advanced nonsmall cell carcinoma of the lung. Int J Radiat Oncol 84:456–463

SEER (2010) Surveillance, epidemiology and end results. US National Institutes of Health, National Cancer Institute, Bethesda, MD

Taylor NA, Liao ZX, Cox JD et al (2004) Equivalent outcome of patients with clinical Stage IIIA non-small-cell lung cancer treated with concurrent chemoradiation compared with induction chemotherapy followed by surgical resection. Int J Radiat Oncol Biol Phys 58:204–212

Tong S, Qin Z, Wan M, Zhang L, Cui Y, Yao Y (2018) Induction chemoradiotherapy versus induction chemotherapy for potentially resectable stage IIIA (N2) non-small cell lung cancer: a systematic review and meta-analysis. J Thorac Dis 10:2428–2436

van Meerbeeck JP, Kramer GW, van Schil PE et al (2007) Randomized controlled trial of resection versus radiotherapy after induction chemotherapy in stage IIIA-N2 non-small-cell lung cancer. J Natl Cancer Inst 99:442–450

Xu Y-P, Li B, Xu X-L et al (2015) Is there a survival benefit in patients with stage IIIA (N2) non- cell lung cancer receiving neoadjuvant chemotherapy and/or radiotherapy prior to surgical resection. A systematic review and meta-analysis. Medicine (Baltimore) 94:e879

Xu X-L, Dan L, Chen W et al (2016) Neoadjuvant chemoradiotherapy or chemotherapy followed by surgery is superior to that followed by definitive chemoradiation or radiotherapy in stage IIIA(N2) nonsmall-cell lung cancer: a meta-analysis and system review. Onco Targets Ther 9:845–853

Ye JC, Ding L, Atay SM et al (2020) Trimodality vs chemoradiation and salvage resection in cN2 stage IIIA non_small cell lung cancer. Semin Thorac Cardiovasc Surg 32:153–159

Yoshino I, Yoshida S, Miyaoka E et al (2012) Surgical outcome of stage IIIAcN2_ pN2 non-small-cell lung cancer patients in Japanese lung cancer registry study in 2004. J Thorac Oncol 7:850–855

Zeng X, Karnon J, Wang S, Wu B, Wan X, Peng L (2012) The cost of treating advanced non-small cell lung cancer: estimates from the Chinese experience. PLoS One 7:e48323

Multimodality Treatment of Stage IIIA/N2 Non-Small Cell Lung Cancer: When YES to Surgery

Sean All and David J. Sher

Contents

1 Introduction 534
2 **Evolution of Neoadjuvant/Induction Therapies** 535
2.1 Neoadjuvant Radiation Therapy Alone 535
2.2 Neoadjuvant Chemotherapy Alone 535
2.3 Neoadjuvant Chemoradiotherapy Alone 537
2.4 Neoadjuvant Chemotherapy Versus Neoadjuvant Chemoradiotherapy 539
3 **Neoadjuvant CRT (Trimodality) Versus Definitive CRT** 541
4 **Stage IIIA/N2 NSCLC: When YES to Surgery** 542
5 **Future Directions/Immunotherapy** 543
6 **Conclusion** 544
References 544

Abstract

Stage III non-small cell lung cancer (NSCLC) is comprised of a heterogeneous cohort of patient presentations that are broadly considered as "locally advanced disease," but stage IIIA/N2 further selects a subset of this category with a potentially improved prognosis. These individuals may have ipsilateral mediastinal and/or subcarinal lymph node involvement, varying tumor size (up to 7 cm), and possible invasion of surrounding mediastinal structures. Multimodality treatment is universally accepted as the standard-of-care for their management, and historically, definitive concurrent chemoradiotherapy (CRT) has been the preferred paradigm. However, because it has been long recognized that long-term survival is feasible in a small but non-trivial and growing group of these patients, there has been considerable controversy about intensifying their local therapy by using surgical resection. In fact, there are some data that support improved locoregional control and hence progression-free and even overall survival with trimodality therapy potentially warranting the increase in morbidity. This chapter will focus on reviewing the published evidence supporting the incorporation of surgery into the multimodality treatment of stage IIIA/N2 NSCLC patients.

S. All · D. J. Sher (✉)
Department of Radiation Oncology, University of Texas Southwestern Medical Center,
Dallas, TX, USA
e-mail: David.Sher@utsouthwestern.edu

1 Introduction

It is well-known that patients with stage III, locally advanced non-small cell lung cancer (LA-NSCLC) have poor overall outcomes. The 5-year overall survival (OS) for all stage IIIA patients has been estimated to be around 36% (Goldstraw et al. 2016), but for patients with clinical N2 disease at the time of diagnosis, the 5-year OS decreases to 23% (Asamura et al. 2015). Due to the wide variability of disease burden at presentation—both locoregional and micrometastatic—in stage IIIA patients, delineating the most effect therapeutic approach has been controversial. Early surgical series established that surgery alone was clearly inadequate for N2 disease, with only 21% of patients surviving past 5 years after undergoing complete resection (Mountain 1990). Other surgical series found improvements in long-term survival ranging from 25 to 40% with complete resection of N2 disease followed by adjuvant radiation to the mediastinum (Martini et al. 1981; Martini and Flehinger 1987). Yet they also found high rates of locoregional recurrences and distant failures, indicating the prevalence of residual microscopic and micrometastatic disease.

At the same time of these surgical experiences, early studies were being performed on the effectiveness of definitive radiation alone for LA-NSCLC. Radiation Therapy Oncology Group (RTOG) 7301 was a prospective randomized dose escalation study using definitive radiation to treat unresectable or medically inoperable NSCLC patients (Perez et al. 1987). Patients were randomized to four different regimens: 4000 cGy split course, or continuous daily fractionation to total doses of 4000 cGy, 5000 cGy, or 6000 cGy. The intrathoracic failure rates within the irradiated field ranged from 27% to 48%, with the higher doses having lower rates of failure. For the entire group, the failure rate in the non-irradiated lung was 25% to 30% and the incidence of distant failure was 75% to 80%, highlighting how unimodality therapy is inadequate for this disease.

Subsequent trials explored the effectiveness and superiority of combined modality treatment. Two prospective randomized trials, CALGB 8433 and RTOG 8808, established that sequential chemoradiation improved OS versus radiation alone (Dillman et al. 1996; Sause et al. 1995). A meta-analysis compared sequential versus concurrent chemoradiation in this population and found 3- and 5-year absolute OS benefits of 5.7% and 4.5%, respectively, favoring concurrent treatment (Aupérin et al. 2010). This OS benefit was due to improved locoregional control, with the tradeoff of increased acute esophageal toxicity. In the landmark RTOG 9410 study, Curran et al. demonstrated that concurrent chemoradiation was superior to sequential therapy, establishing concurrent chemoradiotherapy as the standard-of-care treatment for unresectable stage III NSCLC (Curran Jr. et al. 2011). Despite these demonstrated improvements in OS, the concurrent chemoradiation arm had a first failure rate of 29% (at the primary site), 12% (thoracic lymph nodes infield), and 4% (thoracic lymph nodes out of field), showing unacceptably high locoregional failure rates. To answer the question of whether radiation dose escalation could improve these results, RTOG 0617 randomized patients between 6000 cGy and 7400 cGy, finding no improvement with dose escalation (Bradley et al. 2020). Importantly, there was no statistically significant difference in the rates of locoregional failure with higher dose radiation, with 5-year locoregional failures at 49.7% in the standard dose arm and 55.4% in the high dose arm. This succession of clinical trials established the benefit of combined concurrent therapy for LA-NSCLC but despite these advances, the locoregional failure rates remained discouragingly high.

These results have continuously raised the obvious question of how to improve locoregional control and therefore survival in LA-NSCLC, specifically in the stage IIIA population that has a more favorable prognosis. Efforts to incorporate surgical resection as a method of improving thoracic control signaled the next step in the evolution of the treatment paradigm. This chapter will serve to review the literature regarding the neoadjuvant/induction strategies prior to surgery as well as the evidence supporting resection in medically operable patients. It will summarize with a discussion on which stage IIIA patients may benefit from the addition of surgery to their multimodality treatment regimen as well as future directions with the expanding use of immunotherapy.

2 Evolution of Neoadjuvant/Induction Therapies

The treatment approach of integrating neoadjuvant or induction therapy prior to surgical resection for stage IIIA disease remains a hotly debated topic in thoracic oncology. The strategic benefits of neoadjuvant therapy include decreasing the burden of micrometastatic disease upfront, improving the resectability of tumors, and sterilizing the mediastinum, the latter of which may be beneficial either therapeutically or as a predictive marker. This induction strategy has been studied primarily in patients deemed resectable at diagnosis, those with low volume N2 disease, and in those with advanced local tumor burden upfront for whom initial resection is not technically feasible (superior sulcus tumors, T4 N0-N1). Retrospective studies have suggested that patients with complete nodal clearance after CRT experience improved overall survival with surgical resection, whereas those who have residual nodal burden had no obvious benefit over CRT alone (Ziel et al. 2015). The fundamental concept is that patients with a sterilized mediastinum are most likely to have had eradicated micrometastatic disease, and thus improved local control with surgical resection is most likely to translate into a survival advantage. Several therapeutic modalities have been used, either alone or in combination, in the neoadjuvant setting prior to surgery.

2.1 Neoadjuvant Radiation Therapy Alone

Preoperative radiation alone as a neoadjuvant therapy prior to surgical resection was examined in early studies. A study from 1975 randomized patients between upfront surgery or preoperative radiation to the primary tumor and mediastinum with a dose of 4000 cGy followed by surgery, finding no difference in any outcome (Warram 1975). A subsequent randomized phase II study from 1994 looked at preoperative radiation alone (44 Gy in 22 fractions to primary tumor and mediastinum) versus preoperative chemotherapy in stage III NSCLC patients (Wagner Jr. et al. 1994). Of the 67 total patients included, 31 were randomized to the preoperative radiation alone arm. There was only one pathologic complete response from this group, with three toxic postoperative deaths. Based on these studies, radiation is not recommended as a sole induction modality prior to surgical resection in LA-NSCLC.

2.2 Neoadjuvant Chemotherapy Alone

In contrast to preoperative radiotherapy, neoadjuvant systemic therapy provides immediate treatment of micrometastatic disease, and it does not compromise the surgical field with fibrosis. Many phase I and phase II studies have evaluated the role of chemotherapy alone in the preoperative setting. There is a great degree of variation among inclusion criteria, treatment regimens and documentation of stage III disease, making cross-trial comparisons difficult, but results do suggest improved outcomes with induction chemotherapy. Several phase III randomized control trials (Table 1) have been published comparing surgery alone versus preoperative chemotherapy followed by surgery.

M.D. Anderson Cancer Center (MDACC) conducted a prospective, randomized trial that included 60 potentially resectable stage IIIA/N2 NSCLC patients (Roth et al. 1994). Patients were treated with either cyclophosphamide, etoposide, or cisplatin followed by surgery or surgery alone. Among the neoadjuvant patients, if documented tumor regression at time of surgery, an additional 3 cycles were delivered postoperatively. Postoperative radiation was used for residual or unresectable disease. The perioperative chemotherapy arm showed a marked 3-year overall survival benefit over the surgery alone arm at interim

Table 1 Reported phase III trials of surgery with or with induction chemotherapy in resectable stage IIIA NSCLC

Trial	No. of patients	Stages included	Treatment regimen	Resection rates	Local control	Progression-free survival	Overall survival	Toxicity (grade 5)
MDACC (Roth et al. 1994)	60	IIIA/N2; few IIIB	CEP × 3 ® surgery ® CEP × 3 vs surgery alone (RT used for residual or unresectable dz)	61% chemo vs 66% surgery alone; Complete resection: 39% chemo vs 31% surgery alone	NR	Median EFS: Not reached for chemo arm vs 9 months for surgery alone ($p = 0.015$)	Median OS: 64 months chemo vs 11 months surgery ($p = 0.008$) 3-year OS: 56% chemo vs 15% surgery	Surgery alone: 2 pts. (6%) vs chemo: 1 pt. (3%)
Spain (Rosell et al. 1994)	60	IIIA/N2	MIP × 3 ® surgery ® RT vs surgery ® RT	Complete resection: 85% chemo vs 90% surgery alone	LRF: 54% chemo vs 55% surgery alone	Median DFS: 20 months vs 5 months favoring chemo ($p < 0.001$)	Median OS: 26 months vs 8 months favoring chemo ($p < 0.001$)	Overall mortality rate: 7% 2 pts. in chemo vs 2 pts. in surgery alone
FTCG (Depierre et al. 2002)	355	I (except T1N0), II, IIIA	MIP × 2 ® surgery ® MIP × 2 vs Surgery alone (RT used for pT3/pN2 disease in both arms)	Complete resection: 92% chemo arm vs 86% surgery alone	NR	Median DFS: 26.7 months vs 12.9 months favoring chemo 3-year DFS: 44% vs 33% favoring chemo	Median OS: 37 months vs 26 months favoring chemo ($p = 0.15$/NS)	Chemo: 16 pts. Surgery alone: 9 pts

Abbreviations: *MDACC* MD Anderson Cancer Center, *FTCG* French Thoracic Cooperative Group, *C* cyclophosphamide, *E* etoposide, *P* cisplatin, *RT* radiotherapy, *Dz* disease, *chemo* chemotherapy, *pts* patients, *vs* versus, *OS* overall survival, *NR* not reported, *M* mitomycin, *I* ifosfamide, *DFS* disease free survival, *LRF* locoregional failure, *NS* not significant analysis, 56% vs 15%, respectively, resulting in closure of the trial early (Roth et al. 1998). Resection rates were similar between the two groups, revealing both the poor sensitivity of preoperative staging for resectability as well as the inability for this chemotherapy regimen to render more patients operable. There was a similar rate of local recurrences between the two arms, indicating that the apparent benefit in neoadjuvant chemotherapy was from systemic control.

Another study from Spain randomized 60 patients with stage IIIA NSCLC to surgery alone versus 3 cycles of mitomycin, ifosfamide, and cisplatin preoperatively followed by resection and postoperative mediastinal irradiation (Rosell et al. 1994). The results reported a statistically significant difference in median survival and median disease free survival favoring the preoperative chemotherapy group, with 2-year OS probabilities of 30% vs 0%. The bulk of the failures were metastatic in the surgery alone cohort although both arms had similar rates of locoregional failures.

Finally, a larger randomized trial performed by the French Thoracic Cooperative Group enrolled 355 patients with stage IB-IIIA NSCLC (Depierre et al. 2002). Again, the patients were randomized between preoperative chemotherapy with 2 cycles of mitomycin, ifosfamide, and cisplatin with two additional cycles postoperatively for responders versus primary surgery alone. In both arms, postoperative thoracic radiation was delivered if patients were found to have pT3 or pN2 disease. Improvement in overall survival was noted in the chemotherapy plus surgery arm over the surgery alone arm, but they were unable to find a benefit in the subset of N2 positive patients.

Taken together, these studies identified a benefit of neoadjuvant chemotherapy followed by surgery over surgery alone in locally advanced NSCLC, recognizing that both the MDACC and Spanish studies were quite small, making it difficult to draw concrete conclusions from their results. The Spanish Lung Cancer Group phase II study reported encouraging results with approximately 13% of stage IIIA/N2 patients achieving pathologic complete response with induction chemotherapy (Garrido et al. 2007). Still, there were high rates of locoregional recurrence identified. Efforts to intensify locoregional control, resectability, and pathologic complete response led to the investigation of adding radiation to chemotherapy in the neoadjuvant setting (Table 2).

2.3 Neoadjuvant Chemoradiotherapy Alone

Southwestern Oncology Group (SWOG) 8805 was one of the earliest studies to assess the potential benefit of neoadjuvant chemoradiotherapy following by surgery, often labeled trimodality therapy (Albain et al. 1995). Patients with biopsy proven N2 (IIIA), N3, or T4 primary lesions (IIIB) were eligible for enrollment. Induction chemotherapy was given with 2 cycles of cisplatin and etoposide plus concurrent radiation to 4500 cGy to the chest followed by attempted resection for responders or those with stable disease. Of the evaluable patients, 59% had an objective response to induction CRT (CR in 2 patients and PR in 72 patients) and 29% (37 patients) had stable disease. Based on response to induction CRT, 111 patients were ultimately eligible for surgery with 85% stage IIIA patients and 80% stage IIIB undergoing resection. A pathologic complete response was achieved in 21% of all patients, notably higher than the results with induction chemotherapy alone. Moreover, in patients who underwent resection with clinically stable disease after induction CRT, 46% had either no residual tumor or microscopic foci. A complete response was achieved in 15%, partial response in 57%, and stable disease in 13% of patients.

A total of 65 of the original 126 patients (51.6%) had a relapse. Only 11% had a solitary locoregional failure, 43% had a distant failure in a single site, 18% had distant failures in multiple sites, and 28% had both local and distant failures. The median survival time and 3-year survival rate for the 48 patients with pathologically clear mediastinal lymph nodes were significantly improved compared to all others (Table 2), remarkable outcomes in this era. Mediastinal

Table 2 Selected phase II trials of neoadjuvant therapy (chemotherapy or CRT) followed by surgery

Trial	No. of patients	Stages included	Treatment regimen	Resection rates	Local control	Progression-free survival	Overall survival	Toxicity (grade 5)
Neoadjuvant chemotherapy								
Spanish LCG trial 9901 (Garrido et al. 2007)	136	IIIA/N2, IIIB	PGT × 3 ® surgery	90 pts. underwent surgery: Overall complete resection rate: 68.9% pCR: 8.9% pCR (N2 ® N0): 27.3%	NR	Median EFS: 9.9 months	Median OS: 15.9 months 3, 5-year OS: 36.8%, 21.1% Median OS for complete resection: 48.5 months 3, 5-year OS for complete resection: 60.1%, 41.4%	7 pts. (7.8%)
Neoadjuvant chemoradiotherapy								
SWOG 8805 (Albain et al. 1995)	126	IIIA/N2, IIIB	PE × 2 with concurrent RT (45Gy) ® surgery	89 pts. resected; Overall pCR:21%; Nodal pCR: 56.5%	LRF: 11%	NR	2, 3-year OS for IIIA/N2: 37%, 27% Median and 3-year OS (nodal pCR vs all others): 30 months, 41% vs 9 months, 11% (p = 0.003)	13 pts. total; 2 during induction; 8 in postoperative period
GLCCG (Eberhardt et al. 1998)	94	IIIA/N2, IIIB	PE × 3 ® CRT(45Gy BID fractionation + PE × 1) ® surgery	62 pts. resected Complete resection: 67% pCR: 39%	LRF: 28%	Actuarial 3-year EFS for completely resected pts.: 49%	Median and 4-year OS for completely resected pts.: 42 months and 46%	6 pts. total; 2 from induction, 4 in postoperative period
RTOG 0229 (Suntharalingam et al. 2012)	57	IIIA/N2, IIIB/N3	CRT (61.2Gy + TC × 6) ® surgery	37 pts. resected; Complete resection: 76% pCR mediastinum: 63%	NR	Median and 2-year PFS: 12.9 months, 33%; pCR median and 2-year PFS: 19 months, 56%	Median and 2-year OS: 26.6 months, 54%; pCR 2-year OS: 75%	1 pt. in postoperative period

Abbreviations: *LCG* Lung Cancer Group, *SWOG* Southwestern Oncology Group, *GLCCG* German Lung Cancer Cooperative Group, *RTOG* Radiation Therapy Oncology Group, *P* cisplatin, *G* gemcitabine, *T* docetaxel, *pCR* pathologic complete response, *OS* overall survival, *EFS* event free survival, *NR* not reported, *E* etoposide, *RT* radiotherapy, *LRF* locoregional failure, *CRT* concurrent chemoradiotherapy, *Gy* gray, *BID* twice daily, *T* paclitaxel, *C* carboplatin clearance was the only significant predictor of long-term survival in these patients. In a subset analysis of 74 patients with initial positive N2 disease who were completely resected, there was a significant improvement in survival for the patients with mediastinal sterilization (median 30 vs 9 months, and 41% vs 11%, respectively, $p = 0.003$), and only three patient experienced any local relapse. These results drive home the importance that sterilization of nodal disease with induction therapy dramatically improves overall survival and appears to improve locoregional control.

The surgical morbidity and mortality outcomes from this trimodality study are of great importance as well. Ten percent of patient deaths were attributable to treatment: two during induction and 8 out of 13 during postoperative days 1–31. Of the 13 treatment related deaths that occurred postoperatively, 6 underwent pneumonectomy.

Now that a clear connection had been established between pathologic clearance of nodal disease with induction CRT and improved outcomes, other phase II studies attempted to further increase sterilization rates in the mediastinum (Table 2). A German phase II trial used an altered dose-fractionation scheme in unfavorable stage III disease (Eberhardt et al. 1998), delivering 3 cycles of cisplatin and etoposide followed by CRT using hyperfractionated accelerated radiation. At the end of induction therapy, approximately two-thirds of patients ultimately proceeded to resection. Pathologic complete response was achieved in 26% of all patients or 39% of all patients operated on. Of the 63 patients that underwent repeat mediastinoscopy after completion of induction therapy, there was a trend towards significant median and 4-year survival in the patients that had no residual disease versus those with residual N2/N3 disease (30 vs 17.5 months, 38% vs 15%, $p = 0.11$), and importantly, only one patient experienced a local failure at the resection stump. Four patients had a regional recurrence and thus only five operated patients had a locoregional recurrence.

RTOG 0229 was a multi-institutional phase II study with a primary endpoint to evaluate mediastinal nodal clearance in patients with stage III NSCLC (Suntharalingam et al. 2012). The goal of the study was to assess if definitive full-dose CRT (61.2 Gy total dose with concurrent carboplatin and paclitaxel) would affect rates of mediastinal sterilization and impact outcomes without untoward toxicity. Sixty-two percent of patients ultimately underwent resection. There was a single grade 5 toxicity related to postoperative pulmonary edema in a patient after a pneumonectomy, but only three patients needed a pneumonectomy. The rate of mediastinal clearance was 63% after full-dose CRT. The 2-year overall survival rate was 75% for those with nodal clearance, 52% for those with residual nodal disease, and 23% for those who were not offered resection ($p = 0.0002$). This study was vital because it showed that full-dose CRT is safe and effective to deliver prior to lobectomy, and patients achieving mediastinal clearance have, for stage III NSCLC, a remarkable outcome.

2.4 Neoadjuvant Chemotherapy Versus Neoadjuvant Chemoradiotherapy

The final comparison in the evolution of neoadjuvant treatment modalities is induction chemotherapy versus induction CRT (Table 3). The German Lung Cancer Cooperative Group (GLCCG) conducted a large multi-institutional, randomized phase III trial directly comparing these two induction strategies in marginally resectable disease (Thomas et al. 2008). The radiotherapy arm of this trial was the same as their previously discussed phase II trial, and the chemotherapy arm included the same 3 cycles of induction chemotherapy with cisplatin and etoposide alone followed by surgery. Patients in the control arm all received postoperative radiation to the chest. The primary endpoint of the trial was progression-free survival with secondary endpoints of overall survival and proportion of patients undergoing surgery. There was no difference in the likelihood of undergoing surgery between the arms, but of those patients undergoing surgery, complete resection was achieved in

Table 3 Reported phase III Trials of neoadjuvant therapy followed by surgical resection

Trial	No. of patients	Stages included	Treatment regimen	Resection rates	Local control	Progression-free survival	Overall survival	Toxicity (grade 5)
Neoadjuvant chemotherapy vs neoadjuvant CRT								
GLCCG (Thomas et al. 2008)	558	IIIA, IIIB	PE × 3 ⓘ HFX CRT (45Gy BID + CV) ⓘ surgery vs PE × 3 ⓘ surgery ⓘ RT	142 CRT resected vs 154 chemo resected; R0: 69% vs 55% favoring CRT ($p = 0.01$); Mediastinal down staging: 46% vs 29% favoring CRT ($p = 0.02$)	LRF: 34% CRT vs 40% chemo	Median PFS all resections: 19.6 months CRT vs 21.3 months chemo ($p = 0.64$); Median PFS R0 resection: 23.3 months CRT vs 44.4 months chemo ($p = 0.73$)	Median OS all resections: 32.4 months CRT vs 33.0 months chemo ($p = 0.54$); Median OS R0 resection: 43.1 months CRT vs 55.6 months chemo ($p = 0.82$)	CRT: 17 pts. (2 with chemo, 2 with RT, 13 with surgery); Chemo: 14 pts. (3 with chemo, 5 with post op RT, 6 with surgery)
SAKK (Pless et al. 2015)	232	IIIA/N2	PT × 3 ⓘ RT (44Gy/22fx) ⓘ surgery vs PT × 3 ⓘ surgery	99 CRT resected vs 94 chemo resected; R0: 91% CRT vs 81% chemo ($p = 0.06$); pCR: 16% CRT vs 12% chemo	LRF: 15% CRT vs 28% chemo	Median EFS: 12.8 months CRT vs 11.6 months chemo ($p = 0.67$)	Median OS: 37.1 months CRT vs 26.2 months chemo (NS)	CRT: 0 pts.; Chemo: 3 pts. in postoperative period
Trimodality (neoadjuvant CRT + surgery) vs definitive CRT								
EORTC 08941 (van Meerbeeck et al. 2007)	332	IIIA/N2	3 cycles platinum-based chemo ⓘ RT (60Gy) vs surgery alone	154 pts. resected; pCR: 5%; R0: 50%; ypN0: 25%	LRF: 55% RT vs 32% surgery	Median and 2-year PFS: RT: 11.3 months and 24%; Surgery: 9 months and 27%	Median and 5-year OS: RT: 17.5 months and 14%; Surgery: 16.4 months and 15.7%	1 pt. due to RT pneumonitis; 6 pts. in postoperative period
INT 0139 (Albain et al. 2009)	396	IIIA/N2	CRT (PE × 2 + 45Gy) ⓘ surgery ⓘ PE × 2 vs Definitive CRT alone (PE × 2 + 61Gy) ⓘ PE x2	164 pts. resected; ypN0: 46.3%	LRF: 10% CRT/S vs 22% CRT	Median PFS: 12.8 months CRT/S vs 10.5 months CRT ($p = 0.017$); 5-year PFS: 22% CRT/S vs 11% CRT	Median OS: 23.6 months CRT/S vs 22.2 months CRT ($p = 0.24$)	CRT/S: 17 pts. (14 pts. after pneumonectomy); CRT: 3 pts
ESPATUE (Eberhardt et al. 2015)	246	IIIA/N2, IIIB	PT × 3 ⓘ HFX CRT (45Gy BID + P/vinorelbine) ⓘ curgery vs CRT boost (65-71Gy)	70 pts. resected; R0: 94.3%; pCR: 33%	NR	5-year PFS: 35% CRT vs 32% CRT/S (NS)	5-year OS: 40% CRT vs 44% CRT/S (NS)	CRT: 2 pts.; CRT/S: 6 pts. (5 pts. in postoperative period)

Abbreviations: *EORTC* European Organization for Research and Treatment of Cancer, *chemo* chemotherapy, *RT* radiotherapy, *Gy* gray, *R0* complete resection, *pCR* pathologic complete response, *ypN0* pathologic complete response in mediastinum, *LRF* locoregional failure, *PFS* progression-free survival, *OS* overall survival, *CRT* concurrent chemoradiotherapy, *GLCCG* German Lung Cancer Cooperative Group, *INT* North American Intergroup, *P* cisplatin, *E* etoposide, *HFX* hyperfractionated, *BID* twice daily, *C* carboplatin, *V* vindesine, *T* docetaxel, *CRT/S* concurrent chemoradiotherapy + surgery, *T* paclitaxel

69% of patients in the induction CRT arm compared to 55% in the control arm ($p = 0.01$). There was a statistically significant difference between the proportion of those with mediastinal down staging (N2–3 to N0–1) between treatment groups (interventional group: 46%; control group: 29%; $p = 0.02$) and the proportion of patients with major histopathological response (CRT vs. chemotherapy, 60% vs. 20%; $p < 0.0001$). Those who had complete resection and successful mediastinal down staging after initial N2-N3 disease had better PFS and OS compared to those with persistent mediastinal disease, but despite these favorable pathologic results, there was no difference in progression-free survival (PFS) or overall survival (OS) between the two arms.

The SAKK Lung Cancer Project Group Trial was another large ($n = 232$), multicenter, randomized phase III study that compared neoadjuvant CRT and neoadjuvant chemotherapy alone followed by surgery in pathologically proven stage IIIA/N2 NSCLC patients (Pless et al. 2015). Those in the CRT arm received 3 cycles of neoadjuvant chemotherapy (cisplatin and docetaxel) followed by radiation (4400 cGy in 22 fractions delivered over 3 weeks with a concomitant boost technique), and those in the control arm received neoadjuvant chemotherapy alone. High rates of complete resection were achieved in both arms, but favoring the CRT arm. Nodal down staging (to N1 or N0) was observed in 64% and 53% of patients in the CRT and chemotherapy alone arms, respectively, but these differences were not significant. There were no statistically significant improvements in event free or overall survival, nor were there significant differences in postoperative complications.

Taken together, these two studies both suggest that complete resection is more feasible with the addition of radiotherapy, and nodal down staging may be more likely, although the choice of chemotherapy regimen may be important in this comparison. Yet while there was no dramatically worsened toxicity with the addition of preoperative radiotherapy, there was no clear oncologic benefit either. The last natural question is whether the morbidity of the surgical resection grants the patient a meaningful oncologic victory given its costs.

3 Neoadjuvant CRT (Trimodality) Versus Definitive CRT

Prior to studies comparing trimodality therapy and definitive CRT head to head, the European Organization for Research and Treatment of Cancer (EORTC) 08941 randomized control trial sought to establish surgical resection as the superior modality over radiation for locoregional control following response to induction therapy (van Meerbeeck et al. 2007). Patients with pathologically confirmed, unresectable stage IIIA/N2 NSCLC received 3 cycles of platinum-based induction chemotherapy and responders were randomized to undergo surgical resection or thoracic radiation. The primary endpoint was overall survival, with progression-free survival and toxicity as secondary endpoints. With an overall response rate of 61% to induction chemotherapy, approximately 330 patients were randomized with the study closing early due to slow accrual. Median OS and PFS were similar between the two groups. The radiation arm had significantly more locoregional failures as the first site of relapse compared to the surgery arm (absolute increase over 20%), with more distant failures occurring in the surgery arm (39% vs 61%).

Two randomized control trials looked to further establish a role for surgery and trimodality therapy in the management of stage IIIA/N2 NSCLC patients (Table 3). The first was the North American Intergroup 0139 (INT 0139) trial which compared trimodality therapy to definitive CRT (Albain et al. 2009). Patients with resectable, pathologically confirmed N2 disease were randomized to receive either concurrent CRT with 2 cycles of cisplatin and etoposide plus 4500 cGy followed by surgery or to continue with definitive CRT uninterrupted to full dose (6100 cGy). Two additional cycles of cisplatin and etoposide were given in each arm. Approximately 400 patients were enrolled in this study, and the median OS was not significantly different between the two arms. However, there was a 5-year progression-free survival benefit in the trimodality group, primarily because the CRT cohort had twice the risk of local failure. Patients who had a complete pathologic nodal response displayed an increased median OS (34.4 months vs 26.4 months) compared to those with residual nodal disease (T (any) N1–3). One critical finding in this study was 14 out of 54 patients undergoing a pneumonectomy died from the procedure.

This high number of deaths prompted the authors to perform an unplanned, exploratory OS analysis. Patients who underwent pneumonectomy and lobectomy were each matched 1:1 with patients in the CRT arm based on age, sex, performance status, and clinical T stage. Among patients in the lobectomy comparison, surgery significantly improved overall survival at 5 years (36% vs 18%, $p = 0.002$), without a similar advantage among the pneumonectomy cohort. Although this finding has been argued to support resection if the patient can undergo a lobectomy, such an interpretation is fallacious, because we do not know the correct comparator among the definitive CRT cohort. Patients were not stratified for randomization by expected surgery type, and those who were able to undergo lobectomy may have been responders or had smaller volume disease at diagnosis, both of which are potent confounders for survival when comparing to a non-selected CRT population.

The second trial, ESPATUE, again compared trimodality therapy versus definitive CRT with OS as the primary endpoint (Eberhardt et al. 2015). Patients with pathologically proven N2 disease and selected IIIB patients (who formed the majority of the population) received 3 cycles of induction chemotherapy with cisplatin and paclitaxel alone followed by neoadjuvant hyperfractionated CRT with concurrent cisplatin and vinorelbine. Patients who remained resectable were then randomized to surgery or a CRT boost. The primary endpoint was overall survival. The trial only accrued approximately half (246 patients) of its planned total, thus leaving it underpowered to detect an OS benefit. After induction therapy was complete, only 161 of the 246 patients were randomized (81 to undergo surgery and 80 to receive CRT boost). Pathologic complete response was seen in 27 (33%) of 81 randomized patients, but there were no significant differences in 5-year overall or progression-free survival; failure patterns were not reported.

A total of five (7%) patients experienced a grade 5 toxicity after surgery, but only one of those patients underwent pneumonectomy. Nevertheless, it is important to note that most of these patients had IIIB disease and they were heavily pre-selected prior to randomization, both with the addition of neoadjuvant chemotherapy and a pre-randomization tumor board that defined operability.

4 Stage IIIA/N2 NSCLC: When YES to Surgery

The data presented in this review reflect the extant prospective literature on the incorporation of surgical resection into the treatment of stage IIIA/N2 NSCLC. The one obvious conclusion from the randomized data is that many patients, if not most, will not benefit from trimodality therapy over definitive chemoradiotherapy. The results of the two critical randomized studies are clear that the typical patient does not gain an overall survival advantage from resection. Yet the large improvement in PFS seen in Intergroup 0139 is intriguing, and the *potentially significant reduction in local failure with resection* highlights the subgroup that may gain the most from this intensified local treatment.

A conceptual paradigm for the use of surgical resection after chemoradiotherapy can be designed by considering the competing risks of recurrence in this disease—locoregional versus distant—as well as the most salient signal we have of successful eradication of micrometastatic disease, nodal down staging (Table 4). Consider three hypothetical scenarios of the patient's disease status following neoadjuvant chemoradiotherapy. If the patient has experienced a pathologic CR in both the primary and nodes, the utility of surgical resection to clear residual dis-

Table 4 Conceptual framework for the integration of surgery into the management of stage IIIA/N2 non-small cell lung cancer

	Scenario 1	Scenario 2	Scenario 3
Mediastinal pathologic response (presumed)	−	+	−
Primary pathologic response (presumed)	−	±	+
Predicted locoregional control	Controlled	Not controlled	Not controlled
Predicted distant control	Controlled	Not controlled	Controlled
Recommendation	*No surgery*	*No surgery*	*Surgery*

ease is nil; there is nothing viable in the resection specimen to save from future recurrence. If on the other hand, the patient has residual disease in both the primary site and mediastinum while surgery may improve locoregional control by extirpating treatment-resistant cancer, the likelihood of remaining micrometastatic disease is so high that a survival advantage from the surgery is highly unlikely. Finally, consider the scenario in which the patient has sterilized the mediastinum but has persistent primary disease; in this subgroup, micrometastatic disease may have been successfully treated but there is disease left in the chest that will ultimately prove to be a first recurrence. For this key population, surgical resection is not just a reasonable approach but one that is supported by the data, provided a right-sided pneumonectomy would not be the required operation. That said, barring supernatural insight, one will not know the final pathology results prior to the surgery itself, and thus this proposed approach hinges on adequate preoperative restaging, which may include any combination of mediastinal sampling (preferred, (Muthu et al. 2018)) or radiologic imaging such as PET-CT (Kremer et al. 2016).

Whether a stage IIIA/N2 patient should undergo neoadjuvant chemotherapy alone is a more challenging question, because as seen in multiple studies, the true likelihood of resectability is closer to 60–70%, and patients may have received unnecessary induction chemotherapy and even an aborted surgery prior to moving forward with definitive chemoradiotherapy. Yet there is clearly a smaller cohort of patients with smaller volume primary disease and mediastinal lymphadenopathy that is clearly operable, and for these highly resectable individuals who may gain the benefit of early systemic therapy, chemotherapy followed by surgery is an appropriate paradigm.

5 Future Directions/Immunotherapy

In recent years, immunotherapy has led to a sea of change in the management of NSCLC. Initially used in the metastatic setting, the literature is growing on its uses in the consolidative and definitive settings. The results of the PACIFIC study, a phase III randomized trial using durvalumab after definitive CRT immediately changed the standard-of-care for unresectable stage III NSCLC (Antonia et al. 2017). The addition of adjuvant durvalumab significantly improved progression-free and overall survival. On the recent 3-year update, the addition of adjuvant immunotherapy improved OS by a remarkable 14%, 57% vs 43.5% (Gray et al. 2020); this 3-year OS result after durvalumab is superior or on par with almost any surgical study. Yet the locoregional failure risk was still approximately 20%, and the benefit to immunotherapy was limited to PD-L1 expressing tumors, leaving approximately 20% of individuals non-responsive to this adjuvant treatment.

Yet just like all is fair in love and war, so too may immunotherapy transform the use of surgery as well as chemoradiotherapy in stage IIIA/N2 disease. Preliminary studies using neoadjuvant immunotherapy followed by resection in this population have shown encouraging responses. For example, Forde et al. delivered 2 doses of nivolumab alone to patients with resectable stage I-IIIA NSCLC, and major pathologic responses were seen in 9 of 20 patients, and T-cell clones in both tumor and blood were also seen in almost all evaluated patients (Forde et al. 2018). The addition of neoadjuvant chemo-immunotherapy is also promising, with one prospective study finding an 87% resectability rate and 57% major pathologic response among 30, mostly stage IIIA, patients treated with neoadjuvant carboplatin, nab-paclitaxel, and atezolizumab (Shu et al. 2020).

With improved systemic control from immune checkpoint inhibition, the survival impact of superior locoregional control becomes more prominent. Yet it remains to be seen whether more successful treatment of micrometastatic disease warrants increased surgical risk or if a synchronous improvement in locoregional control with immunotherapy further minimizes any potential gain with thoracic resection.

6 Conclusion

Identifying which stage IIIA/N2 patients would benefit from surgical resection is difficult and requires input from a multidisciplinary thoracic oncology team, in part because of the heterogeneity of disease burden and prognoses incorporated under this stage. There is evidence to suggest that through careful and rigorous patient selection, there is a subset of stage IIIA patients with N2 disease who would be optimal candidates for surgical intervention. In particular, individuals whose mediastinum is pathologically sterilized by neoadjuvant therapy but have residual primary disease are ideal candidates for safe surgical resection. The introduction of immunotherapy into this paradigm has been groundbreaking, but whether it tilts the balance towards surgical resection for stage IIIA/N2 patients is an open question.

References

Albain KS, Rusch VW, Crowley JJ, Rice TW, Turrisi AT 3rd, Weick JK et al (1995) Concurrent cisplatin/etoposide plus chest radiotherapy followed by surgery for stages IIIA (N2) and IIIB non-small-cell lung cancer: mature results of southwest oncology group phase II study 8805. J Clin Oncol 13(8):1880–1892

Albain KS, Swann RS, Rusch VW, Turrisi AT 3rd, Shepherd FA, Smith C et al (2009) Radiotherapy plus chemotherapy with or without surgical resection for stage III non-small-cell lung cancer: a phase III randomised controlled trial. Lancet (London, England) 374(9687):379–386

Antonia SJ, Villegas A, Daniel D, Vicente D, Murakami S, Hui R et al (2017) Durvalumab after chemoradiotherapy in stage III non-small-cell lung cancer. N Engl J Med 377(20):1919–1929

Asamura H, Chansky K, Crowley J, Goldstraw P, Rusch VW, Vansteenkiste JF et al (2015) The International Association for the Study of Lung Cancer Lung Cancer Staging Project: proposals for the revision of the N descriptors in the forthcoming 8th edition of the TNM classification for lung cancer. J Thorac Oncol 10(12):1675–1684

Aupérin A, Le Péchoux C, Rolland E, Curran WJ, Furuse K, Fournel P et al (2010) Meta-analysis of concomitant versus sequential radiochemotherapy in locally advanced non-small-cell lung cancer. J Clin Oncol 28(13):2181–2190

Bradley JD, Hu C, Komaki RR, Masters GA, Blumenschein GR, Schild SE et al (2020) Long-term results of NRG oncology RTOG 0617: standard- versus high-dose chemoradiotherapy with or without cetuximab for unresectable stage III non-small-cell lung cancer. J Clin Oncol 38(7):706–714

Curran WJ Jr, Paulus R, Langer CJ, Komaki R, Lee JS, Hauser S et al (2011) Sequential vs. concurrent chemoradiation for stage III non-small cell lung cancer: randomized phase III trial RTOG 9410. J Natl Cancer Inst 103(19):1452–1460

Depierre A, Milleron B, Moro-Sibilot D, Chevret S, Quoix E, Lebeau B et al (2002) Preoperative chemotherapy followed by surgery compared with primary surgery in resectable stage I (except T1N0), II, and IIIa non-small-cell lung cancer. J Clin Oncol 20(1):247–253

Dillman RO, Herndon J, Seagren SL, Eaton WL Jr, Green MR (1996) Improved survival in stage III non-small-cell lung cancer: seven-year follow-up of cancer and leukemia group B (CALGB) 8433 trial. J Natl Cancer Inst 88(17):1210–1215

Eberhardt W, Wilke H, Stamatis G, Stuschke M, Harstrick A, Menker H et al (1998) Preoperative chemotherapy followed by concurrent chemoradiation therapy based on hyperfractionated accelerated radiotherapy and definitive surgery in locally advanced non-small-cell lung cancer: mature results of a phase II trial. J Clin Oncol 16(2):622–634

Eberhardt WE, Pöttgen C, Gauler TC, Friedel G, Veit S, Heinrich V et al (2015) Phase III study of surgery versus definitive concurrent chemoradiotherapy boost in patients with resectable stage IIIA(N2) and selected IIIB non-small-cell lung cancer after induction chemotherapy and concurrent chemoradiotherapy (ESPATUE). J Clin Oncol 33(35):4194–4201

Forde PM, Chaft JE, Smith KN, Anagnostou V, Cottrell TR, Hellmann MD et al (2018) Neoadjuvant PD-1 blockade in resectable lung cancer. N Engl J Med 378(21):1976–1986

Garrido P, González-Larriba JL, Insa A, Provencio M, Torres A, Isla D et al (2007) Long-term survival associated with complete resection after induction chemotherapy in stage IIIA (N2) and IIIB (T4N0-1) non small-cell lung cancer patients: the Spanish lung cancer group trial 9901. J Clin Oncol 25(30):4736–4742

Goldstraw P, Chansky K, Crowley J, Rami-Porta R, Asamura H, Eberhardt WE et al (2016) The IASLC lung cancer staging project: proposals for revision of the TNM stage groupings in the forthcoming (eighth) edition of the TNM classification for lung cancer. J Thorac Oncol 11(1):39–51

Gray JE, Villegas A, Daniel D, Vicente D, Murakami S, Hui R et al (2020) Three-year overall survival with durvalumab after chemoradiotherapy in stage III NSCLC-update from PACIFIC. J Thorac Oncol 15(2):288–293

Kremer R, Peysakhovich Y, Dan LF, Guralnik L, Kagna O, Nir RR et al (2016) FDG PET/CT for assessing the resectability of NSCLC patients with N2 disease after neoadjuvant therapy. Ann Nucl Med 30(2):114–121

Martini N, Flehinger BJ (1987) The role of surgery in N2 lung cancer. Surg Clin North Am 67(5):1037–1049

Martini N, Flehinger BJ, Zaman MB, Beattie EJ (1981) Results of surgical treatment in N2 lung cancer. World J Surg 5(5):663–666

Mountain CF (1990) Expanded possibilities for surgical treatment of lung cancer. Survival in stage IIIa disease. Chest 97(5):1045–1051

Muthu V, Sehgal IS, Dhooria S, Aggarwal AN, Agarwal R (2018) Efficacy of endosonographic procedures in mediastinal restaging of lung cancer after neoadjuvant therapy: a systematic review and diagnostic accuracy meta-analysis. Chest 154(1):99–109

Perez CA, Pajak TF, Rubin P, Simpson JR, Mohiuddin M, Brady LW et al (1987) Long-term observations of the patterns of failure in patients with unresectable non-oat cell carcinoma of the lung treated with definitive radiotherapy. Report by the radiation therapy oncology group. Cancer 59(11):1874–1881

Pless M, Stupp R, Ris HB, Stahel RA, Weder W, Thierstein S et al (2015) Induction chemoradiation in stage IIIA/N2 non-small-cell lung cancer: a phase 3 randomised trial. Lancet (London, England) 386(9998):1049–1056

Rosell R, Gómez-Codina J, Camps C, Maestre J, Padille J, Cantó A et al (1994) A randomized trial comparing preoperative chemotherapy plus surgery with surgery alone in patients with non-small-cell lung cancer. N Engl J Med 330(3):153–158

Roth JA, Fossella F, Komaki R, Ryan MB, Putnam JB Jr, Lee JS et al (1994) A randomized trial comparing perioperative chemotherapy and surgery with surgery alone in resectable stage IIIA non-small-cell lung cancer. J Natl Cancer Inst 86(9):673–680

Roth JA, Atkinson EN, Fossella F, Komaki R, Bernadette Ryan M, Putnam JB Jr et al (1998) Long-term follow-up of patients enrolled in a randomized trial comparing perioperative chemotherapy and surgery with surgery alone in resectable stage IIIA non-small-cell lung cancer. Lung Cancer (Amsterdam, Netherlands) 21(1):1–6

Sause WT, Scott C, Taylor S, Johnson D, Livingston R, Komaki R et al (1995) Radiation therapy oncology group (RTOG) 88-08 and eastern cooperative oncology group (ECOG) 4588: preliminary results of a phase III trial in regionally advanced, unresectable non-small-cell lung cancer. J Natl Cancer Inst 87(3):198–205

Shu CA, Gainor JF, Awad MM, Chiuzan C, Grigg CM, Pabani A et al (2020) Neoadjuvant atezolizumab and chemotherapy in patients with resectable non-small-cell lung cancer: an open-label, multicentre, single-arm, phase 2 trial. Lancet Oncol 21(6):786–795

Suntharalingam M, Paulus R, Edelman MJ, Krasna M, Burrows W, Gore E et al (2012) Radiation therapy oncology group protocol 02-29: a phase II trial of neoadjuvant therapy with concurrent chemotherapy and full-dose radiation therapy followed by surgical resection and consolidative therapy for locally advanced non-small cell carcinoma of the lung. Int J Radiat Oncol Biol Phys 84(2):456–463

Thomas M, Rübe C, Hoffknecht P, Macha HN, Freitag L, Linder A et al (2008) Effect of preoperative chemoradiation in addition to preoperative chemotherapy: a randomised trial in stage III non-small-cell lung cancer. Lancet Oncol 9(7):636–648

van Meerbeeck JP, Kramer GW, Van Schil PE, Legrand C, Smit EF, Schramel F et al (2007) Randomized controlled trial of resection versus radiotherapy after induction chemotherapy in stage IIIA-N2 non-small-cell lung cancer. J Natl Cancer Inst 99(6):442–450

Wagner H Jr, Lad T, Piantadosi S, Ruckdeschel JC (1994) Randomized phase 2 evaluation of preoperative radiation therapy and preoperative chemotherapy with mitomycin, vinblastine, and cisplatin in patients with technically unresectable stage IIIA and IIIB non-small cell cancer of the lung. LCSG 881. Chest 106(6 Suppl):348s–354s

Warram J (1975) Preoperative irradiation of cancer of the lung: final report of a therapeutic trial. A collaborative study. Cancer 36(3):914–925

Ziel E, Hermann G, Sen N, Bonomi P, Liptay MJ, Fidler MJ et al (2015) Survival benefit of surgery after chemoradiotherapy for stage III (N0-2) non-small-cell lung cancer is dependent on pathologic nodal response. Jo Thorac Oncol 10(10):1475–1480

Combined Radiation Therapy and Chemotherapy as an Exclusive Treatment Option in Locally Advanced Inoperable Non-small Cell Lung Cancer

Branislav Jeremić, Pavol Dubinsky, Slobodan Milisavljević, and Ivane Kiladze

Contents

1 Introduction 548
2 Radiation Therapy Alone 548
3 Induction Chemotherapy Followed by Radiation Therapy 550
4 Concurrent Radiochemotherapy 552
5 Neoadjuvant (Induction) Chemotherapy Followed by Radiation Therapy Versus Concurrent Radiochemotherapy 555
6 Optimization of Concurrent Radiochemotherapy 557
7 New Approaches in Radiation Therapy and Chemotherapy of Locally Advanced Non-small Cell Lung Cancer 560
8 Conclusions 562
References 563

B. Jeremić (✉)
School of Medicine, University of Kragujevac, Kragujevac, Serbia
e-mail: nebareje@gmail.com

P. Dubinsky
University Hospital to East Slovakia Institute of Oncology, Kosice, Slovakia

S. Milisavljević
Department of Thoracic Surgery, University Clinical Center, Kragujevac, Serbia

I. Kiladze
Department of Clinical Oncology, Caucasus Medical Center, Tbilisi, Georgia

Abstract

Locally advanced non-small cell lung cancer is one of the major battlegrounds in clinical research in lung cancer. Improved diagnostic and staging opportunities were not followed by increased efforts in a systematic way, e.g., prospective randomized studies which could have helped us optimize our treatment approaches. Although limited prospects for all of the treatment options remain nowadays, the vast minority of patients are treated with surgery in combination with other treatment modalities. The remaining one, and they represent the vast majority of cases treated either alone with radiation therapy or systemic therapy or various combinations in both curative and palliative setting. In curative setting, though, evidence accumulated over the past 3 decades supports superiority of concurrent radiochemotherapy over other existing treatment options. It is expected that with novel radiotherapy technologies and new generations of drugs overall results in this disease are further improved.

1 Introduction

Approximately one-third of all patients with non-small cell lung cancer (NSCLC) present with a locally advanced disease. Patients falling into this group represent a heterogeneous group of patients. According to staging systems used in the past 35 years (Mountain 1986, 1997; Golsdstraw et al. 2007; Goldstraw et al. 2016), this remains almost synonymous to stage III. The most recent attempt of the International Association for the Study of Lung Cancer (Rami-Porta et al. 2014; Goldstraw et al. 2016) provided additional step in a continuous evolution of the staging principles in lung cancer. Both previous and current staging systems were nevertheless surgical, focused exclusively the size of the tumor, its location, and invasion of neighboring structures. These systems even nowadays, unfortunately, never took into account tumor volumes. That said, a major principle of anticancer action of both radiation therapy (RT) and chemotherapy (CHT), and that is log cell kill, is not considered at all. This is an extremely important issue, tumors could have had similar tumor volume, but which could have been designed a different stage in case of different location or invasion of neighboring structures. This is especially important in stage III NSCLC which has also underwent a change in the most recent staging revision. If we exclude all existing, that is, eight, T and N combinations belonging to stage IIIA, a focus of two previous chapters, still, however, remaining stage IIIB and IIIC, respectively, have a total of nine different T and N combinations, ranging from T3N2 to T4N3. The contribution of T and N component, to a particular sub/stage obviously greatly varies. Although stage subgroupings mostly reflect similar prognosis, one crucial issue remained unanswered: is there even more specific "effect trade-off" when adverse effect of an increasing T substage is, perhaps, leveled-off with decreasing N substage, or which one of these two descriptors of substages may be more important than the other one and if so, then exactly when? Finally, since volumes of these descriptors could also vary (depending on their size, multiplicity, and/or location), the nature of non-surgical cell kill (i.e., log cell kill) favors the volume use, importance of which in relation to treatment outcome will be discussed in detail further in this chapter.

2 Radiation Therapy Alone

Locally advanced NSCLC has frequently been treated with RT alone in the past 50 years since the early reports showed that it led to an improvement in survival over the best supportive care (Roswit et al. 1968), in spite of shortcomings from the early studies (outdated techniques of diagnosis/staging, RT treatment planning, and execution). In the landmark trial, continuous course RT with doses of 50–60 Gy has been shown to be superior to 40 Gy given either split-course or continuous course (Perez et al. 1986). The 60 Gy-continuous course schedule has subsequently been adopted as the standard RT. However, the results obtained with RT alone were unsatisfactory, since the median survival time (MST) was approximately 9–10 months and the overall survival (OS) rate at 5 years was only 3–6% in prospective randomized trials (Holsti and Matson 1980; Petrovich et al. 1981; Perez et al. 1987). Since various retrospective and prospective randomized studies have revealed that both local and systemic failure play an important role in the poor survival of these patients (Petrovich et al. 1977; Cox et al. 1979; Perez et al. 1986), various means of improving local and systemic control of this disease were sought.

Altered fractionation regimens have also been used to improve local control (Cox et al. 1990, 1993; Saunders and Dische 1990; Byhardt et al. 1993). The Radiation Therapy Oncology Group (RTOG) (Cox et al. 1990) has investigated hyperfractionated (Hfx) RT with 1.2 Gy b.i.d. fractions and reported improved survival in a subgroup of patients with favorable prognostic factors treated with doses ≥69.6 Gy compared to that obtained with the standard treatment (60 Gy/30 fractions/6 weeks). Continuous hyperfractionated accelerated radiation therapy (CHART) was tested against standard fractionation RT in inoperable NSCLC and it was shown be beneficial (Saunders et al. 1999). This treatment design was, unfortunately, extremely complicated for daily clinical practice preventing it from widespread use. Several attempts to modify it included the omission of weekend days or neoadjuvant CHT, both of which effectively destroyed its underlying principle and that was accelerated fractionated RT to combat accelerated tumor clonogen proliferation. It was then not surprising that the CHART Weekend-less CHARTWEL trial which compared 66 Gy in 33 daily fractions with 60 Gy in 40 fractions in 18 treatment days (t.i.d.) has not found a survival advantage for accelerated regimen (Baumann et al. 2005). Recent years also brought attempts to combined acceleration and hyperfractionation in less demanding regimen, such as Hyperfractionated Accelerated Radiation Therapy (HART) (Mehta et al. 1998) which also proven to be effective in this setting. A decade ago, Zhang et al. (2012) performed a meta-analysis comparing conventional and non-conventional RT. Their analysis included 13 randomized controlled trials with a total of 2206 patients and showed that the non-conventional RT group could significantly improve the overall response rate (ORR) (OR 1.68, 95% confidence intervals (CI) 1.19–2.37) and 1–5 year OS as well as 1–3 year local control compared with the conventional RT group. With regard to the side effects, non-conventional RT was more likely to result in grade 3 and 4 RT-induced esophagitis, but there was no significant difference in the incidence of RT-induced pneumonitis. In the subgroup analysis they found late course accelerated Hfx RT improving 1–3 year OS and ORR.

Studies using altered fractionated regimens reconfirmed the duality of patterns of failure in patients treated with RT alone. This fact again stressed the need to add CHT to the overall treatment plan, to improve both local/regional control and combat possible distant (microscopic) spread, the latter not addressed by the RT. Unfortunately, the results of early studies designed with that aim were neither encouraging nor different from that obtained with RT alone. Timing of CHT administration was usually adjuvant (i.e., post-RT) and it consisted of non-platinum based drugs (Reynolds and O'Dell 1978; White et al. 1982). RT-induced fibrotic changes in lungs that prevented successful blood/drug perfusion and, therefore, drug supply to the tumor-bearing area, were likely the main reason for such an observation. Inefficiency of then-available drugs, mostly considered as first-generation CHT drugs, originating in the pre-cisplatin era (Reynolds and O'Dell 1978; White et al. 1982) was also implicated as important additional reason.

Contrary to this, RT and platinum-based CHT have been increasingly practiced around the world in the past four decades. A number of possible combinations have arisen, largely exploiting different aspects of such combination, frequently focusing on the issue of timing/scheduling, and mostly being cisplatin based. Induction (neoadjuvant) CHT followed by radical RT (Dillman et al. 1990; Sause et al. 1995), "sandwich" CHT, and RT (Le Chevalier et al. 1992) as well as concurrent RT-CHT (Schaake-Koning et al. 1992; Jeremic et al. 1995, 1996, 1998) have all gained widespread use. Sometimes very similar results were obtained with these approaches, obtained with quite different radiobiological background. To further obscure the overall picture, both RT and CHT have evolved over the years. A number of different time/dose/fractionation RT regimens have been used (Cox et al. 1990; Byhardt et al. 1993; Saunders and Dische 1990). They paralleled the introduction of the third generation of CHT drugs, namely paclitaxel (Johnson et al. 1996; Herscher et al. 1998), docetaxel (Millward et al. 1996; Mauer et al. 1998), vinorelbine (LeChevalier et al. 1994; Masters et al. 1998), gemcitabine (Manegold et al. 1997; Vokes et al. 1998), irinotecan (Fukuoka et al. 1992; Oshita et al. 1997), and topotecan (Lynch et al. 1994; Perez-Soler et al. 1996). In most recent years, a number of new CHT agents as well as targeted agents and finally the immunotherapy drug have been introduced into the clinical research in this disease.

3 Induction Chemotherapy Followed by Radiation Therapy

Major aims of this type of combined RT and CHT are (1) to decrease tumor burden, which may permit delivery of RT to a reduced tumor volume and (2) to combat micrometastatic disease, believed to be present at the time of starting the treatment. Increased drug delivery with less overall toxicity (especially those expected to occur within the RT treatment field) may also be one of the possible advantages when compared to concurrent administration. Potential disadvantages of induction treatment include (1) prolonged overall treatment time, (2) significant toxicity due to CHT preventing or delaying the delivery of full RT dose, (3) tumor cell resistance induced by CHT which results in reduced RT efficacy, as well as (4) accelerated tumor clonogen repopulation which occurs during the CHT (Byhardt et al. 1998; Byhardt 1999).

Several phase III trials have demonstrated a survival benefit for induction CHT over RT alone. The Cancer and Leukemia Group B (CALGB) 8433 was the landmark trial comparing sequential RT-CHT vs. RT alone in the treatment of patients with locally advanced NSCLC (Dillman et al. 1990). Induction CHT consisted of cisplatin and vinblastine. RT to a total dose of 60 Gy in 30 fractions was given in both arms and began on day 50 in the combined modality arm. Although there were no treatment-related deaths on either arm, the addition of CHT increased the number of hospital admissions for vomiting (5% vs. 0%) and infection (7% vs. 3%). In the initial report (Dillman et al. 1990), induction CHT improved MST (13.8 vs. 9.7 months, $p = 0.0066$) and 3-year survival (23% vs. 11%). Seven year follow-up of that study confirmed superiority of induction CHT (MST, 13.7 vs. 9.6 months, $p = 0.012$) over RT alone (Dillman et al. 1996).

The Radiation Therapy Oncology Group/ Eastern Cooperative Oncology Group (RTOG/ ECOG) trial was a trial which randomized 458 patients with good performance status (PS), and minimal weight loss to receive either once daily RT to 60 Gy in 2 Gy fractions or the same RT with two cycles of induction cisplatin and vinblastine (Sause et al. 1995), or the RT given twice daily (1.2 Gy b.i.d.) to a total dose of 69.6 Gy. The MST was statistically superior ($p = 0.03$) for the combined modality arm (13.8 months) vs. either the standard RT arm (11.4 months) or the twice daily RT arm (12.3 months). Prolonged follow-up of this study reconfirmed superiority of combined modality therapy. However, long-term survival rates remained less than 10% (Sause et al. 2000).

French phase III trial tested RT alone vs. combined RT-CHT (Le Chevalier et al. 1991). In this trial, 353 patients with unresectable locally advanced squamous cell or large cell lung carcinoma were randomized to either RT alone (65 Gy in 2.5 Gy fractions) or three monthly cycles of cisplatin-based CHT followed by the same RT regimen and followed again by the same CHT. A significant decrease in distant metastases for the combined modality arm was observed and the MST (12.0 vs. 10.0 months) and 2-year survival rates (21% vs. 14%, $p = 0.02$) were improved as well (Le Chevalier et al. 1992). Long-term follow-up provided, unfortunately, more sobering facts: only 8% of patients had continued local control at 5 years (Arriagada et al. 1997), while 5-year survival rates remained poor at 6% and 3% (for the two arms), likely a consequence of the high rate of local failure on both arms. An intriguing question remained unanswered: was improvement in the distant metastasis control a consequence of starting the treatment with induction CHT or it was a mere reflection of higher total doses being given (due to a post-RT CHT also being given)?

The Medical Research Council also performed a trial which randomized 447 eligible patients with good PS and localized, inoperable NSCLC to receive either RT alone or cisplatin-based induction CHT followed by the same RT (Cullen et al. 1997). On both arms, the median RT dose in both arm was rather low, 50 Gy. The MST was improved with the addition of CHT (13.0 vs. 9.9 months, $p = 0.056$) although this difference was of borderline (in)significance.

What these trials have demonstrated is that the addition of platinum-based induction CHT to RT resulted in improved survival over that obtained with the same RT given alone. While this certainly holds true for short-term survival, long-term survival figures remained to be dismal, indicating that only modest improvements in long-term survival have been achieved. Three large meta-analyses have demonstrated a small but consistent survival benefit for the addition of induction CHT to RT for locally advanced NSCLC (Non-small Cell Lung Cancer Collaborative Group 1995; Marino et al. 1995; Pritchard and Anthony 1996).

Since it became obvious that patterns of failure after induction CHT followed by conventionally fractionated radical RT shifted focus towards more locoregional failures, investigators made efforts to offer more intensive latter (i.e., RT) part of the combined treatment. By doing so, Clamon et al. (1999) compared the standard induction CHT consisting of cisplatin/vinblastine followed by standard RT (60 Gy in 30 daily fractions). RT was given either with or without concurrently given weekly carboplatin as radiosensitizer. No difference in OS (MST: 13.4 vs. 13.5 months; 4-year survival: 13% vs. 10%; $p = 0.74$) was found between the radiosensitized and non-radiosensitized groups of patients. These results showed that induction cisplatin/vinblastine followed by conventionally fractionated radical RT and concurrent CHT is not consistently reproduced, being inferior in the study of Clamon et al. (1999) to what was expected from previous two studies (Dillman et al. 1990; Sause et al. 1995). They have shown that even when sensitized by carboplatin, standard fraction RT cannot compensate for accelerated proliferation of surviving tumor clonogens which occur during the induction (CHT) phase of treatment. Furthermore, the results of the study of Clamon et al. (1999) were not different from those obtained by Hfx RT alone in the Radiation Therapy Oncology Group/Eastern Cooperative Oncology Group study 8808 (Sause et al. 1995) or the same Hfx RT (69.6 Gy using 1.2 Gy twice daily) in the study of Jeremic et al. (1996).

In an attempt to additionally intensify the second part (i.e., RT) of the combined treatment even more, Vokes et al. (2002) reported on randomized phase II study of CALGB 9431 which used two cycles of induction CHT (cisplatin/gemcitabine or cisplatin/paclitaxel or cisplatin/vinorelbine) followed by the two cycles of the same CHT concurrently with conventionally fractionated radical RT (66 Gy). While the MST for all patients was 17 months, 3-year survival rates for the three groups were 28%, 19%, and 23%, respectively. Although authors suggested that this approach led to improvement in outcome when compared to previous CALGB experience (Dillman et al. 1990, 1996; Clamon et al. 1999), it seemed it did not improve the outcome when compared to what concurrent RT-CHT offered. Several subsequent studies of the similar design only reconfirmed these observations. They have clearly shown that *ANY* intensification of the latter/major part of the combined treatment approach via concurrent RT-CHT was not effective, once the treatment had started with induction CHT, as there was no compensation for insufficient start (Clamon et al. 1999; Vokes et al. 2002; Akerley et al. 2005; Socinski et al. 2008). Other attempts, such as the use of three daily fractions of RT (Belani et al. 2005a, b), also proved to be ineffective. In that trial which compared standard fractionation RT vs. HART, all patients in both arms received induction CHT with carboplatin/paclitaxel. Concurrent CHT was not used during the RT course. Unfortunately, the study did not meet its accrual goals and was closed early; nonetheless the results were not significantly different (MST and 3-year survival: 22.2 months, and 20% vs. 13.7 months, and 15%, respectively) (Belani et al. 2005a, b). All in all, whatever you do after you start with CHT, failure is inevitable and comes fast. With this approach, you can only achieve more toxicity (Vokes et al. 2002; Socinski et al. 2008) and even if you use the modern RT tools such as three-dimensional radiation therapy (3D RT) and attempt treatment intensification by escalating the total dose, again, one cannot achieve better outcome. Indeed, impressive 12% mortality in CALGB attempt (Socinski et al. 2008) to combine induction CHT with subsequently given concurrent RT-CHT led investigators to early stopping the trial. Other authors reached the same conclusion in studies which induction CHT was followed by several concurrent RT-CHT regimens using different drugs and different RT regimens (Nyman et al. 2009; Hatton et al. 2011).

Radiobiological principles can easily serve the purpose of identifying reasons of never-achieved improvement in local control in locally advanced NSCLC treated with induction CHT followed by either conventionally fractionated radical RT or RT-CHT. The study of El Sharouni et al. (2003) has compared CT scans pre- and post-induction CHT, focusing on the time from the last induction CHT cycle to the time of RT treatment planning CT was actually done. They have been able to measure an increase in gross tumor volumes (GTVs) and subsequently define volume doubling times. During the waiting period (for the planning of CT scan and start of RT), a total of 41% of all tumors became incurable, with the ratio of GTVs being in the range of 1.1–81.8. Tumor doubling times ranged 8.3–171 days, with the median of 29 days. In other words, even if one may have thought that CT-defined response occurs (and that it matters), there is actually an opposite development, with surviving tumor clonogens repopulating fast, leading tumors to regrow to the state of incurability. Recent confirmation of these observations came from Bozcuk et al. (2010) who attempted to correlate the benefit from induction CHT before RT in NSCLC using a meta-analytical approach with meta-regression analysis. They have used thirteen randomized clinical trials including 2776 patients. Time to RT was inversely associated with the benefit from induction CHT at 2- ($p = 0.050$) and 3-years ($p = 0.093$). This meta-analysis highlighted the importance of shorter time to RT to maximize NSCLC patients' survival.

4 Concurrent Radiochemotherapy

This combined modality approach denotes the administration of both modalities at the same time, meaning that CHT is given during the course of radical, curative RT. A number of variations exist, including CHT being administered on a 3-weekly, bi-weekly, weekly, or daily basis although concurrent RT-CHT employing third-generation drugs (e.g., paclitaxel) also witnessed administration of the drug twice or trice weekly. Whatever was the design of concurrent RT-CHT, its main aim is to address the issue of locoregional and distant disease at the same time, from the start of the treatment as intensively as possible. This, unfortunately, may lead to increased toxicity (mostly acute) which may require dose reductions or treatment interruptions, both adversely influencing treatment outcome. On the other side, with this approach two of radiobiological premises, namely independent cell kill and synergistic action, as postulated by Steel and Peckham (1979), can be exploited.

Concurrent RT-CHT was compared to RT alone, the former aiming mostly on an improvement at local tumor control. A number of prospective randomized phase III studies investigated this issue (Soresi et al. 1988; Schaake-Koning et al. 1992; Trovo et al. 1992; Blanke et al. 1995; Jeremic et al. 1995, 1996; Bonner et al. 1998; Ball et al. 1999; Groen et al. 2004). Relatively low total RT dose (Soresi et al. 1988; Trovo et al. 1992) and CHT being given in an insufficient total dose (Soresi et al. 1988) were likely reasons for suboptimal results. All three positive studies, however, used protracted CHT dosing. While an European Organization for Research and Treatment of Cancer study (Schaake-Koning et al. 1992) tested both daily and weekly cisplatin with split-course RT, showing superior outcome for daily cisplatin/RT, Jeremic et al. first used bi-weekly and weekly (Jeremic et al. 1995) and then daily (Jeremic et al. 1996) carboplatin/etoposide with Hfx RT doses of 64.8 (Jeremic et al. 1995) and then 69.6 Gy (Jeremic et al. 1996). The best results were obtained with low-dose daily CHT given during the Hfx RT course, with 4–5 year survival rates being at the order of 20% (Jeremic et al. 1995, 1996). Survival advantage in these three studies was a consequence of an advantage at local tumor level, confirming radiobiological expectations that low-dose daily CHT has acted synergistically with RT, and enhanced its effects on local tumor level. Also as expected, no influence on distant metastasis control was noted. Ulutin et al. (2000) reported on a three-armed study which compared sequential and concurrent RT-CHT. Each treatment arm consisted of 15 patients with histologically confirmed stage III NSCLC. In group 1, the main treatment approach was split-course RT alone. In group 2, cisplatin was applied daily and concurrently with split-course RT. In group 3, two cycles of etoposide, ifosfamide, and cisplatin, which ended 3 weeks before split-course RT, were applied. Overall response rates were 40%, 66%, and 53% in groups 1–3, respectively. Median survival was 10, 11, and 10 months for groups 1–3, respectively. Recently, another study from Turkey (Cakir and Egehan 2004) provided additional evidence that concurrent RT (64 Gy in 32 daily fractions) and cisplatin (20 mg/sqm, days 1–5, weeks 2 and 6) offer survival advantage over the same RT alone (3-year survival, 10% vs. 2%). Combined treatment approach also offered better locoregional control ($p = 0.0001$) and disease-free survival (DFS) ($p = 0.0006$). Most recently, West Japan Thoracic Oncology Group (Yamamoto et al. 2010) presented the data from a phase III trial of concurrent RT-CHT (WJTOG0105) which was conducted to compare third-generation CHT with second-generation CHT in patients with unresectable stage III NSCLC. Eligible patients received the following treatments: A (control), four cycles of mitomycin/vindesine/cisplatin plus thoracic RT 60 Gy (treatment break for 1 week); B, weekly irinotecan/carboplatin for 6 weeks plus thoracic RT 60 Gy, followed by two courses of irinotecan/carboplatin; C, weekly paclitaxel/carboplatin for 6 weeks plus thoracic RT 60 Gy, followed by two courses of paclitaxel/carboplatin. The MST and 5-year survival rates were 20.5, 19.8, and 22.0 months and 17.5, 17.8, and 19.8% in arms A–C, respectively. While no significant differences in OS were apparent among the treatment arms, noninferiority of the experimental arms was not achieved. The incidences of grade 3–4 neutropenia, febrile neutropenia, and gastrointestinal disorder were significantly higher in arm A than in arm B or C ($p < 0.001$). CHT interruptions were more common in arm B than in arm A or C. Arm C was equally efficacious and exhibited a more favorable toxicity profile among three arms. This study confirmed effectiveness of third-generation CHT and concurrent RT in this setting. In a similar study, also coming from Japan, Segawa et al. (2010) reported on a phase III trial comparing docetaxel and cisplatin with mitomycin, vindesine, and cisplatin both given with concurrent thoracic RT. The survival time at 2 years, a primary end point, was favorable to the docetaxel and cisplatin arm ($p = 0.059$ by a stratified log-rank test as a planned analysis and $p = 0.044$ by an early-period, weighted log-rank as an unplanned analysis). There was a trend toward improved response rate, 2-year survival rate, median progression-free survival (PFS) time, and MST in the docetaxel and cisplatin arm (78.8, 60.3%, 13.4, and 26.8 months, respectively) compared with the mitomycin, vindesine, and cisplatin arm (70.3, 48.1%, 10.5, and 23.7 months, respectively) although not statistically significant ($p > 0.05$). Grade 3 febrile neutropenia occurred more often in the mitomycin, vindesine, and cisplatin arm than in the docetaxel and cisplatin arm (39% vs. 22%, respectively; $p = 0.012$), and grade 3–4 radiation esophagitis was likely to be more common in the docetaxel and cisplatin arm than in the mitomycin, vindesine, and cisplatin arm (14% vs. 6%, $p = 0.056$). This study showed that docetaxel and cisplatin given with concurrent RT may be seen as an alternative to mitomycin, vindesine and cisplatin given with concurrent RT in patients with locally advanced NSCLC.

Important observation from clinical trials is that studies/arms which used high-dose CHT (mimicking classic CHT administration and necessarily given with more split between the consecutive CHT cycles) concurrently with RT neither had any impact on distant metastasis control, nor did so on local level. Beside the overall treatment success, another advantage of low-dose concurrent CHT over high-dose CHT and concurrent RT is that the former type of concurrent RT-CHT leads to less high-grade acute toxicity and, consequently, better treatment compliance, less treatment interruptions, which influence on treatment outcome (Cox et al. 1993). Recently,

Harada et al. (2009) retrospectively compared the survival and toxicities associated with RT-CHT using full-dose and weekly regimens in patients with stage III NSCLC. In both univariate and multivariate analyses, treatment with weekly regimens was associated with a better OS than that with full-dose regimens (2-year survival rates: 75% for weekly regimens vs. 41% for full-dose regimens). The toxicities and compliance in the two groups were comparable. These results indirectly supported previous observations that low-dose daily CHT (Schaake-Koning et al. 1992; Jeremic et al. 1995, 1996, 2005) provides good treatment results with lower toxicity than that observed with high-dose RT and concurrent high-dose CHT.

In an attempt to improve local control, radiation dose escalation with conventional fractionation and concurrent CHT was performed (Rosenman et al. 2002; Belani et al. 2005a, b; Lee 2006; Bradley et al. 2010). Results of these trials established 74 Gy as the maximum tolerated dose and subsequently led to the multi-institutional randomized phase III trial RTOG 0617. In this 2 × 2 factorial design trial, all patients received weekly carboplatin and paclitaxel with concurrent RT in 2 Gy per once daily fraction followed by two cycles of consolidative CHT after the completion of RT. Patients were randomized to receive either 60 or 74 Gy and to receive this with or without cetuximab. At the first interim analysis, the trial had crossed the futility boundary with respect to the 74 Gy arm, and this high-dose arm was closed. The trial continued accruing only at the 60 Gy arm. At the third interim analysis, the cetuximab arm had also crossed the futility boundary. There was a significantly increased rate of death in the 74 Gy arm. The MST was 28.7 months in the 60 Gy arm vs. 19.5 months in the 74 Gy arm (HR 1.56, 95% CI: 1.19–2.06; $p = 0.0007$) (Bradley et al. 2015). There was a 37% increased risk of local failure in the high-dose arms (HR 1.37, 95% CI: 0.99–1.89; $p = 0.0319$). There was no difference in overall grade ≥ 3 toxicity, in severe pulmonary events specifically, or in severe RT-induced pneumonitis between the RT dose groups. Severe RT-induced esophagitis was more common in the high-dose group (21% vs. 16%, $p < 0.0001$). Long-term results (Bradley et al. 2020) reconfirmed previous findings. The MST was 28.7 vs. 20.3 months ($p = 0.0072$) in the 60 Gy and 74 Gy arms, respectively, 5-year OS and PFS rates were 32.1% and 23% and 18.3% and 13% ($p = 0.055$), respectively. Factors associated with improved OS on multivariable analysis were standard radiation dose, tumor location, institution accrual volume, esophagitis/dysphagia, planning target volume, and heart V5. The use of cetuximab conferred no survival benefit at the expense of increased toxicity.

The poor survival in the high RT dose group in RTOG0617 has been extensively discussed. Treatment-related deaths were more common in the 74 Gy group than in the 60 Gy group although this was not of statistical significance. Protocol non-compliance was significantly more pronounced in the 74 Gy group, 26% vs. 17% ($p = 0.02$), as were treatment delays. RT planning was more likely to be non-compliant in the 74 Gy group, and planning target volume coverage by the 95% isodose line was poorer in the group. Concerns that non-compliance in the 74 Gy group produced these results led to analysis of OS only in those patients with RT plans compliant with the protocol which changed nothing; OS remained better in the 60 Gy group. It strongly suggested that it was not only dose to tumor that should be considered in future studies. Finally, a factor that was subsequently discussed, and the one secondary analysis of RTOG 0617 clearly emphasized with important implication for future studies was that patients treated at centers with low accrual had inferior survival, higher esophageal and heart doses, and more lethal events (Eaton et al. 2016).

Another attempt to bring more clarity into the issue of RT dose and its effectiveness in the setting of concurrent RT-CHT was recently provided by Schild et al. (2018) who collected individual patient data from 3600 patients with locally advanced NSCLC which participated in 16 cooperative group trials of concurrent RT-CHT. Beside the field design strategy, the primary RT parameters examined included total dose and Biologically Effective Dose (BED). RT doses ranged from 60 to 74 Gy with most treatments administered once daily. Patients were divided into 3 dose groups: low total dose (60 Gy), medium total dose (>60 Gy–66 Gy), and high total dose (>66 Gy–74 Gy). Compared to a reference of the low-dose group, the multivariable HRs were 1.08 for the medium dose group (95% CI = 0.93–1.25) and 1.12 for the high-dose group (CI = 0.97–1.30). The univariate $p = 0.054$ and multivariable $p = 0.17$ were reached. BED was grouped as follows: low (<55.5 Gy_{10}), medium (=55.5 Gy_{10}), or high (>55.5 Gy_{10}). Compared to the reference of the low BED group, the HR was 1.00 (95% CI = 0.85–1.18) for the medium BED group and 1.10 (95% CI = 0.93–1.31) for the high BED group. The univariable $p = 0.076$ and multivariable $p = 0.16$ were observed. This study showed that lowest radical RT dose (60 Gy) and lowest BED value RT (< 55 Gy_{10}) were not inferior to higher dose and higher BEDs, respectively, in the setting of concurrent RT-CHT as used in clinical trials nowadays. Institutions worldwide now almost unequivocally use 60 Gy given once daily as preferred RT when given with concurrent CHT in the setting of locally advanced NSCLC.

5 Neoadjuvant (Induction) Chemotherapy Followed by Radiation Therapy Versus Concurrent Radiochemotherapy

The studies using induction CHT followed by radical RT showed a survival advantage for the combined approach owing to the improvement in the distant metastasis control. It is a finding opposite to that of the studies using concurrent RT-CHT, which unequivocally showed improvement in survival owing to the improvement in locoregional tumor control. Considered from the standpoint of exploitable mechanisms of combined RT and CHT (Steel and Peckham 1979), the induction regimens enabled the therapeutic benefit due to spatial cooperation only. Neither independent cell kill nor enhancement of tumor response could be noted because there was no significant difference in locoregional tumor control, as one may expect if the two mechanisms of action would have happened. Contrary to that, in concurrent studies, spatial cooperation did not work, while both independent cell kill and enhancement of tumor response may have occurred. In the low-dose (daily) CHT arms of the concurrent studies, however, it seems unlikely that independent cell kill occurred (and if so, then to a much lesser degree due to lower daily and total doses of CHT), leaving, thus, enhancement of tumor response as the only and likely alternative.

In order to compare induction CHT followed by radical RT to concurrent RT-CHT, several clinical trials were performed. Beside the aforementioned CALGB study (Clamon et al. 1999), Furuse et al. (1999, 2000) compared mitomycin, cisplatin, and vindesine given as either induction followed by continuous course radical RT (56 Gy) with the same mitomycin, cisplatin, and vindesine given concurrently with split-course RT of the same total dose. First publication showed superior results (the MST, 16.5 vs. 13.3 months; 5-year survival, 16% vs. 9%; $p = 0.039$) for concurrent RT-CHT (Furuse et al. 1999). Subsequent data analysis showed that an improvement in local tumor control (median time, 10.6 vs. 8.0 months; 5-year, 34% vs. 20%; $p = 0.0462$) is the reason for an improvement in survival (Furuse et al. 2000). More recently, Curran et al. (2011) reported on RTOG 9410 study which compared (1) induction CHT followed by RT, same as CALGB 8433 (Dillman et al. 1990) and RTOG 8808/ECOG 4508 (Sause et al. 1995) with concurrent either (2) standard fraction RT (60 Gy) and cisplatin/etoposide or (3) Hfx RT (69.6 Gy) and cisplatin/etoposide. Both standard RT-CHT and Hfx RT-CHT arm had better MST than the induction arm (17.0 vs. 16.0 vs. 14.6 months) although only standard RT-CHT was statistically significantly better than induction CHT (Curran et al. 2011). Pattern of failure analysis showed that the best local control was in the Hfx RT-CHT, confirming indirectly the observations of Jeremic et al. (1995, 1996) that high-dose Hfx RT-CHT is an advantageous approach. Furthermore and contrary to studies using low-dose CHT concurrently with high-dose RT, it was shown again that high-dose CHT carried a significant risk of acute toxicity when given with high-dose standard RT or Hfx RT. This finding was not just limited to RTOG 9410 but was also seen in similar studies (Byhardt et al. 1995; Lee et al. 1996; Komaki et al. 1997). Groupe Lyon-Saint-Etienne d'Oncologie Thoracique-Groupe Français de Pneumo-Cancérologie (Fournel et al. 2005) randomly assigned 205 patients to receive either induction cisplatin and vinorelbine, followed by RT at a dose of 66 Gy in 33 fractions or the same RT (started on day 1) with two concurrent cycles of cisplatin and; patients then received consolidation therapy with cisplatin and vinorelbine. There were six toxic deaths in the induction arm and 10 in the concurrent arm. The MST was 14.5 months in the induction arm and 16.3 months in the concurrent arm ($p = 0.24$). Two-, 3-, and 4-year survival rates were better in the concurrent arm (39, 25, and 21%, respectively) than in the induction arm (26%, 19%, and 14%, respectively). Esophageal toxicity was significantly more frequent in the concurrent arm than in the induction arm (32% vs. 3%). Although not statistically significant, differences in the median, 2-, 3-, and 4-year survival rates which were observed were clinically meaningful, with a trend in favor of concurrent RT-CHT, suggesting that is the optimal strategy in this setting. Belderbos et al. (2007) reported on EORTC study in which patients were randomized to receive two courses of gemcitabine and cisplatin prior to, or daily low-dose cisplatin (6 mg/sqm) concurrent with RT, consisting of 24 fractions of 2.75 Gy in 32 days, with a total dose of 66 Gy. Acute hematological toxicity grade 3/4 was more pronounced in the induction arm (30% vs. 6%), oesophagitis grade 3/4 more frequent in the concurrent arm (5% vs. 14%). No difference in late toxicity was observed. Because of the poor power of the study no significant differences in MST (induction, 16.2, concurrent, 16.5 months, respectively) and 3-year OS (induction, 22%, concurrent, 34%) could be detected.

Although discussed clinical trials have clearly shown that concurrent RT-CHT should be considered as standard treatment option in, at least favorable (good PS, less pronounced weight loss), patients with locally advanced NSCLC, last three decades continued to be the time of continuous discussions regarding this issue. To solve major scientific and clinical question, three meta-analyses/systematic reviews were performed.

O'Rourke et al. (2010) identified 19 randomized studies (totaling 2728 participants) of RT and concurrent CHT vs. RT alone. RT and concurrent CHT significantly reduced overall risk of death (HR 0.71, 95% CI 0.64–0.80; 1607 participants) and overall PFS at any site (HR 0.69, 95% CI 0.58–0.81; 1145 participants). Incidence of acute oesophagitis, neutropenia, and anemia was significantly increased with RT and concurrent CHT. Six trials (1024 patients) of RT and concurrent CHT vs. induction CHT and RT were included. A significant benefit of CHT was shown in OS (HR 0.74, 95% CI 0.62–0.89; 702 participants). This represented a 10% absolute survival benefit at 2 years. More treatment-related deaths (4% vs. 2%) were reported in the RT and concurrent CHT arm without statistical significance (RR 2.02, 95% CI 0.90–4.52; 950 participants). There was increased severe oesophagitis with RT and concurrent CHT (RR 4.96, 95% CI 2.17–11.37; 947 participants).

Liang et al. (2010) performed a systematic review of 11 trials (2043 patients; concurrent—1019, induction—1024) comparing RT and concurrent CHT with induction CHT followed with RT. Results confirmed that RT and concurrent CHT led to a statistically significant increase in MST (16.3 vs. 13.9 months; pooled median ratios = 1.17, 95% CI 1.09–1.26), response rate (64.0% vs. 56.3%; odds ratio = 1.38, 95% CI 1.10–1.72), and tumor-relapse control (odds ratio = 0.82, 95% CI 0.69–0.97), though at the expense of increased hematological toxicity (neutropenia and thrombocytopenia) and non-hematological toxicity (nausea/vomiting, stomatitis, and esophagitis). Similar results were obtained from the sensitivity analysis of all Phase-III trials designed to evaluate the primary end point of OS. Subgroup analysis revealed that concurrent approach was mainly associated with improved locoregional control (odds ratio = 0.68, 95% CI 0.52–0.87). However, no difference in PFS was shown. While careful interpretation of their conclusions was required because of potential bias, authors concluded that further improvements will be obtained by optimizing the conditions for a concurrent regimen.

Finally, Aupérin et al. (2010) used updated individual patient data to address the same question. The primary outcome was OS; secondary outcomes were PFS, cumulative incidences of locoregional and distant progression, and acute toxicity. Of seven eligible trials, data from six trials were received (1205 patients, 92% of all randomly assigned patients). Median follow-up was 6 years. There was a significant benefit of RT and concurrent CHT on OS (pooled HR, 0.84; 95% CI 0.74–0.95; $p = 0.004$), with an absolute benefit of 5.7% (from 18.1% to 23.8%) at 3 years and 4.5% at 5 years. For PFS, the pooled HR was 0.90 (95% CI 0.79–1.01; $p = 0.07$). RT and concurrent CHT decreased locoregional progression (pooled HR, 0.77; 95% CI 0.62–0.95; $p = 0.01$); its effect was not different from that of induction treatment on distant progression (pooled HR, 1.04; 95% CI 0.86–1.25; $p = 0.69$). RT and concurrent CHT increased acute esophageal toxicity (grade 3–4) from 4 to 18% with a relative risk of 4.9 (95% CI 3.1–7.8; $p < 0.001$). There was no significant difference regarding acute pulmonary toxicity. Identically to a previous conclusions of two meta-analyses, here, too, RT and concurrent CHT improved survival of patients with locally advanced NSCLC, primarily because of a better locoregional control, but at the cost of manageable increased acute esophageal toxicity.

These three meta-analyses firmly established superiority of RT and concurrent CHT over the induction CHT followed by radical RT and helped the majority of institutions world-wide accepting the highest level of evidence and introduced it in daily clinical practice. In addition to it, two recent meta-analyses found the same. Hung et al. (2019) used randomized a total of 13 controlled trials and two-armed prospective studies ($n = 1936$) that compared combined RT + CHT with RT alone in patients with locally advanced (stage III) nonresectable NSCLC. However, they excluded studies that evaluated two types of CHT, those designed to compare dose and sequence of RT (e.g., sequential vs concurrent), as well as those that did not report quantitatively outcomes of interest. Pooled 1- and 2-year data clearly showed that RT-CHT achieved higher OS and higher PFS. Investigating the place and role of CHT given either before RT-CHT, concurrent to RT or after RT-CHT in stage III NSCLC, Ying et al. (2019) performed a systematic review and meta-analysis of 12 studies. The ORR and disease control rate (DCR) were not different among the three treatment options. Importantly, induction CHT followed by RT-CHT did not have significant survival benefits compared with RT-CHT alone. Similar was observed when comparing RT-CHT followed by consolidation CHT with RT-CHT alone. Furthermore, induction CHT followed by RT-CHT was not associated with improved survival compared to RT-CHT followed by consolidation CHT with respect to OS and PFS. The findings of this meta-analysis clearly showed limited effects of any (induction, consolidation) CHT when added to RT-CHT.

6 Optimization of Concurrent Radiochemotherapy

In order to optimize combined modality approach in patients with locally advanced NSCLC several new attempts have been undertaken. While Jeremic et al. (1998) tested the addition of weekend carboplatin/etoposide to concurrent Hfx RT (69.6 Gy) and low-dose daily carboplatin/etoposide in phase II study leading to promising MST of 29 months and 5-year survival in 25%, the results of their subsequent prospective randomized trial showed no advantage for weekend chemotherapy CHT when compared to no-weekend CHT (the MST, 22 vs. 20 months; 5-year survival, 23% vs. 20%; $p = 0.57$) (Jeremic et al. 2001). In their continuous efforts to optimize RT and concurrent CHT, Jeremic et al. (2005) pioneered a combined modality approach consisting of Hfx RT and concurrent low-dose daily paclitaxel and carboplatin. In order to increase likelihood of successfully combating accelerated proliferation of tumor clonogens, they have adapted their initial standard regimen (69.6 Gy in 58 fractions of 1.2 Gy given b.i.d) in 6 weeks to 67.6 Gy in 52 fractions of 1.3 Gy given also b.i.d., but in a 5-week total treatment time, saving approximately 1 week. In 64 patients with stage III NSCLC very promising MST of 28 months and a 5-year survival rate of 26% were obtained, accompanied with low incidence of high-grade toxicity, reconfirming effectiveness and low toxicity of Hfx RT and concurrent low-dose daily CHT. Most recently, Dieleman et al. (2018) reported on 154 consecutive patients staged with PET-CT and treated with daily low-dose cisplatin (6 mg/m^2) combined with a total dose of 66 Gy given in 24 fractions of 2.75 Gy. The MST was 36 months and 5-year survival rate was 40%. The local relapse-free survival at 5 years was 55% and metastasis-free survival at 5 years was 53%. Grade 3 radiation-induced esophagitis was 8.4% and grade 3 radiation-induced pneumonitis was 1.3%. These excellent results not only reconfirmed that radical RT and low-dose daily CHT are very effective and low-toxic approach, but reconfirmed results of previous studies done in the pre-PET era (Schaake-Koning et al. 1992; Jeremic et al. 1995, 1996, 2005). They also reconfirmed findings of the review done almost 10 years ago which showed that concurrent RT and low-dose CHT regimens resulted in a favorable toxicity profile compared RT and high-dose single- or multi-agent CHT with comparable treatment results (Koning et al. 2013).

The most recent studies have also undertaken efforts to optimize this approach by testing different drugs given concurrently with RT (Segawa et al. 2010; Shimokawa et al. 2021), and even non-CHT drugs, such as cartilage shark (AE-941) thought to have radiosensitizing properties (Lu et al. 2010) all without much success and apparent advantage over "classical approach" in RT-CHT, as described above. The most common CHT regimens used concurrently with RT in this setting are cisplatin or carboplatin–paclitaxel, cisplatin–etoposide, cisplatin–vinorelbine and carboplatin with pemetrexed, but currently there is no consensus regarding which CHT is best in combination with concurrent RT in the curative setting. Santana-Davilla et al. (2015) analyzed Veterans Administration Health Data to observe that no difference in efficacy between cisplatin–etoposide and carboplatin–paclitaxel doublets was given concurrently with RT although cisplatin–etoposide was more toxic. In a systematic review, Steuer et al. (2017) investigated the same combinations in 31 studies including 3090 patients to observe similar efficacy and more toxicity for cisplatin–etoposide. In the recent secondary reanalysis of the data for patients enrolled into a prospective randomized study which investigated RT target volume concepts in the context of concurrent RT-CHT for locally advanced NSCLC, various CHT regimens were used. Cisplatin–vinorelbine regimens achieved superior results when compared to carboplatin–vinorelbine regimen but only in univariate analysis (Gkika et al. 2020), becoming insignificant one in the multivariate analysis. Toxicity was more pronounced in cisplatin–vinorelbine regimens. This seems to hold true in elderly population as the analysis of a Surveillance, Epidemiology and End Results-Medicare registry comparing cisplatin vs. carboplatin-based CHT, showed similar long-term survival but lower rates of toxicity for the latter (Ezer et al. 2014). Contrary to these, two Chinese studies observed advantage for cisplatin–etoposide. Wang et al. (2012) reported a small randomized phase II study evaluating the activity and safety of weekly paclitaxel–carboplatin compared with cisplatin–etoposide with concurrent RT. A significantly better OS was found in the cisplatin–etoposide arm than in the paclitaxel–carboplatin arm ($p = 0.04$). Based on these results, same investigators proceeded to a phase III trial which included 191 patients (Liang et al. 2017). The 3-year OS was significantly higher in the cisplatin–etoposide arm than that of the paclitaxel–carboplatin arm. The estimated difference was 15.0% ($p = 0.024$). The MSTs were 23.3 months in the cisplatin–etoposide arm and 20.7 months in the paclitaxel–carboplatin arm (HR 0.76, 95% CI 0.55–1.05; $p = 0.095$). Grade 2 RT pneumonitis was more frequent in the paclitaxel–carboplatin arm (33.3% vs. 18.9%, $p = 0.036$) while the incidence of grade 3 esophagitis was higher in the cisplatin–etoposide arm (20.0% vs. 6.3%, $p = 0.009$). Inconclusive results and institutional preferences continue to play a major role in the decision-making process in this setting.

Past 25 years witnessed a particular approach aimed to optimize concurrent RT-CHT. By adding more CHT after the end of concurrent RT-CHT, labeled as either maintenance or consolidation CHT, better treatment of microscopic disease is sought. Initially, most studies used the same CHT given in concurrent and consolidation phase of the treatment (LePechoux et al. 1996; Albain et al. 2002; Sakai et al. 2004; Belani et al. 2005a, b; Davies et al. 2006; Jain et al. 2009; Movsas et al. 2010; Choy et al. 2013; Kawano et al. 2018; Sasaki et al. 2018) but many following studies used different drugs (so-called switch approach) (Gandara et al. 2003; Keene et al. 2005; Sekine et al. 2006; Hanna et al. 2008; Gadgeel et al. 2011; Fournel et al. 2016; Hasegawa et al. 2016) based on the assumption that consolidation drugs should be more effective and with different toxicity profile if different from those given during the concurrent phase. Finally, following the events and results coming from metastatic NSCLC, thoracic oncologists started introducing both targeted agents (Kelly et al. 2008; Blumenschein et al. 2011; Bradley et al. 2015; Wozniak et al. 2015; Levy et al. 2017), vaccine (Brunsvig et al. 2011; Butts et al. 2014), and immunotherapy (Antonia et al. 2017; Durm et al. 2020) in both concurrent and consolidation phase of the treatment. More than 10 years had passed since various phase II studies brought promising results until more sobering results started appearing, but requested confirmation in a phase II study design. Hosier Oncology Group (Hanna et al. 2008) randomized patients to receive cisplatin and etoposide concurrently with RT to 59.40 Gy. Patients who did not experience progression were randomly assigned to docetaxel for three cycles vs. observation. Grade 3–5 toxicities during docetaxel included febrile neutropenia (10.9%) and pneumonitis (9.6%); 28.8% of patients were hospitalized during docetaxel (vs. 8.1% in observation arm), and 5.5% died as a result of docetaxel. The MST was 21.2 months for docetaxel arm compared with 23.2 months for observation arm ($p = 0.883$), showing that consolidation docetaxel resulted in increased toxicities but did not improve survival compared with RT and concurrent cisplatin/etoposide alone. Kelly et al. (2008) reported on a study that used targeted agents in consolidation phase. Untreated patients received cisplatin plus etoposide for two cycles with concurrent RT (1.8–2.0 Gy fractions per day; total dose, 61 Gy) followed by three cycles of docetaxel. Patients whose disease did not progress were randomly assigned to gefitinib or placebo until disease progression, intolerable toxicity, or the end of 5 years. An unplanned interim analysis led to rejecting the alternative hypothesis of improved survival and the study was closed. The MST was 23 months for gefitinib vs. 35 months for placebo ($p = 0.013$). The toxic death rate was 2% with gefitinib compared with 0% for placebo. This study showed that gefitinib did not improve survival, and that decreased survival was a result of tumor progression and not gefitinib toxicity. It also showed not only inefficiency of targeted agent gefitinib, but also reconfirmed inefficiency of consolidation CHT approach in locally advanced NSCLC.

These disappointing results challenged the use of consolidation CHT in this disease. While studies outlined overall results, relapse-free-survivals, and clearly documented toxicity, this did not happen with the patterns of failure. Some studies presented very detailed pattern of failure in general, but this was done for the whole time period of the study (treatment plus follow-up). This way we only learned about the total patterns of failure and not about which type of failure was observed when, i.e., after concurrent or after consolidation part, and particularly in which patients after the concurrent part, although some studies mandated consolidation CHT in non-progressing patients.

There may be several reasons why exact pattern of failure is important. First, there are several types of patients observed after the concurrent RT-CHT, easily separated regarding the response. While it is extremely unlikely that those achieving a stable disease (SD) would benefit from the consolidation CHT, those with either a complete response (CR) or a partial response (PR) seem as likely candidates to benefit from the consolidation CHT. Separation, therefore, of pattern of failure occurring in likely (CR and PR) and unlikely (SD) candidates could be used for further studies using similar design with respect to, e.g., eligibility criteria. Second, a distinction should be made between those achieving CR and those achieving PR after concurrent RT-CHT, since different mechanisms (precisely, different location) of action of consolidation CHT could be expected. In the CR patients, consolidation CHT would target microscopic disease both intrathoracically and extrathoracically, while in the PR patients, it would have to deal with clinically overt intrathoracic disease and a microscopic one extrathoracically. It is obvious that pattern of failure in these two distinct groups of patients would then clearly show how and where consolidation CHT are actually acting and to what extent (clinical vs. subclinical).

Unfortunately, no study investigated treatment outcome per various responses observed after receiving consolidation part of the treatment, specifically OS, LPFS, and DMFS. The only study which provided only a hint towards this issue was PACIFIC study (Antonia et al. 2017) which showed benefit for both patients with PR or SD for the immunotherapy, and with the similar outcome for these response categories. Also, no study ever provided exact patterns of failure of patients receiving concurrent RT-CHT, in particular concerning the three non-PD patients. As a consequence, treatment outcome per pattern of failure occurring in one of these response categories remained unknown. Although identifying pattern of failure in patients achieving different response after concurrent RT-CHT would require additional efforts, it would eventually be rewarding. This way we would be able to discriminate between different patients and different options and to proceed (or not) with a consolidation therapy in one or more patient subsets, ultimately improving patient-tailored treatment.

7 New Approaches in Radiation Therapy and Chemotherapy of Locally Advanced Non-small Cell Lung Cancer

Some of the newer approaches regarding the CHT have been mentioned above. It is also expected that more new drugs will become more readily available in the future and that the process of their initial clinical testing (phase I–II) includes testing for their radioenhancing potentials which would go in parallel to its testing for systemic anticancer effects. This way, we would be able earlier to learn about drug properties, both alone or in combination with RT and to address important issues of optimal sequencing RT and CHT in locally advanced disease.

Regarding RT, wide application of powerful computers made a substantial impact on treatment planning and delivery. Three-dimensional (3D) conformal RT became standard practiced worldwide in the past 30 years. It enabled RT doses at the order of ≥ 80 Gy to be used with increased efficacy and acceptable toxicity (Armstrong et al. 1993; Robertson et al. 1997). Intensity-modulated radiotherapy (IMRT) has increasingly been used and potential advantages of IMRT became evident when one compares the 3D RT and IMRT plans (Yorke 2001). With IMRT, in majority of cases the prescription dose could be increased. This was coupled with the decreased lung dose and improved planning target volume uniformity, as well as significantly reducing cumulative RT dose to the esophagus while maintaining the same or higher dose to gross disease (Giraud et al. 2001). Data on the use of IMRT in locally advanced NSCLC accumulated over the past 20 years. While some (Bezjak et al. 2012) showed its favorable effect, albeit of potential for increased low-dose toxicity, others could not demonstrate its superiority over 3D RT (Harris et al. 2014; Chen et al. 2014). Recently, Koshy et al. (2017) used the data from the NCDB which included patients treated with definitive RT-CHT to 60–63 Gy. Out of 7492 patients, 10% received IMRT. The MST for non-IMRT vs. IMRT was 18.2 months vs. 20 months ($p < 0.0001$). Use of IMRT predicted for a decreased likelihood of RT interruptions (OR, 0.84, $p = 0.04$). On multivariate analysis for OS, IMRT remained independent prognosticator ($p = 0.01$), associated with small but significant survival advantage for patients treated with RT-CHT.

However, it should be clearly emphasized that proper selection of patients remains prerequisite for the use of these new technologies in locally advanced and/or metastatic NSCLC. On the other side, proper selection of patients suitable for any form of combined RT and CHT may enable using the two modality approach also in non-curative approach. In such one study, Nawrocki et al. (2010) reported on a randomized phase II study using palliative RT alone (30 Gy/10 fractions) vs. two cycles of cisplatin and vinorelbine followed by the same palliative RT together with third cycle in patients with stage IIIA to IIIB NSCLC not eligible for radical (tumor >8 cm and/or forced expiratory volume ≤ 40%, PS 0–2, and existing tumor-related chest symptoms). The MST was 9.0 vs. 12.9 months, $p = 0.0342$; and median PFS was 4.7 vs. 7.3 months, $p = 0.046$, in RT vs. RT-CHT, respectively. There were no deaths during treatment in RT alone arm and six deaths in RT-CHT arm; no hematological grade 3–4 toxicities in RT alone arm and 14 toxicities in RT-CHT arm. Symptom control was high and similar in both arms. Induction CHT combined with palliative RT/CHT seemed as a suitable treatment option in the subpopulation of patients not amenable for definitive RT-CHT. Strøm et al. (2013) performed a subgroup study of a previously randomized study focusing on poor prognosis patients with bulky stage III locally advanced NSCLC deemed unsuitable for concurrent RT-CHT to explore how tumor size influenced OS and health-related quality of life (HRQOL). This subset study offered comparison of patients having tumors >7 cm ($n = 108$) vs. tumors ≤7 cm ($n = 76$). Among those with tumors >7 cm, the MST in the CHT vs. RT-CHT arm was 9.7 and 13.4 months, respectively ($p = 0.001$). The 1-year survival was 33% and 56%, respectively ($p = 0.01$). HRQOL was maintained in the CRT arm, regardless of tumor size. The RT-CHT group had significantly more esophagitis and hospitalizations because of side effects regardless of tumor size. Except for PS 2, patients with tumors >7 cm apparently benefited from RT-CHT. In the largest study, Ball et al. (2013) used the data available from the IASLC staging project database on 868 patients. Primary tumor size was categorized according to tumor, node, metastasis of seventh edition. On univariate analysis, the following factors were prognostic for survival: age (continuous) ($p = 0.0035$); performance status of 1 or more ($p = 0.0021$); weight loss less than 5% ($p < 0.0001$); CHT ($p = 0.0189$); and primary tumor size (continuous) ($p = 0.0002$). Sex and clinical nodal stages were not significant. On multivariate analysis, age and weight loss remained significant factors for survival, as was tumor size <3 cm. They concluded that in patients treated with RT with or without CHT, tumor size <3 cm was associated with longer survival than larger tumors.

Besides the tumor size, the past 20 years brought increasing emphasis on the importance of tumor volume and its impact on treatment outcome. Bradley et al. (2002) used multiple sections from a treatment planning CT scans in which tumor targets were contoured in and 3D treatment volumes and normal structures reconstructed. Outcome was analyzed by prognostic factors for NSCLC including various pretreatment patient parameters including the gross tumor volume (GTV) in cm^3. OS, cause-specific survival (CSS), and local tumor control were most highly correlated with the GTV in cm^3. On multivariate analysis the independent variable most predictive of survival was the GTV. Traditional staging such as T, N, and overall clinical staging were not independent prognostic factors, indicating that GTV as determined by CT and 3D RT-CHT planning was highly prognostic for OS, CSS, and local tumor control and may be important in stratification of patients in prospective therapy trials. Similarly, Basaki et al. (2006) identified the primary tumor and nodal volume in pretreatment CT scans and univariate and multivariate analyses were used to evaluate the impact of tumor volume on survival after RT. The 2-year OS was 23%, with a MST of 14 months. The MSTs were 10 months and 19 months with large primary tumor volume more than median volume and smaller primary tumor volume, respectively. At a univariate analysis, the total tumor volume (TTV) ($p < 0.0003$) and the primary tumor volume ($p < 0.00008$) were significant and the nodal volume was not. At multivariate analyses, both the TTV and the primary tumor volume were significant prognostic factors. In order to improve its ability to predict survival in patients treated with RT with or without CHT in stage I-IIIB NSCLC, Dehinge-Obeije et al. (2008) investigated the prognostic value of tumor volume and N status, assessed by PET. The final multivariate Cox model consisted of number of positive lymph node stations (PLNSs), and gross tumor volume (i.e., volume of the primary tumor plus lymph nodes), in addition to sex, WHO PS, and equivalent RT dose corrected for time, while N stage was not significant. Authors suggested that these factors should be taken into account when risk stratification is done in future studies. Using the data from patients enrolled into a RTOG phase I-II dose-escalation study, Werner-Wasik et al. (2008) used a multivariate analysis to show that only a smaller GTV (≤ 45 cm^3) was a significant prognostic factor for improved MST and PFS (HR, 2.12, $p = 0.0002$; and HR, 2.0, $p = 0.0002$, respectively). The GTV as a continuous variable was also significantly associated with the MST and PFS (HR, 1.59, $p < 0.0001$; and HR, 1.39, $p < 0.0001$, respectively), indicating that it can be used in the stratification process in future studies. Alexander et al. (2011) investigated whether primary tumor and nodal volumes defined on RT planning scans were correlated with outcome (survival and recurrence) after RT-CHT. In addition to tumor and nodal volume measurements, various clinical factors were investigated. Both nodal volume (HR, 1.09; $p < 0.01$) and tumor volume (HR, 1.03; $p < 0.01$) were associated with OS on multivariate analysis as well as they both were on local tumor control (HR, 1.10; $p < 0.01$; HR, 1.04; $p < 0.01$, respectively), but not on distant metastases. This information may be helpful in determining prognosis and identifying groups of patients for which RT-CHT is warranted. Lee et al. (2012) used metabolic tumor volume (MTV) as an independent prognosticator of OS and PFS. Higher MTV was significantly associated with worse OS ($p = 0.00075$) and PFS ($p = 0.00077$) in entire cohort of patients. When MTV was analyzed as a binary value above or below the median value in definitively treated patients, 2-year PFS and 2-year OS were marginally insignificant, but when MTV was analyzed as a continuous variable, multivariate analysis demonstrated a trend to worse PFS and significantly worse OS with increasing MTV. Tumor burden as assessed by MTV may provide prognostic information on survival beyond that of established prognostic factors in patients with NSCLC treated definitively and should be taken into account in future studies when stratifying patients.

8 Conclusions

Locally advanced NSCLC continues to be one of the major battlefields in clinical research in lung cancer. The past several decades witnessed progress in both RT and CHT and it is reasonable to expect that this will continue in the future and will bring us to the exiting era of more successful clinical research, leading ultimately to better outcome in this disease. However, *the* future seems to have already begun. Several years ago, the results of the prospective randomized phase III study widely known as PACIFIC (Antonia et al. 2017) have seemingly changed the landscape of treatment options in a combined modality approach. Patients received durvalumab or placebo every 2 weeks for up to 12 months. The study drug was administered 1–42 days after the patients had received RT-CHT. Of a total of 713 randomized patients, 709 received consolidation therapy (473 received durvalumab and 236 received placebo). The median PFS from randomization was 16.8 months (95% CI, 13.0–18.1) with durvalumab vs. 5.6 months (95% CI, 4.6–7.8) with placebo (stratified HR for disease progression or death, 0.52; 95% CI, 0.42–0.65; $p < 0.001$); the 12-month PFS was 55.9% vs. 35.3%, and the 18-month PFS was 44.2% vs. 27.0%. The response rate was higher with durvalumab than with placebo (28.4% vs. 16.0%; $p < 0.001$), and the median duration of response was longer (72.8% vs. 46.8% of the patients had an ongoing response at 18 months). The median time to death or distant metastasis was longer with durvalumab than with placebo (23.2 months vs. 14.6 months; $p < 0.001$). Grade 3 or 4 adverse events occurred in 29.9% of the patients who received durvalumab and 26.1% of those who received placebo; the most common adverse event of grade 3 or 4 was pneumonia (4.4% and 3.8%, respectively). A total of 15.4% of patients in the durvalumab group and 9.8% of those in the placebo group discontinued the study drug because of adverse events. With the PFS being significantly longer with durvalumab than with placebo, the secondary end points also favored durvalumab, while safety was similar between the groups. Longer follow-up (Antonia et al. 2018) reconfirmed superiority of durvalumab. The 24-month OS was 66.3% (95% CI, 61.7–70.4) in the durvalumab group, as compared with 55.6% (95% CI, 48.9–61.8) in the placebo group (two-sided $p = 0.005$). Durvalumab significantly prolonged OS, as compared with placebo (stratified HR for death, 0.68; 99.73% CI, 0.47–0.997; $p = 0.0025$). Updated analyses regarding PFS were similar to those previously reported, with a median PFS of 17.2 months in the durvalumab group and 5.6 months in the placebo group (stratified HR for disease progression or death, 0.51; 95% CI, 0.41–0.63). The median time to death or distant metastasis was 28.3 months in the durvalumab group and 16.2 months in the placebo group (stratified HR, 0.53; 95% CI, 0.41–0.68). A total of 30.5% of the patients in the durvalumab group and 26.1% of those in the placebo group had grade 3 or 4 adverse events of any cause; 15.4% and 9.8% of the patients, respectively, discontinued the trial regimen because of adverse events. Important aspect of this study was that clinical benefit with durvalumab was attained without compromising patient reported outcomes (PROs) (Hui et al. 2019). Between baseline and 12 months, the prespecified longitudinal PROs of interest, cough, dyspnoea, chest pain, fatigue, appetite loss, and global health status or quality of life remained stable with both treatments, with no clinically relevant changes from baseline. The same held true for differences between the two groups in aforementioned items from baseline to 12 months which were not clinically relevant.

These results established durvalumab as the part of a combined treatment that is now considered by many as "new standard" treatment option in patients with locally advanced NSCLC. Many ongoing studies continue evaluating various systemic therapies, focusing on immunotherapy principles and their respective agents in this setting, results of which should help us further refine our treatment approaches in the second decade of the twenty-first century.

References

Akerley W, Herndon JE Jr, Lyss AP et al (2005) Induction paclitaxel/carboplatin followed by concurrent chemoradiation therapy for unresectable stage III non-small-cell lung cancer: a limited-access study—CALGB 9534. Clin Lung Cancer 7:47–53

Albain KS, Crowley JJ, Turrisi AT III et al (2002) Concurrent cisplatin, etoposide, and chest radiotherapy in pathologic stage IIIB non-small-cell lung cancer: a southwest oncology group phase II study, SWOG 9019. J Clin Oncol 20:3454–3460

Alexander BM, Othus M, Caglar HB, Allen AM (2011) Tumor volume is a prognostic factor in non-small-cell lung cancer treated with chemoradiotherapy. Int J Radiat Oncol Biol Phys 79:1381–1387

Antonia SJ, Villegas A, Daniel D et al (2017) Durvalumab after chemoradiotherapy in stage III non-small-cell lung cancer. N Engl J Med 377:1919–1929

Antonia SJ, Villegas A, Daniel D et al (2018) Overall survival with durvalumab after chemoradiotherapy in stage III NSCLC. N Engl J Med 379:2342–2350

Armstrong JG, Burman C, Leibel SA et al (1993) Three-dimensional conformal radiation therapy may improve the therapeutic ratio of high dose radiation therapy for lung cancer. Int J Radiat Oncol Biol Phys 26:685–689

Arriagada R, Le Chevalier T, Rekacewicz C et al (1997) Cisplatin-based chemotherapy (CT) in patients with locally advanced non-small cell lung cancer (NSCLC): late analysis of a French randomized trial. Proc Am Soc Clin Oncol 16:16. (abstract)

Aupérin A, Le Péchoux C, Rolland E et al (2010) Meta-analysis of concomitant versus sequential radiochemotherapy in locally advanced non-small-cell lung cancer. J Clin Oncol 28:2181–2190

Ball D, Bishop J, Smith J et al (1999) A randomised phase III study of accelerated or standard fraction radiotherapy with or without concurrent carboplatin in inoperable non-small cell lung cancer: final report of a multi-Centre trial. Radiother Oncol 52:129–136

Ball D, Mitchell A, Giroux D, Rami-Porta R, The IASLC Staging Committee and Participating Institutions (2013) Effect of tumor size on prognosis in patients treated with radical radiotherapy or chemoradiotherapy for non–small cell lung cancer an analysis of the staging project database of the International Association for the Study of Lung Cancer. J Thorac Oncol 8:315–321

Basaki K, Abe Y, Aoki M, Kondo H, Hatayama Y, Nakaji S (2006) Prognostic factors for survival in stage III non-small-cell lung cancer treated with definitive radiation therapy: impact of tumor volume. Int J Radiat Oncol Biol Phys 64:449–454

Baumann M, Hermann T, Koch R (2005) Continuous hyperfractionated accelerated radiotherapy weekendless versus conventionalloy fractionated (CF) in non-small cell lung cancer (NSCLC): first results of a phase III randomzied multicentre trial (ARO 97-91). Eur J Cancer 3(Suppl):S323

Belani CP, Wang W, Johnson DH (2005a) Phase III study of the eastern cooperative oncology group (ECOG 2597): induction chemotherapy followed by either standard thoracic radiotherapy or hyperfractionated accelerated radiotherapy for patients with unresectable stage IIIA and B non-small-cell lung cancer. J Clin Oncol 23:3760–3767

Belani CP, Choy H, Bonomi P et al (2005b) Combined chemoradiotherapy regimens of paclitaxel and carboplatin for locally advanced non-small-cell lung cancer: a randomized phase II locally advanced multi-modality protocol. J Clin Oncol 23:5883–5891

Belderbos J, Uitterhoeve L, van Zandwijk N, EORTC LCG and RT Group et al (2007) Randomised trial of sequential versus concurrent chemo-radiotherapy in patients with inoperable non small cell lung cancer (EORTC 08972-22973). Eur J Cancer 43:114–121

Bezjak A, Rumble RB, Rodrigues G et al (2012) Intensity-modulated radiotherapy in the treatment of lung cancer. Clin Oncol (R Coll Radiol) 24:508–520

Blanke C, Ansari R, Mantravadi R et al (1995) Phase III trial of thoracic irradiation with or without cisplatin for locally advanced unresectable non-small cell lung cancer: a Hoosier oncology group protocol. J Clin Oncol 13:1425–1429

Blumenschein GR Jr, Paulus R, Curran WJ et al (2011) Phase II study of cetuximab in combination with chemoradiation in patients with stage IIIA/B non-small-cell lung cancer: RTOG 0324. J Clin Oncol 29:2312–2318

Bonner JA, McGinnis WL, Stella PJ et al (1998) The possible advantage of hyperfractionated thoracic radiotherapy in the treatment of locally advanced non small cell lung cancer. Results of a north central cancer treatment group phase III study. Cancer 82: 1037–1048

Bozcuk H, Artac M, Ozdogan M (2010) Correlates of benefit from neoadjuvant chemotherapy before radiotherapy in non-small cell lung cancer: a meta-analytical approach with meta-regression analysis. J BUON 15:43–50

Bradley JD, Ieumwananonthachai N, Purdy JA et al (2002) Gross tumor volume, critical prognostic factor in patients treated with three-dimensional conformal radiation therapy for non-small-cell lung carcinoma. Int J Radiat Oncol Biol Phys 52:49–57

Bradley JD, Bae K, Graham MV et al (2010) Primary analysis of the phase II component of a phase I/II dose intensification study using three-dimensional conformal radiation therapy and concurrent chemotherapy for patient with inoperable non-small-cell lung cancer: RTOG 0117. J Clin Oncol 28:2475–2480

Bradley JD, Paulus R, Komaki R et al (2015) Standard-dose versus high-dose conformal radiotherapy with concurrent and consolidation carboplatin plus paclitaxel with or without cetuximab for patients with stage IIIA or IIIB non-small-cell lung cancer (RTOG 0617): a randomised, two-by-two factorial phase 3 study. Lancet Oncol 16:187–199

Bradley JD, Hu C, Komaki R et al (2020) Long-term results of NRG oncology RTOG 0617: standard- versus high-dose chemoradiotherapy with or without cetuximab for unresectable stage III non-small-cell lung cancer. J Clin Oncol 38:706–t14

Brunsvig PF, Kyte JA, Kersten C et al (2011) Telomerase peptide vaccination in NSCLC: a phase II trial in stage III patients vaccinated after chemoradiotherapy and an 8-year update on a phase I/II trial. Clin Cancer Res 17:6847–6857

Butts C, Socinski MA, Mitchell PL et al (2014) Tecemotide (L-BLP25) versus placebo after chemoradiotherapy for stage iii nonsmall- cell lung cancer (start): a randomised, double-blind, phase 3 trial. Lancet Oncol 15:59–68

Byhardt RW (1999) Toxicities in RTOG combined-modality trials for inoperable non-small-cell lung cancer. Oncology (Huntingt) 13(10 Suppl 5):116–120

Byhardt RW, Pajak TF, Emami B, Herskovic A, Doggett RS, Olsen LA (1993) A phase I/II study to evaluate accelerated fractionation via concomitant boost for squamous, adeno, and large cell carcinoma of the lung: report of radiation therapy oncology group 84-07. Int J Radiat Oncol Biol Phys 26:459–468

Byhardt RW, Scott CB, Ettinger DS et al (1995) Concurrent hyperfractionated irradiation and chemotherapy for unresectable nonsmall cell lung cancer. Results of radiation therapy oncology group 90-15. Cancer 75:2337–2344

Byhardt RW, Scott C, Sause WT et al (1998) Response, toxicity, failure patterns, and survival in five radiation therapy oncology group (RTOG) trials of sequential and/or concurrent chemotherapy and radiotherapy for locally advanced non-small-cell carcinoma of the lung. Int J Radiat Oncol Biol Phys 42:469–478

Cakir S, Egehan I (2004) A randomized clinical trial of radiotherapy plus cisplatin versus radiotherapy alone in stage III non-small cell lung cancer. Lung Cancer 43:309–316

Chen AB, Li L, Cronin A et al (2014) Comparative effectiveness of intensity-modulated versus 3D conformal radiation therapy among medicare patients with stage III lung cancer. J Thorac Oncol 9:1788–1790

Choy H, Schwartzberg LS, Dakhil SR et al (2013) Phase 2 study of pemetrexed plus carboplatin, or pemetrexed plus cisplatin with concurrent radiation therapy followed by pemetrexed consolidation in patients with favorable-prognosis inoperable stage IIIA/B non-small-cell lung cancer. J Thorac Oncol 8:1308–1316

Clamon G, Herndon J, Cooper R, Chang AY, Rosenman J, Green MR (1999) Radiosensitization with carboplatin for patients with unresectable stage III non-small-cell lung cancer: a phase III trial of the cancer and leukemia group B and the eastern cooperative oncology group. J Clin Oncol 17:4–11

Cox JD, Yesner R, Mietlowski W, Petrovich Z (1979) Influence of cell type on failure pattern after irradiation for locally advanced carcinoma of the lung. Cancer 44:94–98

Cox JD, Azarnia N, Byhardt RW, Shin KH, Emami B, Pajak TF (1990) A randomized phase I/II trial of hyperfractionated radiation therapy with total doses of 60.0 Gy to 79.2 Gy: possible survival benefit with >69.6 Gy in favorable patients with radiation therapy oncology group stage III non-small cell lung carcinoma: report of radiation therapy oncology group 83-11. J Clin Oncol 8:1543–1555

Cox JD, Pajak TF, Asbell S et al (1993) Interruptions of high-dose radiation therapy decrease long-term survival of favorable patients with unresectable non-small cell carcinoma of the lung: analysis of 1244 cases from 3 radiation therapy oncology group (RTOG) trials. Int J Radiat Oncol Biol Phys 27:493–498

Cullen MH, Billingham LJ, Woodroffe CM et al (1997) Mitomycin, ifosfamide and cisplatin (MIC) in non-small cell lung cancer (NSCLC): 1. Results of a randomised trial in patients with localised, inoperable disease. Lung Cancer 18(Suppl 1):5. (abstract 10)

Curran WJ Jr, Paulus R, Langer CJ et al (2011) Sequential vs. concurrent chemoradiation for stage III non-small cell lung cancer: randomized phase III trial RTOG 9410. J Natl Cancer Inst 103:1452–1460

Davies AM, Chansky K, Lau DH et al (2006) Phase II study of consolidation paclitaxel after concurrent chemoradiation in poor-risk stage III non-small-cell lung cancer: SWOG S9712. J Clin Oncol 24:5242–5246

Dehing-Oberije C, De Ruysscher D, van der Weide H et al (2008) Tumor volume combined with number of positive lymph node stations is a more important prognostic factor than TNM stage for survival of non-small-cell lung cancer patients treated with (chemo)radiotherapy. Int J Radiat Oncol Biol Phys 70:1039–1044

Dieleman EMT, Apollonia LJ, Uitterhoeve ALJ, van Hoek MW et al (2018) Concurrent daily cisplatin and high-dose radiation therapy in patients with stage III non-small cell lung cancer. Int J Radiation Oncol Biol Phys 102:543–551

Dillman RO, Seagren SL, Propert KJ et al (1990) A randomized trial of induction chemotherapy plus high-dose radiation versus radiation alone in stage III non-small-cell lung cancer. N Engl J Med 323:940–945

Dillman RO, Herndon J, Seagren SL, Eaton WL Jr, Green MR (1996) Improved survival in stage III non-small-cell lung cancer: seven-year follow-up of cancer and leukemia group B (CALGB) 8433 trial. J Natl Cancer Inst 88:1210–1215

Durm GA, Jabbour SK, Althouse SK et al (2020) A phase 2 trial of consolidation pembrolizumab following concurrent chemoradiation for patients with unresectable stage III non-small cell lung cancer: Hoosier cancer research network LUN14-179. Cancer 126:4353–4361

Eaton BR, Pugh SL, Bradley JD et al (2016) Institutional enrollment and survival among NSCLC patients receiving chemoradiation: NRG oncology radiation therapy oncology group (RTOG) 0617. J Natl Cancer Inst 108:djw034

El Sharouni SY, Kal HB, Battermann JJ (2003) Accelerated regrowth of non-small-cell lung tumors after induction chemotherapy. Br J Cancer 89:2184–2189

Ezer N, Smith CB, Galsky MD et al (2014) Cisplatin vs. carboplatin-based chemoradiotherapy in patients >65 years of age with stage III non-small cell lung cancer. Radiother Oncol 112:272–278

Fournel P, Robinet G, Thomas P, Groupe Lyon-Saint-Etienne d'Oncologie Thoracique-Groupe Français de Pneumo-Cancérologie et al (2005) Randomized phase III trial of sequential chemoradiotherapy compared with concurrent chemoradiotherapy in locally advanced non-small-cell lung cancer: Groupe Lyon-saint-Etienne d'Oncologie Thoracique-Groupe Français de Pneumo-Cancérologie NPC 95-01 study. J Clin Oncol 23:5910–5917

Fournel P, Vergnenegre A, Robinet G, GFPC and IFCT Team et al (2016) Induction or consolidation chemotherapy for unresectable stage III non-small-cell lung cancer patients treated with concurrent chemoradiation: a randomized phase II trial GFPC—IFCT 02-01. Eur J Cancer 52:181–187

Fukuoka M, Niitani H, Suzuki A et al (1992) Phase II study of CPT-11, a new derivative of camptothecin for previously untreated non-small cell lung cancer. J Clin Oncol 10:16–20

Furuse K, Nishikawa H, Takada Y et al (1999) Phase III study of concurrent versus sequential thoracic radiotherapy in combination with mitomycin, vindesine and cisplatin in unresectable stage III non-small-cell lung cancer. J Clin Oncol 17:2692–2699

Furuse K, Hosoe S, Masuda N (2000) Impact of tumor control on survival in unresectable stage III non-small cell lung cancer (NSCLC) treated with concurrent thoracic radiotherapy (TRT) and chemotherapy (CT). Proc Am Soc Clin Oncol 19(Abstract 1893)

Gadgeel SM, Ruckdeschel JC, Patel BB et al (2011) Phase II study of pemetrexed and cisplatin, with chest radiotherapy followed by docetaxel in patients with stage III non-small cell lung cancer. J Thorac Oncol 6:927–933

Gandara DR, Chansky K, Albain KS et al (2003) Consolidation docetaxel after concurrent chemoradiotherapy in stage IIIB non-small-cell lung cancer: phase II southwest oncology group study S9504. J Clin Oncol 21:2004–2010

Giraud P, Rosenzweig KE, Yorke E (2001) Radiotherapy for lung cancer: can IMRT decrease the risk of esophagitis? Proc Am Soc Ther Radiol Oncol (ASTRO). San Francisco, Int J Radiat Oncol Biol Phys, pp 355–356 (abstr. #2250)

Gkika E, Lenz S, Schimek-Jasch T et al (2020) Efficacy and toxicity of different chemotherapy protocols for concurrent chemoradiation in non-small cell lung cancer—a secondary analysis of the PET plan trial. Cancers 12:3359

Goldstraw P, Crowley J, Chansky K, Giroux DJ, Groome PA (2007) The IASLC lung cancer staging project: proposals for the revision of the TNM stage groupings in the forthcoming (seventh) edition of the TNM classification of malignant tumours. J Thorac Oncol 2:706–714

Goldstraw P, Chansky K, Crowley J et al (2016) The IASLC lung cancer staging project: proposals for revision of the TNM stage groupings in the forthcoming (eighth) edition of the TNM classification for lung cancer. J Thorac Oncol 11:39–51

Groen HJG, van de Leest AHW, Fokkema E et al (2004) Phase III study of continuous carboplatin over 6 weeks with radiation versus radiation alone in stage III non small cell lung cancer. Ann Oncol 15:427–432

Hanna N, Neubauer M, Yiannoutsos C, Hoosier Oncology Group, US Oncology et al (2008) Phase III study of cisplatin, etoposide, and concurrent chest radiation with or without consolidation docetaxel in patients with inoperable stage III non-small-cell lung cancer: the Hoosier oncology group and U.S. oncology. J Clin Oncol 26:5755–5760

Harada H, Yamamoto N, Takahashi T et al (2009) Comparison of chemotherapy regimens for concurrent chemoradiotherapy in unresectable stage III non-small cell lung cancer. Int J Clin Oncol 14:507–512

Harris JP, Murphy JD, Hanlon AL et al (2014) A population-based comparative effectiveness study of radiation therapy techniques in stage III non-small cell lung cancer. Int J Radiat Oncol Biol Phys 88:872–884

Hasegawa T, Futamura Y, Horiba A et al (2016) Phase II study of nab-paclitaxel plus carboplatin in combination with thoracic radiation in patients with locally advanced non–small-cell lung cancer. J Radiat Res 57:50–54

Hatton M, Nankivell M, Lyn E et al (2011) Induction chemotherapy and continuous hyperfractionated accelerated radiation therapy (CHART) for patients with lo9cally advanced inoperable non-small-cell lung cancer: the MRC INCH randomized trial. Int J Radiation Oncol Biol Phys 81:712–718

Herscher LL, Hahn SM, Kroog G et al (1998) Phase I study of paclitaxel as a radiation sensitizer in the treatment of mesothelioma and non-small-cell lung cancer. J Clin Oncol 16:635–641

Holsti LR, Matson K (1980) A randomized study of splitcourse radiotherapy of lung cancer: long term results. Int J Radiat Oncol Biol Phys 6:977–981

Hui R, Özgüroğlu M, Villegas A et al (2019) Patient-reported outcomes with durvalumab after chemoradiotherapy in stage III, unresectable non-small-cell lung cancer (PACIFIC): a randomised, controlled, phase 3 study. Lancet Oncol 20:1670–1680

Hung M-S, Wu Y-F, Chen Y-C (2019) Efficacy of chemoradiotherapy versus radiation alone in patients with inoperable locally advanced non–small-cell lung cancer. A meta-analysis and systematic review. Medicine 98:27. (e16167)

Jain AK, Hughes RS, Sandler AB et al (2009) A phase II study of concurrent chemoradiation with weekly docetaxel, carboplatin, and radiation therapy followed by consolidation chemotherapy with docetaxel and carboplatin for locally advanced inoperable non-small cell lung cancer (NSCLC). J Thorac Oncol 4:722–727

Jeremic B, Shibamoto Y, Acimovic L, Djuric L (1995) Randomized trial of hyperfractionated radiation therapy with or without concurrent chemotherapy for stage III non-small-cell lung cancer. J Clin Oncol 13:452–458

Jeremic B, Shibamoto Y, Acimovic LJ, Milisavljevic S (1996) Hyperfractionated radiation therapy with or without concurrent low-dose daily carboplatin/etoposide for stage III non-small-cell lung cancer: a randomized study. J Clin Oncol 14:1065–1070

Jeremic B, Shibamoto Y, Milicic B, Nikolic N, Dagovic A, Milisavljevic S (1998) Concurrent radiochemotherapy for patients with stage III non-small cell lung cancer (NSCLC). Long-term results of a phase II study. Int J Radiat Oncol Biol Phys 42:1091–1096

Jeremic B, Shibamoto Y, Acimovic LJ et al (2001) Hyperfractionated radiation therapy and concurrent low-dose, daily carboplatin/etoposide with or without week-end carboplatin/etoposide chemotherapy in stage III non-small-cell lung cancer: a randomized trial. Int J Radiat Oncol Biol Phys 50:19–25

Jeremic B, Milicic B, Acimovic L, Milisavljevic S (2005) Concurrent hyperfractionated radiotherapy and low-dose daily carboplatin/paclitaxel in patients with stage III non-small cell lung cancer (NSCLC). Long-term results of a phase II study. J Clin Oncol 23:1144–1151

Johnson DH, Paul DM, Hande KR et al (1996) Paclitaxel plus carboplatin in advanced non-small-cell lung cancer: a phase II trial. J Clin Oncol 14:2054–2060

Kawano Y, Sasaki T, Yamaguchi H et al (2018) Phase I/II study of carboplatin plus nab-paclitaxel and concurrent radiotherapy for patients with locally advanced non–small cell lung cancer. Lung Cancer 125:136–141

Keene KS, Harman EM, Knauf DG, McCarley D, Zlotecki RA (2005) Five-year results of a phase II trial of hyperfractionated radiotherapy and concurrent daily cisplatin chemotherapy for stage III non-small-cell lung cancer. Am J Clin Oncol 28:217–222

Kelly K, Chansky K, Gaspar LE et al (2008) Phase III trial of maintenance gefitinib or placebo after concurrent chemoradiotherapy and docetaxel consolidation in inoperable stage III non-small-cell lung cancer: SWOG S0023. J Clin Oncol 26:2450–2456

Komaki R, Scott C, Ettinger D et al (1997) Randomized study of chemotherapy/radiation therapy combinations for favorable patients with locally advanced inoperable nonsmall cell lung cancer: radiation therapy oncology group (RTOG) 92-04. Int J Radiat Oncol Biol Phys 38:149–155

Koning CC, Wouterse SJ, Daams JG, Uitterhoeve LL, van den Heuvel MM, Belderbos JS (2013) Toxicity of concurrent radiochemotherapy for locally advanced non–small-cell lung cancer: a systematic review of the literature. Clin Lung Cancer 14:481–487

Koshy M, Malik R, Spiotto M, Mahmood U, Rusthovend CG, Sher DJ (2017) Association between intensity modulated radiotherapy and survival in patients with stage III non-small-cell lung cancer treated with chemoradiotherapy. Lung Cancer 108:222–227

Le Chevalier T, Arriagada R, Quoix E et al (1991) Radiotherapy alone versus combined chemotherapy and radiotherapy in nonresectable non-small-cell lung cancer: first analysis of a randomized trial in 353 patients. J Natl Cancer Inst 83:417–423

Le Chevalier T, Arriagada R, Tarayre M et al (1992) Significant effect of adjuvant chemotherapy on survival in locally advanced non-small cell lung carcinoma. J Natl Cancer Inst 84:58

Le Chevalier T, Brisgand D, Douillard J-Y et al (1994) Randomized study of vinorelbine and cisplatin versus vindesine and cisplatin versus vinorelbine alone in advanced non-small-cell lung cancer: results of a European multicenter trial including 612 patients. J Clin Oncol 12:360–367

Le Péchoux C, Arriagada R, Le Chevalier T et al (1996) Concurrent cisplatin vindesine and hyperfractionated thoracic radiotherapy in locally advanced nonsmall cell lung cancer. Int J Radiat Oncol Biol Phys 35:519–525

Lee C (2006) High-dose 3D chemoradiotherapy in stage III non-small cell lung cancer (NSCLC) at the University of North Carolina: Long-term follow up and late complications. Pro Amer Soc Clin Oncol 24:7145

Lee JS, Scott C, Komaki R et al (1996) Concurrent chemoradiation therapy with oral etoposide and cisplatin for locally advanced inoperable non-small-cell lung cancer: radiation therapy oncology group protocol 91-06. J Clin Oncol 14:1055–1064

Lee P, Bazan JG, Lavori PW et al (2012) Metabolic tumor volume is an independent prognostic factor in patients treated definitively for non–small-cell lung cancer. Clin Lung Cancer 13:52–58

Levy A, Bardet E, Lacas B et al (2017) A phase II open-label multicenter study of gefitinib in combination with irradiation followed by chemotherapy in patients with inoperable stage III non-small cell lung cancer. Oncotarget 8:1529–1533

Liang HY, Zhou H, Li XL, Yin ZH, Guan P, Zhou BS (2010) Chemo-radiotherapy for advanced non-small cell lung cancer: concurrent or sequential? It's no longer the question: a systematic review. Int J Cancer 127:718–728

Liang J, Bi N, Wu S et al (2017) Etoposide and cisplatin versus paclitaxel and carboplatin with concurrent thoracic radiotherapy in unresectable stage III non-small cell lung cancer: a multicenter randomized phase III trial. Ann Oncol 28:777–783

Lu C, Lee JJ, Komaki R et al (2010) Chemoradiotherapy with or without AE-941 in stage III non–small cell lung cancer: a randomized phase III trial. J Natl Cancer Inst 102:1–7

Lynch TJ Jr, Kalish L, Strauss G et al (1994) Phase II study of topotecan in metastatic non-small-cell lung cancer. J Clin Oncol 12:347–352

Manegold C, Bergman B, Chemaissani A et al (1997) Single-agent gemcitabine versus cisplatin-etoposide: early results of a randomized phase II study in locally-advanced or metastatic non-small cell lung cancer. Ann Oncol 8:525–529

Marino P, Preatoni A, Cantoni A (1995) Randomized trials of radiotherapy alone versus combined chemotherapy and radiotherapy in stages IIIa and IIIb nonsmall cell lung cancer. A meta-analysis. Cancer 76:593–601

Masters GA, Haraf DJ, Hoffman PC et al (1998) Phase I study of vinorelbine, cisplatin and concomitant thoracic radiation in the treatment of advanced chest malignancies. J Clin Oncol 16:2157–2163

Mauer AM, Masters GA, Haraf DJ et al (1998) Phase I study of docetaxel with concomitant thoracic radiation therapy. J Clin Oncol 16:159–164

Mehta MP, Tannehill SP, Adak S et al (1998) Phase II trial of hyperfractionated accelerated radiation therapy for nonresectable non-small-cell lung cancer: results of eastern cooperative oncology group 4593. J Clin Oncol 16:3518–3523

Millward MJ, Zalcberg J, Bishop JF et al (1996) Phase I trial of docetaxel and cisplatin in previously untreated patients with advanced non-small cell lung cancer. J Clin Oncol 14:750–758

Mountain CF (1986) A new international staging system for lung cancer. Chest 89:225S–233S

Mountain CF (1997) Revisions in the international system for staging lung cancer. Chest 111:1710–1717

Movsas B, Langer CJ, Ross HJ et al (2010) Randomized phase II trial of cisplatin, etoposide, and radiation followed by gemcitabine alone or by combined gemcitabine and docetaxel in stage III a/B unresectable non-small cell lung cancer. J Thorac Oncol 5:673–679

Nawrocki S, Krzakowski M, Wasilewska-Tesluk E et al (2010) Concurrent chemotherapy and short course radiotherapy in patients with stage IIIA to IIIB non-small cell lung cancer not eligible for radical treatment: results of a randomized phase II study. J Thorac Oncol 5:1255–1262

Non-small Cell Lung Cancer Collaborative Group (1995) Chemotherapy in non-small cell lung cancer: a meta-analysis using updated data on individual patients from 52 randomised clinical trials. Brit Med J 311:899–909

Nyman J, Friesland S, Hallqvist A et al (2009) How to improve loco-regional control in stages IIIa-b NSCLC? Results of a three-armed randomized trial from the Swedish lung cancer study group. Lung Cancer 65:62–67

O'Rourke N, Roqué I, Figuls M, Farré Bernadó N, Macbeth F (2010) Concurrent chemoradiotherapy in non-small cell lung cancer. Cochrane Database Syst Rev 6:CD002140

Oshita F, Noda K, Nishiwaki Y et al (1997) Phase II study of irinotecan and etoposide in patients with metastatic non-small-cell lung cancer. J Clin Oncol 15: 304–309

Perez CA, Bauer M, Edelstein S, Gillespie BW, Birch R (1986) Impact of tumor control on survival in carcinoma of the lung treated with irradiation. Int J Radiat Oncol Biol Phys 12:539–547

Perez CA, Pajak TF, Rubin P et al (1987) Long term observations of the patterns of failure in patients with unresectable non-oat cell carcinoma of the lung treated with definitive radiotherapy. Report by the radiation therapy oncology group. Cancer 59:1874–1881

Perez-Soler R, Fossella FV, Glisson BS et al (1996) Phase II study of topotecan in patients with advanced non-small-cell lung cancer previously untreated with chemotherapy. J Clin Oncol 14:503–513

Petrovich Z, Mietlowski W, Ohanian M, Cox J (1977) Clinical report on the treatment of locally advanced lung cancer. Cancer 40:72–77

Petrovich Z, Stanley K, Cox JD, Paig C (1981) Radiotherapy in the management of locally advanced lung cancer of all cell types: final report of randomized trial. Cancer 48:1335–1340

Pritchard RS, Anthony SP (1996) Chemotherapy plus radiotherapy compared with radiotherapy alone in the treatment of locally advanced, unresectable, non-small-cell lung cancer: a meta-analysis. Ann Intern Med 125:723–729

Rami-Porta R, Bolejack V, Giroux DJ, International Association for the Study of Lung Cancer Staging and Prognostic Factors Committee et al (2014) Advisory board members and participating institutions. The IASLC lung cancer staging project: the new database to inform the eighth edition of the TNM classification of lung cancer. J Thorac Oncol 9:1618–1624

Reynolds RD, O'Dell S (1978) Combination modality therapy in lung cancer: a survival study showing beneficial results of AMCOF (adriamycin, methotrexate, cyclophosphamide, oncovin and 5-fluorouracil). Cancer 42:385–389

Robertson JM, Ten Haken RK, Hazuka MB (1997) Dose escalation for non small cell lung cancer using conformal radiation therapy. Int J Radiat Oncol Biol Phys 37:1079–1085

Rosenman JG, Halle JS, Socinski MA et al (2002) High-dose conformal radiotherapy for treatment of stage IIIA/B non-small cell lung cancer: technical issues and results of a phase I/II trial. Int J Radiat Oncol Biol Phys 54:348–356

Roswit B, Patno ME, Rapp R et al (1968) The survival of patients with inoperable lung cancer: a large-scale randomized study of radiation therapy versus placebo. Radiology 90:688–697

Sakai H, Yoneda S, Kobayashi K et al (2004) Phase II study of bi-weekly docetaxel and carboplatin with concurrent thoracic radiation therapy followed by consolidation chemotherapy with docetaxel plus carboplatin for stage III unresectable non-small cell lung cancer. Lung Cancer 43:195–201

Santana-Davila R, Devisetty K, Szabo A et al (2015) Cisplatin and etoposide versus carboplatin and paclitaxel with concurrent radiotherapy for stage III non-small-cell lung cancer: an analysis of veterans health administration data. J Clin Oncol 33:567–574

Sasaki T, Seto T, Yamanaka T et al (2018) A randomised phase II trial of S-1 plus cisplatin versus vinorelbine plus cisplatin with concurrent thoracic radiotherapy for unresectable, locally advanced non-small cell lung cancer: WJOG5008L. Br J Cancer 119: 675–682

Saunders MI, Dische S (1990) Continuous, hyperfractionated, accelerated radiotherapy (CHART) in non-small cell carcinoma of the bronchus. Int J Radiat Oncol Biol Phys 19:1211–1215

Saunders M, Dische S, Barrett A, Harvey A, Griffiths G, Palmar M (1999) Continuous hyperfractionated accelerated radiotherapy (CHART) versus conventional radiotherapy in non-small cell lung cancer: mature data from the randomised multicentre trial. Radiother Oncol 52:137–148

Sause WT, Scott C, Taylor S et al (1995) Radiation therapy oncology group 88-08 and eastern cooperative oncology group 4588: preliminary results of a phase III trial in regionally advanced, unresectable nonsmall cell lung cancer. J Natl Cancer Inst 87:198–205

Sause W, Kolesar P, Taylor S IV et al (2000) Final results of phase III trial in regionally advanced unresectable non-small cell lung cancer: radiation therapy oncology group, eastern cooperative oncology group, and southwest oncology group. Chest 117:358–364

Schaake-Koning C, van den Bogaert W, Dalesio O et al (1992) Effects of concomitant cisplatin and radiotherapy on inoperable non-small cell lung cancer. N Engl J Med 326:524–530

Schild SE, Fan W, Stinchcombe TE et al (2018) Exploring radiotherapy targeting strategy and dose: a pooled analysis of cooperative group trials of combined modality therapy for stage III non-small cell lung cancer. J Thorac Oncol 13:1171–1182

Segawa Y, Kiura K, Takigawa N et al (2010) Phase III trial comparing docetaxel and cisplatin combination chemotherapy with mitomycin, vindesine, and cisplatin combination chemotherapy with concurrent thoracic radiotherapy in locally advanced non-small-cell lung cancer: OLCSG 0007. J Clin Oncol 28:3299–3306

Sekine I, Nokihara H, Sumi M et al (2006) Docetaxel consolidation therapy following cisplatin, vinorelbine, and concurrent thoracic radiotherapy in patients with unresectable stage III non-small cell lung cancer. J Thorac Oncol 1:810–815

Shimokawa T, Yamada K, Tanaka H et al (2021) Randomized phase II trial of S-1 plus cisplatin or docetaxel plus cisplatin with concurrent thoracic radiotherapy for inoperable stage III non-small cell lung cancer. Cancer Med 10:626–633

Socinski MA, Blackstock AW, Bogart JA et al (2008) Randomized phase II trial of induction chemotherapy followed by concurrent chemotherapy and dose escalated thoracic conformal radiotherapy (74 Gy) in stage III non-small-cell lung cancer: CALGB 30105. J Clin Oncol 26:2457–2463

Soresi E, Borghini U, Zucali R et al (1988) A randomized clinical trial comparing radiation therapy versus radiation therapy plus cis-Dichlorodiamine platinum (II) in the treatment of locally advanced non small cell lung cancer. Semin Oncol 15(Suppl 7):20–25

Steel GG, Peckham MJ (1979) Exploitable mechanisms in combined radiotherapy–chemotherapy. Int J Radiat Oncol Biol Phys 5:85–91

Steuer CE, Behera M, Ernani V et al (2017) Comparison of concurrent use of thoracic radiation with either carboplatin-paclitaxel or cisplatin-etoposide for patients with stage III non–small-cell lung cancer. A systematic review. JAMA Oncol 3:1120–1129

Strøm HH, Bremnes RM, Sundstrøm SH, Helbekkmo H, Fløtten Ø, Aaseb U (2013) Concurrent palliative chemoradiation leads to survival and quality of life benefits in poor prognosis stage III non-small-cell lung cancer: a randomised trial by the Norwegian lung cancer study group. Br J Cancer 109:1467–1475

Trovo MG, Minatel E, Franchin G et al (1992) Radiotherapy versus radiotherapy enhanced by cisplatin in stage III non small cell lung cancer. Int J Radiat Oncol Biol Phys 24:11–15

Ulutin HC, Guden M, Oysul K, Surenkok S, Pak Y (2000) Split-course radiotherapy with or without concurrent or sequential chemotherapy in non-small cell lung cancer. Radiat Med 18:93–96

Vokes EE, Gregor A, Turrisi AT (1998) Gemcitabine and radiation therapy for non-small cell lung cancer. Semin Oncol 25(Suppl 4):66–69

Vokes EE, Herndon JE II, Crawford J et al (2002) Randomized phase II study of cisplatin with gemcitabine or paclitaxel or vinorelbine as induction chemotherapy followed by concomitant chemoradiotherapy for stage IIIB non-small-cell lung cancer: cancer and leukemia group B study 9431. J Clin Oncol 20:4191–4198

Wang L, Wu S, Ou G et al (2012) Randomized phase II study of concurrent cisplatin/ etoposide or paclitaxel/carboplatin and thoracic radiotherapy in patients with stage III non-small cell lung cancer. Lung Cancer 77:89–96

Werner-Wasik M, Swann RS, Bradley J et al (2008) Increasing tumor volume is predictive of poor overall and progression-free survival: secondary analysis of the radiation therapy oncology group 93-11 phase I-II radiation dose-escalation study in patients with inoperable non-small-cell lung cancer. Int J Radiat Oncol Biol Phys 70:385–390

White JE, Chen T, Reed R et al (1982) Limited squamous cell carcinoma of the lung: a southwest oncology group randomised study of radiation with or without doxorubicin chemotherapy and with or without levamisole immunotherapy. Cancer Treat Rep 66:1113–1120

Wozniak AJ, Moon J, Thomas CR Jr et al (2015) A Pilot trial of cisplatin/etoposide/radiotherapy followed by consolidation docetaxel and the combination of bevacizumab (NSC-704865) in patients with inoperable locally advanced stage III non-small-cell lung cancer: SWOG S0533. Clin Lung Cancer 16:340–347

Yamamoto N, Nakagawa K, Nishimura Y et al (2010) Phase III study comparing second- and third-generation regimens with concurrent thoracic radiotherapy in patients with unresectable stage III non-small-cell lung cancer: West Japan thoracic oncology group WJTOG0105. J Clin Oncol 28:3739–3745

Ying M, Liu J, Zhou W, Weng K, Long B, Wang Y (2019) The role of additional chemotherapy in combination with concurrent chemoradiotherapy for locally advanced inoperable non-small cell lung cancer, a systematic review and meta-analysis of 12 randomized trials. Cancer Investig 37:376–386

Yorke E (2001) Advantages of IMRT for dose escalation in radiation therapy for lung cancer. Med Phys 28:1291–1294

Zhang Q-N, Wang D-L, Wang X-H et al (2012) Non-conventional radiotherapy versus conventional radiotherapy for inoperable non-small-cell lung cancer: a meta-analysis of randomized clinical trials. Thorac Cancer 3:269–279

Optimizing Drug Therapies in the Maintenance Setting After Radiochemotherapy in Non-small Cell Lung Cancer

Steven H. Lin and David Raben

Contents

1. Introduction 571
2. Improving Outcomes with Maintenance ICI After CRT 572
3. Further Enhancements of ICI Combinations in the Maintenance Setting ... 574
   3.1 ICI + Stereotactic Body Radiotherapy (SBRT) 575
   3.2 ICI + Angiogenesis Inhibitors 575
   3.3 Anti-CTLA-4 and Anti-PD-1 575
   3.4 Anti-PD-L1 and Anti-TIGIT 576
   3.5 ICI and DNA Damage Repair Inhibitors 576
   3.6 ICI and Anti-TGF-β 577
   3.7 ICI and Anti-CD73 or Anti-NKG2A 577
4. Oncogene-Driven Tumors 577
5. Conclusion 578

References 579

S. H. Lin (✉)
The University of Texas MD Anderson Cancer Center, Houston, TX, USA
e-mail: SHLin@mdanderson.org

D. Raben (✉)
Department of Radiation Oncology,
University of Colorado Health, Aurora, CO, USA
e-mail: david.raben@cuanschutz.edu

1 Introduction

While only around a quarter of the patients with a diagnosis of non-small cell lung cancer present with stage III disease, majority of patients are deemed unresectable due to medical or technical reasons (Duma et al. 2019). The curative intent approach is concomitant chemotherapy with radiotherapy, established over decades of clinical trials that demonstrated that adding chemotherapy before radiotherapy improved outcomes over radiotherapy alone (Dillman et al. 1996) and the benefit of concomitant chemotherapy and radiotherapy at the expense of enhanced toxicities (Curran et al. 2011; Koning et al. 2013). Locoregional failures can reach 30–40%, but the greatest risk is still systemic recurrence, with more than 80% of recurrences after CRT observed to be distant metastatic failures, with or without locoregional recurrences (Taugner et al. 2020). Enormous efforts were made in numerous clinical trials testing the role of induction chemotherapy (Vokes et al. 2007), different concurrent chemotherapy regimens (Senan et al. 2016), consolidation chemotherapy (Tsujino et al. 2013), or even adding epidermal growth factor receptor-tyrosine kinase inhibitors (EGFR-TKI) in maintenance after CRT and chemotherapy (Kelly et al. 2008), none of which demonstrated any survival benefit, if not a detriment in some trials, over

CRT alone. The PACIFIC trial, adding anti-PD-L1 monoclonal antibody durvalumab as maintenance therapy after CRT, was the first trial in the history of the treatment of unresectable NSCLC where the addition of a single modality of therapy improved survival by greater than 10%, larger than any of the previous advances in this disease (Antonia et al. 2017). Importantly, no significant increases in toxicity were observed signifying a critical inflexion point for an improved therapeutic ratio. The PACIFIC results with the most recent 4-year update certainly have established a new bar in improved survival outcomes; however, a significant number of patients will still relapse and die from their disease (Faivre-Finn et al. 2021). While ongoing clinical trials are evaluating if outcomes could improve by bringing immune checkpoint inhibitors (ICI) earlier even before starting CRT or during CRT, many are building on the current PACIFIC paradigm and applying additional agents or approaches that could potentially synergize with consolidation ICI. This chapter focuses on optimizing maintenance therapy after CRT to prevent systemic disease recurrence. Combination approaches to enhance CRT are mentioned in other chapters.

2 Improving Outcomes with Maintenance ICI After CRT

Arguably, the most impactful study for the field of unresectable NSCLC in the modern era was the PACIFIC trial (NCT02125461). This was a global phase III double-blind, placebo-controlled, randomized trial that evaluated 713 patients who did not demonstrate progression or pneumonitis after CRT and randomized 2:1 to durvalumab vs. placebo. Durvalumab was given intravenously (IV) at 10 mg/kg every 2 weeks up to 1 year. The co-primary endpoints were progression-free survival and overall survival, along with post-CRT treatment-related toxicity. The first report on PFS already demonstrated a median PFS of 16.8 months vs. 5.6 and 18 months of 44.2% vs. 27.0%, for the durvalumab vs. placebo arms, respectively (Antonia et al. 2017). While adverse events were numerically slightly higher with durvalumab, most of the AEs were of low grade, and higher grade toxicities of concern such as pneumonitis were not significantly higher in the durvalumab group. Shortly after the publication of these results, in February 2018, the US FDA granted approval for the use of durvalumab as consolidation therapy in patients who have not progressed after CRT. A year later, the overall survival results were released, demonstrating a 24-month OS rate of 66.3% vs. 55.6%, with a HR of 0.68 ($p = 0.0025$) (Antonia et al. 2018). The distant metastatic relapse rate was substantially reduced with durvalumab, with a median time to death or DM of 28.3 vs. 16.2 months (HR 0.53; 95% CI, 0.41–0.68). The most frequent AEs that led to trial discontinuation were pneumonitis in 4.8% in the durvalumab group vs. 2.6% in the placebo group, but most of the differences were attributable to expected low levels of drug-induced pneumonitis, as the severe radiation pneumonitis only occurred in 1.3% in both groups. The OS results have been updated, with a median follow-up of 34.2 months, median OS of 47.5 vs. 29.1 months, and estimated 4-year OS rate of 49.6% vs. 36.3%, for the durvalumab vs. the placebo groups, respectively. The 4-year PFS remained statistically significant at 35.3% vs. 19.5%, and median PFS was 17.2 vs. 5.8 months, for the two groups, respectively.

A single-arm trial in 93 patients was conducted by the Hoosier Oncology Group (LUN14-179) using maintenance pembrolizumab after CRT (Hoosier Cancer Research Network) (NCT02343952) (Durm et al. 2020). With a median follow-up of 32.2 months, the time to distant metastatic disease or death was 30.7 months, with a median PFS of 18.7 months and OS of 35.8 months. The 1-, 2-, and 3-year OS estimates were 81.2%, 62.0%, and 48.5%, respectively. While these numbers were more or less similar to the durvalumab arm of the PACIFIC trial, both trials convincingly demonstrated that adding ICI in the maintenance setting was critical to improve survival outcomes that greatly exceeded historical rates seen from RTOG 0617, which previously set the benchmark for the best survival outcomes in the modern era with CRT alone using the standard dose of 60 Gy in 30 fractions with concurrent chemotherapy. The trial showed a median PFS of 12 months, median OS of 28.7 months, and 5-year OS of 32.1%. These numbers were a step-up from the results seen in RTOG 9410 with CRT alone but paled in comparison to the studies that added maintenance ICI.

Three smaller single-arm studies combined ICI with concurrent CRT followed by maintenance ICI, mostly to assess the safety of such combination but also preliminary efficacy, with the hopes that adding concomitant ICI with CRT should further enhance outcomes over just ICI giving in maintenance. In a phase I study of 21 stage III unresectable NSCLC (NCT02621398), pembrolizumab (200 mg IV Q3weeks) was added concurrently with chemoradiation followed by maintenance pembrolizumab for up to 1 year (Jabbour et al. 2020). The regimen was well tolerated with grade 3 immune-related adverse events seen in 18%, with one grade 5 pneumonitis. For patients who received at least one dose of pembrolizumab ($N = 21$), the median PFS was 18.7 and 12-month PFS was 69.7%. With at least two doses ($N = 19$), the median PFS was 21 months.

In the phase II single-arm DETERRED trial (NCT02525757), atezolizumab (1500 mg IV Q3weeks) was given in two parts: part 1 in 10 patients as maintenance therapy given concomitantly with two cycles of carboplatin/paclitaxel followed by atezolizumab monotherapy up to 1 year. In part 2 in 30 patients, concurrent atezolizumab was given with chemoradiation followed by two cycles of carboplatin/paclitaxel/atezolizumab followed by atezolizumab maintenance (Lin et al. 2020). For part 1, grade 3 immune-related adverse events were 30% and grade 2+ pneumonitis was 10%. For part 2, grade 3 immune-related adverse events were 20%, and grade 2+ pneumonitis was 16% (no grade 5 pneumonitis). For part 1, the median PFS was 18.6 months and OS was 22.8 months. For part 2, the median PFS was 13.2 months, and the OS was not reached.

Combination of nivolumab with CRT followed by nivolumab maintenance was tested in the phase II single-arm NICOLAS study (NCT02434081) (Peters et al. 2021). The study enrolled 79 patients with unresectable stage IIIA/B (per AJCC 7th edition) NSCLC, and they were treated with three cycles of platinum-based chemotherapy and concurrent radiotherapy to 66 Gy in 33 fractions, with nivolumab administered at 360 mg IV Q3weeks. Nivolumab was given as maintenance therapy at 480 mg IV Q4weeks up to 1 year. With a median follow-up time of 21 months, the 1-year PFS was 53.7% and median PFS was 12.7 months. At a longer median follow-up of 32.6 months, the median OS was 38.8 months, and the 2-year OS was 63.7%.

The aforementioned trials that combined concurrent ICI with CRT followed by maintenance ICI were small studies that had demonstrated the safety of combining ICI with CRT. However, given the small size of the studies and heterogeneity in the patient population, it is difficult to provide a meaningful comparison to PACIFIC or LUN14-179 in terms of relative efficacy, but the early signal for the concurrent ICI studies does not suggest a substantial improvement over ICI maintenance alone. This is corroborated with the disappointing results from JAVELIN Head and Neck 100 (NCT02952586), which compared anti-PD-L1 monoclonal antibody avelumab added to concurrent chemoradiation and maintenance avelumab for 1 year to placebo-controlled chemoradiation alone and in maintenance for locally advanced head and neck squamous cell carcinoma (Lee et al. 2021). With 697 patients enrolled, there was no improvement with the addition of avelumab in PFS or OS, and it even trended in favor of the control chemoradiation arm. The only explanation for these unexpected findings is the possible antagonism to the effectiveness of ICI with chemoradiation as well as the possibility that treating large fields with radiation including uninvolved lymph node basins over 6–7 weeks may have led to increased immunosuppression. Whether such antagonism will also be seen with

NSCLC will need to wait for the completion of EA5181, an ongoing phase III randomized trial testing the efficacy of concurrent durvalumab with CRT followed by maintenance durvalumab vs. the PACIFIC regimen (NCT04092283).

At this point in time, the PACIFIC regimen is still considered the standard of care, but it is expected that only a subset of patients will benefit from maintenance durvalumab. Using circulating tumor DNA (ctDNA) minimal residual disease (MRD) assessment after CRT and before durvalumab, Max Diehn and colleagues demonstrated that detectable ctDNA after CRT portended to rapid progression of disease (Chaudhuri et al. 2017). Importantly, patients who had no evidence of ctDNA detected MRD after CRT did extremely well, with patients treated with CRT alone and undetectable ctDNA having the same clinical outcomes as patients treated with consolidation durvalumab and undetectable ctDNA. In the MRD analysis of a small number of patients with detectable ctDNA after CRT, a decline in ctDNA levels after starting durvalumab predicted for long-term survival for these patients (Moding et al. 2020). Patients without any decline in ctDNA levels with durvalumab had rapid progression of disease. This suggests that the benefit of maintenance therapy with durvalumab could be predicted by ctDNA MRD analysis and that treatment intensification may be important for patients with +MRD after CRT (Hellmann et al. 2020). This idea is currently being tested in a trial where chemotherapy is added to durvalumab in MRD+ disease after CRT as a potential treatment intensification to help convert nonresponders to responders (NCT04585490). While this is clearly an important step toward augmenting ICI effectiveness after CRT, more targeted or personalized approaches are needed, to rationally combine agents with ICI in the maintenance setting to improve cures after CRT in unresectable NSCLC.

For patients unable to receive standard CRT regimens, SWOG 1933 has sought to evaluate the safety and utility of treating stage II–III NSCLC patients with hypofractionated RT (60 Gy in 15 fractions) followed by atezolizumab (NCT04310020).

3 Further Enhancements of ICI Combinations in the Maintenance Setting

Enhancement of maintenance therapy after CRT will build on consolidation ICI. Any approaches to combine additional agents should have the biologic rationale that will enhance the effectiveness of ICI but also not substantially increase the toxicity of the combination. While ICI in the maintenance setting can benefit a subset of patients, its activity is primarily acting as an effective systemic therapy as a single agent that will be effective against certain tumors, but any synergy with CRT is unlikely to be present since the start of durvalumab is far removed enough in time to not exert any additive/synergistic interactions. There is some indication that the earlier durvalumab starts relative to the end of CRT, particularly <14 days, the point estimate of PFS seems to be better than >14 days (Antonia et al. 2017). So much like in some preclinical models, adding radiation with or shortly before the start of ICI could promote inflammation, upregulate PD-L1, and enhance combination effect of ICI (Lhuillier et al. 2019). Besides radiation itself, many factors within the tumor cells and the tumor microenvironment could be modulated to help enhance the inflammatory response when immune checkpoint is blocked. The potential approaches for combination strategies are vast, which may be easier to conduct without the need in most cases for a phase I study since many of the combinations have already been conducted in stage IV settings with well-established toxicity profiles. There may be concern that radiation pneumonitis could be exacerbated by adding combination drug therapy. Safety run-in in a single-arm phase II trial will be an effective way to accelerate the development of novel combination therapies, with efficacy using PFS and toxicity as co-primary endpoints. Determining the most favorable combinations to test in the maintenance setting would leverage efficacy signals seen in stage IV settings in lung cancer. We will highlight some of the currently open trials that are examining some of these approaches, with the anticipation that many more will be proposed in the future as more novel therapies and combinations are being discovered.

3.1 ICI + Stereotactic Body Radiotherapy (SBRT)

Since local recurrence is common after CRT, and residual disease within the primary lesion after CRT is potentially a source of resistant clones that could confer treatment resistance, annihilating residual primary disease after CRT could improve recurrence-free survival and possibly contribute to overall survival. There is also potential synergy of giving ablative doses of radiation to areas of residual disease with administration of ICI afterwards. Interestingly, Wei et al. recently published preclinical data showing that the timing of radiation and anti-PD-1 therapy influenced abscopal responses with the greatest benefit noted when anti-PD-1 was administered AFTER radiation, resulting in the expansion of CD8 T cells. In contrast, anti-PD-1 therapy PRIOR to radiation suppressed any strong immune response and destruction of CD8 T cells (Wei et al. 2021). A single-arm phase I/II study is assessing the safety and efficacy of consolidative SBRT boost after CRT in a phase I dose escalation study starting with 6.5 Gy × 2 fractions up to 10 Gy × 2 fractions to the residual primary lung mass delivered 1–2 months after CRT and with adjuvant durvalumab (NCT04748419). An additional 32 patients will be treated at the MTD. The primary endpoints are safety of combining boost SBRT in phase I and 12-month PFS in phase II. Another similar study in 25 patients will deliver two doses at 10 Gy × 2 SBRT to the primary tumor over 1–2 weeks after completing CRT and between the first and second doses of durvalumab (10 mg/kg Q2weeks) (NCT03589547).

3.2 ICI + Angiogenesis Inhibitors

Intratumoral hypoxia commonly seen in solid tumors increases HIF-alpha expression, which leads to increases in VEGF levels. This can trigger angiogenesis, but also exerts immunosuppressive effects in the TME by inhibition of dendritic cell maturation; recruiting of Tregs, MDSCs, and tumor-associated macrophages; macrophage polarization from M1 to M2; and upregulation of PD-1 on CD8 T cells and Tregs. Clinical trials in advanced-stage renal cell carcinoma have already demonstrated the benefit of combining VEGFR inhibitors with ICI. In IMmotion151 trial, atezolizumab and bevacizumab as compared to sunitinib demonstrated significantly prolonged PFS with the atezo/bev combination (HR 0.74; 95% CI, 0.57–0.96). In the JAVELIN Renal 101 phase III trial comparing avelumab and axitinib vs. sunitinib in previously untreated stage IV RCC, the combination prolonged PFS (HR 0.69; 95% CI, 0.56–0.84). In nonsquamous carcinoma of the lung, the IMpower150 trial showed that atezo/bev in combination with carboplatin/paclitaxel is superior than either atezo/carboplatin/paclitaxel or bev/carboplatin/paclitaxel (HR 0.76; 95% CI, 0.63–0.93). While adding bev with durvalumab is not yet developed, a study is combining camrelizumab (anti-PD-1 agent from Jiangsu Hengrui Medicine Co., China) with apatinib, a TKI that selectively inhibits VEGF-R2, in a single-arm phase II open-label trial (NCT04749394).

3.3 Anti-CTLA-4 and Anti-PD-1

Targeting CTLA-4 with PD-1 enhances antitumor immunity by blocking immune checkpoint protein on antigen-presenting cells and also depletes Tregs that express high levels of CTLA-4. Due to the phase III CheckMate 227 trial, combining ipilimumab and nivolumab was recently FDA approved for use in advanced NSCLC in the first-line setting who had PD-L1 expression of ≥1%. Given the safety of the NICOLAS study of combining nivolumab with CRT and in maintenance, CheckMate 73L (NCT04026412) is a phase III trial in which 888 patients with untreated stage III NSCLC and stratified by age, PD-L1 expression, and disease stage will be randomized 1:1:1 to one of the three arms: (1) concurrent nivolumab and CRT followed by nivolumab; (2) concurrent nivolumab and CRT followed by nivolumab + ipilimumab; and (3) CRT followed by durvalumab. Primary endpoints are PFS and OS comparing arm 1 vs. 3, with secondary endpoints of PFS comparing arm 2 vs. 1 or 3, objective response rate, time to response, duration of response, time to distant metastasis, and safety.

3.4 Anti-PD-L1 and Anti-TIGIT

T-cell immunoreceptor with Ig and ITIM domains (TIGIT) is a cell surface protein present on T and NK cells. TIGIT binds to CD155 on antigen-presenting cells or tumor cells to suppress T- and NK-cell functions (Johnston et al. 2014; Yu et al. 2009). Combining dual blockade of TIGIT and PD-1/L-1 can augment immune-stimulated antitumor response in preclinical models (Hung et al. 2018), and this is also seen in advanced NSCLC in the CITYSCAPE trial in first-line metastatic NSCLC (NCT03563716) (Rodriguez-Abreu et al. 2020). In this phase II double-blind, placebo-controlled, randomized trial, the combination of anti-TIGIT tiragolumab and anti-PD-L1 atezolizumab vs. atezolizumab alone significantly improved overall treatment response (37% vs. 21%) and resulted in a 42% lowered risk of disease worsening or death. This is even more significant in the high PD-L1-expressing tumors, with a response rate of 66% vs. 24%, respectively. Importantly, minimal additional toxicity was noted with the addition of tiragolumab. Because of this trial, tiragolumab in combination with atezolizumab was granted breakthrough therapy designation by the US FDA on January 5, 2021, for the first-line treatment of people with metastatic NSCLC. Currently, this combination is being tested in the maintenance setting after CRT without evidence of progression in stage III unresectable NSCLC compared to durvalumab in the phase III SKYSCRAPER-03 trial (NCT04513925). Eight-hundred patients are randomized in this open-label trial with no crossover. This trial stratifies by PD-L1 expression, staging using AJCC 8th edition (IIIA vs. IIIB vs. IIIC), histology, and performance status, and excludes ALK and EGFR+ patients.

3.5 ICI and DNA Damage Repair Inhibitors

DNA-damaging agents hold the promise to synergize with ICI by enhancing inflammatory response triggered by intrinsic cytosolic free DNA-sensing pathways such as STING/cGAS. This triggers release of type I interferon, which can induce PD-L1 but also serves as a chemoattractant to pull in T cells to the TME (Pantelidou et al. 2019). PARP inhibitors can also increase mutations during DNA replication and increase neoantigen load, which can also trigger antigen-specific response. Poly-ADP-ribose polymerase (PARP)-1 inhibitors have single-agent antitumor efficacy DNA damage repair (DDR)-deficient tumors like in BRCA1/2-mutant breast and ovarian cancers, as well as tumors that carry somatic mutations in other DDRs such as ATM, ATR, BARD1, BRIP1, CHK1, CHK2, PALB2, RAD51, and FANC. PARP-1 inhibitors with ICI have been combined in BRCA-mutant breast and ovarian cancer trials, with promising overall response rates. Besides direct impact on genetically susceptible tumors, PARP-1 regulates the immune system, directs the expression of immunosuppressive FoxP3 on Tregs (Zhang et al. 2013a), and modulates the expression of the immunosuppressive transforming growth factor-β (TGF-β) receptors on T cells (Zhang et al. 2013b). Blocking PARP-1 could potentially reverse immunosuppressive mechanisms to enhance ICI response. The MK-7339-012/KEYLYNK-012 (NT04380636) is a phase III randomized trial in a head-to-head comparison to see if the combination of PARP-1 inhibitor olaparib with anti-PD-1 pembrolizumab will be superior to the PACIFIC regimen. The trial will randomize 870 patients with stage III NSCLC to one of the three arms: (1) pembrolizumab with concurrent CRT followed by pembrolizumab maintenance and olaparib placebo; (2) pembrolizumab with concurrent CRT followed by pembrolizumab + olaparib; and (3) concurrent CRT followed by maintenance durvalumab (PACIFIC). Co-primary endpoints are PFS and OS with superiority of arm 1 vs. arm 3, and arm 2 vs. arm 3.

3.6 ICI and Anti-TGF-β

TGF-β is an immunosuppressive cytokine released by tumor cells or inflammatory or stromal cells from within the TME to suppressive effector T and NK cells and antigen-presenting cells, causes expansion of Tregs, and polarizes macrophages to the anti-inflammatory M2 phenotype (Batlle and Massagué 2019). This results in the ability for cancer cells to block immune surveillance and abrogate the effectiveness of ICI. M7824 is a novel bifunctional antibody that is a fusion protein linked to the extracellular domain of the TGF-β receptor 2 protein that serves to sequester free TGF-β and the monoclonal light-chain region that specifically binds to PD-L1. There is a strong preclinical rationale to reduce TGF-β signaling to optimize the effectiveness of anti-PD-L1 therapy (Lan et al. 2018). This is currently being tested head-to-head comparing M7824 given concurrently with CRT followed by maintenance M7824 vs. PACIFIC regimen (NCT03840902) in this double-blind, placebo-controlled, multicenter randomized trial. Up to 350 stage III unresectable NSCLC will be randomized to one of the two arms. For the experimental arm, M7824 will be given IV Q2weeks at 1200 mg concurrent with 60 Gy/30-fraction intensity-modulated radiation therapy and chemotherapy (with three chemotherapy choices of carboplatin/paclitaxel, cisplatin/etoposide, or cisplatin/pemetrexed) as well as in maintenance up to 1 year. For the control arm, the same standard chemoradiation will be given with placebo IV Q2weeks followed by durvalumab IV Q2week at 10 mg/kg.

3.7 ICI and Anti-CD73 or Anti-NKG2A

AstraZeneca has a phase II master protocol called COAST which builds on the PACIFIC regimen but combines potential immunomodulatory agents with durvalumab (NCT03822351). There are two experimental arms combining either anti-CD73 antibody (oleclumab) targeting the adenosine signaling pathway or anti-NKG2A antibody (monalizumab) in combination with durvalumab vs. durvalumab alone in the maintenance setting. CD73 is a glycosylphosphatidylinositol-anchored cell surface enzyme also known as ecto-5′-nucleotidase, which converts AMP to adenosine and phosphate. Since AMP is generated under conditions of hypoxia, the resulting adenosine binds to G-protein-coupled adenosine receptors on various immune cells in the TME to suppress NK and T cells and causes a distinct adenosine-differentiated dendritic cell type that secretes a number of immune-suppressive molecules such as VEGF, IL-8, IL-10, COX-2, TGF-β, and indoleamine 2,3-dioxygenase-1. CD73 expression has been linked to poor prognosis in multiple tumor types. Blocking of CD73 has been shown to have antitumor effects and enhance immune response in combination with ICI in preclinical models. NKG2A is a novel inhibitory immune checkpoint protein expressed on NK cells, NK-T cells, and subset of CD8+ T cells. NKG2A dimerizes with CD94, couples to HLA-E, and inhibits activation of T-NK cells. Tumor cells not only promote the expression of high levels of NKG2A and CD94 on CD8 T cells, but also aberrantly display HLA-E molecules, leading to NKG2A immune resistance (Creelan and Antonia 2019). Blocking NKG2A along with anti-PD-1/L-1 agents can significantly promote effector T- and NK-cell antitumor response (André et al. 2018).

4 Oncogene-Driven Tumors

NSCLC tumors harbor a number of oncogene driver mutations that could be targeted, namely EGFR, ALK, ROS, BRAF, RET, MET, NTRK, and more recently KRAS G12C subset. As a whole, EGFR mutation is the most commonly seen, with rates as high as 50% in Asia countries. For stage III NSCLC treated in the PACIFIC trial, the small subset of patients with EGFR mutation appears to be an outlier in the subset of patients who do not seem to benefit from maintenance ICI

(Antonia et al. 2017). Although the small number of patients that had known EGFR mutation preclude any definitive conclusion about the lack of efficacy of durvalumab maintenance, there has been some indication in the metastatic setting on the relative efficacy of ICI in patients with EGFR mutation. A number of studies have shown that tumors harboring EGFR mutation tend to be immune cold and have also shown relative lack of efficacy from first- or second-line ICI. Although a preclinical study has indicated that adding EGFR-TKI to ICI may enhance combined efficacy in EGFR-mutant tumors, the high incidence of grade 3–4 adverse events when EGFR-TKI is combined with ICI makes this approach very difficult. Recently, a multi-institutional report on stage III patients with EGFR mutation treated with durvalumab had much shorter PFS compared to non-EGFR-mutant tumors. This data supports an alternative approach for EGFR-mutant tumors. The benefit of adjuvant EGFR-TKI with osimertinib after surgical resection has been proven in resectable stage II–III NSCLC in the ADAURA trial (Wu et al. 2020). PFS was substantially improved in these EGFR-mutant patients, with or without adjuvant chemotherapy. Intracranial relapse was also significantly reduced in the osimertinib group, demonstrating the drug's ability to cross the blood-brain barrier. Adding osimertinib as maintenance therapy after CRT in stage III NSCLC is being tested in the LAURA trial (NCT03521154), a phase III double-blind, randomized, placebo-controlled, clinical trial to assess the efficacy and safety of osimertinib following chemoradiation in stage III unresectable EGFR-TKI sensitizing mutant (Exon19del and L858R) NSCLC. Up to 200 patients will be enrolled in this global trial. PFS is the primary endpoint, with other secondary endpoints including OS and time to CNS relapse. This approach offers a very exciting option for patients who otherwise might not respond to ICI in the locally advanced setting.

Besides EGFR mutations, other oncogene drivers could also be targeted in the maintenance setting after CRT with the myriad of FDA-approved small-molecule orally bioavailable drugs: (1) ALK-fusion: alectinib, brigatinib, ceritinib, lorlatinib, and crizotinib; (2) RET rearrangement: cabozantinib, pralsetinib, selpercatinib, and vandetanib; (3) ROS1 rearrangement: ceritinib, entrectinib, lorlatinib, and crizotinib; (4) MET exon 14 skipping mutation: capmatinib and crizotinib; (5) NTRK fusion: entrectinib and larotrectinib; and (6) BRAFV600E: dabrafenib (and in combination with trametinib) and vemurafenib. Although not yet FDA approved, KRAS G12C can now be targeted with the small molecules sotorasib (AMG510) and adagrasib (MRTX849), in the CodeBreak 100 and KRYSTAL-1 trials, respectively, in heavily previously treated, advanced NSCLC patients. Both agents show remarkable activity in these KrasG12C-mutated patients, especially in the STK-11 subset of double-mutant tumors, which normally fare poorly with chemotherapy and do not respond well to ICIs. Bringing these highly active drugs from the metastatic setting to the maintenance setting in locally advanced NSCLC after CRT where patients are known to be at high risk for micrometastatic disease should therefore further enhance the potential cure rates for these patients. These are fruitful areas of research for many years to come.

5 Conclusion

Maintenance therapy in locally advanced NSCLC after CRT is an important area of research, since improvement of micrometastatic disease control or elimination could make a very significant stride in enhancing cure rates for these patients. The PACIFIC trial of incorporating the single anti-PD-L1 durvalumab antibody significantly improved OS by 13% compared to CRT alone seen in the placebo group and even compared to the best arm of RTOG 0617. While almost 50% of patients are considered disease free and "cured" by 5 years, a substantial portion of patients are still dying from this disease. Many of the improvements that are needed to enhance this further may come in the form of combination therapies with consolidation SBRT radiation to the tumor, DDR targeting, or immune modulatory agents. Whether adding ICI concurrently with CRT will significantly enhance CRT alone followed by durvalumab maintenance is currently being tested in NSCLC. For oncogene-driven tumors, maintenance therapy with oncogene-targeted small-molecule inhibitors could be quite promising since ICIs are typically not suitable to treat these tumors, and micrometastatic disease is also much easier to treat and less likely to develop treatment resistance compared to widespread metastatic disease. Finally, expanding our knowledge of emerging biomarkers and ctDNA may offer an even more customized approach for our patients with locally advanced disease and determine rapidly who may not respond or catch early progressors to allow for agile pivots in cancer management. While we are still quite early in the development of these strategic approaches, the current pace of discoveries and innovations in the metastatic setting will also greatly impact the cures seen in patients with locally advanced NSCLC.

References

André P, Denis C, Soulas C et al (2018) Anti-NKG2A mAb is a checkpoint inhibitor that promotes antitumor immunity by unleashing both T and NK cells. Cell 175:1731–1743.e13

Antonia SJ, Villegas A, Daniel D et al (2017) Durvalumab after chemoradiotherapy in stage III non-small-cell lung cancer. N Engl J Med 377:1919–1929

Antonia SJ, Villegas A, Daniel D et al (2018) Overall survival with durvalumab after chemoradiotherapy in stage III NSCLC. N Engl J Med 379:2342–2350

Batlle E, Massagué J (2019) Transforming growth factor-β signaling in immunity and cancer. Immunity 50:924–940

Chaudhuri AA, Chabon JJ, Lovejoy AF et al (2017) Early detection of molecular residual disease in localized lung cancer by circulating tumor DNA profiling. Cancer Discov 7:1394–1403

Creelan BC, Antonia SJ (2019) The NKG2A immune checkpoint—a new direction in cancer immunotherapy. Nat Rev Clin Oncol 16:277–278

Curran WJ Jr, Paulus R, Langer CJ et al (2011) Sequential vs. concurrent chemoradiation for stage III non-small cell lung cancer: randomized phase III trial RTOG 9410. J Natl Cancer Inst 103:1452–1460

Dillman RO, Herndon J, Seagren SL et al (1996) Improved survival in stage III non-small-cell lung cancer: seven-year follow-up of cancer and leukemia group B (CALGB) 8433 trial. J Natl Cancer Inst 88:1210–1215

Duma N, Santana-Davila R, Molina JR (2019) Non-small cell lung cancer: epidemiology, screening, diagnosis, and treatment. Mayo Clin Proc 94:1623–1640

Durm GA, Jabbour SK, Althouse SK et al (2020) A phase 2 trial of consolidation pembrolizumab following concurrent chemoradiation for patients with unresectable stage III non-small cell lung cancer: Hoosier Cancer Research Network LUN 14-179. Cancer 126:4353–4361

Faivre-Finn C, Vicente D, Kurata T et al (2021) Four-year survival with durvalumab after chemoradiotherapy in stage III NSCLC—an update from the PACIFIC trial. J Thorac Oncol 16:860–867

Hellmann MD, Nabet BY, Rizvi H et al (2020) Circulating tumor DNA analysis to assess risk of progression after long-term response to PD-(L)1 blockade in NSCLC. Clin Cancer Res 26:2849–2858

Hung AL, Maxwell R, Theodros D et al (2018) TIGIT and PD-1 dual checkpoint blockade enhances antitumor immunity and survival in GBM. Oncoimmunology 7:e1466769

Jabbour SK, Berman AT, Decker RH et al (2020) Phase 1 trial of pembrolizumab administered concurrently with chemoradiotherapy for locally advanced non-small cell lung cancer: a nonrandomized controlled trial. JAMA Oncol 6:848–855

Johnston RJ, Comps-Agrar L, Hackney J et al (2014) The immunoreceptor TIGIT regulates antitumor and antiviral CD8(+) T cell effector function. Cancer Cell 26:923–937

Kelly K, Chansky K, Gaspar LE et al (2008) Phase III trial of maintenance gefitinib or placebo after concurrent chemoradiotherapy and docetaxel consolidation in inoperable stage III non-small-cell lung cancer: SWOG S0023. J Clin Oncol 26:2450–2456

Koning CC, Wouterse SJ, Daams JG et al (2013) Toxicity of concurrent radiochemotherapy for locally advanced non-small-cell lung cancer: a systematic review of the literature. Clin Lung Cancer 14:481–487

Lan Y, Zhang D, Xu C et al (2018) Enhanced preclinical antitumor activity of M7824, a bifunctional fusion protein simultaneously targeting PD-L1 and TGF-β. Sci Transl Med 10:eaan5488

Lee NY, Ferris RL, Psyrri A et al (2021) Avelumab plus standard-of-care chemoradiotherapy versus chemoradiotherapy alone in patients with locally advanced squamous cell carcinoma of the head and neck: a randomised, double-blind, placebo-controlled, multicentre, phase 3 trial. Lancet Oncol 22:450–462

Lhuillier C, Rudqvist NP, Elemento O et al (2019) Radiation therapy and anti-tumor immunity: exposing immunogenic mutations to the immune system. Genome Med 11:40

Lin SH, Lin Y, Yao L et al (2020) Phase II trial of concurrent atezolizumab with chemoradiation for unresectable NSCLC. J Thorac Oncol 15:248–257

Moding EJ, Liu Y, Nabet BY et al (2020) Circulating tumor DNA dynamics predict benefit from consolidation immunotherapy in locally advanced non-small-cell lung cancer. Nat Cancer 1:176–183

Pantelidou C, Sonzogni O, De Oliveria TM et al (2019) PARP inhibitor efficacy depends on CD8(+) T-cell recruitment via intratumoral STING pathway activation in BRCA-deficient models of triple-negative breast cancer. Cancer Discov 9:722–737

Peters S, Felip E, Dafni U et al (2021) Progression-free and overall survival for concurrent nivolumab with standard concurrent chemoradiotherapy in locally advanced stage IIIA-B NSCLC: results from the European Thoracic Oncology Platform NICOLAS phase II trial (European Thoracic Oncology Platform 6-14). J Thorac Oncol 16:278–288

Rodriguez-Abreu D, Johnson ML, Hussein MA et al (2020) CITYSCAPE: primary analysis of a randomized, double-blind, phase II study of the anti-TIGIT antibody tiragolumab plus atezolizumab versus placebo plus atezolizumab as 1L treatment in patients with PD-L1-selected NSCLC. J Clin Oncol 38:9503

Senan S, Brade A, Wang LH et al (2016) PROCLAIM: randomized phase III trial of pemetrexed-cisplatin or etoposide-cisplatin plus thoracic radiation therapy followed by consolidation chemotherapy in locally advanced nonsquamous non-small-cell lung cancer. J Clin Oncol 34:953–962

Taugner J, Eze C, Käsmann L et al (2020) Pattern-of-failure and salvage treatment analysis after chemoradiotherapy for inoperable stage III non-small cell lung cancer. Radiat Oncol 15:148

Tsujino K, Kurata T, Yamamoto S et al (2013) Is consolidation chemotherapy after concurrent chemoradiotherapy beneficial for patients with locally advanced non-small-cell lung cancer? A pooled analysis of the literature. J Thorac Oncol 8:1181–1189

Vokes EE, Herndon JE 2nd, Kelley MJ et al (2007) Induction chemotherapy followed by chemoradiotherapy compared with chemoradiotherapy alone for regionally advanced unresectable stage III non-small-cell lung cancer: Cancer and Leukemia Group B. J Clin Oncol 25:1698–1704

Wei J, Montalvo-Ortiz W, Yu L et al (2021) Sequence of αPD-1 relative to local tumor irradiation determines the induction of abscopal antitumor immune responses. Sci Immunol 6:eabg0117

Wu YL, Tsuboi M, He J et al (2020) Osimertinib in resected EGFR-mutated non-small-cell lung cancer. N Engl J Med 383:1711–1723

Yu X, Harden K, Gonzalez LC et al (2009) The surface protein TIGIT suppresses T cell activation by promoting the generation of mature immunoregulatory dendritic cells. Nat Immunol 10:48–57

Zhang P, Maruyama T, Konkel JE et al (2013a) PARP-1 controls immunosuppressive function of regulatory T cells by destabilizing Foxp3. PLoS One 8:e71590

Zhang P, Nakatsukasa H, Tu E et al (2013b) PARP-1 regulates expression of TGF-β receptors in T cells. Blood 122:2224–2232

Prophylactic Cranial Irradiation in Non-small Cell Lung Cancer

Hina Saeed, Monica E. Shukla, and Elizabeth M. Gore

Contents

1 Introduction... 581
2 Risk Factors for Brain Metastasis Development... 582
2.1 Age... 582
2.2 Disease Stage... 582
2.3 Histology and Grade... 582
2.4 Molecular/Genetic Factors... 583
2.5 Chemotherapy... 583
2.6 Targeted Therapy... 584
3 Morbidity and Mortality Associated with Brain Metastases... 584
4 Randomized Controlled Trials of PCI for NSCLC... 585
5 PCI and the Incidence of Brain Metastases (BM)... 587
6 PCI and Time to Brain Metastases (BMs)... 588
7 PCI and Survival... 589
8 PCI Toxicity... 590
9 Quality of Life (QoL)... 591
10 Neurocognitive Function (NCF)... 591
11 Best PCI Regimen... 593
12 Summary... 593
References... 593

H. Saeed · M. E. Shukla · E. M. Gore (✉)
Department of Radiation Oncology, Medical College of Wisconsin, Milwaukee, WI, USA
e-mail: egore@mcw.edu

Abstract

The incidence of brain metastases following definitive intent treatment for locally advanced non-small cell lung cancer (LA-NSCLC) is high. Failures in the brain are associated with poor prognosis, impaired function, and poor quality of life. Brain failures are particularly devastating when the disease is otherwise cured. PCI has consistently been shown to decrease brain failures although it is not the standard of care. There has been a sustained, although unsuccessful, interest over the last several decades to demonstrate that PCI improves overall survival in appropriately selected patients with LA-NSCLC. This chapter provides a comprehensive updated review of the risks of brain metastases and the potential role of PCI in LA-NSCLC with a review of seven prospective randomized trials.

1 Introduction

Development of brain metastases is a devastating complication of non-small cell lung cancer, often leading to debilitating neurologic symptoms, deterioration in quality of life, and reduced survival. Approximately 10% of patients with newly diagnosed NSCLC present with brain metastases (Waqar et al. 2018a, b), and up to 50% will develop brain metastases during the course of their disease (Strauss et al. 2005; Law et al.

1997). The majority are within 1 year of diagnosis (Schouten et al. 2002). Thirty percent of patients experience brain as one of the first sites of relapse following locoregional treatment for stage I–III NSCLC. Prophylactic cranial irradiation or treatment of micrometastatic disease in the brain may change the course of disease in appropriately selected patients by delaying or preventing brain failures.

In the setting of small cell lung cancer (SCLC) with response to systemic therapy, prophylactic cranial irradiation (PCI) has been shown to significantly reduce the incidence of brain metastases by approximately 50%. In a meta-analysis of patients with limited-stage disease, PCI improved overall survival at 3 years by 5.4% (PCIOCG 2018).

Despite the high incidence of brain metastases in patients with LA-NSCLC, the role of PCI has not been established. There have been six published randomized controlled trials (RCTs) of PCI versus no PCI in patients with LA-NSCLC following locoregional treatment (Cox et al. 1981; Umsawasdi et al. 1984; Russell et al. 1991; Miller et al. 1998; Gore et al. 2011; DeRuyyscher et al. 2018).

This chapter reviews the literature on PCI for LA-NSCLC with specific reference to these trials and other relevant publications.

2 Risk Factors for Brain Metastasis Development

2.1 Age

Data from several retrospective studies show that younger patients have a proportionally higher incidence of brain metastases. In a retrospective multicenter analysis of consecutively treated stage III NSCLC (with either sequential or concurrent chemoradiotherapy), patients developing brain metastases were significantly younger with mean age of 59 versus 63 years (Hendriks et al. 2016). Similar findings were noted by Ceresoli and colleagues. In this study, following multimodality treatment for locally advanced non-metastatic lung cancer, brain was the first site of failure in 22% of the study population. This was seen more commonly in patients younger than 60 years of age as compared to their older counterparts. This finding has also been noted in studies by Carolan et al. (2005), and Westeel (2003).

2.2 Disease Stage

Larger primary tumor size and greater extent of nodal involvement have both been correlated with higher incidence of brain metastasis. A retrospective review of NSCLC patients who had undergone diagnostic imaging studies of the chest and brain found that the predicted probability of metastatic disease to the brain correlated positively with the size of the primary tumor and lymph node stage (Majoomdar et al. 2007). Among over 1200 patients receiving curative surgery at the National Cancer Center in South Korea between 2001 and 2008, brain metastases as the first relapse were higher in patients with a higher pT and pN stage (Won et al. 2015). Others have reported on higher incidence of brain metastases with bulky (≥2 cm) mediastinal lymph nodes (Ceresoli et al. 2002), presence of N3 nodal involvement (Lee et al. 2015), and involvement of multiple mediastinal nodal stations (Wang, et al. 2009).

2.3 Histology and Grade

Multiple studies have shown a proportionally higher incidence of brain metastases in patients with adenocarcinoma, large cell carcinoma, and poorly or undifferentiated carcinoma in comparison to those with squamous cell carcinoma. Three-year incidence of brain metastases in a group of patients following definitive treatment for lung cancer at Sun Yat-sen University was 45% vs. 28.6% in those with non-squamous vs. squamous histology, respectively (Wang et al. 2009). A similarly higher incidence of brain metastases was noted in patients with nonsquamous histology in a large review of the US National Cancer Database (Waqar et al. 2018a, b) as well as in other retrospective reviews from the United States/Canada (Majoomdar et al. 2007) and the Netherlands (Hendriks et al. 2016).

Two analyses from the US Surveillance, Epidemiology, and End Results (SEER) and National Cancer Database (NCDB) showed a higher incidence of brain metastases in patients with greater than grade 2 histology (Waqar et al. 2018a, b (SEER); Waqar et al. 2018a, b (NCDB)).

2.4 Molecular/Genetic Factors

A growing body of data is shedding light on the molecular and genetic underpinnings of lung cancer and their influence on patterns of recurrence including intracranial relapse. In lung adenocarcinoma, presence of an EGFR mutation is associated with a higher incidence of brain metastasis at presentation and development of brain metastases following curative-intent treatment for non-metastatic disease (Shin et al. 2014). In a retrospective study reviewing 522 consecutive NSCLC patients tested for EGFR mutations, there was a nearly twofold higher incidence of EGFR mutations in patients with brain metastases at diagnosis. In the overall group, patients with brain metastases at presentation had a significantly shorter overall survival (OS); however, in the cohort of patients harboring an EGFR mutation, the OS between patients with and without brain metastases was not statistically significant, 20.8 vs. 25.1 months, $p = 0.11$, respectively (Bhatt et al. 2016). A proposed pathobiology for higher rate of brain relapse in this population is deregulation of MET pathway, which can lead to abnormal activation of invasive signaling that promotes epithelial-mesenchymal transition (EMT), increased cell motility, migration, angiogenesis, and invasion (Benedettini et al. 2010; Buonato and Lazzara 2014). A similar higher propensity for intracranial relapse was seen in patients harboring an anaplastic lymphoma kinase (ALK) gene rearrangement in a cohort of patients at the Mayo Clinic (Yang et al. 2012), although this association was not seen in a cohort studied at the University of Colorado (Doebele et al. 2012).

2.5 Chemotherapy

Establishment of combined modality therapy (combinations of surgery, chemotherapy, and radiotherapy) as the standard of care for locally advanced NSCLC in the 1990s led to significant improvements in locoregional and distant tumor control and overall survival. With improved systemic control and greater longevity, an increase in the incidence of intracranial relapse was seen, often as the sole site of failure. Gustave Roussy Institute reported on relapse patterns in 109 patients with N2 disease treated with neoadjuvant chemotherapy prior to surgery compared to 185 patients treated with primary surgical resection (Andre et al. 2001). Brain metastases occurred in 32% of patients in the combined modality group vs. 18% in surgery-alone group; brain was the isolated site of failure in 22% and 11% of patients, respectively. In a similar study of stage III–N2 NSCLC treated with surgical resection at Sun Yat-sen University, receipt of postoperative platinum-based chemotherapy (vs. observation) improved median survival from 25.4 to 33.4 months, but also increased frequency of brain metastasis at 1, 2, and 3 years. Frequency of brain metastasis as the first site of failure at 1 year in the adjuvant chemotherapy group was 22% vs. 5.5% in the observation group (Wang et al. 2009). These findings were explained by the lack of traditional chemotherapeutics crossing the blood-brain barrier (BBB). As systemic disease came under better control and patients were living longer, it allowed time for tumor progression in the brain as a sanctuary site. Those patients not receiving chemotherapy experienced overall disease progression at much higher rates and succumbed to extracranial metastases or locoregional progression prior to experiencing brain failures.

2.6 Targeted Therapy

Available options for the treatment of brain metastases have expanded significantly over the past couple of decades. In addition to surgery and radiotherapy, systemic therapy can also be an important component of management. Whereas traditional cytotoxic chemotherapies are ineffective intracranially due to poor BBB penetration, small molecule tyrosine kinase inhibitors (TKIs) that target driver mutations such as EGFR, ALK, and ROS-1 can cross the BBB and have been shown to stabilize and prevent the progression of intracranial metastatic disease. In a phase II study of patients diagnosed with EGFR-mutated NSCLC with metastatic brain tumors receiving either erlotinib or gefitinib, 83% had at least a partial response (Park et al. 2012). After cessation of therapy, 50% went on to receive local therapy (whole-brain RT or radiosurgery), allowing for a local therapy-free interval of just over 12 months. Since that time, two additional generations of EGFR-TKIs have been developed, which address acquired resistance that usually develops within 8–12 months on the first/second-line therapy. Third-generation EGFR-TKI, osimertinib, has shown excellent CNS objective response rate (ORR) in patients with asymptomatic or stable intracranial metastatic disease. In a subgroup analysis of the FLAURA study, CNS ORR was 91% as compared with 68% in the standard EGFR-TKI (erlotinib or gefitinib) arm (Reungwetwattana et al. 2018).

Although there is some debate regarding a higher propensity to develop brain metastases in the ALK-mutated population, there is agreement that the brain is a common site of disease progression (up to 60%) following treatment with the first-generation ALK TKI, crizotinib. Next-generation ALK agents have since been approved and show improved intracranial activity. Alectinib, a second-generation agent, showed a higher overall CNS response rate as compared to crizotinib (86% vs. 71%) and also significantly delayed time to CNS progression (Gadgeel et al. 2018). Other approved ALK agents such as ceritinib, brigatinib, and lorlatinib have also shown good intracranial efficacy.

3 Morbidity and Mortality Associated with Brain Metastases

Development of brain metastases is a devastating complication of non-small cell lung cancer leading to significantly reduced survival. Median survival for locally advanced, nonmetastatic lung cancer following modern concurrent chemoradiotherapy is around 29 months (Bradley et al. 2019), equating to a 2-year OS rate of around 60%. Addition of consolidative immunotherapy in this group of patients has further improved 2-year OS rate to around 66%; median survival has not yet been reached/reported (Antonia et al. 2018). In contrast to these impressive outcomes, in a large US National Cancer Database review of patients diagnosed with NSCLC between 2010 and 2012, median OS for patients presenting with stage IV disease with brain metastases was 6 months (Waqar et al. 2018a, b). In 2017, an update to the diagnosis-specific Graded Prognostic Assessment (ds-GPA) for Lung Cancer was published (Sperduto et al. 2017) called the Lung-molGPA. In addition to the four factors identified on the original ds-GPA found to be predictive of survival in lung cancer patients with brain metastases (age, Karnofsky performance status, presence of extracranial metastases, and number of brain metastases), two new factors were added—presence/absence of EGFR and ALK alterations in patients with adenocarcinoma. Using these six factors, survival of lung cancer patients with brain metastases can be stratified into groups with an estimated median survival time from 5.3 months to 46.8 months, with the two factors predicting for a significantly longer survival due to presence of genetic driver mutations (EGFR and ALK).

The morbidity of brain metastases is often associated with debilitating neurologic symptoms and associated deterioration in quality of life. Depending on location, brain metastases can lead to significant impairments in motor, balance, visual, speech production/comprehension, memory, integrative, and executive functions. Impairments in motor, balance, and visual function can lead to loss of independence due to increasing need for assistance from others when performing instrumental activities of daily living (e.g., transportation, preparing meals, managing finances) as well as the more basic activities of daily living (e.g., toileting, bathing, feeding). Impaired cognitive function can lead to impaired concentration, poor memory, and decreased ability to effectively communicate with others, often leading to isolation and depression. Meyers et al. (2004) reported on neurologic, neurocognitive function (NCF), and survival outcomes of 401 patients with brain metastases of varying histologies (predominantly NSCLC) treated with whole-brain radiation therapy with or without motexafin gadolinium (a radiosensitizer). At baseline (pretreatment), nearly all (91%) of the patients had impairment in one or more neurocognitive tests with 42% having impairments in four or more tests. This study also showed that NCF at baseline was predictive of overall survival regardless of treatment arm. In a study done on 208 patients enrolled on PCI-P120-9801 study, patients were followed and their NCF and QoL were measured over time. Decline in NCF during earlier visits was predictive of deterioration in the ability to perform ADLs and QoL at future visits. These findings underscore the importance of preventing intracranial recurrence which, in and of itself, leads to decreased NCF, QoL, and OS. It is essential that prevention is effective with limited toxicity.

4 Randomized Controlled Trials of PCI for NSCLC

There have been seven published randomized controlled trials (RCTs) of PCI versus no PCI in patients with locally advanced non-small cell lung cancer (LA-NSCLC) following locoregional treatment, which are summarized in Table 1 (Cox et al. 1981; Umsawasdi et al. 1984; Russell et al. 1991; Mira et al. 1990; Miller et al. 1998; Gore et al. 2011; Sun et al. 2019; Li et al. 2015; DeRuyyscher et al. 2018). The seven studies included different patient groups. Four studies (Miller et al. 1998; Gore et al. 2011; Li et al. 2015; DeRuyyscher et al. 2018) included stage III NSCLC patients only; two studies (Umsawasdi et al. 1984; Russell et al. 1991) included stage I, II, and III patients; and in one study (Cox et al. 1981), staging was unclear. The studies varied widely in the local therapies used and PCI dose fractionation schedules. Dosing of cranial irradiation ranged from 20 to 37.5 Gy (10 fractions of 2 Gy to 15 fractions of 2.5 Gy). Brain imaging was mainly done by a radionuclide scan in two studies (Cox et al. 1981; Umsawasdi et al. 1984). One study (Russell et al. 1991) used CT scans, three more recent studies (Gore et al. 2011; Li et al. 2015; DeRuyyscher et al. 2018) used MRI, and in one study (Miller et al. 1998) the technology of brain imaging was unclear.

All seven trials required histological confirmation of the diagnosis. In four trials (Cox et al. 1981; Umsawasdi et al. 1984; Russell et al. 1991; Miller et al. 1998), patients were randomized to PCI or observation irrespective of the thoracic response to treatment; in others, patients needed to have nonprogressive disease after local treatment (Gore et al. 2011; Li et al. 2015; DeRuyyscher et al. 2018).

1. VALG (Cox et al. 1981): The VALG trial randomized 410 evaluable male patients not considered suitable for surgical resection with no spread beyond the regional nodes to one of the two radical chest radiation therapy (RT) regimens: 50 Gy in 25 fractions over 5 weeks or 42 Gy in 15 fractions over 3 weeks. No chemotherapy was used. Overall, 323 patients were evaluable. In the PCI arm, patients received 20 Gy in 10 fractions over 2 weeks. The primary endpoint was the rate of brain metastases (BM).

2. MDACC (Umsawasdi et al. 1984): One hundred patients with LA-NSCLC of any cell type were randomized, and 97 patients were evaluable. Of these, 87% were stage III and 13% were stage I–II. The thoracic treatment received was not clearly stated for all patients. Sixty-three patients received radical chemo-RT (thoracic RT dose 50 Gy in 25 fractions over 5 weeks), and 34 patients received differing combinations of surgery, RT, and chemotherapy. PCI patients received 30 Gy in 10

Table 1 Published RCTs of PCI in LA-NSCLC

RCT	No.	Patient selection	Thoracic treatment	PCI dose	Brain metastasis incidence (PCI vs. no PCI)	Survival (PCI vs. no PCI)
VALG (1981)	410	Inoperable disease	RT: 50 Gy/25F/5 weeks or 42 Gy/15F/3 weeks	20 Gy/10F	6% vs. 13% (S)	35.4 vs. 41.4 weeks (NS)[a]
MDACC (1984)	100	Stage I–III (87% stage III)	Chemo-RT (50 Gy/25F/5 weeks), or combinations of surgery, RT, and chemo	30 Gy/10F	4% vs. 27% (S)	22% vs. 23.5% at 3 years
RTOG 8403 (1991)	187	Adenocarcinoma or large cell carcinoma	RT: 55–60 Gy/30F/6 weeks Post-op: 50 Gy/25F/5 weeks	30 Gy/10F	9% vs. 19% (NS)	8.4 vs. 8.1 months (NS)[a]
SWOG (1990,1998)	254	Inoperable stage III	Primary RT: 58 Gy/29F or neoadjuvant chemo, then RT, and adjuvant chemo	37.5 Gy/15F or 30 Gy/15F	1 vs. 11% (S)	8 vs. 11 months (S)[a]
RTOG 0214 (2011, 2019)	356	Stage III without progression after definitive management	RT alone ($\geq$30 Gy) or combinations of surgery, RT, and chemo	30 Gy/15F	17% vs. 28% (S) at 10 years	17.6% vs. 13.3% (NS) at 10 years
Li et al. (2015)	156	Resected N2	No RT Adjuvant chemo alone	30 Gy/10F	20 vs. 50% (S) at 5 years	31.2 vs. 27.4 months (NS)[a]
NVALT-11 (2018)	175	Stage III without progression after definitive management	Concurrent or sequential chemo-RT ± surgery	36 Gy/18F, 30 Gy/12F, 30 Gy/10F	7% vs. 27% (S) at 2 years	24.2 vs. 21.9 months (NS)[a]

No. number of patients, RT radiotherapy, PCI prophylactic cranial irradiation, F fractions, chemo chemotherapy, S significant NS not significant
[a]Median survival

fractions over 2 weeks. The primary endpoint was the rate of BM.
3. RTOG 8403 (Russell et al. 1991): RTOG 8403 randomized 187 patients with inoperable or unresectable adenocarcinoma or large cell carcinoma confined to the chest and resected carcinomas of the same cell types. Patients received primary RT 55–60 Gy in 30 fractions over 6 weeks or 50 Gy in 25 fractions over 5 weeks to the mediastinum and hilar areas following surgical resection. PCI patients received 30 Gy in 10 fractions over 2 weeks. The primary endpoint was the time to BM.
4. SWOG (Miller et al. 1998; Mira et al. 1990): The SWOG trial randomized 254 patients with inoperable stage III NSCLC. Patients were first randomized to either chest RT (58 Gy in 29 fractions) or neoadjuvant chemotherapy followed by chest RT and adjuvant chemotherapy. The first 34 patients in the PCI arm received 37.5 Gy in 15 fractions, but this was changed to 30 Gy in 15 fractions soon after the trial began recruiting due to concerns about early deaths in the PCI arm. The primary endpoint was overall survival.
5. RTOG 0214 (Gore et al. 2011; Sun et al. 2019): RTOG 0214 randomized 356 patients with stage III NSCLC without disease progression after surgery and/ or RT with or without chemotherapy. Local treatment was extremely variable; patients could have RT alone (>30 Gy) or RT with neoadjuvant, concurrent, or adjuvant chemotherapy; surgery alone; or surgery with pre- or postoperative chemotherapy, RT, or both. RTOG 0214 had planned to recruit 1058 patients but closed early due to poor recruitment. The PCI schedule used was 30 Gy in 15 fractions. The primary endpoint was overall survival.
6. Li et al. (2015): This trial randomized 156 patients with stage III NSCLC with resected confirmed N2 disease and without disease progression after adjuvant platinum-based chemotherapy. This study was terminated early as a result of slow accrual. The PCI schedule used was 30 Gy in 10 fractions. The primary endpoint was disease-free survival.
7. Dutch NVALT-11/DKCRG02 (DeRuyyscher et al. 2018): In NVALT-11 study, 175 patients with stage III NSCLC and without disease progression after concurrent or sequential chemoradiotherapy with or without surgery were randomized. The PCI schedule used was left to the physician: 36 Gy in 18 fractions, 30 Gy in 12 fractions, or 30 Gy in 10 fractions. The primary endpoint was the rate of symptomatic BM.
8. PRoT-BM trial (Arrieta et al. 2021): Randomized phase II study of patients with stage IIIB/IV NSCLC with an EGFR mutation, an ALK rearrangement or elevated CEA level at diagnosis, but without brain metastases (per MRI) who were given systemic therapy according to molecular status. Those without progression were randomized between further standard of care therapy (SoC) and SoC + PCI. Primary outcome was cumulative incidence of brain metastases (CMB). Eighty-four patients were enrolled. At 24 months, CBM was lower in the SoC + PCI arm at 7% (vs. 38% in the SoC alone arm).

5 PCI and the Incidence of Brain Metastases (BM)

PCI significantly reduced the incidence of BMs in six of the seven published randomized trials (Cox et al. 1981; Umsawasdi et al. 1984; Miller et al. 1998; Gore et al. 2011; Li et al. 2015; DeRuyyscher et al. 2018). The results from RTOG 8403, although not statistically significant, also strongly support the effectiveness of PCI in reducing the incidence of BMs (Russell et al. 1991).

In the VALG study, the two thoracic RT schedules used were combined for statistical analysis (Cox et al. 1981). The incidence of BMs was significantly lower in the PCI arm compared to the observation arm (6% vs. 13%, $p = 0.038$). Subgroup analysis showed that the only specific cell type in which PCI was significantly more effective in reducing the incidence of BMs was adenocarcinoma (0% vs. 29%, $p = 0.04$). It might be expected that any benefit from PCI is more likely to be seen in patients with adenocarcinoma, as these patients have a higher incidence of BMs (Perez et al. 1987).

In MDACC trial (Umsawasdi et al. 1984), the incidence of BMs in the PCI arm was 4% compared to 27% in the observation arm ($p = 0.02$). Multivariate analysis suggested that the beneficial effect of PCI was only significant in female patients with a good performance status, weight loss less than 6%, squamous histology, and stage III disease. The benefit for squamous cancers only is counterintuitive as BMs are more common in patients with adenocarcinoma (Perez et al. 1987). Only 97 patients in total were evaluable, so sample sizes in the subgroup analysis may have been too small to reliably estimate differences.

In the SWOG trial, the incidence of BMs in the PCI arm was 1% compared to 11% in the observation arm ($p = 0.003$) (Miller et al. 1998). No subgroup analysis was published.

RTOG 0214 was the first trial to include regular brain imaging as part of the follow-up protocol (Gore et al. 2011). CT head was required at 6 and 12 months and then yearly after radiation. The incidence of BMs was lower in the PCI arm compared to the control arm at 6 months (3.3% vs. 10.7%, $p = 0.004$) and 1 year (7.7% vs. 18%, $p = 0.004$). Long-term follow-up (Sun et al. 2019) showed that 5- and 10-year BM rates were 16.7% and 28.3% for PCI vs. observation, which were significantly different ($p = 0.003$). Patients in the PCI arm were 57% less likely to develop BMs than those in the observation arm. Subgroup analysis showed that younger patients (<60 years) and patients with nonsquamous disease had higher rates of BMs.

In Li trial (Li et al. 2015), PCI was associated with a decrease in the risk of BMs (the actuarial 5-year BM rate, 20.3% versus 49.9%; $p < 0.001$). The actuarial and crude 5-year brain relapse as the first site of recurrence rates were 15.6% and 9.9% for PCI versus 45.3% and 33.3% for observation, respectively ($p = 0.001$, $p < 0.001$).

In NVALT-11, PCI decreased the cumulative incidence of symptomatic BMs. Seven percent in the PCI arm and 27% in the control group ($p < 0.001$) developed symptomatic brain metastases at 2 years after therapy (DeRuyyscher et al. 2018). A post hoc subgroup analysis showed that older (>61 years) patients had a statistically significantly lower risk of developing symptomatic BMs compared to younger (≤61 years) patients (Witlox et al. 2019).

In RTOG 8403, PCI did not significantly reduce the incidence of BMs compared to the observation arm (9% vs. 19%, $p = 0.10$) (Russell et al. 1991). The prevalence of BMs at 24 months for PCI was 15% versus 31% in the observation arm. Again, this result was not statistically significant, but RTOG 8403 results strongly suggest that PCI reduces the incidence of BMs and that this benefit is maintained 2 years after PCI.

Looking at the results of all seven RCTs together, it is clear that PCI is effective at reducing the incidence of BMs in patients with LA-NSCLC given locoregional treatment for their disease. Attempts to define particular subgroups, which may derive proportionally more benefit from PCI, have been largely unsuccessful due to the relatively small size of the trials carried out.

6 PCI and Time to Brain Metastases (BMs)

In the VALG trial, the median time to development of BMs was 34 weeks in the PCI group and 29 weeks in the observation group (Cox et al. 1981). The statistical significance of this result was not reported, but the difference is clearly not a large one. In MDACC trial (Umsawasdi et al. 1984), PCI significantly prolonged the median time to BMs (50.5 vs. 23 weeks, $p = 0.002$). Moreover, PCI use was also stated to delay the onset of BMs in RTOG 8403 (Russell et al. 1991), but no further information on the duration of delay was provided in their study. The SWOG, RTOG 0214, and Li et al. trials did not report on the time to BMs (Miller et al. 1998; Gore et al. 2011; Li et al. 2015). In the NVALT-11 trial, PCI was stated to significantly increase the time to develop symptomatic BMs ($p = 0.0012$), but this was not the case for brain metastasis-free survival

(DeRuyyscher et al. 2018). Although it cannot be conclusively stated, there is a hint that PCI delays the time to brain metastases.

7 PCI and Survival

To date, no trial has reported a survival advantage with PCI over observation despite impressive reductions in the incidence of BMs in all published RCTs. The median survival figures for PCI versus observation in the VALG trial were 35.4 weeks versus 41.4 weeks ($p = 0.5$), and in RTOG 8403, 8.4 months versus 8.1 months ($p = 0.36$) (Cox et al. 1981; Russell et al. 1991). RTOG 8403 also reported no significant difference between PCI and observation in 1- and 2-year survival rates (40% vs. 44% and 13% vs. 21%, $p = 0.36$) (Russell et al. 1991). In MDACC trial (Umsawasdi et al. 1984), 3-year survival rates in the PCI and control groups were 22% and 23.5%, respectively. No statistical analysis of the survival data was reported, but it is highly unlikely that there was a real difference between the arms. In the SWOG trial, median survival was actually significantly shorter in the PCI arm (8 vs. 11 months, $p = 0.004$) (Miller et al. 1998). In this study, the first 34 patients in the PCI arm received 37.5 Gy in 15 fractions, but this was changed to 30 Gy in 15 fractions soon after the trial began recruiting due to concerns about early deaths in the PCI arm. The remaining patients who were randomized to PCI received 30 Gy in 15 fractions but had a similar median survival to the 37.5 Gy group. It was not clear to the investigators why there was a shorter life expectancy in the PCI arm. Some hypothesize that PCI with concurrent thoracic RT may have resulted in increased toxicity and contributed to the reduced survival.

The more recent RCTs (Gore et al. 2011; Li et al. 2015; DeRuyyscher et al. 2018) required patients to have at least stable disease after locoregional treatment. It is reasonable to assume that any survival advantage with PCI is far more likely to be seen in patients with controlled thoracic disease. Patients who have progressive or metastatic disease after locoregional treatment will have a short life expectancy and are likely to die from extracranial disease complications before any benefit from PCI can be seen. Despite this, there was no difference in the 1-year overall survival rate in RTOG 0214 (75.6% for PCI vs. 76.9% for controls) (Gore et al. 2011). Long-term follow-up (Sun et al. 2019) similarly showed that the OS for PCI was not significantly better than observation (5- and 10-year rates, 24.7% and 17.6% vs. 26.0% and 13.3%, respectively, $p = 0.12$). Li et al. (2015) showed that the median OS was 31.2 months in the PCI group and 27.4 months in the control group ($p = 0.310$). The 3-year and 5-year OS rates were, respectively, 44.5% and 27.4% with PCI and 38.7% and 22.8% with observation. In NVALT-11 trial, there was no significant difference in overall survival between the two arms (DeRuyyscher et al. 2018). Median OS was slightly longer in the PCI arm than in the control arm (24.2 months versus 21.9 months, respectively), but this difference was not statistically significantly different ($p = 0.56$).

The lack of survival advantage in these RCTs is not necessarily surprising. RTOG 0214 was initially planned to randomize 1058 patients; this was the number of patients needed to detect a 20% difference in the overall survival with 80% statistical power (Gore et al. 2011). The trial closed early due to poor recruitment with only 340 evaluable patients enrolled, so any true benefit is unlikely to have been seen. Applying the same statistical logic to the other six RCTs, it is clear that none of the studies were large enough to detect a survival benefit from PCI if one truly exists—the largest study was the VALG study and this only included 410 evaluable patients (Cox et al. 1981).

The experience with PCI in small cell lung cancer (SCLC) is also important to consider and continues to evolve. Although PCI significantly decreases the risk of BMs in both limited- and extensive-stage SCLC, its role in improving survival is less clear especially in the era of modern imaging. The ongoing SWOG 1827 (NCT04155034) trial will address the role of PCI in the setting of modern staging and therapy. It is not logical to extrapolate these results to NSCLC patients as SCLC is a more radiosensitive disease with a higher incidence of BMs, but it may be that a large enough RCT with modern imaging would demonstrate a survival advantage not seen in the relatively small trials reported to date.

In addition, the locoregional treatment for many patients in these RCTs was variable and would not be considered optimal by today's standards. In RTOG 0214, patients were eligible having had as little as 30 Gy RT to the chest (Gore et al. 2011). This is not a tumoricidal RT dose and is unlikely to achieve long-term local disease control. Patients would then be at risk of disease relapse and early death before any PCI benefit could be seen. The disease-free survival (DFS) at 1 year was not significantly different between the two arms in RTOG 0214 despite a significant decrease in the incidence of brain metastases with PCI suggesting that patients are relapsing systemically and dying, possibly before any PCI benefit can be seen. However, long-term follow-up (Sun et al. 2019) did show improved DFS rates at 5 and 10 years (19.0% and 12.6% vs. 16.1% and 7.5% for PCI vs. observation, $p = 0.03$).

Similarly, Li et al. (2015) showed that PCI group had significantly lengthened DFS compared with the control group, with a median DFS of 28.5 months versus 21.2 months ($p = 0.037$). The 3- and 5-year DFS rates were, respectively, 42.0% and 26.1% with PCI and 29.8% and 18.5% with observation. In NVALT-11, the details of the delivered treatments are missing. The trial showed slightly longer median progression-free survival in the PCI arm than in the control arm (12.3 versus 11.5 months, respectively), but this difference was not statistically significantly different ($p = 0.17$) (DeRuyyscher et al. 2018).

Summarizing the above, no RCT had shown a survival benefit from PCI in locally advanced NSCLC despite all showing a reduction in the incidence of brain metastases. The reasons for this may in part be due to trial design; individual trials had relatively few participants, included some patients with early-stage disease, and had suboptimal and variable locoregional treatment.

8 PCI Toxicity

Toxicity data collection and subsequent publication were poor in four of the seven trials. The VALG trial did not report on PCI-related toxicity (Cox et al. 1981). RTOG 8403 reported no acute toxicity other than epilation and skin reactions and no late toxicity (Russell et al. 1991). The MDACC and SWOG trials reported no excessive toxicity with PCI compared to the observation arm, but it was not stated in either trial how or what data were collected (Umsawasdi et al. 1984; Miller et al. 1998).

RTOG 0214 was one of the first RCTs to include detailed prospective toxicity data collection (Gore et al. 2011). The trial reported that PCI resulted in generally mild toxicity. Grade 3 and 4 toxicities occurred in 4% and 1% of patients, respectively. Grade 3 toxicities reported were acute fatigue, dyspnea, ataxia, and depression. One patient reported acute grade 4 mood alteration/depression. Four patients reported grade 3 late toxicity including dyspnea, syncope, weakness, and fatigue.

Li et al. reported that for patients in the PCI arm, the main acute toxicities (within 90 days) included headache in 27% (grade 1, 20%; grade 2, 6%; grade 3, 1%), nausea or vomiting in 23% (grade 1, 17%; grade 2, 6%), fatigue in 22% (grade 1, 11%; grade 2, 9%; grade 3, 2%), skin toxicity in 5% (grade 1, 1%; grade 2, 4%), and insomnia in 2% (grade 2). The main late toxicities (after 90 days) of the brain included mild headache or slight lethargy (22.2%), moderate headache or great lethargy (11.1%), and severe headaches (2.5%). Other grade 3 late toxicities included skin atrophy in one patient and fatigue in one patient (Li et al. 2015).

Detailed toxicity data was collected by NVALT-11 trial (DeRuyyscher et al. 2018). Grade 1 and 2 neurologic adverse events, as scored by the physicians, occurred numerically more frequently in the PCI group. Only grade 1 and 2 memory impairment (26 of 86 versus 7 of 88 patients) and cognitive disturbance (16 of 86 versus 3 of 88 patients) were significantly increased in the PCI arm. The number of grade 3–5 toxicities was low in both arms. Among the non-neurologic adverse events, alopecia, fatigue, and headache were significantly more frequent in the PCI arm, occurring in 36 of 86 patients versus 5 of 88 patients, 55 of 86 patients versus 30 of 88 patients, and 33 of 86 patients versus 12 of 88 patients, respectively. Severe toxicity was rare in both study arms. Patient-reported adverse events included dizziness, headache, hypersomnia, memory impairment, and vomiting. These adverse events were numerically higher in the PCI arm than in the observation arm, but only headache occurred significantly more frequently in the PCI arm (55 of 87 patients versus 36 of 88 patients, respectively). Grade ≥3 adverse effects were rare in both study arms. Unsurprisingly, patient and physician scoring were not always concordant. With the exception of vomiting, all events were underreported by physicians. Fatigue and memory impairment were more reported by patients compared with physicians in the observation arm versus the PCI arm. Of note, although physician-scored both neurologic and non-neurologic events were more frequent in PCI-treated patients than in the observation arm, neurologic events tended to increase over time after PCI, whereas non-neurologic events were the highest during PCI and decreased continuously over time. Overall, the toxicities were mild, and it is reasonable to say that PCI is generally well tolerated.

9 Quality of Life (QoL)

RTOG 0214 was the first RCT to conduct a prospective quality-of-life (QoL) assessment. QoL was assessed using the European Organization for Research and Treatment of Cancer (EORTC) Quality of Life Questionnaire (QLQ) C30 and BN20 questionnaires (Gore et al. 2011). In total, 340 patients were evaluable in RTOG 0214. At baseline, 95% of patients completed QoL assessments, but compliance to testing declined rapidly during the study. At 3 months, only 43% of potentially evaluable patients completed the assessments, and this fell further to 34% at 12 months. There were no significant differences between the two arms in change in QoL scores from baseline at 6 and 12 months. In the trial, subgroup analysis was carried out to try and identify patients at higher risk of experiencing a decline in QoL. No clear differences emerged in any of the subgroups tested.

In the trial by Li et al. (2015), assessable QoL data were available for 83% (129 of 156) of all randomized patients, including 70 with PCI and 59 without PCI. The total QoL compliance was 96.2% at baseline and dropped to 59% at 1 year and 43.3% at 2 years. No significant differences were noted in the deterioration rate for QoL and symptoms between the two groups, as assessed by the Functional Assessment of Cancer Therapy-Lung (FACT-L) total score ($p = 0.81$), the FACT-L Trial Outcome Index (TOI) ($p = 0.73$), and the FACT-L Lung Cancer Subscale (LCS) ($p = 0.94$).

In NVALT-11 study, QoL (as measured by the EORTC QLQ C30, EuroQol 5D, and QLQ-BN20) was similar between both arms at baseline. At 3 months after PCI, QoL was worse in the PCI arm, particularly in physical functioning (median scores: PCI, 73; observation, 87; $p = 0.0017$). At 6, 12, and 18 months, QoL was similar between both arms, but in the long term (24, 36, and 48 months), there was a slight, nonsignificant advantage in QoL in the observation arm (DeRuyyscher et al. 2018). A subsequent update reported on generalized linear mixed effects (GLM) model approach to assess the impact of PCI compared to observation over time on health-related quality of life (HRQoL) metrics and found that none of the metrics were clinically relevant or statistically significantly different (Witlox et al. 2019).

In general, it seems that PCI may cause a transient impairment in QoL but is unlikely to result in a permanent detriment on QoL. Confirmatory research is needed, and more robust and longer follow-up data is essential to reach a conclusive statement.

10 Neurocognitive Function (NCF)

RTOG 0214 was the only RCT to collect detailed prospective data on the long-term effects of PCI on neurocognitive function

(NCF) (Gore et al. 2011). NCF was assessed using the Mini-Mental State Examination (MMSE), Hopkins Verbal Learning Test (HVLT), and Activities of Daily Living Scale (ADLS). The change in MMSE scores from baseline to 3 months showed significantly more patients reporting a decline in the PCI arm than in the control arm (36% vs. 21%, $p = 0.04$). A similar trend was seen in the HVLT, with significantly more patients in the PCI arm reporting deterioration in immediate recall (45% vs. 13%, $p < 0.001$) and delayed recall (44% vs. 10%, $p < 0.001$). At the 6-month time point, the differences in both MMSE and HVLT had disappeared. Interestingly, at the 12-month time point, there remained no difference in the MMSE scores, but immediate recall (26% vs. 7%, $p = 0.03$) and delayed recall (32% vs. 5%, $p = 0.008$) in the HVLT were again significantly worse in the PCI arm.

It is likely that the decline in recall is a consequence of PCI; the differences seen in the tests may be because HVLT has better sensitivity than MMSE for detecting early dementia (Wade 1992). What is not known is whether this decline stabilizes or continues to deteriorate. Longer term NCF data in the setting of PCI may help to answer this question.

In a pooled secondary analysis of RTOG 0212 (high (36 Gy in 18 daily or 24 Gy twice-daily fractions) versus low dose (25 fractions in 10 daily fractions) PCI in limited-stage small cell lung cancer) and RTOG 0214 (PCI versus observation in locally advanced NSCLC), Gondi et al. reported on tested and self-reported cognitive functioning (SRCF) (Gondi et al. 2013). The former was assessed by Hopkins Verbal Learning Test (HVLT)-Recall and -Delayed Recall and the latter by EORTC QLQ-C30. PCI was associated with a higher risk of decline in SRCF at 6 months ($p < 0.0001$) and 12 months ($p < 0.0001$). Decline on HVLT-Recall at 6 and 12 months was also associated with PCI ($p = 0.002$ and $p = 0.002$, respectively) but was not closely correlated with decline in SRCF at the same time points ($p = 0.05$ and $p = 0.86$, respectively). This suggests that they may represent distinct elements of the cognitive spectrum.

Decline in NCF has been studied more extensively in the setting of whole-brain radiation therapy (WBRT). Several factors have been linked to this decline after WBRT. The NRG CC001 trial compared hippocampal-avoidance WBRT with conventional WBRT (Brown et al. 2020). The report included a multivariable Cox proportional hazards model for time to cognitive failure, which found that younger age (≤ 61 versus >61) was a significant predictor of reduced risk of cognitive failure ($p = 0.0016$). In addition, age was shown to predispose patients to a higher risk of new neurocognitive impairment with 36 Gy, compared to 25 Gy prophylactic cranial irradiation (PCI) in the RTOG 0212 trial (Wolfson et al. 2011). In a multivariable model, age over 60 predicted for a decline in the Hopkins Verbal Learning Test-Delayed Recall (HVLT) at 12 months in Gondi's RTOG 0212 and 0214 analyses (Gondi et al. 2013). A small study by Sabsevitz et al. (2013) found that pretreatment white matter hyperintensity was a predictor for worse white matter changes after WBRT. The same group also published a secondary analysis of NRG Oncology's Radiation Therapy Oncology Group 0933 phase II clinical trial of HA-WBRT showing that a higher baseline volume of white matter hyperintensity on MRI before radiation therapy (RT) predicted for worse memory decline on HVLT-Revised at 4 months (Bovi et al. 2019). Whether greater white matter hyperintensity on pre-treatment imaging increases the risk of global cognitive decline after WBRT or PCI remains a question. These white matter changes are considered to be a metric of physiologic age and tend to increase with it (Chan et al. 2020). Additional risk factors for cognitive decline include smoking history (McDuff et al. 2013) and receipt of chemotherapy (Wefel et al. 2010).

Major randomized trials have shown worse NCF in patients treated with WBRT than in patients treated with stereotactic radiosurgery (SRS); thus, modern practice has shifted toward increasing SRS utilization to treat a higher number of BMs (Chang et al. 2009; Brown et al. 2016, 2017). Other randomized trials have shown success in reducing the cognitive impairment from WBRT with drugs such as memantine and techniques such as hippocampal avoidance (Brown et al. 2013, 2017). Pulsed reduced dose rate and genu-sparing techniques are being currently explored to reduce radiation-associated toxicity.

11 Best PCI Regimen

Various PCI regimens were used in the seven RCTs (Table 1), but the small number of patients in each trial, differences in inclusion criteria, and locoregional treatment make any comparison between the trials inappropriate. In addition, no randomized trial has compared these (or any other) PCI regimens head-to-head. Therefore, it is not possible to establish which PCI regimen is superior.

12 Summary

PCI is effective at preventing the progression of subclinical brain metastases. Prevention of brain metastases is essential for cure and for sustained quality of life in patients with extracranial disease. PCI has not reliably been shown to translate into improvement in survival and is associated with measurable toxicity; therefore, it is not considered standard of care. However, it is important to have informed conversations with patients about the risk of brain metastases. Given the hypothetical choices for PCI, patients would accept PCI even without a survival benefit if there was a reduction in brain metastases (Lehman et al. 2016). The conversation about employing PCI is becoming increasingly complex. On the one hand, in favor of PCI, there is improved understanding of who is at the highest risk of brain failures. Additionally, data has shown that it is possible to mitigate the side effects of brain radiotherapy (Brown 2020). On the other hand, early detection of asymptomatic metastases amenable to local treatment and development of new agents that cross the blood-brain barrier that address disease with limited toxicity may obviate the need for prevention. Identifying and studying the appropriate population with LA-NSCLC that will benefit from PCI are increasingly difficult.

References

Andre F, Grunenwald D, Pujol JL et al (2001) Patterns of relapse of N2 non-small cell lung carcinoma patients treated with preoperative chemotherapy: should prophylactic cranial irradiation be reconsidered? Cancer 91:2394–2400

Antonia SJ, Villegas A, Daniel D et al (2018) Overall survival with durvalumab after chemoradiotherapy in stage III NSCLC. NEJM 379:2342–2350

Arrieta O, Maldonado F, Turcott JG, Zatarain-Barrón ZL, Barrón F, Blake-Cerda M, Cabrera-Miranda LA, Cardona AF, de la Garza JG, Rosell R (2021) Prophylactic cranial irradiation reduces brain metastases and improves overall survival in high-risk metastatic non-small cell lung cancer patients: a randomized phase 2 study (PRoT-BM trial). Int J Radiat Oncol Biol Phys 110(5):1442–1450. https://doi.org/10.1016/j.ijrobp.2021.02.044

Benedettini E, Sholl LM, Peyton M et al (2010) Met activation in nonsmall cell lung cancer is associated with de novo resistance to EGFR inhibitors and the development of brain metastasis. Am J Pathol 177(1):415–423

Bhatt VR, D'Souza SP, Smith LM et al (2016) Epidermal growth factor receptor mutational status and brain metastases in non-small-cell lung cancer. J Glob Oncol 3:208–217

Bovi JA, Pugh SL, Sabsevitz D et al (2019) Pretreatment volume of MRI-determined white matter injury predicts neurocognitive decline after hippocampal avoidant whole-brain radiation therapy for brain metastases: secondary analysis of NRG oncology radiation therapy oncology group 0933. Adv Radiat Oncol 4(4):579–586. https://doi.org/10.1016/j.adro.2019.07.006

Bradley JD, Hu C, Komaki RR et al (2019) Long-term results of NRG Oncology RTOG 0617: standard- versus high-dose chemoradiotherapy with or without cetuximab for unresectable stage III non–small-cell lung cancer. J Clin Oncol 38:706–713

Brown PD, Pugh S, Laack NN et al (2013) Memantine for the prevention of cognitive dysfunction in patients receiving whole-brain radiotherapy: a randomized, double-blind, placebo-controlled trial. Neuro-Oncology 15(10):1429–1437. https://doi.org/10.1093/neuonc/not114

Brown PD, Jaeckle K, Ballman KV et al (2016) Effect of radiosurgery alone vs radiosurgery with whole brain radiation therapy on cognitive function in patients with 1–3 brain metastases: a randomized clinical trial. JAMA 316(4):4019. https://doi.org/10.1001/jama.2016.9839

Brown PD, Ballman KV, Cerhan JH et al (2017) Postoperative stereotactic radiosurgery compared with whole brain radiotherapy for resected metastatic brain disease (NCCTG N107C/CEC.3): a multicentre, randomised, controlled, phase 3 trial. Lancet Oncol 18(8):1049–1060. https://doi.org/10.1016/S1470-2045(17)30441-2

Brown PD, Gondi V, Pugh S et al (2020) Hippocampal avoidance during whole-brain radiotherapy plus memantine for patients with brain metastases: phase III trial NRG oncology CC001. J Clin Oncol 38(10):1019–1029. https://doi.org/10.1200/JCO.19.02767

Buonato JM, Lazzara MJ (2014) ERK1/2 blockade prevents epithelial-mesenchymal transition in lung cancer cells and promotes their sensitivity to EGFR inhibition. Can Res 74(1):309–319

Carolan H, Sun AY, Bezjak A et al (2005) Does the incidence and outcome of brain metastases in locally advanced nonsmall cell lung cancer justify prophylactic cranial irradiation or early detection? Lung Cancer 49:109–115

Ceresoli GL, Reni M, Chiesa G et al (2002) Brain metastases in locally advanced non-small cell lung carcinoma after multimodality treatment: risk factors analysis. Cancer 95:605–612

Chan M, Ferguson D, Ni Mhurchu E et al (2020) Patients with pretreatment leukoencephalopathy and older patients have more cognitive decline after whole brain radiotherapy. Radiat Oncol 15:271. https://doi.org/10.1186/s13014-020-01717-x

Chang EL, Wefel JS, Hess KR et al (2009) Neurocognition in patients with brain metastases treated with radiosurgery or radiosurgery plus whole-brain irradiation: a randomised controlled trial. Lancet Oncol 10(11):1037–1044. https://doi.org/10.1016/S1470-2045(09)70263-3

Cox JD, Stanley K, Petrovich Z et al (1981) Cranial irradiation in cancer of the lung of all cell types. JAMA 245:469–472

DeRuyyscher DD, Dingemans AMC, Pragg J et al (2018) Prophylactic cranial irradiation versus observation in radically treated stage III Non-small-cell lung cancer: a randomized phase III NVALT-11/DLCRG-02 study. JCO 36:2366–2377

Doebele RC, Lu X, Sumey C et al (2012) Oncogene status predicts patterns of metastatic spread in treatment-naive nonsmall cell. Lung Cancer 118(18):4502–4511

Gadgeel S, Peters S, Mok T et al (2018) Alectinib versus crizotinib in treatment-naive anaplastic lymphoma kinase-positive (ALK+) non-small-cell lung cancer: CNS efficacy results from the ALEX study. Ann Oncol 29:2214–2222

Gondi V, Paulus R, Bruner DW et al (2013) Decline in tested and self-reported cognitive functioning after prophylactic cranial irradiation for lung cancer: pooled secondary analysis of radiation therapy oncology group randomized trials 0212 and 0214. Int J Radiat Oncol Biol Phys 86(4):656–664. https://doi.org/10.1016/j.ijrobp.2013.02.033

Gore EM, Bae K, Wong SJ et al (2011) Phase III comparison of prophylactic cranial irradiation versus observation in patients with locally advanced non-small-cell lung cancer: primary analysis of radiotherapy oncology group study RTOG 0214. J Clin Oncol 29:272–278

Hendriks LEL, Brouns AJWM, Amini M et al (2016) Development of symptomatic brain metastases after chemoradiotherapy for stage III non-small cell lung cancer: does the type of chemotherapy regimen matter? Lung Cancer 101:68–75

Law A, Daly B, Madsen M et al (1997) High incidence of isolated brain metastases following complete response in advanced non-small cell lung cancer: a new challenge. Lung Cancer 18:65s

Lee H, Jeong SH, Jeong BH et al (2015) Incidence of brain metastasis at the initial diagnosis of lung squamous cell carcinoma on the basis of stage, excluding brain metastasis. J Thorac Oncol 11:426–431

Lehman M et al (2016) Patient preferences regarding prophylactic cranial irradiation: a discrete choice experiment. Radiother Oncol 121(2):225–231

Li N, Zeng Z-F, Wang S-Y, Ou W, Ye X, Li J et al (2015) Randomized phase III trial of prophylactic cranial irradiation versus observation in patients with fully resected stage IIIA-N2 nonsmall-cell lung cancer and high risk of cerebral metastases after adjuvant chemotherapy. Ann Oncol 26:504–509. https://doi.org/10.1093/annonc/mdu567

Majoomdar A, Austin JHM, Malhotra R et al (2007) Clinical predictors of metastatic disease to the brain from non-small cell lung carcinoma: primary tumor size, cell type, and lymph node metastases. Radiology 242:882–888

McDuff SGR et al (2013) Neurocognitive assessment following whole brain radiation therapy and radiosurgery for patients with cerebral metastases. J Neurol Neurosurg Psychiatry 84(12):1384–1391

Meyers CA, Smith JA, Bezjak A et al (2004) Neurocognitive function and progression in patients with brain metastases treated with whole-brain radiation and motexafin gadolinium: results of a randomized phase III trial. J Clin Oncol 22:157–165

Miller TP, Crowley JJ, Mira J, Schwartz JG, Hutchins L, Baker L (1998) A randomized trial of chemotherapy and radiotherapy for stage III non-small cell lung cancer. Cancer Ther 1(229–36):11

Mira JG, Miller TP, Crowley JJ (1990) Chest irradiation vs. chest irradiation plus chemotherapy with or without prophylactic brain radiotherapy in localized nonsmall lung cancer: a Southwest Oncology Group Study. Int J Radiat Oncol Biol Phys 19:145. https://doi.org/10.1016/0360-3016(90)90693-E10

Park SJ, Kim HR, Lee DH et al (2012) Efficacy of epidermal growth factor receptor tyrosine kinase inhibitors for brain metastasis in non-small cell lung cancer patients harboring either exon 19 or 21 mutation. Lung Cancer 77:556–560

PCIOCG (The Prophylactic Cranial Irradiation Overview Collaborative Group) (2018) Cranial irradiation for preventing brain metastases of small cell lung cancer in patients in complete remission. Cochrane

Database Syst Rev 2018(2):CD002805. https://doi.org/10.1002/14651858.CD002805

Perez CA, Pajak TF, Rubin P et al (1987) Long term observations of the patterns of failure in patients with unresectable non-oat cell carcinoma of the lung treated with definitive radiotherapy. Cancer 59:1874–1881

Reungwetwattana T, Nakagawa K, Cho BC et al (2018) CNS response to osimertinib versus standard epidermal growth factor receptor tyrosine kinase inhibitors in patients with untreated EGFR-mutated advanced non-small-cell lung cancer. J Clin Oncol 36:3290–3297

Russell AH, Pajak TE, Selim HM et al (1991) Prophylactic cranial irradiation for lung cancer patients at high risk for development of cerebral metastasis: results of a prospective randomised trial conducted by the radiation therapy oncology group (RTOG 84-03). Int J Radiat Oncol Biol Phys 21:637–643

Sabsevitz DS, Bovi JA, Leo PD et al (2013) The role of pre-treatment white matter abnormalities in developing white matter changes following whole brain radiation: a volumetric study. J Neuro-Oncol 114(3):291–297. https://doi.org/10.1007/s11060-013-1181-8

Schouten LJ, Rutten J, Huveneers HA et al (2002) Incidence of brain metastases in a cohort of patients with carcinoma of the breast, colon, kidney, and lung and melanoma. Cancer 94(10):2698–2705

Shin DY, Na II, Kim CH et al (2014) EGFR mutation and brain metastasis in pulmonary adenocarcinomas. J Thorac Oncol 9:195–199

Sperduto PW, Yang J, Beal K et al (2017) Estimating survival in patients with lung cancer and brain metastases an update of the graded prognostic assessment for lung cancer using molecular markers (Lung-molGPA). JAMA Oncol 3:827–831

Strauss GM, Herndon JE, Sherman DD et al (2005) Neoadjuvant chemotherapy and radiotherapy followed by surgery in stage III non-small cell carcinoma of the lung: a report of a cancer and leukemia group B phase II study. J Clin Oncol 10:1237–1244

Sun A et al (2019) Prophylactic cranial irradiation vs observation in patients with locally advanced non-small cell lung cancer: A long-term update of the NRG Oncology/RTOG 0214 phase 3 randomized clinical trial. JAMA Oncol 5(6):847–855

Umsawasdi T, Valdivieso M, Chen TT et al (1984) Role of elective brain irradiation during combined chemo-radiotherapy for limited disease non-small cell lung cancer. J Neuro-Oncol 2:253–259

Wade DT (1992) Measurement in neurological rehabilitation. Oxford University Press, NY

Wang SY, Xiong Y, Ou W et al (2009) Risk of cerebral metastases for postoperative locally advanced non-small-cell lung cancer. Lung Cancer 64:238–243

Waqar SN, Sampson PP, Robinson CG et al (2018a) Non-small cell lung cancer with brain metastases at presentation. Clin Lung Cancer 19:e373–e379

Waqar SN, Waqar SH, Trinkaus K et al (2018b) Brain metastases at presentation with non-small cell lung cancer. Am J Clin Oncol 41:36–40

Wefel JS et al (2010) Acute and late onset cognitive dysfunction associated with chemotherapy in women with breast cancer. Cancer 116(14):3348–3356

Westeel V (2003) Risk of brain metastases in non-metastatic non-small cell lung cancer. Lung Cancer 41:21s

Witlox WJA, Ramaekers BLT, Groen HJM, Dingemans AM, Praag J, Belderbos J, van der Noort V, van Tinteren H, Joore MA, De Ruysscher DKM (2019) Factors determining the effect of prophylactic cranial irradiation (PCI) in patients with stage-III nonsmall cell lung cancer: exploratory subgroup analyses of the NVALT-11/DLCRG-02 phase-III study. Acta Oncol 58(10):1528–1531. https://doi.org/10.1080/0284186X.2019.1629016

Wolfson AH, Bae K, Komaki R et al (2011) Primary analysis of a phase II randomized trial radiation therapy oncology group (RTOG) 0212: impact of different total doses and schedules of prophylactic cranial irradiation on chronic neurotoxicity and quality of life for patients with limited-disease small-cell lung cancer. Int J Radiat Oncol Biol Phys 81(1):77–84. https://doi.org/10.1016/j.ijrobp.2010.05.013

Won YW, Joo J, Yun T et al (2015) Clinical predictors of metastatic disease to the brain from non-small cell lung carcinoma: primary tumor size, cell type, and lymph node metastases. Lung Cancer 88:201–207

Yang P, Kulig K, Boland JM et al (2012) Worse disease-free survival in never-smokers with ALK+ lung adenocarcinoma. J Thorac Oncol 7:90–97

Palliative External Beam Thoracic Radiation Therapy of Non-small Cell Lung Cancer

Stein Sundstrøm

Contents

1 Introduction 597
2 Symptoms 597
3 Palliative Radiotherapy: Definition 598
4 Prognostic Factors for Selecting Treatment 598
5 Radiotherapy Technique 599
5.1 Defining the Radiotherapy Volume 599
5.2 Dose and Fractionation 599
6 Palliative Radiotherapy Studies (Period 1990–2005) 599
6.1 Phase III Studies (Low Dose Versus Normo-Dose) 599
6.2 Phase III Studies (Normo-Dose Versus High Dose) 600
6.3 Side Effects 600
6.4 Special Consideration 601
6.5 Interpretation 601
7 How to Treat Stage III–IV NSCLC Patients After Better Staging and in the Area of Molecular Profiling? 601
8 When Is Palliative Radiotherapy Indicated? 602
9 Treatment Recommendations 602
10 Summary 603
References 603

S. Sundstrøm (✉)
St Olav University Hospital, Trondheim, Norway
e-mail: Stein.Harald.Sundstrom@stolav.no

1 Introduction

Lung cancer is still the leading cause of cancer-related deaths worldwide, however with a significant decline in the industrialized nations in the last decades (Barta et al. 2019). About two-thirds of patients with non-small cell lung cancer (NSCLC) are diagnosed with localized stage III or metastatic stage IV disease (Bryan et al. 2018). Of these, 30% have stage III disease. During the last 5–10 years, the effect of systemic therapy, either a tyrosine kinase inhibitor, immunotherapy alone, or immunotherapy combined with chemotherapy, can give considerable prolonged survival, challenging the distinction between curative or palliative treatment goal. Many patients will have symptoms from intrathoracic tumor at diagnosis or will develop symptoms in the near future (Hopwood and Stephens 1995; Lutz et al. 2001). Radiotherapy is effective in reducing intrathoracic symptoms. Due to advanced disease and limited prognosis, intervention should have effective palliation avoiding unacceptable toxicity as the major goal.

2 Symptoms

Common symptoms from tumors in the chest are dyspnea, cough, and hemoptysis. Other symptoms are chest pain, compression of large vessels (superior vena cava syndrome), nerve infiltration causing hoarseness or Horner syndrome, and dysphagia due to compression of esophagus. These latter symptoms indicate advanced tumors. Approximately 70% of patients with advanced disease have one or more symptoms from intrathoracic tumor at diagnosis requiring treatment intervention (Hopwood and Stephens 1995; Lutz et al. 2001). In symptomatic patients, palliative radiotherapy is an efficient strategy for relieving symptoms.

3 Palliative Radiotherapy: Definition

Palliative radiotherapy is defined as radiotherapy given with less than radical doses, perceived as a total dose less than 50 Gy. A great variation in treatment schedules considering dose, fractionation, and overall treatment time is used. The different regimens vary due to tradition, preference, and radiotherapy capacity (Fraser et al. 2019). The selection for fractionation and dose requires a thorough clinical evaluation of the individual patient before decision. A division in good or poor prognostic group is practical and recommended.

4 Prognostic Factors for Selecting Treatment

Stage of the disease, weight loss in the last 3–6 months, and performance status (WHO, ECOG) are the most robust prognostic factors in NSCLC (Brundage et al. 2002). Disease stage is most powerful (Goldstraw et al. 2016). Patients with metastatic disease have shorter survival than those with stage III disease. Good prognostic stage III patients have better survival than poor prognostic stage III patients. However, even when good prognostic stage III patients are treated with high-dose chemoradiotherapy, the survival is not favorable.

After stage, performance status (PS) is next (Buccheri and Ferrigo 2004). Patients with WHO PS status 0–1 will experience a meaningful effect of all kinds of treatment, chemotherapy, radiotherapy, targeted therapy, and immunotherapy. Patients in WHO PS 2 are a borderline group; they achieve less effect of treatment, and often with considerably toxicity. Patients with WHO PS status of 3–4 should not be offered systemic treatment, except in treatment-naïve patients harboring a gene alteration appropriate for a specific tyrosine kinase inhibitor.

Involuntary weight loss developed over the last 3–6 months before diagnosis is a consistent negative prognosticator in lung cancer (Morel et al. 2018). Self-reported appetite loss is also related to a poorer prognosis compared with those with normal appetite (Sundstrøm et al. 2006).

Large tumors have less probability of eradication by radiotherapy due to hypoxia in the tumor. There is no accepted consensus as to what maximum tumor size or volume precludes a radical strategy. The pivotal study from RTOG in 1982 showed a clear relation to less effect in tumors larger than 6 cm in diameter (Perez et al. 1982). Other studies show the same picture (Bradley et al. 2002; Dehing-Oberije et al. 2008). Therefore, larger tumors (>10–12 cm) are treated by most with a palliative intent. However, recent reports challenge this practice (Ball et al. 2013a, b). In patients within stage II–III disease treated with not-radical radiotherapy, there is no clear association with volume (tumor and lymph nodes) and effect on survival (Nieder et al. 2021; Ball et al. 2013a, b). Better staging with PET/CT and more precise radiotherapy with IMRT/VMAT and use of 3D/4D CRT technique challenge this perception even more.

Overall, in the heterogeneous stage III group patients, selection to curative or palliative schedule should be based on a conscientious evaluation of the factors outlined in Table 1. Occurrence of one or more of the poor prognostic factors should conduct a palliative treatment strategy. Patients in

Table 1 Prognostic factors in stage III patients

Good prognostic factors	Poor prognostic factors
WHO PS status 0–1	WHO PS status ≥2
Tumor volume <10–12 cm in largest diameter	Tumor volume >12 cm in largest diameter
Weight loss <10% in the last 3 months	Weight loss ≥10% in the last 3 months

stage IV disease should be treated with a palliative intent, except in rare situations with oligometastatic disease.

5 Radiotherapy Technique

Given the palliative treatment goal intending to reduce symptoms, the radiotherapy should be simple to set up and to perform and less time consuming for the patient.

Modern radiotherapy including palliative schedules is based on CT scan and computer planning. However, a conventional two-dimensional radiotherapy (2D RT) using an X-ray beam simulator is sufficient in most cases and is still in use in countries with limited radiotherapy resources. Shielding of uninvolved lung tissue reducing side effects is advised. If computerized IMRT/VMAT is available, this technique is time sparing even in palliative schedules. Previously, 40 Gy/20 fractions were considered to be maximal spinal cord tolerance. Updates confirm 50 Gy using conventional fractionation as safe to the thoracic spine (Kirkpatrick et al. 2010). If a more protracted schedule with higher palliative dose is planned, a three-dimensional conformal radiotherapy (3D CRT) technique based on CT scan should be preferred. This will better define the tumor volume and organs at risk. High-energy photon beams with 5–15 MeV are recommended.

5.1 Defining the Radiotherapy Volume

The tumor with disease-related lymph nodes should be incorporated in the field plan. Elective lymph node irradiation will only add toxicity with no impact on local control or survival (Yan et al. 2007).

When high-dose palliative radiotherapy is considered, a standard margin with GTV and CTV/PTV including tumor- and disease-related nodes should be defined. According to international guidelines, a setup margin of 1 cm from GTV to CTV, and 0.5 cm from CTV to PTV, is recommended. Larger margins in the craniocaudal direction due to respiration movements might be necessary. Reduced margins are desirable if the treated volume enlarges >200 cm^2 in field size.

If low-dose palliative radiotherapy is advised, the treated volume should include the symptomatic part of the tumor. In most cases, the volume can be confined to the symptomatic area avoiding unnecessary radiotherapy to nonsymptomatic lung tissue, even though these parts may include tumor spread. The central airways with mediastinum and hilus on the affected side will be an adequate volume. Margins from the tumor border to CTV and PTV should not be stressed. Close margins or even margins set up in the tumor are acceptable, if the volume becomes large. Due to palliation, radiotherapy side effects should be focused. In that respect, smaller volumes are more desirable than large volumes encompassing the complete tumor extension.

5.2 Dose and Fractionation

A large variety of fractionation schemes and radiotherapy schedules are in use for palliative treatment, from single fraction of 8–10 Gy up to subradical doses of 50–60 Gy. Until the first study from the UK Medical Research Council was published in 1991 (MRC Lung Cancer Working Party 1991), a typical course was 30 Gy in ten fractions.

6 Palliative Radiotherapy Studies (Period 1990–2005)

6.1 Phase III Studies (Low Dose Versus Normo-Dose)

Since the MRC I study published in 1991, eight other randomized phase III trials (Medical Research Council Lung Cancer Working Party 1992, 1996; Rees et al. 1997; Bezjak et al. 2002; Sundstrøm et al. 2004; Erridge et al. 2005; Kramer et al. 2005; Senkus-Konefka et al. 2005) comparing a strict hypofractionated schedule

Table 2 Different phase III trials using low-dose hypofractionated palliative TRT in advanced NSCLC

Study	N	Regimens	Stage III–IV (%)	WHO PS	Palliation	Survival
MRC I (1991)	369	17 Gy/2 vs. 30 Gy/10	68–32	0–2(3)	Equal	Equal
MRC II (1992)	235	10 Gy/1 vs. 17 Gy/2	71–29	2–4	Equal	Equal
MRC III (1996)	509	17 Gy/2 vs. 39 Gy/13	100–0	0–2	Equal	39 Gy better
Rees (1997)	216	17 Gy/2 vs. 22.5 Gy/5	Not reported	0–3	Equal	Equal
Bezjak (2002)	230	10 Gy/1 vs. 20 Gy/5	76–24	0–3	Equal	20 Gy better
Sundstrøm (2004)	407	17 Gy/2 vs. 42 Gy/15 vs. 50 Gy/25	78–22	0–3	Equal	Equal
Erridge (2005)	148	10 Gy/1 vs. 30 Gy/10	Not reported	0–3	30 Gy better	Equal
Kramer (2005)	297	16 Gy/2 vs. 30 Gy/10	52–48	0–3(4)	30 Gy better	30 Gy better
Senkus-Konefka (2005)	100	16 Gy/2 vs. 20 Gy/5	84–16	1–3(4)	Equal	16 Gy better

versus a normo-fractionated regimen have been published, as outlined in Table 2. No new studies since 2005 have been published. More than 2500 patients were included in these trials. All trials have either a single (8 or 10 Gy) or two large fractions (17 Gy/2 or 16 Gy/2) as the short-course experimental arm. The comparative arms were fractionated schedules with a range of 20–50 Gy. The trials included patients up to WHO PS 3 with the majority of stage III patients. One trial (Medical Research Council Lung Cancer Working Party 1992) included poor-performance-status patients only (WHO PS 2–4) comparing a single fraction versus 17 Gy/2 fractions. All trials reported the effect on symptoms assessed by patients through self-reported questionnaires and physicians' evaluation of symptoms, as well as overall survival. In two trials (Bezjak et al. 2002; Kramer et al. 2005), the effect on symptoms is in favor of the higher dose, in the others the effect on symptoms is equal. In three trials (MRC III 1996; Bezjak et al. 2002; Kramer et al. 2005), the survival is in favor of the high-dose arm: 39 Gy/13 fractions, 30 Gy/10 fractions, and 30 Gy/10 fractions, respectively. One trial (Senkus-Konefka et al. 2005) reports a survival benefit for the low-dose arm: 16 Gy/2 fractions versus 20 Gy/5 fractions. In one three-armed trial (Sundstrøm et al. 2004) comparing 17 Gy/2 fractions versus two high-dose arms, 42 Gy/15 fractions and 50 Gy/25 fractions, no difference in median survival was found.

6.2 Phase III Studies (Normo-Dose Versus High Dose)

Five randomized phase III studies (Simpson et al. 1985; Teo et al. 1987; Abratt et al. 1995; Reinfuss et al. 1999; Nestle et al. 2000) have compared different normo- to high-dose regimens, including more than 1000 patients, as shown in Table 3. Also in this setting, no new studies have been published since 2000. Nearly all had stage III localized disease with a reasonable good performance status WHO PS 0–2. Four of five studies have assessed the effect on symptoms. One has used patient self-reported questionnaires (Nestle et al. 2000). In the other studies, the physicians assessed the effect on symptoms. One study reports better palliation in the high-dose arm (Teo et al. 1987). Four studies have data on survival, equal in three and better in one in the high-dose arms (Reinfuss et al. 1999). This study by Reinfuss is special since one arm in this three-armed trial was a "wait-and-see" arm: 40 Gy/10 (split) versus 50 Gy/25 versus "wait and see." The survival in this "wait-and-see" arm was inferior compared to the two actively treated arms.

6.3 Side Effects

All studies reporting side effects show that esophagitis and dysphagia were the most frequent in the high-dose arms, although dysphagia was also detectable in the hypofractionated low-

Table 3 Different phase III trials using normal-high-dose palliative TRT in advanced NSCLC

Study	N	Regimens	Stage III–IV (%)	WHO PS	Palliation	Survival
Simpson (1985)	316	20 Gy/20 vs. 30 Gy/10 vs. 40 Gy/20 split	100–0	0–2	Equal	Equal
Teo (1997)	291	31.2 Gy/4 vs. 45 Gy/18	90–3	0–3	45 Gy better	Equal
Abratt (1995)	84	35 Gy/10 vs. 45 Gy/15	100–0	0–2	Equal	Not reported
Reinfuss (1999)	240	40 Gy/10 (split 4 weeks) vs. 50 Gy/25 vs. wait and see	100–0	0–2	Not reported	Better 40/50 Gy
Nestle (2000)	152	32 Gy/16 (twice/day) vs. 60 Gy/30	79–21	1–2	Equal	Equal

dose arms. Onset and duration of dysphagia were earlier and shorter in the hypofractionated arms compared to high-dose arms. Rare cases of radiation-induced myelopathy are reported, usually mild and temporary (Sundstrøm et al. 2004; Erridge et al. 2005). The incidence is estimated to be 2% at 2-year survival for hypofractionated schedules.

6.4 Special Consideration

The abovementioned studies included mostly stage III patients. The staging procedure in these study periods was simple with no use of PET/CT scan and brain MRI for detecting nonsymptomatic brain metastasis. These studies were also completed in the prechemotherapy area, and in that perspective can be interpreted as purely radiotherapy studies, studying the local effect of radiotherapy only.

6.5 Interpretation

Palliation: Most studies show that the effect on symptoms is similar regardless of dose and fractionation. A trend of more rapid relief of symptoms in favor of low-dose hypofractionation schedule is noticed.

Survival: No difference in median survival is observed in patients with advanced disease not candidates for systemic treatment. Some patients with localized stage III disease may have better survival with a protracted high-dose schedule. As seen in Tables 2 and 3, the majority of patients in the trials had localized stage III disease. In one trial (MRC I 1991), there was some evidence that higher dose could give some long-term survivors in stage III, even though median survival was equal. Therefore, MRC III study (MRC III 1996) was set up including only stage III disease and good performance status, comparing 17 Gy/2 fractions (F1) versus high-dose 39 Gy/13 fractions (F2). The median survival increased from 7 to 9 months in the F2 arm, although not significant, with 1- and 2-year survival rates of 31% and 9% versus 36% and 12% in the F1 and F2 arms, respectively. In the other study (Sundstrøm et al. 2004) comparing strict low-dose to high-dose schedules, a trend in better survival in the high-dose arms was found. Later exploration of this study restricted to stage III patients only (Sundstrøm et al. 2006) revealed 3- and 5-year survival rates in the three arms (17 Gy/2, 42 Gy/15, 50 Gy/25) of 1%, 8%, and 6%, versus 0%, 4%, and 3%, respectively. With the overall interpretation concerning survival, patients with metastatic disease can safely be treated with a hypofractionated schedule.

Side effects: Acute toxicity with dysphagia is mild, temporary, and manageable. Late toxicity is rare and sporadic with low severity.

7 How to Treat Stage III–IV NSCLC Patients After Better Staging and in the Area of Molecular Profiling?

Modern staging of lung cancer involves the use of PET scan and MRI brain, unless the primary investigation reveals metastatic disease. For more accurate-stage investigated patients, palliative low-dose radiotherapy is inferior for secure stage III. There is, however, no validated criteria to define which stage III NSCLC patients are eligible for a curative or a palliative treatment schedule. Nevertheless, the prognostic criteria outlined in Table 1 suggest that a pragmatic distinction between curative or palliative fractionation and dose provided adequate investigation. Recent guidelines and studies recommend that patients with stage III disease not deemed for radical treatment should be treated with chemotherapy and high-dose palliative schedule (Moeller et al. 2018; Strom et al. 2013).

Novel treatment with tyrosine kinase treatment in subgroups of metastatic NSCLC patients harboring specific gene alterations, mono-immunotherapy, or immunotherapy combined with chemotherapy can give considerable survival benefit for some patients (Maemondo et al. 2010; Gandhi et al. 2018). Patients considered candidates for such treatment, and are in need for radiotherapy palliation, will be recommended by most clinicians a more high-dose palliative schedule (Jumeau et al. 2019).

8 When Is Palliative Radiotherapy Indicated?

Most patients diagnosed with locally advanced or metastatic NSCLC will suffer from or develop symptoms in the near future from the chest tumor. One of the issues is whether to irradiate an asymptomatic patient or wait for symptoms to appear. One randomized trial, completed before systemic effective treatment was recognized in patients unsuitable for resection or curative radiotherapy, did not show any difference for immediate or delayed treatment in minimally symptomatic patients concerning symptoms and survival (Falk et al. 2002). A subanalysis from a randomized trial restricted to stage III patients stratified in nonsymptomatic or symptomatic revealed that nonsymptomatic patients developed more symptoms and side effects, while symptomatic patients experienced symptom relief (Sundstrøm et al. 2005). Immediate treatment is therefore likely to give unnecessary side effects in otherwise symptom-free patients and does not prevent the development of later symptoms. A wait-and-see procedure is therefore advocated until the patient develops disease-related symptoms.

9 Treatment Recommendations

Updated Cochrane reviews and ASTRO Guidelines focusing on palliative thoracic radiotherapy in lung cancer conclude that there is no strong evidence that higher dose gives a better outcome concerning symptom relief and survival and that a hypofractionated regimen is an option for most patients (Stevens et al. 2015; Moeller et al. 2018). Due to large heterogeneity concerning dose and fractionation in performed studies, no meta-analysis has been initiated. However, patients with accurate stage III disease with a reasonable performance status should be treated with a protracted or high-dose fractionated regimen 30–45 Gy. Patient selection to short- or long-course palliative radiotherapy should be based on the factors outlined in Table 1. Stage IV patients can be treated safely with a hypofractionated technique in almost all cases, unless they harbor gene alterations predictive for targeted therapy with a high chance for response. Some selected cases with single metastasis can be treated more radically provided a radical strategy for the metastatic site. Before treatment decision is made, a thorough clinical evaluation of the individual patient should be mandatory in all cases, elucidating the patient into a good or poor prognostic group.

Of special interest is the fact that palliative radiotherapy in lung cancer unexpectedly can generate some long-term survivors (Sundstrøm et al. 2006; Mac Manus et al. 2005). Approximately 1–3% of patients with localized disease have been found with 5-year survival after palliative high-dose radiotherapy. This can be explained by unpredictable high radiotherapy sensitivity of some lung tumors.

10 Summary

- Hypofractionated and moderately high-dose palliative radiotherapy gives equal effect on symptoms and survival in advanced non-small cell lung cancer.
- Stage III patients not candidates for a curative strategy with favorable prognostic factors should be treated with a fractionated schedule to a dose of 30–45 Gy combined with chemotherapy.
- Stage IV patients can safely be treated with a strict hypofractionated schedule.
- Advanced treatment-naïve NSCLC patients harboring specific gene alterations or with predictive factors for the effect of immunotherapy should be treated with systemic therapy up front, delaying palliative radiotherapy.
- Palliative thoracic radiotherapy should not be administrated to patients without symptoms present.

References

Abratt RP, Shepherd LJ, Mameena Salton DG (1995) Palliative radiation for stage 3 non-small cell lung cancer. A prospective study of two moderately high dose regimens. Lung Cancer 13:137–143

Ball D, Mitchell A, Giroux D et al (2013a) Effect of tumour size on prognosis in patients treated with radical radiotherapy or chemotherapy for non-small cell lung cancer. Journ Thorc Oncol 8:315321

Ball D, Fisher R, Burmeister BH et al (2013b) The complex relationship between lung tumour and survival in patients with non-small cell lung cancer treated by definitive radiotherapy: a prospective, observational prognostic factor study of the Trans-Tasman Radiation Oncology Group (TROG 99.05). Radiother Oncol 106:305–311

Barta JA, Pwell CA, Wisnievsky (2019) Global epidemiology of lung cancer. Ann Glob Health 85(1):8., 1–16

Bezjak A, Dixon P, Brundage M et al (2002) Randomized phase III trial of single versus fractionated thoracic radiation in the palliation of patients with lung cancer (NCIC CTG SC.15). Int J Radiat Oncol Biol Phys 54:719–728

Bradley JF, Ieumwananonthachai N, Purdy JA et al (2002) Gross tumor volume, critical prognostic factor in patients treated with three-dimensional conformal radiation therapy for non-small-cell lung carcinoma. Int J Radiat Oncol Biol Phys 52:49–57

Brundage MD, Davies D, Mackillop WJ (2002) Prognostic factors in non-small cell lung cancer. Chest 122:1037–1057

Bryan S, Masoud H, Weir HK et al (2018) Cancer in Canada: stage at diagnosis • Health Brief. Statistics Canada, Catalogue no. 82–003-X. Health Rep 29(12):21–25

Buccheri G, Ferrigo D (2004) Prognostic factors in lung cancer, tables and comments. Eur Respir J 7:1350–1354

Dehing-Oberije C, de Ruysscher D, van der Weide H et al (2008) Tumor volume combined with number of positive lymph node stations is a more important prognostic factor than TNM stage for survival of non-small-cell lung cancer patients treated with (chemo)radiotherapy. Int J Radiat Oncol Biol Phys 70:1039–1044

Erridge SC, Gaze MN, Price A et al (2005) Symptom control and quality of life in people with lung cancer: a randomised trial of two palliative radiotherapy fractionation schedules. Clin Oncol 17:61–67

Falk S, Girling DJ, White RJ et al (2002) Immediate versus delayed palliative thoracic radiotherapy in patients with unresectable locally advanced non-small cell lung cancer and minimal thoracic symptoms: randomised controlled trial. BMJ 325:465–468

Fraser I, Lefresne S, Regan J et al (2019) Palliative thoracic radiotherapy near the end of life in lung cancer: a population-based analysis. Lung Cancer 135:97–103

Gandhi L, Rodrigues-Abreu S, Gadgeel E et al (2018) Pembrolizumab plus chemotherapy in metastatic non-small-cell lung cancer. N Engl J Med 31(378):2078–2092

Goldstraw P et al (2016) The IASCLC lung cancer staging project. Proposals for revision of the TNM stage groupings in the forthcoming (eight) edition of the TNM classification for lung cancer. J Thorac Oncol 11:39–51

Hopwood P, Stephens RJ (1995) Symptoms at presentation for treatment in patients with lung cancer: implications for the evaluation of palliative treatment. Br J Cancer 71:663–666

Jumeau R, Vilotte F, Durham AD et al (2019) Current landscape of palliative radiotherapy for non-small-cell lung cancer. Transl Lung Cancer Res 8(Suppl. 2):S192–S201

Kirkpatrick JP, van der Kogel AJ, Schultheiss TE (2010) Radiation dose-volume effects in the spinal cord. Int J Radiat Oncol Biol Phys 76(Suppl):S42–S49

Kramer G, Wanders SL, Noordijk EM et al (2005) Results of the Dutch National Study of the palliative effect of irradiation using two different treatment schemes for non-small-cell lung cancer. J Clin Oncol 13:2962–2970

Lutz S, Norrell R, Bertucio C et al (2001) Symptom frequency and severity in patients with metastatic or locally recurrent lung cancer: a prospective study using Lung Cancer Symptom Scale in a community Hospital. J Palliat Med 4:157–165

Mac Manus MP, Matthews JP, Wada M et al (2005) Unexpected long-term survival after low-dose palliative radiotherapy for nonsmall cell lung cancer. Cancer 116:1110–1116

Maemondo M, Inoue A, Kobayashi K, Sugawara S, Oizumi S, Isobe H et al (2010) Gefitinib or chemotherapy for non-small-cell lung cancer with mutated EGFR. N Engl J Med 362(25):2380–2388

Medical Research Council Lung Cancer Working Party (1992) A Medical Research Council (MRC) randomised trial of palliative radiotherapy with two fractions or a single fraction in patients with inoperable non-small cell lung cancer (NSCLC) and poor performance status. Br J Cancer 65:931–941

Medical Research Council Lung Cancer Working Party (1996) Randomised trial of palliative 2-fraction versus more intensive 13-fraction radiotherapy for patients with inoperable non-small cell lung cancer and good performance status. Clin Oncol 1996(8):167–175

Moeller B, Balagamwala EH, Chen A et al (2018) Palliative thoracic radiation therapy for non-small cell lung cancer: 2018 Update of an American Society for Radiation Oncology (ASTRO) Evidence-Based Guideline. Pract Radiat Oncol 8:245–250

Morel H et al (2018) Prediagnosis weight loss, a stronger factor than BMI, to predict survival in patients with lung cancer. Lung Cancer 126:55–63

MRC Lung Cancer Working Party (1991) Inoperable non-small-cell lung cancer (NSCLC): a Medical Research Council randomised trial of palliative radiotherapy with two fractions or ten fractions. Br J Cancer 63:265–270

Nestle U, Nieder C, Walter K et al (2000) A palliative accelerated irradiation regimen for advanced non-small-cell lung cancer vs conventionally fractionated 60 Gy: results of a randomized equivalence study. Int J Radiat Oncol Biol Phys 48:195–203

Nieder C, Imingen KS, Mannsaker B et al (2021) Palliative thoracic radiotherapy for non-small cell lung cancer: is there any impact of target volume size on survival? Anticancer Res 41:355–358

Perez CA, Stanley K, Grundy G et al (1982) Impact of irradiation technique and tumor extent in tumor control and survival of patients with unresectable non-oat cell carcinoma of the lung. Cancer 50:1091–1099

Rees GJG, Devrell CE, Barley VL et al (1997) Palliative radiotherapy for lung cancer: two versus five fractions. Clin Oncol (R Coll Radiol) 9:90–95

Reinfuss M, Glinski B, Kowalska T et al (1999) Radiothérapie du cancer bronchique non á petites cellules de stade III inopérable asymptomatique. Résultats définitifs d'un essai prospectif randomisé (240 patients). Cancer Radiother 3:475–479

Senkus-Konefka E, Dziadziuszko R, Bednaruk-Mlynski E et al (2005) A prospective randomised study to compare two palliative radiotherapy schedules for non-small-cell cancer (NSCLC). Br J Cancer 92:1038–1045

Simpson JR, Francis ME, Perez-Tamayo R et al (1985) Palliative radiotherapy for inoperable carcinoma of the lung: final report of a RTOG multi-institutional trial. Int J Radiat Oncol Biol Phys 11:751–758

Stevens R, MacBeth F, Toy E et al (2015) Cochrane Database Syst Rev 1(1):CD002143. https://doi.org/10.1002/14651858.CD002143.pub4

Strom HH, Bremnes RM, Sundstrom SH et al (2013) Concurrent palliative chemoradiation leads to survival and quality of life benefits in poor prognosis stage III non-small-cell lung cancer: A randomised trial by the Norwegian Lung Cancer Study Group. Br J Cancer 109:1467–1475

Sundstrøm S, Bremnes R, Aasebø U et al (2004) Hypofractionated palliative radiotherapy (17 Gy per two fractions) in advanced non-small-cell lung carcinoma is comparable to standard fractionation for symptom control and survival: a national phase III trial. J Clin Oncol 22:801–810

Sundstrøm S, Bremnes R, Brunsvig P et al (2005) Immediate or delayed radiotherapy in advanced non-small cell lung cancer (NSCLC)? Data from a prospective randomised study. Radiother Oncol 75:141–148

Sundstrøm S, Bremnes R, Brunsvig P et al (2006) Palliative thoracic radiotherapy in locally advanced non-small cell lung cancer: Can quality-of-life assessments help in selection of patients for short- or long-course radiotherapy? J Thorac Oncol 1:816–824

Teo P, Tai TH, Choy D et al (1987) A randomized study on palliative radiation therapy for inoperable non-small cell carcinoma of the lung. Int J Radiat Oncol Biol Phys 14:867–871

Yan S, Sun X, Li MH et al (2007) A randomized study of involved field irradiation versus elective nodal irradiation in combination with concurrent chemotherapy for inoperable stage III non-small cell lung cancer. Am J Clin Oncol 30:239–244

Intraoperative Radiotherapy in Lung Cancer: Methodology (Electrons or Brachytherapy), Clinical Experiences, and Long-Term Institutional Results

Felipe A. Calvo, Javier Aristu, Javier Serrano, Mauricio Cambeiro, Rafael Martinez-Monge, and Rosa Cañón

Contents

1 Introduction 606
2 Tissue Tolerance Studies of IORT 607
3 Technical Considerations: IOERT 608
4 Clinical Indications: IOERT 609
5 **International Intraoperative Electron Radiotherapy (IOERT) Clinical Experiences and Results** 610
5.1 National Cancer Institute Experience 610
5.2 University Medical School of Graz Experience 610
5.3 Montpellier Regional Cancer Centre Experience 611
5.4 The Allegheny University Hospital of Philadelphia Experience 611
5.5 Madrid Institute of Oncology (Grupo IMO) Experience 611
5.6 USP Hospital San Jaime Experience 611
5.7 The University Clinic of Navarra Experience 612
5.8 Tomsk Cancer Research, National Research Medical Center, Russia Experience 614
6 **International LDR-IORT and HDR-IORT Clinical Experiences and Results** 615
6.1 Stage I–II Disease 615
6.2 Stage III Disease 616
6.3 Superior Sulcus Tumors (SST) 617
7 **Summary and Final Considerations** 618
References 619

F. A. Calvo (✉) · J. Aristu · J. Serrano · M. Cambeiro
Department of Oncology, Clínica Universidad de Navarra, Madrid, Spain
e-mail: fcalvom@unav.es

R. Martinez-Monge
Department of Oncology, Clínica Universidad de Navarra, Pamplona, Spain

R. Cañón
Department of Radiation Oncology, Hospital San Jaime, Torrevieja, Spain

Abstract

Intraoperative radiotherapy is a feasible technical modality to improve precision and dose escalation in high-local-risk lung cancer patients. Methodology is described regarding the use of high-energy electron beams or brachytherapy. Results of normal tissue tolerance in experimental animal models and in clinical experiences are analyzed in detail. Characteristics of clinical experiences using IORT electrons or brachytherapy are reported and clinical outcome results are discussed. Ten IORT brachytherapy and six electron-based publications are identified proving the adaptability of IORT to the clinical-therapeutic scenario of lung cancer, its feasibility, and the promotion of high local control rates in the context of dose escalation trials. The context of therapeutic potential of these high-precision irradiation techniques evolves with the advances in imaging, staging techniques, molecular biology, and improved systemic therapy (Calvo, Radiat Oncol 12:36–39, 2017).

1 Introduction

Lung cancer is the leading cause of cancer-related mortality worldwide, with nearly 1.4 million deaths each year (Jemal et al. 2010). Lung cancer is diagnosed at an advanced stage in a majority of patients, which is the primary reason behind the high mortality rate associated with this disease (Ramalingam et al. 2011). Adjuvant immunotherapy has significantly impacted progression-free survival after chemoradiation in stage III patients (Antonia et al. 2017).

The dose-response relationship in non-small cell lung cancer (NSCLC) has been questioned (Bradley et al. 2020). RTOG 0617 has reported the long-term results (with a median follow-up of 5 years). Locoregional failures were 49% (60 Gy) versus 55% (74 Gy). This data builds up in the controversy of the role of radiation dose in the therapeutic index in NSCLC. In previous studies of Rengan et al. (2004) the median survival time described for patients treated with 64 Gy or higher was 20 months versus 15 months for those treated with less than 64 Gy and a 10 Gy increase in dose resulted in a 36.4% decreased risk of local failure. A phase I–II RTOG 9311 study confirmed a safety of dose escalation to 83.8 Gy with three-dimensional conformal techniques (Bradley et al. 2005). In terms of relevant prognostic factors for overall survival (Dong-Soo et al. 2011) clinical tumor response after concurrent chemoradiation in locally advanced, recurrent, and postoperative gross residual NSCLC has been identified.

Pattern of failure data shows that 40–70% of the patients with non-small cell lung cancer stages II–IIIB are expected to relapse locally (Kumar et al. 1996). A dose-dependent pattern of failure in a NSCLC was suggested by Sura et al. (2008). Seventy-five percent of patients with NSCLC who received <60 Gy had failure within GTV and 25% had disease relapse at the GTV margin while among patients who received ≥60 Gy 33% and 61% had relapse within GTV and at the margin of GTV, respectively. This data has to be reconsidered at present: adjuvant immunotherapy after chemoradiation has reduced to 16% in the long-term locoregional recurrence rate (Antonia et al. 2017).

Local control in NSCLC continues to being an unresolved issue and the introduction of new radiation techniques to intensify the local dose is justified. Intraoperative radiation (IORT) is a sophisticated radiation modality well explored in the treatment of abdominopelvic tumors but is scarcely used in thoracic tumors. The therapeutic gain in IORT procedures is obtained with the displacement of radiosensitive organs away from the electron beam or with the shielding of fixed structures with lead sheets. Target definition is done after the surgical resection jointly with the thoracic surgery team.

IORT has been integrated into multidisciplinary programs as a boosting modality that completes the total dose given with fractionated external beam radiation therapy (ISIORT 1998). This treatment has the advantage of the radiobiological effects of fractionation over the primary volume that includes the primary tumor and the draining areas while the tumor bed is boosted with single-dose electrons. The growing interest for hypofractionated EBRT schemes is compatible with IORT strategies. Together dose-dense radiotherapy can be explored with the potential to modulate radio-immunogenicity (Rodriguez-Ruiz et al. 2019) without compromising normal tissue tolerance.

The current review describes methodology and clinical results of retrospective analyses including the prognostic factors related with local control and survival in large institutional experiences generated in NSCLC patients treated with IOERT or intraoperative brachytherapy components within multidisciplinary treatment programs.

2 Tissue Tolerance Studies of IORT

The tolerance of mediastinal structures to IORT with high-energy electron beams (IOERT) are based in animal studies. In a dose escalation study (Barnes et al. 1987) delivering 20, 30, and 40 Gy to two separated intrathoracic IOERT fields which included collapsed right upper lobe, esophagus, trachea, phrenic nerve, right atrium, and blood vessels. Pathologic changes were observed at 30 Gy in the trachea and esophagus, with severe ulceration and peribronchial and perivascular chronic inflammation in the normal lung. At a dose of 20 Gy medial and adventitial fibrosis, obliterative endarteritis of the vasa vasorum, and severe coagulative necrosis were observed. Acute pneumonitis was seen at all doses, and changes in the contralateral lung were detected using 12 MeV electrons.

De Boer et al. (1989) studied the effects of 20, 25, and 30 Gy in mediastinal structures. The bronchial stump healed in all dogs. Severe tissue damage was seen at all doses and included bronchovascular and esophagoaortic fistulas and esophageal stenosis.

At the National Cancer Institute, an experimental program evaluated the tolerance of surgically manipulated mediastinal structures to IOERT in 49 adult foxhounds. Tolerance of normal tissues was also evaluated in a limited phase I clinical trial (four patients with stage II or III NSCLC). Normal healing of the bronchial stump was found after pneumonectomy at IOERT doses of 20, 30, and 40 Gy, but there were late changes with tracheobronchial irradiation damage at all doses (5–10 months after treatment). Two out of four patients receiving 20 Gy developed esophageal ulceration at 6 months without late stricture. In dogs given 30 and 40 Gy, esophageal damage was severe (esophagoaortic fistula and stenosis) and one dog developed carinal necrosis. The same institution reported the results of five dogs reserved for long-term studies and one stage II NSCLC patient alive at 5 years. They concluded that IOERT in the mediastinum may be safe at dose levels that do not exceed 20 Gy (Tochner et al. 1992).

Additional experimental analysis of canine esophagus tolerance to IOERT has been reported by the NCI investigators (Sindelar et al. 1992). After right thoracotomy with mobilization of the intrathoracic esophagus, IOERT was delivered to include a 6 cm esophageal segment using a 9 MeV electron beam with escalating single doses of 0, 20, and 30 Gy. Dogs were followed clinically with endoscopic and radiologic studies and were electively sacrificed at 6 weeks or 3, 12, or 60 months after treatment. Transient mild dysphagia and mild esophagitis were observed in all dogs receiving 20 Gy, without major clinical or pathological sequelae, except in one dog that developed achalasia requiring a liquid diet. At a dose of 30 Gy, changes in the esophagus were pronounced with ulcerative esophagitis and chronic ulcerative esophagitis inducing gross stenosis after 9 months.

Zhou et al. (1992) analyzed the acute responses of the mediastinal and thoracic viscera in nine canines that were sacrificed after they received single IOERT doses of 25, 35, and 45 Gy. No pathological changes were found in the spinal cord and vertebra. Microscopic examination of trachea, esophagus, and lung showed mild or severe histological changes at 30 days at the level of 25 Gy versus 35–45 Gy, respectively. Severe and unrepaired histologic changes were found in the heart and aorta receiving 35–45 Gy.

Morpho-functional changes in the bronchial mucosa were studied in 33 patients with stage III NSCL treated with 15 Gy IORT with or without cisplatin (Kritskaia et al. 2006). No degenerative changes in the bronchial epithelium were

Table 1 Clinical and pathologic findings observed in animal experimental models (Barnes et al. 1987; De Boer et al. 1989; Tochner et al. 1992; Sindelar et al. 1992; Zhou et al. 1992; Kritskaia et al. 2006)

IORT doses (Gy)	Bronchial stump	Esophageal damage	Lung damage	Pathologic changes in heart and vessels
20	Normal healing	Transient mild dysphagia	Mild	Moderate
30	Normal healing	Chronic ulcerative esophagitis	Moderate	Moderate-severe
40	Normal healing	Esophageal perforation / Esophageal stricture	Severe	Severe

found 2 weeks after IORT. Basal cell proliferation was observed, goblet cells were reduced in size, and basement membrane was thickened and twisted. Epithelial reparation due to pronounced local basal cell proliferation was observed 3 months later. A year later, the mucosa was covered with the multinuclear cylindrical epithelium and the cover of ciliated cells was preserved. The functional activity of goblet cells was in the normal range and scanty lymphoplasmocytic infiltration was found in the stroma. In patients treated with IORT without radiosensitization, the damaged epithelium was regenerated due to the reserved cells coming from the damaged margins with the formation of an epidermoid regenerative layer and subsequent cell differentiation. Moderate sclerosis occurred in the stroma. A year later the bronchial epithelium was characterized by moderate goblet cell hyperplasia with preserved functional activity. The authors concluded that IORT caused mucosal damage as alteration, dystrophy, and desquamation of the epithelium. Subsequently, the bronchial epithelium recovered through reparative regeneration.

Based on these data, active clinical programs using thoracic IOERT agree that 20 Gy is the upper single-dose limit that can be safely tolerated by mediastinal and thoracic viscera (Table 1) with IOERT alone. There are no reported experimental normal tissue tolerance studies of IOERT used in combination with EBRT.

3 Technical Considerations: IOERT

IOERT requires the adaptation of linear accelerator with multi-energetic electron beam capability (energies recommended from 6 to 20 MeV), through the development of specially designed applicators for electron beam conformation (cone sizes recommended from 5 to 12 cm diameter). The clinical program combines the efforts of surgeons, anesthesiologists, physicists, and radiation oncologists to adequately select patients for IOERT indications; perform the surgical procedure (tumor resection plus normal tissue protection); monitor the patient during intraoperative irradiation; and finally decide the radiotherapeutic parameters for treatment prescription (Fig. 1). In general, IOERT during lung cancer surgery involves the coordination of 10–15 health professionals, prolongs the surgical time for approximately 30–45 min. Miniaturized and mobile linear accelerator operates at energies in the range of 4–12 MeV (Figs. 2 and 3) (Calvo et al. 2013).

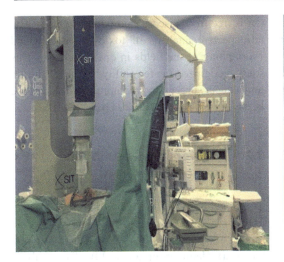

Fig. 1 General view of an IOERT procedure setup

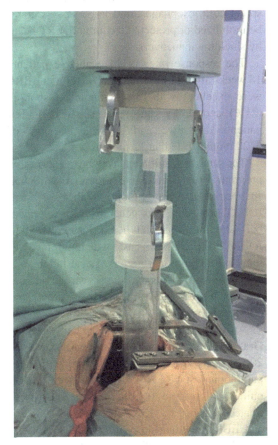

Fig. 2 IOERT procedure with a miniaturized linear accelerator (Liac HD) in a lung cancer patient. Vascularized flap is prepared and ready to cover the bronchial stump

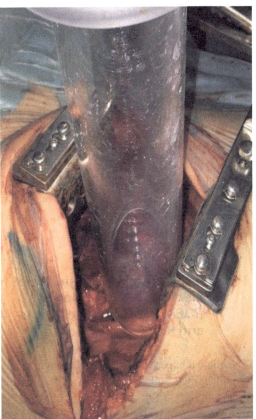

Fig. 3 Normal lung and vascularized flap are displaced and not included in the target IOERT region

4 Clinical Indications: IOERT

IOERT at the time of thoracotomy for a surgical approach to lung cancer has been employed in three different situations:

- Treatment of unresectable hilar and/or mediastinal disease
- Treatment of postresected residual disease (chest wall, mediastinum, and/or bronchial stump)
- Adjuvant treatment of mediastinum

Conceptual indications for IOERT in thoracic surgery have been the treatment of residual disease at the primary site and/or nodal regions, or adjuvant treatment of high risk of recurrence without proven cancer residue after induction therapy and surgery. IOERT is a super-selective radiation boost component available for integration in conventional radiotherapy programs for lung cancer. Lung parenchyma is the normal tissue that may benefit the most from IOERT.

Esophagus, trachea, aorta, and heart are difficult to displace from the IOERT beam, particularly in the treatment of mediastinal regions or left lower chest cavity. In the case that the bronchial stump is included in the IOERT field, tissue coverage with a vascularized pleural or pericardial flap is recommended to promote bronchial healing.

5 International Intraoperative Electron Radiotherapy (IOERT) Clinical Experiences and Results

The clinical experience of IOERT in lung cancer is still limited and the available data regarding treatment of NSCLC were obtained in phase I–II trials in a small series of patients. Abe and colleagues in the initial Japanese experience did not use IOERT in lung neoplasms because of the early systemic dissemination of disease (Abe and Takahashi 1981).

5.1 National Cancer Institute Experience

Based on a previous canine experimental model involving the use of pneumonectomy and IOERT doses of 0, 20, 30, and 40 Gy, a limited phase I National Cancer Institute (NCI) clinical trial demonstrated considerable toxicity with 25 Gy of IOERT to two separated fields encompassing the superior and inferior mediastinum following pneumonectomy (Pass et al. 1987). Early complications were described in three out of four patients: one case of bronchial stump dehiscence, one bronchopleural fistula, and one case of reversible esophagitis. Three patients with late complications showed one case of irreversible radiation esophagitis. Only one long-term survivor is free from disease (more than 3 years). The retrospective analysis of toxic events detected overlapping of the fields in one toxic case. This study recognized the feasibility of IOERT during lung cancer surgery and recommended a decrease in the IOERT dose to 15–20 Gy.

5.2 University Medical School of Graz Experience

Combined IOERT (10–20 Gy) and postoperative EBRT (46–56 Gy) were used in 21 inoperable tumors at the University Medical School of Graz (Austria) (Jeuttner et al. 1990). The analysis included 12 patients with N0 disease. The radiosensitive mediastinal structures such as the heart, spinal cord, esophagus, and large vessels could be mobilized or protected from the IOERT beam by shielding maneuvers.

The response rates in 14 evaluable patients 18 weeks after they completed IOERT and EBRT were excellent with three complete responses (21%) and ten partial responses (71%). Ten patients are alive and well at a range of 5–20 months (median 12 months).

The same institution updated the results of this program in two consecutive studies (Arian-Schad Juellner et al. 1990; Smolle et al. 1994). The IOERT procedure was generally well tolerated, but fatal intrabronchial hemorrhage related to IOERT occurred in two cases with tumor involvement of the pulmonary artery. Local failure was seen in three patients and the 5-year overall and recurrence-free survival rates were 15% and 53%, respectively.

An expanded series from the University of Graz has been recently published (Jakse et al. 2007). Fifty-two patients with predominantly pathological stage I NSCLC (76%) with limited pulmonary reserve (median FEV1: 1.3) were treated with surgery, IORT (median dose 20 Gy), and EBRT (median dose 46 Gy). The actuarial overall survival and disease-specific survival at 3 years were 37% and 48%, respectively. Females had a significantly better disease-specific survival than males. Causes of death were unrelated to tumor in 17% and tumor related in 54% of patients. Two patients died from second cancers and 25% are alive without evidence of tumor progression. Overall locoregional tumor control was 73% at 12 months and 68% at 24 and 36 months, respectively. IORT and EBRT were well tolerated without serious treatment-related acute or late side effects.

5.3 Montpellier Regional Cancer Centre Experience

The Centre Regional De Lutte Contre Le Cancer in Montpellier (France) reported results in 17 patients: three stage I, seven stage II, and seven stage IIIA (Carter et al. 2003). The treatment protocol involved the use of IOERT with doses in the range of 10–20 Gy and 45 Gy EBRT in 20–25 fractions with or without a 3-week rest period following a complete surgical excision. Microscopic residual disease in the mediastinal nodes or pleura-chest wall was seen in 12 and 5 patients, respectively. The median follow-up time for the entire group of patients alive was 59 months, with follow-up ranging from 40 to 120 months.

Disease control and survival results were as follows. Local control was obtained in 13 out of 17 patients (76%) and central recurrence in the IOERT field has been demonstrated in four patients. Three patients are alive without disease at 5.5, 8, and 11 years. Fourteen patients are dead: 7 from distant metastases, 4 from locoregional recurrence, 1 patient developed a second cancer, and 2 patients had a local recurrence in the EBRT field. The median survival time for the entire group was 36 months and the actuarial survival rate is 18% projected at 11 years.

5.4 The Allegheny University Hospital of Philadelphia Experience

This unique experience in the USA was preliminarily reported in 1994 (Fisher et al. 1994). The last update (Aristu et al. 1999) includes 21 patients treated from 6/92 to 9/97 as part of a pilot feasibility experience for stage I ($n = 1$), II ($n = 2$), and III ($n = 18$) NSCLC patients managed by surgical resection, IOERT (10 Gy), and EBRT (45.0–59.4 Gy, 16 preoperatively and 5 postoperatively). Chemotherapy was administered to all patients. The median survival time for the alive patients is 33 months. Patterns of relapse have shown 3 (14%) thoracic and 12 (55%) systemic. Actuarial 5-year survival rate was 33%.

5.5 Madrid Institute of Oncology (Grupo IMO) Experience

In the Instituto Madrileño de Oncología (Grupo IMO) in Madrid from February 1992 to July 1997, 18 patients with stage III non-small cell lung cancer (11 Pancoast's tumors) received IOERT as part of a multidisciplinary program including surgical resection in all cases, chemotherapy in 13, preoperative EBRT in 7, and postoperative EBRT in 7. Tumor residue at the time of surgery was macroscopic (gross) in eight cases. The median survival time for the entire series is 14 months. Intrathoracic recurrence has been identified in two patients. Five-year actuarial survival is projected as 22% (cause-specific 33%). Long-term toxicity observed included neuropathy (two cases) and esophageal structure (one case) (Calvo et al. 1999).

5.6 USP Hospital San Jaime Experience

Between June 2004 and October 2008 in the USP Hospital San Jaime in Torrevieja, Spain, eight patients were treated with IORT using the Mobetron mobile linear accelerator: two women and six men, with a median age of 53 years (range 45–66 years). All patients had locally advanced non-small cell lung cancer (NSCLCs), stage IIA ($n = 1$), stage IIIA ($n = 1$), stage IIIB ($n = 4$), and stage IV ($n = 1$, a woman with T2N2 and brain metastases), and one patient with local relapse after surgery and radiotherapy.

All patients received preoperative radiochemotherapy: 50 Gy with conventional fractionation, except two patients: one patient with local relapse after radiochemotherapy and then treated with hypofractionation (10 Gy for four sessions, 2 days a week) and one patient stage IV, who received 66 Gy with a radical intention and systemic chemotherapy. There were three ypT0, five ypTmicroscopic, five ypN0, one ypNmicro, and two ypN1 pathologic responses in the surgical specimens.

The median dose of IOERT administered was 10 Gy (range 6–10 Gy), using a cone of 4.5 cm of diameter (range 3.5–6 cm) and 9 MeV (range 4–9 MeV) electron beam and with a median time for the procedure of 35 min, with a range of 15–60 min.

At a median follow-up of 36.5 months (range 2–66 months), one patient is lost for follow-up; two died free of disease; one died with local and brain relapse; three are alive free of disease 36, 37, and 53 months after the IOERT; and one is alive with pleural and mediastinal relapse 2 years after the IOERT and 1 year after suprarenalectomy for metastasis. Two patients died 1.5 months after the IOERT where the first patient who had received 66 Gy of radiotherapy died for lung complication, and the second patient with local relapse after radiochemotherapy and treated with hypofractionation died from massive bleeding.

The median overall survival is 22 months and the disease-free survival is 12 months. Patterns of failure are as follows: one patient with local relapse was rescued with reirradiation. After 6 months he progressed with brain metastases and died with disease. The second patient had adrenal gland metastases 11 months after surgery which were rescued with suprarenalectomy and 13 months after he developed pleural and mediastinal relapse.

5.7 The University Clinic of Navarra Experience

During the period from November 1984 to November 1993 104 patients with histologically confirmed non-small cell lung cancer stage III were treated with IOERT as a treatment component of multidisciplinary management at the University Clinic of Navarra in Pamplona (Spain) (Calvo et al. 1990, 1991, 1992; Aristu et al. 1997, 1999; Martínez-Monge et al. 1994). Twenty-two patients were treated with surgery, IOERT, and postoperative EBRT; 82 patients received neoadjuvant chemotherapy and were treated depending on tumor response as follows: 46 responders with respectable tumor were managed with surgery, IOERT, and postoperative EBRT and nonresponders with unresectable disease (17 patients) or Pancoast's tumor (19 patients) received preoperative chemoradiotherapy, surgery, and IOERT boost.

The neoadjuvant chemotherapy consisted of cisplatin 120 mg/m^2 i.v. on day 1, mitomycin C 8 mg/m^2 i.v. on day 1, and vindesine 3 mg/m^2 (maximum dose 5 mg/m^2) i.v. on days 1 and 14 (MVP) or the same treatment regimen where the cisplatin administration was replaced by intraarterial carboplatin 150 mg/m^2. The cycles of chemotherapy were repeated every 28 days for 3–5 treatments until maximum response was achieved (3–5 cycles). Patients who documented a clinical response or stable disease and who were considered resectable were referred to surgical resection including the primary tumor and mediastinal lymphadenectomy 4–5 weeks after the last cycle of neoadjuvant chemotherapy. The bronchial stump was protected with a pleural or pericardial flap in order to prevent anastomotic leak. After surgical resection IOERT was applied over the surgical bed, hilar, and mediastinal regions depending on the tumor location. Total dose administered varied between 10 and 15 Gy depending on the amount of residual tumor. A detailed description of the IOERT methodology for thoracic tumors has been published previously (Calvo et al. 1990, 1992; Aristu et al. 1997; Martínez-Monge et al. 1994). Postoperative external beam radiation therapy was started 4–5 weeks after surgical resection. Treatment was delivered with a linear accelerator employing AP–PA technique to encompass the treatment volume which included bronchial stump, ipsilateral hilum, bilateral mediastinal, and supraclavicular lymph nodes. A dose of 46 Gy in 23 fractions was applied.

Tumors that were not considered resectable after neoadjuvant chemotherapy were treated with preoperative external beam radiation therapy using the same total dose and fractionation than with postoperative external beam radiation therapy described above. All patients received concurrent chemotherapy with preoperative radiation using the same chemotherapy combination used as neoadjuvant or with cisplatin 20 mg/m^2 or carboplatinum 55 mg/m^2 combined with five fluorouracil 1000 mg/m^2 (maximum daily dose 1500 mg) during 3–5 days over the first and last weeks of external beam radiation therapy. Four to six weeks after the completion of the preoperative chemoradiation course the patients were referred for surgical resection and IOERT, when feasible.

The local control rates observed in patients with microscopic residual disease (R0 or R1 resection) were 18/24 (75%), 4/14 (29%), and 11/12 (92%) for stage IIIA, IIIB, and Pancoast's tumors, respectively. Local control rates in patients with macroscopic residual disease (R2 resection) were 3/7 (43%), 7/30 (23%), and 5/5 (100%) for stage IIIA, IIIB, and Pancoast's tumors, respectively. Table 2 describes the patterns of failure according to the treatment group.

At the time of analysis 16 patients (15%) were alive and free of disease. Five-year OS for the entire group was 40% for stage IIIA and 18% for stage IIIB patients ($p = 0.01$). Five-year disease-free survival (DFS) regarding the amount of residual disease is as follows: 69% and 42% for microscopic (R1) or no residual disease (R0) for stages IIIA and IIIB, respectively, and 58% and 41% for macroscopic (gross) residual disease (R2) for stages IIIA and IIIB, respectively. Anecdotally, 19 patients survived for more than 5 years after IOERT with a follow-up range from 64 to 107 months. Among patients surviving for more than 5 years there were 3 s tumors (colon, esophagus, and head and neck) and one cancer-unrelated death.

Table 2 Patterns of failure according to disease stage and surgical residue in the University Clinic of Navarra Experience

Surgical residue	Local control[a]	Distant failure[b]
Micro/absent		
IIIA	18/24 (75%)	7/24 (29)
IIIB	4/14 (29%)	4/14 (29)
Pancoast's tumors	11/12 (92%)	2/12 (17)
Macroscopic/unresected		
IIIA	3/7 (43%)	6/7 (86)
IIIB	7/30 (23%)	12/30 (40)
Pancoast's tumors	5/5 (100%)	1/5 (20)

[a] No local or distant failure
[b] Distant failure alone or distant and local failure

Regarding treatment toxicity and complications, four patients died in the postoperative period due to possible IOERT-related toxicity: two bronchopleural fistulas and two pulmonary hemorrhages. The first bronchopleural fistula occurred in a lobectomized patient, in whom the bronchial stump was not included into the IOERT field. Another patient died 3 months after surgery due to a bronchopleural fistula in a microscopic tumor involved in bronchial stump. One patient developed fatal massive hemoptysis at 2 months following IOERT because of pulmonary artery rupture. This latter patient had prior hemoptysis and a left hilar unresected tumor treated by tumor exposure and 15 Gy (20 MeV) IOERT plus 46 Gy postoperative EBRT. The autopsy study showed a necrotic cavity in the primary tumor with no viable residual tumor cells and a fistulous tract communicating between the pulmonary artery and the bronchial tree. A nonresected patient treated with three cycles of MVP regimen, preoperative EBRT (44 Gy), and IORT of 15 Gy died early in the postoperative period from pulmonary hemorrhage.

Esophagitis grade 3–4 was noted in 26 (25%) patients and esophageal damage with ulcerated or necrotic tissue was observed in two patients. One out of two patients who developed esophageal ulcer died 8 months after surgery from fatal hemorrhage. This patient had a T4 tumor infiltrating the descending portion of the aorta and the esophagus. He was treated with three cycles of MVP chemotherapy regimen, preoperative EBRT (46 Gy), surgery (atypical resection plus chest wall resection), and 10 Gy IORT boost (12 MeV). No viable microscopic tumor was encountered in the resected specimen and the necropsy findings revealed a connection between the esophagus and the aorta without histological evidence of tumor cells.

Symptomatic radiation acute pneumonitis was observed in six patients. Seven patients were diagnosed with severe long-term fibrosis and required chronic cortico-therapy administration. Neurologic toxicity was noted only in patients treated with IOERT which included the thoracic apex or chest wall. Six patients developed transient neuropathy (four Pancoast's tumors) with pain and paresthesia in the superior ipsilateral extremity or chest wall. Severe infectious complications were seen in 11 patients. Six of these patients were diagnosed with simultaneous thoracic tumor progression coexisting with an abscess.

5.8 Tomsk Cancer Research, National Research Medical Center, Russia Experience

A recent contribution from the University of Tomsk colleagues (Pankova et al. 2020) has reported 171 patients with locally advanced (T 1–4, N 0–3, M0) NSCLC (104 squamous cell, 67 adenocarcinoma) treated in the period 2000–2015. Neoadjuvant chemotherapy (carboplatin + Taxol) was given to 90 patients (52%), observing 42% partial responses and in which 37 (41%) radical surgeries were performed. In 36 patients IOERT was delivered (using doses inferior to 15 Gy with a 6 MeV electron beam) over the high-risk postsurgical resection bed. Cisplatin was given pre-IOERT to 14 patients. Recurrent disease was developed at 5 years as follows: 0% of the (15) patients treated with neoadjuvant chemotherapy and IOERT; 39% of patients treated with a component of IOERT alone; and 83% not receiving none of the mentioned components (chemotherapy or IOERT). Outcomes in terms of overall survival were significantly superior for the cohort treated with neoadjuvant chemotherapy and IOERT (75% at 5 years).

A summary of NSCLC IOERT clinical experiences from different institutions is presented in Table 3.

Table 3 IOERT international clinical experiences in NSCLC

Authors (reference)	Number of patients	Stage	Treatment protocol	Local control	5-Year survival
University Medical School of Graz[a] (Smolle et al. 1994)	24	12 I 1 II 10 IIIA	IORT 10–20 Gy + EBRT 46–56 Gy	19/23 (83%)	15%
Montpellier Regional Cancer Centre (Carter et al. 2003)	17	3 I 7 II 7 IIIA	S + IORT (10–20 Gy) + EBRT 45 Gy	13/17 (76%)	18%
University Clinic of Navarra in Pamplona (Calvo et al. 1990, 1991, 1992; Aristu et al. 1997, 1999; Martínez-Monge et al. 1994)	104	19 IIIA (N0) 29 IIIA (N2) 56 IIIB	Multidisciplinary treatment (see text) with IORT 10–20 Gy + EBRT (46 Gy) ± CT	48/92 (52%)	40% (IIIA) 18% (IIIB)
The Allegheny University Hospital of Philadelphia (Aristu et al. 1999)	21	1 I 2 II 15 IIIA 3 IIIB	Neoadjuvant CT ± pre-op EBRT + S + IORT ± post-op EBRT	18/21 (86%)	33%
Madrid Institute of Oncology (Grupo IMO) (Calvo et al. 1999)	18	11 IIIA 6 IIIB 1 IV	Neoadjuvant CT ± pre-op EBRT + S + IORT ± post-op EBRT	16/18 (90%)	22%
USP Hospital San Jaime in Torrevieja (Cañon et al. 2008)	8	1 IIA 1 IIIA 4 IIIB 1 IV 1 local relapse	Preoperative EBRT 50 Gy + S + IORT 6–10 Gy	6/8 (75%)	Median OS 22 m, DFS 12 m
Tomsk Cancer Research (Pankova et al. 2020)	171	I 14 IIA 9 IIB 34 IIIA 84 IIIB 30	NAC (90) +/− IOERT (36) +/− AC (26) +/−	100% NAC + IORT 39% IORT 83% No NAC	75% 57% 39%

CT Chemotherapy, *NAC* neoadjuvant chemotherapy, *AC* adjuvant chemotherapy, *m* months
[a] Inoperable patients

6 International LDR-IORT and HDR-IORT Clinical Experiences and Results

Intraoperative brachytherapy using low-dose rate (LDR-IORT) or high-dose rate (HDR-IORT) is a radiation treatment alternative in lung cancer patients who are technically operable but cannot tolerate the operative procedure and the expected reduction in lung function after resection or conventional EBRT. LDR-IORT/HDR-IORT can also be used as a radiation boost technique in patients with residual disease after chemoradiation or in previously irradiated patients diagnosed with recurrent disease.

The LDR-IORT/HDR-IORT technique to be used depends on the tumor location and volume of residual disease after resection (R0, R1, and R2). Resectable but inoperable tumors, R2 resections, and recurrent tumors may be treated by a permanent implant using iodine-125 (I-125) or palladium-103 (Pd-103) seeds. Unresectable chest wall lesions and R1 resections may be treated intraoperatively by either a temporary iridium-192 (Ir-192) implant or a permanent I-125 implant imbedded in absorbable polyglactin (Vicryl) sutures and directly sutured onto the target area (d'Amato et al. 1998) or it may be treated by employing I-125 seeds imbedded into an absorbable gelatin sponge (Gelfoam) plaque (Nori et al. 1995). Perioperative high-dose-rate brachytherapy (PHDRB) using Ir-192 administered over the immediate postoperative period has been mainly used in R0–R1 tumor resections. Intraoperative implantation of plastic catheters into the tumor bed after surgical resection for PHDRB has several theoretical advantages over other types of radiation boosting techniques, including (1) accurate real-time definition of the clinical target volume (CTV) surrounding the tumor bed and other high-risk areas (with the assistance of the surgical team); (2) CT scan-based treatment planning; (3) risk-adapted brachytherapy dose selection based upon the amount of residual disease described in the final pathology report; and (4) early delivery of fractionated radiation during the immediate postoperative period.

6.1 Stage I–II Disease

The largest experience with IOBT has been published in patients with stage I–II lung cancer who are unfit for surgery and radical EBRT. The majority of the studies are retrospective and come from single institutions. The MSKCC experience has been reported by Hilaris and Mastoras (1998). The study included 55 patients treated with thoracotomy and interstitial I-125 implantation ± moderate doses of EBRT. There were no operative or postoperative deaths. Locoregional control at 5 years was 100% in T1N0 lesions, 70% of patients with T2N0 tumors, and 71% in T1–2N1 tumors. The 5-year OS was 32% and DFS was 63%. The median survival was better in patients with cancer in the right lung but no difference in survival could be demonstrated among patients with squamous versus adenocarcinoma, T1 versus T2 tumors, or those who did or did not receive postoperative EBRT.

Fleischman et al. (1992) have published the results of 14 medically inoperable stage I patients treated with I-125 implantation at thoracotomy. Doses ranged from 80 Gy at the periphery to 200 Gy at the center. There was one operative mortality and two postoperative complications. With a minimum follow-up of 1 year, the local control was 71% and the median survival was 15 months.

A retrospective multicenter study of 291 patients with T1N0 disease was done comparing the outcomes after sub-lobar resection (124 patients) and lobar resection (167 patients) (Fernando et al. 2005). Brachytherapy (100–120 Gy to a 0.5 cm depth) was used in 60 patients with sub-lobar resection. With a mean follow-up of 34.5 months, brachytherapy decreased the local recurrence rate significantly among patients undergoing sub-lobar resection from 17.2% to 3.3%. There was no difference in survival between sub-lobar resection and lobar resection in tumors smaller than 2 cm. However, for tumor ranging from 2 to 3 cm, median survival was significantly better in the lobar resection group.

The experience of the New England Medical Center in Boston is based on the implantation of radioactive I-125 seeds along the resection margin in 35 patients with stage I lung cancer treated with limited resection (not candidates for lobectomy) (Lee et al. 2003). Two patients developed local recurrence at the resection margin and six patients developed regional recurrences in the mediastinum or chest wall. The 5-year OS was 67% and 39% for patients with T1N0 and T2N0 tumors, respectively.

Investigators of the University of Pittsburgh Cancer Institute reported a trial exploring the feasibility and outcomes of 125-I Vicryl mesh brachytherapy after sub-lobar resection (open or video-assisted thoracoscopic procedure) in stage I non-small cell lung cancer patients with poor pulmonary function (Chen et al. 1999; Voynov et al. 2005). The implant was introduced through the surgical incision and sutured to the visceral pleura. A prescribed dose of 100–120 Gy was delivered to a volume within 0.5 cm from the plane of the implant. There were four local recurrences in the 110 patients treated and the estimated 5-year local control, locoregional control, and OS rates were 90%, 61%, and 18%, respectively.

A randomized adjuvant post-sub-lobar resection trial including or not a brachytherapy component has been designed by the American College of Surgeons Z4032 trial. Preliminary analysis has reported equivalent pulmonary function and dyspnea at 3-month follow-up in patients evaluated (Fernando et al. 2011).

6.2 Stage III Disease

In the University of Navarra investigators initiated a prospective, nonrandomized, controlled phase II clinical trial to determine whether perioperative high-dose-rate brachytherapy (PHDRB) using Ir-192 administered over the immediate postoperative period is feasible and tolerable and may improve locoregional control rates in lung cancer patients with residual disease after chemoradiation or recurrent disease after previous radiation therapy (Valero et al. 2007). In R0–R1 lung cancer resections the tumor bed was implanted with plastic catheters for PHDRB. The brachytherapy dose was 4 Gy b.i.d. × 4–10 fractions (16–40 Gy total dose). Selected technically unfeasible cases for PHDRB were treated using a silicone mold in which plastic catheters are inserted and a single dose of 10–12.5 Gy was administered. Macroscopic residual unresectable tumors (R2 resections) were implanted with I-125 or Pd-103 seeds to deliver a minimum tumor dose of 90–110 Gy. Between 2001 and 2006 period, 20 patients have been treated, 15 patients had residual disease, and 5 patients had recurrent disease. Two patients developed grade three complication with thoracic abscess. Nine patients are alive: seven without disease, one without disease after radiosurgery for brain metastases, and one patient alive with disease. The local, locoregional, and systemic control rates are 89%, 84%, and 70%, respectively. After a median follow-up of 20 months (6–78 months) the 6-year OS and DFS are 36% and 27%, respectively.

The MSKCC treated 322 patients considered unresectable at thoracotomy and treated with brachytherapy (Hilaris and Nori 1987). Patients without mediastinal node metastases achieved 71% local control versus 63% in patients with affected mediastinal nodes. The 2- and 3-year OS in N0 and N2 patients were 20/15% and 10/3%, respectively. A subgroup of 100 patients with positive mediastinal nodes were treated with surgical resection when feasible, brachytherapy (temporary Ir-192 implantation in patients with close or positive margins or I-125 implantation in patients with residual gross disease), and postoperative EBRT (median dose 40 Gy). There was no postoperative mortality and local control obtained in 76% of patients (77% for patients with no residual disease and 72% in patients who had incomplete or no resection) (Hilaris et al. 1983, 1985).

The same institution presented a later experience including 225 patients with thoracotomy and IOBT when need in primary non-small cell lung invading only the mediastinum (T3-4N0-2) (Burt et al. 1987). The authors encountered a positive correlation between prolongation of survival and extent of resection/IORT. Forty-nine patients had complete resection without IORT and fared no better than a cohort group of 33 patients who underwent pulmonary resection with simultaneous iodine-125 interstitial implantation or iridium-192 delayed afterloading to areas of unresectable primary or nodal disease. The median survival and 3- and 5-year survival rates were 17 months and 21% and 5%, respectively, with incomplete resection, and 12 months and 22% and 22% with incomplete resection and brachytherapy. One hundred and one patients underwent interstitial implantation without resection, with a median survival of 11 months, 3-year survival of 9%, and no 5-year survivors. The perioperative mortality was 2.7% and the nonfatal complication rate 13%.

Researchers in the New York Hospital Medical Center of Queens in New York investigated the safety, reproducibility, and effectiveness of intraoperative I-125 or Pd-103 Gelfoam plaque implant technique in 12 patients as a treatment complement for resected stage III patients with positive surgical margin. All patients received preoperative or postoperative EBRT (45–60 Gy) and four patients received chemotherapy. There were no early or late complications due to brachytherapy or EBRT. The local control and 2-year OS and cause-specific survival were 82%, 45%, and 56%, respectively (Nori et al. 1995).

6.3 Superior Sulcus Tumors (SST)

The Erasmus Medical Cancer Center Experience in SST has been recently reported (van Geel et al. 2003). Twenty-six patients with cytologically or histologically proven NSCLC (T3N0-1 or T4N0) arising in the pulmonary apex were treated with preoperative EBRT (46 Gy in 23 fractions, 2 Gy per fraction, 5 fractions per week), surgery, and HDR-IORT using a flexible intraoperative template (FIT). FIT is a 5 mm thick silicone mold in which afterloader catheters are inserted parallel to each other at a fixed distance of 1 cm and is used to deliver a homogeneous dose to a surface to which the shape of the mold is adjusted. A single radiation fraction of 10 Gy was administered specified in a plane parallel to the surface of the FIT at 1 cm distance with HDR Ir-192. EBRT (12×2 Gy) was indicated for unresectable tumors during thoracotomy. Three patients progressed during the preoperative treatment and were excluded. In two patients HDR-IORT was not considered because the tumors had no chest wall invasion. Finally, 21 patients underwent the entire programmed treatment protocol. One patient (4%) died in the postoperative period due to a cardiac failure. Another patient died 7 weeks after surgery with a bronchopleural fistula and sepsis. Two patients had a prolonged hospital stay of more than 3 weeks because of ARDS and pleural empyema recovering after intensive conservative treatment. With a median follow-up of 18 months, 8 patients were alive (37%), of which 7 had no evidence of disease and 18 patients (85%) were free from locoregional relapse. The median survival for patients without and with distant failure was 14 months and 6 months, respectively.

Hilaris et al. (1974, 1987) presented the results of 129 patients with SST treated with thoracotomy (in bloc excision of the involved lung and chest wall when feasible) interstitial IORT using either permanent implantation of I-125 seeds or temporary implantation of Ir-192, and postoperative EBRT in patients who had received no preoperative EBRT or when the implant presented unacceptable dose distribution requirements. The authors describe a 0.8% of postoperative death and 17 patients (13%) presented nonfatal complications including wound infection, empyema with or without bronchopleural fistula, bleeding, atelectasis or pneumonia, and phlebitis. The 5-year OS was 25% and patients with negative mediastinal nodes fared better than patients with positive mediastinal nodes showing a 5-year OS of 29% and 10%, respectively.

A summary of NSCLC LDR-IORT and HDR-IORT clinical experiences from different centers is presented in Tables 4 and 5.

Table 4 LDR-HDR-IORT international clinical experiences in stage I–II NSCLC

Authors (reference)	Number of patients	Stage	Treatment protocol	Local control	Time point
Hilaris and Mastoras (1998)	55	T1-2N0-1	S + I-125 (160 Gy) ± EBRT	100% (T1N0) 70% (T2N0) 71% (T1-2N1)	32% 5-year OS
Fleischman et al. (1992)	14	T1N0	S + I-125 (80–200 Gy)	10/14 (71%)	MS 15.1 m
Fernando et al. (2005)	291	T1N0	Lobar resection (LR) versus sub-lobar resection (SR) ± I-125 (100–120 Gy)	96.5% (LR)[a] 95.6% (SR)[a]	MS 68.7 m (LR)[a] 50.6 m (SR)[a]
Lee et al. (2003)	33	T1-2N0	Limited resection + I-125	31/33 (94%)	5-year OS 67% (T1N0) 39% (T2N0)
Voynov et al. (2005)	110	T1-2N0	Limited resection + I-125 (100–120 Gy) S + I-125 (117 Gy)	106/110 (96%) 5-year LC 90%	5-year OS 22% (T1N0)
Colonias et al. (2011)	145	I		96% LC	12% (T2N0) 35% OS 5 years

S surgery, *EBRT* external beam radiation therapy, *MS* median survival, *OS* overall survival, *m* months
[a] Local recurrence and survival rates for the 2–3 cm tumors

Table 5 LDR-HDR-IORT international clinical experiences in stage III NSCLC

Authors (reference)	Number of patients	Stage	Treatment protocol	Local control	Time point
Valero et al. (2007)	20	III	S + PHDRB (16–40 Gy) or IOBT (10.12.5 Gy) or I-125/Pd-103 seeds (90–110 Gy)	89%	36% 6-year OS
Burt et al. (1987)	225	III	S ± I-125[a]/Ir-192	10/14 (71%)	MS 12 m[b] 22% 5-year OS[b]
Hilaris and Nori (1987)	322	Unresectable	Thoracotomy + I-125 (160 Gy)	71% (N0) 63% (N2)	15% 3-year OS (N0) 3% 3-year OS (N +)
Hilaris et al. (1985)	100	IIIN2	I-125 (160 Gy)/Ir-192 (30 Gy) ± S + EBRT (30–40 Gy)	89% (R0) 53% (R1) 72% (R2)	22% 5-year OS 22% 5-year OS (R2)
Nori et al. (1995)	12	III (PSM)	± EBRT (45–60 Gy) + S + I-125/Pd-103 Gelfoam implant ± EBRT (45–60 Gy)	82%	45% 2-year OS

S surgery, *EBRT* external beam radiation therapy, *MS* median survival, *OS* overall survival, *PHDRB* perioperative high-dose-rate brachytherapy, *IOBT* intraoperative brachytherapy using a silicone mold in which plastic catheters are inserted, *PSM* gross and microscopic positive surgical margins, *m* months
[a] 125-I in patients with incomplete resections
[b] Patients with incomplete resection and brachytherapy

7 Summary and Final Considerations

The modern developments in the treatment of localized NSCLC confirm the oncology tendency to bio-intensify systemic and local treatment to promote cancer control. In the past century a large number of patients with stage III NSCLC died of systemic disease and local failure remained a substantial problem. CALGB reported patterns of disease failure in stage IIIA patients treated with induction chemotherapy, surgery, and thoracic irradiation (Kumar et al. 1996). The study found that 52 out of 74 patients had failures and the thorax was the first site of isolated or combined local failure in 36 patients (69%).

Unfortunately, less than 20% of stage III patients have disease that is resectable for cure at diagnosis and the optimal management of patients with unresectable disease remains controversial. In spite of improvement in resectability rates with neoadjuvant approaches, stage III NSCLC patients have a relevant incidence of local recurrence. Based on these observations, higher tumor doses may result in improved local control, and several trials have emerged in an attempt to promote thoracic control by escalating total radiation doses exploring altered fractionation or precision delivery radiotherapy including volumetric modulated photon therapy, proton therapy, and three-dimensional molecular guided radiation planning (Rengan et al. 2004; Bradley et al. 2005; Sura et al. 2008; Mesko and Gomez 2018).

IORT/IOBT has been integrated into the multidisciplinary management of NSCLC in several small prospective single-institution pilot trials as a sophisticated electron, LDR, or HDR boost of radiation, confirming the feasibility of IORT procedure during surgical exploration of NSCLC patients. IORT doses between 10 and 15 Gy combined with EBRT (46–50 Gy) induce acute and late toxic events at a clinically acceptable level. Tables 3, 4, and 5 show summarized international IORT clinical trials regarding local control and survival data in NSCLC.

Definitive conclusions based on the available experiences discussed in this chapter cannot be established. In stage I or II NSCLC, IOERT and IOBT have been used for medically inoperable patients with excellent rates of local control (70–100%). Alternatively, stereotactic body radiotherapy (SBRT) has emerged as a well-tolerated technique in this subgroup of patients with high rates of local control (Fakiris et al. 2009; Lo et al. 2008). IOBT may be reserved to complex central T1-2 tumors or unsuspected surgical findings.

Thoracic control seems to be related to tumor stage and location, surgical residue, and neoadjuvant treatment in locally advanced NSCLC. In the twenty-first century thoracic control has also been impacted by the use of immunotherapy (particularly in the adjuvant setting) with locoregional recurrence rates below 20% (Antonia et al. 2017). Local control rates in Pancoast's and stage IIIA tumors with microscopic residual disease are in continuous improvement by optimized multimodal approaches.

The effect of IORT on the group of patients presenting with stage IIIB appears to be favorable. This point is illustrated by the fact that patients with macroscopic residual disease or unresected disease achieved modest rates of local control (23%), but a few long-term survivors are identified. The high rates of metastatic disease in locally advanced NSCLC may conceal the definitive long-term local control but the introduction of novel systemic agents generating more long-term survivors will clarify this question.

Further confirmatory trials will be necessary to define the implication of IORT/IOBT in thoracic control and survival of patients with NSCLC. IORT/IOBT as a component of treatment can be integrated in phase III trials with treatment strategies that may include surgical thoracic exploration. Multimodal therapy and interdisciplinary knowledge are key in the progress of lung cancer treatment (Takeda et al. 2019). Efforts to generate evidence on intraoperative irradiation potential adapted to precision medicine and personalized oncology will require international cooperation among expert IORT institutions.

References

Abe M, Takahashi M (1981) Intraoperative radiotherapy: the Japanese experience. Int J Radiat Oncol Biol Phys 7(7):863–868

Antonia SJ, Villegas A, Daniel DN et al (2017) Durvalumab after chemoradiotherapy in stage III non-small-cell lung cancer. N Engl J Med 377:1919–1929

Arian-Schad Juellner FM, Ratzenhofer B et al (1990) Intraoperative plus external beam irradiation in non-resectable lung cancer: assessment of local response and therapy-relate side effects. Radiother Oncol 119:137–144

Aristu J, Rebollo J, Martínez-Monge R, Aramendía JM et al (1997) Cisplatin, mitomycin, and vindesine followed by intraoperative and postoperative radiotherapy for stage III non-small-cell lung cancer: final results of a phase II study. Am J Clin Oncol 20:276–281

Aristu JJ, Calvo FA, Martínez R, Dubois JB, Santos M, Fisher S, Azinovic I (1999) Lung cancer: EBRT with or without IORT. In: Gunderson LL, Willet CG, Harrison LB, Calvo FA (eds) Intraoperative irradiation. Techniques and results. Humana, Totowa, pp 437–453

Barnes M, Pass H, De Luca A et al (1987) Response of mediastinal and thoracic viscera of the dog to intraoperative radiation therapy (IOERT). Int J Radiat Oncol Biol Phys 13:371–378

Bradley J, Graham MV, Winter K, Purdy JA, Komaki R, Roa WH et al (2005) Toxicity and outcome results of ROG 9311: a phase I–II dose-escalation study using three-dimensional conformal radiotherapy in patients with inoperable non-small-cell lung carcinoma. Int J Radiat Oncol Biol Phys 61:318–328

Bradley JD, Hu C, Komaki RR, Masters GA et al (2020) Long-term results of NRG Oncology RTOG 0617: Standard- versus high-dose chemoradiotherapy with or without cetuximab for unresectable stage III non-small-cell lung cancer. J Clin Oncol 38:706–714

Burt ME, Pomerantz AH, Bains MS et al (1987) Results of surgical treatment of stage III lung cancer invading the mediastinum. Surg Clin North Am 67:987–1000

Calvo FA, Ortiz de Urbina D, Abuchaibe O et al (1990) Intraoperative radiotherapy during lung cancer surgery: technical description and early clinical results. Int J Radiat Oncol Biol Phys 19:103–109

Calvo FA, Santos M, Ortiz de Urbina D (1991) Intraoperative radiotherapy in thoracic tumors. Front Radiat Ther Oncol 25:307–316

Calvo FA, Ortiz de Urbina D, Herreros J, and Llorens R (1992) Lung cancer, In: Calvo FA, Santos M, Brady LW (eds) Intraoperative radiotherapy. Clinical experiences and results. Springer Berlin pp. 43–50

Calvo FA, Aristu JJ, Moreno M et al (1999) Intraoperative radiotherapy for lung cancer. In: Van Houte P (ed) Progress and perspectives in the treatment of lung cancer. Springer, Berlin, pp 173–182

Calvo FA, Sallabanda M, Sole CV et al (2013) Intraoperative radiation therapy opportunities for clinical practice normalization: data recording and innovative development. Rep Pract Oncol Radiother 19:246–252

Cañon R, Azinovic I, Ramis B et al (2008) Intraoperative radiation therapy using mobile linear accelerator in the multimodality approach to lung cancer. Rev Cancer (Madrid) 22:27

Carter YM, Jablons DM, DuBois JB et al (2003) Intraoperative radiation therapy in the multimodality approach to upper aerodigestive tract cancer. Surg Oncol Clin N Am 12:1043–1063

Chen A, Galloway M, Landreneau R et al (1999) Intraoperative 125I brachytherapy for high-risk stage I non-small-cell lung carcinoma. Int J Radiat Oncol Biol Phys 44:1057–1063

Colonias A, Betler J, Trombetta M et al (2011) Mature follow-up for high-risk stage I non-small-cell lung carcinoma treated with sublobar resection and intraoperative iodine-125 brachytherapy. Int J Radiat Oncol Biol Phys 79:105–109

d'Amato TA, Galloway M, Szydlowski G et al (1998) Intraoperative brachytherapy following thoracoscopic wedge resection of stage I lung cancer. Chest 114:1112–1115

De Boer WJ, Mehta DM, Oosterhius JW et al (1989) Tolerance of mediastinal structures to intraoperative radiotherapy after pneumonectomy in dogs. Strahlenther Oncol 165:768

Dong-Soo L, Yeon-Sil K, Jin-Hyoung K, Sang-Nam L, Young-Kyoun K, Myung-Im A et al (2011) Clinical responses and prognostic indicators of concurrent chemoradiation for non-small-cell lung cancer. Cancer Res Treat 43(1):32–41

Fakiris AJ, McGarry RC, Yiannoutsos CT et al (2009) Stereotactic body radiation therapy for early-stage non-small-cell lung carcinoma: four-year results of a prospective phase II study. Int J Radiat Oncol Biol Phys 75(3):677–682

Fernando HC, Santos RS, Benfield JR et al (2005) Lobar and sublobar resection with and without brachytherapy for small stage IA non-small-cell lung cancer. J Thorac Cardiovasc Surg 129:261–267

Fernando HC, Landreneau RJ, Mandrekar SJ et al (2011) The impact of adjuvant brachytherapy with sublobar resection on pulmonary function and dyspnea in high-risk patients with operable disease: preliminary results from the American College of Surgeons Oncology Group Z4032 trial. J Thorac Cardiovasc Surg 142:554–562

Fisher S, Fallahnejad M, Lisker S et al (1994) Role of intraoperative radiation therapy (IORT) for stage III non-small-cell lung cancer. Hepatogastroenterology 41:15

Fleischman EH, Kagan AR, Streeter OE et al (1992) Iodine125 interstitial brachytherapy in the treatment of carcinoma of the lung. J Surg Oncol 49:25–28

Hilaris BS, Mastoras DA (1998) Contemporary brachytherapy approaches in non-small-cell lung cancer. J Surg Oncol 69:258–264

Hilaris BS, Nori D (1987) The role of external radiation and brachytherapy in unresectable non-small-cell lung cancer. Surg Clin North Am 67:1061–1071

Hilaris BS, Martini N, Luomanen RK et al (1974) The value of preoperative radiation therapy in apical cancer of the lung. Surg Clin North Am 54:831–840

Hilaris BS, Nori D, Beattie EJ Jr et al (1983) Value of perioperative brachytherapy in the management of non-oat cell carcinoma of the lung. Int J Radiat Oncol Biol Phys 9:1161–1166

Hilaris BS, Gomez J, Nori D et al (1985) Combined surgery, intraoperative brachytherapy, and postoperative external radiation in stage III non-small-cell lung cancer. Cancer 55:1226–1231

Hilaris BS, Martini N, Wong GY et al (1987) Treatment of superior sulcus tumor (Pancoast tumor). Surg Clin North Am 67:965–977

ISIORT'98 (1998) Proceedings of the 1st congress of the International Society of Intraoperative Radiation Therapy, 6–9 Sep, Pamplona, España, Rev Med Univ Navarra vol XLII: n extraordinario, pp 13–68

Jakse G, Kapp KS, Geyer E et al (2007) IORT and external beam irradiation (EBI) in clinical stage I-II NSCLC patients with severely compromised pulmonary function: an 52-patient single-institutional experience. Strahlenther Onkol 183(2):24–25

Jemal A, Center MM, DeSantis C, Ward EM (2010) Global patterns of cancer incidence and mortality rates and trends. Cancer Epidemiol Biomarkers Prev 19:1893–1907

Jeuttner FM, Arian-Schad K, Porsch G et al (1990) Intraoperative radiation therapy combined with external irradiation in non resectable non-small-cell lung cancer: preliminary report. Int J Radiat Oncol Biol Phys 18:1143–1150

Kritskaia NG, Dobrodeev AI, Zav'ialov AA et al (2006) Morphofunctional changes in the bronchial epithelium in combined therapy for lung cancer. Arkh Patol 68:10–14

Kumar P, Herndon J, Langer M, Kohman LJ, Elias AD, Kass FC et al (1996) Patterns of disease failure after trimodality therapy of non-small-cell lung carcinoma pathologic stage IIIA (N2). Analysis of cancer and leukemia group b protocol 8935. Cancer 77(11):2393–2399

Lee W, Daly BD, DiPetrillo TA et al (2003) Limited resection for non-small-cell lung cancer: observed local control with implantation of I-125 brachytherapy seeds. Ann Thorac Surg 75:237–242

Lo SS, Fakiris AJ, Papiez L et al (2008) Stereotactic body radiation therapy for early-stage non-small-cell lung cancer. Expert Rev Anticancer Ther 8:87–98

Martínez-Monge R, Herreros J, Aristu JJ, Aramendía JM, Azinovic I (1994) Combined treatment in superior sulcus tumor. Am J Clin Oncol 17:317–322

Mesko S, Gomez D (2018) Proton therapy in non-small cell lung cancer. Curr Treat Options Oncol 19:76–84

Nori D, Li X, Pugkhem T (1995) Intraoperative brachytherapy using Gelfoam radioactive plaque implants for resected stage III non-small-cell lung cancer with positive margin: a pilot study. J Surg Oncol 60:257–261

Pankova OV, Rodionov EO, Miller SV (2020) Neoadjuvant chemotherapy combined with intraoperative radiotherapy is effective to prevent recurrence in high-risk non-small cell lung cancer (NSCLC) patients. Transl Lung Cancer Res 9:988–999

Pass HI, Sindelar WF, Kinsella TJ et al (1987) Delivery of intraoperative radiation therapy after pneumonectomy: experimental observations and early clinical results. Ann Thorac Surg 44:14–20

Ramalingam SS, Owonikoko TK, Khuri FR (2011) Lung cancer: new biological insights and recent therapeutic advances. CA Cancer J Clin 61:91–112

Rengan R, Rosenzweig KE, Venkatraman E, Koutcher LA, Fox JL, Nayak R et al (2004) Improved local control with higher doses of radiation in large-volume stage III non-small-cell lung cancer. Int J Radiat Oncol Biol Phys 60:741–747

Rodriguez-Ruiz ME, Rodriguez I, Leaman O et al (2019) Immune mechanisms mediating abscopal effects in radioimmunotherapy. Pharmacol Ther 196:195–203

Sindelar WF, Hoekstra HJ, Kinsella TJ et al (1992) Response of the canine esophagus to intraoperative electron beam radiotherapy. Int J Radiat Oncol Biol Phys 25:663–669

Smolle J, Geyer E, Kapp KS et al (1994) Evaluating intraoperative radiation therapy (IORT) and external beam radiation therapy (EBRT) in non-small-cell lung cancer (NSCLC). Eur J Cardiothorac Surg 8:511–516

Sura S, Greco C, Gelblum D, Yorke ED, Jackson A, Rosenzweig KE (2008) 18F-fluorodeoxyglucose positron emission tomography-based assessment of local failure patterns in non-small-cell lung cancer treated with definitive radiotherapy. Int J Radiat Oncol Biol Phys 70:1397–1402

Takeda T, Takeda S, Uryu K et al (2019) Multidisciplinary Lung Cancer Tumor Board connecting eight general hospitals in Japan via a high-security communication line. JCO Clin Cancer Inform 3:1–7

Tochner ZA, Pass HI, Sindelar WF et al (1992) Long term tolerance of thoracic organs to intraoperative radiotherapy. Int J Radiat Oncol Biol Phys 22(1):65–69

Valero J, Martinez-Monge R, Pagola M et al (2007) Rescate quirúrgico con técnicas de braquiterapia intraoperatoria en cáncer de pulmón con enfermedad residual tras tratamiento quimiorradioterápico o con enfermedad recurrente tras radioterapia previa. Clin Transl Oncol 9(Ext 3):5 (a618)

van Geel AN, Jansen PP, van Klaveren RJ et al (2003) High relapse-free survival after preoperative and intraoperative radiotherapy and resection for sulcus superior tumors. Chest 124:1841–1846

Voynov G, Heron DE, Lin CJ et al (2005) Intraoperative (125)I Vicryl mesh brachytherapy after sublobar resection for high-risk stage I non-small-cell lung cancer. Brachytherapy 4:278–285

Zhou GX, Zeng DW, Li WH (1992) Acute responses of the mediastinal and thoracic viscera of canine to intraoperative irradiation. In: Schildberg FW, Wilich N, Krämling HJ (eds) Intraoperative radiation therapy, proceedings 4th international symposium, Munich, pp 50–52

Further Reading

Calvo FA (2017) Intraoperative irradiation: precision medicine for quality cancer control promotion. Radiat Oncol 12:36–39

Brachytherapy for Lung Cancer

Raul Hernanz de Lucas, Teresa Muñoz Miguelañez,
Alfredo Polo, Paola Lucia Arrieta Narvaez,
and Deisy Barrios Barreto

Contents

1 Introduction... 623
2 **Procedure for Lung Brachytherapy**............ 624
2.1 Endobronchial High-Dose-Rate
Brachytherapy... 624
2.2 Interstitial Brachytherapy.............................. 625
3 **Clinical Results**.. 625
3.1 Endobronchial Brachytherapy with Radical
Intention... 625
3.2 Endobronchial Brachytherapy
with Palliative Intention................................. 627
3.3 Interstitial Brachytherapy.............................. 630
3.4 Toxicity.. 631
4 **Conclusion**... 632
References... 632

Abstract

Brachytherapy is a radiation modality treatment where a radioactive source is placed inside or close to the tumor; this procedure is minimally invasive and in lung cancer is generally used for non-small cell lung cancer. The targets of brachytherapy treatment in lung cancer are diverse: we can use it with radical intention only if surgery or external beam radiotherapy cannot be realized, as an adjuvant to surgery in case of close or positive margins, as a boost to external beam radiotherapy, or with palliative intention in the case that the symptoms are related to intraluminal component of the lung cancer. Attending to the different brachytherapy techniques, we can refer to endoluminal, interstitial, or intraoperative. Technological advances in the last two decades have helped in the development of brachytherapy, but most of our knowledge is based on historical and retrospective studies.

R. H. de Lucas · T. M. Miguelañez · A. Polo (✉)
Servicio oncologia radioterapica H universitario
Ramon y Cajal Madrid, Madrid, Spain
e-mail: J.A.Polo-Rubio@iaea.org

P. L. A. Narvaez · D. B. Barreto
Servicio neumologia H universitario Ramon y Cajal
Madrid, Madrid, Spain

1 Introduction

Radiotherapy is one of the main options of treatment for lung cancer, which is the most diagnosed cancer in the world and the principal cause of cancer-related death. Early diagnosis can help in success, but at diagnosis, only near 20% of the lung cancers are confined to primary site, 25% are locally advanced disease, and more than 50% are in a metastatic situation.

Radiotherapy can be delivered using external beam radiation, which can be used alone or combined with chemotherapy and/or immunotherapy. Stereotactic body radiotherapy (SBRT) is one modality inside external radiotherapy that is specially used when a radical surgery cannot be realized in early-stage tumors (Ettinger et al. 2020).

Brachytherapy is a specific form of radiotherapy; it is based on the placement of radioactive sources directly into or close to the tumor, and it is used for primary, secondary, and recurrent tumors in most of the tumor localizations in the body (Gaspar 1998; Gauwitz et al. 1992; Mendiondo et al. 1983; Moylan et al. 1983; Nag et al. 2001; Qiu et al. 2020).

One of the advantages of this treatment is the possibility of delivering a high dose of radiation limiting the dose in the organs next to the tumor that is very helpful in lung cancer, where several studies indicated that it can improve local control and survival.

Endoluminal high-dose-rate brachytherapy is used for curative and palliative treatment when the endoluminal component of the tumor induces respiratory symptoms. Endoluminal brachytherapy can be used in combination with external beam radiotherapy for dose escalation as part of the radical approach or it can be used like rescue after the failure of primary radical treatments.

Interstitial brachytherapy can be performed in an intraoperative moment or by a percutaneous procedure. Intraoperative permanent ^{125}I seed implantation can be used in lung cancer treatment when resection margins are close to or involved with tumor, and it has been described by Stewart. Percutaneous implantation of radiation seeds in early stages of lung cancer with CT-guided approach has been reported by Martinez-Monge. Due to the low energy of ^{125}I, the falloff in the dose allows a high conformal dose and optimal sparing of normal tissues surrounding the implant.

In 1920, the initial use of brachytherapy in lung cancer was described; the sources have changed from those early times to the present: radium, gold-198, and iodine-125 were replaced by a rigid bronchoscope. These early techniques were not popular due to the risk of severe complications and poor dosimetric control.

From the 1950s, the development of afterloading techniques was essential for the widespread application of brachytherapy (Henschke et al. 1964). Afterloading techniques facilitate intraluminal brachytherapy using cesium-137, cobalt-60, and iridium-192. ^{192}Ir became the isotope of choice for brachytherapy. In the last two decades, new ways to place the seeds with the use of polyethylene catheters and new rules of implantation and dose calculation have made brachytherapy in lung cancer an easier technique, with the possibility to realize with local anesthesia and flexible bronchoscopy.

2 Procedure for Lung Brachytherapy

2.1 Endobronchial High-Dose-Rate Brachytherapy

The procedure starts with the introduction of one or more flexible plastic vectors (5-6F closed-end plastic tube) into the patient's airway. The number of catheters depends on the size and localization of the tumor inside the bronchial tree.

The catheters are connected to an afterloader device holding an iridium or cobalt source that is going to travel through the catheter to the position desired thanks to a computerized dosimetric system.

The procedure must be realized by a multidisciplinary medical team: First of all, the anesthesiologist makes brachytherapy possible with sedation of the patient. Then the pulmonologist introduces the bronchoscope in the affected bronchus, and in case of local obstruction that does not allow the bronchoscope to progress, the pulmonologist can make recanalization of the way prior to brachytherapy. When the bronchoscope is in position near the tumor, the catheter is inserted through the bronchoscope working channel and must advance distal to the gross tumor volume (GTV) under direct visualization.

Endoluminal irradiation should be delivered with a "safety margin" at both ends of GTV to cover microscopic disease (clinical target volume—CTV) and catheter movement (planning target volume—PTV).

After the placement of catheters, one or several, we can make a new parallel bronchoscope to be sure of the right procedure. Finally, the catheter is fixed to the nose in its way out.

The patient can suffer from some acute side effects by the placement of catheters like severe coughing, which can be minimized by the instillation of topical anesthesia and codeine pill treatment before the procedure. Some other severe adverse effects are bleeding and pneumothorax but are very rare (Speiser and Spratling 1993b).

The treatment can be delivered in a diverse number of fractions, depending on the status of the patient, the response of the tumor, or the local toxicity interfraction and the intention of the treatment (Mehta et al. 1992). It is usually delivered with 1–6 fractions in 1–3 weeks, and the prescription dose ranges between 3 and 20 Gy at 0.5–1 cm from the source axis.

2.2 Interstitial Brachytherapy

The interstitial technique varies depending on the type of implantation used, if it is permanent or temporary. Seeds can be placed into a tumor as a volume implant or can be meshed in a grid pattern in a planar implant (Stewart et al. 2009).

The first step is to delineate the area to be treated (GTV) and the microscopic disease margins (CTV). Image studies before the implant can be useful, but the real moment to determine the volumes is after the thoracotomy. The second step is to make a provisional dosimetry to calculate the number of seeds needed, and after that, insert the needles and afterload with the calculated number of seeds (Du et al. 2017; Tselis et al. 2011; Wang et al. 2011).

In some occasions in surgical treatments, tumors are large and the margins are positive. Critical vessels, bones, or other visceral structures are close to the tumor, and a safety margin cannot be realized. In this case, an intraoperative implant can be performed by different techniques; it can be permanent with ^{125}I or ^{103}Pd seeds suturing the mesh to the region of interest (Trombetta et al. 2008). Also, it can be performed with a temporary mesh with ^{192}Ir that is removed after the high-dose-rate treatment.

Another technique is percutaneous CT-guided approach although it is infrequent because there is not a big tradition about that and the number of possible candidates is small (Martinez-Monge et al. 2008; Sider et al. 1988; Heelan et al. 1987). It is performed in a TC room with general anesthesia that reduces the lung movement and the risk of pneumothorax (Chatzikonstantinou et al. 2019; Doggett et al. 2019). The TC is used to optimize the introduction of the needles required and to determine the volumes of treatment. Like the intraoperative technique, it can be permanent or temporary and the prescription dose ranges are between 125 Gy for ^{103}Pd and 100–160 Gy for ^{125}I (Li et al. 2013; Yan et al. 2017).

3 Clinical Results

3.1 Endobronchial Brachytherapy with Radical Intention

There are different scenarios where endobronchial brachytherapy has an important role: in cases where there is an exclusive endoluminal tumor, the exclusive radical brachytherapy is the right treatment. *Another case is* after a surgery where it is known that the margins are close or microscopically affected and also when after an external beam radiotherapy treatment there is still an intraluminal component.

Brachytherapy as an ablative treatment has been reported in numerous studies, where tumor control rate is over 80% and tracheal obstruction remission rate is about 60–80% (Knox et al. 2018) (Table 1).

The effect of brachytherapy as an exclusive treatment is based mostly on retrospective studies with a very important component of heterogeneity about doses, fraction schemes, and overall treatment time. The results have been observed by different groups using exclusively endobronchial

Table 1 Definitive brachytherapy alone: clinical results

Author	n	EBRT (Gy)	BT technique	Total dose (dose per fraction/number of fractions)	MFU (months)	LC (%)	CSS (%)	OS (%)	MST
Hilaris et al. (1987)	55	44% EBRT mediastinum	LDR/HDR		54	63	NA	32	NA
Schraube et al. (1993)	13	–	HDR	5–30 (3–5/1–6)	NA	NA	NA	NA	9 months
Sutedja et al. (1994)	2	–	HDR	30 (10/3)	40	NA	100	NA	NA
Tredaniel et al. (1994)	29	–	HDR	42 (7/6)	23	NA	NR	NA	Not reached
Aumont-le Guilcher et al. (2011)	226	–	HDR	24–35 (5–7/4–6)	30.4	68 (2 years)	81 (2 years)	57 (2 years)	28.6 months
Perol et al. (1997)	19	–	HDR	35 (7/5)	28	75 (1 years)	78 (1 years) 58 (2 years)	NA	28 months
Taulelle et al. (1998)	23	–	HDR	24–40 (8–10/3–4)	32	NA	46 (2 years)	NA	17 months
Stout et al. (2000)	49	–	HDR	15 (15/1)	NA	NA	NA	2	250 days
	50	30	–	–				10 $p = 0.04$	287 days $p = 0.04$
Peiffert et al. (2000)	33	No EBRT (18p)	HDR	30 (5/6)	14	NA	53 (2 years)	80 (2 years)	23 months
		50–60 (15p)	HDR	10–20 (5/2–4)					
Marsiglia et al. (2000)	34	–	HDR	30 (5/6)	29	85 (2 years)	NA	78 (2 years)	NA
Hennequin et al. (2007)	106	–	HDR	30–42 (5–7/6)	48	60.3 (2 years) 51.6 (5 years)	67.9 (2 years) 48.5 (5 years)	47.4 (2 years) 24 (5 years)	21.4 months
Soror (2019)	126	–	sORO	15	67	86.6	NA	23.6	NA

EBRT: external beam radiotherapy; BT: brachytherapy; HDR: high-dose rate; LDR: low-dose rate; MFU: median follow-up; LC: local control; CSS: cancer-specific survival; OS: overall survival; MST: median survival time; NA: not available brachytherapy with curative intent (Hilaris et al. 1987; Schraube et al. 1993; Sutedja et al. 1994; Tredaniel et al. 1994; Perol et al. 1997; Taulelle et al. 1998; Stout et al. 2000; Peiffert et al. 2000; Marsiglia et al. 2000; Hennequin et al. 2007; Aumont-le Guilcher et al. 2011), with the largest retrospective study with 266 patients treated with endobronchial brachytherapy showing 93.6% of overall response at 3 months and 2- and 5-year survival rates of 57% and 29%, respectively.

The results of brachytherapy as the treatment of isolated endobronchial tumor recurrence are good, with a complete local response rate of 86.5%, disease-free survival rate of 41.4%, and overall survival rate of 23.6% at 5 years in a retrospective review by Soror T.

The results of the addition of endoluminal brachytherapy external beam radiotherapy with the intention of dose escalation and higher local control are not very clear. Like in the case of exclusive brachytherapy, the studies are heterogeneous. Table 2 lists the clinical outcomes observed in studies in this field (Aygun et al. 1992; Cotter et al. 1993; Nori et al. 1993; Speiser and Spratling 1993a; Kohek et al. 1994; Fuwa et al. 2000; Nomoto et al. 1997; Huber et al. 1997; Furuta et al. 1999; Muto et al. 2000; Saito et al. 2000; Langendijk et al. 2001; Ozkok et al. 2008). In a prospective, randomized trial performed by Huber et al. (1997) including a total of 98 patients, two groups were compared. One group was treated with external radiotherapy alone (planned dose 60 Gy), and the second group received an additional boost of HDR brachytherapy (4.8 Gy scheduled, at 10 mm from the source axis) before and after external irradiation. In patients with squamous cell carcinoma, the HDR brachytherapy group showed a borderline advantage in median survival and a better local tumor control Huber et al. (1995).

The combination of brachytherapy and other treatment modalities, like cryotherapy, laser, electrocautery, or photodynamic therapy, is another aspect that can help in bulky disease (Freitag et al. 2004; Schray et al. 1985).

One study about the combination of brachytherapy and photodynamic therapy has been conducted by Freitag with 32 patients, without severe toxicity, and has obtained excellent therapeutic efficacy. Moreover, 28/32 patients (87.5%) were free of residual tumor and local recurrence at a mean follow-up of 24 months.

The combination of Nd-YAG laser and HDR endobronchial brachytherapy has also been explored when central airway is involved being superior than the only use of laser (8.5 vs. 2.8 months, $p < 0.05$) and also in terms of disease's progression-free period (7.5 vs. 2.2 months, $p < 0.05$) and number of further endoscopic treatments (3 vs. 15, $p < 0.05$).

Finally, EBB has also been used as an adjunctive treatment to radical surgery (Skowronek et al. 2013). The presence of microscopic disease in the surgical resection margin of the bronchial stump is a known risk factor for local recurrence. The study by McKenna et al. (2008) discusses their experience in the use of EBB as an adjuvant treatment after surgery.

3.2 Endobronchial Brachytherapy with Palliative Intention

Endoluminal brachytherapy is a good alternative to reduce the symptoms associated with endobronchial component of tumor, like persistent cough and hemoptysis; the procedure is quick and simple, but the patient should not present an active bleeding and the tumor must allow the passage of the catheter (Stewart et al. 2016).

Like in the radical intention, the series of studies are heterogeneous and combine different techniques and radiation treatments making it difficult to establish a definitive role for palliative treatment (Schray et al. 1988). Table 3 shows the results of symptomatic improvement observed in studies involving more than 50 patients using EBB as palliative treatment.

There are no differences among different schedules of palliative treatments, with similar rates of survival. Skrowonek included 648 patients with advanced lung cancer (303 patients received a total dose of 22.5 Gy in three fractions once a week, and 345 patients received a single fraction of 10 Gy). The impact of the fractionation schedule on survival was not statistically significant in a multivariate analysis ($p = 0.853$).

Another trial comparing twice 7.2 Gy application was found superior to four times 3.8 Gy

Table 2 Definitive brachytherapy boost with external beam radiotherapy: clinical results

Author	n	EBRT (Gy)	BT technique	Total dose (dose per fraction/number of fractions)	MFU	LC (%)	CSS (%)	OS (%)	MST (months)
Aygun et al. (1992)	62	50–60	HDR	15–25 (5/3–5)	18 months	NA	NA	NA	13
Cotter et al. (1993)	65	55–66	LDR	6–35	NA	NA	NA	23 (2 years)	8
Nori et al. (1993)	17	50*	HDR	15 (5/3)	14.5 months	88 (6 months)	NA	NA	17.5
Speiser and Spratling (1993a)	50	60	HDR	22.5–30 (7.5–10/3)	NA	NA	NA	NA	11
Kohek et al. (1994)	39	50–70	HDR	5–25 (5/1–5)	NA	NA	NA	NA	13
Fuwa et al. (2000)	41	50	LDR	22	0–60 months	NA	NA	61 (CR)	NA
Nomoto et al. (1997)	9	40–60	HDR	18 (6/3)	NA	NA	NA	64 (3 years)	NA
Huber et al. (1997)	56	60	HDR	9.6 (4.8/2)	2.5 years	12 weeks	NA	25 (1 year)	10
	42	60	–	–		21 weeks		19 (1 year)	8 ($p = 0.09$)
Furuta et al. (1999)	5	40	HDR	18 (6/3)	36 months	100 (CR)	80 (CR)	60 (CR)	NA
Muto et al. (2000)	320	60	HDR	10–15 (5–10/1–3)	5–36 months	NA	NA	NA	11
Saito et al. (2000)	64	40	LDR	25	44 months	87 (5 years)	96 (5 years)	72 (5 years)	NA
Langendijk et al. (2001)	48	30–60	HDR	15 (7.5/2)	12 months	NA	NA	9 (CR)	7
	47	30–60	–	–				15 (CR)	8.5
Ozkok et al. (2008)	43	60	HDR	15 (5/3)	NA	NA	NA	25.5 (2 years)	11
BT and Surgery									
McKenna et al. (2008)	48	Wedge resection	HDR	24.5 (3.5/7)	13.5	92 (CR)	NA	83 (CR)	NA

EBRT: external beam radiotherapy; BT: brachytherapy; HDR: high-dose rate; LDR: low-dose rate; MFU: median follow-up; LC: local control; CSS: cancer-specific survival; OS: overall survival; MST: median survival time; CR: crude rate; NA: not available

Table 3 Palliative brachytherapy: clinical results

Author	n	Prior treatments	BT technique	BT schedule	Symptomatic response
Lo et al. (1992)	77	Laser	LDR	45–60 Gy	Overall: 54%
Gollins et al. (1996)	322	EBRT, laser	HDR	15 Gy × 1	Stridor: 92%
				20 Gy × 1	Hemoptysis: 88%
					Cough: 62%
					Dyspnea: 60%
					Pain: 50%
					Pulmonary collapse: 46%
Speiser and Spratling (1993a)	109	Laser	HDR	7.5 Gy × 3	Overall: 70%
				5 Gy × 3	Hemoptysis: 99%
					Pneumonia: 99%
					Dyspnea: 86%
					Cough: 85%
Delclos et al. (1996)	81	EBRT	HDR	15 Gy × 2	Overall: 84%
Ornadel et al. (1997)	117	EBRT, laser	HDR		Cough: 62–77%
					Dyspnea: 32–56%
					Hemoptysis: 78–97%
Stout et al. (2000)	50	None	EBRT	30 Gy (3.75 × 8)	Improved symptom palliation for EBRT (83%) versus HDR (59%), $p = 0.03$
	49		HDR	15 Gy × 1	
Kelly et al. (2000)	175	EBRT, laser	HDR	15 Gy × 1	Overall: 66%
Celebioglu et al. (2002)	95	EBRT	HDR	7.5 Gy × 3	Overall: 100%
				10 Gy × 2	
Mallick et al. (2007)	95	NA	HDR	10 Gy × 1	Dyspnea: 92.5%
				8 Gy × 2	Cough: 81%
				15 Gy × 1	Hemoptysis: 97%
					Pneumonia: 91%
Kubaszewska et al. (2008)	270	EBRT, BT	HDR	8 Gy × 1	Overall: 80%
				10 Gy × 1	Dyspnea: 76%
					Cough: 77%
					Hemoptysis: 92%
					Pneumonia: 82%
Skowronek et al. (2009)	648	EBRT	HDR	7.5 Gy × 3 (303p)	Overall: 88%; no differences between schedules
				10 Gy × 1 (345p)	
Niemoeller et al. (2013)	142	–	HDR	4 × 3.8 Gy	Overall no differences
				2 × 7.2 Gy	Local response higher in 2 × 7.2 Gy

EBRT: external beam radiotherapy; BT: brachytherapy; HDR: high-dose rate; LDR: low-dose rate; NA: not available

application per week with a 3 weeks' interval schedule at the time of local tumor response (median 12 vs. 6 weeks; $p < 0.015$); however, there was no significant difference in survival (median 18 vs. 19 weeks, p = n.s.) and fatal hemoptysis between groups (12.2% vs. 18.3%, respectively, $p = 0.345$) (Niemoeller et al. 2013).

Furthermore, quality of life and complications were found to be better in a combination treatment arm with external beam radiotherapy 30 Gy/10 fractions and two sessions of HDR brachytherapy 8 Gy, each one compared with the same external treatment but with only a single dose of 10 Gy and with another arm.

In general, in different studies, between 40% and 90% of hemoptysis is resolved and around 50% of cough and dyspnea are controlled after 6 months of treatment (Marsiglia et al. 2000).

Comparing external beam radiation and endobronchial brachytherapy with palliative intention, when external treatment has not been realized before there are two systematical reviews (Ontario

Cancer Care clinical guidelines and Cochrane Review in 2008) determine that external radiotherapy is more effective and is no clear the result of the addition of the brachytherapy. Hans L et al. reported in a randomized study that a higher rate of re-expansion of the collapsed lung was observed in EBRT plus endobronchial BT (57%) compared to endobronchial BT alone (35%) ($p < 0.01$).

In a Cochrane review of 953 patients, there was no difference between both modalities about symptom relief (Reveiz et al. 2012).

When the obstruction of the airway is complicated with acute dyspnea, endoluminal brachytherapy should not be the first treatment; instead, laser resection and electrocautery should be preferred.

A novel approach is the use of tracheobronchial stent loaded with iodine-125 seeds (Wang et al. 2017, 2018); there is a study by Gao-Jun Teng in 66 patients with malignant airway obstruction in a randomized controlled trial (RCT). Restenosis of the stent was significantly reduced, and patients' overall survival was improved compared with a conventional stent (170 days vs. 123 days, $p < 0.05$), with no significant difference in the incidence of complications between groups ($p < 0.05$).

The American Society for Radiation Oncology (ASTRO) published an evidence-based clinical practice guideline about the palliative thoracic treatment and endobronchial brachytherapy and described it like an option especially when the patient has received external beam radiotherapy before Rodrigues et al. (2011).

3.3 Interstitial Brachytherapy

Another technique is interstitial brachytherapy; in the surgery act or when an image procedure is being realized, the radiation oncologist places the radiative source inside or in the proximity of the target volume (Kim and Hilaris 1975; Lewis Jr et al. 1990).

^{125}I seed implantation is an alternative with excellent results (Wei et al. 2012); clinical guidelines have been realized by Chinese expert consensus for primary and metastatic lung tumors (Zhang & Wang 2019).

There are different ways of implementation, guided by TC (Zhang et al. 2007), ultrasound, or RMN, depending on the depth of the lesion or whether the localization of the tumor is central by fibro-bronchoscope; another situation is when the tumor is near large vessels, heart, or hilus; then it can be placed during the surgery when it can be performed (Ji et al. 2020; Jiang et al. 2015; Jiao et al. 2017).

It is the major form to treat early-stage tumors in patients where surgery is not possible or cannot tolerate external beam radiotherapy.

In different trials, PD is between 100 and 120 Gy and the local control is about 80–100%; survival rates at 1 and 2 years are 90–95% and 70–80%, respectively.

Complications like pneumothorax, hemoptysis, and hemorrhage are not frequent, 10–60%, and are variable (Kou et al. 2019).

Li W et al. published one trial comparing external beam radiotherapy and interstitial brachytherapy in unresectable tumor stage III–IV. The local control rate was higher with brachytherapy than with external beam radiotherapy (97.1% and 80%, respectively, $p < 0.05$), and RSI-BT significantly increased the 1- and 2-year survival rates (82.8% vs. 41.6%, 37.1% vs. 11.1%, respectively, $p < 0.05$) (Li et al. 2015).

Zhang et al. published one meta-analysis on advanced lung cancer comparing interstitial brachytherapy and chemotherapy with a better local control rate and overall response in the brachytherapy arm; also, in the trials that combined chemotherapy and interstitial brachytherapy, there was an improvement in the quality of life and survival, with results in the combination regimen reported to be 83.35%, 25.57%, and 11.34%, respectively, for local tumor control at 1, 3, and 5 years (Table 4).

For recurrent lung cancer after surgery, brachytherapy can be used in different localizations. Huo et al. published one retrospective trial evaluating the effectiveness and safety of brachytherapy guided by TAC, and the results after 2 months showed 50%, 37%, and 8% of complete response, partial response, and progressive disease, respectively.

Table 4 Interstitial brachytherapy: clinical results

Author	n	Disease stage (AJCC)	BT technique	Total dose (Gy)	LC (%)	OS (%)
Hilaris and Martini (1979)	470	I–III	^{125}I	160	80 (5 years, stages I, II) 80 (5 years, stage III)	7 (5 years)
Hilaris and Martini (1988)	88	T1–3 N2	^{125}I; HDR	160; 30	76 (2 years)	51 (2 years)
	225	T3N0				22 (2 years)
Ginsberg et al. (1994)	102	I–III, close/ positive margins	^{125}I HDR	160 10–20	NA	41 (5 years)
Brach et al. (1994)	20	I, tumor 2 cm	HDR	10–20	NA	75% (CR, 3–30 months)
Chen et al. (1999)	23	I	^{125}I	100–120	100 (CR)	83 (CR)
Santos et al. (2003)	203	IA–B	^{125}I (101p) –(102p)	100–120 –	98 (CR) 81 (CR)	60 (4 years) 67 (4 years)
Lee et al. (2003)	33	I	^{125}I	125–140	94 (5 years)	47 (5 years)
Voynov et al. (2005)	118	IA–B	^{125}I	85–129	87 (5 years)	18 (5 years)
Birdas et al. (2006)	167	IB	Sublobar resection ^{125}I (41p) Lobectomy (126p)	100–120 –	95.2 (CR) 96.8 (CR)	54 (4 years) 52 (4 years)
Colonias et al. (2011)	145	IA–B	^{125}I	120	NA	35 (5 years)
Wei Li (2015)	71	III–IV	^{125}I vs. EBRT		97% vs. 80%	82.8% vs. 41.6% (1 year) 37.1% vs. 11.1% (2 years)

BT: brachytherapy; HDR: high-dose rate; LC: local control; OS: overall survival; CR: crude rate; NA: not available, EBRT: external beam radiotherapy

Median overall survival was 21 months, and the rates of 2-year overall survival, progression-free survival, and local tumor control were 47.4%, 39.5%, and 83.5%, respectively. D90 was a significant prognostic factor for survival.

The presurgery idea of an incomplete resection or close or positive margins is the occasion when the surgeon refers the patient to the radiation oncologist for planning interstitial brachytherapy. Sometimes, the collateral health condition of the patient makes you think about an insufficient surgery.

3.4 Toxicity

Brachytherapy in lung cancer is a routine treatment for an expert multidisciplinary team; usually, it is not more difficult than a diagnostic flexible bronchoscopy, but it is possible to find acute toxicity related to the procedure. Exacerbation of cough during a short period of time after brachytherapy is the most frequent side effect, and it is relatively easy to control, but there could be other side effects that can be worse for the patient like hemoptysis. The incidence of this complication ranges between 0% and 32% of patients treated with a prevalence of approximately 10% (Vergnon et al. 2006; Bedwinek et al. 1992). There is not a clear factor related with this side effect, perhaps in tumors close to pulmonary artery (Aygun and Blum 1995). The progression of the tumor can also be the origin of hemoptysis. Prior treatments, radiation dose higher than 15 Gy, and reirradiation are factors that increase the risk. Stout et al. compared a sole treatment of 15 Gy with brachytherapy with another by external beam radiation in eight fractions with a total dose of 30 Gy, and the risk was the same 7%.

Radiation in all its techniques can cause inflammation in minor or major grade, and this inflammation can cause late fibrosis. Depending on the clinical relevance of these effects, we must use different treatments like steroids, balloon dilatation, and endobronchial prosthesis (Vergnon et al. 2006).

Endobronchial brachytherapy is a well-tolerated procedure with a low incidence of toxicity and a good palliative chance.

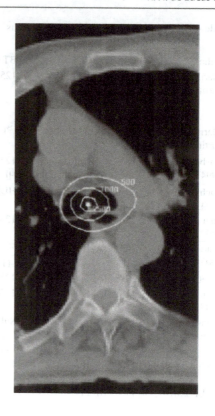

4 Conclusion

Brachytherapy is a multidisciplinary modality of radiation treatment that can be used with radical or palliative intention, with good results in small intraluminal tumors. It can be used alone or associated with other techniques, like surgery, external beam radiotherapy, cryotherapy, or chemotherapy.

The optimal dose and the fractionation schemes are not clear due to the absence of a large number of studies that can support consistent conclusions.

Toxicity associated with brachytherapy is low, but we must stay vigilant, especially when it is not used as *a stand-alone treatment*.

More clinical trials must be performed to document the appropriate role of brachytherapy in lung cancer treatment.

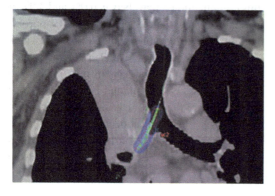

References

Aumont-le Guilcher M, Prevost B, Sunyach MP et al (2011) High-dose-rate brachytherapy for non-small-cell lung carcinoma: a retrospective study of 226 patients. Int J Radiat Oncol Biol Phys 79:1112–1116

Aygun C, Blum JE (1995) Treatment of unresectable lung cancer with brachytherapy. World J Surg 19:823–827

Aygun C, Weiner S, Scariato A, Spearman D, Stark L (1992) Treatment of non-small cell lung cancer with external beam radiotherapy and high dose rate brachytherapy. Int J Radiat Oncol Biol Phys 23:127–132

Bedwinek J, Petty A, Bruton C, Sofield J, Lee L (1992) The use of high dose rate endobronchial brachytherapy to palliate symptomatic endobronchial recurrence of previously irradiated bronchogenic carcinoma. Int J Radiat Oncol Biol Phys 22:23–30

Birdas TJ, Koehler RP, Colonias A et al (2006) Sublobar resection with brachytherapy versus lobectomy for stage Ib nonsmall cell lung cancer. Ann Thorac Surg 81:434–438. discussion 438–439

Brach B, Buhler C, Hayman MH, Joyner LRJ, Liprie SF (1994) Percutaneous computed tomography-guided fine needle brachytherapy of pulmonary malignancies. Chest 106:268–274

Bray F, Ferlay J, Soerjomataram I et al (2018) Global cancer statistics 2018: GLOBOCAN estimates of incidence and mortality worldwide for 36 cancers in 185 countries. CA Cancer J Clin 68:394–424

Celebioglu B, Gurkan OU, Erdogan S et al (2002) High dose rate endobronchial brachytherapy effectively palliates symptoms due to inoperable lung cancer. Jpn J Clin Oncol 32:443–448

Chatzikonstantinou G, Zamboglou N, Baltas D et al (2019) Image-guide interstitial high-dose-rate brachytherapy for dose escalation in the radiotherapy treatment of locally advanced lung cancer: a single institute experience. Brachytherapy 18:829–834

Chen A, Galloway M, Landreneau R et al (1999) Intraoperative 125I brachytherapy for high-risk stage I non-small cell lung carcinoma. Int J Radiat Oncol Biol Phys 44:1057–1063

Colonias A, Betler J, Trombetta M et al (2011) Mature follow-up for high-risk stage I non-small-cell lung carcinoma treated with sublobar resection and intraoperative iodine-125 brachytherapy. Int J Radiat Oncol Biol Phys 79:105–109

Cotter GW, Lariscy C, Ellingwood KE, Herbert D (1993) Inoperable endobronchial obstructing lung cancer treated with combined endobronchial and external beam irradiation: a dosimetric analysis. Int J Radiat Oncol Biol Phys 27:531–535

Delclos ME, Komaki R, Morice RC, Allen PK, Davis M, Garden A (1996) Endobronchial brachytherapy with high-dose-rate remote afterloading for recurrent endobronchial lesions. Radiology 201:279–282

Doggett SW, Chino S, Lempert T (2019) A novel approach for salvage treatment of non-small-cell lung cancer: Percutaneous CT fluoroscopy-guided permanent seed brachytherapy for salvage treatment of lung cancer: long-term results of a case series. J Contemp Brachyther 11:174–179

Du P, Xiao Y, Lu W (2017) Modified fan-shaped distribution technology for computed tomography (CT)-Guided radioactive seed implantation in lung cancer patients with lung dysfunction. Med Sci Monit 23:4366–4375

Ettinger DS, Gettinger S, Ng T et al (2020) NCCN Guidelines: non-small cell lung cancer, version 8.2020. National Comprehensive Cancer Network

Freitag L, Ernst A, Thomas M et al (2004) Sequential photodynamic therapy (PDT) and high dose brachytherapy for endobronchial tumour control in patients with limited bronchogenic carcinoma. Thorax 59:790–793

Furuta M, Tsukiyama I, Ohno T et al (1999) Radiation therapy for roentogenographically occult lung cancer by external beam irradiation and endobronchial high dose rate brachytherapy. Lung Cancer 25:183–189

Fuwa N, Ito Y, Matsumoto A, Morita K (2000) The treatment results of 40 patients with localized endobronchial cancer with external beam irradiation and intraluminal irradiation using low dose rate (192)Ir thin wires with a new catheter. Radiother Oncol 56:189–195

Gaspar LE (1998) Brachytherapy in lung cancer. J Surg Oncol 67:60–70

Gauwitz M, Ellerbroek N, Komaki R et al (1992) High dose endobronchial irradiation in recurrent bronchogenic carcinoma. Int J Radiat Oncol Biol Phys 23:397–400

Ginsberg RJ, Martini N, Zaman M et al (1994) Influence of surgical resection and brachytherapy in the management of superior sulcus tumor. Ann Thorac Surg 57(1440–1):445

Gollins SW, Ryder WD, Burt PA, Barber PV, Stout R (1996) Massive haemoptysis death and other morbidity associated with high dose rate intraluminal radiotherapy for carcinoma of the bronchus. Radiother Oncol 39:105–116

Heelan RT, Hilaris BS, Anderson LL et al (1987) Lung tumors: percutaneous implantation of I-125 sources with CT treatment planning. Radiology 164:735–740

Hennequin C, Bleichner O, Tredaniel J et al (2007) Long-term results of endobronchial brachytherapy: a curative treatment? Int J Radiat Oncol Biol Phys 67:425–430

Henschke UK, Hilaris BS, Mahan GD (1964) Remote after loading with intracavitary applicators. Radiology 83:344–345

Hilaris BS, Martini N (1979) Interstitial brachytherapy in cancer of the lung: a 20 year experience. Int J Radiat Oncol Biol Phys 5:1951–1956

Hilaris BS, Martini N (1988) the current state of intraoperative interstitial brachytherapy in lung cancer. Int J Radiat Oncol Biol Phys 15:1347–1354

Hilaris BS, Martini N, Wong GY, Nori D (1987) Treatment of superior sulcus tumor (Pancoast tumor). Surg Clin North Am 67:965–977

Huber RM, Fischer R, Hautmann H et al (1995) Palliative endobronchial brachytherapy for central lung tumors. A prospective, randomized comparison of two fractionation schedules. Chest 107:463–470

Huber RM, Fischer R, Hautmann H, Pollinger B, Haussinger K, Wendt T (1997) Does additional brachytherapy improve the effect of external irradiation? A prospective, randomized study in central lung tumors. Int J Radiat Oncol Biol Phys 38:533–540

Ji Z, Jiang Y, Guo F et al (2020) Safety and efficacy of CT-guided radioactive iodine-125 seed implantation assisted by a 3D printing template for the treatment of thoracic malignancies. J Cancer Res Clin Oncol 146:229–236

Jiang G, Li Z, Ding A et al (2015) Computed tomography-guided iodine-125 interstitial implantation as an alternative treatment option for lung cancer. Indian J Cancer 51:e9ee12

Jiao D, Ren K, Li Z et al (2017) Clinical role of guidance by C-arm CT for (125)I brachytherapy on pulmonary tumors. Radiol Med 122:829–836

Kelly JF, Delclos ME, Morice RC, Huaringa A, Allen PK, Komaki R (2000) High-dose-rate endobronchial brachytherapy effectively palliates symptoms due to airway tumors: the 10-year M. D. Anderson cancer center experience. Int J Radiat Oncol Biol Phys 48:697–702

Kim JH, Hilaris B (1975) Iodine 125 source in interstitial tumor therapy. Clinical and biological considerations. Am J Roentgenol Radium Ther Nucl Med 123:163–169

Knox MC, Bece A, Bucci J et al (2018) Endobronchial brachytherapy in the management of lung malignancies: 20 years of experience in an Australian center. Brachytherapy 17:973–980

Kohek PH, Pakisch B, Glanzer H (1994) Intraluminal irradiation in the treatment of malignant airway obstruction. Eur J Surg Oncol 20:674–680

Kou F, Gao S, Liu S et al (2019) Preliminary clinical efficacy of iodine-125 seed implantation for the treatment of advanced malignant lung tumors. J Cancer Res Ther 15:1567–1573

Kubaszewska M, Skowronek J, Chichel A, Kanikowski M (2008) The use of high dose rate endobronchial brachytherapy to palliate symptomatic recurrence of previously irradiated lung cancer. Neoplasma 55:239–245

Langendijk H, de Jong J, Tjwa M et al (2001) External irradiation versus external irradiation plus endobronchial brachytherapy in inoperable non-small cell lung cancer: a prospective randomized study. Radiother Oncol 58:257–268

Lee W, Daly BD, DiPetrillo TA et al (2003) Limited resection for non-small cell lung cancer: observed local control with implantation of I-125 brachytherapy seeds. Ann Thorac Surg 75:237–242. discussion 242–3

Lewis JW Jr, Ajlouni M, Kvale PA et al (1990) Role of brachytherapy in the management of pulmonary and mediastinal malignancies. Ann Thorac Surg 49:728–732. Discussion 732e723

Li J, Yu M, Xiao Y et al (2013) Computed tomography fluoroscopy-guided percutaneous (125)I seed implantation for safe, effective and real-time monitoring radiotherapy of inoperable stage T1-3N0M0 nonsmall-cell lung cancer. Mol Clin Oncol 1:1019–1024

Li W, Guan J, Yang L, Zheng X, Yu Y, Jiang J (2015) Iodine-125 brachytherapy improved overall survival of patients with inoperable stage III/IV non-small cell lung cancer versus the conventional radiotherapy. Med Oncol 32:395.

Li W, Guan J, Yang L et al (2015) Iodine-125 brachytherapy improved overall survival of patients with inoperable stage III/IV non-small cell lung cancer versus the conventional radiotherapy. Med Oncol 32:395

Lo TC, Beamis JFJ, Weinstein RS et al (1992) Intraluminal low-dose rate brachytherapy for malignant endobronchial obstruction. Radiother Oncol 23:16–20

Mallick I, Sharma SC, Behera D (2007) Endobronchial brachytherapy for symptom palliation in non-small cell lung cancer–analysis of symptom response, endoscopic improvement and quality of life. Lung Cancer 55:313–318

Marsiglia H, Baldeyrou P, Lartigau E et al (2000) High-dose-rate brachytherapy as sole modality for early-stage endobronchial carcinoma. Int J Radiat Oncol Biol Phys 47:665–672

Martinez-Monge R, Pagola M, Vivas I, Lopez-Picazo JM (2008) CT-guided permanent brachytherapy for patients with medically inoperable early-stage non-small cell lung cancer (NSCLC). Lung Cancer 61:209–213

McKenna RJJ, Mahtabifard A, Yap J et al (2008) Wedge resection and brachytherapy for lung cancer in patients with poor pulmonary function. Ann Thorac Surg 85:S733–S736

Mehta M, Petereit D, Chosy L et al (1992) Sequential comparison of low dose rate and hyperfractionated high dose rate endobronchial radiation for malignant airway occlusion. Int J Radiat Oncol Biol Phys 23:133–139

Mendiondo OA, Dillon M, Beach LJ (1983) Endobronchial brachytherapy in the treatment of recurrent bronchogenic carcinoma. Int J Radiat Oncol Biol Phys 9:579–582

Moylan D, Strubler K, Unal A, Mohiuddin M, Giampetro A, Boon R (1983) Work in progress. Transbronchial brachytherapy of recurrent bronchogenic carcinoma: a new approach using the flexible fiberoptic bronchoscope. Radiology 147:253–254

Muto P, Ravo V, Panelli G, Liguori G, Fraioli G (2000) High-dose rate brachytherapy of bronchial cancer: treatment optimization using three schemes of therapy. Oncologist 5:209–214

Nag S, Kelly JF, Horton JL, Komaki R, Nori D (2001) Brachytherapy for carcinoma of the lung. Oncology (Williston Park) 15:371–381

Niemoeller OM, Pollinger B, Niyazi M et al (2013) Mature results of a randomized trial comparing two fractionation schedules of high dose rate endoluminal brachytherapy for the treatment of endobronchial tumors. Radiat Oncol 8:8

Nomoto Y, Shouji K, Toyota S et al (1997) High dose rate endobronchial brachytherapy using a new applicator. Radiother Oncol 45:33–37

Nori D, Allison R, Kaplan B, Samala E, Osian A, Karbowitz S (1993) High dose-rate intraluminal irradiation in bronchogenic carcinoma. Technique and results. Chest 104:1006–1011

Ornadel D, Duchesne G, Wall P, Ng A, Hetzel M (1997) Defining the roles of high dose rate endobronchial brachytherapy and laser resection for recurrent bronchial malignancy. Lung Cancer 16:203–213

Ozkok S, Karakoyun-Celik O, Goksel T et al (2008) High dose rate endobronchial brachytherapy in the management of lung cancer: response and toxicity evaluation in 158 patients. Lung Cancer 62:326–333

Peiffert D, Spaeth D, Menard O, Winnefeld J (2000) High dose endobronchial brachytherapy: a curative treatment. Cancer Radiother 4:197–201

Perol M, Caliandro R, Pommier P et al (1997) Curative irradiation of limited endobronchial carcinomas with high-dose rate brachytherapy. Results of a pilot study. Chest 111(5):1417–1423

Qiu B, Jiang P, Ji Z, Huo X, Sun H, Wang J (2020) Brachytherapy for lung cancer. Brachytherapy S1538-4721(20):30253-30251. https://doi.org/10.1016/j.brachy.2020.11.009. Epub ahead of print. PMID: 33358847

Reveiz L, Rueda JR, Cardona AF (2012) Palliative endobronchial brachytherapy for non-small cell lung cancer. Cochrane Database Syst Rev 12:CD004284

Rodrigues G, Videtic GM, Sur R (2011) Palliative thoracic radiotherapy in lung cancer: an American Society for Radiation Oncology evidence-based clinical practice guideline. Pract Radiat Oncol:60–71

Saito M, Yokoyama A, Kurita Y, Uematsu T, Tsukada H, Yamanoi T (2000) Treatment of roentgenographically occult endobronchial carcinoma with external beam radiotherapy and intraluminal low-dose-rate brachytherapy: second report. Int J Radiat Oncol Biol Phys 47:673–680

Santos R, Colonias A, Parda D et al (2003) Comparison between sublobar resection and 125Iodine brachytherapy after sublobar resection in high-risk patients with Stage I non-small-cell lung cancer. Surgery 134:691–697. discussion 697

Schraube P, Fritz P, Becker HD, Wannenmacher M (1993) The results of the endoluminal high-dose-rate irradiation of central non-small cell bronchial carcinomas. Strahlenther Onkol 169:228–234

Schray MF, McDougall JC, Martinez A, Edmundson GK, Cortese DA (1985) Management of malignant airway obstruction: clinical and dosimetric considerations using an iridium-192 afterloading technique in conjunction with the neodymium-YAG laser. Int J Radiat Oncol Biol Phys 11:403–409

Schray MF, McDougall JC, Martinez A, Cortese DA, Brutinel WM (1988) Management of malignant airway compromise with laser and low dose rate brachytherapy. The Mayo Clinic experience. Chest 93:264–269

Sider L, Mittal BB, Nemcek AAJ, Bobba VS (1988) CT-guided placement of iodine-125 seeds for unresectable carcinoma of the lung. J Comput Assist Tomogr 12:515–517

Skowronek J, Kubaszewska M, Kanikowski M, Chichel A, Mlynarczyk W (2009) HDR endobronchial brachytherapy (HDRBT) in the management of advanced lung cancer—comparison of two different dose schedules. Radiother Oncol 93:436–440

Skowronek J, Piorunek T, Kanikowski M et al (2013) Definitive high-dose-rate endobronchial brachytherapy of bronchial stump for lung cancer after surgery. Brachytherapy 12:560–566

Soror T, Kovacs G, Furschke V et al (2019) Salvage treatment with sol high-dose-rate endobronchial interventional radiotherapy (brachytherapy) for isolated endobronchial tumor recurrence in nonsmall-cell lung cancer patients: a 20-year experience. Brachytherapy 18:727–732

Speiser BL, Spratling L (1993a) Remote after loading brachytherapy for the local control of endobronchial carcinoma. Int J Radiat Oncol Biol Phys 25:579–587

Speiser BL, Spratling L (1993b) Radiation bronchitis and stenosis secondary to high dose rate endobronchial irradiation. Int J Radiat Oncol Biol Phys 25:589–597

Stewart AJ, Mutyala S, Holloway CL, Colson YL, Devlin PM (2009) Intraoperative seed placement for thoracic malignancy—a review of technique, indications, and published literature. Brachytherapy 8:63–69

Stewart A, Parashar B, Patel M et al (2016) American Brachytherapy Society consensus guidelines for thoracic brachytherapy for lung cancer. Brachytherapy 15:1–11

Stout R, Barber P, Burt P et al (2000) Clinical and quality of life outcomes in the first United Kingdom randomized trial of endobronchial brachytherapy (intraluminal radiotherapy) vs. external beam radiotherapy in the palliative treatment of inoperable non-small cell lung cancer. Radiother Oncol 56:323–327

Sutedja G, Baris G, van Zandwijk N, Postmus PE (1994) High-dose rate brachytherapy has a curative potential in patients with intraluminal squamous cell lung cancer. Respiration 61:167–168

Taulelle M, Chauvet B, Vincent P et al (1998) High dose rate endobronchial brachytherapy: results and complications in 189 patients. Eur Respir J 11:162–168

Tredaniel J, Hennequin C, Zalcman G et al (1994) Prolonged survival after high-dose rate endobronchial radiation for malignant airway obstruction. Chest 105:767–772

Trombetta MG, Colonias A, Makishi D et al (2008) Tolerance of the aorta using intraoperative iodine-125 interstitial brachytherapy in cancer of the lung. Brachytherapy 7:50–54

Tselis N, Ferentinos K, Kolotas C et al (2011) Computed tomography guided interstitial high-dose-rate brachytherapy in the local treatment of primary and secondary intrathoracic malignancies. J Thorac Oncol 6:545–552

Vergnon JM, Huber RM, Moghissi K (2006) Place of cryotherapy, brachytherapy and photodynamic therapy in therapeutic bronchoscopy of lung cancers. Eur Respir J 28:200–218

Voynov G, Heron DE, Lin CJ et al (2005) Intraoperative (125) I Vicryl mesh brachytherapy after sublobar resection for high-risk stage I non-small cell lung cancer. Brachytherapy 4:278–285

Wang ZM, Lu JJ, Liu T et al (2011) CT-guided interstitial brachytherapy of inoperable non-small cell lung cancer. Lung Cancer 74:253–257

Wang Y, Guo JH, Zhu GY et al (2017) A novel self-expandable, radioactive airway stent loaded with (125) I seeds: a feasibility and safety study in healthy beagle dog. Cardiovasc Intervent Radiol 40:1086–1093

Wang Y, Lu JJ, Guo JH et al (2018) A novel tracheobronchial stent loaded with (125)I seeds in patients with malignant airway obstruction compared to a conventional stent: a prospective randomized controlled study. EBioMedicine 33:269–275

Wei W, Shen XH, Sun HH et al (2012) The short term therapeutic effects of radioactive (125)I seeds implantation for treatment of non-small cell lung cancer. Zhonghua Nei Ke Za Zhi 51:978–981

Yan WL, Lv JS, Guan ZY et al (2017) Impact of target area selection in (125) Iodine seed brachytherapy on locoregional recurrence in patients with non-small cell lung cancer. Thorac Cancer 8:147–152

Zhang F, Wang J (2019) Chinese expert consensus workshop report: guideline for permanent iodine-125 seed implantation of primary and metastatic lung tumors. Thoracic Cancer 10(2):388–394. ISSN 1759-7706

Zhang FJ, Li CX, Wu PH et al (2007) CT guided radioactive 125I seed implantation in treating localized advanced pulmonary carcinoma. Zhonghua Yi Xue Za Zhi 87:3272–3275

Oligometastatic Disease: Basic Aspects and Clinical Results in NSCLC

Gukan Sakthivel, Deepinder P. Singh, Haoming Qiu, and Michael T. Milano

Contents

1 Introduction 638
2 Definition of OMD 639
3 Clinical Studies 640
3.1 Select Prospective Nonrandomized Studies of SBRT of OMD from NSCLC 640
3.2 Select Phase II Randomized Studies of SBRT of OMD 641
4 Meta-analysis 643
5 Selected Other Studies 643
6 Molecular Studies 643
7 Ongoing Studies and Future Directions 644
8 Conclusions 645
References 645

Abstract

Oligometastatic disease (OMD) represents a unique subset of metastatic disease that is limited in extent, with a generally accepted definition being metastatic disease confined to one or a few sites. Such limited metastatic disease can be amenable to resection or ablative doses of radiation. OMD treated with stereotactic ablative radiotherapy (SABR)/stereotactic body therapy (SBRT) has been shown to be associated with a survival advantage in prospective randomized phase II clinical studies, including studies specific to patients with non-small cell lung cancer. Currently, there are ongoing phase III studies around the world validating the initial findings in these studies. There are limitations to our understanding of OMD. For example, there are no validated molecular biomarkers to stratify the patients who would benefit most from SBRT/SABR. Furthermore, the definition of the oligometastatic state is limited by the currently available imaging modalities' ability to identify sites of metastatic disease. With new advances on the horizon in imaging and molecular markers, the study of OMD is burgeoning. Future endeavors to further substratify oligometastatic state, and possible expansion of the definition for more patients to benefit from the survival advantage, are also on the horizon.

G. Sakthivel · D. P. Singh · H. Qiu · M. T. Milano (✉)
Department of Radiation Oncology,
University of Rochester, Rochester, NY, USA
e-mail: Gukan_Sakthivel@URMC.Rochester.edu;
Deepinder_Singh@URMC.Rochester.edu;
Haoming_Qiu@URMC.Rochester.edu;
Michael_Milano@URMC.Rochester.edu

1 Introduction

Metastases develop at organs and tissues distant from the primary site of cancer. The local-regional as well as distant spread of cancer depends on the specific tumor biology and receptiveness of specific organs. Oligometastases imply few (oligo) sites of metastases in a patient. While the concept of limited metastases being a potentially discrete clinical entity dates back many decades (Rubin and Green 1968; Rubin 1968; Peters et al. 1983; Milano et al. 2021), the term oligometastatic disease (OMD) was proposed initially by Hellman and Weichselbaum to be a distinct cancer state between locally confined and extensive disease in 1995 (Hellman and Weichselbaum 1995). Their spectrum theory proposed that cancer can exist in intermediate states of metastatic disease. At one extreme is widely metastatic cancer, while at the other extreme is metastatic cancer limited in extent to a single distant site. The spectrum theory lies between Fisher's concept of cancer being metastatic at inception, even in patients with clinically localized cancer (i.e., micrometastatic disease without clinical/radiographic evidence of metastases), and Halstead's theory that there is an orderly spread of cancer, from localized cancer, direct extension of the cancer, and regional nodal metastatic progression to distant progression. Hellman and Weichselbaum argued against such a sharp dichotomy, postulating that metastatic cancer can exist between these extremes. Along the spectrum is OMD, a state of cancer progression which is amenable to potentially curative metastasis-directed therapy. Metastasis-directed treatment can result in prolonged overall survival (OS) in what historically has been considered an incurable disease (Aujla et al. 2019). In the case of non-small cell lung cancer (NSCLC), patients with OMD with indolent disease courses may be cured or rendered disease free for long durations of time with aggressive local and systemic therapy (Bergsma et al. 2015, 2017).

Hellman and Weichselbaum also described, in their landmark paper, two very different clinical scenarios of OMD. De novo OMD describes tumors early in the chain of progression with metastases limited in number and location. Induced OMD also known as oligopersistent disease can occur in patients with widespread metastases that were mostly eradicated by systemic agents, with either (1) systemic therapy having failed to destroy select sites with significant disease burden; (2) persistent tumors with the presence of drug-resistant cells; or (3) tumors being in a pharmacologically privileged site.

Historically, metastasectomy (resection of metastatic disease) was utilized for select patients with discrete metastases amenable to resection. With the advent of more sophisticated radiation planning and delivery technology in recent decades, targeted radiotherapy has been increasingly utilized. Select patients have fared well with respect to overall and progression-free survival after metastasis-directed therapy. Patients with oligometastatic NSCLC (i.e., stage IV) appear to have outcomes similar to those with nonmetastatic locally advanced NSCLC (Cheruvu et al. 2011). Notably, the American Joint Committee on Cancer (AJCC) 8th edition introduced M1b as a unique M stage for NSCLC—with a single extrathoracic metastasis in a single organ.

In recent decades, stereotactic body radiation therapy (SBRT, also referred to as or LAT (locally ablative therapy)) for primary lung cancer and oligometastases from lung cancer has been studied, and the safety and efficacy have been well established. The features of SBRT that are important for its safety and efficacy include motion management, daily image guidance, multiple beams for conformal radiation delivery, steep dose gradient, small tumor volumes, high dose per fraction with high biological effective dose delivery >100Gy. These treatment planning and delivery attributes make SBRT/SABR well suited for the definitive treatment of discrete lesions from cancer and have ultimately led to >90% tumor control rates with primary NSCLC (Lee et al. 2021) and oligometastatic lesions (Salama and Milano 2014), with acceptable rates of toxicity (Milano et al. 2008).

Further, SABR/SBRT for more limited and widespread NSCLC, combining immunotherapy with SBRT to potentiate the immune response, is an active area of investigation with promising results in preliminary studies. Two analyses have shown that, for patients with 1–5 oligometastatic lesions, SABR is cost effective compared with standard of care (Qu et al. 2021; Kumar et al. 2021). Other methodologies being used clinically, that require further study, include radiofrequency ablation and cryoablation. SBRT/SABR was recently approved by the British NHS as a cost-effective means of treating oligometastatic disease (Chalkidou et al. 2021).

2 Definition of OMD

In recent years, there have been efforts directed at refining the definition of OMD. Most published studies and clinical trials have defined oligometastases as the presence of up to three or five metastatic lesions.

The consensus recommendation for classifying oligometastatic disease by the European Society for Medical Oncology (ESMO) and the European Organization for Research and Treatment of Cancer (EORTC) included number of metastases as a quantitative characteristic of oligometastatic cancer but did not provide a definitive cutoff.

The European Society for Radiotherapy and Oncology (ESTRO) and the American Society for Radiation Oncology (ASTRO) convened a committee to establish consensus definition of OMD and define gaps in current evidence (Lievens et al. 2020). They performed a systematic review of the literature that focused on metastatic directed radiotherapy for OMD. The consensus was that the oligometastatic state is independent of the primary tumor, metastatic location, and presence or length of disease-free interval. There was also consensus for extra-cranial OMD being limited to a maximum of 5 metastatic lesions off-protocol. The group also supported the consensus that, due to the lack of validated biomarkers, the ability to deliver safe and clinically meaningful radiotherapy was a minimum requirement for OMD for radiation therapy planning.

There have been attempts at further classifying oligometastatic disease states, to characterize and risk stratify prognosis. This is important, as synchronous oligometastatic disease has been associated with a more aggressive disease phenotype and a worse prognosis than metachronous oligometastatic disease (Palma et al. 2015). Ashworth and colleagues, in their meta-analysis of outcomes and prognostic factors after treatment of oligometastatic NSCLC, stratified patients into low-risk metachronous metastatic disease (5-year overall survival rate of 47.8%), intermediate-risk synchronous metastases with N0 (5-year overall survival rate of 36.2%), and high-risk synchronous metastases N1/N2 (5-year overall survival rate of 13.8%) (Ashworth et al. 2013, 2014).

OMD can be further subclassified based on how and when it presents in relation to initial diagnosis and response to intervening therapy. If OMD presents at initial diagnosis, it is classified as synchronous/de novo oligometastatic disease. Oligorecurrence is a metachronous presentation of limited disease after definitive treatment for initial disease. A patient with initial presentation of widespread/poly-metastatic disease, left with limited OMD after receiving systemic therapy, may be referred to as having oligoresistance/induced oligometastases/oligoprogressive disease. The term oligoprogression has also been used to describe patients with widespread disease that is controlled but with few sites of progression. This may be seen with patients receiving tyrosine kinase inhibitors or targeted therapy, perhaps representing mutational changes in select sites that confer resistance to that therapy in those select sites.

Guckenberger and colleagues proposed an oligometastatic disease classification system that breaks down the oligometastatic state into eight subtypes (Guckenberger et al. 2020). The two broad categories were a genuine oligometastatic state and an induced oligometastatic state. The first genuine oligometastatic state is divided into synchronous/de novo OMD, metachronous oligorecurrence, and repeat oligorecurrence/persistence/progression. The induced state is subdivided into oligorecurrence, induced oligopersistence, or induced oligoprogression. Overall, the goal with these eight subdivisions is to test these states of oligometastatic disease in OligoCare prospective cohort trial NCT0318503, to risk stratify the disease, and to further clarify which patients with OMD might benefit from treatment.

It is worth emphasizing that currently without any other markers for validating the OMD, the consensus statement and staging for OM-NSCLC are limited by the quality of imaging modality. In the case of lung cancer, whole-body ^{18}F-FDG-PET/CT has been shown to be the most reliable imaging technique in assessing extracranial disease (Madsen et al. 2016). Furthermore, PET/CT imaging has shown that approximately 15% of NSCLC patients initially thought to be lower staged were upstaged to stage IV with the use of PET/CT in addition to CT imaging alone. PET/CT staging is associated with improved OS as outlined by several studies (Li et al. 2013; Tönnies et al. 2016). However, there are limitations to PET; PET is less reliable for adenocarcinoma histology, lesions <1 cm, lesions with the appearance of ground-glass opacity CT, and central tumors. Ashworth and colleagues, in their meta-analysis, also noted worse survival with adenocarcinoma vs. squamous cell histology among patients with OMD from NSCLC. Highlighting the need to overcome imaging limitations to have meaningful clinical benefit.

3 Clinical Studies

Clinical data for the aggressive treatment of OMD emerged in the 2000s. Select studies are summarized here.

3.1 Select Prospective Nonrandomized Studies of SBRT of OMD from NSCLC

A phase II prospective trial included 39 patients with synchronous OM-NSCLC (≤5 lesions) who were amenable for radical therapy to all tumor sites including the primary site (De Ruysscher et al. 2012). Treatment modalities included surgery, stereotactic radiosurgery, SBRT, and fractionated radiotherapy to a dose of 60 Gy. The vast majority of patients had a single metastatic focus, approximately 95% were treated with up-front chemotherapy, and approximately half had brain metastases. They reported a median progression-free survival of 12.1 months and overall survival of 13.5 months. Fifteen percent of the patients experienced grade 3 toxicity.

A prospective study from Belgium reported on 26 patients with synchronous OM-NSCLC patients with up to five metastases treated with SBRT (50 Gy in 10 fractions) (Collen et al. 2014). Notably, patients with uncontrolled primary tumors, intracranial sites, and multiorgan involvement were eligible; 65% of the patients received induction chemotherapy. The primary endpoint was complete metabolic response (CMR) on PET (3 months post-SBRT). Seventeen patients underwent SBRT after up-front chemotherapy, and the remaining underwent SBRT (to all sites) as primary treatment. Sixty percent of patients achieved metabolic response, with half of them reaching CMR. The median progression-free survival was 11.2 months and median overall survival 23 months. Fifteen percent of the patients experienced grade 2 toxicity and 8% had pulmonary toxicity. The inferior results of this study relative to the study by De Ruysscher et al. (2012) may be related to the larger proportion of patients with brain metastases, as well as few patients receiving systemic therapy, in their study.

An international multicenter phase II prospective trails assessed the role of SABR for oligometastatic cancer (Sutera et al. 2019). Patients with limited disease between one and five lesions were prospectively recruited. Patients must have had biopsy-proven oligometastatic or recurrent cancer defined on PET/CT imaging within 8 weeks of enrollment. Patient follow-up occurred within 6 weeks of completion of SABR and at 3-month intervals. A total of 147 patients with oligometastatic cancer were analyzed. The median age was 66.4 years. The most common primary tumors were lung (21.8%, NSCLC; $n = 29$, small-cell lung cancer: $n = 3$). With a median follow-up of 41.3 months, the median overall survival was 42.3 months (95% confidence interval: 27.4 months–not reached) with

5-year overall survival rate of 43%. Five-year local progression-free survival and distant progression-free survival were 74% and 17%, respectively. Acute grade 2+ and 3+ toxicities were 7.5% and 2.0%, respectively, and late grade 2+ and 3+ toxicities were both 1.4%. There was no significant change in quality of life at completion and 6 weeks, 3 months, and 9 months after treatment. Further, at 6 and 12 months, patients were found to have statistically significant improvement in patient-reported quality of life.

The University of Pennsylvania recently published their single-arm phase II trial that evaluated whether the addition of pembrolizumab after locally ablative therapy improves outcomes for patients with oligometastatic NSCLC (Bauml et al. 2019). A total of 51 patients with ≤4 lesions were enrolled and received up-front pembrolizumab, which was continued for 8 cycles, with provision to continue to 16 cycles in the absence of progressive disease or toxic effects. The primary endpoints were progression-free survival from the start of locally ablative therapy (progression-free survival-L) and progression-free survival from the start of pembrolizumab (progression-free survival-P). The secondary endpoints were overall survival. They reported a median progression-free survival-L of 19.1 months and progression-free survival-P of 18.7 months and 1-year overall survival of 90.9% at 12 months and 77.5% at 24 months. This is notably much improved compared to the value of 6.6 months that the authors used for their historical median survival.

3.2 Select Phase II Randomized Studies of SBRT of OMD

In 2019 SABR-COMET study, a phase II randomized open-label, controlled trial enrolled 99 patients with OMD from any cancer (Palma et al. 2019, 2020). Patients were assigned to the SABR group 66 (67%) or control group 33 (33%). All patients had to have a controlled primary tumor, one to five metastatic lesions, ECOG performance status score 0–1, and life expectance of >6 months. The main exclusions were serious medical comorbidities, bone metastasis in the femoral bone, and presence of one to three brain metastases with no extracranial disease. Eighteen percent of patients had lung cancer. The study reported that grade 2 or worse toxicity occurred in 3 of 33 (9%) controls and 19 of 66 patients (29%) in SABR group. Treatment-related death occurred in 3 of 66 patients (4.5%) after SABR. The median overall survival was 28 months (95% CI, 19–33 months) in the control group versus 41 months (26–not reached) in the SABR group (hazard ratio 0.57, 95% CI, 0.30–1.10; $p = 0.090$).

Gomez and colleagues conducted a randomized phase II trial in all patients with histologically confirmed stage IV NSCLC, with three for fewer OMD sites after first-line systemic therapy, with ECOG performance status of 0–2 (Gomez et al. 2016, 2019). Patients were randomized to receive or not receive local consolidative therapy—radiation or resection of all lesions (including primary sites). Patients in both arms were able to receive maintenance systemic therapy. The initial reports were released in 2016 and final results in 2019. The trial was closed early after 49 patients were randomly assigned because of a significant progression-free survival benefit in the local consolidative therapy arm. Initial reports showed progression-free survival of 11.9 months compared with 3.9 months. In an updated analysis, with a median follow-up of 38.8 months (range 28.3–61.4 months), the difference remained significant with a median progression-free survival of 14.2 months [95% CI, 7.4–23.1 months] with local consolidative therapy versus 4.4 months [95% CI, 2.2–8.3 months] with maintenance therapy/observation ($p = 0.022$). Consistent with SABR-COMET was an OS benefit in the local consolidative therapy arm (median 41.2 months [95% CI, 18.9 months to not reached] with local consolidative therapy vs. 17.0 months [95% CI, 10.1–39.8 months] with MT/O; $p = 0.017$). No additional grade 3 or greater toxicities were observed.

Iyengar and colleagues conducted another randomized phase II trial evaluating whether intervening with noninvasive stereotactic ablative therapy leads to improvements in progression-free survival (Iyengar et al. 2018). Patients who did not have ALK/EGFR mutation and those that achieved partial response or stable disease were randomized to SBRT + maintenance chemotherapy vs. maintenance chemotherapy. SBRT/SABR was delivered to all sites of gross disease. A total of 29 patients (9 women and 20 men) with NSCLC and up to 5 OMD lesions were enrolled. The trial was stopped early due to significant improvements with the addition of SBRT (progression-free survival 9.7 vs. 3.5 months, $p = 0.01$). Toxicities were similar in both arms. Overall consolidative SBRT prior to maintenance chemotherapy tripled progression-free survival with no difference in toxicity that was noted. Tables 1 and 2 summarize the studies by Gomez and Iyengar.

Table 1 Summary of key characteristics of randomized phase II studies by Gomez et al. (2019) and Iyengar et al. (2018)

Institutions	MDACC, U Colorado, London (ON)	UTSW
Study authors	Gomez et al.	Iyengar et al.
Patients		
• Planned	94	36
• Enrolled	74 (**49 randomized**)	**29**
Eligibility	1–3 metastatic lesions • Thoracic lymph nodes = 1 siteLesions with CR to chemo not counted No progression on systemic therapy	1–5 metastatic lesions • 1–3 lesions in lung (or liver) – *No* GI or skin metastases; CNS only if controlled No progression on systemic therapy
Stratification	# Sites (0–1, 2–3) Stable disease vs. partial response N stage (N0–1, N2–3) Oncogene (EGFR or ALK) driven	
Systemic therapy	4+ cycles of platinum doublet therapy *or* 3+ months of EGFR TKI *or* *3*+ months of crizotinib	4–6 cycles of platinum-based chemotherapy
Standard arm	Observation or maintenance systemic therapy	Maintenance systemic therapy
Radiotherapy arm	SBRT or 15-fraction RT to primary site SBRT to metastases → Observation or maintenance therapy	SBRT or 15-fraction RT to primary site SBRT to metastases (1, 3, or 5 fraction) → Maintenance systemic therapy

Table 2 Summary of patient characteristics and outcomes from the randomized phase II studies by Gomez et al. (2019) and Iyengar et al. (2018)

	MDACC, U Colorado, London (ON)		UTSW	
	+SBRT	No SBRT	+SBRT	No SBRT
#	25	24	14	15
Characteristics				
• No driver mutations	20 (80%)	21 (88%)	*All patients*	*All patients*
• Brain metastases	7 (28%)	6 (25%)	8 (57%)	10 (67%)
• PR/CR	9 (36%)	9 (38%)	Not reported	Not reported
• SD	16 (64%)	15 (62%)		
• Synchronous	24 (96%)	22 (92%)	Not reported	Not reported
• Metachronous	1 (4%)	2 (8%)		
Outcomes				
• Median OS	41.2 M	17 M ($p = 0.017$)	Not reached	17 M
• Median progression-free survival	14.2 M	4.4 M ($p = 0.022$)	9.7 M	3.5 M ($p = 0.01$)
• Time to new metastases	11.9 M	5.7 M ($p = 0.050$)		

M months

4 Meta-analysis

Lehrer and colleagues analyzed single- or multi-arm prospective trials that included patients with 1–5 extracranial lesions, treated with SBRT/SABR with fractional doses greater than 5 Gy, with 8 fractions or less (Lehrer et al. 2021). Overall, 21 studies comparing 943 patients and 1290 oligometastatic sites were included. The median age of patients was 63.8 years and median follow-up 16.9 months. The most common primary sites were prostate (22.9%), colorectal (16.6%), breast (13.1%), and lung (12.8%). The rate of acute grade 3–5 toxicity (using random effects models) was 1.2%, and the rate of grade 3–5 late toxicity was 1.7%. The estimate for 1-year local control was 94.7% (95% CI, 88.6–98.6%). The estimate for 1-year overall survival was 85.4% (95% CI, 77.1–92.0%) and 51.4% for 1-year progression-free survival (95% CI, 42.7–60.1%). The authors concluded that SABR/SBRT is safe in OMD with excellent local control, OS, and progression-free survival.

5 Selected Other Studies

A prospective registry-based cohort study, conducted by the National Health Service in England, also analyzed the use of SABR for patients with OMD (Chalkidou et al. 2021). A total of 1422 patients from 17 radiation therapy centers in England were included. The median age of the patients was 69 years; a variety of histological lesions were included the most common primary tumor was prostate cancer 28.6%, and 4.5% of patient has lung cancer in this study. The study specifically looked at the use of SABR with metachronous oligometastatic lesions, defined as those sites that developed more than 6 months after a primary cancer diagnosis. The only exception was for synchronous metastases from colorectal cancer. All oligometastatic lesions were limited to a maximum size of 6 cm. After a median follow-up of 13 months, the overall survival was 92.3% at 1 year and 79.2% at 2 years, specifically for lung cancer OS at 1 and 2 years are 80.2%, 64.4% respectively. A low rate of overall toxicity were noted, the most common grade 3 event was fatigue experienced in 2% of the study population (2.0% of patients), Rates of grade 3 pneumonitis, and pericarditis were <1%; no grade 4 lung or heart toxicities were noted.

6 Molecular Studies

There has been less progress made in understanding and defining oligometastatic disease based upon tumor biology. The classic "seed and soil" hypothesis recognized the complex interplay between "seed"—tumor biology—and "soil," which constitutes the complex micro- and macro-environment that cancer cells maneuver to establish the metastatic state.

It is generally well accepted that the tumor "seed" goes through a series of sequential steps that must be taken prior to metastatic spread. There is usually a loss of cell adhesion, dedifferentiation, increased migration kinetics, adhesion and invasion of circulatory vessels, extravasation, and colonization of distant sites. These processes are reliant on changes at the genetic and epigenetic level and interaction with micro- and macro-environment (Gupta and Massagué 2006; Nguyen and Massagué 2007; Chiang and Massagué 2008). These processes also in part hide the tumor cells from the immune surveillance. Further, there is a large heterogeneity within the tumor cell population, which can produce cells with increased metastatic potential, so-called clonogenic cells (Shindo-Okada et al. 2001; Li et al. 2001).

There have been various genetic studies to identify genes responsible for the transition to oligometastatic state. For NSCLC, there is still work being done to identify genes responsible for OMD.

In the area of epigenetics, microRNAs (miRNAs) have a role in evaluating patients with oligometastatic disease. microRNAs are noncoding segments of RNA that post-translationally regulate RNA expression. A study from the University of Chicago demonstrated, in mouse xenograft models, that miR-200 family overexpression correlated with progression from oligometastatic to poly-metastatic lung disease (Lussier et al. 2011, 2012). The miR-200 family is known to maintain the epithelial phenotype, and overexpression is correlated with the transition to mesenchymal state required for metastatic progression. However, understanding of the role of miR-200 is evolving (Dykxhoorn et al. 2009). Other studies have validated miR-200c conferring cellular morphology for metastases; the miR-200 family overall has also been shown to maintain the epithelial phenotype (Gregory et al. 2008; Elson-Schwab et al. 2010).

Researchers at the University of Chicago examined the molecular markers in a cohort of 61 treated patients with SBRT, 17 of whom had samples that allowed for molecular analysis (Wong et al. 2016). They showed that miR23b was over expressed in those treated with SBRT with survival >3 years, and miR-449a and mirR-499b were overexpressed in those living <3 years. However, of the three genes identified, none were statistically significant, thus requiring independent validation.

In the seed and soil hypothesis, the concept of soil acknowledges the role of the immune system, and the tumor milieu in which the tumor operates plays an important role in the metastatic state. There has been a multitude of proposed mechanisms that SBRT may enhance immune function, altering tumor stroma, promoting antigen presentation (Schreiber et al. 2011; Weichselbaum et al. 2017; Pitroda and Weichselbaum 2019; Pitroda et al. 2019; Brooks and Chang 2019). Much of the data currently is preliminary and limited to the realm of hypothesis generating.

7 Ongoing Studies and Future Directions

There has been considerable progress made since initially defining the oligometastatic state for NSCLC. Clearer definition of subsets of patients from the effort by ESTRO and EORTC (Guckenberger et al. 2020) will facilitate more refined studies based upon the subclassifications of OMD. Following that effort, the intention of ESTRO and EORTC is to use this classification system to prospectively evaluate patients in the OligoCare study.

Although the results from recent randomized phase II data for patients with OMD from NSCLC are strong, phase III trials are still needed. There are currently multiple trials underway examining in a multitude of regions around the world.

In the United Kingdom, two phase III trials are underway. SARON (NCT02417662) is a large, randomized controlled, multicenter (approximately 30 sites) phase III trial for patients with oligometastatic NSCLC (1–3 sites of synchronous metastatic disease, one of which must be extracranial). Patients with NSCLC with driver mutations of EGFR, ALK, or ROS1 are excluded. Eligible patients will be randomized to either standard-doublet chemotherapy or standard chemotherapy followed by SABR to primary and SABR/SRS to all other sites. The primary endpoint is overall survival; the study is powered to detect an improvement in median survival from 9.9 months in the control arm to 14.3 months in the investigational arm with 85% power and two-sided 5% significance level. The secondary endpoints are LC, progression-free survival, new distant metastasis-free survival, toxicity, and quality of life. Unlike other phase II studies for NSCLC, SARON includes patients with intracranial metastases. Patients will be stratified based on whether or not they received both conventional radiotherapy for their primary cancer in addition to SBRT for metastatic sites.

Another phase III study from the United Kingdom is the conventional care versus radioablation (stereotactic body radiotherapy) for extracranial oligometastases (NCT02759783; CORE). This is a multicenter, nonblinded, randomized trial conducted by the Institute of Cancer Research in the United Kingdom and in collaboration with researchers from Australia. The trial will enroll patients with NSCLC primary cancer (other histologies allowed included breast and prostate) with ≤3 extracranial, metachronous, oligometastases, all suitable for SBRT, and compare standard of care with or without SBRT for extracranial metastases.

Standard of care includes systemic therapy, palliative radiotherapy, or observation at investigators' discretion. Patients who are randomized to receive SBRT with SOC will receive a dose and fractionation regimen dependent on the site of OMD and constraints of the organs at risk.

In Canada, there are two phase III studies extending on the SABR-COMET study: SABR-COMET 3 (NCT03862911) (2020) recruiting patients with up to three metastases and SABR-COMET 10 (NCT03721341) (2019) with 4–10 metastases. These studies will provide further evidence on the effect of number of metastases on the survival in patients with oligometastatic cancer. In both SABR-COMET 3 and 10, patients are required to have SBRT treatment planning before randomization to demonstrate the safety and feasibility of SBRT in that patient. The doses have also been adjusted relative to the original SABR study, such that the preferred doses are 20 Gy × 1 fraction, 30 Gy in 3 fractions, and 35 Gy in 5 fractions so that they all have relatively similar biologically effective values of 60 Gy (using linear-quadratic model with an alpha-beta ratio of 10). These are lower than the ablative doses used in the initial SABR-COMET study (Palma et al. 2019). The ARREST study is examining whether SABR can be used in the poly-metastatic setting (>10 metastases).

In the United States, NRG-LU002 study (NCT03137771) is being conducted to evaluate maintenance systemic therapy with vs. without local consolidative therapy for NSCLC, with a target accrual of 378 patients. Patients are stratified based upon the histology and receipt of immunotherapy. Eligible patients have 1–3 sites of metastases, at least one of which is amenable to SBRT, and all amenable to SBRT or resection. Patients with synchronous or metachronous metastases are eligible. For those with synchronous metastases, the primary sites are treated with 15-fraction radiotherapy or SBRT. Primary objectives are progression-free survival (for the phase IIR component) and overall survival (phase III component). Secondary endpoints include in-field recurrence, development of new lesions, toxicity, duration of maintenance therapy, quality-of-life measures, and circulating DNA analyses.

8 Conclusions

SBRT for patients with OMD from NSCLC is an emerging technique, with compelling evidence of improved outcomes vs. standard-of-care therapy alone. The treatment paradigm for metastatic NSCLC is continually evolving with immunotherapy greatly improving survival outcomes and becoming standard of care. It is worth emphasizing that as improvements in survival for NSCLC from more effective systemic therapy evolve, metastasis-directed local therapy may become more important. The Norton-Simon hypothesis postulates that a given systemic therapy at a given dose is less effective in terms of cell kill as the overall tumor burden increases. Metastasis-directed therapy can therefore effectively reduce this burden. Finally, improvements in imaging modalities, characterizing molecular signatures, and refining and subclassifying OMD are on the horizon. A deeper understanding of the molecular biology of OMD, and how molecular signatures can correlate with outcomes and response to SBRT, is needed.

References

Ashworth A, Rodrigues G, Boldt G, Palma D (2013) Is there an oligometastatic state in non-small cell lung cancer? A systematic review of the literature. Lung Cancer 82(2):197–203. https://doi.org/10.1016/j.lungcan.2013.07.026. Epub 2013 Aug 20

Ashworth AB, Senan S, Palma DA, Riquet M, Ahn YC, Ricardi U, Congedo MT, Gomez DR, Wright GM, Melloni G, Milano MT, Sole CV, De Pas TM, Carter DL, Warner AJ, Rodrigues GB (2014) An individual patient data meta-analysis of outcomes and prognostic factors after treatment of oligometastatic non-small-cell lung cancer. Clin Lung Cancer 15(5):346–355. https://doi.org/10.1016/j.cllc.2014.04.003. Epub 2014 May 15

Aujla KS, Katz AW, Singh DP, Okunieff P, Milano MT (2019) Hypofractionated stereotactic radiotherapy for non-breast or prostate cancer oligometastases: a tail of survival beyond 10 years. Front Oncol 9:111. https://doi.org/10.3389/fonc.2019.00111

Bauml JM, Mick R, Ciunci C, Aggarwal C, Davis C, Evans T, Deshpande C, Miller L, Patel P, Alley E, Knepley C, Mutale F, Cohen RB, Langer CJ (2019) Pembrolizumab after completion of locally ablative therapy for oligometastatic non-small cell lung cancer: a phase 2 trial. JAMA Oncol 5(9):1283–1290. https://

doi.org/10.1001/jamaoncol.2019.1449. Epub ahead of print

Bergsma DP, Salama JK, Singh DP, Chmura SJ, Milano MT (2015) The evolving role of radiotherapy in treatment of oligometastatic NSCLC. Expert Rev Anticancer Ther 15(12):1459–1471. https://doi.org/10.1586/14737140.2015.1105745. Epub 2015 Nov 4

Bergsma DP, Salama JK, Singh DP, Chmura SJ, Milano MT (2017) Radiotherapy for oligometastatic lung cancer. Front Oncol 7:210. https://doi.org/10.3389/fonc.2017.00210

Brooks ED, Chang JY (2019) Time to abandon single-site irradiation for inducing abscopal effects. Nat Rev Clin Oncol 16(2):123–135. https://doi.org/10.1038/s41571-018-0119-7

Chalkidou A, Macmillan T, Grzeda MT, Peacock J, Summers J, Eddy S, Coker B, Patrick H, Powell H, Berry L, Webster G, Ostler P, Dickinson PD, Hatton MQ, Henry A, Keevil S, Hawkins MA, Slevin N, van As N (2021) Stereotactic ablative body radiotherapy in patients with oligometastatic cancers: a prospective, registry-based, single-arm, observational, evaluation study. Lancet Oncol 22(1):98–106. https://doi.org/10.1016/S1470-2045(20)30537-4

Cheruvu P, Metcalfe SK, Metcalfe J, Chen Y, Okunieff P, Milano MT (2011) Comparison of outcomes in patients with stage III versus limited stage IV non-small cell lung cancer. Radiat Oncol 6:80. https://doi.org/10.1186/1748-717X-6-80

Chiang AC, Massagué J (2008) Molecular basis of metastasis. N Engl J Med 359(26):2814–2823. https://doi.org/10.1056/NEJMra0805239

Collen C, Christian N, Schallier D, Meysman M, Duchateau M, Storme G, De Ridder M (2014) Phase II study of stereotactic body radiotherapy to primary tumor and metastatic locations in oligometastatic nonsmall-cell lung cancer patients. Ann Oncol 25(10):1954–1959. https://doi.org/10.1093/annonc/mdu370. Epub 2014 Aug 11

De Ruysscher D, Wanders R, van Baardwijk A, Dingemans AM, Reymen B, Houben R, Bootsma G, Pitz C, van Eijsden L, Geraedts W, Baumert BG, Lambin P (2012) Radical treatment of non-small-cell lung cancer patients with synchronous oligometastases: long-term results of a prospective phase II trial (Nct01282450). J Thorac Oncol 7(10):1547–1555. https://doi.org/10.1097/JTO.0b013e318262caf6

Dykxhoorn DM, Wu Y, Xie H, Yu F, Lal A, Petrocca F, Martinvalet D, Song E, Lim B, Lieberman J (2009) miR-200 enhances mouse breast cancer cell colonization to form distant metastases. PLoS One 4(9):e7181. https://doi.org/10.1371/journal.pone.0007181

Elson-Schwab I, Lorentzen A, Marshall CJ (2010) MicroRNA-200 family members differentially regulate morphological plasticity and mode of melanoma cell invasion. PLoS One 5(10):e13176. https://doi.org/10.1371/journal.pone.0013176

Gomez DR, Blumenschein GR Jr, Lee JJ, Hernandez M, Ye R, Camidge DR, Doebele RC, Skoulidis F, Gaspar LE, Gibbons DL, Karam JA, Kavanagh BD, Tang C, Komaki R, Louie AV, Palma DA, Tsao AS, Sepesi B, William WN, Zhang J, Shi Q, Wang XS, Swisher SG, Heymach JV (2016) Local consolidative therapy versus maintenance therapy or observation for patients with oligometastatic non-small-cell lung cancer without progression after first-line systemic therapy: a multicentre, randomised, controlled, phase 2 study. Lancet Oncol 17(12):1672–1682. https://doi.org/10.1016/S1470-2045(16)30532-0. Epub 2016 Oct 24

Gomez DR, Tang C, Zhang J, Blumenschein GR Jr, Hernandez M, Lee JJ, Ye R, Palma DA, Louie AV, Camidge DR, Doebele RC, Skoulidis F, Gaspar LE, Welsh JW, Gibbons DL, Karam JA, Kavanagh BD, Tsao AS, Sepesi B, Swisher SG, Heymach JV (2019) Local consolidative therapy vs. maintenance therapy or observation for patients with oligometastatic non-small-cell lung cancer: long-term results of a multi-institutional, phase II, randomized study. J Clin Oncol 37(18):1558–1565. https://doi.org/10.1200/JCO.19.00201. Epub 2019 May 8

Gregory PA, Bert AG, Paterson EL, Barry SC, Tsykin A, Farshid G, Vadas MA, Khew-Goodall Y, Goodall GJ (2008) The miR-200 family and miR-205 regulate epithelial to mesenchymal transition by targeting ZEB1 and SIP1. Nat Cell Biol 10(5):593–601. https://doi.org/10.1038/ncb1722. Epub 2008 Mar 30

Guckenberger M, Lievens Y, Bouma AB, Collette L, Dekker A, deSouza NM, Dingemans AC, Fournier B, Hurkmans C, Lecouvet FE, Meattini I, Méndez Romero A, Ricardi U, Russell NS, Schanne DH, Scorsetti M, Tombal B, Verellen D, Verfaillie C, Ost P (2020) Characterisation and classification of oligometastatic disease: a European Society for Radiotherapy and Oncology and European Organisation for Research and Treatment of Cancer consensus recommendation. Lancet Oncol 21(1):e18–e28. https://doi.org/10.1016/S1470-2045(19)30718-1

Gupta GP, Massagué J (2006) Cancer metastasis: building a framework. Cell 127(4):679–695. https://doi.org/10.1016/j.cell.2006.11.001

Hellman S, Weichselbaum RR (1995) Oligometastases. J Clin Oncol 13(1):8–10. https://doi.org/10.1200/JCO.1995.13.1.8

Iyengar P, Wardak Z, Gerber DE, Tumati V, Ahn C, Hughes RS, Dowell JE, Cheedella N, Nedzi L, Westover KD, Pulipparacharuvil S, Choy H, Timmerman RD (2018) Consolidative radiotherapy for limited metastatic non-small-cell lung cancer: a phase 2 randomized clinical trial. JAMA Oncol 4(1):e173501. https://doi.org/10.1001/jamaoncol.2017.3501. Epub 2018 Jan 11

Kumar A, Straka C, Courtney PT, Vitzthum L, Riviere P, Murphy JD (2021) Cost-Effectiveness Analysis of Stereotactic Ablative Radiation Therapy in Patients With Oligometastatic Cancer. Int J Radiat Oncol Biol Phys. 109(5):1185–1194. https://doi.org/10.1016/j.ijrobp.2020.09.045. Epub 2020 Sep 28. PMID: 33002541.

Lee P, Loo BW Jr, Biswas T, Ding GX, El Naqa IM, Jackson A, Kong FM, LaCouture T, Miften M, Solberg T, Tome WA, Tai A, Yorke E, Li XA (2021) Local control after stereotactic body radiation therapy for stage I non-small cell lung cancer. Int J Radiat Oncol Biol Phys 110(1):160–171

Lehrer EJ, Singh R, Wang M, Chinchilli VM, Trifiletti DM, Ost P, Siva S, Meng MB, Tchelebi L, Zaorsky NG (2021) Safety and survival rates associated with ablative stereotactic radiotherapy for patients with oligometastatic cancer: a systematic review and meta-analysis. JAMA Oncol 7(1):92–106. https://doi.org/10.1001/jamaoncol.2020.6146

Li Y, Tang ZY, Ye SL, Liu YK, Chen J, Xue Q, Chen J, Gao DM, Bao WH (2001) Establishment of cell clones with different metastatic potential from the metastatic hepatocellular carcinoma cell line MHCC97. World J Gastroenterol 7(5):630–636. https://doi.org/10.3748/wjg.v7.i5.630

Li J, Xu W, Kong F, Sun X, Zuo X (2013) Meta-analysis: accuracy of 18FDG PET-CT for distant metastasis staging in lung cancer patients. Surg Oncol 22(3):151–155. https://doi.org/10.1016/j.suronc.2013.04.001. Epub 2013 May 9

Lievens Y, Guckenberger M, Gomez D, Hoyer M, Iyengar P, Kindts I, Méndez Romero A, Nevens D, Palma D, Park C, Ricardi U, Scorsetti M, Yu J, Woodward WA (2020) Defining oligometastatic disease from a radiation oncology perspective: an ESTRO-ASTRO consensus document. Radiother Oncol 148:157–166. https://doi.org/10.1016/j.radonc.2020.04.003. Epub 2020 Apr 22

Lussier YA, Xing HR, Salama JK, Khodarev NN, Huang Y, Zhang Q, Khan SA, Yang X, Hasselle MD, Darga TE, Malik R, Fan H, Perakis S, Filippo M, Corbin K, Lee Y, Posner MC, Chmura SJ, Hellman S, Weichselbaum RR (2011) MicroRNA expression characterizes oligometastasis(es). PLoS One 6(12):e28650. https://doi.org/10.1371/journal.pone.0028650. Epub 2011 Dec 13

Lussier YA, Khodarev NN, Regan K, Corbin K, Li H, Ganai S, Khan SA, Gnerlich JL, Darga TE, Fan H, Karpenko O, Paty PB, Posner MC, Chmura SJ, Hellman S, Ferguson MK, Weichselbaum RR (2012) Oligo- and polymetastatic progression in lung metastasis(es) patients is associated with specific microRNAs. PLoS One 7(12):e50141. https://doi.org/10.1371/journal.pone.0050141. Epub 2012 Dec 10. Erratum in: PLoS One. 2013;8(6). https://doi.org/10.1371/annotation/2489ae5e-3650-4897-8df6-3e974ca585c4. Gnerlich, Jennifer [corrected to Gnerlich, Jennifer L]

Madsen PH, Holdgaard PC, Christensen JB, Hoilund-Carlsen PF (2016) Clinical utility of F-18 FDG PET-CT in the initial evaluation of lung cancer. Eur J Nucl Med Mol Imaging 43:2084–2097

Milano MT, Constine LS, Okunieff P (2008) Normal tissue toxicity after small field hypofractionated stereotactic body radiation. Radiat Oncol 3:36. https://doi.org/10.1186/1748-717X-3-36

Milano MT, Biswas T, Simone CB II, Lo SS (2021) Oligometastases: history of a hypothesis. Ann Palliat Med 10(5):5923–5930

Nguyen DX, Massagué J (2007) Genetic determinants of cancer metastasis. Nat Rev Genet 8(5):341–352. https://doi.org/10.1038/nrg2101

Palma DA, Louie AV, Rodrigues GB (2015) New strategies in stereotactic radiotherapy for oligometastases. Clin Cancer Res 21(23):5198–5204. https://doi.org/10.1158/1078-0432.CCR-15-0822

Palma DA, Olson R, Harrow S, Gaede S, Louie AV, Haasbeek C, Mulroy L, Lock M, Rodrigues GB, Yaremko BP, Schellenberg D, Ahmad B, Griffioen G, Senthi S, Swaminath A, Kopek N, Liu M, Moore K, Currie S, Bauman GS, Warner A, Senan S (2019) Stereotactic ablative radiotherapy versus standard of care palliative treatment in patients with oligometastatic cancers (SABR-COMET): a randomised, phase 2, open-label trial. Lancet. 393(10185):2051–2058. https://doi.org/10.1016/S0140-6736(18)32487-5. Epub 2019 Apr 11. PMID: 30982687.

Palma DA, Olson R, Harrow S, Gaede S, Louie AV, Haasbeek C, Mulroy L, Lock M, Rodrigues GB, Yaremko BP, Schellenberg D, Ahmad B, Senthi S, Swaminath A, Kopek N, Liu M, Moore K, Currie S, Schlijper R, Bauman GS, Laba J, Qu XM, Warner A, Senan S (2020) Stereotactic Ablative Radiotherapy for the Comprehensive Treatment of Oligometastatic Cancers: Long-Term Results of the SABR-COMET Phase II Randomized Trial. J Clin Oncol. 38(25):2830–2838. https://doi.org/10.1200/JCO.20.00818. Epub 2020 Jun 2. PMID: 32484754; PMCID: PMC7460150

Peters LJ, Milas L, Fletcher GH (1983) The role of radiation therapy in the curative treatment of metastatic disease. Symp Fundam Cancer Res 36:411–420

Pitroda SP, Weichselbaum RR (2019) Integrated molecular and clinical staging defines the spectrum of metastatic cancer. Nat Rev Clin Oncol 16(9):581–588. https://doi.org/10.1038/s41571-019-0220-6

Pitroda SP, Chmura SJ, Weichselbaum RR (2019) Integration of radiotherapy and immunotherapy for treatment of oligometastases. Lancet Oncol 20(8):e434–e442. https://doi.org/10.1016/S1470-2045(19)30157-3. Epub 2019 Jul 29

Qu XM, Chen Y, Zaric GS, Senan S, Olson RA, Harrow S, John-Baptiste A, Gaede S, Mulroy LA, Schellenberg D, Senthi S, Swaminath A, Kopek N, Liu M, Warner A, Rodrigues GB, Palma DA, Louie AV (2021) Is SABR Cost-Effective in Oligometastatic Cancer? An Economic Analysis of the SABR-COMET Randomized Trial. Int J Radiat Oncol Biol Phys. 109(5):1176–1184. https://doi.org/10.1016/j.ijrobp.2020.12.001. Epub 2020 Dec 10. PMID: 33309977.

Rubin P (1968) Comment: Are metastases curable? JAMA 204(7):612–613

Rubin P, Green J (1968) Solitary metastases. C. C. Thomas, Springfield, IL

SABR-COMET 3: Olson R, Mathews L, Liu M, Schellenberg D, Mou B, Berrang T, Harrow S, Correa RJM, Bhat V, Pai H, Mohamed I, Miller S, Schneiders F, Laba J, Wilke D, Senthi S, Louie AV, Swaminath A, Chalmers A, Gaede S, Warner A, de Gruijl TD, Allan

A, Palma DA (2020) Stereotactic ablative radiotherapy for the comprehensive treatment of 1-3 Oligometastastic tumors (SABR-COMET-3): study protocol for a randomized phase III trial. BMC Cancer. 20(1):380. https://doi.org/10.1186/s12885-020-06876-4. PMID: 32370765; PMCID: PMC7201684.

SABR COMET 10: Palma DA, Olson R, Harrow S, Correa RJM, Schneiders F, Haasbeek CJA, Rodrigues GB, Lock M, Yaremko BP, Bauman GS, Ahmad B, Schellenberg D, Liu M, Gaede S, Laba J, Mulroy L, Senthi S, Louie AV, Swaminath A, Chalmers A, Warner A, Slotman BJ, de Gruijl TD, Allan A, Senan S (2019) Stereotactic ablative radiotherapy for the comprehensive treatment of 4-10 oligometastatic tumors (SABR-COMET-10): study protocol for a randomized phase III trial. BMC Cancer. 19(1):816. https://doi.org/10.1186/s12885-019-5977-6. PMID: 31426760; PMCID: PMC6699121.

Salama JK, Milano MT (2014) Radical irradiation of extracranial oligometastases. J Clin Oncol 32(26):2902–2912. https://doi.org/10.1200/JCO.2014.55.9567. Epub 2014 Aug 11

Schreiber RD, Old LJ, Smyth MJ (2011) Cancer immunoediting: integrating immunity's roles in cancer suppression and promotion. Science 331(6024):1565–1570. https://doi.org/10.1126/science.1203486

Shindo-Okada N, Takeuchi K, Nagamachi Y (2001) Establishment of cell lines with high- and low-metastatic potential from PC-14 human lung adenocarcinoma. Jpn J Cancer Res 92(2):174–183. https://doi.org/10.1111/j.1349-7006.2001.tb01080.x

Sutera P, Clump DA, Kalash R, D'Ambrosio D, Mihai A, Wang H, Petro DP, Burton SA, Heron DE (2019) Initial results of a multicenter phase 2 trial of stereotactic ablative radiation therapy for oligometastatic cancer. Int J Radiat Oncol Biol Phys 103(1):116–122. https://doi.org/10.1016/j.ijrobp.2018.08.027. Epub 2018 Aug 25

Tönnies S, Tönnies M, Kollmeier J, Bauer TT, Förster GJ, Kaiser D, Wernecke KD, Pfannschmidt J (2016) Impact of preoperative 18F-FDG PET/CT on survival of resected mono-metastatic non-small cell lung cancer. Lung Cancer 93:28–34. https://doi.org/10.1016/j.lungcan.2015.12.008. Epub 2015 Dec 30

Weichselbaum RR, Liang H, Deng L, Fu YX (2017) Radiotherapy and immunotherapy: a beneficial liaison? Nat Rev Clin Oncol 14(6):365–379. https://doi.org/10.1038/nrclinonc.2016.211. Epub 2017 Jan 17

Wong AC, Watson SP, Pitroda SP, Son CH, Das LC, Stack ME, Uppal A, Oshima G, Khodarev NN, Salama JK, Weichselbaum RR, Chmura SJ (2016) Clinical and molecular markers of long-term survival after oligometastasis-directed stereotactic body radiotherapy (SBRT). Cancer 122(14):2242–2250. https://doi.org/10.1002/cncr.30058. Epub 2016 May 20

Part VI

Current Treatment Strategies in Small Cell Lung Cancer

Radiation Therapy in Limited Disease Small Cell Lung Cancer

Branislav Jeremić, Ivane Kiladze, Pavol Dubinsky, and Slobodan Milisavljević

Contents

1 Introduction 651
2 RT in "EARLY" LD SCLC 652
3 RT in LD SCLC 653
4 Specific Aspects of TRT IN LD SCLC 659
5 What Is Practiced and Recommended Nowadays? 660
6 Future Aspects 661
References 662

B. Jeremić (✉)
School of Medicine, University of Kragujevac, Kragujevac, Serbia
e-mail: nebareje@gmail.com

I. Kiladze
Department of Clinical Oncology, Caucasus Medical Center, Tbilisi, Georgia

P. Dubinsky
University Hospital to East Slovakia Institute of Oncology, Kosice, Slovakia

S. Milisavljević
Department of Thoracic Surgery, University Clinical Center, Kragujevac, Serbia

Abstract

Patients with limited disease small cell lung cancer (LD SCLC) represent one-third of all patients with SCLC. Accumulated evidence over the past several decades points to as early concurrent thoracic radiation therapy (TRT) and platinum-etoposide (PE) as possible (cycle 1 or 2). TRT dose and fractionation favor hyperfractionated accelerated TRT using 45 Gy in 30 fractions in 15 days, but researchers and groups/societies still recommend conventionally fractionated TRT doses to 60–70 Gy. Increased evidence of efficacy of various immunotherapy agents in non-small cell lung cancer led to a number of prospective clinical trials investigating same compounds as part of combined modality approach in LD SCLC.

1 Introduction

Small cell lung cancer (SCLC) is the most aggressive histological subtype of all lung cancers and is characterized by having a rapid doubling time and high growth rate, early dissemination with over 70% of patients being diagnosed with metastatic disease at the time of diagnosis (Govindan et al. 2006; Yin et al. 2019;

National Cancer Institute 2020) and frequently rapid symptom onset (Van Meerbeeck et al. 2011). It comprises about 15% of all lung cancer cases (Govindan et al. 2006). While the incidence of SCLC is strongly associated with cigarette smoking, fewer new cases of SCLC are being diagnosed overall as smoking prevalence has decreased in Western world. Contrary to that, however, the incidence has increased in women, accounting for 50% of new cases, reflecting changes in smoking habits (Kalemkerian et al. 2013; Bray et al. 2018). Histologically, it is a high-grade neuroendocrine tumor, characterized by small round blue malignant cells that stain positive for chromogranin A, synaptophysin and having a high Ki-67 index (Taneja and Sharma 2004; Pelosi et al. 2014; Kalemkerian et al. 2018).

In the 1950s, the Veterans Administration Lung Study Group (VALSG) developed a staging system for SCLC that split the disease into limited disease (LD SCLC) and extensive disease (ED SCLC) (Micke et al. 2002). LD SCLC is defined as the disease confined to the hemithorax of origin along with the involved regional lymph nodes (hilar and mediastinal), with or without ipsilateral supraclavicular lymph nodes. It can also be considered as a disease which can be incorporated within a single, tolerable radiation therapy (RT) treatment field, and may include patients with contralateral, mediastinal, or hilar lymph nodes. What has created confusion and still does it is the term "tolerable RT treatment field." It was not always easy to denote and compare it between clinicians, especially radiation oncologists. Overall, less than one-third of patients with SCLC are diagnosed with LD. On the other hand, the classic oncological staging system, which uses tumor, node, and metastases (TNM) descriptors, has only recently been applied to SCLC. Several studies examining SCLC and TNM staging confirmed a correlation between TNM stage and survival, which was later on seen as strong tool for both clinical and pathological staging (Shepherd et al. 2007; Vallieres et al. 2009). More frequent use of the TNM staging system in recent years was seen as a welcome, albeit slow, shift towards improved staging precision, reporting and communication. This seems to be of particular importance when discussing the place and role of surgery in early LD SCLC.

Surgery was almost completely abandoned after the data of the Medical Research Council trial in the 1960s became available, which showed better overall survival (OS) for RT compared to surgery (Miller et al. 1969) as well as those of the study by The Lung Cancer Study Group 832 phase III randomized clinical trial, which also found no survival benefit with surgery for LS-SCLC (median OS, 15.4 vs. 18.6 months; $p = 0.78$) (Lad et al. 1994). A recent Cochrane analysis based on these two trials and another for all lung cancer histologies was inconclusive with respect to the role of surgery for clinical Stage I SCLC (Barnes et al. 2017). The past 2 decades, however, brought some evidence, albeit being of single-institutional or large data bases retrospective analysis, supporting surgery in early LD SCLC (Inoue et al. 2000; Brock et al. 2005; Combs et al. 2015; Ahmed et al. 2017). Beside further studies focusing on surgery alone, prospective randomized trials comparing surgery to RT alone (conventional or stereotactic ablative radiotherapy—SABR) with or without chemotherapy (CHT) should be considered as one of the priorities for thoracic oncologists in this setting.

2 RT in "EARLY" LD SCLC

Patients with early (Stage I and II) LD SCLC have frequently been lumped with those of more advanced LD SCLC, i.e., Stage III LD SCLC in various retrospective and prospective studies, hence, specific data per stage was frequently missing. In one recent study, however, Salem et al. (2019) reported on a subgroup analysis of patients enrolled during CONVERT trial where 16.9% patients had TNM Stage I to II disease. Patients with Stage I to II disease achieved longer overall median survival time (MST) (50 vs 25 months; hazard ratio, 0.60, 95% CI, 0.44–0.83; $p = 0.001$) compared with patients with Stage III disease. Similarly to overall results of that trial, in patients with Stage I to II disease, no significant survival difference was found between the trial arms. The incidences of acute and late toxic effects were not significantly different, but there was lower incidence of acute esophagitis in patients with Stage I to II disease compared with patients with Stage III disease (grade ≥ 3, 11.3% vs 21.1%; $p < 0.001$).

Largely due to excellent results achieved in early non-small cell lung cancer (NSCLC), SABR has been increasingly used in these patients, with CHT being given in 50–100% patients. Several retrospective studies, single (Videtic et al. 2013; Ly et al. 2014) or multi-institutional (Shioyama et al. 2013; Verma et al. 2017) or those using the data from large databases (Stahl et al. 2017), mostly reporting on a limited number of patients, documented MSTs up to 24 months, 3-year OS up to 70%, and 3-year disease-free survival (DFS) up to 85%. Quite similar to experience in early NSCLC, local control was 95–100% (Videtic et al. 2013; Shioyama et al. 2013; Verma et al. 2017). In a single center, prospective phase II study, Li et al. (2014) reconfirmed these results in LD SCLC patients which received 4–6 cycles of standard cisplatin–etoposide (PE) at 3 weekly intervals. SABR at a dose of 40–45 Gy in 10 fractions was given concurrently with CHT starting on day 1. Twenty-nine patients were followed up for a median duration of 19 (range, 10–85) months. The MST was 27 months and the median PFS was 12 months. Grade 3 adverse events occurred in 13.8% patients. Neutropenia of any grade was observed in 15% patients, with grade 3 neutropenia only seen in only 3.4% patients. No grade 4 adverse events were observed.

While prospective randomized studies are lacking, accumulated experience seems to favor SABR with additional CHT in early LD SCLC when surgery is contraindicated, but patients can still stand CHT. Besides "technical" questions (dose, fractionation, volumes), questions whether SABR could be used in highly selected cases as postoperative RT, or whether CHT could or should be replaced or augmented by immunotherapy remain unanswered today. Almost certainly these questions request multi-institutional cooperation, having in mind that very few percent of LD SCLC cases would continue falling into a Stage I and II category.

3 RT in LD SCLC

While CHT was traditionally considered the mainstay of the treatment, however, it leads to intrathoracic failure rates in up to 80% when given alone, leading to a median survival of 10–14 months (Cohen et al. 1979). RT was increasingly practiced in the seventies and the eighties of the last century and showed it can significantly decrease locoregional failures. However, RT became an indispensible part of the combined modality approach only when results of two meta-analyses appeared almost simultaneously two decades ago (Pignon et al. 1992; Warde and Payne 1992). These two analyses showed small but significant improvement in 2-year and 3-year survival, averaging 5–7% and an improvement in local control rates in 25% of cases when thoracic RT (TRT) was used. While many CHT agents achieve response rates of $\geq 30\%$ in SCLC (Sandler 2003), studies done in the last four decades established PE as preferred regimen to combine with TRT due to its activity and low toxicity shown more than 30 years ago (Einhorn et al. 1988). These results were reconfirmed by prospective randomized trials (Sundstrøm et al. 2002) and systematic reviews and meta-analyses (Mascaux et al. 2000; Pujol et al. 2000) but opposite results challenged it (Amarasena et al. 2008). Although majority of investigators continue to consider PE and TRT as the mainstay of concurrent treatment today, carboplatin (C) was sometimes used instead of P (Kosmidis et al. 1994; Jeremic et al. 1997). It was used in combination with etoposide (i.e., CE) due to a similar response and survival as PE but with less kidney and ear toxicity than PE (Kosmidis et al. 1994; Jeremic et al. 1997). Other drugs were also attempted to incorporate into the treatment plan (Woo et al. 2000; Hanna et al. 2002).

Irinotecan–cisplatin (IC) tended to have better survival in comparison to PE/CE likely due to several reasons. CE regimens were more frequently used in studies where patients had worse PS and more comorbidities, negatively affecting its outcome. As a confirmation for this observation, there was no difference in the efficacy of P and C in a systematic review of individual patient data between the two (MST, 9.6 months and 9.4 months for P and C, respectively) (Rossi et al. 2012). Also, the majority of I—containing studies have been conducted in Asia where it has more favorable outcomes (Lima et al. 2010). Outside of Asia, however, there is limited evidence for its superiority over E (Lara Jr et al. 2010). A systematic review which included many Asian studies/patients concluded that I improved survival by 1–2 months compared to PE/CE (Lima et al. 2010). These results were recently confirmed by Jones et al. (2020) in the most comprehensive systematic review done so far, including 160 studies in both LD SCLC and ED SCLC. Contrary to that, a study in Caucasians found no differences in survival between E- and I-containing CHT (Lara Jr et al. 2010). Another prospective randomized trial (Kubota et al. 2014) tested 3 cycles of PE vs IP given in non-progressive disease (PD) patients, all of which initially received concurrent one cycle of PE and ACC HFX RT (45 Gy in 30 fractions in 15 treatment days). In the PE group, MST was 3.2 years while in the IC group it was 2.8 years. OS did not differ between the two groups ($p = 0.70$), and no difference was seen regarding the toxicity, except more thrombocytopenia in PE and more diarrhea in the IC group. The authors concluded that PE and TRT remained standard approach in this setting.

Various CHT intensification efforts unequivocally failed such as prolonged administration (Woods and Levi 1984; Cullen et al. 1986; Bleehen et al. 1989; Lebeau et al. 1992; Giaccone et al. 1993; Beith et al. 1996; Sculier et al. 1996; Byrne et al. 1989) or increase in the number of induction CHT courses (Spiro et al. 1989) or intensification of the CHT dose (Leyvraz et al. 2008). Last two decades also brought investigation of the place and the role of the third generation drugs, but with disappointing results (Schiller et al. 2001; Mavroudis et al. 2001; Niell et al. 2002; Edelmen et al. 2004; Sandler et al. 2000).

Beside the issue of target volumes (to be discussed in another chapter) and prophylactic cranial irradiation (also discussed in another chapter), two major issues remain in focus of clinical investigations in LD SCLC: timing of combined RT and CHT, and total RT dose and fractionation. When timing of combined RT and CHT is considered, one must also take into consideration whether the combination is depicted as either concurrent, or sequential or alternating. Although some studies showed promising results for alternating RT and CHT, this approach is largely abandoned today. With the remaining two modes of administration the main question is whether any portions of TRT and CHT overlap and, if so, when overlapping actually occurs. Some concurrent TRT and CHT studies used non-P-based regimens, or alternated it with PE, while more recent ones were exclusively P-based regimens. Some studies (Perry et al. 1987; Schultz et al. 1988; Work et al. 1997) suggested that TRT delayed until the fourth cycle of CHT (Perry et al. 1987) or until day 120 (Schultz et al. 1988) may be superior to initial TRT or suggested no difference when compared to early TRT and CHT (Work et al. 1997). Marked reduction of CHT dose in the Cancer and Leukemia Group B (Perry et al. 1987) and the Danish trial when TRT was applied early was seen as the major reason. Importantly, the Danish trial (Work et al. 1997) should not be considered as a concurrent study because sequential TRT was used before and after CHT. More recent studies using PE (Jeremic et al. 1997; Takada et al. 2002) or PE alternating with cyclophosphamide/doxorubicin/vincristine (Murray et al. 1993) showed clear superiority for early administration of TRT (concurrently given during the first or the second cycle of CHT). These studies have also reconfirmed in clinical practice an original Goldie and Coldman (1979) theoretical considerations that an early administration of both treatment modalities leads to the best outcome on both local and distant level. Early concurrent TRT and PE were capable of achieving 5-year survival of >20%, while late TRT usually obtained only about 10%. Therefore, it became a common practice to offer as early as possible (cycle one or two of CHT) TRT with curative doses worldwide. Others have also proved that this is indeed the fact even outside the clinical trial, e.g., in an institutional setting. Kamath et al. (1998) showed that early concurrent TRT/PE offers advantage over sequential CHT and TRT in terms of OS and decreased distant metastasis in patients with LD SCLC. Several meta-analyses and systematic reviews addressed this issue by putting all then-existing evidence into a perspective of timing of combined TRT and CHT in LD SCLC. Huncharek and McGarry (2004) observed significantly superior survival at both 2- and 3-years for early TRT and CHT. Fried et al. (2004) observed a significantly higher 2-year survival in the early group and there was a suggestion of a similar trend at 3 and 5 years. Contrary to these, Pijls-Johannesma et al. (2005) did not find any advantage for early TRT and CHT. Spiro et al. (2006) found no difference between the early and the late administration of the two regimens. However, they documented that test for heterogeneity was significant ($p = 0.0002$), which indicated that hazard ratios estimates likely differed from overall estimates. To correct these ambiguities, they have performed Forest plot analysis for treatment effect. When they focused on cases which received all CHT cycles, they have found better survival for patients in early group if patients received similar percentage of CHT in both arms, contrary to cases when there was less percentage in early arm, leading to better survival in late group. Similarly, positive effect of hyperfractionated (Hfx) RT was found in early group, but not in late, as well as when P-based CHT was used, early group was better and when not, late was better. These four analyses (Huncharek and McGarry 2004; Fried et al. 2004; Pijls-Johannesma et al. 2005; Spiro et al. 2006) brought somewhat conflicting results which were result of: (a) different definition of LD SCLC, (b) different definition of "early" and "late" administration, (c) inclusion of "grey literature," (d) different patient number, and (e) lack of individual patient data. In an attempt to resolve the matter, Jeremic (2006) performed "meta -analysis" of the meta-analyses, identifying common findings in existing analyses, which included the following: (a) there was more leucopoenia in late group, (b) there was a favorable effect of short ($\leq$30 days) overall treatment time, (c) there was a favorable effect of Hfx, (d) there was a favorable effect of PE CHT, and (e) there was negative effect of split-course RT. Overall, prevailing evidence 15 years ago was that using "standard" approach consisting of Hfx RT and 4 courses of PE, early administration seems favorable and should be practiced as standard approach. Reports showing that prolonged (e.g., 4–6 cycles) sequential administration of CHT followed by radical TRT is inferior treatment approach when compared to early and concurrent TRT/CHT continue to be documented (El Sharouni et al. 2009; Yilmaz et al. 2010).

Past decade brought several important studies focused on the issue of timing of administration of TRT and CHT in LD SCLC. In a prospective randomized study, Sun et al. (2013) randomized 222 eligible patients with LD SCLC to receive either TRT administered concurrently with the first cycle (early TRT) or the third cycle (late TRT) of CHT, the latter consisting of four cycles of PE given every 3 weeks. Total dose TRT was 52.5 Gy with 2.1 Gy per fraction in once a day and five times a week for consecutive 5 weeks. Late TRT achieved results similar to early TRT in terms of the complete response rate (early versus late; 36.0% versus 38.0%), MST [24.1 versus 26.8 months; hazard ratio (HR) 0.90; 95% CI 0.18–1.62], and PFS (median, 12.4 versus 11.2 months; HR 1.10; 95% CI 0.37–1.84). While investigation of the pattern of treatment failures numerically favored early TRT, the difference was not significant ($p = 0.14$). However, neutropenic fever occurred more commonly in the early TRT arm than the late TRT arm (21.6% versus 10.2%; $p = 0.02$). Authors concluded that contrary to widespread beliefs of superiority of early TRT, later (cycle 3) TRT and PE should not easily be discarded from daily clinical practice. Second study was meta-analysis based on individual patient data (De Ruysscher et al. 2016) from nine trials and 2,305 patients being available for analysis. The median follow-up was 10 years. When all trials were analyzed together, "earlier or shorter" (TRT initiated before 9 weeks after randomization and before the third cycle of CHT) versus "later or longer" TRT did not affect OS. However, the HR for OS was significantly in favor of "earlier or shorter" TRT among trials with a similar proportion of patients who were compliant with CHT (defined as having received 100% or more of the planned CHT cycles) in both arms (HR 0.79, 95%CI 0.69–0.91). It was in favor of "later or longer" TRT among trials with different rates of CHT compliance (HR 1.19, 1.05–1.34, interaction test, $p < 0.0001$). The absolute gain between "earlier or shorter" versus "later or longer" TRT in 5-year OS for similar and for different CHT compliance trials was 7.7% (95% CI 2.6–12.8%) and − 2.2% (−5.8% to 1.4%), respectively. However, "earlier or shorter" TRT was associated with a higher incidence of severe acute oesophagitis than "later or longer" TRT. These results mirrored those of meta-analysis of Spiro et al. (2006) and favored early administration of TRT and CHT, and were most recently reconfirmed by Jones et al. (2020).

Second question is that of dose and fractionation pattern of TRT. Total TRT doses ranged from as low as 30 Gy to as high as 70 Gy. In addition, many studies have used some form of hyperfractionation (b.i.d.). Regardless of fractionation regimen, major site of recurrence continues to be in-field (about 30% are isolated and additional 20% are combined with systemic progression). Majority of available studies are retrospective in nature, with one study (Choi and Carey 1989) observing a better local control for doses 40–50 Gy than with doses <40 Gy (>50 vs. 30%), indicating, therefore, potential dose–response relationship. Another study indicated excellent local control of 97% after 60 Gy (Papac et al. 1987). The Cancer and Leukemia Group B (Choi et al. 1998) performed a trial to identify at least 70 Gy (using standard fractionation) as the maximum tolerated dose (MTD) for combination with CHT. Subsequently, Bogart et al. (2004) reported that 70 Gy was feasible and effective when given concurrently with 3 cycles of CE, following an induction with 2 cycles of paclitaxel and topotecan. The MST was 19.8 months with a 1-year survival rate of 70% and the median failure-free survival was 12.9 months. Group study results were also confirmed in a single-institutional setting. Miller et al. (2003) retrospectively evaluated the data of 65 patients from the Duke University in which 58–66 Gy, standard fractionation was used with either concurrent ($n = 32$) or sequential ($n = 33$) CHT. Somewhat lower (30%) 2-year survival rate was explained by less than one-half of patients receiving concurrent TRT/CHT and with only 26% receiving prophylactic cranial irradiation (PCI). The toxicity of their regimen was low. Similarly, Roof et al. (2003) observed that OS, local control, and DFS obtained with >50 Gy compared favorably with the historic controls which were using lower doses. Most recently, Komaki et al. (2005) reported on Radiation Therapy Oncology Group 9,712 study which was a phase I dose-escalation study of TRT/PE in LD SCLC. TRT was given 1.8 Gy daily to 36 Gy followed by boost delivered with escalations of 1.8 Gy b.i.d. during the final days which permitted doses of up to 64.8 Gy to be given. The MTD was determined to be 61.2 Gy in 34 fractions of 1.8 Gy when given concurrently with 2 cycles of PE and followed by 2 additional cycles of PE.

Hypofractionated RT regimens were also used, which was thought to cause more damage to SCLC cells (Murray et al. 1993; Spiro et al. 2006). More recently, Xia et al. (2015) treated 59 patients with 55 Gy at 2.5 Gy per fraction over 30 days given on the first day of the second or third cycle of PE regimen which was given to 4 to 6 cycles. Patients who had a good response to initial treatment were offered PCI. The 2-year PFS rate was 49.0%, the MST was 28.5 months, and the 2-year OS rate was 58.2%. The 2-year local control rate was 76.4%. Grade 3 or 4 hematologic toxicities were leukopenia (32%), neutropenia (25%), and thrombocytopenia (15%). Acute esophagitis and pneumonitis of grade ≥ 3 occurred in 25% and 10% of the patients, respectively. In another study, shifting from such hypofractionated to conventionally fractionated TRT did not alter outcomes, the survival, local control, and toxicity rates were all similar (Videtic et al. 2003).

Of altered fractionated regimens, accelerated hyperfractionation was the logical choice due to a high sensitivity of SCLC to RT, sparing effect of twice-daily fractionation and possible effect of the dose acceleration to combat rapid proliferation thought to occur in SCLC. In the Intergroup study (Johnson et al. 1996a, b; Turrisi et al. 1999), 45 Gy given in 30 fractions in 3 weeks (b.i.d.) was compared with the same dose given once-daily, both with concurrent PE. While a survival was significantly better in the b.i.d. arm (5-year, 26% vs. 19%), this was, however, achieved with somewhat higher incidence of acute toxicity. Another study investigating this issue was a North Central Cancer Treatment Group study which compared concurrent two cycles of PE with either b.i.d., split-course TRT (48 Gy in a total of 5.5 weeks), or once-daily TRT (50.4 Gy), both given after 3 cycles of PE (Bonner et al. 1999). There was no difference in a 3-year overall and locoregional control. After 5 years (Schild et al. 2003), the median and 5-year survival were 20.4 months and 22% for b.i.d. versus 20.5 months and 21% for once-daily TRT, respectively ($p = 0.7$). Having these two studies together, possible explanation may lie either in inferiority of split-course regimen (which undermined the effect of b.i.d.) or effects of acceleration outweighing those of b.i.d. (in other words, b.i.d. given with a split equals conventional, once-daily fractionation, providing total dose and treatment duration being similar if not the same). Extending overall treatment time, therefore, which allows tumor cell regeneration, may have been the reason for this finding due to a delay in TRT either by long lasting induction CHT or by split-course protocol for TRT. A quality-adjusted reanalysis of a that phase III trial (Bonner et al. 1999; Schild et al. 2003) comparing once-daily TRT versus b.i.d TRT in patients with LD SCLC using Quality Time Without Symptoms or Toxicity methodology showed no difference in survival after adjusting for toxicity and progression (Sloan et al. 2002).

While accelerated hyperfractionated TRT was practiced with increasing evidence in the past 25 years, the accumulated data show different outcome (Johnson et al. 1996a, b; Ali et al. 1998; Mennecier et al. 2000; Segawa et al. 2003; Chen et al. 2005) and toxicity profile. Recent clinical studies and meta-analysis directly comparing b.i.d. to once-daily fractionation brought some answers about optimal total dose and fractionation regimen preferentially used. One single-institutional report (Watkins et al. 2010) compared two RT regimens with planned doses of (1) ≥59.4 Gy at 1.8–2.0 Gy per once-daily fraction or (2) ≥45 Gy at 1.5 Gy b.i.d. with concurrent platinum-based CHT. A total of 71 patients were included in the study with patient, tumor, staging, and treatment factors being similar between the two treatment groups. Acute toxicities were similar between the groups. The 2-year OS was similar at 43% and 49% for the once-daily versus b.i.d. groups, respectively. Isolated in-field failures were similar between the two groups. While this analysis did not detect a statistically significant difference in acute toxicities, disease control, or survival outcomes in LD SCLC patients treated with concurrent CHT and once-daily versus b.i.d. RT, it should not be forgotten that other regimens of b.i.d. irradiation (e.g., 54 Gy in 36 fractions in 18 treatment days in 3.5 weeks) have been successfully implemented in practice concurrently with low-dose CHT in both LD (Jeremic et al. 1997) and extensive disease SCLC (Jeremic et al. 1999), providing not only excellent results, but also leading to low toxicity. Gronberg et al. (2015) reported on the first prospective randomized phase II trial comparing b.i.d and hypofractionated (once-daily, OD) TRT in LD SCLC. Patients received four courses of PE and were randomized to TRT of 42 Gy in 15 fractions (OD) or 45 Gy in 30 fractions (b.i.d.) between the second and third PE course. Good responders received PCI of 30 Gy in 15 fractions. One hundred and fifty-seven patients were enrolled, of which 72% had Stage III disease and 11% non-malignant pleural effusion. While the response rates were similar, more b.i.d. patients achieved a complete response (OD: 13%, b.i.d.: 33%; $p = 0.003$). There was no difference in 1-year PFS (OD: 45%, b.i.d.: 49%; $p = 0.61$) or median PFS (OD: 10.2 months, b.i.d.: 11.4 months; $p = 0.93$). The MST in the b.i.d. arm was 6.3 months longer (OD: 18.8 months, b.i.d.: 25.1 months; $p = 0.61$). There were no differences in grade 3–4 esophagitis

(OD: 31%, b.i.d.: 33%, $p = 0.80$) or pneumonitis (OD: 2%, b.i.d.: 3%, $p = 1.0$). Patients on the b.i.d. arm reported slightly more dysphagia at the end of the TRT. The authors concluded that b.i.d. resulted in significantly more complete responses and a numerically longer MST, but no firm conclusions about efficacy could be drawn from this phase II trial.

In a CONVERT trial (Faivre-Finn et al. 2017), EORTC evaluated 66 Gy using standard fractionation with the b.i.d. fractionation as used in the intergroup study (45 Gy in 30 fractions in 15 treatment days in 3 weeks), both starting on day 22 after commencing PE (given as four to six cycles every 3 weeks in both groups). Of 547 enrolled patients, b.i.d. was employed in 274 patients and OD in 273 patients. At a median follow-up of 45 months the MST was 30 months for b.i.d. versus 25 months for OD (hazard ratio for death in the once-daily group 1.18, 95% CI 0.95–1.45; $p = 0.14$). Two-year OS was 56% in b.i.d. and 51% in the OD (absolute difference between the treatment groups 5.3% [95% CI −3.2% to 13.7%]). Most CHT-related toxicities were similar between the groups, except there was significantly more grade 4 neutropenia with b.i.d. (49% vs 38%; $p = 0.05$). For TRT-related toxicity, there was no difference in grade 3–4 oesophagitis and grade 3–4 radiation pneumonitis between the groups. Because survival outcomes did not differ between b.i.d. and OD TRT/CHT, and toxicity was similar and lower than expected with both regimens and because the trial was designed to show superiority of OD TRT and was not powered to show equivalence, the authors concluded that b.i.d. should continue to be considered the standard of care in this setting. Mature data from joint CALGB 30610/RTOG 0538 study, similar to the EORTC study, should supplement existing ones and hopefully give better perspective about fractionation issue.

Focusing on fractionation issue and comparing b.i.d. to OD, Wu et al. (2020) performed a meta-analysis by screening 1,499 articles and including 5 RCTs with 1,421 patients. They found that b.i.d. TRT/CHT improved OS (hazard ratio, HR = 0.88, 95% CI 0.78–0.99, $p = 0.03$), the 1-year OS rate (risk ratio, RR = 1.07, 95%CI 1.01–1.13, $p = 0.03$), and OS at 4 years (RR = 1.22, 95%CI 1.03–1.43, $p = 0.02$), with better trends in OS at 2 years, 3 years, and 5 years, respectively, compared to OD TRT/CHT. In addition, TRT/CHT had a higher complete response (CR, RR = 1.31, 95%CI 1.01–1.70, $p = 0.04$) than OD TRT/CHT. PFS (HR = 0.92, 95%CI 0.79–1.07, $p = 0.29$), annual PFS rate, ORR (RR = 0.99, 95%CI 0.93–1.05, $p = 0.72$), and adverse events (AEs) for all grades (RR = 1.00, 95%CI 0.98–1.01, $p = 0.57$), and grades 3–5 (RR = 1.02, 95%CI 0.95–1.09, $p = 0.60$) were similar between the two arms. Conclusion of this analysis was that b.i.d. TRT/CHT appeared to be better than OD TRT/CHT for LD SCLC, with better antitumor effects (OS and CR) and similar AEs.

Another issue which was evaluated in this setting was the TRT dose, using BED approach to differentiate various studies in a systematic review by Zhu et al. (2016). The background for their analysis was that the efficacy of TRT could be closely related to the TRT dose, but that any attempt to achieve clear dose–response relationship remained poorly documented in clinical practice. Currently, total doses that range from 45 to 50 Gy OD and 45 to 54 Gy b.i.d. have been used in order to minimize toxicity but maintain the efficacy. Data from a number of PRCTs, however, were associated with a high rate of locoregional failure. Attempts have been made to administer high-dose TRT, but unfortunately, CALGB 39808, 30,002, and 30,202 failed to demonstrate the superiority of high-dose (70 Gy) RT (Salama et al. 2013). Some experts ascribed this to the prolonged overall radiation time (ORT) of the 70 Gy dose. In fact, several factors including single dose, fraction scheme, as well as the ORT may have an impact on the outcome. In their attempt, Zhu et al. (2016) investigated the correlations between the biological effective dose (BED) and MST, MPFS, 1-, 3-, and 5-year OS as well as local relapse (LR). In this study, 2,389 patients in 19 trials were included. Among the trials, seven were conducted in Europe, eight were conducted in Asia, and four were conducted in the USA. The 19 trials that were included consisted of 29 arms with 24 concurrent and 5 sequential TRT arms. For all included studies, the results showed that a higher BED prolonged the MST ($p < 0.001$) and the MPFS ($p < 0.001$). Increased BED improved the 1-, 3-, and 5-year OS. A 10-Gy increment added a 6.3%, a 5.1%, and a 3.7% benefit for the 1-, 3-, and 5-year OS, respectively. Additionally, BED was negatively correlated with LR ($p < 0.001$). A subgroup analysis of concurrent TRT showed that a high BED prolonged the MST ($p < 0.001$) and the MPFS ($p < 0.001$), improved the 1-, 3-, and 5-year OS ($p < 0.001$) and decreased the rate of LR ($p < 0.001$).

Finally, the last effort of a Scandinavia group (Grønberg et al. 2021) represented one of the final steps and the most meaningful attempts in optimization of treatment approaches in LD SCLC. They have performed a PRCT using a phase II design to directly compare 45 Gy b.i.d. with the same b.i.d. of 60 Gy, evaluating the dose response with significantly different BED Gy_{10} (51.75 vs. 69.00). Treatment included four courses of standard cisplatin or carboplatin and etoposide. TRT was given to the primary lung tumor and PET-CT positive lymph node metastases starting 20–28 days after the first CHT course. Responders also received PCI of 25–30 Gy. One hundred and seventy patients were randomly assigned to 60 Gy ($n = 89$) or 45 Gy ($n = 81$). Two-year OS was 74.2% (95% CI 63.8–82.9) in the 60 Gy group, compared with 48.1% (36.9–59.5) in the 45 Gy group (odds ratio, 3.09; $p = 0.0005$). No difference in toxicity and treatment-related mortality was seen between the two groups. The authors concluded that the higher 60 Gy BID resulted in a substantial survival improvement compared with 45 Gy b.i.d., without increased toxicity, suggesting that b.i.d. RT of 60 Gy is an alternative to existing schedules.

4 Specific Aspects of TRT IN LD SCLC

While many older studies combined patients with various T and N designations in LD SCLC, some investigated more specific staging descriptors. Salem et al. (2019) were the first to provide a post-hoc analysis of the CONVERT trial (Faivre-Finn et al. 2017) trying to explore different outcome in patients with Stage I–II vs Stage III (LD) SCLC. There were 86 patients with Stage I–II and 423 patients with Stage III (LD) SCLC. Patients with Stage I-II achieved the MST of 50 months and 5-year OS of 49% while corresponding figures for Stage III patients were 25 months and 28%, respectively. In patients with Stage I–II, no significant survival difference was found between the two trial arms (MST, 39 months in the OD arm vs 72 months in the b.i.d. arm; $p = 0.38$). There was a lower incidence of acute esophagitis in patients with Stage I–II compared with patients with Stage III (grade ≥ 3, 11.3% vs 21.1%; $p < 0.001$), but the incidences of other acute and late toxic effects were not significantly different. More recently, Valan et al. (2018) explored the impact of various N3 disease subcategories on the outcome of 144 patients with LD SCLC enrolled during the study which tested hypofractionated OD versus b.i.d. TRT in LD SCLC (Grønberg et al. 2016). They have shown that the MST was 23.3 months in the whole cohort, with N3-patients ($n = 37$) having shorter MST than those with N0-2 (16.7 vs. 33.0 months; $p < 0.001$). There were no significant differences in OS between the N3 subcategories, but patients with metastases to two or more N3 regions had shorter survival than other N3 patients (MST: 13.4 vs. 19.9 months; $p = 0.011$). The authors concluded that due to no survival differences between the N3 subcategories, all N3 disease should be considered as LD.

The same group (Halvorsen et al. 2016) investigated the place and role of an early assessment of response to the first course of CHT in an attempt to optimize treatment in LD SCLC. Patients recruited to their, previously reported study (Grønberg et al. 2016) which tested b.i.d. (45 Gy/30 fractions) with hypofractionated OD (42 Gy/15 fractions) TRT, given concurrently with four courses of PE ($n = 157$) were subjects of this study. Tumor size was assessed on CT scans at baseline and planning scans for TRT according to RECIST v.1.0 criteria. CT scans were available for 135 patients

(86%). Ninety-four percent had a reduction in tumor size after the first CHT course. Eighty-two percent had stable disease, and 18% had partial response. Reduction in the sum of diameters was significantly associated with complete response at first follow-up (OR: 1.05, 95% CI 1.01–1.09; $p = 0.013$), PFS (HR: 0.97, 95% CI 0.96–0.99; $p = 0.001$), and OS (HR: 0.98, 95% CI 0.96–1.00; $p = 0.010$). This study provided evidence that response from the first course of CHT had a significant positive association with outcomes from TRT/PE, and might be used to stratify and randomize patients in future studies.

5 What Is Practiced and Recommended Nowadays?

While majority of practicing radiation oncologists try to follow existing data, either using original study data or recommendations coming from professional group/society guidelines, little is known about actual practices. Surveys of such practices have been undertaken to bring more light into what is actually delivered to patients in this setting. In one such attempt, Shahi et al. (2016) created a survey to assess patterns of practice and clinical decision-making in the management of SCLC by Canadian radiation oncologists. They have created a 35-item survey which included questions about the role of RT, its dose and timing, target delineation, and use of PCI in both LD SCLC and ED SCLC. Responses were received from 52 eligible radiation oncologists. For LD SCLC, the most common dose and fractionation schedule was 40–45 Gy in 15 daily fractions (40%). Preferred management of clinical T1/2aN0 SCLC was primary TRT/CHT (64%). If surgery was to be offered first, 36% of radiation oncologists would offer some form of adjuvant TRT especially if pathologic N2 disease was to be found (17%) or if a positive margin had been reported (15%). Most of the radiation oncologists indicated that they would offer TRT concurrently with PE (98%), most often initiating the TRT during cycle 1 or 2 of CHT (94%) rather than during cycle 3 or 4 (2%), after CHT (2%), or at any point provided that total treatment time was 30 days or fewer (2%). More recently, a similar survey was undertaken in the USA. Farrell et al. (2018) focused on the issue of timing of administration of TRT in LD SCLC. They surveyed 309 US radiation oncologists with questions covering treatment recommendations, self-rated knowledge of trials, and demographics. Ninety-eight percent of respondents recommend concurrent TRT/CHT over sequential. Seventy-one percent recommended starting TRT in cycle 1 of CHT, and 25% recommended starting in cycle 2. In actual practice, however, it started most commonly in cycle 2 (48%) and cycle 1 (44%). Potential explanations for this discordance included the logistical complexity of modern treatment planning, the desire to begin CHT urgently, and the advantages of starting TRT during later cycles of CHT to allow tumor shrinkage to better meet treatment planning parameters. Half of respondents (54%) believed that starting in cycle 1 improved survival compared to cycle 3. It must, however, be stressed out that the most recent phase III randomized controlled trial on this topic from Korea (Sun et al. 2013), which more than half of respondents were not familiar with, showed that late TRT in cycle 3 of CHT was non-inferior to early TRT in cycle 1. When, however, self-assessed knowledge of the Korean trial was documented, it unequivocally supported late start of TRT in cycle 3. Those familiar with the trial were more likely to show flexibility and be willing to start RT later in actual practice than they preferred to do under ideal circumstances. It is entirely possible that the results of the Korean randomized trial provided enough reassurance to US radiation oncologists that delay would not affect OS.

Current NCCN guidelines (Version 2.21 – January 11, 2021) recommend a variety of treatment options in "early" LD SCLC (Stage I-IIA: T1-2, N0, M0). They range from lobectomy with mediastinal lymph node dissection or sampling in cases of pathologically negative mediastinal staging, followed then by either a systemic therapy (N0) or systemic therapy with or without TRT (N0-1). Postoperative TRT is also recommended in cases of pathologic N2 disease. In inoperable cases or whenever surgery is not to be pursued, SABR followed by a systemic therapy or concurrent RT/CHT is recommended. In more advanced cases of LD SCLC, i.e., Stage IIB-IIIC (T3-4, N0, M0 and T1-4, N1-3, M0), it recommends either a concurrent or sequential TRT and systemic therapy, depending on the PS, but not active oncological treatment in cases of PS3-4. TRT is recommended to start concurrently with cycles 1 or 2 of CHT. In spite of higher doses of OD TRT, i.e., 60–70 Gy and clear inconveniences to both patients and hospitals, these guidelines still consider it appropriate, together with b.i.d. TRT of 45 Gy in 30 fractions in 15 treatment days.

National Institute for Health and Care Excellence (NICE) recommends almost the same regarding all categories of LD SCLC. However, it states as preferred TRT b.i.d. regimen, and allows OD only in cases when b.i.d. is impossible to undertake or patients declines it. (NICE Pathways; Treating Small Cell Lung Cancer; http://pathways.nice.org.uk/pathways/lung-cancer, NICE Pathway last updated: 27 January 2021)

6   Future Aspects

There is obvious necessity to address many important issues in domain of LD SCLC through prospective clinical trials, ranging from better definition of the place and role of surgery in "early" LD SCLC, to attempts to better define various TRT- and/or CHT-related aspects in the setting of combined treatment approach in LD SCLC. However, the landscape of combined treatments is rapidly changing with the wide introduction of immunotherapy, largely owing to encouraging, though sporadic, studies showing its advantage in ED SCLC.

In spite of numerous ongoing studies which include TRT and immunotherapy, there is a general lack of solid evidence for superiority of this novel approach. Only recently, Welsh et al. (2020) reported on a first ever phase I/II trial of concurrent TRT/CHT and pembrolizumab in patients with LS-SCLC or other neuroendocrine tumors and good performance status (ECOG ≤2). Concurrent TRT/CHT consisted of PE with 45 Gy RT, 30 Gy being given via b.i.d. PCI (25 Gy in 10 daily fractions) was given at the physician's discretion. Pembrolizumab was started concurrently with TRT/CHT and continued for up to 16 cycles. All of the 40 enrolled patients completed RT and received ≥1 cycle of pembrolizumab. There were no grade 5 toxicities, and three grade 4 events (2 neutropenia, 1 respiratory failure). Grade 2 + 3 pneumonitis rate was 15%. All 17 (42.5%) esophagitis events were grades 1–2. At median follow-up time of 23.1 months, the MPFS time was 19.7 months and MST was 39.5 months. This combination was well tolerated and yielded favorable outcomes, providing a good starting point for future randomized studies. By comparing their study results with those of CONVERT study (Faivre-Finn et al. 2017) they observed fewer grade 4 or 5 events as well as all other side effects. In addition, they have judged their treatment efficacy as superior to CONVERT, while reasoning that more sophisticated TRT techniques (namely, intensity modulated radiation therapy) played likely reason for this.

Several clinical trials are underway in this domain. They can broadly be separated into two major pathways. In the first, checkpoint inhibitors can complement standard TRT/CHT as sequential consolidation therapy. In the second, checkpoint inhibitors are incorporated in the standard concurrent regimen. NCT04189094 is investigating induction sintilimab (PD-1 inhibitor) with standard PE (2 cycles). Concurrent TRT/CHT will utilize PE alone, followed by maintenance sintilimab. The STIMULI trial (NCT02046733), similarly to Checkmate-451, is evaluating the efficacy of N1I3 when given after standard concurrent TRT/CHT. ADRIATIC (NCT03703297) is similar to STIMULI but uses durvalumab and tremelimumab. Contrary to induction or maintenance strategies alone, NCT03811002 compares TRT/CHT with or without atezolizumab offered for the whole treatment duration (being offered during the concurrent with TRT, too). In NCT02402920, patients with LD SCLC (patients with ED SCLC are also eligible for this trial) will receive pembrolizumab beginning with concurrent TRT.

It is expected that studies focused on immune checkpoint inhibitors, together with other immunotherapy approaches produce high level evidence which should help define place and role of these treatments in the new era in thoracic oncology.

References

Ahmed Z, Kujtan L, Kennedy KF et al (2017) Disparities in the management of patients with stage I Small Cell Lung Carcinoma (SCLC): a Surveillance, Epidemiology and End Results (SEER) Analysis. Clin Lung Cancer 18:e315–e325

Ali MA, Kraut MJ, Valdivieso M, Herskovic AM, Du W, Kalemkerian GP (1998) Phase II study of hyperfractionated radiotherapy and concurrent weekly alternating chemotherapy in limited-stage small cell lung cancer. Lung Cancer 22:39–44

Amarasena IU, Walters JA, Wood-Baker R, Fong K (2008) Platinum versus non-platinum chemotherapy regimens for small cell lung cancer. Cochrane Database Syst Rev 4:CD006849

Barnes H, See K, Barnett S et al (2017) Surgery for limited-stage small-cell lung cancer. Cochrane Database Syst Rev 4:CD011917

Beith JM, Clarke SJ, Woods RL, Bell DR, Levi JA (1996) Long-term follow-up of a randomised trial of combined chemoradiotherapy induction treatment, with and without maintenance chemotherapy in patients with small cell carcinoma of the lung. Eur J Cancer 32A:438–443

Bleehen NM, Fayers PM, Girling DJ, Stephens RJ (1989) Controlled trial of twelve versus six courses of chemotherapy in the treatment of small-cell lung cancer. Br J Cancer 59:584–590

Bogart JA, Herndon JE, Lyss AP, Cancer and Leukemia Group B study 39808 et al (2004) 70 Gy thoracic radiotherapy is feasible concurrent with chemotherapy for limited-stage small-cell lung cancer: analysis of cancer and leukemia group B study 39808. Int J Radiat Oncol Biol Phys 59:460–468

Bonner JA, Sloan JA, Shanahan TG et al (1999) Phase III comparison of twice-daily split-course irradiation versus once-daily irradiation for patients with limited stage small-cell lung carcinoma. J Clin Oncol 17:2681–2691

Bray F, Ferlay J, Soerjomataram I, Siegel RL, Torre LA, Jemal A (2018) Global Cancer Statistics 2018: GLOBOCAN estimates of incidence and mortality worldwide for 36 cancers in 185 countries. CA Cancer J Clin 68:394–424

Brock MV, Hooker CM, Syphard JE et al (2005) Surgical resection of limited disease small cell lung cancer in the new era of platinum chemotherapy: its time has come. J Thorac Cardiovasc Surg 129:64–72

Byrne MJ, Van Hazel G, Trotter J et al (1989) Maintenance chemotherapy in limited small cell lung cancer: a randomised controlled clinical trial. Br J Cancer 59:584–590

Chen G-Y, Jiang G-L, Wang L-J et al (2005) Cisplatin/etoposide chemotherapy combined with twice daily thoracic radiotherapy for limited small-cell lung cancer: a clinical phase II trial. Int J Radiation Oncol Biol Phys 61:70–75

Choi NC, Carey RR (1989) Importance of radiation dose in achieving improved locoregional tumor control in small-cell lung carcinoma: an update. Int J Radiat Oncol Biol Phys 17:307–310

Choi N, Herndon J, Rosenman J et al (1998) Phase I study to determine the maximum tolerated dose of radiation in standard daily and accelerated twice daily radiotherapy schedules with concurrent chemotherapy for limited stage small cell lung cancer: CALGB 8837. J Clin Oncol 16:3528–3536

Cohen MH, Ihde DC, Bunn PA Jr et al (1979) Cyclic alternating combination chemotherapy for small cell bronchogenic carcinoma. Cancer Treat Rep 62:163–170

Combs SE, Hancock JG, Boffa DJ et al (2015) Bolstering the case for lobectomy in stages I, II, and IIIA small-cell lung cancer using the National Cancer Data Base. J Thorac Oncol 10:316–323

Cullen M, Morgan D, Gregory W et al (1986) Maintenance chemotherapy for anaplastic small cell carcinoma of the bronchus: a randomised, controlled trial. Cancer Chemother Pharmacol 17:157–160

De Ruysscher D, Lueza B, Le Péchoux C, on behalf of the RTT-SCLC Collaborative Group et al (2016) Impact of thoracic radiotherapy timing in limited-stage small-cell lung cancer: usefulness of the individual patient data meta-analysis. Ann Oncol 27:1818–1828

Edelmen MJ, Chansky K, Gaspar LE et al (2004) Phase II trial of cisplatin/etoposide and concurrent radiotherapy followed by paclitaxel/carboplatin consolidation for limited small-cell lung cancer: southwest Oncology Group 9713. J Clin Oncol 22:127–132

Einhorn LH, Crawford J, Birch R, Omura G, Johnson DH, Greco FA (1988) Cisplatin plus etoposide consolidation following cyclophosphamide, doxorubicin, and vincristine in limited small-cell lung cancer. J Clin Oncol 6:451–456

El Sharouni SY, Kal HB, Barten-Van Rijbroek A, Struikmans H, Battermann JJ, Schramel FM (2009) Concurrent versus sequential chemotherapy and radiotherapy in limited disease small cell lung cancer: a retrospective comparative study. Anticancer Res 29:5219–5224

Faivre-Finn C, Snee M, Ashcroft L, for the CONVERT Study Team et al (2017) Concurrent once-daily versus twice-daily chemoradiotherapy in patients with limited-stage small-cell lung cancer (CONVERT): an open-label, phase 3, randomised, superiority trial. Lancet Oncol 18:1116–1125

Farrell MJ, Yahya JB, Degnin C et al (2018) Timing of thoracic radiation therapy with chemotherapy in limited-stage small cell lung cancer: survey of US radiation oncologists on current practice patterns. Clin Lung Cancer 19(6):e815–e821

Fried DB, Morris DE, Poole C et al (2004) Systematic review evaluating the timing of thoracic radiation therapy in combined modality therapy for limited-stage small-cell lung cancer. J Clin Oncol 22:4837–4845

Giaccone G, Dalesio O, McVie GJ et al (1993) Maintenance chemotherapy in small-cell lung cancer: long-term results of a randomized trial. J Clin Oncol 11:1230–1240

Goldie JG, Coldman AJ (1979) A mathematical model for relating the drug sensitivity of tumors to their spontaneous mutation rate. Cancer Treat Rep 63:1727–1735

Govindan R, Page N, Morgensztern D et al (2006) Changing epidemiology of small-cell lung cancer in the United States over the last 30 years: analysis of the surveillance, epidemiologic, and end results database. J Clin Oncol 24:4539–4544

Grønberg B, Halvorsen TO, Fløtten Ø, on behalf of the Norwegian Lung Cancer Study Group et al (2016) Randomized phase II trial comparing twice daily hyperfractionated with once daily hypofractionated thoracic radiotherapy in limited disease small cell lung cancer. Acta Oncol 55(5):591–597

Grønberg BH, Killingberg KT, Fløtten Ø et al (2021) High-dose versus standard-dose twice-daily thoracic radiotherapy for patients with limited stage small-cell lung cancer: an open-label, randomised, phase 2 trial. Lancet Oncol 22:321–331

Halvorsen TO, Herje M, Levin N et al (2016) Tumour size reduction after the first chemotherapy-course and outcomes of chemoradiotherapy in limited disease small-cell lung cancer. Lung Cancer 102:9–14

Hanna N, Ansari R, Fisher W, Shen J, Jung S-H, Sandler A (2002) Etoposide, ifosfamide and cisplatin (VIP) plus concurrent radiation therapy for previously untreated limited small cell lung cancer (SCLC) : a Hoosier oncology group (HOG) phase II study. Lung Cancer 35:293–297

Huncharek M, McGarry R (2004) A meta-analysis of the timing of chest irradiation in the combined modality treatment of limited-stage small cell lung cancer. Oncologist 9:665–762

Inoue M, Miyoshi S, Yasumitsu T et al (2000) Surgical results for small cell lung cancer based on the new TNM staging system. Thoracic Surgery Study Group of Osaka University, Osaka, Japan. Ann Thorac Surg 70:1615–1619

Jeremic B (2006) Timing of concurrent radiotherapy and chemotherapy in limited-disease small-cell lung cancer: "meta-analysis of meta-analyses". Int J Radiat Oncol Biol Phys 64:981–982

Jeremic B, Shibamoto Y, Acimovic L, Milisavljevic S (1997) Initial versus delayed accelerated hyperfractionated radiation therapy and concurrent chemotherapy in limited small cell lung cancer. J Clin Oncol 15:893–900

Jeremic B, Shibamoto Y, Nikolic N, Milicic B, Milisavljevic S, Dagovic A, Aleksandrovic J, Radosavljevic-Asic G (1999) Role of radiation therapy in the combined-modality treatment of patients with extensive disease small-cell lung cancer: a randomized study. J Clin Oncol 17:2092–2099

Johnson BE, Bridges JD, Sobezeck M et al (1996a) Patients with limited-stage small-cell lung cancer treated with concurrent twice-daily chest radiotherapy and etoposide/cisplatin followed by cyclophosphamide, doxorubicin, and vincristine. J Clin Oncol 14:806–813

Johnson DH, Kim K, Sause W (1996b) Cisplatin (p), etoposide (e) + thoracic radiotherapy (TRT) administered once or twice daily (bid) in limited stage (LS) small cell lung cancer (SCLC): final report of intergroup trial 0096. Proc Am Soc Clin Oncol 15:374

Jones GS, Elimian K, Baldwin DR, Hubbard RB, McKeever TM (2020) A systematic review of survival following anti-cancer treatment for small cell lung cancer. Lung Cancer 141:44–55

Kalemkerian GP, Akerley W, Bogner P et al (2013) Small cell lung cancer. J Natl Compr Cancer Netw 11:78–98

Kalemkerian GP, Loo BW, Akerley W et al (2018) NCCN guidelines insights: small cell lung cancer, version 2.2018 featured updates to the NCCN guidelines. JNCCN J Natl Compr Cancer Netw 16:1171–1182

Kamath SS, McCarley DL, Zlotecki RA (1998) Decreased metastasis and improved survival with early thoracic radiotherapy and prophylactic cranial irradiation in combined modality treatment of limited-stage small cell lung cancer. Radiat Oncol Investig 6:226–232

Komaki R, Swann S, Ettinger DS et al (2005) Phase I study of thoracic radiation dose escalation with concurrent chemotherapy for patients with limited small-cell lung cancer: Report of Radiation Therapy Oncology Group (RTOG) protocol 97-12. Int J Radiat Oncol Biol Phys 62:342–350

Kosmidis P, Samantas E, Fountzilas G, Pavlidis N, Apostolopoulou F, Skarlos D (1994) Cisplatin/etoposide vs carboplatin/etoposide and irradiation in small-cell lung cancer: a randomized phase III study. Semin Oncol 21(Suppl. 6):23–30

Kubota K, Hida T, Ishikura S, on behalf of the Japan Clinical Oncology Group et al (2014) Etoposide and cisplatin versus irinotecan and cisplatin in patients with limited-stage small-cell lung cancer treated with etoposide and cisplatin plus concurrent accelerated hyperfractionated thoracic radiotherapy (JCOG0202): a randomised phase 3 study. Lancet Oncol 15:106–113

Lad T, Piantadosi S, Thomas P et al (1994) A prospective randomized trial to determine the benefit of surgical resection of residual disease following response of small cell lung cancer to combination chemotherapy. Chest 106:320S–323S

Lara PN Jr, Chansky K, Shibata T et al (2010) Common arm comparative outcomes analysis of phase 3 trials of cisplatin + irinotecan versus cisplatin + etoposide in extensive stage small cell lung cancer: final patient-level results from Japan Clinical Oncology Group 9511 and Southwest Oncology Group 0124. Cancer 116(24):5710–5715

Lebeau B, Chastang CL, Allard P, Migueres J, Boita F, Fichet D (1992) Six vs twelve cycles for complete responders to chemotherapy in small cell lung cancer: definitive results of a randomised clinical trial. Eur Respir J 5:286–290

Leyvraz S, Pampallona S, Martinelli G, Solid Tumors Working Party of the European Group for Blood and Marrow Transplantation et al (2008) A threefold dose intensity treatment with ifosfamide, carboplatin, and etoposide for patients with small cell lung cancer: a randomized trial. J Natl Cancer Inst 100:533–541

Li C, Xiong Y, Zhou Z et al (2014) Stereotactic body radiotherapy with concurrent chemotherapy extends survival of patients with limited stage small cell lung cancer: a single-center prospective phase II study. Med Oncol 31:369

Lima JP, dos Santos LV, Sasse EC, Lima CS, Sasse AD (2010) Camptothecins compared with etoposide in combination with platinum analog in extensive stage small cell lung cancer: systematic review with meta-analysis. J Thorac Oncol 5(12):1986–1993

Ly NB, Allen PK, Lin SH (2014) Stereotactic body radiation therapy for stage I small cell lung cancer: a single institutional case series and review of the literature. J Radiat Oncol 3:285–291

Mascaux C, Paesmans M, Berghmans T, European Lung Cancer Working Party (ELCWP) et al (2000) A systematic review of the role of etoposide and cisplatin in the chemotherapy of small cell lung cancer with methodology assessment and meta-analysis. Lung Cancer 30:23–36

Mavroudis D, Papadakis E, Veslemes M et al (2001) A multicenter randomized clinical trial comparing paclitaxel-cisplatin-etoposide versus cisplatin-etoposide as first-line treatment in patients with small-cell lung cancer. Ann Oncol 12:463–470

Mennecier B, Jacoulet P, Dubiez A et al (2000) Concurrent cisplatin/etoposide chemotherapy plus twice daily thoracic radiotherapy in limited stage small cell lung cancer: a phase II study. Lung Cancer 27: 137–143

Micke P, Faldum A, Metz T et al (2002) Staging small cell lung cancer: Veterans Administration Lung Study Group versus International Association for the Study of Lung Cancer—what limits limited disease? Lung Cancer 37:271–276

Miller AB, Fox W, Tall R (1969) Five-year follow-up of the Medical Research Council comparative trial of surgery and radiotherapy for the primary treatment of small-celled or oat-celled carcinoma of the bronchus. Lancet 2:501–505

Miller KL, Marks LB, Sibley GS et al (2003) Routine use of approximately 60 Gy once-daily thoracic irradiation for patients with limited-stage small-cell lung cancer. Int J Radiat Oncol Biol Phys 56:355–359

Murray N, Coy P, Pater J et al (1993) Importance of timing for thoracic irradiation in the combined modality treatment of limited stage small cell lung cancer. J Clin Oncol 11:336–344

National Cancer Institute. (2020) SEER explorer: an Interactive Website for SEER Cancer Statistics. Surveill Res Progr.

NCCN Guidelines: version 2.21 – January 11, 2021. (Assessed on March 1, 2021 at https://www.nccn.org/professionals/physician_gls/pdf/sclc.pdf)

NICE Pathways; Treating Small Cell Lung Cancer.; http://pathways.nice.org.uk/pathways/lung-cancer, NICE Pathway last updated: 27 January 2021; assessed on March 1, 2021)

Niell HB, Herndon JE, Miller AA (2002) Randomized phase III intergroup trial (CALGB 9732) of etoposide and cisplatin with or without paclitaxel and G-CSF in patients with extensive stage small cell lung cancer. Proc Am Soc Clin Oncol 21:293a

Papac RJ, Son Y, Bien R, Tiedemann D, Keohane M, Yesner R (1987) Improved local control of thoracic disease in small-cell lung cancer with higher dose thoracic irradiation and cyclic chemotherapy. Int J Radiat Oncol Biol Phys 13:993–998

Pelosi G, Rindi G, Travis WD, Papotti M (2014) Ki-67 antigen in lung neuroendocrine tumors: unraveling a role in clinical practice. J Thorac Oncol 9: 273–284

Perry MC, Eaton WL, Propert KJ, Ware JH, Zimmer B, Chahinian AP, Skarin A, Carey RW, Kreisman H, Faulkner C (1987) Chemotherapy with or without radiation therapy in limited small-cell carcinoma of the lung. N Engl J Med 316:912–918

Pignon JP, Arriagada R, Ihde DC et al (1992) A meta-analysis of thoracic radiotherapy for small-cell lung cancer. N Engl J Med 327:1618–1627

Pijls-Johannesma MC, De Ruysscher D, Lambin P, Rutten I, Vansteenkiste JF (2005) Early versus late chest radiotherapy for limited stage small cell lung cancer. Cochrane Database Syst Rev 1:CD004700

Pujol JL, Carestia L, Daurès JP (2000) Is there a case for cisplatin in the treatment of small-cell lung cancer? A meta-analysis of randomized trials of a cisplatin-containing regimen versus a regimen without this alkylating agent. Br J Cancer 83:8–15

Roof KS, Fidias P, Lynch TJ, Ancukiewicz M, Choi NC (2003) Radiation dose escalation in limited-stage small-cell lung cancer. Int J Radiat Oncol Biol Phys 57:701–708

Rossi A, Di Maio M, Chiodini P et al (2012) Carboplatin- or cisplatin-based chemotherapy in first-line treatment of small-cell lung cancer: the COCIS meta-analysis of individual patient data. J Clin Oncol:1692–1698

Salama JK, Hodgson L, Pang H et al (2013) A pooled analysis limited-stage small-cell lung cancer patients treated with induction chemotherapy followed by concurrent platinum-based chemotherapy and 70 Gy daily radiotherapy: CALGB 30904. J Thorac Oncol 8:1043–1049

Salem A, Mistry H, Hatton M (2019) Association of chemoradiotherapy with outcomes among patients with stage I to II vs stage III small cell lung cancer. Secondary Analysis of a Randomized Clinical Trial. JAMA Oncol 5(3):e185335

Sandler AB (2003) Chemotherapy for small cell lung cancer. Sem Oncol 30:9–25

Sandler A, Declerck L, Wagner H (2000) A phase II study of cisplatin plus etoposide plus paclitaxel and concurrent radiation therapy for previously untreated limited stage small cell lung cancer (E2596): an eastern cooperative oncology group trial. Proc Am Soc Clin Oncol 19:491a. (Abstract 1920)

Schild S, Brindle JS, Geyer SM (2003) Long-term results of a phase III trial comparing once a day radiotherapy (QD RT) or twice a day radiotherapy (BID RT) in limited stage small cell lung cancer (LSCLC). Proc Am Soc Clin Oncol 21. (Abstract 2536)

Schiller JH, Adak S, Cella D, DeVore RF 3rd, Johnson DH (2001) Topotecan versus observation after cisplatin plus etoposide in extensive-stage small-cell lung cancer: E7593—a phase III trial of the eastern cooperative oncology group. J Clin Oncol 19:2114–2122

Schultz HP, Nielsen OS, Sell A (1988) Timing of chest radiation with respect to combination chemotherapy in small cell lung cancer, limited disease. Lung Cancer 4:153. (Abstract)

Sculier JP, Paesmans M, Bureau G et al (1996) Randomized trial comparing induction chemotherapy versus induction chemotherapy followed by maintenance chemotherapy in small-cell lung cancer. J Clin Oncol 14:2337–2344

Segawa Y, Uoeka H, Kiura K et al (2003) Phase I/II study of altered schedule of cisplatin and etoposide administration and concurrent accelerated hyperfractionated thoracic radiotherapy for limited-stage small-cell lung cancer. Lung Cancer 41:13–20

Shahi J, Wright JR, Gabos Z, Swaminath A (2016) Management of small-cell lung cancer with radiotherapy—a pan-Canadian survey of radiation oncologists. Curr Oncol 23:184–195

Shepherd FA, Crowley J, Van Houtte P et al (2007) The International Association for the Study of Lung Cancer lung cancer staging project: proposals regarding the clinical staging of small cell lung cancer in the forthcoming (seventh) edition of the tumor, node, metastasis classification for lung cancer. J Thorac Oncol 2:1067–1077

Shioyama Y, Nakamura K, Sasaki T et al (2013) Clinical results of stereotactic body radiotherapy for Stage I small-cell lung cancer: a single institutional experience. J Radiat Res 54:108–112

Sloan JA, Bonner JA, Hillman SL et al (2002) A quality-adjusted reanalysis of a phase III trial comparing once-daily thoracic radiation vs twice-daily thoracic radiation in patients with limited-stage small-cell lung cancer. Int J Radiat Oncol Biol Phys 52:371–381

Spiro SG, Souhami RL, Geddes DM et al (1989) Duration of chemotherapy in small cell lung cancer: a cancer research campaign trial. Br J Cancer 59:578–583

Spiro SG, James LE, Rudd RM et al (2006) London lung cancer group early compared with late radiotherapy in combined modality treatment for limited disease small-cell lung cancer: a London lung cancer group multicenter randomized clinical trial and meta-analysis. J Clin Oncol 24:3823–3830

Stahl JM, Corso CD, Verma V et al (2017) Trends in stereotactic body radiation therapy for stage I small cell lung cancer. Lung Cancer 103:11–16

Sun J-M, Ahn YC, Choi EK et al (2013) Phase III trial of concurrent thoracic radiotherapy with either first- or third-cycle chemotherapy for limited-disease small-cell lung cancer. Ann Oncol 24(8):2088–2092

Sundstrøm S, Bremnes RM, Kaasa S et al (2002) Norwegian lung cancer study group cisplatin and etoposide regimen is superior to cyclophosphamide, epirubicin, and vincristine regimen in small-cell lung cancer: results from a randomized phase III trial with 5 years' follow-up. J Clin Oncol 20:4665–4467

Takada M, Fukuoka M, Kawahara M et al (2002) Phase III study of concurrent versus sequential thoracic radiotherapy in combination with cisplatin and etoposide for limited-stage small-cell lung cancer: results of the Japan clinical oncology group study 9104. J Clin Oncol 20:3054–3060

Taneja TK, Sharma SK (2004) Markers of small cell lung cancer. World J Surg Oncol 2:1–5

Turrisi AT, Kim K, Blum R et al (1999) Twice-daily compared with once-daily thoracic radiotherapy in limited small-cell lung cancer treated concurrently with cisplatin and etoposide. N Engl J Med 340:264–271

Valan CD, Slagsvold JE, Halvorsen TE et al (2018) Survival in limited disease small cell lung cancer according to N3 lymph node involvement. Anticancer Res 38:871–876

Vallières E, Shepherd FA, Crowley J et al (2009) The IASLC Lung Cancer Staging Project: proposals regarding the relevance of TNM in the pathologic staging of small cell lung cancer in the forthcoming (seventh) edition of the TNM classification for lung cancer. J Thorac Oncol 4:1049–1059

Van Meerbeeck JP, Fennell DA, De Ruysscher DK (2011) Small-cell lung cancer. Lancet 378:1741–1755

Verma V, Simone CB 2nd, Allen PK et al (2017) Multi-institutional experience of stereotactic ablative radiation therapy for stage I small cell lung cancer. Int J Radiat Oncol Biol Phys 97:362–371

Videtic GMM, Truong PT, Dar AR, Yu EW, Stitt LW (2003) Shifting from hypofractionated to "conventionally" fractionated thoracic radiotherapy: a single institution's 10-year experience in the management of limited-stage small-cell lung cancer using concurrent chemoradiation. Int J Radiat Oncol Biol Phys 57:709–716

Videtic GM, Stephans KL, Woody NM et al (2013) Stereotactic body radiation therapy-based treatment model for stage I medically inoperable small cell lung cancer. Pract Radiat Oncol 3:301–306

Warde P, Payne D (1992) Does thoracic radiation improve survival and local control in limited-stage small cell carcinoma of the lung? J Clin Oncol 10:890–895

Watkins JM, Fortney JA, Wahlquist AE et al (2010) Once-daily radiotherapy to > or = 59.4 Gy versus twice-daily radiotherapy to > or = 45.0 Gy with concurrent chemotherapy for limited-stage small-cell lung cancer: a comparative analysis of toxicities and outcomes. Jpn J Radiol 28:340–348

Welsh JW, Heymach JV, Guo C et al (2020) Phase I/II trial of pembrolizumab and concurrent chemoradiation therapy for limited-stage small cell lung cancer. J Thorac Oncol 15:266–273

Woo IS, Park YS, Kwon SH et al (2000) A phase II study of VP-16-ifosfamide-cisplatin combination chemotherapy plus early concurrent thoracic irradiation for previously untreated limited small cell lung cancer. Jpn J Clin Oncol 30:542–546

Woods RL, Levi JA (1984) Chemotherapy for small cell lung cancer (SCLC): A randomised study of maintenance therapy with cyclophosphamide, adriamycin and vincristine (CAV) after remission induction with cis-platinum (CIS-DDP), VP 16–213 and radiotherapy. Proc Am Soc Clin Oncol 3:214

Work E, Nielsen O, Bentzen S, Fode K, Palshof T (1997) Randomized study of initial versus late chest irradiation combined with chemotherapy in limited-stage small cell lung cancer. J Clin Oncol 15:3030–3037

Wu Q, Xiong Y, Zhang S et al (2020) A meta-analysis of the efficacy and toxicity of twice-daily vs. once-daily concurrent chemoradiotherapy for limited-stage small cell lung cancer based on randomized controlled trials. Front Oncol 9:1460

Xia B, Hong L-Z, Cai X-W et al (2015) Phase 2 study of accelerated hypofractionated thoracic radiation therapy and concurrent chemotherapy in patients with limited-stage small-cell lung cancer. Int J Radiation Oncol Biol Phys 91:517–523

Yilmaz U, Anar C, Korkmaz E, Yapicioglu S, Karadogan I, Ozkök S (2010) Carboplatin and etoposide followed by once-daily thoracic radiotherapy in limited disease small-cell lung cancer: unsatisfactory results. Tumori 96:234–240

Yin X, Yan D, Qiu M, Huang L, Yan SX (2019) Prophylactic cranial irradiation in small cell lung cancer: a systematic review and meta-analysis. BMC Cancer 19:95

Zhu L, Zhang S, Xu X et al (2016) Increased biological effective dose of radiation correlates with prolonged survival of patients with limited-stage small cell lung cancer: a systematic review. PLoS One 11(5):e0156494

Role of Thoracic Radiation Therapy in Extensive Disease Small Cell Lung Cancer

Branislav Jeremić, Mohamed El-Bassiouny, Ramy Ghali, Ivane Kiladze, and Sherif Abdel-Wahab

Contents

1 Introduction 668
2 Thoracic Radiation Therapy (TRT) in ED SCLC 668
3 Specific Aspects of TRT in ED SCLC 671
4 What Is Practiced and What Is Recommended Nowadays 673
5 Future Aspects 673
References 674

Abstract

Of all patients with small cell lung cancer (SCLC), approximately two-thirds have extensive disease (ED SCLC) which represents the disease that spreads beyond confines of the thorax (M1), but includes as well patients whose disease has traditionally been described as "too large to be encompassed with a tolerable radiation port." Over the past several decades, chemotherapy (CHT) has been considered standard treatment option and only recently immunotherapy was introduced as additional ingredient to the standard treatment option. The vast majority of the data gathered from the past studies, however, is coming from CHT era where patterns of failure after CHT alone revealed substantial percentage failures occurring in the chest. It is, therefore, that curative, high-dose thoracic radiation therapy (TRT) was considered potentially useful tool capable of improving chest disease control and, hence, improved survival. Three important and prospective randomized studies and many retrospective studies showed potential for TRT in this setting, with, sometimes, confusing results. These have largely influenced existing practices and differing recommendations and guidelines worldwide. This chapter summarizes important aspects of TRT in ED SCLC and highlights existing controversies.

B. Jeremić (✉)
School of Medicine, University of Kragujevac, Kragujevac, Serbia
e-mail: nebareje@gmail.com

M. El-Bassiouny · R. Ghali · S. Abdel-Wahab
Department of Clinical Oncology, Ain Shams University, Cairo, Egypt

I. Kiladze
Department of Clinical Oncology, Caucasus Medical Center, Tbilisi, Georgia

1 Introduction

Small cell lung cancer (SCLC) accounts for 13–15% of all new lung cancer cases (Janne et al. 2002). It has a distinct tendency to disseminate early, which leads to the fact that 80–85% of patients present with advanced or extensive disease (ED SCLC) at diagnosis (Simon and Wagner 2003). In spite of significant efforts and refinements in staging system (Nicholson et al. 2015), this designation, however, includes not only metastatic patients, but also patients whose disease has traditionally been described as "too large to be encompassed with a tolerable radiation port," according to the Veterans' Affairs Lung Study Group (VALSG) classification (Kalemkerian 2011).

The standard treatment option for patients with ED SCLC remains chemotherapy (CHT). When given alone, it provides the median survival time (MST) of 9–12 months and 5-year survivals of 1–3% (Bunn Jr et al. 1977; Beck et al. 1988; Jeremic et al. 1999). In spite of the fact that up to 90% of patients experience response following initial CHT, it remains the disease with very poor prognosis because most of patients subsequently relapse. In order to improve dismal prognosis, many approaches aiming intensification of the treatment were attempted. Many of them including maintenance CHT (given after 4–6 cycles of initial CHT) (Splinter 1989; Bunn Jr 1992; Schiller et al. 2001) and higher doses of CHT (Ihde et al. 1994; Leyvraz et al. 2008) brought nothing in this setting. Only recently, immunotherapy added to CHT offered improved treatment results. Two studies, first-ever in this setting, IMpower 133 (Horn et al. 2018) and CASPIAN (Paz-Ares et al. 2019), showed an improvement in overall survival (OS) with the addition of immunotherapy to first-line CHT.

However, vast majority of existing knowledge and observations about the natural course and events in this setting come from CHT alone era. It was observed that even in patients achieving a complete intrathoracic response after initial CHT relapses are frequent and occur fast. This prompted speculation about the place and role of thoracic radiation therapy (TRT) which can be used to improve intrathoracic tumor control which, hopefully, can then translate into an improvement in the overall survival (Jeremic et al. 1999).

2 Thoracic Radiation Therapy (TRT) in ED SCLC

More than 20 years ago Jeremic et al. (1999) opened the new era in modern treatment of ED SCLC which included TRT. They have tested, in a prospective randomized Phase III fashion, TRT added to standard treatment option (CHT) versus the same CHT given alone, with a prophylactic cranial irradiation (PCI) given in both arms. This trial's premises included: (1) failure of second line CHT to control fast tumor recurrences, (2) these failures likely becoming the source of subsequent and lethal metastatic disease (in patients with previous non-metastatic ED SCLC), (3) TRT could hopefully control intrathoracic tumor, (4) if successful to a certain magnitude (both improved and prolonged intrathoracic tumor control), and (5) if the latter becomes a significant issue, then lead to an improvement in OS. The overshadowing question was which ED SCLC patients may benefit from TRT in ED SCLC?

In the Jeremic et al. trial (1999) patients initially received 3 cycles of cisplatin/etoposide (PE), after which patients were reevaluated and restaged at local and the distant level. Randomized were only patients with either a complete response (CR) at both local and distant level (CR/CR) or those who achieved a partial response (PR) within the thorax accompanied with the CR elsewhere (PR/CR). They received either accelerated hyperfractionated radiation therapy (Acc Hfx RT) or concurrent low-dose daily CHT, followed by PCI and then by additional 2 cycles of PE (group I) or 4 additional cycles of PE and PCI (Group II). Total tumor dose was 54 Gy in 36 fractions, 1.5 Gy BID, while PCI dose was 25 Gy in 10 daily fractions. TRT added to CHT offered superior median survival time (MST) and 5-year survival rates (17 vs. 11 months; $p = 0.041$, and

9.1 and 3.7%, respectively) and local recurrence-free survival (the median time to local recurrence, 30 vs. 22 months, and 5-year local recurrence-free survival, 20% vs. 8.1%, respectively; $p = 0.062$), but without effect on the distant metastasis-free survival ($p = 0.35$). Importantly, adding the fourth and the fifth cycle of CHT after Acc Hfx RT barely improved response in TRT group, and similarly to it, the sixth and seventh cycles of PE in CHT alone group brought only a few percent increase in response rates. These results question the need for more than 3–4 CHT cycles in this patient population, and may be seen as possible food for thoughts for future trials. An analysis of various pretreatment prognostic factors showed that higher Karnofsky performance status (KPS) score and no significant weight loss were strong prognosticators of improved treatment outcome. As a potential guide for future studies, the number of metastases independently influenced survival. It was shown that metastatic tumor burden should be taken into account since patients with ≥2 metastases had significantly worse outcome than those with only one metastasis. Since approximately 90% of all patients in the study of Jeremic et al. (1999) had 1–2 metastases, subsequent discussions in this field frequently labeled this disease extent as "limited" extensive disease.

Community of thoracic oncologists took years to digest these pioneering study results and more than 15 years passed until the next study was published in this setting. EORTC (Slotman et al. 2015) prospective phase III study included patients with performance status (PS) 0–2 and confirmed ED SCLC without clinical evidence of brain, leptomeningeal, or pleural metastases, who achieved any response to 4–6 cycles of PE who were treated with either TRT (30 Gy in 10 fractions) or no TRT, with all patients receiving PCI. Overall survival was longer in the TRT arm ($p = 0.066$), and 12-, 18-, and 24-month OS in the 2 arms was 33%, 16%, and 13% vs. 28%, 16%, and 3%, respectively. While the trial was negative for the primary endpoint of 1-year OS, it, however, became positive at 18 months ($p = 0.03$) and it remained so at 24 months ($p = 0.004$). Progression-free survival (PFS) was longer in the TRT arm ($p = 0.001$), while intrathoracic progression was seen more frequently in the CHT alone arm. Importantly, almost 50% reduction in intrathoracic recurrences (80% vs. 44%, respectively; $p = 0.001$) was observed for patients treated with TRT.

The Jeremic et al. (1999) and EORTC (Slotman et al. 2015) study characteristics greatly differed although EORTC study (Slotman et al. 2015) reconfirmed the importance of local control as initially suggested by Jeremic et al. (1999). However, owing to a more intensive TRT given with concurrent CHT in a shorter overall treatment time by Jeremic et al. (1999), faster improvement in local control was observed which led to faster improvement in the OS. When considering the 2 studies' characteristics and the magnitude of the difference in the treatment outcome (Jeremic 2015; Jeremic et al. 2017), which one may perhaps see as being at the two extremes, there seems to have been a necessity to fill in the existing gap with more clinical research.

The Radiation Therapy Oncology Group (RTOG) study 0937 (Gore et al. 2017) included patients with 1–4 extracranial metastases deemed eligible after achieving either CR or PR achieved after initial CHT. Patients received the PCI alone or PCI + TRT to the thorax and metastases. PCI was given with 25Gy in 10 daily fractions in 2 weeks, while TRT was given with 45Gy in 15 daily fractions in 3 weeks. Unfortunately, this study crossed the futility boundary for OS and was closed at planned interim analysis. One-year OS was similar between the groups: 60.1% for no-TRT and 50.8% for TRT ($p = 0.21$). One-year rates of progression were 79.6% for no-TRT, and 75% for TRT. Time to progression favored TRT group ($p = 0.01$). While OS exceeded predictions for both arms and TRT delayed progression it did not improve the 1-year OS. This trial reconfirmed that the first site of failure after CHT is likely to be in sites of presenting disease, that RT to these sites alters failure patterns, and that oligometastatic ED SCLC survival seems to have again approached that of LD SCLC, confirming the postulates and results of Jeremic et al. (1999).

The authors suggested that a more appropriate treatment for the patients with low volume systemic disease could have been early RT concurrent with cycle three or four of CHT in patients with a favorable response to cycles one and two of CHT followed by PCI, similar to the Jeremic trial (Jeremic et al. 1999).

Due to somewhat confusing results of these prospective studies, three recent meta-analyses attempted to bring clarity to this matter. While Palma et al. (2016) and Rathod et al. (2019) used only 2 (Palma et al. 2016) or 3 (Rathod et al. 2019) prospective randomized studies, Zhang et al. (2017) used 2 prospective and three retrospective studies. Each of these meta-analyses showed significant impact of TRT when added to standard treatment option (CHT alone) in terms of OS and PFS, although in the study of Rathod et al. (2019), the hazard ratio (HR) of 0.88 for OS did not significantly favor TRT. However, it clearly showed significant impact of TRT on reducing the risk of thoracic progression as the first site of progression with a relative risk of 0.52 (95% CI: 0.44–0.61).

Several studies, both of phase II design and retrospective nature reconfirmed important place and role of TRT in this setting (Zhu et al. 2011; Giuliani et al. 2011; Yee et al. 2012). In addition, several authors used propensity score matching (PSM) analysis to compare TRT/CHT with CHT alone in ED SCLC (Xu et al. 2017; Zhang et al. 2017; Deng et al. 2019; Tian et al. 2019; Qi et al. 2019). While some evaluated relatively small patient numbers (Xu et al. 2017; Qi et al. 2019; Deng et al. 2019) other used large data bases such as those of The National Cancer data Base (NCDB) (Zhang et al. 2017; Tian et al. 2019). Regardless of this difference, all of these studies unequivocally showed that OS and PFS were significantly improved by the addition of TRT and multivariate analyses used in some of these studies reconfirmed these findings.

All of the studies discussed above addressed TRT in a more "general" patient ED SCLC population. However, since the majority of ED SCLC patients are over 65-years-old, and few elderly patients are included in clinical trials, it remained poorly documented whether TRT can improve OS in elderly ED SCLC patients (Eskandar et al. 2015). Some authors specifically addressed the issue of effectiveness of TRT in this setting. An et al. (2017) reported on 118 patients >65 years with distant metastasis who were treated either with TRT/CHT or CHT alone. The MST and 3-year OS rates in the TRT/CHT group were significantly higher than those in the CHT alone group (17.0 months vs. 11.7 months; 18.1% vs. 14.9%; $p = 0.014$). In a similar patient population of a total of 93 patients, Qi et al. (2019) performed a PSM analysis with 40 patients each in TRT/CHT and CHT alone group. One-year OS, PFS, and local progression-free survival (LPFS) were all significantly better for TRT/CHT (55% vs. 25%, 32.1% vs. 0%, and 31% vs. 2.6%, respectively). MVA reconfirmed independent influence of TRT on OS.

Besides its effectiveness, TRT in ED SCLC has another proven and positive aspect, being cost-effective treatment option. Patrice et al. (2018) used cost-utility analysis and compared TRT/CHT versus CHT alone. The base case time horizon was 24 months; consistent with the maximum PFS reported in the CREST study (Slotman et al. 2015). OS was partitioned into two health states: PFS and post-progression survival. Costs were from a United States health care payer perspective and utilities were derived from the literature. Incremental cost-effectiveness ratios (ICERs) were calculated per quality-adjusted life year (QALY). In the base case, adding TRT to CHT was both cost-saving and more effective thereby strongly dominating CHT alone. At willingness-to-pay thresholds of $50,000, $100,000, and $200,000/QALY, TRT was preferred 68%, 81%, and 96% of the time, respectively. In the lifetime scenario analysis, the TRT ICER increased to $194,726/QALY. Having in mind that other studies showed much greater benefit than CREST did, with both longer survivals and more patients surviving prolonged periods of post-treatment, it is reasonable to assume, even without formal analysis, that cost-effectiveness of TRT in ED SCLC would be much higher and, therefore, preferable for both patients and health care systems.

3 Specific Aspects of TRT in ED SCLC

Both prospective and retrospective studies have used virtually all dose and fractionation TRT regimens. Both palliative and radical TRT, standard fraction, hypofractionated and hyperfractionated TRT had all been used in the past, without clear consensus of how practicing radiation oncologist should decide about it. Importantly, the *TRT dose* itself brought discussion in the light of existing data from the literature and several studies addressed that issue. Yoon et al. (2019) investigated this issue in 85 patients treated between 2008 and 2017 which received TRT with a biologically effective dose (BED) of >30 Gy_{10}. In univariate analysis, a BED >50 Gy_{10} was a significant prognostic factor for OS (40.8% vs. 12.5%, $p = 0.006$), PFS (15.9% vs. 9.6%, $p = 0.004$), and intrathoracic PFS (IT-PFS) (39.3% vs. 20.5%, $p = 0.004$) at 1 year. In multivariate analysis, a BED >50 Gy_{10} remained a significant prognostic factor for OS, PFS, and IT-PFS (HRs: 0.502; 0.453; 0.331), respectively. Xu et al. (2017) focused on 306 patients with ED SCLC and used a PSM analysis to compare TRT/CHT versus CHT alone. After matching, (113 cases for each group), the rates of OS, PFS, and local control (LC) at 2 years were 21.4%, 7.7%, and 34.5% for TRT/CHT and 10.3% ($p < 0.001$), 4.6% ($p < 0.001$), and 6.3% for CHT alone ($p < 0.001$), respectively. To investigate the effect of TRT dose, and considering the time efficiencies, they have introduced a concept of the time-adjusted BED (tBED) formula. Among PSM patients, 56 cases for each group received the high dose (tBED > 50 Gy) TRT and received low-dose (tBED < 50 Gy) TRT. Two-year OS, PFS, and LC rates were 32.3%, 15.3%, and 47.1% for the high dose compared with 17.0% ($p < 0.001$), 12.9% ($p = 0.097$), and 34.7% ($p = 0.029$) for low-dose TRT. Finally, Hasan et al. (2018) used the data from the NCDB and performed a PSM analysis on 3,280 M1 ED SCLC patients comparing TRT dose of >45 Gy to <45 Gy. The higher TRT dose was independent prognosticator of superior OS together with the female gender, age < 65 years, lower comorbidity score, absence of brain/liver/bone metastasis and starting the TRT 12 weeks after CHT. Propensity adjusted regression model showed a persistent correlation between a higher TRT dose and OS. These results reconfirm the necessity of administering as high TRT dose as possible in selected patients with ED SCLC, which was already brought to attention by a simple comparison of BED Gy_{10} in prospective studies of Jeremic et al. (1999), Slotman et al. (2015), and Gore et al. (2017): the best results were achieved in the study of Jeremic et al. (1999) having the highest BED Gy_{10}.

Another issue of importance may well be the *timing of TRT administration*. While universally accepted reasoning call for administration of TRT after all CHT had showed its effect, exactly when this is, remained unexplored. Simple observation of the start of TRT, i.e., after how many cycles of CHT it had been given, points to large differences between studies. While some mandated its start after a minimum of 6 cycles of PE (Slotman et al. 2015), other had shortened that period to 3–4 (Jeremic et al. 1999). Another issue connected to it, although rather obliquely, is whether administered TRT was given sequentially post-CHT (Slotman et al. 2015) or concurrently with CHT (Jeremic et al. 1999), whenever it actually started. Beside the effectiveness, the latter aspect should also bring into the focus existing toxicities these seemingly different approaches could bring. In one study (Luo et al. 2017), timing of administration of TRT post-CHT was investigated as "early" (<3 cycles) versus "late" (>3 cycles) CHT. PSM analysis was used to show no difference among the total of 56 patients in two groups although "early" group achieved numerically though not statistically significant superiority in OS and locoregionally relapse free survival, but not the PFS. Another loose connection with this issue seems to be the total number of CHT cycles to be given during the whole course on combined treatment. In spite of widely spread belief that 6 cycles of CHT should be considered as minimal, Jeremic et al. (1999) provided an intriguing data when evaluating the temporal aspects of achieving the response between TRT/CHT and CHT alone groups. Analysis of response rates provided the local complete response (CR) rates in two groups at weeks 9, 15, and 21. At week 9 (i.e., after 3 cycles of induction PE rate) and before the randomization, the difference was not observed (47 vs. 44%, $p = 0.77$). At week 15 (when either TRT/CHT or two additional cycles of PE were administered), the CR rate was significantly higher for TRT/CHT than in CHT alone (96 vs. 61%, $p = 0.000007$), and it persisted until week 21 when actual response rates for these two groups were 96 and 66%, respectively ($p = 0.00005$). Looking at both absolute increase in percent responders and the tempo of its achievement, the fourth and the fifth cycles of CHT add nothing to the response achieved in TRT/CHT patients after TRT had been added to 3 cycles of PE. Furthermore, the sixth and seventh cycles of PE in the CHT alone group brought only a few percent increase in response rates. Therefore, it seems that after 3 cycles of induction CHT followed by TRT, no gain was observed with additional CHT in the TRT/CHT alone group. Similarly, addition of sixth and seventh cycle of CHT altogether question the duration (number of cycles) of CHT as it is mostly nowadays.

Among many prognostic factors investigated, recent years brought focused interest in *location and the extent of the tumor spread*. In the study of Fukui et al. (2016), the number of metastatic sites (12.9 months for single sites vs. 7.1 months for multiple sites, $p = 0.015$) was prognosticator in univariate analysis, while MVA reconfirmed that the OS was significantly worse in multiple metastatic sites (HR 1.81, 95% CI 1.08–3.04; $p = 0.026$). When focused on 51 cases without pleural dissemination, the number of metastatic sites was associated with thoracic progression after initial CHT (65% for single sites vs. 36% for multiple sites, $p = 0.036$). Mahmoud et al. (2016) compared the benefits of TRT on OS between the intrathoracic (T-ED SCLC) and metastatic (M-ED SCLC) groups using the Surveillance Epidemiology and End Results (SEER) database. The 2-year OS was 13% in the TRT group compared to 4.1% in the no-TRT group ($p \leq 0.001$). In the M-ED SCLC group, the 2-year OS was 4.4% in the TRT group compared to 2.8% in the no-TRT group ($p < 0.001$). MVA confirmed that TRT was significant prognostic factor of OS in both groups. Hasan et al. (2018) used another large database (NCDB) and used MVA to show that the absence of brain/liver/bone metastases was significant and independent prognostic factor of improved outcome ($P < 0.01$). Zhang et al. (2019) evaluated the role of TRT in a selected patient population with oligometastatic ED SCLC without brain or liver involved. While for patients with oligometastasis ($n = 118$), TRT offered significant improvement in PFS (16.5 months vs. 9.1 months, $p = 0.005$) and OS (19.2 months vs. 15.6 months, $p = 0.039$), however, for patients with brain/liver/multimetastasis, the PFS and OS were not improved with TRT ($p = 0.49$; $p = 0.811$). The results of these studies should be seen in the context of previous findings (Jeremic et al. 1999; Slotman et al. 2017) who identified patients with 1–2 metastases as the likely candidates for successful employment of TRT in ED SCLC.

While widely adopted policy was and still is to offer TRT to patients responding to initial CHT, the question remains how *response to initial CHT* should govern us in that matter, having in mind that patients could experience both CR and PR at local/intrathoracic level, and the same at distant sites (in cases of M1 disease). Subgroup analyses of the CREST trial suggest that patients with residual intrathoracic disease benefited the most from TRT, with a statistically significant difference in OS (HR = 0.81, 95% CI 0.66–0.98, $p = 0.03$) when compared to patients with an intrathoracic CR after initial CHT had been given (Slotman and van Tinteren 2015; Slotman et al. 2017). This is in contrast with our own experience (Jeremic, unpublished data) which showed no difference in outcome between CR and PR patients when TRT is offered to both groups. Even more, they contradict the data coming from CHT alone studies which showed that even in patients who achieved CR, significant percentage of them eventually experienced intrathoracic recurrence, majority of these events occurring in the first year after treatment.

4 What Is Practiced and What Is Recommended Nowadays

Past decade brought several publications all aiming at existing practices regarding the use of TRT in ED SCLC (Ou et al. 2009; Mitin et al. 2016; Shahi et al. 2016; Post et al. 2017). They have all indicated that in a significant percentage of cases, practicing radiation oncologists used it in daily clinical practice in their centers. Importantly, it seems that this percentage rose from one-third (Ou et al. 2009) when non-specific data was used, to 88% (Shahi et al. 2016) and even to 96% when radiation oncologists with interest and significant practice in lung cancer were surveyed (Mitin et al. 2016). Impact of EORTC study (Slotman et al. 2015) and unfounded fear of toxicity seems to have driven respondents to adopt not curative but palliative TRT dose/fractionation of 30 Gy in 10 daily fractions in 2 weeks as the preferred TRT approach (Shahi et al. 2016).

Information coming from existing guidelines mirrors these. North American (US and Canada) guidelines differ a little in that regard with Canadian one (Sun et al. 2018) not recommending TRT but allowing its use in case-by-case basis to reduce intrathoracic recurrence. Besides ASTRO guidelines (Simone 2nd et al. 2020), endorsed by ASCO (Daly et al. 2021), various national medical oncology societies also recommend TRT (Dómine et al. 2020). Probably the most frequently both used and cited guidelines, those of The National Comprehensive Cancer Network (NCCN Guidelines 2021) from the USA, currently (Version. 2.21; January 2021) recommend initial systemic therapy with or without symptomatic therapy and, if needed, RT to extrathoracic sites, including brain RT. If response evaluation after initial therapy disclosed either CR or PR, TRT is recommended with optional PCI. Interestingly, in cases of SD after initial therapy, NCCN does not suggest TRT, in spite of the fact that it was shown to be feasible and effective in this setting (Jeremic et al. 1999). TRT dose/fractionation ranges from 30 Gy in 10 daily fractions to conventionally fractionated 60–70 Gy, but allows other regimens of similar efficacy. National Institute for Health and Care Excellence (NICE) in the UK guidelines for ED SCLC mirrors those of NCCN, but allow TRT to be given also in cases of PR achieved intrathoracically after 6 cycles of systemic therapy (NICE Pathways; Treating Small Cell Lung Cancer; http://pathways.nice.org.uk/pathways/lung-cancer, NICE Pathway last updated: 27 January 2021).

5 Future Aspects

CHT alone remained the mainstay of treatment in ED SCLC for decades and only recently immunotherapy was established as indispensible part of combined treatment approach. Two studies, IMpower 133 (Horn et al. 2018) and CASPIAN (Paz-Ares et al. 2019) showed very modest improvement with the MST improved by 2–3 months for both trials. Not to be forgotten, these trials did not include definitive TRT due to a limited data regarding safety of TRT and immunotherapy. As a result, there is currently uncertainty around if and how to integrate TRT into the chemo-immunotherapy backbone for ED SCLC. However, both preclinical data (Tang et al. 2014; Dovedi et al. 2017) and retrospective clinical data from non-small cell lung cancer studies (Shaverdian et al. 2017) showed synergy of radiation and immune check point inhibitors, establishing sound rationale for clinical use in SCLC. Indeed, initial results for the combination of immunotherapy and TRT in ED SCLC showed that combination of TRT and concurrent pembrolizumab was well tolerated, with no grade 4/5 toxicities, while only 6% patients experienced grade 3 toxicity (Welsh et al. 2020). Also, the combination of nivolumab plus ipilimumab combined with palliative TRT (30 Gy in 10 fractions) following standard CHT was evaluated in a Phase I/II study. This study attempted to enroll 52 ED SCLC patients to establish the recommended dose of immunotherapy when combined with TRT (part I), whereas Part II was planned to estimate PFS. Unfortunately, the study was prematurely closed after the first 21 patients were enrolled due to reported immune related adverse events (IRAEs), with 19.1% patients experiencing grade ≥ 3 pulmonary IRAEs. Six months PFS estimate was 24%, which was quite similar to that obtained with historic controls. Importantly, the toxicity profile of immunotherapy and TRT seemed consistent with those usually attributed to the two immunotherapy drugs given alone (Perez et al. 2021).

Several ongoing clinical trials aim at incorporation of TRT and chemo/immunotherapy in ED SCLC. In NCT02934503, pembrolizumab is added to standard CHT and TRT. Pembrolizumab begins, depending on the arm, with either the Cycle 1 or 2 of standard CHT, following completion of induction CHT or following completion of CHT and TRT. In NCT02402920, patients with ED SCLC will be given pembrolizumab following CHT and starting with TRT. Both NCT03923270 and NCT03043599 are exploring combination of CTLA-4 and PD-1/PD-L1 inhibition with TRT. In NCT03043599, ipilimumab is administered concurrently with TRT and given every 3 weeks for four doses. This is then followed by nivolumab maintenance. NCT03923270 explores administration of durvalumab monotherapy, tremelimumab with durvalumab, or durvalumab with olaparib after the completion of TRT. These studies and without any doubt, more of similar to come in the very near future, should help us define the place and role of chemo/immunotherapy and TRT in the setting of ED SCLC.

References

An C, Jing W, Zhang Y, Liu S, Wang H, Zhu K, Kong L, Guo H, Hui Z (2017) Thoracic radiation therapy could give survival benefit to elderly patients with extensive-stage small-cell lung cancer. Future Oncol 13:1149–1158

Beck LK, Kane MA, Bunn PA Jr (1988) Innovative and future approaches to small cell lung cancer treatment. Semin Oncol 15:300–314

Bunn PA Jr (1992) Clinical experience with carboplatin (paraplatin) in lung cancer. Semin Oncol 19(suppl 2):1–11

Bunn PA Jr, Cohen MH, Ihde DC, Fossieck BE Jr, Matthews MJ, Minna JD (1977) Advances in small cell bronchogenic carcinoma: a commentary. Cancer Treat Rep 61:333–342

Daly ME, Ismaila N, Decker RH et al (2021) Radiation therapy for small-cell lung cancer: ASCO guideline endorsement of an ASTRO guideline. J Clin Oncol 39(8):931–939. https://doi.org/10.1200/JCO.20.03364

Deng L, Zhou ZM, Xiao ZF et al (2019) Impact of thoracic radiation therapy after chemotherapy on survival in extensive-stage small cell lung cancer: a propensity score-matched analysis. Thorac Cancer 10:799–806

Dómine M, Moran T, Isla D et al (2020) SEOM clinical guidelines for the treatment of small-cell lung cancer (SCLC) (2019). Clin Transl Oncol 22:245–255

Dovedi SJ, Cheadle EJ, Popple AL et al (2017) Fractionated radiation therapy stimulates antitumor immunity mediated by both resident and infiltrating polyclonal T-cell populations when combined with PD-1 blockade. Clin Cancer Res 23:5514–5526

Eskandar A, Ahmed A, Daughtey M, Kenderian S, Mahdi F, Khan A (2015) Racial and sex differences in presentation and outcomes of small cell lung cancer in the United States: 1973 to 2010. Chest 147:e164–e165

Fukui T, Itabashi M, Ishihara M et al (2016) Prognostic factors affecting the risk of thoracic progression in extensive-stage small cell lung cancer. BMC Cancer 16:197

Giuliani ME, Atallah S, Sun A et al (2011) Clinical outcomes of extensive stage small cell lung carcinoma patients treated with consolidative thoracic radiotherapy. Clin Lung Cancer 12:375–379

Gore EM, Hu C, Sun AY et al (2017) Randomized phase II study comparing prophylactic cranial irradiation alone to prophylactic cranial irradiation and consolidative extracranial irradiation for extensive-disease small cell lung cancer (ED SCLC): NRG oncology RTOG 0937. J Thorac Oncol 12:1561–1570

Hasan S, Renz P, Turrisi A, Colonias A, Finley G, Wegner RE (2018) Dose escalation and associated predictors of survival with consolidative thoracic radiotherapy in extensive stage small cell lung cancer (SCLC): a National Cancer Database (NCDB) propensity-matched analysis. Lung Cancer 124:283–290

Horn L, Mansfield AS, Szczesna A, IMpower133 Study Group et al (2018) First-line atezolizumab plus chemotherapy in extensive-stage small-cell lung cancer. N Engl J Med 379:2220–2229

Ihde DC, Mulshine JL, Kramer BS et al (1994) Prospective randomized comparison of high-dose and standard-dose etoposide and cisplatin chemotherapy in patients with extensive-stage small cell lung cancer. J Clin Oncol 12:2022–2034

Janne PA, Freidlin B, Saxman S et al (2002) Twenty-five years of clinical research for patients with limited stage small cell lung carcinoma in North America. Cancer 95:1528–1538

Jeremic B (2015) Thoracic radiation therapy (TRT) in extensive disease small cell lung cancer (ED SCLC). Int J Radiat Oncol Biol Phys 93:7–9

Jeremic B, Shibamoto Y, Nikolic N et al (1999) The role of radiation therapy in the combined modality treatment of patients with extensive disease small-cell lung cancer (ED SCLC): a randomized study. J Clin Oncol 17:2092–2099

Jeremic B, Gomez-Caamano A, Dubinsky P, Cihoric N, Casas F, Filipovic N (2017) Radiation therapy in extensive stage small-cell lung cancer. Front Oncol 7:169

Kalemkerian GP (2011) Staging and imaging of small cell lung cancer. Cancer Imaging 11:253–258

Leyvraz S, Pampallona S, Martinelli G et al (2008) Solid tumors working party of the European group for blood and marrow transplantation. A threefold dose intensity treatment with ifosfamide, carboplatin, and etoposide for patients with small cell lung cancer: a randomized trial. J Natl Cancer Inst 100:533–541

Luo J, Xu L, Zhao L et al (2017) Timing of thoracic radiotherapy in the treatment of extensive-stage small-cell lung cancer: important or not? Radiat Oncol 12:42

Mahmoud O, Kwon D, Greenfield B, Wright JL, Samuels MA (2016) Intrathoracic extensive-stage small cell lung cancer: assessment of the benefit of thoracic and brain radiotherapy using the SEER database. Int J Clin Oncol 21:1062–1070

Mitin T, Jain A, Degnin C, Chen Y, Henderson M, Thomas CR Jr (2016) Current patterns of care for patients with extensive stage small cell lung cancer: survey of US radiation oncologists on their recommendations regarding thoracic consolidation radiotherapy. Lung Cancer 100:85–88

NCCN Guidelines: version 2.21 – January 11, 2021. https://www.nccn.org/professionals/physician_gls/pdf/sclc.pdf. Assessed 1 March 2021

NICE Pathways; Treating Small Cell Lung Cancer; NICE Pathway last updated: 27 January 2021. http://pathways.nice.org.uk/pathways/lung-cancer. Assessed 1 March 2021

Nicholson AG, Chansky K, Crowley J, on behalf of the Staging and Prognostic Factors Committee, Advisory Boards, and Participating Institutions et al (2015) The International Association for the Study of Lung Cancer Lung Cancer Staging Project: proposals for the revision of the clinical and pathologic staging of small cell lung cancer in the forthcoming eighth edition of the TNM classification for lung cancer. J Thorac Oncol 11:300–311

Ou S-H, Ziogas A, Zell JA (2009) Prognostic factors for survival in extensive stage small-cell lung cancer (ED-SCLC). The importance of smoking history, socioeconomic and marital statuses, and ethnicity. J Thorac Oncol 4:37–43

Palma DA, Warner A, Louie AV, Senan S, Slotman B, Rodrigues GB (2016) Thoracic radiotherapy for extensive stage small-cell lung cancer: a meta-analysis. Clin Lung Cancer 17:239–244

Patrice GI, Lester-Coll NH, Yu JB, Amdahl J, Delea TE, Patrice SJ (2018) Cost-effectiveness of thoracic radiotherapy for extensive stage small cell lung cancer using evidence from the CREST trial. Int J Radiat Oncol Biol Phys 100:97–106

Paz-Ares L, Dvorkin M, Chen Y, CASPIAN investigators et al (2019) Durvalumab plus platinum-etoposide versus platinum-etoposide in first-line treatment of extensive-stage small-cell lung cancer (CASPIAN): a randomised, controlled, open-label, phase 3 trial. Lancet 394:1929–1939

Perez BA, Kim S, Wang M et al (2021) Prospective single-arm phase 1 and 2 study: ipilimumab and nivolumab with thoracic radiation therapy after platinum chemotherapy in extensive-stage small cell lung cancer. Int J Radiat Oncol Biol Phys 109:425–435

Post CM, Verma V, Mitin T, Simone CB II (2017) Practice patterns of thoracic radiotherapy for extensive-stage small cell lung cancer: survey of United States academic thoracic radiation oncologists. Clin Lung Cancer 18:310–315.e1

Qi J, Xu L, Sun J, Wang X, Zhao L (2019) Thoracic radiotherapy benefits elderly extensive-stage small cell lung cancer patients with distant metastasis. Cancer Manag Res 11:10767–10775

Rathod S, Jeremic B, Dubey A, Giuliani M, Bashir B, Chowdhury A, Liang Y, Pereira S, Agarwal JP, Koul R (2019) Role of thoracic consolidation radiation in extensive stage small cell lung cancer: a systematic review and meta-analysis of randomised controlled trials. Eur J Cancer 110:110–119

Schiller JH, Adak S, Cella D, DeVore RF 3rd, Johnson DH (2001) Topotecan versus observation after cisplatin plus etoposide in extensive-stage small-cell lung cancer: E7593–a phase III trial of the eastern cooperative oncology group. J Clin Oncol 19:2114–2122

Shahi J, Wright JR, Gabos Z, Swaminath A (2016) Management of small-cell lung cancer with radiotherapy-a pan-Canadian survey of radiation oncologists. Curr Oncol 23:184–195

Shaverdian N, Lisberg AE, Bornazyan K et al (2017) Previous radiotherapy and the clinical activity and toxicity of pembrolizumab in the treatment of non-small-cell lung cancer: a secondary analysis of the KEYNOTE-001 phase 1 trial. Lancet Oncol 18:895–903

Simon GR, Wagner H (2003) Small cell lung cancer. Chest 123(1 Suppl):259S–271S

Simone CB 2nd, Bogart JA, Cabrera AR et al (2020) Radiation therapy for small cell lung cancer: an ASTRO clinical practice guideline. Pract Radiat Oncol 10:158–173

Slotman BJ, van Tinteren H (2015) Which patients with extensive stage small-cell lung cancer should and should not receive thoracic radiotherapy? Transl Lung Cancer Res 4:292–294

Slotman BJ, Van Tinteren H, Praag JO et al (2015) Use of thoracic radiotherapy for extensive stage small-cell lung cancer: a phase 3 randomised controlled trial. Lancet 385:36–42

Slotman BJ, Faivre-Finn C, van Tinteren H et al (2017) Which patients with ES-SCLC are most likely to benefit from more aggressive radiotherapy: a secondary analysis of the phase III CREST trial. Lung Cancer 108:150–153

Splinter TAW (1989) Chemotherapy of small cell lung cancer (SCLC): duration of treatment. Lung Cancer 5:186–196

Sun A, Durocher-Allen LD, Ellis PM et al (2018) Guideline for the initial management of small cell lung cancer (limited and extensive stage) and the role of thoracic radiotherapy and first-line chemotherapy. Clin Oncol (R Coll Radiol) 30:658–666

Tang C, Wang X, Soh H et al (2014) Combining radiation and immunotherapy: a new systemic therapy for solid tumors? Cancer Immunol Res 2:831–838

Tian S, Zhang X, Jiang R et al (2019) Survival outcomes with thoracic radiotherapy in extensive-stage small-cell lung cancer: a propensity score-matched analysis of the national cancer database. Clin Lung Cancer 20(6):484–493.e6

Welsh JW, Heymach JV, Chen D et al (2020) Phase I trial of pembrolizumab and radiation therapy after induction chemotherapy for extensive-stage small cell lung cancer. J Thorac Oncol 15:266–273

Xu LM, Cheng C, Kang M et al (2017) Thoracic radiotherapy (TRT) improved survival in both oligo- and polymetastatic extensive stage small cell lung cancer. Sci Rep 7:9255

Yee D, Butts C, Reiman A et al (2012) Clinical trial of post-chemotherapy consolidation thoracic radiotherapy for extensive-stage small cell lung cancer. Radiother Oncol 102:234–238

Yoon HG, Noh JM, Ahn YC, Oh D, Pyo H, Kim H (2019) Higher thoracic radiation dose is beneficial in patients with extensive small cell lung cancer. Radiat Oncol J 37(3):185–192

Zhang X, Yu J, Zhu H et al (2017) Consolidative thoracic radiotherapy for extensive stage small cell lung cancer. Oncotarget 8:22251–22261

Zhang H, Deng L, Wang X, Wang D, Teng F, Yu J (2019) Metastatic location of extensive stage small-cell lung cancer: implications for thoracic radiation. J Cancer Res Clin Oncol 145:2605–2612

Zhu H, Zhou Z, Wang Y et al (2011) Thoracic radiation therapy improves the overall survival of patients with extensive-stage small cell lung cancer with distant metastasis. Cancer 117:5423–5431

Prophylactic Cranial Irradiation in Small Cell Lung Cancer

William G. Breen and Yolanda I. Garces

Contents

1 Introduction 677
2 **Studies Evaluating Prophylactic Cranial Irradiation** 678
2.1 Rationale and Initial Studies of Prophylactic Cranial Irradiation 678
2.2 Early Randomized Trials 678
2.3 Meta-analyses 679
2.4 Extensive-Stage Small Cell Lung Cancer 680
3 **Treatment Schedule** 681
3.1 Dose and Fractionation 681
3.2 Timing of PCI 681
4 **Neurotoxicity and Quality of Life** 682
4.1 Retrospective Studies 682
4.2 Prospective Trials 682
4.3 Hippocampal Avoidance Prophylactic Cranial Irradiation 683
5 **Patterns of Care and Modern Perspectives** 684
6 **Conclusions** 685
References 685

W. G. Breen · Y. I. Garces (✉)
Department of Radiation Oncology, Mayo Clinic Alix School of Medicine, Rochester, MN, USA
e-mail: breen.william@mayo.edu;
garces.yolanda@mayo.edu

Abstract

Prophylactic cranial radiation (PCI) has been used to prevent or delay the development of brain metastases in patients with small cell lung cancer, given the propensity for disease relapse in the brain. Several older studies demonstrated that PCI reduces the rate of brain metastases and improves survival. However, the use of PCI in the modern era of routine MRI imaging is controversial due to conflicting evidence of efficacy and toxicities. Modern techniques such as hippocampal avoidance are being tested in hopes of decreasing toxicity. Prospective clinical trials addressing these issues are ongoing and will help guide modern treatment.

1 Introduction

Small cell lung cancer (SCLC) comprises 15% of all lung cancer cases. Disease spread to the central nervous system (CNS) is unfortunately common in patients with SCLC. Up to 15% of SCLC patients have brain metastases present at the time of diagnosis. Additionally, approximately 30–70% of small cell lung cancer patients will ultimately develop clinical evidence of brain metastases (Aupérin et al. 1999; Takahashi et al. 2017). Autopsy series report even higher incidence of brain metastases, at 65–80% (Nugent et al. 1979; Hirsch et al. 1982; Komaki et al. 1981). Standard cytotoxic chemotherapy has difficulty crossing the blood-brain barrier, and therefore methods to prevent CNS progression and death are needed.

Treatment of the whole brain with radiotherapy prior to the diagnosis of brain metastases, with the intent of preventing future development of brain metastases, is referred to as prophylactic cranial irradiation (PCI). PCI has previously been established as a standard of care for patients with limited-stage SCLC responding to initial treatment, as it was demonstrated to decrease the incidence of brain metastases and improve overall survival (Aupérin et al. 1999). However, the use of PCI in the modern management of small cell lung cancer has become increasingly controversial due to conflicting evidence of efficacy and toxicities in the modern era of MRI imaging and advancing treatment techniques.

2 Studies Evaluating Prophylactic Cranial Irradiation

2.1 Rationale and Initial Studies of Prophylactic Cranial Irradiation

PCI for SCLC was first proposed in 1973 by Hansen and colleagues to address the high rate of brain metastasis development in SCLC patients experiencing prolonged survival after the use of novel chemotherapeutic agents (Hansen 1973). In an early retrospective study evaluating the role of PCI in the management of SCLC, Komaki and colleagues analyzed the impact of PCI use on the incidence of brain metastases in patients with SCLC. Of 131 patients included, 57 received PCI and 74 did not. Patients who received PCI were significantly less likely to experience CNS failure at 12 and 24 months compared to those who did not receive PCI (11% vs. 28%, and 11% vs. 58%, respectively; $p < 0.01$) (Komaki et al. 1981).

Similarly, prospective studies from the 1970s also concluded that PCI decreased the incidence of brain metastases in patients with SCLC but did not result in an overall survival benefit for the entire SCLC population (Cox et al. 1978; Jackson Jr et al. 1977). Later, clinical trials from the 1990s demonstrated that patients experiencing a complete response to chemoradiotherapy may indeed experience a survival benefit with the use of PCI (Arriagada et al. 1995; Gregor et al. 1997; Laplanche et al. 1998; Shaw et al. 1994; Ohonoshi et al. 1993).

2.2 Early Randomized Trials

Several randomized trials have been performed in an attempt to better define the role of PCI in the management of SCLC (Table 1). A French prospective randomized trial (PCI-85) was performed to evaluate the effect of PCI on the incidence of brain metastases, overall survival, and late toxic effects of treatment. A total of 300 patients with SCLC in complete remission were enrolled at 21 centers from March 1985 to March 1993. Patients with extensive-stage SCLC comprised 20% of the study population. Randomization was to PCI at a dose of 24 Gray in 8 fractions (24 Gy/8 Fx) ($n = 149$) vs. no PCI ($n = 151$). PCI was given at the time of determination of complete remission. No chemotherapy was allowed from 1 week before PCI until 1 week after PCI (Arriagada et al. 1995). The incidence of brain metastasis at 2 years was significantly decreased in the arm receiving PCI (40% vs. 67%, $p < 10^{-13}$), which translated into a non-statistically significant improvement in 2-year overall survival (29% vs. 21.5%, $p = 0.14$). A follow-up study (PCI-88) was closed early based on the interim analysis showing such a significant decrease in the incidence of brain metastasis that most investigators felt that PCI should be administered to all patients (Laplanche et al. 1998).

An early Japanese trial evaluating 46 patients with SCLC in complete remission showed a significant decrease in the rate of brain metastasis with the use of PCI (Ohonoshi et al. 1993). The incidence of CNS relapse in the group receiving PCI was 22% versus 52% in those who did not receive PCI. A trend toward improved median

Table 1 Characteristics of studies examining the role of PCI in SCLC

Study	N	PCI dose[a]	Brain metastasis PCI	Brain metastasis No PCI	Overall survival PCI	Overall survival No PCI
Arriagada et al. (1995)	300	24 Gy/8 Fx	40% 2 years	67% 2 years	29% 2 years	21.5% 2 years
Laplanche et al. (1998)	211	24 Gy/8 Fx	44% 4 years	51% 4 years	22% 4 years	16% 4 years
Ohonoshi et al. (1993)	46	40 Gy/20 Fx	22%	52%	22% 5 years	13% 5 years
Gregor et al. (1997)	314	30 Gy/10 Fx	30% 2 years	38% 2 years	25% 2 years	19% 2 years
Aupérin et al. (1999)	987	24–25 Gy/8–12 Fx	33.3% 3 years	58.6% 3 years	20.7% 3 years	15.3% 3 years
Slotman et al. (2007)	286	20 Gy/5 Fx	14.6% 1 year	40.4% 1 year	27.1% 1 year	13.3% 1 year
Takahashi et al. (2017)	224	25 Gy/10 Fx	32.9% 1 year	59.0% 1 year	48.4% 1 year	53.6% 1 year

PCI prophylactic cranial radiation, *Gy* gray, *Fx* fractions
[a] Most common dose

overall survival (21 vs. 15 months) was also seen in the group receiving PCI. The 5-year overall survival rate for patients receiving PCI or no PCI was 22% and 13%, respectively.

A three-arm trial performed by the UKCCCR and EORTC was designed to randomize 314 patients to either PCI at a dose of 36 Gy/18 Fx or 24 Gy/12 Fx versus no PCI (Gregor et al. 1997). Poor accrual rates after initiation of the trial led to a trial redesign that allowed treating physicians to select the PCI dose regimen. Most physicians chose 30 Gy/10 Fx ($n = 61$) or 8 Gy/1 Fx ($n = 25$). Consistent with other studies, PCI was associated with a significant reduction in brain metastases (38% vs. 54%, HR = 0.44, 95% CI: 0.29–0.67), as well as an improvement in metastasis-free survival (HR = 0.75, 95% CI: 0.58–0.96). No difference in overall survival was observed between the group receiving PCI and those not receiving PCI, with median survival durations of 305 days and 300 days, respectively.

As in SCLC, the use of PCI after complete remission in patients with non-small cell lung cancer (NSCLC) has also been studied and demonstrated to reduce the incidence of brain metastases, but without overall survival benefit. Recently, long-term results were reported from the NRG Oncology/RTOG 0214 phase III randomized clinical trial comparing PCI versus observation in patients with stage III NSCLC without progression after definitive therapy (Gore et al. 2011; Sun et al. 2019). At a median follow-up time of 9.2 years for living patients and 2.1 years for all patients, patients who received PCI were 57% less likely to develop brain metastases. No difference was observed in the overall survival between groups, with 5- and 10-year survival rates of 24.7% and 17.6% for patients receiving PCI, compared to 26.0% and 13.3% for those who did not receive PCI (HR for death with PCI: 0.82, 95% CI: 0.63–1.06, $p = 0.12$).

2.3 Meta-analyses

Given the suggestions of improved survival with PCI for SCLC patients with limited-stage disease who have responded to initial treatment, a pivotal meta-analysis was performed by Auperin and colleagues. This study included 7 prospective trials containing 987 patients with limited-stage SCLC in complete remission after primary chemoradiotherapy (Aupérin et al. 1999). As was demonstrated in the original trials, the use of PCI significantly reduced the incidence of brain metastasis at 3 years (33.3% vs. 58.6% at 3 years, $p < 0.001$). More strikingly, an absolute 3-year overall survival benefit of 5.4% was also detected (15.3% vs. 20.7%, $p = 0.01$) favoring the use of PCI. While this study has influenced treatment guidelines and practice, there have been criticisms of the methodology employed. Over half of the trials included (4 of 7) enrolled less than 100 patients, and approximately 15% of patients had extensive-stage disease. Furthermore, the dose fractionation regimens were not uniform among the trials.

A subsequent meta-analysis by Meert and colleagues, which included 12 randomized trials and 1547 patients, drew a similar conclusion: PCI reduces the incidence of brain metastases and improves overall survival (Meert et al. 2001). In this analysis, a decrease in the incidence of metastatic brain lesions was seen for all patients given PCI (HR 0.48; 95% CI: 0.39–0.60), and an improvement in overall survival was seen for patients in complete remission given PCI (HR 0.82; 95% CI: 0.71–0.96). This meta-analysis also has limitations, as only 5 of the 12 trials consisted exclusively of patients known to be in complete remission after primary therapy, meaning cranial radiation may have been treating clinically detectable brain metastases in the other trials. In the other trials, five included patients given PCI at the time of induction chemotherapy, and two included patients given PCI at the end of induction chemo without any restaging.

As a result of the randomized trials and meta-analyses described, PCI for limited-stage SCLC after complete or partial response became a standard of care, earning a Category 1 NCCN recommendation which remains in modern guidelines (Small Cell Lung Cancer 2021).

2.4 Extensive-Stage Small Cell Lung Cancer

Two major randomized clinical trials have examined the role of PCI in extensive-stage small cell lung cancer. The EORTC trial included 286 patients with extensive-stage SCLC and any response to 4–6 cycles of chemotherapy (Slotman et al. 2007). Patients in this trial were randomized to either PCI (20 Gy/5 Fx or 30 Gy/12 Fx) or no radiotherapy. Cumulative risk of brain metastasis at 1 year was decreased in the group that received PCI (14.8% vs. 40.4%, $p < 0.001$), and progression-free survival was also improved with PCI at 14.7 vs. 12 weeks ($p = 0.02$). Although not a primary endpoint of the trial, overall survival at 1 year was also improved in patients receiving PCI compared to the no-radiotherapy group (27% vs. 13%, respectively, $p = 0.003$). This trial is not without valid criticisms. Most notably, all patients did not receive staging MRI prior to PCI. This could result in a number of patients with potentially clinically detectable brain metastases, who therefore received therapeutic whole-brain radiation rather than true PCI.

A more modern phase III randomized clinical trial of PCI for extensive-stage SCLC was performed in Japan, and it required MRI for every patient prior to PCI (Takahashi et al. 2017). This study randomized 224 patients with extensive-stage disease who had any response to chemotherapy and no brain metastases on MRI to PCI (25 Gy in 10 fractions) versus no PCI. Patients were stratified by age, performance status, and response to chemotherapy. This study was terminated early for futility to detect a difference in the primary endpoint of overall survival, and final analysis showed median survival of 11.6 months for PCI vs. 13.7 months for no PCI (HR: 1.27, 95% CI: 0.96–1.68, $p = 0.094$). PCI was associated with decreased brain metastasis development, with cumulative incidence of brain metastases at 12 months 32.9% (95% CI: 24.3–41.7%) for those who received PCI, compared to 59.0% (95% CI: 49.1–67.6%) for those who did not receive PCI.

A meta-analysis by Yin and colleagues incorporated these more recent PCI studies (Yin et al. 2019). They included seven studies with 2114 total patients, including the EORTC and Japanese studies described above. They again demonstrated that PCI decreased the rate of brain metastasis development (HR: 0.45, 95% CI: 0.38–0.55, $p < 0.001$) and improved OS (HR 0.81, 95% CI: 0.67–0.99, $p < 0.001$). However, they noted high heterogeneity in their findings attributable to whether patients had brain imaging after initial chemoradiotherapy. In studies where patients had brain imaging after chemoradiotherapy, there was no survival benefit to PCI (HR: 0.94, 95%

CI: 0.74–1.18), while a survival benefit remained in studies that did not incorporate post-chemoradiotherapy brain imaging (HR: 0.70, 95% CI: 0.57–0.85).

These more recent studies, particularly the Japanese trial by Takahashi and colleagues, indicating that patients who undergo routine MRI surveillance do not have a survival benefit from PCI have influenced clinical practice and led many clinicians to decrease the utilization of PCI (Gjyshi 2019). Still, these findings were in patients with extensive-stage disease, and as indicated by the NCCN guidelines, it is important that clinicians continue to engage patients in shared decision-making regarding risks and benefits of PCI. We await the results of the ongoing SWOG MAVERICK phase III clinical trial comparing PCI vs. MRI surveillance for further insights (NCT04155034).

3 Treatment Schedule

3.1 Dose and Fractionation

The UKCCCR/EORTC study indicated a potential dose-response to PCI, as patients receiving 24 Gy/12 Fx PCI had no difference in the incidence of brain metastasis compared to those patients not receiving any PCI, while those who received 36 Gy in 18 Fx appeared to have more benefit (Gregor et al. 1997). A dose-response was also seen in the meta-analysis performed by the Prophylactic Cranial Irradiation Overview Collaborative Group (Aupérin et al. 1999).

Conflicting data comes from Canadian investigators who reported the results of a retrospective review of 163 patients with limited-stage SCLC given PCI (Tai et al. 2003). No difference in outcomes based on dosing schedule was seen among the patients in this study. Additionally, a higher biologically equivalent dose (BED) did not significantly decrease the incidence of brain metastases. On further analysis, the 5-year overall survival rate was improved in patients that received a BED of <39 Gy_{10} compared to those receiving a BED of ≥39 Gy_{10} (22.3% vs. 13.3%, $p = 0.03$). It is worthwhile to note, however, that only a small number of patients ($n = 6$) in this review actually received a dose ≥39 Gy.

A large intergroup trial attempted to address this question by enrolling 720 patients with limited-stage SCLC in a randomized trial comparing standard PCI dose (25 Gy/10 Fx) versus a higher dose PCI (36 Gy/18 Fx or 36 Gy/24 BID Fx). Patients in this trial were required to have a documented complete remission prior to enrollment. Patients from 157 different treatment centers in 22 different countries were represented (Le Pechoux et al. 2009). No significant difference in the incidence of brain metastasis at 2 years was detected between the high- and low-dose groups (23% and 29%, respectively, $p = 0.18$). An increased 5-year overall survival rate was seen in the high-dose arm compared to the low-dose arm (42% vs. 37%, $p = 0.05$), but of note, survival was not the primary endpoint of the trial. The authors concluded that 25 Gy in 10 fractions should remain the standard of care.

Altered fractionation has also been evaluated as a potential method to improve control of brain metastasis and promote improved survival. A single-institution phase II trial comparing twice-daily PCI to observation reported a 2-year disease-free and overall survival of 54% and 62%, respectively, in 15 patients who received PCI (Wolfson et al. 2001).

Based on the lack of evidence for increased effectiveness of a higher PCI dose or altered fractionation, 25 Gy in 10 fractions has remained a standard PCI regimen. The currently open NRG CC003 (NCT02635009) trial also uses 25 Gy in 10 fractions.

3.2 Timing of PCI

The large meta-analysis conducted by Aupérin et al. (1999) suggests that control of brain metastases improves as the delay to receiving PCI is decreased. On subgroup analysis, a significant reduction in the risk of brain metastasis was seen as the time between the start of induction therapy and PCI decreased. The relative risk of developing brain metastases compared to a control group was 0.27 in patients receiving PCI <4 months from the start of induction therapy, 0.50 in the 4–6-month group, and 0.69 in the >6-month group ($p = 0.01$) (Aupérin et al. 1999). It should be acknowledged that this study did not require MRI prior to PCI, and more timely PCI may have actually meant more timely whole-brain radiation therapy for clinically detectable brain metastases. In another study, the rate of brain metastases was decreased in patients receiving PCI after 2–3 cycles of chemotherapy compared to after 5–6 cycles (Lee et al. 1987).

A radiobiologic analysis was performed to evaluate the effect of increased cranial radiation dose on brain relapse rate in patients with SCLC (Suwinski et al. 1998). Using data from 42 trials which report the incidence of brain metastases both with and without the use of PCI, these investigators calculated that in patients not receiving PCI, the cumulative incidence of brain metastases was 32%. In the group of patients receiving PCI within 60 days of starting primary therapy, a linear dose-response was established up to a dose of 35 Gy when delivered as daily 2 Gy fractions. The same relationship was not seen, however, if PCI was delayed and delivered after 60 days. Also, in patients receiving early PCI (<60 days), the dose of radiation needed to produce a 50% reduction in the rate of brain metastases was less than that in those receiving late PCI (20 Gy vs. 27 Gy, respectively).

These studies illuminate the importance of timely initiation of PCI in order to optimize results.

4 Neurotoxicity and Quality of Life

4.1 Retrospective Studies

In the large meta-analyses showing improved brain control and survival in patients who received PCI, the neurotoxicity experienced is not well described and data regarding the extent of neurotoxicity induced by PCI is inconclusive (Aupérin et al. 1999; Meert et al. 2001). Data from Mayo Clinic and North Central Cancer Treatment Group indicates a 2- and 5-year risk of severe neurotoxicity of 3% and 10%, respectively, in patients receiving PCI (Shaw et al. 1994).

A retrospective study of 30 patients treated at MD Anderson Cancer Center attempted to better characterize the risks of neurotoxicity from PCI (Komaki et al. 1995). On initial evaluation, 97% of patients had evidence of cognitive dysfunction prior to receiving PCI. The most common deficiencies were in verbal memory, frontal lobe dysfunction, and fine motor coordination. Excluding the patients with underlying medical conditions such as stroke, learning disability, or alcohol abuse, 20 of 21 patients still displayed abnormal testing. Additional testing of 11 patients at 6–20 months after PCI revealed no significant difference in any of the tests compared to baseline. A dose of 25 Gy delivered in 10 fractions was used in all patients analyzed. A corollary study published in 2008 confirms these results (Grosshans et al. 2008). In the 17 patients with extended follow-up (mean 1.5 years), early declines in executive function and expressive language tests were observed. When controlling for disease progression, no differences were seen from pre-PCI testing. Testing at later time points (≥450 days) revealed significant improvements in expressive speech and motor coordination. In another study which showed improved brain control and survival in the group of patients treated with PCI, late neurotoxicity was observed infrequently with only one patient experiencing mild neurological deterioration (Ohonoshi et al. 1993).

4.2 Prospective Trials

The results regarding neuropsychological testing, global health status, and quality-of-life outcomes in patients enrolled in randomized trials are also mixed (Takahashi et al. 2017; Arriagada et al. 1995; Gregor et al. 1997; Slotman et al. 2007).

In the PCI-85 study, patients underwent neuropsychological testing including temporospatial orientation, memory, judgment, language, praxis, and mood status (Arriagada et al. 1995). The tests were performed at randomization and at 6, 18, 30, and 48 months later and if neurological symptoms appeared. At 2 years, no test showed any significant difference from baseline.

In the UKCCCR/EORTC trial, 136 patients participated in extensive psychometric testing that was performed at randomization and every 6 months (Gregor et al. 1997). Up to 41% of patients analyzed had significant abnormalities on individual tests before PCI, and additional impairment was seen at 6 months and 1 year. There were no notable differences, however, between the group receiving PCI and the group that did not. The most common symptoms reported at follow-up were tiredness, lack of energy, irritability, decreased sexual interest, shortness of breath, and cough. These symptoms were moderate or severe more frequently in the group of patients that did not receive PCI, potentially due to increased incidence of brain metastases.

Based on the increased local control in the brain with the use of PCI in SCLC, recent trials have also focused on patients with NSCLC. A prematurely closed, prospective randomized trial enrolled 340 patients without disease progression after completing definitive therapy for NSCLC, and randomized to PCI (30 Gy/15 Fx) versus observation (Sun et al. 2011). Patients had neurocognitive function assessed with Mini-Mental Status Exam (MMSE), Hopkins Verbal Learning Test (HLVT), and Activity of Daily Living Scale (ADLS) and used the same quality-of-life tools as the patients described in the EORTC extensive-stage SCLC study (Slotman et al. 2007, 2009). No significant differences in quality of life, MMSE, or ADLS were observed at 1 year, but patients receiving PCI had decreased scores for immediate and delayed recall ($p = 0.03$ and 0.008, respectively) on HVLT.

The effect of PCI on quality of life has also been studied in patients with extensive-stage lung cancer (Slotman et al. 2007, 2009). In the EORTC trial, two quality-of-life tools (EORTC-QLQ-C30 and BN20) were used to analyze short- and long-term changes in functioning. In a preliminary report, the authors noted that fatigue and hair loss were significantly more severe in patients receiving PCI (Slotman et al. 2007). No significant differences were seen in global health status, role functioning, cognitive functioning, or emotional functioning. A subsequent study showed a limited effect of PCI on these factors, with no cognitive factors reaching the level of clinical significance predefined in the protocol design (Slotman et al. 2009). Patients receiving PCI had an increased rate of severe worsening in global health status (35% vs. 22%) from baseline to 3 months. There was poor compliance with follow-up assessments, dropping from 94% participation rate at baseline to only 60% and 55% at 6 weeks and 3 months, respectively. Furthermore, the median survival of 6 months seen in this cohort was shorter than expected. Both of these factors may have contributed to a lack of power to detect a difference between groups. An exploratory analysis of other symptom scale factors, however, still showed significant worsening in patients receiving PCI in a number of domains including appetite loss, constipation, nausea and vomiting, social functioning, future uncertainty, headaches, motor dysfunction, and weakness of the legs.

The Japanese study by Takahashi and colleagues also included comparisons of toxicity and neurocognitive function between PCI and no PCI (Takahashi et al. 2017). At 3 months after randomization, the most common grade 3+ adverse event was anorexia, noted in 6% of PCI patients compared to 2% of non-PCI patients. Two patients in the PCI arm experienced grade 3+ dermatitis (compared to 0 on the no-PCI arm), and three patients experienced grade 3+ malaise (compared to one on the no-PCI arm). There were no significant differences in neurocognitive function as measured by the Mini-Mental State Exam (MMSE) at baseline, 12 months, or 24 months.

4.3 Hippocampal Avoidance Prophylactic Cranial Irradiation

Techniques have been developed to decrease the potential neurocognitive effects of whole-brain radiotherapy (WBRT). Evidence suggests that radiation disrupts the normal microvascular angiogenesis of the hippocampus and decreases neurogenic cell proliferation in vitro (Monje et al. 2002). Abnormal hippocampal function has been shown to correlate with decreased memory in both humans and animals (Abayomi 1996; Broadbent et al. 2004). As such, the technique of hippocampal avoidance whole-brain radiation therapy (HA-WBRT) for brain metastases was established (Gondi et al. 2010; Gutierrez et al. 2007; Hsu et al. 2010). A second, complementary technique developed to prevent cognitive deterioration is the medication 3,5-dimethyladamantan-1-amine (memantine). Memantine was associated with better cognitive function and delayed time to cognitive decline on a large, randomized clinical trial (Brown et al. 2013).

The NRG CC001 phase III clinical trial randomized 518 patients with brain metastases to HA-WBRT with memantine versus standard WBRT with memantine. Patients who received HA-WBRT had significantly lower risk of cognitive failure, attributable to less deterioration in executive function at 4 months and less deterioration in learning and memory at 6 months. Consistent with other studies, there was no increase in rates of intracranial progression or death for patients who received HA-WBRT compared to standard WBRT.

After the demonstration of the cognitive benefits of HA-WBRT, hippocampal avoidance prophylactic cranial irradiation (HA-PCI) became the subject of several recent and ongoing clinical trials. The Spanish PREMER phase III clinical trial randomized 118 patients to HA-PCI vs. standard PCI, with a primary outcome of neurocognitive function at 3 months using the Free and Cued Selective Reminding Test (FCSRT). Initial results were presented in abstract form in 2019 and showed less decline in FCSRT in patients who received HA-PCI (3 months: 5.1% vs. 21.7%, $p = 0.01$) (De Dios et al. 2019). Publication in manuscript form is awaited for further insights.

Belderbos and colleagues completed another phase III randomized trial of HA-PCI but found a different result. One-hundred sixty-eight patients with limited- or extensive-stage SCLC without evidence of brain metastases on MRI after chemoradiotherapy or chemotherapy were randomized to HA-PCI versus standard PCI. The primary endpoint was total recall on the Hopkins Verbal Learning Test-Revised (HVLT-R) at 4 months. There was no difference in this endpoint between arms, with significant HVLT-R declines in 28% of HA-PCI patients and 29% of standard PCI patients ($p = 1.000$). Importantly, there were no differences in cumulative incidence of brain metastases or survival between treatment arms, indicating that HA techniques are safe and effective in SCLC as well as patients with SCLC were often excluded from previous HA trials.

There are several potential reasons the study by Belderbos did not detect a cognitive benefit to hippocampal avoidance, while other studies including NRG CC001 and PREMER did. First, this study did not utilize memantine, which was used on NRG CC001, and may be synergistic with HA by preventing radiation-induced synaptic remodeling (Duman et al. 2018). Second, as described above, patients with SCLC have impaired baseline cognitive function, blunting the potential benefit of cognitive preservation (Grosshans et al. 2008). Finally, this study did not require real-time pretreatment review, and weekly (rather than daily) image guidance was allowed, potentially decreasing actual dose sparing to the hippocampi.

Results from the NRG CC003 (NCT02635009) clinical trial, comparing HA-PCI to standard PCI, stratified by age, stage, and planned memantine use, will provide further guidance on the benefit of hippocampal avoidance for PCI, and whether it should be utilized outside of a clinical trial.

5 Patterns of Care and Modern Perspectives

Following the results of the Takahashi study and other modern studies examining the benefit of PCI in patients who are able to receive MRI imaging, in clinical practice providers and patients are increasingly opting against PCI and in favor of close observation with MRI imaging. A key point in such discussions with patients is the willingness of the patient to undergo serial MRI imaging, regardless of PCI administration. Another factor that may lead to increased omission of PCI in the future is the ability of modern immunotherapies to potentially cross the blood-brain barrier, unlike cytotoxic chemotherapies (Abid et al. 2019).

One study completed in 2010 included 207 patients without progressive disease after chemotherapy and thoracic radiotherapy and showed that only 61% of patients received PCI (Giuliani et al. 2010). Of the 38% of patients who refused PCI, over half (53%) cited concerns about potential toxicity and another 20% cited excessive toxicity of their prior chemoradiotherapy as a reason to refuse PCI. These numbers have likely increased in more recent years with the Takashi and other factors discussed above.

One alternative to PCI that has been growing in popularity is MRI surveillance followed by salvage stereotactic radiosurgery when indicated, rather than whole-brain radiotherapy (Rusthoven et al. 2020). However, the median survival after SRS is short in this large cohort, at 8.5 months (95% CI: 7.9–9.5 months), bringing into question whether waiting for clinical evidence of brain metastases may be associated with worse outcomes. Stereotactic radiosurgery may be appropriate for a subset of patients with SCLC with brain relapse. We await the results of the ongoing SWOG MAVERICK trial comparing PCI vs. MRI for further guidance (NCT04155034).

6 Conclusions

Prophylactic cranial irradiation remains a Category 1 NCCN recommendation for patients with limited-stage SCLC who have responded to initial chemoradiotherapy, as it has been demonstrated to decrease the rate of brain metastasis development and improve survival. However, more recent studies in extensive-stage disease have indicated that patients undergoing routine MRI imaging may be able to forego PCI without sacrificing survival, albeit at the cost of increased development of brain metastases. Thus, PCI for patients with extensive-stage disease requires careful shared decision-making given the limited survival of these patients and the long-term effects of PCI (Robin et al. 2018). Data is mixed regarding the neurocognitive and quality-of-life impacts of PCI. Techniques such as hippocampal avoidance and memantine may decrease these toxicities. The NCCN now recommends that all patients have regular MRIs of the brain in follow-up regardless of PCI status (Small Cell Lung Cancer 2021). As the survival of patients with SCLC improves, and new treatments such as immunotherapy are incorporated, the role of PCI may continue to evolve. Prospective clinical trials addressing these issues are needed and are ongoing.

References

Abayomi OK (1996) Pathogenesis of irradiation-induced cognitive dysfunction. Acta Oncol 35(6):659–663

Abid H et al (2019) Efficacy of pembrolizumab and nivolumab in crossing the blood brain barrier. Cureus 11(4):e4446

Arriagada R et al (1995) Prophylactic cranial irradiation for patients with small-cell lung cancer in complete remission. J Natl Cancer Inst 87(3):183–190

Aupérin A et al (1999) Prophylactic cranial irradiation for patients with small-cell lung cancer in complete remission. N Engl J Med 341(7):476–484

Broadbent NJ, Squire LR, Clark RE (2004) Spatial memory, recognition memory, and the hippocampus. Proc Natl Acad Sci U S A 101(40):14515–14520

Brown PD et al (2013) Memantine for the prevention of cognitive dysfunction in patients receiving whole-brain radiotherapy: a randomized, double-blind, placebo-controlled trial. Neuro Oncol 15(10):1429–1437

Cox JD et al (1978) Prophylactic cranial irradiation in patients with inoperable carcinoma of the lung: preliminary report of a cooperative trial. Cancer 42(3):1135–1140

De Dios NR et al (2019) Phase III trial of prophylactic cranial irradiation with or without hippocampal avoidance for SMALL-CELL LUNG cancer. Int J Radiat Oncol Biol Phys 105(1):S35–S36

Duman JG et al (2018) Memantine prevents acute radiation-induced toxicities at hippocampal excitatory synapses. Neuro Oncol 20(5):655–665

Giuliani M et al (2010) Utilization of prophylactic cranial irradiation in patients with limited stage small cell lung carcinoma. Cancer 116(24):5694–5699

Gjyshi O (2019) Prophylactic cranial radiation use in small cell lung cancer declines sharply after trial. Hematology/Oncology. https://www.healio.com/news/hematology-oncology/20190313/prophylactic-cranial-radiation-use-in-small-cell-lung-cancer-declines-sharply-after-trial#:~:text=All%2049%20radiation%20oncologists%20who,results%20were%20published%20(P%20%3C%20

Gondi V et al (2010) Hippocampal-sparing whole-brain radiotherapy: a "how-to" technique using helical tomotherapy and linear accelerator-based intensity-modulated radiotherapy. Int J Radiat Oncol Biol Phys 78(4):1244–1252

Gore EM et al (2011) Phase III comparison of prophylactic cranial irradiation versus observation in patients with locally advanced non–small-cell lung cancer: primary analysis of Radiation Therapy Oncology Group Study RTOG 0214. J Clin Oncol 29(3):272–278

Gregor A et al (1997) Prophylactic cranial irradiation is indicated following complete response to induction therapy in small cell lung cancer: results of a multicentre randomised trial. Eur J Cancer 33(11):1752–1758

Grosshans DR et al (2008) Neurocognitive function in patients with small cell lung cancer. Cancer 112(3):589–595

Gutierrez AN et al (2007) Whole brain radiotherapy with hippocampal avoidance and simultaneously integrated brain metastases boost: a planning study. Int J Radiat Oncol Biol Phys 69(2):589–597

Hansen HH (1973) Should initial treatment of small cell carcinoma include systemic chemotherapy and brain irradiation? Cancer Chemother Rep 3 4(2):239–241

Hirsch FR et al (1982) Intracranial metastases in small cell carcinoma of the lung: correlation of clinical and autopsy findings. Cancer 50(11):2433–2437

Hsu F et al (2010) Whole brain radiotherapy with hippocampal avoidance and simultaneous integrated boost for 1–3 brain metastases: a feasibility study using volumetric modulated arc therapy. Int J Radiat Oncol Biol Phys 76(5):1480–1485

Jackson DV Jr et al (1977) Prophylactic cranial irradiation in small cell carcinoma of the lung. A randomized study. JAMA 237(25):2730–2733

Komaki R, Cox JD, Whitson W (1981) Risk of brain metastasis from small cell carcinoma of the lung related to length of survival and prophylactic irradiation. Cancer Treat Rep 65(9–10):811–814

Komaki R et al (1995) Evaluation of cognitive function in patients with limited small cell lung cancer prior to and shortly following prophylactic cranial irradiation. Int J Radiat Oncol Biol Phys 33(1):179–182

Laplanche A et al (1998) Controlled clinical trial of prophylactic cranial irradiation for patients with small-cell lung cancer in complete remission. Lung Cancer 21(3):193–201

Le Pechoux C et al (2009) Standard-dose versus higher-dose prophylactic cranial irradiation (PCI) in patients with limited-stage small-cell lung cancer in complete remission after chemotherapy and thoracic radiotherapy (PCI 99-01, EORTC 22003-08004, RTOG 0212, and IFCT 99-01): a randomised clinical trial. Lancet Oncol 10(5):467–474

Lee JS et al (1987) Timing of elective brain irradiation: a critical factor for brain metastasis-free survival in small cell lung cancer. Int J Radiat Oncol Biol Phys 13(5):697–704

Meert AP et al (2001) Prophylactic cranial irradiation in small cell lung cancer: a systematic review of the literature with meta-analysis. BMC Cancer 1:5

Monje ML et al (2002) Irradiation induces neural precursor-cell dysfunction. Nat Med 8(9):955–962

Nugent JL et al (1979) CNS metastases in small cell bronchogenic carcinoma: increasing frequency and changing pattern with lengthening survival. Cancer 44(5):1885–1893

Ohonoshi T et al (1993) Comparative study of prophylactic cranial irradiation in patients with small cell lung cancer achieving a complete response: a long-term follow-up result. Lung Cancer 10(1–2):47–54

Robin TP et al (2018) Physician bias in prophylactic cranial irradiation decision making-an opportunity for a patient decision aid. Clin Lung Cancer 19(6):476–483

Rusthoven CG et al (2020) Evaluation of first-line radiosurgery vs whole-brain radiotherapy for small cell lung cancer brain metastases: the FIRE-SCLC cohort study. JAMA Oncol 6(7):1028–1037

Shaw E et al (1994) Prophylactic cranial irradiation in complete responders with small-cell lung cancer: analysis of the Mayo Clinic and North Central Cancer Treatment Group data bases. J Clin Oncol 12(11):2327–2332

Slotman B et al (2007) Prophylactic cranial irradiation in extensive small-cell lung cancer. N Engl J Med 357(7):664–672

Slotman BJ et al (2009) Prophylactic cranial irradiation in extensive disease small-cell lung cancer: short-term health-related quality of life and patient reported symptoms—results of an international phase III randomized controlled trial by the EORTC Radiation Oncology and Lung Cancer Groups. J Clin Oncol 27(1):78–84

Small Cell Lung Cancer (2021) NCCN Guidelines Version 2.2021 [cited 2021 2/15/2021]. https://www.nccn.org/professionals/physician_gls/pdf/sclc.pdf

Sun A et al (2011) Phase III trial of prophylactic cranial irradiation compared with observation in patients with locally advanced non–small-cell lung cancer: neurocognitive and quality-of-life analysis. J Clin Oncol 29(3):279–286

Sun A et al (2019) Prophylactic cranial irradiation vs observation in patients with locally advanced non-small cell lung cancer: a long-term update of the NRG oncology/RTOG 0214 phase 3 randomized clinical trial. JAMA Oncol 5(6):847–855

Suwinski R, Lee SP, Withers HR (1998) Dose-response relationship for prophylactic cranial irradiation in small cell lung cancer. Int J Radiat Oncol Biol Phys 40(4):797–806

Tai P et al (2003) Twenty-year follow-up study of long-term survival of limited-stage small-cell lung cancer and overview of prognostic and treatment factors. Int J Radiat Oncol Biol Phys 56(3):626–633

Takahashi T et al (2017) Prophylactic cranial irradiation versus observation in patients with extensive-disease small-cell lung cancer: a multicentre, randomised, open-label, phase 3 trial. Lancet Oncol 18(5):663–671

Wolfson AH et al (2001) Twice-daily prophylactic cranial irradiation for patients with limited disease small-cell lung cancer with complete response to chemotherapy and consolidative radiotherapy: report of a single institutional phase II trial. Am J Clin Oncol 24(3):290–295

Yin X et al (2019) Prophylactic cranial irradiation in small cell lung cancer: a systematic review and meta-analysis. BMC Cancer 19(1):95